NON-VIRAL GENE THERAPY

Edited by **Xu-bo Yuan**

Non-Viral Gene Therapy
Edited by Xu-bo Yuan

Published by InTech

Janeza Trdine 9, 51000 Rijeka, Croatia

Publishing Process Manager Romina Krebel

Technical Editor Teodora Smiljanic

Cover Designer InTech Design Team

Additional hard copies can be obtained from orders@intechopen.com

Non-Viral Gene Therapy, Edited by Xu-bo Yuan
p. cm.
ISBN 978-953-307-538-9

For EU product safety concerns:
IN TECH d.o.o., Prolaz Marije Krucifikse Kozulić 3, 51000 Rijeka, Croatia,
info@intechopen.com or visit our website at intechopen.com.

Meet the editor

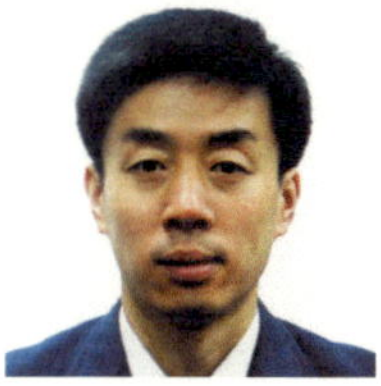

Dr. Xu-bo Yuan, Ph.D., is a nanoparticles (drug and gene delivery) researcher in Tianjin University, China. Dr. Yuan graduated from the Beijing Institute of Science & Technology in 1989 with a degree in Chemical Engineering. He received his M.S. and Ph.D. from Tianjin University in 1995 and 2001, respectively. After doing his poster doctoral work at Institute of Polymer Chemistry, Nankai University, he was an associate professor at Tianjin University, and a visiting scientist in the Department of Chemistry and Biomolecular Engineering at the University of California, Los Angeles. He is currently the professor working on the co-delivery of chemotherapeutant and miRNA in Tianjin University.

Contents

Preface

Gene therapy provides great promises for cancer treatment. Two essential components are absolutely necessary in current gene therapy: an effective therapeutic gene that can be expressed at a target site, and an efficient and safe delivery system.

This book aims to provide an up-to-date report in gene delivery research. With the multidisciplinary contribution in gene delivery, the book covers: (1) various gene delivery systems, like cationic lipids, cationic polymers and silica nanoparticles; (2) methods to enhance delivery, such as ultrasound and microbubble; (3) materials with modification and multifunction for the tumor or tissue targeting.

The book provides an introductory text for nonspecialists in gene delivery, and prepares readers to perform well-controlled experiments with appropriate controls. It illustrates ideas and models with more than 100 figures, including 64 photomicrographs.

Many specialists are not familiar with both drug delivery and the molecular biology of DNA vectors. In this book, molecular biologists will gain a basic knowledge of lipids, liposome, and other gene delivery vehicles and lipids, while drug delivery scientists will better understand DNA, molecular biology, and DNA manipulation.

We acknowledge our contributors and section editors for generously sharing their expertise and scientific skills. We hope this book can help the researchers come up with new ideas and finally bring the gene therapy approaches to the clinical trials.

Xu-bo Yuan
Tianjin University
China

1

Non-Viral Gene Therapy Vectors Carrying Genomic Constructs

George Kotzamanis, Hassan Abdulrazzak, Athanassios Kotsinas and Vassilis G. Gorgoulis
University of Athens, Medical School
Greece

1. Introduction

Gene therapy is the use of genes or DNA for the treatment of diseases. For the treatment of inherited disorders, DNA carrying a functional gene is introduced into the cells of a patient to reverse the defect of the corresponding malfunctioning endogenous gene. Previous genetic characterization of the disease and cloning of the gene that causes it are necessary. In most cases, the cDNA of the therapeutic gene is cloned into a bacterial plasmid under the control of a strong heterologous promoter (often of viral origin). However, such constructs, called mini-genes, lack introns, promoters, enhancers, and long-range controlling elements that precisely control the temporal and spatial expression of the endogenous gene.

For gene therapy of some diseases it is important to achieve expression of the therapeutic gene at specific levels. Expression at lower levels than normal might not be sufficient to correct the defect and at higher levels could result in undesirable effects. In other cases, tissue-specific expression may be very important. The elements responsible for controlled and tissue-specific expression of a gene usually lie within the introns and the sequences before and after the gene. Therefore, the use of genomic constructs which contain the introns and flanking DNA of the therapeutic gene is expected to be more effective than that of mini-gene constructs in gene therapy for certain genetic diseases where precise levels of the gene product are required (reviewed by (Pérez-Luz & Díaz-Nido, 2010)). Bacterial Artificial Chromosomes (BACs), originating from the human genome project, contain genomic loci of approximately 180 kb on average and cover the entire human genome (Osoegawa et al., 2001). These sequenced BACs can accommodate most genes along with their regulatory elements and can serve as tools in gene therapy using genomic constructs.

Gene therapy as a modern therapeutic tool should provide a permanent cure to the patient by long-term maintenance and expression of the administered gene. This can be achieved either by integration of the transgene into the natural chromosomes or by other mechanisms for its replication and nuclear retention.

One of the most important aspects of gene therapy is the choice of the vector that will deliver and express the corrective gene in the appropriate cells. Current vectors fall into two categories: viral and non-viral. Apart from determining the method of delivery, the type of vector also determines the fate of the therapeutic gene within the cells. For instance, the vector may have the ability to remain extra-chromosomally. Non-viral artificial chromosome vectors and adeno-associated viral, adenoviral, Herpes viral and EBV vectors are all examples of this type. In contrast, retroviral and lentiviral vectors integrate into the host genome (reviewed by (Verma & Weitzman, 2005)).

The majority of current gene therapy approaches are based on viral vectors due to their highly efficient delivery into cells. There are some examples of successful viral gene therapy clinical trials which had impressive clinical benefit for the patients (Cavazzana-Calvo et al., 2000). However, viral gene therapy has been subjected to criticism mostly because of two unfortunate events. In one case a patient with ornithine transcarbamylase deficiency treated with an adenoviral vector died due to provocation of an immune response (Raper et al., 2003). This death raised a safety issue that is hard to address, as human immune responses cannot be predicted pre-clinically. In another case, SCID-X1 patients treated with a retroviral vector developed a leukemia-like condition due to disruption of an endogenous oncogene by integration of the vector (Hacein-Bey-Abina et al., 2003a, 2003b). Since vector integration is random and uncontrollable, insertional mutagenesis is a general problem that all integrating viral vectors have.

Ideally, vectors suitable for gene therapy should meet four criteria. Firstly, they should be safe. In this context all vectors that arise from non-human sequences might cause adverse immune responses and are not suitable. Additionally, vectors that integrate into the host genome at random positions are also unsafe. Secondly, they could be efficiently delivered into cells. Viral vectors have an advantage in this respect but recently developed physical methods for non-viral DNA delivery (Reviewed by (Al-Dosari & Gao, 2009)) might prove to be equally effective. Thirdly, they should remain permanently in the cells and provide long-term expression of the transgene they carry. As random integration is excluded due to the first criterion, extra-chromosomally retained or site-specific integrating vectors might be an alternative solution. Fourthly, their cloning capacity should be high enough to allow them to carry fully functional genes with appropriate regulatory elements. Such intact genes, or gene clusters, can be very large and conventional molecular biology techniques will be inadequate for manipulating them. New technologies are therefore needed.

This chapter will focus on non-viral vectors containing entire genomic loci rather than mini-genes. The necessity for using these constructs will become clear through several examples of preclinical work with integrating vectors conferring position independent expression from large transgenes. Key points on delivery of large naked DNA molecules into patients using physical methods will be covered. Emphasis will be given to *ex vivo* transfer of genomic constructs to cultured mammalian cells and nucleofection and bactofection as two promising methods for delivering large constructs will be analyzed. A review of all available vectors that allow extra-chromosomal maintenance of foreign DNA will be provided with an emphasis on the structure and potential application of EBV-based episomes, Human Artificial Chromosomes and Scaffod/Matrix Attachment Region (*S/MAR*) vectors as examples of non-integrating extra-chromosomally retained vectors. In addition, two systems for targeted integration at specific sites not associated with carcinogenesis will be described. The availability of powerful recombination-based methods for manipulating large vectors, a process called recombineering, will also be covered. Finally, an example on the development of genomic DNA containing vectors for gene therapy of Cystic Fibrosis using recombineering will be given.

2. Advantages of use of genomic constructs in gene therapy

The argument for using genomic constructs rather than cDNA in gene therapy is that they contain all the introns and flanking DNA which can confer full control of gene expression.

Inclusion of introns also allows correct function of genes that encode for different products through differential splicing, such as the immunoglobulin genes. Promoters that lie in the flanking DNA could be cloned and used in a cDNA construct. However, the introns and flanking DNA also contain other elements that can participate in the control of chromatin condensation and therefore influence gene expression. The most important of these elements are simple enhancers and locus control regions (LCRs) (Lipps et al., 2003).

Enhancers increase transcription independently of orientation and distance. They can suppress silencing of transgenes that is usually observed when integration occurs in a condensed and therefore repressive heterochromatin region, a phenomenon called position effect (Martin & Whitelaw, 1996). Moreover, they can target transgenes to transcriptionally active nuclear compartments and prevent their localization near heterochromatin (Francastel, et al., 1999). LCRs are more complex and contain enhancers (Li et al., 1999). A general characteristic they have is the presence of DNAse I hypersensitive sites (DHS), where chromatin is not condensed and transcription factors can bind to their cognate sequences allowing transgene expression.

The importance of using genomic constructs rather than cDNA or mini-genes has been shown for several genes, both in cultured cells and in transgenic mice. Generally, the presence of promoters, enhancers, LCRs and other elements, located 5′ or 3′ of the gene or within introns, resulted in position-independent expression of the transgenes in the correct tissue, at proper levels and right times in contrast to the use of small transgenes carrying heterologous promoters. For example transgenic mice generated with long constructs that included all the known DHS 5′ of the class II MHC *Ea* gene showed position-independent, copy number dependent expression of *Ea*. Shorter constructs lacking some of the DHS were subject to position effects (Carson & Wiles, 1993). Similar results were obtained when a 250-kb YAC carrying the genomic locus of the mouse tyrosinase gene was used to generate transgenic mice. The transgene was expressed at levels comparable to the endogenous gene, in the right tissues and proportional to copy number but independent of position (Schedl et al., 1993). Physiological expression of the human Huntington Disease gene has also been achieved from a YAC in transgenic mice containing a targeted disruption of the endogenous gene. Huntigtin is essential for development since its absence is lethal in mice but the human transgene was expressed in the correct tissue, at adequate levels and early enough in development to rescue the mice from embryonic lethality (Hodgson et al., 1996). Likewise, the human Friedrich ataxia (*FRDA*) gene expressed from a 188-kb BAC has been shown to rescue *FRDA* knockout mice from embryonic lethality (Sarsero et al., 2004). Transgenic mice were also generated with constructs covering the human β-globin locus, which is a model system for studying developmental regulation of gene clusters. The locus consists of five genes, ε, Gγ, Aγ, δ and β, the expression of which is tightly regulated both temporally and spatially. ε-globin is expressed at embryonic stages, Gγ- and Aγ- in the fetal liver and δ- and β-globin in the bone marrow of adults. An upstream LCR and a downstream DHS seem to control the expression of the genes. Transgenic mice generated by using a 160-kb BAC containing the entire human β-globin locus, exhibited proper developmental regulation and tissue specific expression of the globin genes (Huang et al., 2000). Interestingly, expression of a human *BCL2L10* (*Boo*) BAC transgene targeted at the *HPRT* locus in transgenic mice, followed the human pattern. Human *Boo* mRNA was detected in organs that had no murine *Boo* mRNA but were known to host *Boo* expression in humans, suggesting that human regulatory elements which were present in the BAC and absent in the mouse endogenous gene could drive tissue-specific expression in the mouse background (Heaney et al., 2004).

Transgenic work has also been carried out with respect to cystic fibrosis (CF). The disease is caused by mutations in the cystic fibrosis transmembrane conductance regulator (*CFTR*) which is normally expressed in specific tissues and shows precisely regulated expression thanks to some DHS that are found as far as 80 kb upstream of the first exon (Smith, et al., 1995). Previous experiments with small mini-gene constructs that obviously could not cover the whole genomic region showed some expression of *CFTR* in transgenic mice (Alton et al., 1993; Hyde et al., 1993) and low levels of transient correction in CF patients (Caplen et al., 1995). However, such constructs were not expressed sufficiently in the appropriate tissues to achieve clinical improvement in patients. A 320-kb YAC carrying the human *CFTR* gene rescued CFTR null mice (Manson et al., 1997). Gene expression followed the wild type mouse pattern except in some tissues such as the pyloric glands, Brunner's glands, epididymis and sublingual glands, presumably due to absence of a distant DHS in the YAC or lack of recognition of the human control elements by mouse transcription factors. More recently, correct temporal and spatial expression of the human *COL6A1* gene (Xing et al., 2007), the human Brain-Derived neurotropic factor (*BDNF*) gene (Koppel et al., 2009) and the porcine Growth Hormone gene (Tong et al., 2010) has been demonstrated in BAC transgenic mice.

The ability of genomic constructs to drive tissue- and time-specific expression, unlike cDNA and mini-genes, has made BAC transgenics an additional tool to knockout transgenics for the identification of potential regulatory elements within the locus of a gene. For instance, an enhancer within the locus of the tyrosinase-related family (*Tyrp1*) gene (Murisier et al., 2006) and a region responsible for tissue-specific expression within the locus of the *Neurogenin1* gene (Quiñones et al., 2010) have been discovered in transgenic mice generated with BACs.

3. Delivery of large DNA molecules

Gene therapy with large genomic constructs cloned on BAC vectors unavoidably raises the issue of delivery into target cells. The majority of recombinant viruses, commonly utilized as carriers for transfer of plasmid DNA, apart from evoking unwanted immune responses, have a maximum packaging capacity and cannot be used to deliver large BACs. An exception to this rule is the *Herpes simplex* virus 1 (HSV-1) -derived amplicon vector, which has been shown to be able to accommodate and deliver large BACs of up to approximately 150 kb in size (Wade-Martins et al., 2003). However, even this promising vector is based on viral sequences and is subject to criticism regarding its safety. Therefore, delivery of genomic loci of therapeutic genes should preferably be non-viral.

Irrespective of their size, naked DNA molecules are difficult to transfect into cells both *in vivo* and *in vitro* due to a series of barriers related to almost all aspects of cellular biology. Such barriers include degradation by nucleases present in the blood and the extracellular matrix, the plasma membrane, transformation of endosomes to digestive lysozomes following endocytosis and the nuclear envelope (Al-Dosari & Gao, 2009). Several physical methods have been employed to facilitate transfer of naked DNA into cells with efficiencies that in some cases resemble those of viral methods. In parallel, chemical methods based mostly on cationic lipids and polymers have been developed and used for *in vitro* and *in vivo* gene transfer. However, the vast majority of published data concern delivery of plasmid DNA and further evaluation of both physical and chemical methods for the delivery of large BACs is required.

3.1 Physical methods for direct delivery to patients

Physical methods facilitate entry of naked DNA into the cells by creating temporary microdisruption of the cell membrane due to physical forces, such as hydrostatic pressure, electric pulse, ultrasound, laser irradiation, magnetic fields and particle bombardment. As of March 2011, naked plasmid DNA has been used in 18.7% (n=319) of clinical gene therapy trials (http://www.wiley.com/legacy/wileychi/genmed/clinical/).

3.1.1 Injection

In early experiments, naked plasmid DNA (or RNA) was injected directly into different organs of different animals and expression of reporter genes was detected at the sites of injection. In mice, this method was used to deliver and express reporter genes in several organs including skeletal muscle (Wolff et al., 1990) and lung (Meyer et al., 1995). Subsequently, expression of therapeutic genes has been achieved using this method and some human clinical trials for limb ischemia (Morishita et al., 2010), erectile dysfunction (Melman et al., 2007), Duchenne/Becker muscular dystrophy (Romero et al., 2004)) have been based on naked DNA injection into tissues. Although these were phase I or IIa trials aiming mostly at assessing safety, some transgene expression and clinical improvement has been shown but the level of expression was low.

A non-invasive alternative to conventional needle injection is jet injection. This technology is based on a high velocity narrow jet of liquid containing the DNA, which is able to penetrate the skin and underlying tissues. It is powered by compressed air and penetration in a specific tissue can be controlled by adjusting the air pressure. So far, the major application of jet injection has been the development of DNA vaccines (Raviprakash & Porter, 2006). Thanks to technical improvements, the efficiency of delivery by jet injection has reached that of other non-viral methods and has been evaluated recently in a clinical trial on patients with melanoma and breast cancer (Walther et al., 2008).

Further progress in the field has led to the development of the so-called hydrodynamic injection, which is considered to be the most efficient non-viral gene delivery method in mice (Al-Dosari & Gao, 2009). According to the hydrodynamic method, a high volume saline solution of plasmid DNA is injected into the tail vein at high velocity. Initial studies have shown that this results in high levels of gene expression in the liver (Liu, et al., 1999; Zhang et al., 1999). The hydrodynamic injection into the tail vain has also been shown to work relatively well with large BAC DNA (Hibbitt et al., 2007; Magin-Lachmann et al., 2004). Moreover, local hydrodynamic delivery into rabbit liver using catheter-assisted perfusion (Eastman et al., 2002) and pressure-mediated delivery to rat kidney (Maruyama et al., 2002) and to limb muscle of mammals (Hagstrom et al., 2004) have been achieved. it remains to be seen whether similar hydrodynamic methods could be deployed in human patients.

3.1.2 Electroporation

In vivo electroporation is the application of electrical pulses following local injection of DNA in the target tissue. This temporarily increases the cell membrane permeability and facilitates DNA uptake by a mechanism that remains unclear. Under optimal conditions the efficiency of plasmid DNA delivery by *in vivo* electroporation can approach that of viral methods but the efficiency decreases when larger DNA molecules are used. By using a variety of electrodes, ranging from needle to surface electrodes, electroporation has been shown to be effective at delivering small in size DNA to several tissues including muscle and lung (Brown et al., 2008; Dean et al., 2003). On the other hand, only few data is available about *in vivo* electroporation of large DNA molecules. In one study, efficient delivery of an 80-kb BAC into electroporated muscle has been achieved but, as expected, reporter gene expression from the BAC was found 5-fold less efficient than from a plasmid (Magin-Lachmann et al., 2004). Increasing knowledge and technological progress in electroporation has resulted in its clinical application in humans for the treatment of melanoma (Daud et al., 2008) and in several ongoing clinical trials for the treatment of other cancers and for DNA vaccination.

3.1.3 Sonoporation

Sonoporation is a technique that uses ultrasound waves of high intensity and low frequency to cause the same effect on the plasma membrane as electroporation that is transient permeabilization in order to facilitate the delivery of DNA into cells. The mechanism is different to electroporation though. Ultrasound is believed to result in acoustic cavitation that can disrupt temporarily the cell membrane. When it is used in combination with microbubbles, which are gas-filled vesicles coated with albumin, polymers or phospholipids, cavitation and therefore local DNA uptake are enhanced (Wells, 2004). Such microbubbles are commercially available and their stability has been shown to affect directly the efficiency of *in vivo* sonoporation (Alter et al., 2009).

Several studies have shown *in vivo* delivery of plasmids carrying either reporter or therapeutic genes to different tissues including lung, heart and muscle (Xenariou et al., 2010; Alter et al., 2009; Sheyn et al., 2008) but comparative data, wherever provided, confirmed that the efficiency of sonoporation was significantly lower than that of electroporation. However, sonoporation is still being considered for clinical application in humans due to its non-invasive nature and lesser tissue damage caused compared to electroporation. Interestingly, a combination of electric pulses and ultrasound waves (electrosonoporation) for gene transfer into the skeletal muscle of mice showed 8-fold and 1.6-fold higher gene expression compared with electroporation and sonoporation alone, respectively (Yamashita et al., 2002).

3.1.4 Other physical methods

Particle bombardment via a gene gun, originally designed for DNA delivery in plants, is a non-viral gene transfer method based on gold particles coated with DNA. The particles are accelerated by pressurized gas and expelled onto tissues. This technique, also referred to as ballistic DNA delivery, has been used to deliver transgenes to skin, liver and muscle tissues of rats and mice (Yang et al., 1990) and DNA vaccines to skin, muscles and tumours in animal models and in human clinical trials. Recently, is has been shown to be efficient at delivering a small reporter gene to mouse liver *in vivo* (Chang et al., 2008). Almost no data is available on the ability of gene gun to deliver large DNA constructs *in vivo*. In just one study, a DNA vaccine containing a 183-kb BAC has been delivered using gene gun and has been shown to confer immune protection to chickens (Tischer et al., 2002).

A new promising method of gene transfer based on the utilization of infrared laser beam has been developed and used to deliver a small transgene to mouse muscle *in vivo* (Zeira et al., 2003). This study reported efficiency of delivery, assessed by measuring the intensity and duration of transgene expression, equal to that by electroporation but with less damage caused to the tissue.

Finally, magnetic fields have been used to enhance *in vivo* targeted gene delivery. In this method, called magnetofection, the DNA is reversibly coupled to superparamagnetic nanoparticles which are directed to the target site, following local injection, via a high-energy magnetic field. *In vivo* magnetofection has been shown to work for small in size plasmid DNA delivery to the gastrointestinal tract of rats and the blood vessels of the ear of pigs (Scherer et al., 2002) and the respiratory epithelium of mice (Xenariou et al., 2006).

3.2 Chemical methods for direct delivery to patients

Chemical vectors used for gene delivery present a broad diversity, with hundreds of different reagents being available (Al-Dosari & Gao, 2009), but generally fall into two main categories: cationic lipids and cationic polymers. These act by forming complexes with the negatively charged DNA, named lipoplexes and polyplexes respectively, which protect the DNA from nucleases and allow its entry into the cells by endocytosis, pinocytarosis or phagocytosis and its transfer into the nucleus by escaping of the complexes from the endosomes following their internalization. The mechanism by which these processes take place are different for lipoplexes and polyplexes and the overall efficiency depends on the chemical structure of the cationic lipids/polymers, the charge ratio between the cationic lipids/polymers and the DNA, the size and structure of the lipoplexes/polyplexes and the inclusion of helper lipids such as DOPE and cholesterol in the complexes (Tros de Ilarduya et al., 2010).

Over the years many cationic lipids showing high transfection efficiency were developed and lipofection has become the most common method for gene transfer *in vitro*. Unfortunately, lipoplexes are not equally good for *in vivo* delivery as most of them are inactivated after interaction with factors present in the blood. However, successful *in vivo* DNA delivery has been reported both with systemic and local administration. A single intravenous injection of lipoplexes into mice has been shown to result in reporter transgene expression in the lung, heart, liver, spleen, and kidney (Song et al., 1997). Impressively, local administration of cationic lipid/*CFTR*-plasmid-DNA complexes in an aerosol formulation to the lungs of cystic fibrosis transgenic mice resulted in correction of the ion transport defect (Hyde et al., 1993). Similar studies in human patients demonstrated some transgene expression but not at sufficient levels to provide a clinical benefit (Griesenbach and Alton, 2009).

Apparently, the choice of the cationic lipid to be used depends on the application and careful optimization of the transfection protocol is required considering that lipoplexes can also induce unwanted immune responses. Lipofection has been used in 6.4% (n=109) of gene therapy clinical trials (http://www.wiley.com/legacy/wileychi/genmed/clinical/).

There has also been an extensive use of cationic polymers in DNA delivery studies with polyethylenimine (PEI) being the most active reagent. Polyplexes are more stable than lipoplexes and their toxicity and transfection activity depend on their molecular weigh (mw). Polymers with low mw are more efficient and less toxic than those with high mw (Fischer et al., 1999). Interestingly, intravenous injection of PEI/BAC-DNA complexes in mice has been found to be less efficient than other non-viral gene delivery methods such as electroporation and hydrodynamic injection (Magin-Lachmann et al., 2004).

3.3 *Ex vivo* delivery to cells

An alternative to *in vivo* delivery of DNA for gene therapy is the *ex vivo* approach. This procedure consists of surgically removing target cells from a patient, transducing them with an appropriate therapeutic gene in culture and then reimplanting them into the body of the donor. Since it involves the use of autologous cells, there is no need for immunosupression following transplantation of the cells back to the patient. In most *ex vivo* gene therapy applications, transplanted cells need to integrate into the appropriate tissue and the efficiency of this "homing" process is tissue type-dependent.

Recent progress in stem cell research has revolutionized *ex vivo* therapy. Stem cells are characterized by their ability to differentiate into a diverse range of cell types when placed in the appropriate environment both *in vitro* and *in vivo* and can therefore be used directly in cell therapy (Abdulrazzak et al., 2010). An *ex vivo* cell therapy approach using Embryonic Stem Cells or foetal Mesenchymal Stem Cells would not involve transfection of a therapeutic gene and would overcome the low gene delivery efficiency hurdle. However, it would have to be used in an allogeneic fashion which would bring the need for using immunosuppressive drugs. A more attractive strategy would be the transfer of a therapeutic gene to patient-derived autologous stem cells such as Mesenchymal Stem Cells (MSCs) which can easily be isolated from the bone marrow or adipose tissue of adults and have been shown to have an excellent differentiation potential (Abdallah & Kassem, 2008) or Induced Pluripotent Stem Cells that can be generated by reprogramming of adult somatic cells (Yu et al., 2007; Takahashi et al., 2007).

Several non-viral methods have been utilized to transfer DNA into MSCs for *ex vivo* gene therapy purposes. The aim of the following sections is to review two of them, nucleofection and bactofection. The criteria for this choice are their ability to deliver very large DNA molecules intact and/or maintain the differentiation potential of the MSCs following transfection.

3.3.1 Nucleofection

Nucleofector technology developed by Amaxa Biosystems is a non-viral method of gene transfer based on electroporation using a combination of electrical parameters and solutions that are specific for each cell type. Unlike other non-viral transfection methods, it facilitates the transfer of DNA directly into the cell nucleus. It is particularly useful for gene transfer into a variety of primary cell types from different species which are normally very difficult to transfect (Gresch et al., 2004).

Nucleofection has been shown to be able to efficiently deliver plasmid DNA carrying a reporter gene to MSCs without impairment of their differentiation capacity (Aluigi et al., 2006). Preliminary data on stable cell lines generated by nucleofection with large BACs suggest that nucleofection can also be used to deliver genomic constructs but does not result in all clones containing intact and unrearranged DNA (Cheung et. al., unpublished data).

3.3.2 Bactofection

Direct delivery of DNA into mammalian cells by invasive bacteria (bactofection) is another potentially useful technique for gene transfer and it may have applications for both *in vitro* and *in vivo* delivery (Larsen et al., 2008). In this method, the DNA is first introduced either in the form of a plasmid or a BAC into bacteria having the ability to invade eukayotic cells and subsequently these bacteria are used to invade and deliver their DNA content into target cells. Several bacterial systems allowing eukaryotic cell invasion have been described. The most convenient is based on the the *E. coli* strain BM4573 (Laner et al., 2005). BM4573 bacteria have been modified to 1) stably express invasin, from the *inv* gene of *Yersinia pseudotuberculosis*, which binds to β1-integrins on mammalian cells leading to internalization, 2) have permanent impaired cell wall synthesis due to diaminopimelic acid (DAP) auxotrophy which causes bacterial lysis following internalization and 3) stably express listeriolysin O, from the *hly* locus of *Listeria monocytogenes*, which is a pore-forming cytolysin that allows escape from the vacuole after bacterial entry and release of the DNA into the cytosol resulting in greater levels of transgene expression (Laner et al., 2005).

One advantage of the method is that there is no need to purify the DNA prior to transfection, which is still a technically challenging procedure for very large DNA molecules. Another advantage is that DNA delivered by bacterial invasion is rarely rearranged. Rearrangements are always an issue of concern when using other DNA delivery methods to transfer large BACs. For instance, although lipofection and electroporation have been used to efficiently deliver large BAC DNA into cultured cells, some of the clones generated have been shown to suffer from rearrangements (Magin-Lachmann et al., 2004; Cheung et al., unpublished data). In contrast, several studies have demonstrated that large BACs are delivered intact by bacterial invasion albeit with low efficiency. In two of them, stable cell lines containing integrations of a ~250-kb BAC carrying the human clotting factor VIII *(FVIII)* gene (Pérez-Luz et al., 2007) and of a ~258-kb BAC carrying the human *CFTR* gene (Kotzamanis et al., 2009) have been generated by bacterial invasion. No clones have been found to contain rearranged DNA in any of the two studies and expression of the respective transgenes has also been shown in both of them. Therefore, bactofection is an attractive method for delivering large genomic DNA containing intact constructs. The ability of the method to deliver large BACs into MSCs without affecting their differentiation potential is yet to be shown.

4. Extra-chromosomal vectors

Regardless of the type and size of the therapeutic gene (small cDNA versus large genomic DNA) and the delivery method (viral versus non-viral) to be used in a gene therapy protocol, efficient retention and long-term expression of the transgene is required so as to eliminate the need for re-administrations. Integration into the host genome has widely been used in gene therapy to fulfil this requirement. However, the dangers of integration due to insertional mutagenesis have become a widely publicised issue as a result of a clinical trial using a retroviral vector to treat X-linked severe combined immune deficiency (SCIDX1). In this trial some patients developed leukaemia due to deregulation of the growth-promoting LIM domain only 2 (*LMO2*) proto-oncogene caused by integration of the vector (Hacein-Bey-Abina et al., 2003a, 2003b). The safety concerns regarding uncontrolled integration of the therapeutic gene into the host genome have been strengthened by observations that there is a preference of integrating vectors for the regulatory regions of transcriptionally active genes (Bushman et al., 2005). Given the need for long-term expression and the problems associated with vector integration, vectors that persist in the nucleus by being maintained episomally without integrating could be highly advantageous. Three different systems have been employed to achieve extra-chromosomal maintenance of the vectors carrying the therapeutic gene: systems based on elements from the Epstein-Barr virus (EBV), artificial chromosomes and systems based on *scaffold/matrix attachment region* (*S/MAR*). All these systems have a high cloning capacity and can be used in combination with large genomic constructs.

4.1 OriP/EBNA-1 episomal vectors

The best characterized system for episomal maintenance is based on sequences derived from the EBV genome. EBV is a member of the herpesvirus family with a 172-kb genome that is latently maintained as an independently replicating episome in a small percentage of infected lymphocytes (Masucci & Ernberg, 1994). During the latent phase of its cycle, DNA replication occurs from the origin of replication *oriP* and only about 10 proteins are produced of which the only protein that is required for replication at *oriP* is the Epstein Barr Nuclear Antigen-1 (EBNA-1) (Yates et al., 1985). The interaction of *oriP* with EBNA-1 also enables the segregation of the viral genome between the daughter cells through the association of EBNA-1 with host metaphase chromosomes (Harris et al., 1985).

These features of the EBV have been exploited to develop a system for episomal maintenance of foreign DNA delivered into cells. It has been shown that plasmids carrying *oriP* and expressing EBNA-1 can replicate autonomously once per cell cycle when delivered into human cells and can segregate by attaching to the host chromosomes (Haase & Calos, 1991). The *oriP*/EBNA-1 system has also been shown to support long-term episomal maintenance without selection and expression of very large human genes, such as the *CFTR* (Huertas et al., 2000), the human hypoxanthine phosphoribosyltransferase (*HPRT*) (Wade-Martins et al., 2000) and the *β-globin* gene (Black & Vos, 2002). Following these promising results, a convenient system for adding the *oriP*/EBNA-1 sequences onto any BAC already containing a therapeutic gene has been developed (Magin-Lachmann et al., 2003) and will be analyzed later on.

The *oriP*/EBNA-1 retention system is easy to use and can provide extra-chromosomal maintenance to foreign DNA of hundred kilobases delivered into cells but has some major disadvantages. It provides random rather than equal segregation of the episomal vector to daughter cells which results in loss of the episomes at a rate of 2-8% per cell division (Sclimenti & Calos, 1998). This, along with the fact that it involves viral sequences particularly from the EBV which has been associated to several types of human malignancies (Cohen, 2000) limits the use of EBV vectors for safe gene therapy.

4.2 Human artificial chromosomes

Human Artificial Chromosomes (HACs) are vectors able to replicate and segregate in parallel with the endogenous chromosomes in human cells. To achieve this, they must contain the minimal elements required for chromosome function, namely an origin of replication, telomeres and centromeres (Pérez-Luz & Díaz-Nido, 2010).

One approach towards constructing HACs, called "top-down", involves fragmentation of already existing chromosomes and generation of smaller mini-chromosomes, where only the three functional chromosomal elements remain. Several studies have shown that mini-chromosomes can host and allow the expression of large therapeutic genes, be transferred between various mouse and human cell lines and be transmitted through the mouse germ line (Kakeda et al., 2005; Shen et al., 2001; Voet et al., 2001). Though mini-chromosomes have useful properties for application in transgenics, their use in gene therapy is restricted to an *ex vivo* approach only.

HACs with a high potential for use in *in vivo* gene therapy are generated by a different approach named the bottom-up. This is similar to the method applied for YAC construction in yeast and involves assembling the functional chromosomal elements and building up a HAC *de novo* in human cells. Different strategies have been followed to generate *de novo* HACs, the most convenient of which is to transfect a BAC carrying only a large array of αsatellite (alphoid) DNA and some marker genes into HT1080 cells. No telomeric sequences or an origin of replication have been shown to be required, probably due to generation of circular HACs and initiation of replication at origins found within the marker genes (Ebersole et al., 2000). HACs generated this way exist as single (or low copy) chromosomes in the nucleus and have a high mitotic stability (close to 100%) in the absence of selection. The potential use of these vectors in gene therapy has been demonstrated by expression of large therapeutic genes from them (Grimes et al., 2001; Mejía & Larin, 2000). Further advance was noted when efficient methods for manipulating large sequences of repetitive nature, such as alphoid DNA, were developed and used to generate HACs, as will be discussed later on (Kotzamanis et al., 2005). Nevertheless, several issues need to be solved before any clinical application. First, HACs have been shown to form efficiently only in HT1080 cells so far. Whether this is due to their inability to form in other cell lines has not been answered yet, but is limiting their use for *in vivo* gene therapy. Second, all HACs produced by *de novo* synthesis in HT1080 cells have been between 1 and 10 Mb in size, definitely smaller than native chromosomes, but larger than the input DNA, suggesting that unpredictable amplifications and rearrangements have occurred during their formation, which is not desired for safe gene therapy vectors. Third, other fates of the input DNA than formation of HACs have been observed and integration has not been excluded (Harrington et al., 1997). This would not be a problem in *ex vivo* therapy where individual clones expressing the gene of interest from a HAC could be isolated, but in *in vivo* gene therapy, any interaction of the input DNA with the endogenous chromosomes could have the same consequences as viral vectors have. Further research is necessary to increase the efficiency of HAC formation so as to ensure that no integration events take place.

4.3 *S/MAR* vectors

S/MARs are diverse sequences found in all eukaryotic genomes where they are involved in many aspects of chromatin function such as organization of chromatin into loops, which seems to be mediated by the interaction between *S/MARs* and the nuclear matrix (Heng et al., 2004). Experiments with a plasmid vector containing an *S/MAR* element isolated from the human interferon *β-* gene has revealed one more feature of *S/MARs*, their ability to provide episomal maintenance of foreign DNA introduced into cells. This vector was able to replicate and remain episomally in CHO cells at low copy number for more than 100 generations in the absence of selection and with a mitotic stability of 98% (Piechaczek et al., 1999). It was later confirmed that the mitotic stability of the vector was provided through the interaction of the *S/MAR* with the nuclear matrix (Baiker et al., 2000). Interestingly, the *S/MAR* used seemed to prevent vectors from integrating into the host genome as integration events were observed in less than 1% of stably transfected clones (Jackson et al., 2006). The ability of the interferon *β S/MAR* to provide replication and episomal retention has been demonstrated in several cell lines and in primary cells (Papapetrou et al., 2006) and also *in vivo* in genetically modified pigs (Manzini et al., 2006). Furthermore, the same *S/MAR* element has been introduced by site-specific homologous recombination to a BAC carrying 135 kb of the human low density lipoprotein receptor *(LDLR)* genomic locus and shown to provide low copy episomal maintenance in CHO *ldlr-/-* cells for more than 100 generations without selection and long-term expression of the transgene at high enough levels to completely restore LDLR function in these cells (Lufino et al., 2007).

In summary, it seems that unlike viral episomal vectors which need to encode viral factors required for their function, S/MAR vectors achieve their replication and segregation by recruiting and interacting with host cell proteins. Moreover, unlike HAC vectors, *S/MAR* vectors do not need to undergo amplifications and rearrangements to function and are therefore of defined structure and composition. These unique safety properties of *S/MARs* make them very attractive for use in gene therapy with large genomic constructs.

5. Vectors integrating at specific sites

An alternative to the use of episomal vectors described above, that still satisfies both requirements for permanent transgene expression and elimination of genotoxic effects is the controlled integration of the therapeutic construct at a specific site in the host genome where no active genes are present. Several vector systems have been developed to achieve this, with each one of them having its own limitations (Voigt et al., 2008). From this variety of available vectors, only two types will be described based on their preference for specific sequences that already exist in the human genome, their potential for *in vivo* use and their ability to support integration of large genomic constructs.

5.1 Phage integrase based vectors

The *Streptomyces* phage ΦC31 integrase is an enzyme that can catalyze site-specific recombination between a phage attachment site (*attP*) and a bacterial attachment site (*attB*) resulting in integration of ΦC31 into the bacterial genome and initiation of the lysogenic phase of its life cycle (Groth & Calos, 2004). This integrase has been shown to be able to irreversibly integrate a single copy of foreign DNA, containing the *attP* site, into the human genome at native pseudo *att* sites found in the intergenic regions on human chromosomes and far from known oncogenes (Chalberg et al., 2005).

A series of studies have validated the potential of ΦC31 integrase-based vector systems in *ex vivo* gene therapy by demonstrating expression of different therapeutic genes in cultured cells including human embryonic stem cells (Thyagarajan et al., 2008) and in *in vivo* gene therapy by showing expression of different therapeutic genes in animal models, like the dystrophin gene in dystrophic mouse muscle (Bertoni et al., 2006). Evidence that the system can be used in gene therapy with genomic constructs has been provided by transgenic work in *Drosophila*, where the ΦC31 integrase has been used to integrate large DNA fragments of up to 133 kb into the genome (Venken et al., 2006). However, other studies have questioned the safety of such vectors by showing that stably expressed ΦC31 integrase could cause numerous chromosomal abnormalities in human cells (Liu et al., 2006) and that in some cases ΦC31-mediated integration is associated with chromosome rearrangements, probably due to recombination between cryptic *att* sites (Ehrhardt et al., 2006). Recently developed mutational derivatives of ΦC31 integrase that have higher integration efficiency and specificity, may eliminate the safety concerns for its use in gene therapy (Keravala et al., 2009).

A very similar approach for site-specific integration is based on the utilization of transposase enzymes, with the *Sleeping beauty* and the *piggyBac* being the most thoroughly studied, which allow for the integration of foreign genes into genomic regions containing transposable elements. (Ivics & Izsvak, 2010). However, such systems are unlikely to prove useful for integration of large genomic constructs as their ability to transpose is significantly decreased when the insert length is increased, a phenomenon called "length-dependence" (Atkinson & Chalmers, 2010).

5.2 Adeno-associated virus based vectors

Some features of the Adeno-associated virus (AAV) can be exploited for site-specific integration of foreign DNA. AAV is a non-pathogenic virus with a 4.7 kb single-stranded DNA genome comprising two genes, *rep* and *cap* flanked by 145 bp palindromic sequences termed inverted terminal repeats (ITRs) (Srivastava et al., 1983). In the presence of a helper virus such as adenovirus or herpes simplex virus, AAV can undergo replication and enter its lytic cycle while in their absence AAV integrates into the human genome and becomes latent. The ITRs contain the sequences required for replication, packaging and integration of the virus and the *rep* gene encodes four regulatory proteins required for catalysis of integration into the human genome during latency. Integration occurs into a specific site on chromosome 19 called the AAVS1 (Kotin et al., 1992).

It has been shown that human transgenes flanked by ITRs can integrate into the AAVS1, with the minimal requirement for expression of viral Rep in cultured human cells (Cortés et al., 2008), and *in vivo* in transgenic mice carrying the human AAVS1 (Liu et al., 2010; Recchia et al., 2004) . The AAV system has also been shown to be able to integrate large genes of 100kb in size into the AAVS1 (Oehmig et al., 2007). These studies have demonstrated the effectiveness of AAV-based vectors but again safety issues have emerged. Integration of small transgenes has been detected in 10-30% of infected human cells in culture with only about half of the integrations occurring specifically at the AAVS1 (Recchia & Mavilio, 2006), suggesting that there would be a 50% probability of insertional mutagenesis in a gene therapy application. In addition, persistent expression of the viral Rep protein is toxic and can cause chromosome instability and mobilisation of the transgene (McCarty et al., 2004).

6. Methods for modification of large DNA molecules

Gene therapy using genomic constructs entails engineering of large DNA fragments often of repetitive nature. For instance, marker genes and other useful sequences, able to confer extra-chromosomal maintenance, need to be added to vectors carrying large genomic fragments, without causing any rearrangements. In other cases, the entire genomic locus of a therapeutic gene may not be available in a single BAC vector and linking of the inserts of two or more BACs is necessary. The technical difficulty in performing such manipulations has hampered progress in this field for a long time. Only recently, efficient engineering methods have been developed allowing the consideration of BACs carrying genomic loci as gene therapy vectors.

6.1 Addition of marker and small genes

In most cases, the cloning of mammalian selectable markers and small reporter genes on the vector region of a BAC carrying a genomic insert by classic molecular biology procedures is limited by lack of convenient cloning sites on the vector, the possible presence of many restriction sites in the insert and the difficulty in manipulating large DNA molecules without affecting their integrity. Alternatives to classic molecular biology techniques using restriction enzymes are therefore required. For adding reporter genes and short sequences onto BACs, site specific homologous recombination mediated by the bacteriophage P1-derived Cre/*loxP* system is such an alternative.

The Cre protein recognizes and catalyses efficiently recombination only between specific *loxP* sites, which are present on all BAC vectors making a modification method based on them generally applicable. As shown in Figure 1, the first step in such a method is the construction of a suitable retrofitting plasmid (pRetro) that carries the gene to be added onto the BAC, a *loxP* site and a selectable marker. Replication of pRetro depends on the high-copy gamma origin (γ-ori) that only operates in an *E. coli* host expressing the π protein (product of the *pir* gene). Following insertion of the plasmid into the BAC in the DH10B *E. coli* host which does not express π, the γ-ori becomes not functional and the BAC remains low-copy. The system shown in Figure 1 uses a separate plasmid to express Cre that is co-transfected with the retrofitting plasmid and then lost once retrofitting has occurred without being involved in the recombination process as it does not have a *loxP* site (Mejía & Larin, 2000). This plasmid contains a LacZ-cre fusion gene so that Cre is expressed after IPTG induction and also a temperature sensitive origin of replication that is functional only at 30ºC. As shown in Figure 1, *in vivo* retrofitting of the BAC with pRetro occurs at 30ºC and then bacteria are grown at 42ºC so that the Cre expressing plasmid is lost to avoid any further unwanted recombination events. Various pRetro plasmids for conveniently adding a G418 mammalian selectable marker, a GFP reporter gene, a luciferase reporter gene and/or an *OriP*/EBNA-1 element onto any BAC have been made available (Magin-Lachmann et al., 2003).

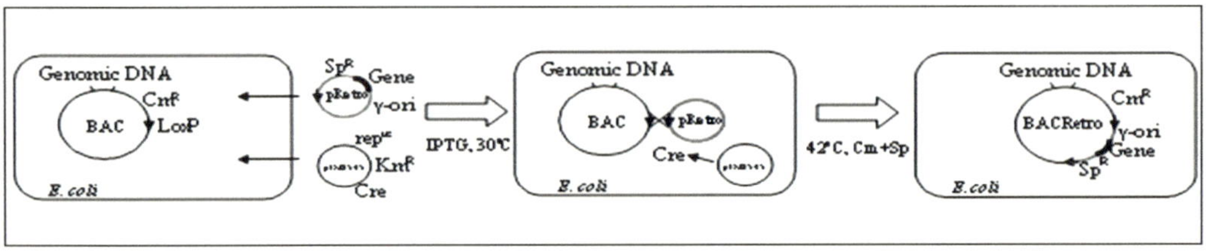

Fig. 1. Addition of small marked/reporter genes onto BACs by Cre/*loxP* recombination

6.2 Addition of large sequences

The construction of a genomic DNA-containing gene therapy vector with the ability to remain extra-chromosomally may involve the addition of large stretches of DNA that are difficult to clone into a pRetro plasmid in order to add them to a BAC by Cre/*loxP* recombination, as described in the previous section. For example, a 70-kb alphoid array has been shown to be required so as to enable a PAC vector to form HACs in HT1080 cells (Ebersole et al., 2000). For such applications, a method for manipulating large segments of DNA, based on homologous recombination in *E. coli* and termed recombineering, has been developed (Copeland et al., 2001). In recombineering, the sequence to be introduced is flanked by two regions of homology to the BAC, the length of which depends on the recombination system that catalyzes the recombination reaction. A selectable marker is also included in most applications so as to allow selection for correctly retrofitted clones in *E. coli*. The phage recombination systems RecET and Red consist of genes encoding proteins involved in homologous recombination of cryptic Rac prophage and bacteriophage λ respectively. These systems are relatively efficient, do not require long homology regions and rarely catalyze unwanted recombination events when used in recombineering (Court et al., 2002; Muyrers et al., 2001). Particularly the Red recombination system has been used to introduce a 70-kb alphoid array into a BAC, carrying a 156-kb genomic insert containing the *HPRT* gene, by recombineering (Figure 2) and expression of the *HPRT* gene from generated HACs has been demonstrated (Kotzamanis et al., 2005). As shown in Figure 2, recombination was targeted to the chloramphenicol resistance gene which is present on all

BACs, allowing for the addition of the 70-kb alphoid array into any BAC and subsequent formation of HACs in the appropriate cells (Kotzamanis et al., 2005).

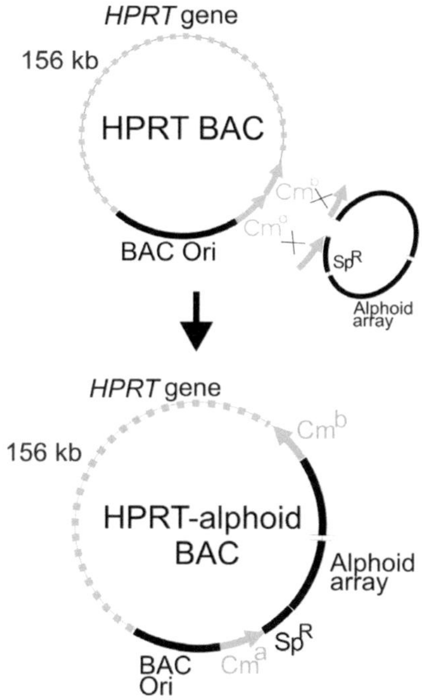

Fig. 2. Addition of large arrays of alphoid DNA onto BACs by recombineering

6.3 Linking of two overlapping BACs

There are many large human genes which are of the same order of size, or larger, than the average insert size of the BAC libraries and for these it is often difficult to find a single BAC spanning the entire gene with all its associated controlling elements. Gene therapy using the genomic loci of such genes would require the assembly of different sequences into a single BAC clone by linking together all available overlapping BAC clones spanning the desired region. Recombineering mediated by the Red system from the λ-prophage has been used to link two overlapping BACs (Kotzamanis & Huxley, 2004; Zhang & Huang, 2003) and linking has been shown to be precise without causing any rearrangements, including shifting of the reading frame of the therapeutic gene (Kotzamanis et al., 2009). As shown in Figure 3, the method comprises two rounds of homologous recombination to link the inserts of two overlapping BACs. In the first round, the inserts of the BACs are subcloned into modified BAC vectors (pBACLink vectors linearized by *Not*I) by homologous recombination at regions indicated as HomA, HomB and HomC (which are PCR amplified and cloned into the pBACLink vectors prior to their linearization). In the second round, one of the modified BACs is linearized by the rare cutting enzyme I-*Ppo*I and introduced into recombination efficient bacteria containing the other modified BAC, resulting in recombination at HomB and Cm^a (part of the chloramphenicol resistance gene present on all BACs) and linking of the two inserts in a single BAC. More overlapping BAC inserts can be added by alternating use of the two pBACLink vectors described in the study (Kotzamanis & Huxley, 2004).

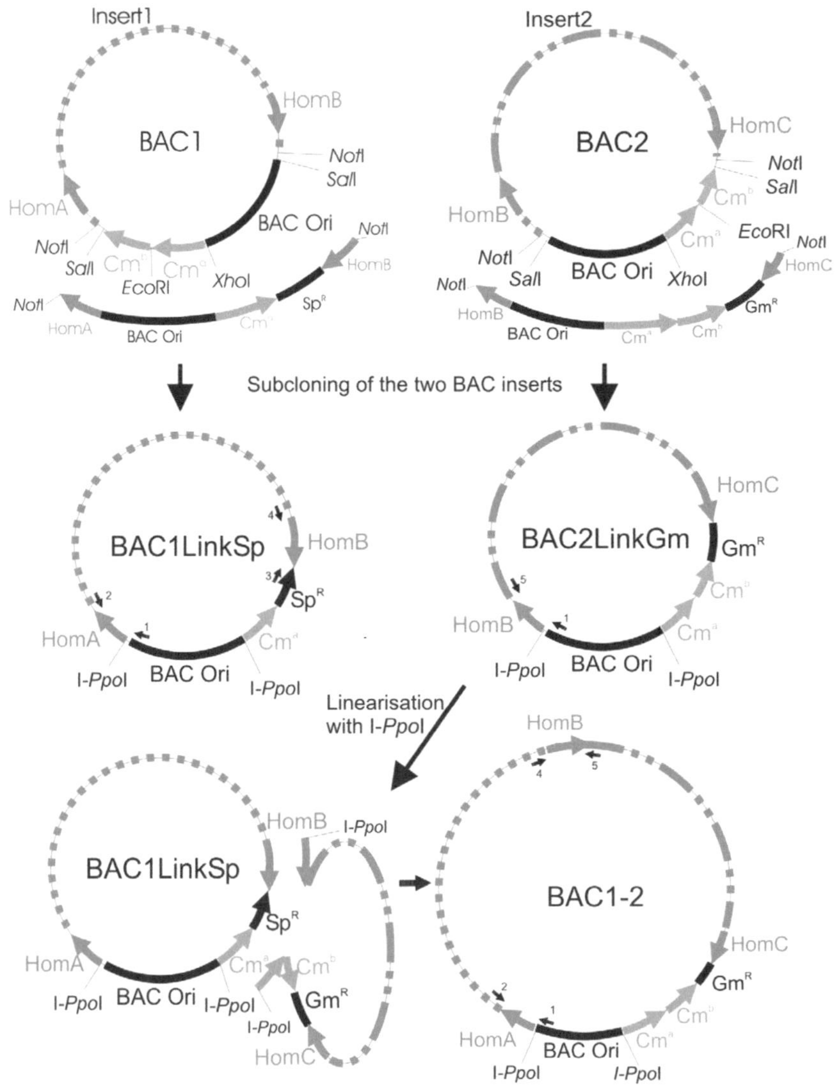

Fig. 3. Linking of two overlapping BACs into a single larger BAC

7. Towards gene therapy of cystic fibrosis using a genomic construct

Cystic Fibrosis is the most common genetic disease in the Caucasians caused by mutations in the *CFTR* gene which is 250 kb long and encodes a cAMP regulated transmembrane Cl- ion channel in epithelial cells of several organs. The most severe implications which eventually lead to death are in the lungs (Boucher, 2002).

For several reasons including the easy access to the respiratory tract without any intervention procedures, the cloning and the characterization of the *CFTR* gene (Riordan et al., 1989; Rommens et al., 1989) and the expectation that even relatively low levels of expression of the gene may have a therapeutic outcome (Dorin et al., 1996), Cystic Fibrosis became an ideal target for gene therapy.

In previous preclinical and clinical studies where *CFTR* cDNA-heterologous promoter systems and different viral vectors were used for the delivery and expression of the transgene, some expression has been shown in transgenic mice and low levels of transient correction of Cl- ion transport deficiency has been observed in patients but no significant clinical improvement has been achieved (Griesenbach & Alton, 2009).

Due to the strict regulation of expression of the *CFTR* gene at specific developmental stages and in specific tissues, controlled by regulatory elements found before, after and within the gene (McCarthy & Harris, 2005), the use of constructs covering the whole genomic locus of the gene may have a better therapeutic potential for Cystic Fibrosis. To date, the only transgene that has fully restored transgenic mice, which did not express endogenous CFTR and would normally die, is the intact gene present on a YAC of approximately 300 kb in length (Manson et al., 1997). However, YAC vectors have the disadvantage of being difficult to shuttle between cells and are inherently unstable and therefore have been replaced by BACs. The *CFTR* gene is one of the large human genes that have not been found to be contained intact in any of the sequenced BACs available from the Human Genome Project. For this reason, the technology described in section 6.3 was developed and used to construct a BAC vector carrying the whole *CFTR* gene and the associated regulatory elements (Kotzamanis et al., 2009). Successful transcription of the gene to a correctly spliced mRNA has been demonstrated in a mouse cell line. This BAC is the only CFTR genomic system available on a convenient vector and may be the basis for non viral gene therapy for Cystic Fibrosis.

Viral approaches to gene therapy for Cystic Fibrosis suffer from gene delivery barriers such as absence of viral receptors in the respiratory epithelium and safety concerns such as provocation of an inflammatory response. This makes either *in vivo* or *ex vivo* non viral gene therapy an attractive avenue of research. However, several issues need to be solved before any clinical application. For instance, the *in vivo* delivery of non viral vectors is limited by the low efficiency, which becomes lower when bigger constructs are used. The demonstration that bone marrow-derived MSCs were able to differentiate to several types of cells including airway epithelial (Wang et al., 2005) indicated a potential application in an *ex vivo* approach but this is limited by poor data on how the *ex vivo* corrected MSCs can be administered and engrafted in the lung of Cystic Fibrosis patients.

Ideally, genetic manipulation with the CFTR BAC whether in the form of *in vivo* or *ex vivo* gene therapy would have to confer permanent transgene expression to avoid repeated gene or cell administration, respectively. In this regard, any of the systems that allow episomal maintenance or targeted integration at non-associated with carcinogenesis regions (described in sections 4 and 5) would have to be added to the CFTR BAC. The methodology required to add small sequences such as the *OriP*/EBNA-1 or the *S/MAR* elements, or large sequences such as the 70-kb alphoid array onto the CFTR BAC is available (see sections 6.1 and 6.2). Moreover, several methods for either *in vivo* or *ex vivo* delivery of the final construct to the respiratory epithelium have been developed and are available for use with the genomic CFTR-locus containing BAC (see section 3).

8. Conclusion

Non-viral gene therapy using the entire genomic locus of the therapeutic gene has two advantages over viral cDNA gene therapy; it is not associated with unwanted immune responses and can confer controlled levels of transgene expression in correct time and tissue. When combined with a system for extra-chromosomal maintenance or targeted integration it can provide permanent transgene expression without causing insertional mutagenesis and is therefore considered to be very safe. Among all available systems, the *S/MAR* element seems to be the most efficient, safe and convenient and may also be utilized *in vivo*. The problem of difficulty in manipulating large segments of DNA and in delivering them into cells *in vitro* or *in vivo*, which has been limiting the use of genomic constructs in gene therapy for years, has started finding its solution by the development of recombineering and of several physical and chemical methods for gene transfer. Apparently, there will not be a delivery system for general use and the choice of the most appropriate delivery method will depend on the specific application and gene therapy strategy.

9. Acknowledgements

This work was funded by the Greek Ministry of Development-GSRT (ENTER 04EP56), the Greek Ministry of Health-KESY (70/3/10295) and the University of Athens (Kapodistrias 70/4/9913).

10. References

Abdallah, BM. & Kassem, M. (2008). Human mesenchymal stem cells: from basic biology to clinical applications. *Gene therapy*, 15(2), pp. 109-16.

Abdulrazzak, H., Moschidou, D., Jones, G. & Guillot PV. (2010). Biological characteristics of stem cells from foetal, cord blood and extraembryonic tissues. *Journal of Royal Society Interface*, 6(7), pp. 689-706

Al-Dosari, MS. & Gao, X. (2009). Nonviral gene delivery: principle, limitations, and recent progress. *AAPS journal*, 11(4), pp. 671-81.

Alter, J., Sennoga, CA., Lopes, DM., Eckersley, RJ. & Wells, DJ. (2009). Microbubble stability is a major determinant of the efficiency of ultrasound and microbubble mediated in vivo gene transfer. *Ultrasound in medicine & biology*, 35(6), pp. 976-84.

Alton, EW, Middleton, PG., Caplen, NJ., Smith, SN., Steel, DM., Munkonge, FM., Jeffery, PK., Geddes, DM., Hart, SL. & Williamson, R. (1993). Non-invasive liposome-mediated gene delivery can correct the ion transport defect in cystic fibrosis mutant mice. *Nature genetics,*Vol. 5, pp. 135-42.

Aluigi, M., Fogli, M., Curti, A., Isidori, A., Gruppioni, E., Chiodoni, C., Colombo, MP., Versura, P., D'Errico-Grigioni, A., Ferri, E., Baccarani, M. & Lemoli, RM. (2006). Nucleofection is an efficient nonviral transfection technique for human bone marrow-derived mesenchymal stem cells. *Stem cells*, 24(2), pp. 454-61.

Atkinson, H. & Chalmers, R. (2010). Delivering the goods: viral and non-viral gene therapy systems and the inherent limits on cargo DNA and internal sequences. *Genetica*, 138, pp. 485–498

Baiker, A., Maercker, C., Piechaczek, C., Schmidt, S. B., Bode, J, Benham, C. & Lipps, H. (2000). Mitotic stability of an episomal vector containing a human scaffold/matrix-attached region is provided by association with nuclear matrix. *Nature cell biology*, 2(3), pp. 182-4.

Bertoni, C., Jarrahian, S., Wheeler, TM., Li, Y., Olivares, EC., Calos, MP. & Rando, TA. (2006). Enhancement of plasmid-mediated gene therapy for muscular dystrophy by directed plasmid integration. *Proceedings of the National Academy of Sciences USA*, 103(2), pp. 419-24.

Black, J., & Vos, JM. (2002). Establishment of an oriP/EBNA1-based episomal vector transcribing human genomic beta-globin in cultured murine fibroblasts. *Gene therapy*, 9(21), pp. 1447-54.

Boucher, RC. (2002). An overview of the pathogenesis of cystic fibrosis lung disease. *Advanced drug delivery reviews*, 54(11), pp. 1359-71.

Brown, PA., Khan, AS., & Draghia-Akli, R. (2008). Delivery of DNA into skeletal muscle in large animals. *Methods in molecular biology*, 423, pp. 215-24.

Bushman, F., Lewinski, M., Ciuffi, A., Barr, S., Leipzig, J., Hannenhalli, S. & Hoffmann, C. (2005). Genome-wide analysis of retroviral DNA integration. *Nature reviews. Microbiology*, 3(11), pp. 848-58.

Caplen, NJ., Alton, EW, Middleton, PG., Dorin, JR., Stevenson, BJ., Gao, X., Durham, SR., Jeffery, PK., Hodson, ME. & Coutelle, C. (1995). Liposome-mediated CFTR gene transfer to the nasal epithelium of patients with cystic fibrosis. *Nature medicine*, 1(1), pp. 39-46.

Carson, S., & Wiles, MV. (1993). Far upstream regions of class II MHC Ea are necessary for position-independent, copy-dependent expression of Ea transgene. *Nucleic acids research*, 21(9), pp. 2065-72.

Cavazzana-Calvo, M, Hacein-Bey, S., Saint Basile, G. de Gross, F., Yvon, E., Nusbaum, P., Seiz, F., Hue, C., Certain, S., Casanova, JL., Bousso, P., Deist, FL. & Fischer, A. (2000). Gene therapy of human severe combined immunodeficiency (SCID)-X1 disease. *Science*, 288(5466), pp. 669-72.

Chang, M.L., Chen, JC., Yeh, CT., Chang, MY., Liang, CK., Chiu, CT., Lin, DY. & Liaw, YF. (2008). Gene gun bombardment with DNA-coated gold particles is a potential alternative to hydrodynamics-based transfection for delivering genes into superficial hepatocytes. *Human gene therapy*, 19(4), pp. 391-5.

Cohen, JI. (2000). Epstein-Barr virus infection. *New England journal of medicine*, 343(7), pp. 481-92.

Copeland, NG, Jenkins, NA, & Court, DL. (2001). Recombineering: a powerful new tool for mouse functional genomics. *Nature reviews. Genetics*, 2(10), pp. 769-79.

Cortés, ML, Oehmig, A., Saydam, O., Sanford, JD., Perry, KF, Fraefel, C. & Breakefield, X. (2008). Targeted integration of functional human ATM cDNA into genome mediated by HSV/AAV hybrid amplicon vector. *Molecular therapy*, 16(1), pp. 81-8.

Court, DL., Sawitzke, JA., & Thomason, LC. (2002). Genetic engineering using homologous recombination. *Annual review of genetics*, 36, pp. 361-88.

Daud, AI., DeConti, RC., Andrews, S., Urbas, P., Riker, A. I., Sondak, V. K., Munster, P., Sullivan, D., Urgen, K., Messina, J. & Heller, R. (2008). Phase I trial of interleukin-12 plasmid electroporation in patients with metastatic melanoma. *Journal of clinical oncology*, 26(36), pp. 5896-903.

Dean, DA., Machado-Aranda, D., Blair-Parks, K., Yeldandi, AV., & Young, JL. (2003). Electroporation as a method for high-level nonviral gene transfer to the lung. *Gene therapy*, 10(18), pp. 1608-15.

Dorin, JR., Farley, R, Webb, S., Smith, SN., Farini, E., Delaney, SJ., Wainwright, B., Alton, EW. & Porteous, DJ. (1996). A demonstration using mouse models that successful gene therapy for cystic fibrosis requires only partial gene correction. *Gene therapy*, 3(9), pp. 797-801.

Eastman, SJ., Baskin, KM., Hodges, BL., Chu, Q., Gates, A., Dreusicke, R., Anderson, S. & Scheule, R. (2002). Development of catheter-based procedures for transducing the isolated rabbit liver with plasmid DNA. *Human gene therapy*, 13(17), pp. 2065-77.

Ebersole, T., Ross, A., Clark, E., McGill, N., Schindelhauer, D., Cooke, H & Grimes, B. (2000). Mammalian artificial chromosome formation from circular alphoid input DNA does not require telomere repeats. *Human molecular genetics*, 9(11), pp. 1623-31.

Ehrhardt, A., Engler, JA., Xu, H., Cherry, A., & Kay, MA. (2006). Molecular analysis of chromosomal rearrangements in mammalian cells after phiC31-mediated integration. *Human gene therapy*, 17(11), pp. 1077-94.

Fischer, D., Bieber, T., Li, Y, Elsässer, H. P., & Kissel, T. (1999). A novel non-viral vector for DNA delivery based on low molecular weight, branched polyethylenimine: effect of molecular weight on transfection efficiency and cytotoxicity. *Pharmaceutical research*, 16(8), pp. 1273-9.

Francastel, C., Walters, MC., Groudine, M., & Martin, DI. (1999). A functional enhancer suppresses silencing of a transgene and prevents its localization close to centrometric heterochromatin. *Cell*, 99(3), pp. 259-69.

Gresch, O., Engel, F. B., Nesic, D., Tran, T., England, H., Hickman, E., Korner, I., Gan, L., Chen, S., Castro-Obregon, S., Hammermann, R., Wolf, J., Muler-Hartmann, H., Nix, M., Siebenkotten, G., Kraus, G. & Lun, K. (2004). New non-viral method for gene transfer into primary cells. *Methods*, 33(2), pp. 151-63.

Griesenbach, U., & Alton, EW. (2009). Cystic fibrosis gene therapy: successes, failures and hopes for the future. *Expert review of respiratory medicine*, 3(4), pp. 363-71.

Grimes, BR., Schindelhauer, D., McGill, NI., Ross, A., Ebersole, TA., & Cooke, HJ. (2001). Stable gene expression from a mammalian artificial chromosome. *EMBO reports*, 2(10), pp. 910-4.

Groth, AC., & Calos MP. (2004). Phage integrases: biology and applications. *Journal of molecular biology*, 335(3), pp. 667-78.

Haase, SB., & Calos, MP. (1991). Replication control of autonomously replicating human sequences. *Nucleic acids research*, 19(18), pp. 5053-8.

Hacein-Bey-Abina, S, Von Kalle, C., Schmidt, M, McCormack, MP., Wulffraat, N, Leboulch, P., (2003). LMO2-associated clonal T cell proliferation in two patients after gene therapy for SCID-X1. *Science*, 302(5644), pp. 415-9.

Hacein-Bey-Abina, S., Von Kalle, C., Schmidt, M., Le Deist, F., Wulffraat, N., McIntyre, E., Radford, I., Villeval, JL., Fraser, C., Cabazzana-Calvo, M. & Fischer, A. (2003). A serious adverse event after successful gene therapy for X-linked severe combined immunodeficiency. *New England journal of medicine*, 348(3), pp. 255-6.

Hagstrom, JE., Hegge, J., Zhang, G., Noble, M., Budker, V., Lewis, DL., Herweijer, H. & Wolf, J. (2004). A facile nonviral method for delivering genes and siRNAs to skeletal muscle of mammalian limbs. *Molecular therapy*, 10(2), pp. 386-98.

Harrington, JJ., Van Bokkelen, G., Mays, RW., Gustashaw, K., & Willard, HF. (1997). Formation of de novo centromeres and construction of first-generation human artificial microchromosomes. *Nature genetics*, 15(4), pp. 345-55.

Harris, A, Young, BD., & Griffin, BE. (1985). Random association of Epstein-Barr virus genomes with host cell metaphase chromosomes in Burkitt's lymphoma-derived cell lines. *Journal of virology*, 56(1), pp. 328-32.

Heaney, JD., Rettew, AN., & Bronson, SK. (2004). Tissue-specific expression of a BAC transgene targeted to the Hprt locus in mouse embryonic stem cells. *Genomics*, 83(6), pp. 1072-82.

Heng, HQ., Goetze, S., Ye, CJ., Liu, G., Stevens, JB., Bremer, SW., Wykes, S., Bode, J. & Krawetz, S. (2004). Chromatin loops are selectively anchored using scaffold/matrix-attachment regions. *Journal of cell science*, 117(Pt 7), pp. 999-1008.

Hibbitt, OC., Harbottle, RP., Waddington, SN., Bursill, CA., Coutelle, C., Channon, KM. &Wade-Martins, R. (2007). Delivery and long-term expression of a 135 kb LDLR genomic DNA locus in vivo by hydrodynamic tail vein injection. *Journal of gene medicine*, 9(6), pp. 488-97.

Hodgson, JG., Smith, DJ., McCutcheon, K., Koide, HB., Nishiyama, K., Dinulos, MB., et al. (1996). Human huntingtin derived from YAC transgenes compensates for loss of murine huntingtin by rescue of the embryonic lethal phenotype. *Human molecular genetics*, 5(12), pp. 1875-85.

Huang, Y., Liu, DP., Wu, L., Li, TC., Wu, M., Feng, DX., et al. (2000). Proper developmental control of human globin genes reproduced by transgenic mice containing a 160-kb BAC carrying the human beta-globin locus. *Blood cells, molecules & diseases*, 26(6), pp. 598-610.

Huertas, D., Howe, S, McGuigan, A., & Huxley, C. (2000). Expression of the human CFTR gene from episomal oriP-EBNA1-YACs in mouse cells. *Human molecular genetics*, 9(4), pp. 617-29.

Hyde, S. C., Gill, D. R., Higgins, C. F., Trezise, A. E., MacVinish, L. J., Cuthbert, A. W., et al. (1993). Correction of the ion transport defect in cystic fibrosis transgenic mice by gene therapy. *Nature*, 362(6417), pp. 250-5.

Ivics, Z. % Izsvak, S. (2010). The expanding universe of transposon technologies for gene and cell engineering. *Mobile DNA*, 1:25

Jackson, D. A., Juranek, S., & Lipps, Hans J. (2006). Designing nonviral vectors for efficient gene transfer and long-term gene expression. *Molecular therapy*, 14(5), pp. 613-26.

Kakeda, M., Hiratsuka, M., Nagata, K., Kuroiwa, Y., Kakitani, M., Katoh, M., et al. (2005). Human artificial chromosome (HAC) vector provides long-term therapeutic transgene expression in normal human primary fibroblasts. *Gene therapy*, 12(10), pp. 852-6.

Keravala, A., Lee, S., Thyagarajan, Bhaskar, Olivares, Eric C, Gabrovsky, V. E., Woodard, L. E., et al. (2009). Mutational derivatives of PhiC31 integrase with increased efficiency and specificity. *Molecular therapy*, 17(1), pp. 112-20.

Koppel, I., Aid-Pavlidis, T., Jaanson, K., Sepp, M., Pruunsild, P., Palm, K., et al. (2009). Tissue-specific and neural activity-regulated expression of human BDNF gene in BAC transgenic mice. *BMC neuroscience*, 10, 68.

Kotin, R. M., Linden, R. M., & Berns, K I. (1992). Characterization of a preferred site on human chromosome 19q for integration of adeno-associated virus DNA by non-homologous recombination. *EMBO journal*, 11(13), pp. 5071-8.

Kotzamanis, G., Abdulrazzak, H., Gifford-Garner, J., Haussecker, PL., Cheung, W., Grillot-Courvalin, C., et al. (2009). CFTR expression from a BAC carrying the complete human gene and associated regulatory elements. *Journal of cellular and molecular medicine*, 13(9A), pp. 2938-48.

Kotzamanis, George, Cheung, W., Abdulrazzak, H., Perez-Luz, S., Howe, Steven, Cooke, Howard, et al. (2005). Construction of human artificial chromosome vectors by recombineering. *Gene*, pp. 351, 29-38.

Kotzamanis, G., & Huxley, C.. (2004). Recombining overlapping BACs into a single larger BAC. *BMC biotechnology*, 4, 1.

Laner, A., Goussard, S., Ramalho, A. S., Schwarz, T., Amaral, M. D., Courvalin, P., et al. (2005). Bacterial transfer of large functional genomic DNA into human cells. *Gene therapy*, 12(21), pp. 1559-72.

Larsen, M. D. B., Griesenbach, U, Goussard, S., Gruenert, D. C., Geddes, D M, Scheule, R K, et al. (2008). Bactofection of lung epithelial cells in vitro and in vivo using a genetically modified Escherichia coli. *Gene therapy*, 15(6), pp. 434-42.

Li, Q., Harju, S., & Peterson, K. R. (1999). Locus control regions: coming of age at a decade plus. Trends in genetics : TIG, 15(10), 403-8.

Lipps, H J, Jenke, A. C. W., Nehlsen, K., Scinteie, M. F., Stehle, I M, & Bode, J. (2003). Chromosome-based vectors for gene therapy. *Gene*, 304, pp. 23-33.

Liu, F., Song, Y., & Liu, D. (1999). Hydrodynamics-based transfection in animals by systemic administration of plasmid DNA. *Gene therapy*, 6(7), pp. 1258-66.

Liu, Q., Perez, C. F., & Wang, Yaming. (2006). Efficient site-specific integration of large transgenes by an enhanced herpes simplex virus/adeno-associated virus hybrid amplicon vector. *Journal of virology*, 80(4), pp. 1672-9.

Liu, R., Li, Yiming, Hu, R., Jin, T., Deng, S., Liang, W., et al. (2010). A site-specific genomic integration strategy for sustained expression of glucagon-like peptide-1 in mouse muscle for controlling energy homeostasis. *Biochemical and biophysical research communications*, 403(2), pp. 172-7.

Lufino, M. M. P., Manservigi, R., & Wade-Martins, Richard. (2007). An S/MAR-based infectious episomal genomic DNA expression vector provides long-term regulated functional complementation of LDLR deficiency. *Nucleic acids research*, 35(15), e98.

Magin-Lachmann, C, Kotzamanis, G, D'Aiuto, L, Cooke, H, Huxley, C, & Wagner, E. (2004). In vitro and in vivo delivery of intact BAC DNA -- comparison of different methods. *Journal of gene medicine*, 6(2), pp. 195-209.

Magin-Lachmann, C., Kotzamanis, G., D'Aiuto, L., Wagner, E., & Huxley, C. (2003). Retrofitting BACs with G418 resistance, luciferase, and oriP and EBNA-1 - new vectors for in vitro and in vivo delivery. *BMC biotechnology*, 3(1), 2.

Manson, A. L., Trezise, A. E., MacVinish, L. J., Kasschau, K. D., Birchall, N., Episkopou, V., et al. (1997). Complementation of null CF mice with a human CFTR YAC transgene. *EMBO journal*, 16(14), pp. 4238-49.

Manzini, S., Vargiolu, A., Stehle, Isa M, Bacci, M. L., Cerrito, M. G., Giovannoni, R., et al. (2006). Genetically modified pigs produced with a nonviral episomal vector. *Proceedings of the National Academy of Sciences USA*, 103(47), pp. 17672-7.

Martin, D. I., & Whitelaw, E. (1996). The vagaries of variegating transgenes. *BioEssays*, 18(11), pp. 919-23.

Maruyama, H., Higuchi, N., Nishikawa, Y., Hirahara, H., Iino, N., Kameda, S., et al. (2002). Kidney-targeted naked DNA transfer by retrograde renal vein injection in rats. *Human gene therapy*, 13(3), pp. 455-68..

Masucci, M. G., & Ernberg, I. (1994). Epstein-Barr virus: adaptation to a life within the immune system. *Trends in microbiology*, 2(4), pp. 125-30.

McCarthy, V. A., & Harris, Ann. (2005). The CFTR gene and regulation of its expression. *Pediatric pulmonology*, 40(1), pp. 1-8.

McCarty, D. M., Young, Samuel M, & Samulski, R Jude. (2004). Integration of adeno-associated virus (AAV) and recombinant AAV vectors. *Annual review of genetics*, 38, pp. 819-45.

Mejía, J. E., & Larin, Z. (2000). The assembly of large BACs by in vivo recombination. *Genomics*, 70(2), pp. 165-70.

Melman, A., Bar-Chama, N., McCullough, A., Davies, K., & Christ, G. (2007). Plasmid-based gene transfer for treatment of erectile dysfunction and overactive bladder: results of a phase I trial. *The Israel Medical Association journal*, 9(3), pp. 143-6.

Meyer, K. B., Thompson, M. M., Levy, M. Y., Barron, L. G., & Szoka, F. C. (1995). Intratracheal gene delivery to the mouse airway: characterization of plasmid DNA expression and pharmacokinetics. *Gene therapy*, 2(7), pp. 450-60.

Morishita, R., Makino, H., Aoki, M., Hashiya, N., Yamasaki, K., Azuma, J., et al. (2010). Phase I/IIa Clinical Trial of Therapeutic Angiogenesis Using Hepatocyte Growth Factor Gene Transfer to Treat Critical Limb Ischemia. *Arteriosclerosis, thrombosis, and vascular biology*.

Murisier, F., Guichard, S., & Beermann, F. (2006). A conserved transcriptional enhancer that specifies Tyrp1 expression to melanocytes. *Developmental biology*, 298(2), pp. 644-55.

Muyrers, J. P., Zhang, Y., & Stewart, A. F. (2001). Techniques: Recombinogenic engineering--new options for cloning and manipulating DNA. *Trends in biochemical sciences*, 26(5), pp. 325-31.

Oehmig, A, Cortés, M L, Perry, K F, Sena-Esteves, M., Fraefel, C., & Breakefield, X O. (2007). Integration of active human beta-galactosidase gene (100 kb) into genome using HSV/AAV amplicon vector. *Gene therapy*, 14(14), pp. 1078-91.

Osoegawa, K., Mammoser, A. G., Wu, C., Frengen, E., Zeng, C., Catanese, J. J., et al. (2001). A bacterial artificial chromosome library for sequencing the complete human genome. *Genome research*, 11(3), pp. 483-96.

Papapetrou, E. P., Ziros, P. G., Micheva, I. D., Zoumbos, N. C., & Athanassiadou, A. (2006). Gene transfer into human hematopoietic progenitor cells with an episomal vector carrying an S/MAR element. *Gene therapy*, 13(1), pp. 40-51.

Piechaczek, C., Fetzer, C., Baiker, A., Bode, J, & Lipps, H J. (1999). A vector based on the SV40 origin of replication and chromosomal S/MARs replicates episomally in CHO cells. *Nucleic acids research*, 27(2), pp. 426-8.

Pérez-Luz, S., Abdulrazzak, H., Grillot-Courvalin, Catherine, & Huxley, Clare. (2007). Factor VIII mRNA expression from a BAC carrying the intact locus made by homologous recombination. *Genomics*, 90(5), pp. 610-9.

Pérez-Luz, S., & Díaz-Nido, J. (2010). Prospects for the use of artificial chromosomes and minichromosome-like episomes in gene therapy. *Journal of biomedicine & biotechnology*, 2010.

Quiñones, H. I., Savage, T. K., Battiste, J., & Johnson, J. E. (2010). Neurogenin 1 (Neurog1) expression in the ventral neural tube is mediated by a distinct enhancer and preferentially marks ventral interneuron lineages. *Developmental biology*, 340(2), pp. 283-92.

Raper, S. E., Chirmule, N., Lee, F. S., Wivel, N. A., Bagg, A., Gao, G.-ping, et al. (n.d.). Fatal systemic inflammatory response syndrome in a ornithine transcarbamylase deficient patient following adenoviral gene transfer. *Molecular genetics and metabolism*, 80(1-2), pp. 148-58.

Raviprakash, K., & Porter, K. R. (2006). Needle-free injection of DNA vaccines: a brief overview and methodology. *Methods in molecular medicine*, 127, pp. 83-9.

Recchia, A., & Mavilio, F. (2006). Site-specific integration into the human genome: ready for clinical application? *Rejuvenation research*, 9(4), pp. 446-9.

Riordan, J. R., Rommens, J. M., Kerem, B., Alon, N., Rozmahel, R., Grzelczak, Z., et al. (1989). Identification of the cystic fibrosis gene: cloning and characterization of complementary DNA. *Science*, 245(4922), pp. 1066-73.

Romero, N. B., Braun, S., Benveniste, O., Leturcq, F., Hogrel, J.-Y., Morris, G. E., et al. (2004). Phase I study of dystrophin plasmid-based gene therapy in Duchenne/Becker muscular dystrophy. *Human gene therapy*, 15(11), pp. 1065-76.

Rommens, J. M., Iannuzzi, M. C., Kerem, B., Drumm, M. L., Melmer, G., Dean, M., et al. (1989). Identification of the cystic fibrosis gene: chromosome walking and jumping. *Science* ,245(4922), pp. 1059-65.

Sarsero, J. P., Li, L., Holloway, T. P., Voullaire, Lucille, Gazeas, S., Fowler, K. J., et al. (2004). Human BAC-mediated rescue of the Friedreich ataxia knockout mutation in transgenic mice. *Mammalian genome*, 15(5), pp. 370-82.

Schedl, A., Montoliu, L., Kelsey, G., & Schütz, G. (1993). A yeast artificial chromosome covering the tyrosinase gene confers copy number-dependent expression in transgenic mice. *Nature*, 362(6417), pp. 258-61.

Scherer, F., Anton, M., Schillinger, U., Henke, J., Bergemann, C., Krüger, A., et al. (2002). Magnetofection: enhancing and targeting gene delivery by magnetic force in vitro and in vivo. *Gene therapy*, 9(2), pp. 102-9.

Sclimenti, C. R., & Calos, M P. (1998). Epstein-Barr virus vectors for gene expression and transfer. *Current opinion in biotechnology*, 9(5), pp. 476-9.

Shen, M. H., Yang, J. W., Yang, J., Pendon, C., & Brown, W. R. (2001). The accuracy of segregation of human mini-chromosomes varies in different vertebrate cell lines, correlates with the extent of centromere formation and provides evidence for a trans-acting centromere maintenance activity. *Chromosoma*, 109(8), pp. 524-35.

Sheyn, D., Kimelman-Bleich, N., Pelled, G., Zilberman, Y., Gazit, D., & Gazit, Z. (2008). Ultrasound-based nonviral gene delivery induces bone formation in vivo. *Gene therapy*, 15(4), pp. 257-66.

Smith, A. N., Wardle, C. J., & Harris, A. (1995). Characterization of DNASE I hypersensitive sites in the 120kb 5′ to the CFTR gene. *Biochemical and biophysical research communications*, 211(1), pp. 274-81.

Song, Y. K., Liu, F., Chu, S., & Liu, D. (1997). Characterization of cationic liposome-mediated gene transfer in vivo by intravenous administration. *Human gene therapy*, 8(13), pp. 1585-94.

Srivastava, A., Lusby, E. W., & Berns, K I. (1983). Nucleotide sequence and organization of the adeno-associated virus 2 genome. *Journal of virology*, 45(2), pp. 555-64.

Takahashi, K., Tanabe, K., Ohnuki, M., Narita, M., Ichisaka, T., Tomoda, K., et al. (2007). Induction of pluripotent stem cells from adult human fibroblasts by defined factors. *Cell*, 131(5), pp. 861-72.

Thyagarajan, Bhaskar, Liu, Y., Shin, S., Lakshmipathy, U., Scheyhing, K., Xue, H., et al. (2008). Creation of engineered human embryonic stem cell lines using phiC31 integrase. *Stem cells*, 26(1), pp. 119-26.

Tischer, B. K., Schumacher, D., Beer, M., Beyer, J., Teifke, J. P., Osterrieder, K., et al. (2002). A DNA vaccine containing an infectious Marek's disease virus genome can confer protection against tumorigenic Marek's disease in chickens. *Journal of general virology*, 83(Pt 10), pp. 2367-76.

Tong, J., Lillico, S. G., Bi, M. J., Qing, T., Liu, X. F., Wang, Yuanyuan, et al. (2010). Tissue-specific and expression of porcine growth hormone gene in BAC transgenic mice. *Transgenic research.*

Tros de Ilarduya, C., Sun, Y., & Düzgüneş, N. (2010). Gene delivery by lipoplexes and polyplexes. *European journal of pharmaceutical sciences*, 40(3), pp. 159-70.

Venken, K. J. T., He, Y., Hoskins, R. A., & Bellen, H. J. (2006). P[acman]: a BAC transgenic platform for targeted insertion of large DNA fragments in D. melanogaster. *Science*, N.Y.), 314(5806), pp. 1747-51.

Verma, I. M., & Weitzman, M. D. (2005). Gene therapy: twenty-first century medicine. *Annual review of biochemistry*, 74, pp. 711-38.

Voet, T., Vermeesch, J., Carens, A., Dürr, J., Labaere, C., Duhamel, H., et al. (2001). Efficient male and female germline transmission of a human chromosomal vector in mice. *Genome research*, 11(1), pp. 124-36.

Voigt, K., Izsvák, Z., & Ivics, Z. (2008). Targeted gene insertion for molecular medicine. *Journal of molecular medicine*, 86(11), pp. 1205-19. .

Wade-Martins, R, White, R. E., Kimura, H., Cook, P. R., & James, M. R. (2000). Stable correction of a genetic deficiency in human cells by an episome carrying a 115 kb genomic transgene. *Nature biotechnology*, 18(12), pp. 1311-4.

Wade-Martins, R., Saeki, Y., & Chiocca, E. A. (2003). Infectious delivery of a 135-kb LDLR genomic locus leads to regulated complementation of low-density lipoprotein receptor deficiency in human cells. *Molecular therapy*, 7(5 Pt 1), pp. 604-12.

Walther, W., Siegel, R., Kobelt, D., Knösel, T., Dietel, M., Bembenek, A., et al. (2008). Novel jet-injection technology for nonviral intratumoral gene transfer in patients with melanoma and breast cancer. *Clinical cancer research*, 14(22), pp. 7545-53.

Wang, G., Bunnell, B. A., Painter, R. G., Quiniones, B. C., Tom, S., Lanson, N. A., et al. (2005). Adult stem cells from bone marrow stroma differentiate into airway epithelial cells: potential therapy for cystic fibrosis. *Proceedings of the National Academy of Sciences USA*, 102(1), pp. 186-91.

Wells, D J. (2004). Gene therapy progress and prospects: electroporation and other physical methods. *Gene therapy*, 11(18), pp. 1363-9.

Wolff, J A, Malone, R. W., Williams, P., Chong, W., Acsadi, G., Jani, A., et al. (1990). Direct gene transfer into mouse muscle in vivo. *Science*, 247(4949 Pt 1), pp. 1465-8.

Xenariou, S, Griesenbach, U, Ferrari, S., Dean, P., Scheule, R K, Cheng, S H, et al. (2006). Using magnetic forces to enhance non-viral gene transfer to airway epithelium in vivo. *Gene therapy*, 13(21), pp. 1545-52.

Xenariou, Stefania, Liang, H.-D., Griesenbach, Uta, Zhu, J., Farley, Raymond, Somerton, L., et al. (2010). Low-frequency ultrasound increases non-viral gene transfer to the mouse lung. *Acta biochimica et biophysica Sinica*, 42(1), pp. 45-51.

Xing, L., Salas, M., Lin, C.-S., Zigman, W., Silverman, W., Subramaniyam, S., et al. (2007). Faithful tissue-specific expression of the human chromosome 21-linked COL6A1 gene in BAC-transgenic mice. *Mammalian genome*, 18(2), pp. 113-22.

Yamashita, Y.-ichi, Shimada, M., Tachibana, K., Harimoto, N., Tsujita, E., Shirabe, K., et al. (2002). In vivo gene transfer into muscle via electro-sonoporation. *Human gene therapy*, 13(17), pp. 2079-84.

Yang, N. S., Burkholder, J., Roberts, B., Martinell, B., & McCabe, D. (1990). In vivo and in vitro gene transfer to mammalian somatic cells by particle bombardment. *Proceedings of the National Academy of Sciences USA*, 87(24), pp. 9568-72.

Yates, J. L., Warren, N., & Sugden, B. (1985.). Stable replication of plasmids derived from Epstein-Barr virus in various mammalian cells. *Nature*, 313(6005), pp. 812-5.

Yu, J., Vodyanik, M. A., Smuga-Otto, K., Antosiewicz-Bourget, J., Frane, J. L., Tian, S., et al. (2007). Induced pluripotent stem cell lines derived from human somatic cells. *Science*, 318(5858), pp. 1917-20.

Zeira, E., Manevitch, A., Khatchatouriants, A., Pappo, O., Hyam, E., Darash-Yahana, M., et al. (2003). Femtosecond infrared laser-an efficient and safe in vivo gene delivery system for prolonged expression. *Molecular therapy*, 8(2), pp. 342-50.

Zhang, G., Budker, V., & Wolff, JA. (1999). High levels of foreign gene expression in hepatocytes after tail vein injections of naked plasmid DNA. *Human gene therapy*, 10(10), pp. 1735-7.

Zhang, XM., & Huang, JD. (2003). Combination of overlapping bacterial artificial chromosomes by a two-step recombinogenic engineering method. *Nucleic acids research*, 31(15), e81.

2

Non-Viral Delivery Systems in Gene Therapy and Vaccine Development

Azam Bolhassani and Sima Rafati
Molecular Immunology and Vaccine Research Laboratory, Pasteur Institute of Iran, Tehran Iran

1. Introduction

Gene therapy is the process of treating a particular disease through the introduction of genetic material in order to elicit a therapeutic benefit [Stone, 2010]. The defective gene of a diagnosed patient can be corrected by a number of different strategies such as "gene replacement", "gene correction", and "gene augmentation" [Katare and Aeri, 2010]. In replacement therapy, a normal gene is inserted somewhere in the genome so that its product could replace that of a defective gene. This approach may be suitable for recessive disorders, which are marked by deficiency of an enzyme or other proteins. Although, the gene functions in the genome providing an appropriate regulatory sequence, the approach may not be successful in treating dominant disorders associated with the production of an abnormal gene product, which interferes with the product of normal gene [Katare and Aeri, 2010]. Corrective gene therapy requires replacement of a mutant gene or a part of it with a normal sequence. This can be achieved by using recombinant technology. Another form of corrective therapy involves the suppression of a particular mutation by a transfer RNA that is introduced into a cell [Katare and Aeri, 2010]. In gene augmentation, introducing a normal genetic sequence into a host genome modifies the expression of mutant gene in defective cell and the defective host gene remains unaltered. In general, the gene therapy recipient cells may be germline cells or somatic cells. Germline cells therapy involves modifying the genes in germ cells which will pass these genetic changes to the future generations. Somatic cells therapy involves the insertion of genes into specific somatic cells like the bone marrow stem cells, fibroblasts, hepatocytes or mycocytes [Katare and Aeri, 2010]. This form of gene therapy is being used at most genetic engineering laboratories throughout the world.

Clearly, gene therapy provides great opportunities for treating diseases from genetic disorders, infections and cancer [Park et al., 2006]. While the genetic mutations underlying various diseases are well understood, delivering a corrective gene to the unhealthy organs/tissues remains a remarkable challenge [Stone, 2010]. To achieve successful gene therapy, development of proper gene delivery systems could be one of the most important factors. Gene delivery systems should be designed to protect the genetic materials from premature degradation in systemic blood stream and to efficiently transfer the therapeutic genes to target cells. Intracellular delivery systems will be required for all molecules that have intracellular function. For example, nucleic acid molecules including encoding genes, oligonucleotides and RNA molecules must enter cells and target the nucleus when transcription is the target. Regardless of the molecules for delivery, a common requirement

is the avoidance of endosomal uptake that may cause degradation and denaturation [Gould and Chernajovsky, 2007]. Several approaches are being developed that can be applied to the delivery of all these types of molecules at disease sites. For the goal to be fully achieved, cell-targeting strategies require still further development.
Currently, a number of older and more recently discovered techniques have been developed for therapeutic gene transfer. A variety of viral and non-viral possibilities are available for basic and clinical researches [Gardlik et al., 2005]. Among these studies, DNA based vaccines are becoming popular. They stimulate the CD4+ T cells of Th1 subset and thereby mediate cellular immune response, which is effective against pathogens. On the other hand, the recombinant protein vaccines stimulate Th2 subset of T cells thereby eliciting a humoral response. The studies showed that DNA vaccines have been successful in protecting animals against influenza, herpes, rabies, malaria and leishmaniasis [Katare and Aeri, 2010]. However, the potential disadvantages of DNA vaccine have reduced the value of the approach. To optimize antigen delivery efficiency as well as vaccine efficacy, the non-viral vector as vaccine carrier has shown particular benefits to avoid the obstacles that both peptide/protein and gene-based vaccines have encountered [Chen and Huang, 2005]. For example, the success of the liposome-based vaccine has been demonstrated in clinical trials and further human trials are also in progress. This chapter summarizes the non-viral delivery routes and methods for gene transfer used in gene therapy and vaccine development.

2. Gene delivery systems

The simplest way of gene delivery is injecting naked DNA encoding the therapeutic protein, but because of low efficiency, there is a need to use special molecules and methods to improve gene delivery. A vector can be described as a system fulfilling several functions, including (a) enabling delivery of genes into the target cells and their nucleus, (b) providing protection from gene degradation, and (c) ensuring gene transcription in the cell. The ideal DNA vehicle should also be suitable for clinical application. It has to be inexpensive and easy to produce and purify in large amounts [Gardlik et al., 2005]. Two kinds of vectors have been employed as vehicles for gene transfer: 1) Viral vectors for gene transduction (e.g., *retroviral, adenoviral, adeno-associated viral* and *lentiviral* vectors), and 2) Non-viral vectors for gene transfection based on lipids, water soluble polycations, non-condensing polymers and nano/ micro-particles [Gardlik et al., 2005; Katare, 2010]. However, each vector has its own advantages and disadvantages.

2.1 Viral vectors (biological delivery systems)

Viral techniques use various classes of viruses as a tool for gene delivery [Gardlik et al., 2005; Stone, 2010]. Viruses introduce their DNA into the cells with high efficiency. Therefore, it is possible to take advantage of this system by introducing a foreign gene into the virus and then using the properties of the virus to deliver this gene with high efficiency into the target cells [Gardlik et al., 2005]. Gene therapy vectors are being developed by genetic modification of *retroviruses, adenoviruses, poxviruses, parvoviruses* (*adeno-associated viruses*), *herpesviruses* etc. [Gardlik et al., 2005; Stone, 2010]. Unlike wild type viruses, these vectors are used to transfer therapeutic genes into target cells and thus are engineered by deleting the essential genes which allow replication, assembling or infection. Replication deficiency ensures the safety of viral vectors, but on the other hand, vectors need to be produced in large amounts of virus particles. For this purpose, there are specialized cell lines called "packaging cell lines" (PCLs) engineered to replace a function of a deleted viral gene and for the production of recombinant viruses [Gardlik et al., 2005]. However, the interaction between a vector and a host-cell genome cannot be completely eliminated. Some disadvantages of viral delivery are addressed in Table 1.

No.	Disadvantage
1	Generation of an immune response to expressed viral proteins that subsequently kill the target cells producing a therapeutic gene product
2	Random integration of some viral vectors into the host chromosome
3	Clearance of viruses delivered systemically
4	Difficulties in engineering viral envelopes or capsids to achieve specific delivery to cells other than those with natural tropism for the virus
5	Possible recombination of the viral vector with DNA sequences in the host chromosome that generates a replication-competent, infectious virus
6	Inability to administer certain viral vectors more than once
7	High costs in producing large amounts of high-titer viral stocks for use in the clinic
8	Limited size of the nucleic acid that can be packaged and used for viral gene therapy

Table 1. Viral delivery system disadvantages [Templeton and Lasic, 1999; Gupta et al., 2004]

Currently, developed Viruses as transfer vectors are divided into two classes, following their different strategies for replication and survival: a) Non-lytic viruses, including *retroviruses* and *lentiviruses*, produce virions from the cellular membrane of an infected cell, leaving the host cell relatively intact; b) Lytic viruses, including human *adenovirus* and *herpes simplex virus* families, destroy the infected cell after replication and virion production. This native nature of the original viruses determines the use of each recombinant replication-defective viral vector in clinical applications [Table 2]. Despite some limitations on the use of viral vectors regarding safety and reproducibility, they are still the most used gene transfer vehicles [Gardlik et al., 2005; Katare, 2010; Gupta et al., 2004].

Vector	Genome	Structure	Properties
Adenoviruses	dsDNA	Capsid	Transient expression, strong immunogenicity
Alphaviruses	RNA	Envelope	Transient, but extreme, expression levels; low immunogenicity
HSV	dsDNA	Envelope	Latent infection, long-term expression, low toxicity (mutant)
Lentiviruses	RNA	Envelope	Genome integration, long term expression, safety concerns low titers, inefficient production
Retroviruses	RNA	Envelope	Genome integration, long-term expression
Adeno-associated viruses (AAV)	ssDNA	Capsid	Slow expression onset, genome integration, long term expression, inefficient large-scale virus production

Table 2. Utilization of viral vectors for gene delivery [Katare and Aeri, 2010]

In clinical studies, a recombinant *vaccinia* virus vector has been developed to express single or multiple T cell co-stimulatory molecules as a vector for local gene therapy in patients with malignant melanoma. This approach generated local and systemic tumor immunity and induced effective clinical responses in patients with metastatic disease [Kim-Schulze and Kaufman, 2009]. Furthermore, PSA-TRICOM vaccine (prostate-specific antigen plus a TRIad of co-stimulatory molecules; PROSTVAC) includes a priming vaccination with recombinant *vaccinia* (rV)-PSA-TRICOM and booster vaccinations with recombinant fowlpox (rF)-PSA-TRICOM. Each vaccine consists of the transgenes for PSA, including an agonist epitope, and three immune co-stimulatory molecules (B7.1, ICAM-1, and LFA3; designated TRICOM) [Kaufman, 2002]. The efficacy of PSA-TRICOM has been evaluated in phase II clinical trials in patients with metastatic hormone-refractory prostate cancer (mHRPC). PANVAC-VF, another poxviral-based vaccine, consists of a priming vaccination with rV encoding CEA (6D), MUC1 (L93), and TRICOM plus booster vaccinations with rF expressing the identical transgenes. CEA (6D) and MUC1 (L93) represent carcinoembryonic antigen and mucin 1 glycoprotein, respectively, with a single amino acid substitution designed to enhance their immunogenicity. This vaccine is currently under evaluation in several different types of CEA or MUC1-expressing carcinomas and in patients with a life expectancy more than three months [Vergati et al., 2010].

2.2 Non-viral vectors (Non-biological gene delivery systems)

In comparison with virus-derived vectors, non-viral vectors have several advantages, such as the safety of administration without immunogenicity, almost unlimited transgene size and the possibility of repeated administration [Gardlik et al., 2005]. Non-viral gene delivery systems generally consist of three categories: (a) naked DNA delivery, (b) lipid-based and (c) polymer-based delivery [Park et al., 2006]. Therapeutic gene can be introduced into the target cell either as an insert in plasmid with regulation sequences, what enables the regulation control of expression (inducible promoter) or as a PCR product. The simplest way of gene introduction is an injection of naked DNA into target cells. Such a naked plasmid DNA was used in several pre-clinical and clinical trials [Gardlik et al., 2005]. For example, some positive results were gained in cancer therapy by intra-tumoral injection of tumor suppressor genes or cytokines. However, this approach does not have the transfection efficiency of viral vectors. Low transfection efficacy and short-term expression still remain the main disadvantages of naked DNA gene transfer compared with viral vectors. Thus, many techniques have been developed to improve the introduction of therapeutic gene. Physical methods like electroporation and gene gun increase the entry of transgene into target cells. In addition, chemical methods like lipoplexes (DNA-liposomes complexes) and polyplexes (DNA-polymers complexes) improve the stability of DNA and also facilitate the entry into the cell [Gardlik et al., 2005]. Main methods of gene delivering systems are summarized in figure 1.

3. Physical delivery systems

A number of methods utilizing various physical techniques have been developed to facilitate the transfer of foreign genes into the host cells [Katare and Aeri, 2010]. Among them, electroporation and gene gun are further involved in preclinical and clinical trials.

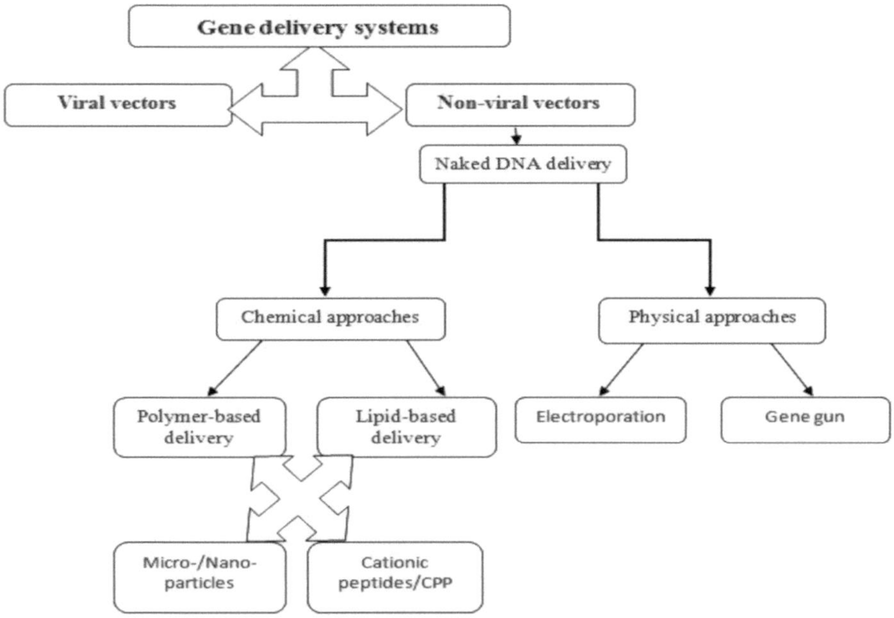

Fig. 1. Summary of the main methods of gene delivery systems

3.1 Electroporation

One of the methods that improve DNA penetration of the cell is electroporation [Lee et al., 2009; , Harrison et al., 1998; Rossini et al., 2002; Ahmad et al., 2009; Collins et al., 2006; Kang et al., 2011;]. *In vivo* use of electroporation is done by injecting naked DNA followed by electric pulses from electrodes that are located *in situ* in the target tissues. Successful use of electroporation was observed in transfecting muscles, brain, skin, liver, and tumors [Gardlik et al., 2005; Garcia-Frigola et al., 2007; Umeda et al., 2004; Babiuk et al., 2006; Harrison et al., 1998; Kang et al., 2011]. Since every tissue is specific and has its own characteristics, there are no generally accepted optimal conditions of electroporation that are suitable for effective transfection. These are dependent both on the amplitude and duration of the electric pulses and on the amount and concentration of DNA [Gardlik et al., 2005]. The generated pulse may be either a high voltage (1.5 kV) rectangular wave pulse for a short duration or a low voltage (350 V) pulse for a longer duration [Katare and Aeri, 2010].

Up to now, several clinical trials have been planned using the electroporation with DNA vaccines for cancer therapy such as: a) Intra-tumoral IL-12 DNA plasmid (pDNA) [ID: NCT00323206, phase I clinical trials in patients with malignant melanoma]; 2) Intratumoral VCL-IM01 (encoding IL-2) [ID: NCT00223899; phase I clinical trials in patients with metastatic melanoma]; 3) Xenogeneic tyrosinase DNA vaccine [ID: NCT00471133, phase I clinical trials in patients with melanoma]; 4) VGX-3100 [ID: NCT00685412, phase I clinical trials for HPV infections], and 5) IM injection prostate-specific membrane antigen (PSMA)/ pDOM fusion gene [ID: UK-112, phase I/II clinical trials for prostate cancer] [Bodles-Brakhop and Draghia-Akli, 2008; Bodles-Brakhop et al., 2009].

Furthermore, Hepatitis C virus DNA vaccine showed acceptable safety when delivered by Inovio Biomedical's electroporation delivery system in phase I/II clinical study at Karolinska University Hospital. ChronVac-C is a therapeutic DNA vaccine being given to individuals already infected with hepatitis C virus with the aim to clear the infection by boosting a cell-mediated immune response against the virus. This vaccination was among the first infectious disease DNA vaccine to be delivered in humans using electroporation-based DNA delivery [Bodles-Brakhop et al., 2009].

3.2 Gold bullet/gene gun

Similar to electroporation, another method, called "gene-gun", does not require the presence of complicated and potentially toxic delivery systems [Gardlik et al., 2005]. The gene transfer is mediated by small particles of gold on which the DNA is bounded. These particles are then shot into the cell under great pressure and speed (with the help of compressed helium) and so pass the membrane barrier [Katare and Aeri, 2010]. At first, the gene-gun was developed for gene transfer into plant cells; then, its use has expanded to gene transfer into the mammalian cells. Effective development of the gene-gun was also achieved in the field of DNA vaccination. The latest clinical experiments focus on cancer vaccines against various human tumors [Gardlik et al., 2005]. This method has been successfully used to deliver DNA *in vivo* into liver, skin, pancreas, muscle, spleen and tumors. Expression of reporter genes (e.g. firefly luciferase and β- galactosidase) or therapeutic genes (human growth hormone) have also been reported by this method [Gardlik et al., 2005]. Recently, gene gun-mediated transgene delivery system has been used for skin vaccination against melanoma using tumor-associated antigen (TAA) human gpl00 and reporter gene assays as experimental systems [Aravindaram and Yang, 2009 S]. In addition, the delivery of HPV DNA vaccines using intradermal administration through gene gun was shown to be the most efficient method of vaccine administration in comparison with routine intramuscular injection [Ogris and Wagner, 2002].

Currently, a HPV16 DNA vaccine encoding a signal sequence linked to an attenuated form of HPV16 E7 (E7 detox) and fused to heat shock protein 70 [(Sig/E7detox/HSP70)] has been used in clinical trials. In a previous study, the immunologic and anti-tumor responses have been evaluated by the pNGVL4a-Sig/ E7 (detox)/ HSP70 vaccine administered using three different delivery methods including needle intramuscular, biojector and gene gun. According to obtained results, DNA vaccine administered via gene gun generated the highest number of E7-specific CD8+ T cells as compared to needle intramuscular and biojector administrations in mice model [Trimble et al., 2003].

4. Chemical delivery systems

In order to facilitate the effective transfer of non-viral DNA into the cells, synthetic vectors improving the DNA admission into the cell and protecting it from undesirable degradation were designed. The most chemical delivery systems were derived from lipids or synthetic polymers [Templeton and Lasic, 1999].

4.1 Lipoplexes (cationic lipids/liposomes)

Plasmid DNA can be covered by lipids into organized structures such as liposomes or micelles [Templeton and Lasic, 1999]. The complex of DNA with lipids is called lipoplex. Lipoplexes can be divided into two types: 1) Anionic and neutral liposomes: At first, these kinds of lipids were used for the construction of synthetic vectors. Although, they were characterized by safety, compatibility with body fluids and the possibility of tissue-specific gene transfer, but the level of transduced cell expression was relatively low. At present, new neutral and anionic liposomes suitable for *in vivo* gene therapy are being constructed [Gardlik et al., 2005; Gupta et al., 2004]; 2) Cationic liposomes: These lipids are naturally produced complexes with negatively charged DNA. Moreover, their positive charge allows interactions with the negatively charged cell membrane and thus penetration into the cell is permitted [Gardlik et al., 2005]. Cationic liposomes ensure effective protection against the degradation of the foreign DNA by the cell. The interactions of liposomes with DNA and the subsequent lipoplex formation are dependent on several physical conditions (pH, charge) as well as structural characteristics of the liposomes. The most frequent use of DNA-liposome complexes is in gene transfer into cancer cells, where the applied genes stimulate anti-tumor immune responses or genes decreasing the activity of oncogenes [Gardlik et al., 2005]. Recent studies revealed the ability of lipoplex gene transfer into the epithelial cells of the respiratory tract, which supports their usage in the therapy of respiratory diseases and cystic fibrosis. Their expression in all main organs, mostly in lungs, was observed after intravenous administration of lipoplexes. Targeted transfection can be gained, to some extent, by the addition of tissue-specific target ligand. It is suggested that the transfection is based on endocytosis of the host cell [Gardlik et al., 2005].

The advantages of using liposomes for gene therapy are included as: 1) lack of immunogenicity; 2) lack of clearance by complement system using improved formulations; 3) unlimited size of nucleic acids that can be delivered, from single nucleotides up to large mammalian artificial chromosomes containing several thousand kilobases; 4) ability to perform repeated administrations *in vivo* without adverse consequences; 5) low cost and relative ease of generating nucleic acid: liposome complexes that deliver therapeutic gene products in large scale; 6) safety, because plasmids used for non-viral delivery contain no-viral sequences, thereby precluding generation of an infectious virus; 7) naked DNA carried by liposome increases its uptake by antigen-presenting cells (APCs); 8) naked DNA carried by liposome enhances both humoral and cellular immunity; 9) naked DNA carried by liposome induces cytotoxic T lymphocyte response [Trimble et al., 2003].

For vaccine development, a general overview of different lipid-based particulate delivery systems, their composition, preparation methods, typical size, route of administration and model antigens has been listed by Myschik J. *et al.*, 2009 [Myschik et al., 2009]. Stimuvax (BLP25 liposome vaccine, L-BLP25, Oncothyreon partnered with Merck KGaA) is a cancer vaccine designed to induce an immune response against the extracellular core peptide of MUC1, a type I membrane glycoprotein widely expressed on many tumors (i.e., lung cancer, breast cancer, prostate cancer and colorectal cancer) [Vergati et al., 2010]. Stimuvax consists of MUC1 lipopeptide BLP25 [STAPPAHGVTSAPDTRPAPGSTAPPK (Pal) G], an immunoadjuvant monophosphoryl lipid A, and three lipids (cholesterol, dimyristoyl phosphatidylglycerol, and dipalmitoyl phosphatidylcholine), capable of enhancing the delivery of the vaccine to APCs. A randomized phase II B clinical trial evaluated the effect of Stimuvax on survival and toxicity in 171 patients with stage III B and IV non-small cell lung cancer (NSCLC), after stable disease or response to first-line chemotherapy. Based on these data, Merck is currently conducting three large phase III clinical trials of Stimuvax. This study will involve more than 1300 patients [Vergati et al., 2010].

Furthermore, a cationic lipid DNA complex (CLDC) consisting of DOTIM/cholesterol liposomes and plasmid DNA, containing immunostimulatory CpG and non-CpG motifs has been designed, with potential immunostimulating and anti-neoplastic activities. Upon systemic administration, TLR-directed cationic lipid-DNA complex JVRS-100 enters dendritic cells (DCs) and macrophages; immunostimulatory DNA binds to and activates

Toll-like receptors (TLRs), which may result in the generation of anti-tumor natural killer (NK) cell and T-cell responses by the innate immune system. In addition, as a vaccine adjuvant, this agent may induce a strong cytotoxic T-lymphocyte (CTL) response to co-administered antigen. The efficacy of JVRS-100 has been evaluated in phase I clinical trials for the treatment of patients with Relapsed or Refractory Leukemia [ID: NCT00860522].

4.2 Polyplex (polysaccharides/cationic polymers)

A wide range of polymeric vectors have been utilized to deliver therapeutic genes *in vivo.* The modification of polymeric vectors has also shown successful improvements in achieving target-specific delivery and in promoting intracellular gene transfer efficiency [Park et al., 2006, Ogris and Wagner, 2002]. Various systemic and cellular barriers, including serum proteins in blood stream, cell membrane, endosomal compartment and nuclear membrane, were successfully avoided by designing polymer carriers having a smart molecular structure [Park et al., 2006; Ogris and Wagner, 2002]. Vectors based on a complex of polymers with DNA are called polyplexes. Most of them consist of cationic polymers and their production is regulated by ionic interactions [Gardlik et al., 2005].

In contrast to lipoplexes, some polyplexes (polylysin) are not able to release intracellular DNA into the cytoplasm [Gardlik et al., 2005]. For this purpose, co-transfection with endosome-lytic agents (inactivated *adenovirus*) is needed. On the other hand, polymers such as polyethylenimine have a mechanism of endosome disruption and there is thus no need for transfection with endosome-lytic agents. Polyethylenimine is used as a vector in aerosol inhalation gene therapy. It is a non-invasive and relatively effective gene transfer, especially into the respiratory tract, with permanent gene expression in this target region without undesirable expression in other tissues [Gardlik et al., 2005]. The size of the polymer determines the transfection efficiency and is specific for each individual gene transfer. Furthermore, the size of the aerosol particles determines the place of action, and thus the specificity of inhalation gene therapy [Gardlik et al., 2005]. An alternative to polyplexes can also be the use of polymer nanoparticles. Two types of such complexes have been characterized as gelatin-DNA and chitosan-DNA. In comparison with naked DNA, transfection using nanoparticles shows increased expression *in vivo* when administrated intratracheally or intramuscularly. Some polymeric vectors are summarized in the following sections:

Poly (L-lysine) (PLL)-based gene delivery systems

PLL has been widely used as a non-viral gene carrier since the formation of polyelectrolyte complexes between PLL and DNA was identified [Park et al., 2006]. Although, PLLs with high molecular weight have some properties suitable for a gene carrier, the PLL/DNA complexes showed a relatively high cytotoxicity and a tendency to aggregate and precipitate depending on the ionic strength. PEGylation [PEG: polyethylene glycol] of cationic polymers is known to greatly improve the problems of cytotoxicity, aggregation and non-specific protein adsorption *in vivo* [Park et al., 2006]. Some examples are mentioned as following:

- **Sugar-conjugated PLL:** Lactose and galactose have been used as conjugation partners with polymeric gene carriers for targeting asialoglycoprotein of hepatocytes. Lac-PEG-PLL showed much less cytotoxicity and higher stability and solubility in a physiological condition compared to PLL [Park et al., 2006].

- **Arterial-wall binding peptide (AWBP)-conjugated PLL:** Arterial-wall binding peptide (AWBP) is a peptide containing the arterial-wall binding domain (1000-1016 amino acids) of apoB-100 protein, a major protein component of LDL. The AWBP was conjugated to PLL via a PEG linkage (AWBP-PEG-g-PLL). When interacted with a plasmid DNA, AWBP-PEG-g-PLL could form spherical shaped complexes with a size of 100 nm and showed dramatic increase of transfection efficiency (150-180-fold), compared to PLL and PEG-g-PLL, in bovine aorta endothelial cells and smooth muscle cells. The presence of free AWBP in the transfection medium reduced the transfection efficiency of AWBP-PEG-g-PLL, suggesting that AWBP-PEG-g-PLL could be used as a tissue-selective gene carrier [Park et al., 2006].
- **Antibody-PLL conjugates:** Antibody-antigen interaction is one of the most specific interactions in biological systems. A monoclonal antibody against leukemia-specific JL-1 antigen (anti-JL-1-Ab) was conjugated with PLL by periodate-mediated oxidation of carbohydrate moiety in the Fc domain of the antibody, followed by reaction with PLL. The anti-JL-1-Ab-PLL conjugate demonstrated significantly higher transfection efficiency than PLL or lipofectin in leukemia (Molt 4) cells [Park et al., 2006].
- **Folate-conjugated PLL:** Folate receptor has been identified as a potential target molecule of various cancer cells. The receptor is up-regulated and over-expressed in a number of rapidly growing malignant tumor cells, resulting in a dramatic promotion of the cellular uptake of folate. Therefore, the conjugation of folate to a variety of polymeric carriers has been chosen as a popular strategy for the target-specific delivery of anti-cancer therapeutics to the folate receptor-bearing tumor cells. A folate-PLL conjugate that incorporates a PEG spacer between folate and PLL (Fol-PEG-PLL) was also synthesized. The Fol-PEG-PLL was coated onto the complexes of PEI/DNA for a receptor-mediated gene transfer. The formulated complexes exhibited much higher transfection efficiency than PEI/DNA or lipofectamine/DNA complexes in the presence of 10% serum, suggesting that the PEG segment of Fol-PEG-PLL could increase the cellular uptake by receptor-mediated endocytosis and efficiently stabilize the complexes by increasing their solubility as well as by reducing the non-specific adsorption of serum proteins. The formulation also showed much lower cytotoxicity than PEI/DNA complexes [Park et al., 2006].
- **The Terplex system:** The Terplex system is a low-density lipoprotein (LDL)-mediated targeting system, where the LDL specifically interacts with the LDL receptors on the cell surface. LDL receptors are membrane-anchored proteins present in many cell types including hepatocytes, endothelial cells and myocytes. The stearyl-PLL conjugate synthesized by N-alkylation of PLL with stearyl bromide interacts with a plasmid DNA to form complexes. The stearyl group could then bind to LDL via hydrophobic interaction to form the supramolecular gene carrier, the terplex. The Terplex system showed efficient *in vitro* transfection in a variety of cells including smooth muscle cells (A7R5), and human lung fibroblasts (CCD-32 Lu). The systemic administration of the Terplex system demonstrated prolonged circulation time compared to naked DNA [Park et al., 2006].

Polyethylenimine (PEI)-based gene carriers

- PEI has been one of the most popularly employed cationic gene carriers due to its superior transfection efficiency in many different types of cells. The buffering property of PEI leads to protect the DNA from degradation in the endosomal compartment during the maturation of the endosome to lysosome, facilitating intracellular trafficking of DNA. High cation density of PEI also contributes to the formation of highly condensed particles by interacting with DNA. However, the property may confer significant cytotoxicity. Studies with linear PEIs showed even higher transfection efficiency and lower cytotoxicity compared to branched PEI [Park et al., 2006]. There are different spectra utilizing PEI as described in following sections:

- **PEI-PEG:** PEI-grafted PEGs (PEI-g-PEG) with different PEG grafting ratios were synthesized to address the cytotoxicity and aggregation problems of PEI. Cell cytotoxicity of PEI-g-PEG was greatly reduced, while the transfection efficiency of PEI-g-PEG was still comparable to that of PEI. Cytotoxicity was independent of molecular weight of PEG but affected by the degree of PEG substitution [Park et al., 2006].
- **PEI conjugates with targeting moieties:** a) PEI-g-PEG-RGD: An angiogenic endothelial cell targeted gene delivery system (PEI-g-PEG-RGD) was developed by incorporating the αvβ3/αvβ5 integrin binding RGD peptide. b) Antibody-conjugated PEIs: A monoclonal antibody against human epidermal growth factor receptor-2 (HER-2) was conjugated to linear PEI for targeted gene transfer to cancer cells. The HER-2 antibody-PEI conjugate showed enhanced transfection efficiency in HER-2 over-expressing human breast adenocarcinoma cells (Sk-Br-3) compared to unmodified PEI [Park et al., 2006].
- **Folate-conjugated PEIs:** Folate-polyethylene glycol-folate-grafted-polyethylenimine (FPF-g-PEI) was synthesized by grafting folate-PEG-folate to PEI. A PEI-PEG-folate (PEI-PEG-FOL) conjugate was used as a carrier for a plasmid encoding small interfering RNA (siRNA) targeting green fluorescence protein (GFP). The complexes between the PEI-PEG-FOL and the siRNA-expressing plasmid showed an efficient suppression of GFP expression compared to unmodified PEI complexes in folate receptor over-expressing cells (KB), which stably expressed GFP [Park et al., 2006].

Water-soluble lipopolymer (WSLP): The water-soluble lipopolymer (WSLP) was synthesized by conjugating chlosteryl chloroformate to a low molecular weight PEI (1.8 kDa). WSLP interacts with DNA to form stable colloidal particles (70 nm). The PEI moiety of WSLP confers a buffering effect, which could facilitate endosomal escape of the WSLP/DNA complex. It was also reported that the dodecylation of PEI enhanced the cellular uptake and transfection efficiency. In a similar way, the hydrophobic cholesterol moiety of WSLP would give a chance to form small and stable complexes, resulting in enhanced cellular uptake and transfection efficiency. WSLP showed higher transfection efficiency and much lower cytotoxicity than 25 kDa PEI, suggesting that WSLP has the advantages from PEI as well as from chlosterol. Intratumoral injection of WSLP/p2CMVmIL-12 complexes to tumor-bearing mice showed a significant improvement in the retardation of tumor growth and survival rate [Park et al., 2006].

Biodegradable polycations

The backbone linkages of most polymeric gene carriers consist of a -C-C- bond or amide bond, which are not degraded in physiological solutions. The non-degradable non-viral carriers are not easily removed by physiological clearance systems and therefore, can possibly accumulate within cells or tissues to elicit further cytotoxicity [Park et al., 2006]. To solve the problems, several biodegradable polycations have been synthesized and evaluated as potential gene carriers. Generally, the biodegradable polycations showed much less cytotoxicity and higher transfection efficiency compared to an unmodified polycations, such as PLL or PEI [Park et al., 2006]. Some examples include: Poly (α-[4-aminobutyl]-L-glycolic acid) (PAGA), a biodegradable PLL analogue; Poly(β-amino ester)s; Poly(2-aminoethyl propylene phosphate) (PPE-EA); Degradable PEIs; The biodegradable PEIs were synthesized by crosslinking low molecular weight PEI (0.8 kDa) with either PEG-bis-succinimidyl succinate or disulfide-containing cross-linkers, such as dithiobis (succinimidylpropionate) (DSP) and dimethyl 3,3′-dithiobispropionimidate (DTBP) [Park et al., 2006].

Neutral and non-condensing polymer-based gene delivery systems

Although, cationic polymers, which electrostatically interact with DNA to neutralize its negative charge and condense DNA into nanosized particles, are generally considered as gene carriers, neutral polymers such as polyvinyl alcohol (PVA) and polyvinyl-pyrolidone (PVP) can also be used for gene transfer. They can protect DNA from enzymatic degradation and facilitate cellular uptake of DNA. These polymers may interact with DNA via hydrogen bonding and/or van der Waals interactions; van der Waals interaction of the hydrophobic vinyl backbones may cover around DNA to make its surface more hydrophobic. In a study, intramuscularly administered PVP/plasmid DNA formulation resulted in a significant increase in the number and distribution of the reporter-gene expressing cells in rat tibialis, compared to naked plasmid [Park et al., 2006].

5. Micro-/nano-particles

Another approach to DNA-vaccine delivery involves microparticle-based technologies to target APCs [Ulmer et al., 2006]. Microencapsulation of DNA, or association of DNA with microcapsules, has led to enhancement of CTL responses to encoded proteins [Doria-Rose and Haigwood, 2003]. Biodegradable, non-antigenic poly-lactide polyglycolide (PLGA or PLG) microspheres offer many advantages as a vaccine delivery system. Both cellular and humoral immune responses can be elicited to antigens encapsulated in, or conjugated onto PLG microspheres. Particles used typically range in size from 1 to 10 μm in diameter, a size that is readily phagocytosed by dendritic cells and other antigen-presenting cells (APCs). Microspheres elicit both CD8+ and CD4+ T cell responses by releasing antigen intracellularly [Doria-Rose and Haigwood, 2003]. Biodegradable PLGA nanoparticles (NPs) have been investigated for sustained and targeted/localized delivery of different agents, including drugs, proteins and peptides and recently, plasmid DNA owing to their ability to protect DNA from degradation in endolysosomes. PLGA-based nanotechnology has been widely used in diagnosis and treatment of cancer. These NPs have been shown to stimulate the immune response as measured by an increase in IL-2 and IFN-γ in spleen homogenates [Lu et al., 2009]. The majority of the existing literature involving PLGA polymers has tended to be focused on PLGA microspheres. In the last 10 years, microspheres have been used extensively for the injectable delivery of vaccine antigens, both for viral and bacterial antigens. Similar to microspheres, PLGA NPs have been shown to effectively enhance immune responses. The major obstacle is providing delivery vehicles with the adequate surface molecules for recognition by the immune system and for more effective targeting. It is likely, therefore, that future studies of PLGA NPs as vaccine candidates will focus on improving these features, as recently tested by grafting RGD peptides (arginine–glycine–aspartic acid-containing synthetic peptides) covalently onto PEG moieties on the surface of PLGA NPs [Lu et al., 2009].

These polymers have been designated as feasible candidates for drug delivery systems, anti-cancer agents and vaccine immunotherapy. For example, DNA vaccine delivery to APCs has been facilitated by microencapsulation of plasmid DNA, which encodes HPV E6/E7 antigenic proteins. The capsule is formed from polymeric PGLA microparticles. These resulting microparticles have a greater propensity toward APC uptake compared to naked DNA. This technique allows HPV DNA plasmid to be condensed inside the microparticle. The physical and chemical properties of the PGLA scaffold make DNA inaccessible to nuclease and preventing degradation, allowing for a sustained release of DNA and enhancing transfection efficiency *in vitro* [Lin et al., 2010]. In mice, microspheres containing HPV plasmid encoding HPV E6/E7 antigens have been shown to elicit a strong antigen-specific cytotoxic T cell response. Using this technology, microencapsulated DNA vaccine termed ZYC-101 encoding multiple HLA-A2 restricted HPV E7 epitopes has undergone Phase I trials in patients with CIN2/3 lesions and high-grade anal intraepithelial neoplasia. In both trials, intramuscularly administered vaccine was well tolerated, and in some patients had resulted in histological regression of the lesions as well as generation of E7-specific IFN-γ expressing T cells. A newer version of the DNA vaccine, ZYC-101a, which encodes HPV16 and HPV18 E6- and E7-derived epitopes has been used in phase II clinical trial in patients with CIN 2/3 lesions [Lin et al., 2010].

The multi-functional nano-devices based on the dendritic polymer or dendrimers are also being applied to a variety of cancer therapies to improve their safety and efficacy. Technical advances have been focused on the development of a linking strategy that allows the dendrimer molecules to be linked via complementary oligonucleotides. At present, further applications of dendrimers in photodynamic therapy, boron neutron capture therapy, and gene therapy for cancer are being examined [Baker, 2009].

Recently, the modified fluorescent nanoparticles have been synthesized as a targeting and delivery system, by conjugating both tumor targeting agent and chemokines to the nanoparticles, in order to attract immune cells toward tumor cells. Biodegradable chitosan nanoparticles encapsulating quantum dots were prepared, with suitable surface modification to immobilize both tumor targeting agent and chemokine on their surfaces [Chatterjee and Zhang, 2007]. Fluorescent chitosan coated quantum dots (QDs) were used to act as bi-functional bridging units between cancer and immune cells. This nanoparticulate form of delivery promises the advantages of enhanced tumor selectivity and longer half-lives, thereby enhancing effectiveness of the immune response and reduction in systemic toxicity [Chatterjee and Zhang, 2007]. Furthermore, the rapid development of Quantum Dots (QDs) technology has already fulfilled some of the hopes of developing new, more effective cancer-imaging probes. First, stable encapsulation of QDs with amphiphilic polymers has prevented the quenching of QD fluorescence in the aqueous *in vivo* environment. Second, QDs are relatively inert and stable. Finally, successful conjugation of QDs with biomolecules has probably made active targeting them to tumors. Despite their success so far in cancer imaging, there are challenges in enhancing sensitivity, maximizing specificity and minimizing toxicity of QDs, which must be undertaken before clinical applications can proceed [Zhang et al., 2008]. A major parameter limiting immune responses to vaccination is the number of activated APCs that capture antigen and migrate to draining lymph nodes. The use of cellular magnetic resonance imaging (MRI) is a promising approach for this purpose [Long et al., 2009]. In a study, an *in vivo* labeling method was described, which relies upon cell-to-cell transfer of super-paramagnetic iron oxide (SPIO) from tumor cells to endogenous APCs, *in situ*, for quantification of APC delivery to lymph nodes in a tumor vaccine model. Mice were immunized with a tumor cell-based vaccine that was labeled with SPIO. APCs that had captured SPIO were imaged over time as they accumulated in lymph nodes. It was indicated that MRI is capable of monitoring, *in vivo*, the trafficking of magnetically labeled APCs inducing a tumor-specific immune response, and that these cells can be magnetically recovered *ex vivo*. Excellent correlation was observed between *in vivo* and *ex vivo* quantification of APCs, with resolution sufficient to detect increased APC trafficking elicited by an adjuvant [Long et al., 2009].

6. Cationic peptides/cell-penetrating peptides (CPP)/trojan peptides

The studies have shown that a number of peptides and proteins are able to penetrate the cell membrane and enter the cell. It has been observed that many cargo molecules that are covalently attached to these peptides will be translocated into the cell. Recently, various natural and/ or synthetic cell-penetrating peptides (CPP) have known as efficient tools in vaccine design as they are capable of delivering therapeutic targets into cellular compartments. In fact, the cell membrane is impermeable to hydrophilic substances and delivery into cells could be facilitated by linking to CPP. Different cargos such as drugs, peptide/ protein, oligonucleotide/ DNA/ RNA, nanoparticles, liposomes, bacteriophages, fluorescent dyes and quantum dots have been linked to CPPs for intracellular delivery with possible use in future vaccine design [Brooks et al., 2010]. Two applications of CPP already validated in vaccine studies are delivery of tumor-associated antigens into antigen-presenting cells (APCs) and use as a non-viral gene delivery vehicle in DNA vaccines. There are two methods for designing CPP incorporating immunogenic antigens: A) chemical linking via covalent bonds B) coupling via recombinant fusion constructs produced by bacterial expression vectors. The orientation of the peptide and cargo and the type of linkage are likely important [Brooks et al., 2010]. In addition, the utilized CPP, attached cargo, concentration and cell type, all significantly affect the mechanism of internalization. The mechanism of cellular uptake and subsequent processing still remains controversial. It is now apparent that CPP mediate intracellular delivery via both endocytic and non-endocytic pathways [Brooks et al., 2010; Jarver and Langel, 2004; Wagstaff and Jans, 2006]. An attractive feature of using polypeptides as gene delivery vectors is incorporating multiple functional domains into one polypeptide chain, such as a DNA-binding domain linked with a receptor-targeting domain. This kind of polypeptides will recognize and bind to cell surface receptors that are unique to target cells and deliver the bound DNA into the cells through receptor-mediated endocytosis. Therefore, this process may ensure the therapeutic effect in desired cells and limit the potential side effects caused by transgene expression into the non-targeted cells [Zeng and Wang, 2005].

Several studies have shown that oligo-deoxynucleotides (ODN) with immune-stimulating sequences (ISS) containing CpG motifs facilitate the priming of MHC class I- restricted CD8+ T cell responses to proteins or peptides. Therefore, ODN/cationic peptide complexes are potent tools for priming CD8+ T cell immunity [Schirmbeck et al., 2003]. The complex formation required electrostatic linkage of the positively charged peptide to the negatively charged ODN. Conjugation of immunostimulatory DNA or ODN to protein antigens facilitates the rapid, long-lasting, and potent induction of cell-mediated immunity. It was shown that ODN (with or without CpG-containing sequences) are potent Th1-promoting adjuvants when bound to cationic peptides covalently linked to antigenic epitopes, a mode of antigen delivery existing in many viral nucleocapsids [Schirmbeck et al., 2003]. Table 3 contains a list of peptides that have been investigated for their ability to penetrate the cell [Futaki, 2005; Brooks et al., 2010].

Class	Protein	Functional peptide	Sequence	Translocation efficiency	Reference
Basic	**TAT [HIV]**	**Tat and related peptides**			Vives et al., 1997
		HIV-1 Tat (48-60)	GRKKRRQRRRPPQ	+++	Futaki, 2005; Brooks et al., 2010
		R9-Tat	GRRRRRRRRRPPQ	+++	Futaki, 2005
Basic		**Arginine-rich RNA binding peptides**			Futaki, 2005; Brooks et al., 2010
		HIV-1 Rev-(34-50)	TRQARRNRRRRWRERQR	+++	Futaki, 2005
		R7W	Fluo-RRRRRRRW-NH_2	+++	Futaki, 2005
		TatP59W	Fluo-GRKKRRQRRRPWQ-NH_2	+++	Futaki, 2005
		FHV Coat-(35-49)	RRRRNRTRRNRRRVR		Futaki, 2005
		BMV Gag-(7-25)	KMTRAQRRAAARRNRWTAR	+++	Futaki, 2005
		HTLV-II REX-(4-16)	TRRQRTRRARRNR	+++	Futaki, 2005
		CCMV Gag-(7-25)	KLTRAQRRAAARKNKRNTR	++	Futaki, 2005
		P22 N-(14-30)	NAKTRRHERRRKLAIER	++	Futaki, 2005
Basic	**VP22 [HSV]**	VP22	DAATATRGRSAASRPTERPRAPARSASRPRRPVE	+++	Cashman et al., 2002
	Human Calcitonin	hCT (9-32)	LGTYTQDFNKFHTFPQTAIGVGAP		Trehin et al., 2004
	Vascular endothelial cadherin [Mouse]	pVEC	LLIILRRRIRKQAHAHSK		Elmquist et al., 2001
	Related to γ-Zein [Maize]	Sweet arrow peptide (SAP)	$(VRLPPP)_3$		Fernandez-Carneado et al., 2004
	Related to γ-Zein [Maize]		$(Tyr\text{-}ZnDPA)_n$		Johnson et al., 2008
Basic/ amphiphilic	**Antennapedia homeodomain [*Drosophila*]**	Antennapedia (43-58) [penetratin]	RQIKIWFQNRRMKWKK	+++	Derossi et al., 1994
		Fluoro-Penetratin	Fluo-RQIKIWFQNRRMKWKK-NH_2		Futaki, 2005

		Pen2W2F	Fluo-RQIKIFFQNRRMKFKK-NH_2		Futaki, 2005
		Model amphipathic peptide	KLALKLALKALKAALKLA-NH_2		Futaki, 2005
		PenArg	Fluo-RQIRIWFQNRRMRWRR-NH_2		Futaki, 2005
		PenLys	Fluo-KQIKIWFQNKKMKWKK-NH_2		Futaki, 2005
		E N-(1-22)	MDAQTRRRERRAEKQAQWKAAN	+	Futaki, 2005
		B21 N-(12-29)	TAKTRYKARRAELIAERR	+	Futaki, 2005
		Yeast PRP6-(129-144)	TRRNKRNRIQEQLNRK	+	Futaki, 2005
		Hum U2AF-(142-153)	SQMTRQARRLYV	-	Futaki, 2005
Chimera (synthetic)	**Galanin/ Mastoparan)**	Transportan	GWTLNSAGYLLGKINLKALAALAKKIL		Pooga et al., 1998
	Galanin/ Mastoparan)	Model amphipathic peptide (MAP)	KLALKLALKALKAALKLA amide		Oehlke et al., 1998
	Hydrophobic-NLS	Pep-1	KETWWETWWTEWSQPKKKRKV		Morris et al., 2001
	Hydrophobic-NLS	CADY	Ac-GLWRALWRLLRSLWRLLWRA-cysteamide		Crombez et al., 2009
	Hydrophobic-NLS	Membrane translocating sequence peptide (MTS)	AAVALLPAVLLALLP		Rojas et al., 2008
	HIVGp41-NLS of SV40 T-antigen	MPG	GALFLGWLGAAGSTMGAPKKKRKV		Morris et al., 2008

Table 3. Protein transduction domains (PTD)

Furthermore, the HIV Tat derived peptide is a small basic peptide that has been successfully shown to deliver a large variety of cargoes, from small particles to proteins, peptides and nucleic acids. The "transduction domain" or region conveying the cell penetrating properties is clearly confined to a small stretch of basic amino acids, with the sequence RKKRRQRRR (residues 49–57) [Riedl et al., 2004; Brooks et al., 2005]. This polycationic nanopeptide is known to be a transfection enhancer of plasmid DNA. The conditions of DNA-peptide complex formation and DNA/Tat ratio have significant impact on the level of transgene expression and degree of DNA protection from nuclease attack [Hellgren et al., 2004]. The conjugation of this peptide to ovalbumin (OVA) resulted in efficient stimulation of MHC class I-restricted T cell responses *in vitro* and, more importantly, the generation of CTLs *in vivo* [Kim et al., 1997]. Also, soluble Tat-antigen conjugates can deliver the antigen directly to the MHC class I processing pathway and thereby increase the generation of antigen-specific CD8+ T cells *in vitro* [Kim et al., 1997; Riedl et al., 2004]. A fusion protein containing the carboxy-terminal end of Tat (amino acids: 49–86) linked to the HPV16 E7 oncoprotein enhanced tumor specific immune responses *in vivo* [Giannouli et al., 2003]. In C57BL/6 mice, E7-Tat mixed with Quil A generated efficient prophylactic and therapeutic suppression of HPV16-positive C3 tumor outgrowth. This study offers a new strategy for improving subunit cancer vaccines [Giannouli et al., 2003]. Particularly, a Tat-derived peptide in combination with a PEG-PEI copolymer could be a promising candidate as gene delivery vehicle intended for pulmonary administration. Tat-PEG-PEI represents a new approach to non-viral gene carrier for lung therapy, comprising protection for plasmid DNA, low toxicity and significantly enhanced transfection efficiency under *in vivo* conditions [Kleemann et al., 2005].

It has been shown that covalent attachment of low molecular weight polyethyleneimine (PEI) improves Tat peptide mediated gene delivery *in vitro* [Alexis et al., 2006; Putnam et al., 2001; Wang, 2006]. In our recent study, two delivery systems including polymer PEI 25 kDa and polymer peptide hybrid as PEI600-Tat conjugate were used to compare their efficiency for HPV16 E7 DNA transfection *in vitro*. Our data indicated that both delivery systems including PEI 25 kDa and PEI600-Tat conjugate are efficient tools for E7 gene transfection. In fact, PEI potency for E7 gene transfection is higher than PEI600-Tat *in vitro*, but its toxicity is obstacle *in vivo* [Bolhassani et al., 2008]. Using HPV16 E7 as a model antigen, the effect of PEI600-Tat conjugate has been evaluated on the potency of antigen-specific immunity in mice model. Assessment of lymphoproliferative and cytokine responses against recombinant E7 protein (rE7) showed that PEI600-Tat/E7DNA complex at certain ratio induces Th1 response. This study has demonstrated that PEI600-Tat conjugate is efficient to improve immune responses *in vivo* [Bolhassani et al., 2009].

Moreover, synthetic peptides containing a nuclear localization signal (NLS) can be bound to the DNA and the resulting DNA-NLS complexes can be recognized as a nuclear import substrate by specific intracellular receptor proteins [53]. For example, conjugation of an NLS to a Minimalistic Immunogenically Defined Gene Expression (MIDGE) vector encoding a truncated and secreted form of BHV-1 glycoprotein D (tgD) improved the tgD expression *in vitro* and induced both humoral and cellular immune responses in mice [Zheng et al., 2006]. This strategy could be applied as an efficient pathway in enhancement of DNA vaccine potency against cancer.

On the other hand, one of the CPPs that have currently received extensive attention in the field of DNA vaccination is the herpes simplex virus (HSV-1) protein VP22 [Brooks et al., 2010]. VP22 can form compacted complexes with short oligonucleotides and form particles of spherical nature with a size range of 0.3 to 1 µm in diameter. These particles entered cells efficiently within 2 to 4 hours. Furthermore, VP22 enables spreading of the antigenic peptide to the cells surrounding the transfected cells [Brooks et al., 2010]. Efforts have been made to increase the potency of DNA vaccines by exploiting the cell-to-cell spreading capabilities of the HSV-1 VP22 protein or the analogous protein from bovin herpesvirus 1 [Ulmer et al., 2006]. The significance of VP22 in intercellular spreading has been demonstrated through *in vitro* studies linking VP22 to p53, thymidine kinase, cytosine deaminase and Green Fluorescent Protein (GFP). These proteins were observed to be distributed to nuclei of surrounding cells [Lin et al., 2010]. Furthermore, vaccination with DNA encoding HPV16E7 linked to the HSV type 1 VP22 elicited the enhanced E7-specific memory CD8+ T lymphocytes and anti-tumor effects against E7-expressing tumor cells [Michel et al., 2002]. Also, VP22 has been used for HPV DNA vaccines targeting the

E6 protein [Lin et al., 2010]. Various groups have demonstrated that DNA constructs which encode fusion proteins of VP22 linked to an antigen increase the immune responses in mice and cattle. Bovine herpesvirus VP22 (BVP22) and Marek's disease virus VP22 (MVP-1) are both closely related by their structural homology to HSV-1 VP22, and can also have a significant role in intercellular spreading. Hung *et al.* has demonstrated that mice vaccinated with DNA encoding MVP22/E7 significantly increased numbers of IFN-γ-secreting, E7-specific CD8+ T cell precursors compared to mice vaccinated with wild-type E7 DNA alone, which directly lead to a stronger tumor prevention response. Similarly, immunization of mice and cattle with DNA vaccine coding for BVP22 linked to truncated glycoprotein D (BVP-tgD) was shown to generate a stronger tgD-specific immune response compared to animals vaccinated with tgD alone. Taken together, DNA vaccine encoding VP22 linked to antigens represents a promising approach to enhance DNA vaccine potency [Lin et al., 2010].

To evaluate the VP22 role in gene therapy of hepatocellular carcinomas (HCCs), the expression vectors were constructed for N- and C-terminal fragments of VP22-p53 fusion proteins and investigated the VP22-mediated shuttle effect in hepatoma cells by co-transfection experiments. VP22-mediated trafficking was not detectable in hepatoma cells *in vitro* by fluorescence microscopy [Zender et al., 2002]. For *in vivo* experiments, the recombinant adenoviruses Ad5CMVp53 and Ad5CMVp53-VP22 were constructed. In contrast to the *in vitro* experiments, intercellular trafficking of VP22-p53 could be observed in subcutaneous tumors of hepatoma cells by fluorescence microscopy, indicating a stronger shuttle effect in solid tumors compared to cell culture experiments [Zender et al., 2002]. In our current study, Herpes simplex virus type 1 (HSV-1) VP22 protein was employed to enhance DNA vaccine potency of *Leishmania major* amastin antigen in BALB/c mice model. Vaccination with the VP22-amastin-EGFP fusion construct elicited significantly higher IFN-gamma response upon antigen stimulation of splenocytes from immunized mice compared to amastin as a sole antigen. These results suggest that the development of DNA vaccines encoding VP22 fused to a target *Leishmania* antigen would be a promising strategy to improve immunogenicity and DNA vaccine potency [Bolhassani et al., 2011].

7. Hybrid vectors

A promising approach to overcome the limitations and develop the advantages of the individual types of vectors is their combination. Several types of hybrid vectors have been known: A) Virosomes are produced by the fusion of lipoplexes (liposomes with DNA) with inactivated HVJ virus (hemagglutinating virus of Japan) or influenza virus [Gardlik et al., 2005]. It was shown that the efficiency of gene transfer into the respiratory tract is higher than cationic liposomes or viral vectors. In addition, they are very well tolerated from the immunological view, so even repeated injection does not influence the efficiency and safety of transfer; B) The second type is represented by hybrids that were generated by mixing cationic liposomes or polymers with adenoviral vector. These are effective mainly in cells which do not have viral receptors. In addition, it was proved that an inactivated adenovirus attachment improves the efficiency of the transfer mediated by cationic liposomes or polymers [Gardlik et al., 2005]; C) Hybrid viruses can be produced by a combination of various types of viral vectors, and they represent a system which employs the main advantages of both viruses [Gardlik et al., 2005].

8. Bacterial delivery systems

The most recent approach in targeting the gene therapy is the use of bacterial systems as vectors for transfer and gene expression in tumor cells. The principle lies in the ability of some anaerobic bacteria to selectively colonize hypoxic areas (e.g., tumors) and replicate there. Therefore, it is possible to achieve selective expression of therapeutic genes specifically in tumors. Currently known and tested bacterial vectors have been divided into two groups: A) Strictly anaerobic bacteria (the species *Clostridium* and *Bifi dobacterium*) are used in *in vivo* experiments. *Clostridium* is the most important bacterial species for use as a vector. On the other hand, the non-pathogenic *Bifi dobacterium*, is naturally present in the human gastrointestinal tract and provides higher safety [Gardlik et al., 2005]. B) The second group consists of attenuated auxotrophic strains of *Salmonella typhimurium* that require the presence of tumor specific nutrition factors for selective replication. They use these factors for their own metabolism, thus prohibiting the tumor cells from utilizing them and growing. In *in vivo* experiments, high levels of *Salmonella* (109 bacteria/g tissue) were obtained. A similar tumor inhibitory effect was shown by application of *Salmonella* producing tymidin-kinase [Gardlik et al., 2005]. Although the above bacteria are characterized by high selectivity in tissue colonization, it is necessary to ensure the maximum level of specificity and therapeutic efficiency of bacterial vectors. For this purpose, promoters inducible by radiation were constructed. The transcription of such promoters is conditioned by irradiation with visible light. Bacteria are known for their resistance to irradiation (having a relatively small genome and effective DNA repair mechanisms). Therefore the localization of a therapeutic gene under the control of a radiation-inducible promoter ensures that cytotoxic proteins are expressed only in bacteria colonizing currently irradiated tissues. This strategy allows eliminating the possibility of expression in non-tumor and hypoxic tissues. The latest approach using prokaryotes in gene therapy is a system of transformed bacteria producing a therapeutic protein *in situ* under exogenous induction regulation [Gardlik et al., 2005].

9. Eukaryotic delivery systems

9.1 *Leishmania tarentolae* as a novel live vector

Although live recombinant vectors (bacterial or viral recombinant vectors) have been known to develop new vaccine strategies against pathogens (e.g., HIV-1), their use as vaccine candidates in human is delayed due to problems related to pre-existing immunity, inefficient antigen delivery or presentation and toxicity issues. Therefore, it is necessary to develop new live-vaccine vectors that are able to enhance antigen presentation and elicit potent immune responses without the risk of developing disease in humans. Recently, a lizard parasitic protozoan that is not pathogenic to humans, *Leishmania tarentolae* (*L. tarentolae)*, has been used as a candidate vaccine against visceral leishmaniasis [Breton et al., 2005], and HIV-1 [Breton et al., 2007]. *L. tarentolae* can elicit T-cell proliferation and the production of gamma interferon (IFN-γ), skewing the T-cell response towards a Th1-cell phenotype, and it provides inflammatory responses for the APC and acts as an immunostimulatory adjuvant. Unlike other pathogenic *Leishmania* strains, *L.tarentolae* lacks the potential to replicate within the targeted APCs and is eliminated after several days from the infected murine host [Breton et al., 2005; Breton et al., 2007]. It has been shown that a single intraperitoneal injection of *L. tarentolae* could elicit a protective immune response against infectious challenge with *L. donovani* in susceptible BALB/c mice [Breton et al., 2005]. Similarly, a single intraperitoneal administration of the A2-recombinant *L. tarentolae* strain could induce high levels of IFN-gamma and protect BALB/c mice against *L. infantum* challenge [Mizbani et al., 2009]. Interestingly, a recombinant *L. tarentolae* vaccine expressing high levels of full-length HIV-1 Gag elicited cell-mediated immunity in mice model and decreased HIV-1 replication in human tonsillar tissue following exposure to HIV-1 infection [Breton et al., 2007]. These data suggest that the use of *L. tarentolae* as a live vaccine vector may represent a promising approach for improving immunity and safety of candidate live vaccines against *Leishmania* infections and likely other intracellular pathogens for which T-cell mediated responses are critical for the development of protective immunity [Breitling et al, 2002; Breton et al., 2005].

9.2 Yeast as an efficient tool in vaccine development

Recent studies have indicated that yeast cell wall components possess multiple adjuvant properties. Interactions between yeast and DCs result in DC maturation, and whole recombinant yeast internalized by DCs can deliver heterologous antigens to both MHC class I and class II pathways and induce potent cell-mediated immunity [Capilla et al., 2009; Bian et al., 2010; Haller et al., 2007]. Vaccination with *Saccharomyces cerevisiae* (*S.cerevisiae)* expressing tumor-associated antigens can induce antigen-specific T-cell responses and protect animals against tumor challenge. In addition, *S. cerevisiae* is inherently nonpathogenic and heat-killed recombinant *S. cerevisiae* shows no toxicity in clinical studies. Yeast can be easily engineered to express multiple antigens and the inherent adjuvant properties of *S. cerevisiae* avoid the need for additional adjuvants. These characteristics make *S. cerevisiae* a potential vaccine vehicle for cancer and infectious diseases [Capilla et al., 2009; Bian et al., 2010; Haller et al., 2007]. There are some limitations and drawback in *S. cerevisiae* expression systems. For example, *S. cerevisiae* has a tendency to hyperglycosylate recombinant proteins, N-linked carbohydrate chains are terminated with alpha-1, 3-linked mannose residues which is considered to be allergenic. Other restriction is that the varieties of carbon sources that can be utilized by this species are limited [Bian et al., 2010]. Currently, two other species including *Hansenula polymorpha* and *Pichia pastoris* belonging to the *Saccharomycetaceae* family, could potentially overcome the described limitations of *S. cerevisiae* [Bazan et al., 2009; Bian et al., 2010]. On the other hand, these two species are broadly used as industrial platforms for heterologous protein production [Maleki et al., 2010; Bian et al., 2010].

10. Conclusion

A number of methods have been and are being invented for the efficient and safe delivery of therapeutic DNA. The perspectives and hopes that are associated with gene therapy support research in this field of molecular biology. Although, clinical trials have already started, there are still various limitations that must be solved before routine clinical use. The major aim in gene therapy is to develop efficient, non-toxic gene carriers that can encapsulate and deliver foreign genetic materials into specific cell types including cancerous cells. Both viral and non-viral vectors were developed and evaluated for delivering therapeutic genes into cancer cells. Many viruses such as *retrovirus*, *adenovirus*, *herpes simplex virus*, *adeno-associated virus* and *pox virus* have been modified to eliminate their toxicity and maintain their high gene transfer capability. Due to the limitations correlated to viral vectors, non-viral vectors have been further focused as an alternative in delivery systems. The main non-viral vectors include cationic polymers, cationic peptides and cationic liposomes. Currently, many modifications to the current delivery systems and novel carrier systems have been developed to optimize the transfection efficiency. Furthermore, the route of immunization can influence the outcome of the immune response through altering the interaction between the vaccine and different APCs at the site of injection. Hence, the routes of administration and formulation of DNA clearly affect the therapeutic response by altering immune pathway. Among the commonly used methods of DNA vaccination, the highest efficacy was achieved after *in vivo* electroporation and gene gun delivery. However, it is critical to further analyze the results of ongoing clinical trials, specifically, in the aspect of their success or failure of certain delivery methodologies for gene therapies.

11. Acknowledgment

Authors acknowledge the financial support by Iran National Science Foundation for experimental works, on following projects: ID#89000588 and ID#87020176

12. References

Ahmad, S.; Casey, G.; Sweeney, P.; Tangney, M. & O'Sullivan G.C. (2009). Prostate stem cell antigen DNA vaccination breaks tolerance to self-antigen and inhibits prostate cancer growth. *Molecular Therapy*, Vol. 17, No. 6, pp. 1101-1108

Alexis, F.; Lo, S.L. & Wang, S. (2006). Covalent attachment of low molecular weight poly (ethyleneimine) improves Tat peptide mediated gene delivery. *Adv. Mater.*, Vol. 18, pp. 2174-2178

Aravindaram, K. & Yang, N.S. (2009). Gene gun delivery systems for cancer vaccine approaches. *Methods Mol. Biol.*, Vol. 542, pp. 167-178

Babiuk, S.; Drunen Little, S. & Babiuk, L.A. (2006). Delivery of DNA vaccines using electroporation. *Methods in Molecular Medicine*, Vol. 127, DNA vaccines: Methods and Protocols

Baker, J.R. (2009). Dendrimer-based nanoparticles for cancer therapy. *Nanotechnology for Hematology*, pp. 708-719

Bazan, S.B.; Chaves, A.A.M.; Aires, K.A.; Cianciarullo, A.M.; Garcea, R.L. & Ho, P.L. (2009). Expression and characterization of HPV16 L1 capsid protein in *Pichia pastoris*. *Arch Virol.*,Vol. 154, pp. 1609-1617

Bian, G.; Cheng, Y.; Wang, Z.; Hu, Y.; Zhang, X.; Wu, M.; Chen, Z.; Shi, B.; Sun, S.; Shen, Y.; Chen, E.; Yao, X.; Wen, Y. & Yuan Z. (2010). Whole recombinant *Hansenula polymorpha* expressing hepatitis B virus surface antigen (yeast-HBsAg) induces potent HBsAg-specific Th1 and Th2 immune responses. *Vaccine*, Vol. 28, pp. 187-194

Bodles-Brakhop, A.M. & Draghia-Akli, R. (2008). DNA vaccination and gene therapy: optimization and delivery for cancer therapy. *Expert Rev. Vaccines*, Vol. 7, pp. 1085-1101

Bodles-Brakhop, A.M.; Heller, R. & Draghia-Akli, R. (2009). Electroporation for the delivery of DNA-based vaccines and immunotherapeutics: current clinical developments. *Molecular Therapy*, Vol. 17, No. 4, pp. 585-592

Bolhassani, A.; Ghasemi, N.; Servis, C.; Taghikhani, M. & Rafati, S. (2008). Comparison of two delivery systems efficiency by using polyethylenimine (PEI) for plasmid HPV16 E7 DNA transfection into COS-7 cells. *Modarres J. Med. Sci.* Vol. 11, pp. 15-19

Bolhassani, A.; Ghasemi, N.; Servis, C.; Taghikhani, M. & Rafati, S. (2009). The efficiency of a novel delivery system (PEI600-Tat) in development of potent DNA vaccine using HPV16 E7 as a model antigen. *Drug Deliv.*, Vol. 16, pp. 196-204

Bolhassani, A.; Gholami, E.; Zahedifard, F.; Moradin, N.; Parsi, P.; Doustdari, F.; Seyed, N.; Papadopoulou, B. & Rafati, S. (2011). *Leishmania major*: Protective capacity of DNA vaccine using amastin fused to HSV-1 VP22 and EGFP in BALB/c mice model. *Experimental Parasitology*, pp. 1-9.

Breitling, R.; Klingner, S.; Callewaert, N.; Pietrucha, R.; Geyer, A.; Ehrlich, G.; Hartung, R.; Muller, A.; Contreras, R.; Beverley, S.M. & Alexandrov, K. (2002). Non-pathogenic trypanosomatid protozoa as a platform for protein research and production. *Protein Expression and Purification*, Vol. 25, pp. 209-218

Breton, M.; Tremblay, M.J.; Ouellette, M. & Papadopoulou B. (2005). Live nonpathogenic parasitic vector as a candidate vaccine against visceral leishmaniasis. *Infection and Immunity*, Vol. 73, No. 10, pp. 6372-6382

Breton, M.; Zhao, C.; Ouellette, M.; Tremblay, M.J. & Papadopoulou, B. (2007). A recombinant non-pathogenic *Leishmania* vaccine expressing human immunodeficiency virus 1 (HIV-1) Gag elicits cell-mediated immunity in mice and decreases HIV-1 replication in human tonsillar tissue following exposure to HIV-1 infection. *Journal of General Virology*, Vol. 88, pp. 217-225

Brooks, N.A.; Pouniotis, D.S.; Tang, C.K.; Apostolopoulos, V. & Pietersz, G.A. (2010). Cell-penetrating peptides: application in vaccine delivery. *Biochimica et biophysica Acta*, Vol. 1805, pp. 25-34

Brooks, H.; Lebleu, B. & Vives, E. (2005). Tat peptide-mediated cellular delivery: back to basics. *Adv. Drug Deliv. Rev.* Vol. 57, pp. 559-577

Brooks, N.A.; Pouniotis, D.S.; Tang, C.K.; Apostolopoulos, V. & Pietersz, G.A. (2010). Cell-penetrating peptides: application in vaccine delivery. *Biochimica et biophysica Acta*, Vol. 1805, pp. 25-34

Capilla, J.; Clemons, K.V.; Liu, M.; Levine, H.B. & Stevens, D.A. (2009). *Saccharomyces cerevisiae* as a vaccine against coccidioidomycosis. *Vaccine*, Vol. 27, pp. 3662-3668

Cashman, S.M.; Sadowski, S.L.; Morris, D.J.; Frederick, J. & Kumar-Singh, R. (2002). Intercellular trafficking of *adenovirus*-delivered HSV VP22 from the retinal pigment epithelium to the photoreceptors-implications for gene therapy. *Mol. Ther.*, Vol. 6, pp. 813-823

Chatterjee, D.K. & Zhang Y. (2007). Multi-functional nanoparticles for cancer therapy. *Science and Technology of Advanced Materials*, Vol. 8, pp. 131-133

Chen, W.C. & Huang, L. (2005). Non-viral vector as vaccine carrier. *Advances in Genetics*, Vol. 54, pp. 315-337

Collins, C.G.; Tangney, M.; Larkin, J.O.; Casey, G.; Whelan, M.C.; Cashman, J.; Murphy, J.; Soden, D.; Vejda, S.; McKenna, S.; Kiely, B.; Collins, J.K.; Barrett, J.; Aarons, S. & O'Sullivan, G.C. (2006). Local gene therapy of solid tumors with GM-CSF and B7-1 eradicates both treated and distal tumors. *Cancer gene Therapy*, Vol. 13, pp. 1061-1071

Crombez, L.; Aldrian-Herrada, G.; Konate, K.; Nguyen, Q.N.; McMaster, G.K.; Brasseur, R.; Heitz, F. & Divita G. (2009). A new potent secondary amphipathic cell-penetrating peptide for siRNA delivery into mammalian cells. *Mol. Ther.*, Vol. 17, pp. 95-103

Doria-Rose, N.A. & Haigwood, N.L. (2003). DNA vaccine strategies: candidates for immune modulation and immunization regimens. *Methods*, Vol. 31, pp. 207-216

Derossi, D.; Joliot, A.H.; Chassaing, G. & Prochiantz, A. (1994). The third helix of the *Antennapedia* homeodomain translocates through biological membranes. *J. Biol.Chem.*, Vol. 269, pp. 10444-10450

Elmquist, A.; Lindgren, M.; Bartfai, T. & Langel, U. (2001). VE-cadherin-derived cell-penetrating peptide, pVEC, with carrier functions. *Exp. Cell. Res.*, Vol. 269, pp. 237-244

Fernandez-Carneado, J.; Kogan, M.J.; Castel, S. & Giralt, E. (2004). Potential peptide carriers: amphipathic proline-rich peptides derived from the N-terminal domain of gamma-zein, Angew. *Chem. Int. Ed. Engl.*, Vol. 43, pp. 1811-1814

Futaki, S. Membrane-permeable arginine-rich peptides and the translocation mechanisms. (2005). *Adv. Drug Deliv. Rev.* Vol. 57, No. 4, pp. 547-58

Garcia-Frigola, C.; Carreres, M.I.; Vegar, C. & Herrera, E. (2007). Gene delivery into mouse retinal ganglion cells by in utero electroporation. *B.M.C. Developmental Biology*, Vol. 7, No. 103, pp. 1-10

Gardlik, R.; Palffy, R.; Hodosy, J.; Lukacs, J.; Turna, J. & Celec P. (2005). Vectors and delivery systems in gene therapy. *Med. Sci. Monit.* Vol. 11, No. 4, pp. RA 110-121

Giannouli, C.; Brulet, J.M.; Gesché, F.; Rappaport, J.; Burny, A.; Leo, O. & Hallez, S. (2003). Fusion of a tumor-associated antigen to HIV-1 Tat improves protein-based immunotherapy of cancer. *Anticancer Res.* Vol. 23, pp. 3523-3532.

Gould, D.J. & Chernajovsky, Y. (2007). Novel delivery methods to achieve immunomodulation. *Curr. Opin. Pharmacol.* Vol. 7, No. 4, pp. 445-450

Gupta, P.N.; Singh, P.; Mishra, V.; Jain, S.; Dubey, P.K. & Vyas, S.P. (2004). Topical immunization: Mechanistic insight and novel delivery systems. *Indian Journal of Biotechnology*, Vol. 3, pp. 9-21

Haller, A.A.; Lauer, G.M.; King, T.H.; Kemmler, C.; Fiolkoski, V.; Lu, Y., Bellgrau, D.; Rodell, T.C.; Apelian, D.; Franzusoff A. & Duke, R.C. (2007). Whole recombinant yeast-based immunotherapy induces potent T cell responses targeting HCV NS3 and Core proteins. *Vaccine*, Vol. 25, pp. 1452-1463

Harrison, R.L.; Byrne, B.J. & Tung, L. (1998). Electroporation-mediated gene transfer in cardiac tissue. *FEBS Letters*, Vol. 435, pp. 1-5

Hellgren, I.; Gorman, J. & Sylven, C. (2004). Factors controlling the efficiency of Tat-mediated plasmid DNA transfer. *J. Drug Target*, Vol. 12; pp. 39-47

Jarver, P. & Langel, U. (2004). The use of cell-penetrating peptides as a tool for gene regulation. D.D.T., Vol. 9, pp. 395-402

Johnson, J.R.; Jiang, H. & Smith, B.D. (2008). Zinc(II)-coordinated oligotyrosine: a new class of cell penetrating peptide. *Bioconjug. Chem.* Vol. 19, pp. 1033-1099

Kang, T.H.; Monie, A.; Wu, L.S.; Pang, X.; Hung, C.F. & Wu, T.C. (2011). Enhancement of protein vaccine potency by *in vivo* electroporation mediated intramuscular injection. *Vaccine*, Vol. 29, No. 5, pp. 1082-9

Katare, D.P. & Aeri, V. (2010). Progress in gene therapy: A Review. *I.J.T.P.R.* Vol. 1, No. 2, pp. 33-41

Kaufman, H.L.; Flanagan, K.; Lee, C.S.; Perretta, D.J. & Horig H. (2002). Insertion of IL-2 and IL-12 genes into *vaccinia* virus results in effective anti-tumor responses without toxicity. *Vaccine*, Vol. 20, pp. 1862-1869

Kim, D.T.; Mitchell, D.J.; Brockstedt, D.G.; Fong, L.; Nolan, G.P.; Fathman, C.G.; Engleman, E.G. & Rothbard, J.B. (1997). Introduction of soluble proteins into the MHC class I pathway by conjugation to an HIV tat peptide. *J. Immunol.*, Vol. 159, pp. 1666-1668

Kim-Schulze, S. & Kaufman, H.L. (2009). Gene therapy for anti-tumor vaccination. Methods in Molecular Biology, *Gene Therapy of Cancer*, Walther, W; Stein, U.S. (eds.), Vol. 542, pp. 515-527

Kleemann, E.; Neu, M.; Jekel, N.; Fink, L.; Schmehl, T.; Gessler, T.; Seeger, W. & Kissel, T. (2005). Nano-carriers for DNA delivery to the lung based upon a TAT-derived peptide covalently coupled to PEG-PEI. *Journal of Controlled Release*, Vol. 109, pp. 299-316

Lee, W.G.; Demirci, U. & Khademhosseini, A. (2009). Microscale electroporation: challenges and perspectives for clinical applications. *Integr. Biol.*, Vol. 1, pp. 242-251

Lin, K.; Roosinovich, E.; Ma, B.; Hung, C.F. and Wu, T.C. (2010). Therapeutic HPV DNA vaccines. *Immunol Res*, pp.1-27

Long, C.M.; van Laarhoven, H.W.M.; Bulte, J.W.M. & Levitsky, H.I. (2009). Magnetovaccination as a novel method to assess and quantify dendritic cell tumor antigen capture and delivery to lymph nodes. *Cancer Res.*, Vol. 69, pp. 3180–3187

Lu, J.M.; Wang, X.; Marin-Muller, C.; Wang, H., Lin, P.H., Yao, Q. & Chen C. (2009). Current advances in research and clinical applications of PLGA-based nanotechnology. *Expert Rev. Mol. Diagn.*, Vol. 9, pp. 325-341

Maleki, A.; Roohvand, F.; Tajerzadeh, H.; Khanahmad, H.; Nobari, M.B.; Beiruti, A. & Rouholamini Najafabadi A. (2010). High expression of methylotrophic yeast-derived recombinant human erythropoietin in a pH-controlled batch system. *Avicenna Journal of Medical Biotechnology*, Vol. 2, No. 4, pp. 197-206.

Michel, N.; Osen, W.; Gissmann, L.; Schumacher, T.N.; Zentgraf, H. & Müller M. (2002). Enhanced immunogenicity of HPV16 E7 fusion proteins in DNA vaccination. *Virology*, Vol. 294, pp. 47-59

Mizbani, A.; Taheri, T.; Zahedifard, F., Taslimi, Y., Azizi, H.; Azadmanesh, K.; Papadopoulou, B. & Rafati, S. (2009). Recombinant *Leishmania tarentolae* expressing the A2 virulence gene as a novel candidate vaccine against visceral leishmaniasis. *Vaccine*, Vol. 28, No. 1, pp. 53-62

Morris, M.C.; Vidal, P.; Chaloin, L.; Heitz, F. & Divita, G. (1997). A new peptide vector for efficient delivery of oligonucleotides into mammalian cells. *Nucleic Acids Res.*, Vol. 25, pp. 2730-2736

Morris, M.C.; Depollier, J.; Mery, J.; Heitz, F. & Divita G. (2001). A peptide carrier for the delivery of biologically active proteins into mammalian cells. *Nat. Biotechnol.* Vol. 19, pp. 1173-1176.

Myschik, J.; Rades, T. & Hook, S. (2009). Advances in lipid-based subunit vaccine formulations. *Current Immunology Reviews*, Vol. 5, pp. 42-48

Oehlke, J.; Scheller, A.; Wiesner, B.; Krause, E.; Beyermann, M.; Klauschenz, E.; Melzig, M. & Bienert, M. (1998). Cellular uptake of an alpha-helical amphipathic model peptide with the potential to deliver polar compounds into the cell interior non-endocytically. *Biochem.Biophys.Acta*, Vol. 1414, pp. 127-139

Ogris, M. & Wagner E. (2002). Targeting tumors with non-viral gene delivery systems. *D.D.T.*, Vol. 7, No. 8, pp. 479-485

Park, T.G.; Jeong, J.H. & Kim, S.W. (2006).Current status of polymeric gene delivery systems. *Advanced Drug Delivery Reviews*, Vol. 58, pp. 467-486

Pooga, M.; Hallbrink, M.; Zorko, M. & Langel, U. (1998). Cell penetration by transportan. F.A.S.E.B. J., Vol. 12, pp. 67-77.

Putnam, D.; Gentry, C.A.; Pack, D.W. & Langer, R. (2001). Polymer based gene delivery with low cytotoxicity by a unique balance of side-chain termini. *Proc. Natl. Acad. Sci.*, Vol. 98, pp. 1200-1205

Riedl, P.; Reimann, J. & Schirmbeck R. (2004). Peptides containing antigenic and cationic domains have enhanced, multivalent immunogenicity when bound to DNA vaccines. *J. Mol. Med.*, Vol. 82, pp. 144-152

Riedl, P.; Reimann, J. & Schirmbeck, R. (2004). Complexes of DNA vaccines with cationic, antigenic peptides are potent, polyvalent CD8+ T cell-stimulating immunogens. *Methods Mol. Med.*,Vol. 127, pp. 159-169

Rojas, M.; Donahue, J.P.; Tan, Z. & Lin, Y.Z. (1998). Genetic engineering of proteins with cell membrane permeability. *Nat. Biotechnol.*, Vol. 16, pp. 370-375

Rossini, K.; Sandri, M. & Dona, M. (2002). High level of gene transfer into adult skeletal muscle by *in vivo* direct electroporation. *Basic Appl. Mol.*, Vol. 12, No. 3, pp. 97-100

Schirmbeck, R.; Riedl, P.; Zurbriggen, R.; Akira, S. & Reimann, J. (2003). Antigenic epitopes fused to cationic peptide bound to oligonucleotides facilitate toll-like receptor 9-dependent, but CD4+ T cell help-independent, priming of CD8+ T cells. *The Journal of Immunology*, Vol. 171, pp. 5198-5207

Stone, D. (2010). Novel viral vector systems for gene therapy. *Viruses*, Vol. 2, pp. 1002-1007

Templeton, N.S. & Lasic D.D. (1999). New directions in liposome gene delivery. *Molecular Biotechnology*, Vol. 11, pp. 175-180

Trehin, R.; Krauss, U.; Muff, R.; Meinecke, M.; Beck-Sickinger, A.G. & Merkle, H.P. (2004). Cellular internalization of human calcitonin derived peptides in MDCK monolayers: a comparative study with Tat (47-57) and penetratin (43-58). *Pharm. Res.*, Vol. 21, pp. 33-42

Trimble, C.; Lin, C.T.; Hung, C.F.; Pai, S.; Juang, J.; He, L.; Gillison, M.; Pardoll, D.; Wu, L. & Wu, T.C. (2003). Comparison of the CD8+ T cell responses and antitumor effects generated by DNA vaccine administered through gene gun, biojector and syringe. *Vaccine*, Vol. 21, pp. 4036–4042.

Ulmer, J.B.; Wahren, B. & Liu, M.A. (2006). Gene-based vaccines: recent technical and clinical advances. *Trends in Molecular Medicine*, Vol. 12, pp. 216-222

Umeda, Y.; Marui, T.; Matsuno, Y.; Shirahashi, K.; Iwata, H.; Takagi, H.; Matsumoto, K.; Nakamura, T.; Kosugi, A.; Mori, Y. & Takemura, H. (2004). Skeletal muscle targeting *in vivo* electroporation-mediated HGF gene therapy of bleomycin-induced pulmonary fibrosis in mice. *Laboratory Investigation*, Vol. 84, pp. 836-844

Vergati, M.; Intrivici, C.; Huen, N.Y.; Schlom, J. & Tsang, K.Y. (2010). Strategies for cancer vaccine development. *Journal of Biomedicine and Biotechnology*, 1-13.

Vives, E.; Brodin, P. & Lebleu, B. (1997). A truncated HIV-1 Tat protein basic domain rapidly translocates through the plasma membrane and accumulates in the cell nucleus. *J. Biol. Chem.*, Vol. 272, pp. 16010-16017

Wagstaff, K.M. & Jans, D.A. (2006). Protein transduction: cell penetrating peptides and their therapeutic applications. *Current Medicinal Chemistry*, Vol. 13, pp. 1371-1387.

Wang, S. (2006). Tat peptide conjugates of low molecular weight polyethylenimine as effective non-viral gene delivery vectors. *Mol. Ther.*, Vol. 13, pp. 76

Zender, L.; Kuhnel, F.; Kock, R.; Manns, M. & Kubicka S. (2002). VP22-mediated intercellular transport of p53 in hepatoma cells *in vitro* and *in vivo*. *Cancer Gene Therapy*, Vol. 9, pp. 489-496.

Zhang, H.; Yee, D. & Wang, C. (2008). Quantum Dots for cancer diagnosis and therapy: biological and clinical perspectives. *Nanomedicine*, Vol. 3, pp. 83-91

Zheng, C.; Juhls, C.; Oswald, D.; Sack, F.; Westfehling, I.; Wittig, B.; Babiuk, L.A. & Hurk S.D.L. (2006). Effect of different nuclear localization sequences on the immune responses induced by a MIDGE vector encoding bovine herpesvirus-1 glycoprotein D. *Vaccine*, Vol. 24, pp. 4625-4629

3

Gene Delivery Systems: Tailoring Vectors to Reach Specific Tissues

Carlos J. Alméciga-Díaz, Rocio Cuaspa and Luis A. Barrera
Institute for the Study of Inborn Errors of Metabolism
Pontificia Universidad Javeriana, Bogotá D.C.
Colombia

1. Introduction

The gene therapy concept was developed more than forty years ago. Edward Tatum in a historic lecture affirmed: "*We can anticipate that viruses will be used effectively for man's benefit, in theoretical studies concerning somatic cell genetics and possibly in genetic therapy... We even can be somewhat optimistic about the long-range possibility of therapy based on the isolation or design, synthesis, and introduction of new genes into defective cells of particular organs*". Two years later Marshall Niremberg predicted that: "*in 25 years it would be possible to program the cells with synthetic messages*", but called to attention that "*it should be postponed until having the sufficient wisdom to use this knowledge for the benefit of mankind*".

Initial efforts to construct vectors were achieved by Rogers and Pfudere in 1968. However, it was not until 1990 that the first gene therapy clinical trial was carried-out in a patient with adenosine deaminase (ADA) deficiency (Friedmann, 1992). Within the last several years, significant advances have been attained in therapies for cancer, AIDS, Parkinson's disease, X-linked severe combined immunedeficiency (X-SCID), hemophilias, cystic fibrosis, Leber's congenital amaurosi, and β-thalassemia, among others. Nonetheless, an adolescent patient suffering from a urea cycle defect died of an anaphylactic reaction a few hours after being injected with an adenoviral vector. Soon after, five children participating in a clinical trial to correct a X-SCID developed a leukemia-like condition due to the activation of an oncogene (Edelstein, 2007). Recently, the tragic death of a volunteer in an clinical trial for rheumatoid arthritis using an adenoassociated virus vector was initially associated to a side effect of the vector (Williams, 2007). However, further studies showed that this was caused by an infection with *Histoplasma capsulatum*, which was produced by an immunosuppression condition induced for a simultaneous systemic anti-TNF-alpha therapy in the form of the drug adalimumab (Williams, 2007). All these failures halted the progress of gene therapy and seriously questioned the efficacy of the procedure. It also prompted the need for more basic studies on the immunogenic aspects and how to make safer, and more efficient vectors.

During the last 35 years a long list of viral and non-viral vectors have been developed to design a vector that allows gene delivery to specific cell types, has a high gene transfer efficiency, produces therapeutic levels of gene expression during long-term periods, and minimizes the generation of side effects (Verma & Weitzman, 2005). Although the field has made great strides in producing an ideal vector, one of the main challenges remains to aim for a cell-specific vector. Most probably a vector left in the general circulation without a specific targeting signal, will be sequestered by the liver or may end-up in cells with no need of the

transfected gene product. In addition, to date gene therapy still encounters two main problems: (i) gene delivery to the central nervous system (CNS), as the gene or its product are naturally blocked by the blood brain barrier; and (ii) gene delivery into poorly circulated tissues such as bone, where up until now, it has only been achieved with low transfection efficiencies.
In this chapter, we will explore the modifications carried out in viral and non-viral vectors to enhance their natural tropism. Regardless of the vector, modification objectives can be summarized in: (i) tropism expansion to permit gene delivery to cells not easily transfected with non-modified vector, (ii) cell-type specific transfection reducing side effects, and (iii) stealth vector improvement to reduce protein interactions or cells that limit its therapeutic activity, e.g. immune system (Yu & Schaffer, 2005).

2. Retroviral vectors

Retroviruses are a family of enveloped, diploid, and positive-stranded RNA virus. This family is formed by alpharetrovirus, betaretrovirus, deltaretrovirus epsilonretrovirus, gammaretrovirus, lentivirus, and spumavirus (foamy virus), from which only the last three have been used as gene therapy vectors (Verma & Weitzman, 2005). The genome basically consists of three genes: (i) *gag*, which encodes for viral matrix, capsid and nucleocapsid proteins, (ii) *pol*, which encodes for protease, reverse transcriptase and integrase, and (iii) *env*, which encodes a bipartite membrane-anchored surface (SF) protein (Escors & Breckpot, 2010). In addition, complex retroviruses (e.g. lentivirus and foamy virus) have accessory genes for the regulation of gene expression, assembly and replication (Escors & Breckpot, 2010). In the viral life cycle, glycoproteins (GPs) play an important role in viral tropism, receptor recognition and cell entry (Liang et al., 2009). The binding of the viral GP to the cellular surface protein induces a conformational change into the viral GP and leads to fusion and insertion of the capsid into the cytoplasm (Yu & Schaffer, 2005). Most of the advantages and limitations of retrovirus targeting are related with this cell entry mechanism.
Retroviral vectors used in gene therapy have properties that allow the transduction of a broad array of cells (Cronin et al., 2005; Frecha et al., 2008). However, the use of targeted retroviral vectors allowing the delivery of the transgene to cells which are not normally transduced, or limiting the delivery to cells which should not be transduced would be advantageous (Cronin et al., 2005; Frecha et al., 2008; Lavillette et al., 2001). In general, retroviral targeting can be achieved by: (i) engineering the GP to produce a vector that recognizes a specific cell surface protein (direct targeting), (ii) pseudotyping with GPs derived from other retrovirus and that recognize specific receptors, (iii) using ligands that block the cell entry of the vector to the cells expressing the receptor for the ligand, while allow the transduction of others cell types (indirect targeting), or (iv) using biospecific antibodies, chemically crosslinking ligands and grafting polymers (Fig. 1) (Lavillette et al., 2001; Verhoeyen & Cosset, 2004; Yu & Schaffer, 2005).

2.1 Retroviral targeting by engineering the glycoproteins

Direct targeting consists of the insertion of ligands or antibody fragments into the viral GP (Fig. 1), which allows recognition of cell surface proteins different from those naturally used by the vector (Lavillette et al., 2001). Direct modification of a GP was first reported in 1990, with the successful fusion of CD4 with the GP of a gammaretroviral vector (Young et al., 1990). Later, a functional murine leukemia virus (MLV) vector bearing a GP protein fused with an antibody fragment against a hapten (4-hidroxy-5-iodo-3-nitrophenacetyl caproate) demonstrated binding of the modified retroviral vector to hapten, and the ability to package a transgene and transduce culture cells (Russell et al., 1993).

After these pioneer works revealed the feasibility of GP engineering, different authors studied the real potential of this targeting approach. The fusion of the erythropoietin polypeptide with the GP of a MLV vector showed for the first time that a chimeric GP was not only correctly incorporated into the virus envelope but also allowed the specific transduction of cells expressing the EPO receptor (Kasahara et al., 1994). A similar result was reported with a gammaretrovirus bearing a GP fused with a single-chain antigen-binding site against a cell surface expressed on human carcinoma cells (Kasahara et al., 1994).

Nevertheless, different studies have exposed the limitations of this approach. The first evidence of this limitation was observed with vectors carrying the Ram-1 phosphate transporter or the epidermal growth factor (EFG) into the GP, which showed a reduced transduction efficiency although the chimeric GPs were correctly expressed, processed, and exposed in the viral envelope (Cosset et al., 1995). A similar observation was reported for a gammaretroviral vector with a GP bearing a peptide binding to the $\alpha_v\beta_3$ integrin (Wu et al., 2000a), or with the stromal cell derived factor 1-alpha (Katane et al., 2002). These low transductions efficiencies were associated with loss or impairment of viral and cell surface proteins binding and subsequent membrane fusion and penetration of the viral core into the cytosol (Frecha et al., 2008; Lavillette et al., 2001; Yu & Schaffer, 2005). In addition, these results strongly suggest that only few set of peptides sequences can be inserted into the GPs without altering the mechanism of retrovirus cell entry (Verhoeyen & Cosset, 2004). The insertion of spacer sequences between the inserted peptide and the GP has proved to overcome this issue, allowing a significant improvement in the transduction efficiency of the modified vectors (Kayman et al., 1999).

2.2 Retroviral targeting by pseudotyping

Pseudotyping involves the production of viral particles bearing GP derived from other enveloped viruses (Fig. 1). This strategy was developed due to the narrow cellular transduction profile observed in vectors with native GPs (Cronin et al., 2005; Yu & Schaffer,

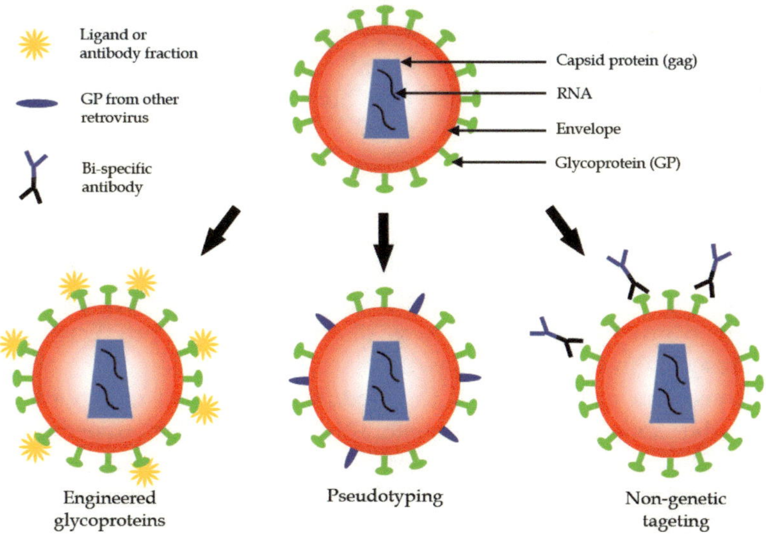

Fig. 1. Strategies for retroviral targeting. Retroviral vectors can be modified by ligand or antibody fraction insertion (engineered glycoproteins), use of glycoprotein (GP) from other retrovirus (pseudotyping), or the use of bi-specific antibodies (non-genetic targeting).

2005). Production of pseudotyped retroviral vectors is a well-established protocol (Bischof & Cornetta, 2010), which in most cases is used to allow virus purification, improve the cellular transduction, extend the range of transduced cells, and reduce cell toxicity (Cronin et al., 2005). However, it should be possible to employ natural tropism in GPs used for pseudotyping to target vectors bearing these proteins.

A large set of GPs has been evaluated for vector pseudotyping, among which vesicular stomatitis virus glycoprotein (VSV-G) is the most used [reviewed in (Bischof & Cornetta, 2010; Cronin et al., 2005)]. However, only a few GPs have allowed the transduction of different cell types compared to those observed VSV-G pseudotyped vectors. The use of a GP derived from rabies virus (RV) for pseudotyping an HIV-1 lentiviral vector allowed the transduction of neurons usually non-transduced with VSV-G vectors, since the RV glycoprotein induced a retrograde transport along axons (Mazarakis et al., 2001). The infusion of an animal model of familial amyotrophic lateral sclerosis (ALS) with a RV-HIV-1 vector carrying the gene of vascular endothelial growth factor (VEGF) delayed the onset of the disease and slowed progression in treated animals. Although treatment was initiated at the onset of paralysis CNS tropism of the vector was still significantly improved (Azzouz et al., 2004).

An interesting tropism was also observed for an HIV-1 vector pseudotyped with a GP from the lymphocytic choriomeningitis virus (LCMV) (Miletic et al., 2004). *In-vitro* and *in-vivo* evaluation of a vector pseudotyped with a LCMV GP showed that it transduced, almost exclusively, astrocytes; while VSV-G pseudotypes vectors infected neurons as well as astrocytes. In addition, LCMV-HIV-1 vector presented a specific transduction of infiltrating tumor cells, while VSV-G-HIV-1 vectors transduced mostly normal brain cells in infiltrating tumor areas. An HIV-1 vector pseudotyped with an Ebola Zaire virus-derived GP appeared useful in the treatment of airway diseases (e.g. cystic fibrosis). This vector allowed *in-vitro* and *in-vivo* transduction of airway epithelial cells, which was not observed with a VSV-G vector (Kobinger et al., 2001).

A recent modification of this approach used an HIV-1 vector pseudotyped with the GP and the fusion protein from a measles virus. The GP had an epidermal growth factor (EGF) or a single chain antibody against CD20 (Funke et al., 2008). The CD20-bearing vector was able to transduce primary and CD20-positive B cells both alone or within a cell mixture, while a VSV-G vector did not transduce these cell types.

2.3 Indirect retroviral targeting

This strategy is based on the finding that inclusion of certain peptides into the GP significantly impairs transduction of some cells. This prohibits gene delivering into cells that should not be transduced and extends viral tropism (Lavillette et al., 2001; Yu & Schaffer, 2005). First evidence of this approach was discovered while producing a MLV vector bearing a GP fused with epidermal growth factor (EGF). Although the chimeric GP was correctly expressed and processed, and the modified vector had the ability to bind to the EGF receptor, this manipulation completely inhibited vector transduction into cells expressing the EGF receptor (Cosset et al., 1995). This transduction inhibition was produced because of the modified vector was directed to the late endosome and destroyed by lysosomal enzymes.

A similar result was observed with a vector carrying the stem cell factor (SCF, a c-Kit receptor ligand), which selectively inhibited vector transduction on c-Kit-expressing cells (Fielding et al., 1998). When a mixture of EGF receptor-positive cancer cells and c-Kit-

positive hematopoietic cells were exposed to the above mentioned vectors, cancer cells were selectively transduced by the SCF-displaying vector, whereas hematopoietic cells were selectively transduced by the EGF-displaying vector. *In-vivo* proof-of-concept of this strategy was established after intravenous infusion of an EGF-displaying HIV-1 vector, showing preferable transduction of spleen with very low levels on EGF-receptor rich tissues (e.g. liver). Furthermore, the VSV-G vector transduced heart, skeletal muscle, lung, brain, kidney, ovaries and bone-marrow (Peng et al., 2001). Transduction inhibition of human and canine cells was also observed for a spleen necrosis virus bearing EFG, which was restored after cleavage via factor Xa at a site located between EFG and GP (Merten et al., 2003).
A variant of this strategy takes advantage of protease-activatable gene delivery vehicles. Matrix metalloproteinases (MMPs) are commonly overexpressed in angiogenesis, inflammation, and cancer invasion. The inclusion of a MMPs-cleavable peptide within an EGF-retroviral vector permitted that in the presence of exogenous MMPs, the infectivity of the MMP-EGF vector but not of the EGF-vector, could be restored. This MMPss-sensitive vector could efficiently discriminate between two different cell types, infecting only MMP-positive cells (Peng et al., 1997).

2.4 Non-genetic retroviral targeting

This strategy involves the use of antibodies or adapter molecules bound to the GP (Fig. 1) (Lavillette et al., 2001; Yu & Schaffer, 2005). This was the first approach used for cell targeting of a gammaretrovirus by using two biotinilated antibodies bridged by streptavidin: one against a GP and the other one against a specific cell membrane marker (Roux et al., 1989). This strategy allowed the specific transduction of cells expressing class I or II major histocompatibility complex (MHC) molecules by using monoclonal antibodies against these MHC molecules and against GP from the retroviral vector (Roux et al., 1989).
For targeting of a retroviral vector to folate receptor-expressing epidermoid carcinoma cells, a myeloproliferative sarcoma retrovirus was modified with folic acid (Reddy et al., 2001). Although receptor binding was observed, this vector was not able to induce gene expression. Similar results were observed for a MLV vector bearing a single chain anti-folate receptor antibody to produce vectors targeting ovarian cancer cells (Pizzato et al., 2001), manifesting the limitations of folate receptor targeting. A modification of this approach combines genetic modification of the GP by inclusion of an IgG-binding domain and the conjugation with an antibody that reacts with specific cell surface molecules expressing the antigen (Ohno et al., 1997). By changing the monoclonal antibody it was possible to transduce efficiently and specifically a variety of cell lines. The potential of this approach was confirmed by *in-vivo* evaluation of modified vectors conjugated with antibodies against surface proteins expressed in cancer cells, indicating that after intravenous infusion the vector preferentially transduced these cells (Liang et al., 2009). This strategy has been used both with gammaretroviral and lentiviral vectors. It represents a powerful tool that can be easily modified to obtain a site-specific gene expression for the treatment of cancers, genetic, infectious and immune diseases.

3. Adenoviral vectors

An adenovirus (AdV) is a non-enveloped virus formed by an icosahedral protein capsid surrounding a lineal double-stranded DNA of 36 kb (Douglas, 2007). The AdV capsid is characterized by the presence of 252 different capsomers and long fibers protruding from each of the twelve vertices. Seven polypeptides form this complex capsid: hexon (II), penton base (III), fiber (IV), IIIa, VI, VIII, and IX (Campos & Barry, 2007; Sharma et al., 2009). The cell receptor depends on the virus subgroup: A, E and F subgroups use the cell surface coxsackievirus B and adenovirus receptor (CAR); B1 and B2 subgroups use CD46, CD80/86, receptor X, or heparan sulfate proteoglycan (HSPG); C subgroup uses CAR, HSPG, MHC-I, vascular cell adhesion molecule-I (VCAM-I), or integrins; and D subgroup uses CAR, sialic acid, or CD46 (Arnberg, 2009; Campos & Barry, 2007; Sharma et al., 2009).

Adenoviral vectors have been used as tools for gene therapy since the late 80s (Friedmann, 1992), and the first clinical trial was started in 1993 (Douglas, 2007). Since then, over 392 clinical trials using AdV vectors have been carried out. Currently AdV are the most used vectors for gene therapy and represent 24% of clinical trials total (Edelstein, 2007). In addition, the first commercially approved gene therapy product, Gendicine, is based on an AdV vector engineered to express p53 for treatment of patients with head and neck squamous cell carcinoma (Peng, 2005).

AdV vectors are mainly derived from serotypes 2 (AdV2) and 5 (AdV5). They have the advantage of inducing high levels of gene expression, are able to infect both diving and non-dividing cells, and can be purified to high titers. Furthermore, AdV2 and AdV5 have high bloodstream stability with a reduced risk of insertional mutagenesis, since their genome remains extrachromosomal (Douglas, 2007; Edelstein, 2007; Volpers & Kochanek, 2004). Nonetheless, several drawbacks have been identified during *in-vivo* evaluation of these vectors: (i) presence of pre-existing antibodies that rapidly neutralize the vector, (ii) after intravenous administration the vector is mainly taken up by liver cells, limiting the vector to reach its target tissue in adequate concentrations, and (iii) use of high doses in an effort to overcome these problems has not proven to be an adequate and safe approach (Arnberg, 2009). Three strategies can be used to solve these issues: (i) use of vectors from other subgroups different from AdV2 and AdV5 (subgroup C), (ii) use of non-human serotypes, and (iii) retargeting of the vector to cells or tissues of interest (Arnberg, 2009). In this section we will explore different strategies for AdV retargeting that include genetic modification of the capsid, use of molecular adaptors and chemical modification of the capsid (Fig. 2) (Campos & Barry, 2007).

3.1 Genetic modification of the AdV capsid

Genetic modification of the viral capsid involves incorporation of foreign peptides into exposed regions of the capsid. In this manner the gene encoding for the peptide is inserted into the vector's genome (Fig. 2) (Campos & Barry, 2007). The possibility of altering the AdV vector capsid was first evaluated by the insertion of octapeptides into the hexon (Crompton et al., 1994) or the fiber knob (Krasnykh et al., 1998). This established the possibility of producing viable vectors with foreign proteins present on the vector capsid surface. Further experiments revealed the possibility of expanding the vector tropism by inserting a heparin-binding domain (Wickham et al., 1996), or an Arg-Gly-Asp (RGD)-containing peptide into the fiber knob (Dmitriev et al., 1998).

Although different studies indicated the feasibility to target vectors to specific cell types, genetic modification often resulted in failure to rescue viable viruses, or in an impaired virus packing, peptide exposure, and vector transduction (Leissner et al., 2001; Wu et al., 2005). Because the insertion of a pre-selected peptide into a fiber knob often fails to generate an adenovirus vector, use of random peptide libraries displayed directly on the AdV capsid allows isolation of viable vectors with high affinity for specific tissues or cells (Miura et al.,

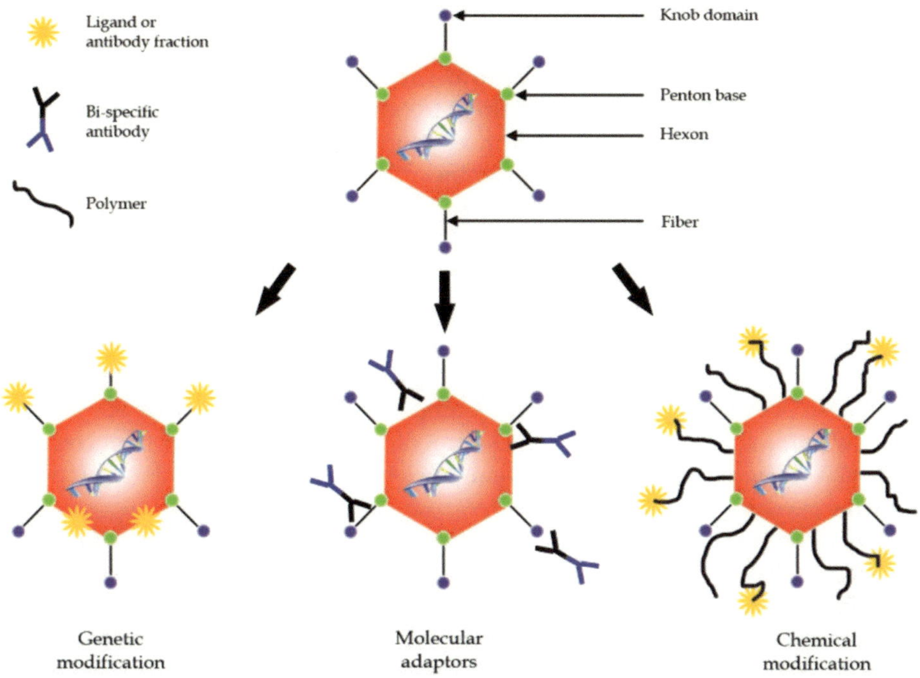

Fig. 2. Strategies for Adenoviral vectors targeting. Adv vectors can be modified by ligand or antibody fraction insertion (genetic modification), use of bi-specific antibodies (molecular adaptors), or conjugation with polymers bearing or not a ligand (chemical modification).

2007). A similar approach involves the pre-selection of peptides by using a phage display peptide library, from which peptides with high affinity for a certain cell type are selected and then inserted into the AdV vector capsid. This has allowed the targeting of AdV vectors to epithelium cells (Nicklin et al., 2001b), tumor cells (Rittner et al., 2007), and neurons (Schmidt et al., 2007).

Most efforts to modify the AdV vector capsid have been on vector targeting to tumor cells (Bachtarzi et al., 2008). Some examples of this approach include: (i) production of an AdV vector bearing a CAR protein fused with EGF producing an enhanced gene transfer efficiency in pancreatic carcinoma cells (Wesseling et al., 2001); (ii) a vector with a polylysine motif in the fiber for a CAR-independent binding to HSPG for specific transduction of different breast cancer cells (Ranki et al., 2007); and (iii) vectors with high affinity for prostate adenocarcinoma (Wu et al., 2010), and human colon carcinoma cells (Rittner et al., 2007).

In addition to cancer cell, genetically modified AdV vectors have been used as tools for gene delivery to other cell types. The insertion of an RGD-modified AdV allowed the production of a vector that mediated cell entry via RGD binding to integrins. Administration into the synovial lining improved the outcome of gene therapy for arthritis (Bakker et al., 2001). Targeting to endothelial cells, an important target in vascular gene therapy, was possible after insertion of the SIGYPLP peptide into the fiber protein in combination with fiber mutations that block natural CAR binding (detargeting) (Nicklin et al., 2001b). For specific kidney gene delivery, the intravenous administration of HTTHREP- and HITSLLS-bearing AdV vectors resulted in selective renal targeting, specifically of tubular epithelium and glomeruli (Denby et al., 2007).

Although genetically modified AdV vectors have been widely studied, most of these modifications have been carried out only into fiber or hexo. Recently it was determined that protein IX in the capsid is a viable platform for the insertion of single-chain variable-fragment antibodies (scFv) or single-domain antibodies (sdAb) for AdV vector retargeting. Even so, only sbAb enhanced virus infection of cells expressing the targeted receptor. Thus, proving that the nature of the ligand can significantly affect vector targeting as already had been observed with fiber and hexo (Poulin et al., 2010).

3.2 Molecular adaptors for AdV targeting

Although genetic modification is the most direct form of vector targeting it has the disadvantage of not all peptides can be inserted into the vector capsid. An approach to overcome this difficulty is to use molecular adaptors consisting of a capsid-binding domain fused with a cell-binding domain (Fig. 2) (Campos & Barry, 2007). This strategy has the advantages of not requiring a correct processing of the cell-binding peptide, since it is not translated with the viral capsid proteins; and that virtually any cell-binding peptide can be fused with the capsid.

The primary adaptor molecules are bi-specific antibodies against a capsid protein and a cellular receptor. The use of a single-chain bi-specific antibody directed against human EGFR and fiber knob significantly increased gene transfer into primary glioma cells and organotypic glioma spheroids, while reducing natural tropism dramatically (Grill et al., 2001). The human epithelial cell adhesion molecule (EpCAM) is highly expressed in malignant lesions of the stomach and esophagus. By using bi-specific antibodies against adenovirus fiber knob protein and EpCAM a specific transduction of gastric and esophageal cancer cell lines was observed with reduced transduction in normal cells (Heideman et al., 2001). For other epithelial tumors, e.g. colon, lung and breast, it was possible to target vectors by using a bi-specific adapter protein, which fused the ectodomain of CAR with a single-chain anti-carcinoembryonic antigen (CEA) antibody. This adaptor molecule allowed the targeting of AdV vectors to CEA-positive epithelial tumor cells in cell culture, in subcutaneous tumor grafts, and in hepatic tumor grafts (Li et al., 2007). A similar strategy was used for vector targeting to pancreatic carcinoma cells by using a vector bearing an EGF peptide fused with CAR (Wesseling et al., 2001). The combination of this adaptor molecule with the insertion of an RGD-containing peptide into the fiber knob resulted in a significant enhancement of gene transfer.

3.3 Chemical modification of the AdV capsid

The third strategy for AdV targeting is the chemical modification of the viral capsid by using primary-amine reactive groups (Fig. 2) (Campos & Barry, 2007). The capsid modification with polyethylene glycol (PEG - PEGylation) is a promising strategy to diminish vector toxicity and immune response. Although other polymers have also been used PEGylation can be employed to modify tropism. Polymer-coated vectors can be targeted to specific cells by incorporation onto the polymer molecules that bind to specific cell-surface proteins (Campos & Barry, 2007; Volpers & Kochanek, 2004).

PEG-modified AdV vectors were conjugated with an anti-HER2/neu monoclonal antibody leading to an enhanced and specific transduction of HER2/neu over-expressed breast cancer cells. Furthermore, a significant reduction of the innate immune response against the vector was accomplished (Jung et al., 2007; Kim et al., 2011). Conjugation of PEG-AdV vectors with an RGD peptide led to a specific $\alpha_v\beta_3$ integrin vector cell entry. This resulted in a significant improvement in transduction and specificity of gene delivery into endothelial cells. These events have implications on the treatment of rheumatoid arthritis, inflammatory bowel disease and epithelial tumors (Eto et al., 2005; Ogawara et al., 2006). Transduction of bone marrow derived human mesenchymal stem cells (MSC) can be significantly improved by using a PEGylated AdV conjugated with a blocked poly-L-lysine. However, modification on vector tropism was not clearly reported in this study (Park et al., 2010).

Although a great part of systemically administrated vector particles is scavenged by Kupffer cells in the liver, the use of a PEG- or a dextran-coated vectors allowed the specific transduction of hepatocytes independent of the presence of Kupffer cells, emphasizing the potential for therapeutic liver-directed gene transfer (Prill et al., 2010). Similar result can be observed by using a multivalent hydrophilic polymer based on poly-[N-(2-hydroxypropyl)methacrylamide] conjugated with EGF or VCAM, producing a CAR-independent binding and uptake into EGF- or VCAM-positive target cells selectively in mixed culture and also in xenografts *in-vivo* (Fisher et al., 2001).

4. Adeno-associated viral vectors

Adeno-associated virus (AAV) are non-enveloped virus belonging to the *Parvoviridae* family that need a helper virus, such as AdV or herpes simplex, for efficient infection and replication (Flotte, 2004). AAV are formed by a single-stranded DNA genome of 4.7 kb that contains two open reading frames (ORFs): (i) *rep*, which encodes for proteins Rep78, Rep68, Rep52 and Rep40, involved in virus genome replication, packing and integration; and (ii) *cap*, which encodes for the capsid proteins VP1, VP2 and VP3 (Wu et al., 2006). These ORFs are flanked by two Inverted Terminal Repeats (ITRs), involved in complementary DNA synthesis, Rep binding proteins, and site-specific genome integration in human chromosome 19 (Wu et al., 2006).

AAV capsid is formed by 60 subunits of VP1, VP2 and VP3 in a 1:1:10 ratio (Michelfelder & Trepel, 2009). These proteins share the C-terminal sequence, while the N-terminal sequences differ according to the start codon, being VP1>VP2>VP3 (Wu et al., 2006). Capsid structure has been elucidated for AAV2, AAV3, AAV4, AAV8 and AAV9 serotypes (Govindasamy et al., 2006; Lerch et al., 2010; Mitchell et al., 2009; Nam et al., 2007; Xie et al., 2002). The difference within capsid proteins allows for each serotype to use a specific receptor: (i) AAV2 and AAV3 use the HSPG, (ii) AAV1, 4 and 5 use glycans with sialic acid ends, and (iii) AAV8 uses the 37/67 kDa laminin receptor (Nam et al., 2007; Summerford & Samulski, 1998; Wu et al., 2006). AAV can infect a wide number of tissues including liver, lung, central nervous system, muscle, and heart; although as a result of the differences in receptor used, each serotype has a characteristic tropism (Flotte, 2004; Verma & Weitzman, 2005).

From the first clinical trial for cystic fibrosis patients with AAV vectors in 1995, over 75 clinical trials have been conducted. Pathologies such as α1-antitrypsin deficiency, Alzheimer's disease, Canavan's disease, hemophilia B, Leber congenital amaurosis, Parkinson's disease and muscular dystrophy; have attained promising results and no direct side effects have been associated with the vector (Warrington & Herzog, 2006). Although AAV vectors have shown to be promising tools for therapeutic gene delivery, they cannot transduce all cell types and could be useful to restrict its transduction to specific cell types. Strategies to modify the natural tropism of AAV vectors include: (i) the insertion of ligands into the viral capsid, (ii) use of chimeric or mosaic capsids, and (iii) conjugation with ligands through non-genetic modifications (Fig. 3) (Choi et al., 2005; Kwon & Schaffer, 2008; Michelfelder & Trepel, 2009).

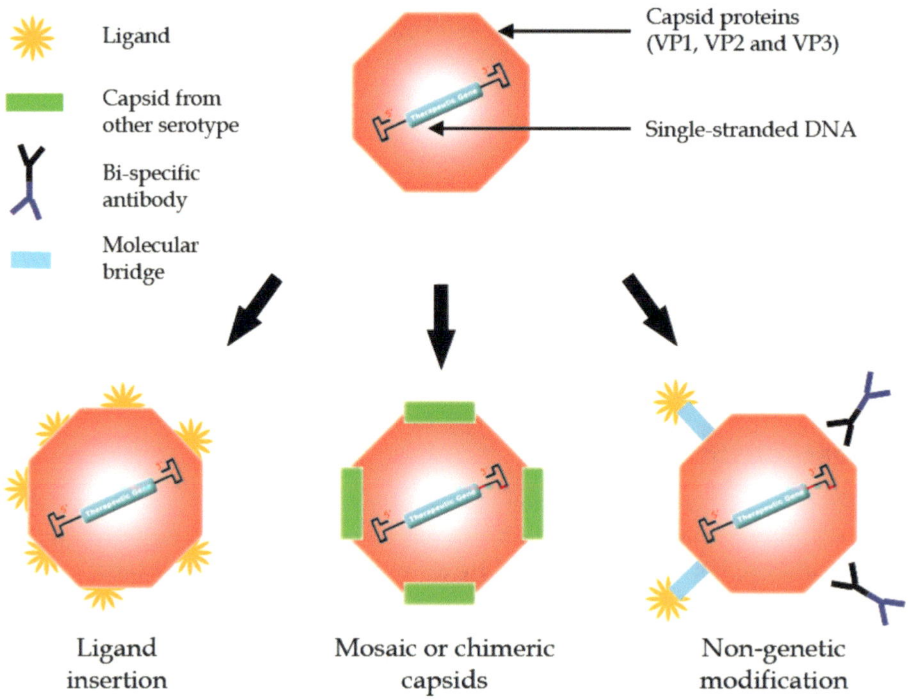

Fig. 3. Strategies for AAV vectors retargeting. AAV vectors can be modified by insertion of ligands into the capsid's proteins (ligand insertion), mixing capsid proteins from different serotypes (mosaic or chimeric capsids), or absorption of molecules onto the capsid using bi-specific antibodies or ligands fused with molecular bridges (non-genetic modification).

4.1 Targeting by ligand insertion

Mutagenesis analysis have permitted the identification of positions within the viral capsid that allow peptide insertion with little or no effect on DNA packaging and virus trafficking. For AAV2-derived vectors, peptides inserted in positions 1, 34, 138, 161, 459, 584, 587 and 588 (relative to VP1 start codon) are displayed on the vector surface, and allow production of vectors with similar viral titers to those observed for unmodified AAV2 vectors (Shi et al., 2001; Wu et al., 2000b). Most of the studies have used positions 138 (VP2 N-terminal), 587 and 588 (HSPG binding domain) to insert peptides ranging from 5 to 272 amino acids (Loiler et al., 2003; Michelfelder et al., 2009; Nicklin et al., 2001a; Perabo et al., 2006; Shi et al., 2001; White et al., 2007; White et al., 2004; Wu et al., 2000b; Yu et al., 2009). Capsid protein modifications have improved gene delivery to lung (Kwon & Schaffer, 2008), endothelial cells (Nicklin et al., 2001a), pancreatic islets (Loiler et al., 2003), vascular tissue (White et al., 2004), atherosclerotic lesions (White et al., 2007), muscle (Yu et al., 2009), myocardium (Yang et al., 2009), and cancer cells (Michelfelder et al., 2009).

Although the therapeutic effect of these vectors still remains to be seen, there is a long list of reports showing different advantages of peptide insertion within different positions of the viral capsid. Insertion after position 588 provided a complete AAV2 retargeting with inhibition of binding to HSPG (Büning et al., 2003; Perabo et al., 2006). AAV vectors designed for vascular tissue targeting were constructed by insertion after position 587 of peptides MSLTTPPAVARP and MTPFPTSNEANL, which showed increased transduction and specificity for venous endothelial cells and reduction of hepatocytes transduction (White et al., 2004). *In-vivo* experiments with these modified AAV vectors demostrated a reduction in liver and kidney transduction, while a significantly higher and specific targeting towards vena cava cells was observed (White et al., 2004). Recently, two new peptides (CAPGPSKSC and CNHRYMQMC) were evaluated for AAV retargeting to atherosclerotic lesions (White et al., 2007). The modified vectors showed higher levels of *in vitro* transduction than those observed for the untagged vector in human, murine, and rat endothelial cells. *In vivo* experiments showed that substantial higher levels of both peptide-modified AAV2 vectors were detected in the brachiocephalic artery (the site of advanced atherosclerotic plaques) and aorta, whereas reduced levels of modified vector were detected in all other organs examined (White et al., 2007). Serpin receptor ligand inserted after position 138 increased by 15-fold the transduction of vector on a lung epithelial cell line expressing the serpin receptor (Wu et al., 2000b). Insertion of a peptide that binds to the luteinizing hormone receptor after position 139 allowed production of a modified vector able to specifically transduce ovarian cancer cells (a luteinizing hormone receptor-bearing cell line) in an HSPG-independent manner (Shi et al., 2001). Insertion after position 138 of the 28-amino acid ApoE-derived ligand led to a 90-fold increase in pancreatic islet cells *in-vitro* transduction. Additionally, a four-fold increase of human antitrypsin expression was observed compared to unmodified AAV vector transduction (Loiler et al., 2003). Viral dose can be reduced 100-fold with similar transduction results as a consequence of ApoE-derived ligand insertion with a critical impact on side effect reduction. Functional AAV-modified vectors with long peptides up to 30 kDa have been reported, yet a laborious producing protocol is necessary to increase yield (Warrington et al., 2004).

Although these studies have demonstrated the feasibility of AAV retargeting, there is only one study evaluating the therapeutic effect of a modified AAV vector. In the study, AAV vectors were designed for brain-endothelial targeting, using peptides identified by phage display (Chen et al., 2009). After intravenous administration of modified vectors in MPS VII mice, there was extensive expression of enzyme in brain, leading to correction of lysosomal storage and reversal of established behavioral deficits (Chen et al., 2009).

During the last years we have worked in the development of a gene therapy strategy for the Mucopolysaccharidosis IV A (Morquio A disease) by using AAV vectors (Alméciga-Díaz et al., 2010; Alméciga-Díaz et al., 2009; Gutierrez et al., 2008). Morquio A disease, as well as other mucopolysaccharidosis, has a marked bone involvement, and an effective therapy should focus on the treatment in these manifestations. Recently, we designed a bone-targeting AAV vector bearing an aspartic acid octapeptide inserted immediately after the N-terminal of the VP2 capsid protein. The vector was designed to interact with hydroxyapatite (HA), a main component of bone (Tomatsu et al., 2010). We observed that the unmodified AAV vector had low bone affinity, while the bone-targeting vector had significantly higher HA affinity with up to 36.6-fold higher vector genome copies in cortical bone compared with the unmodified vector matrix (Alméciga-Díaz CJ, Montaño A, Barrera L, Tomatsu S., unpublished data).

4.2 Chimeric or mosaic capsids

A mosaic capsid AAV is a virion that is composed of a mixture of viral capsid proteins from different serotypes, which are mixed during viral assembly. On the other hand, a chimeric capsid AAV is a vector produced by the insertion of a sequence from another wild-type AAV into the ORF of the capsid gene (Fig. 3) (Choi et al., 2005; Michelfelder & Trepel, 2009). AAV vectors produced by the mixture of capsid proteins of AAV serotypes 1 to 5 led to high-titer viral particles with mixtures of serotype 1, 2, or 3; whereas intermediate titers were observed from AAV5 mixtures (Rabinowitz et al., 2004). Transduction levels varied depending on capsid mixture, producing a synergistic effect in transduction when AAV1 capsids were combined with AAV2 or AAV3 (Rabinowitz et al., 2004). Similar results were observed for a vector produced by the mixture of AAV1 and AAV2 capsid proteins, which exhibited similar titers to those observed for native vectors. The biodistribution profile combined transduction characteristics of both parent vectors (i.e. muscle and liver transduction) (Hauck et al., 2003).

A variant of this strategy uses capsid proteins bearing foreign peptides mixed with wild-type capsids. An AAV2 vector containing wild-type and immunoglobulin-binding Z34C fragment of protein A-bearing capsid proteins; made possible the production of a vector with high virus particle and transduction titers, and the capacity to transduce selectively and efficiently MO7e (human megakaryoblastic leukemia cell line) and Jurkat cells (T lymphocyte cells line) (Gigout et al., 2005). A mosaic vector produced by the mixture of wild-type and integrin-targeted capsid proteins resulted in a vector with a 50 - 100-fold enhancement in endothelial cell gene transfer. This is higher compared to the vector produced only with integrin-targeted capsid (Stachler & Bartlett, 2006).

4.3 Adsorption of receptor ligands

This strategy involves the binding of molecules onto the viral capsid to alter natural tropism of AAV vectors (Fig. 3). Initial approaches used bi-specific antibodies consisting of an anti-AAV antibody cross-linked with another antibody that binds specifically to a cellular receptor (Choi et al., 2005). In the first approach, an anti-AAV antibody was chemically cross-linked to Fab arms of the $\alpha_{II}\beta_3$ integrin binding monoclonal AP-2 antibody, allowing the specific transduction of megakaryocyte cells expressing the integrin (Ponnazhagan et al., 1996).

In a second approach, a high-affinity biotin-avidin interaction was used as a molecular bridge for the adsorption of streptavidin-fused ligands (Ponnazhagan et al., 2002). This strategy did not affect virus production and allowed the vector to be specifically targeted to EGFR- or fibroblast growth factor receptor (FGFR)-positive cells after conjugation of EGF or FGF onto the biotinilated capsid. Recently the exogenous glycation of the viral capsid was presented as a potential alternative to redirect vectors from liver to skeletal and cardiac muscle after systemic administration in mice (Horowitz et al., 2011).

5. Non-viral vectors

Non-viral vectors for gene delivery offer several advantages over viral vectors, since these include lack of an immune response, simple synthesis, and low scale-up production cost (Niidome & Huang, 2002). Non-viral vectors may include lipoplexes (DNA-liposome complex), polyplexes (DNA-polymer complex), lipopolyplexes (DNA-liposome-polymer complex) and peptide-based complexes (Douglas, 2008); which can be mixed with physical methods (e.g. electroporation, ultrasound, gene gun or hydrodynamic infusion) to improve the gene delivery (Niidome & Huang, 2002). In addition, most used non-viral vectors do not integrate into the host genome reducing the risk of mutagenic events in the transfected cells

(Kim et al., 2010). However, transduction efficiencies are significantly lower than that of viral vectors (Douglas, 2008). The reader is referred to other chapters in this book edition for more thorough treatises of non-viral vectors.

Although some physical methods allow gene delivery to a specific cell type, we will only consider some strategies developed to modify vector tropism. It is important to note that although most of these studies have been evaluated exclusively *in-vitro*, they constitute proof-of-concept.

5.1 Lipoplexes

Lipoplexes are the result of a complex formation between cationic liposomes (artificial closed vesicles of lipid bilayer membranes) and genetic material. They can be considered a synthetic means of encapsulating genetic material until it reaches its cellular target (Tros et al., 2010). The main strategies for targeting of lipoplexes involve use of chelator lipids that bind metal-bearing ligands, or the modification with polymers bearing a ligand (Fig. 4).

The insertion of the chelator lipid 3 (nitrilotriacetic acid)-ditetradecylamine (NTA(3)-DTDA) in a lipoplex preparation allowed the engraftment of a His-tagged vascular epidermal growth factor (VEGF) ligand and specific transfection of cells expressing the VEGF receptor (Fig. 4) (Herringson et al., 2009). A similar approach was used to target small iRNAs to B lymphocytes by using a lipoplex bearing the NTA(3)-DTDA chelator lipid engrafted with a His-tagged CD4 or to cells expressing the receptor for tumor necrosis factor alpha (TNFα) by engrafting with a His-tagged TNFα ligand (Herringson & Altin, 2009).

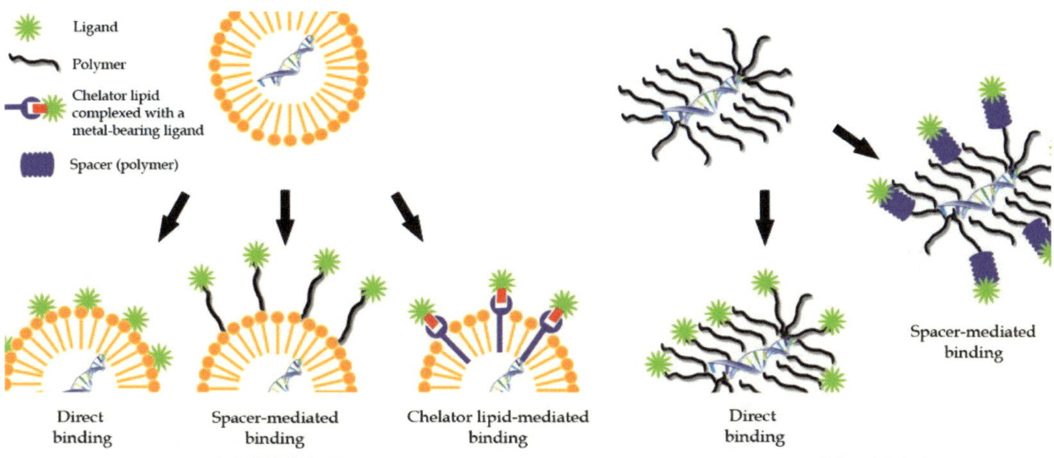

Fig. 4. Modification of lipoplexes and polyplexes. Ligands can be bound to non-viral vectors through direct binding, spacer (polymer)-mediated binding, or chelator lipid-mediated binding (ligand should be fused with a metal).

To improve hepatic specific delivery of a lipoplex after systemic administration, PEG molecules were added to the complex and galactose molecules were covalently affixed at the distal end of the PEG chain to allow an active targeting to the asialoglycoprotein-receptor present on hepatocytes. This resulted in an 18-fold increase in hepatic gene expression (Morille et al., 2009). Inclusion of a PEG conjugated with a nuclear localization signal (NLS) and added to a lipoplex preparation permitted transfection of endothelial cells in the presence of serum. This method was used as a model for transfection of blood-brain barrier cells considered difficult targets for non-modified viral and non-viral vectors (Zhang et al., 2009). A similar strategy was used for targeting of a lipoplex to tumor cells expressing the tumor-associated glycoprotein (TAG)-72 (Kim et al., 2008). In this work, a Fab' fragment from an anti-TAG-72 monoclonal antibody was conjugated with PEG and included within the lipoplex, providing specific gene delivery to TAG-expressing tumor cells both *in-vitro* and *in-vivo*, while non-targeted lipoploxes did not produce the transfection of those cells.

Ligands can be also directly conjugated with liposome molecules (Fig. 4). A hyaluronic acid-liposome conjugate resulted in an increased gene delivery to breast cancer cells with high CD44 levels. Conversely, cells with low CD44 levels were not transfected (Surace et al., 2009). Conjugation of the peptide 4-fluorobenzoyl-RR-(L-3-(2-naphthyl)alanine)-CYEK-(L-citrulline)-PYR-(L-citrulline)-CR with a liposome permitted targeting of a lipoplex to CXCR4-expressing cells, with transfection efficiency depending upon CXCR4 expression levels (Driessen et al., 2008). Conjugation of a liposome with transferrin presented a significant increment in iRNA delivery to hepatocarcinoma cells, with reduced toxicity and enhanced specific gene silencing compared to non-modified lipoplexes (Cardoso et al., 2007). Transferin-conjugated lipoplexes were also used to evaluate specific gene delivery to a metastatic mammary carcinoma cell line, although the results did not demonstrate a significant increase in cytotoxicity with modified lipoplexes in comparison with non-modified lipoplex (Lopez-Barcons et al., 2005).

Another strategy based on *ex-vivo* gene therapy assessed the challenge of nuclear entry by using plasmids transfected with a cationic lipid vector in MSC (Hoare et al., 2010). To enhance gene expression in MSC, they used NLS peptides to direct the plasmid to the nucleus. A significant increase was observed in reporter gene delivery compared to non-modified plasmid. They also noticed the lipid had a protective impact on the plasmid-NLS complex. Differentiation potential was not affected by NLS peptides.

5.2 Polyplexes

Polyplexes are non-viral vectors formed by genetic material coupled with cationic polymers including polylysine (PLL), polyarginine, PEG, polyethylenimine (PEI), polyamidoamine (PAMAM), dendrimers, and chitosan. The mechanism involves interaction between negatively charged DNA or iRNA molecules with positively charged molecules within the polymer (Tros et al., 2010). To target polyplexes to specific cells, they can be modified by incorporation of ligands as small molecules, vitamins, carbohydrates, peptides, or proteins (Wagner et al., 2005).

PEG-derived vectors are widely used as gene therapy tools as a result of their well-known capacity to enhance gene delivery and induce a longer DNA half-life time (Midoux et al., 2008). Due to the possibility to bind ligands in the terminal ends of the polymer (Fig. 4), PEG-derived vectors are commonly used for cell specific gene delivery using non-viral vectors (Hughes & Rao, 2005). PEG polyplexes have been conjugated with a transferrin peptide to target vectors to receptor-expressing cells in two prostate cancer cell lines (Nie et al., 2011). In addition they have been conjugated with EGFR ligand or lactose for specific transfection of human hepatocarcinoma cell lines (Klutz et al., 2011; Oishi et al., 2007).

PEG has also been used as a spacer to bind ligands to polyplexex (Fig. 4), although it has been associated in some cases with reduced transfection efficiencies. A complex of DNA and the HIV-derived TAT protein (which has important translocation abilities due to its strong

cell surface adherence) was conjugated with an ICAM-1 ligand by using a PEG spacer allowing an efficient and specific transfection of ICAM-1 expressing cells (Khondee et al., 2011). Similarly, a PEI-derived polyplex was engineered for enhanced and specific delivery of VEGF iRNA in prostate cancer cells. The conjugation with prostate cancer-binding peptide via a PEG spacer, showed a significantly higher VEGF inhibition than with the unmodified PEI polyplex in human prostate carcinoma cells (Kim et al., 2009). Anionic liposomes and cationic polymers do not display an efficient targeting to liver or tumors cells. Thus, a lipopolyplex was constructed with a liposome. A PEI polymer and a PEG polymer bearing a monoclonal antibody permitted an *in-vitro* and *in-vivo* transfection of tumor cells (Hu et al., 2010). A similar strategy was used to target an iRNA to tumor cells expressing the EGFR by using this lipopolyplex bearing the EGFR ligand (Hu et al., 2011).
Direct binding of ligands in other polyplexes has also been evaluated. Conjugation of folic acid with the aminomethacrylate-phosphoryl-choline based copolymer, allowed transfection of cells overexpressing the receptor for folic acid in some human tumors cells (Lam et al., 2009). A PEI-derived polyplex conjugated with an Arg-Gly-Asp peptide, which binds to the $\alpha_v\beta_3$ integrin receptor, resulted in efficient transfection of HeLa cells with low and high densities of $\alpha_v\beta_3$ integrin (Ng et al., 2009). As observed in viral vectors and lipoplexes, antibodies can be also conjugated with polyplexes to target genetic material to specific cell types. A successful overexpression of the human epidermal growth factor receptor-2 (HER2) by transfection with a polyplex conjugated with an anti-HER2 monoclonal antibody has been reported for a breast cancer cell line (Chiu et al., 2004). Another approach in adult MSCs used a modification of a PLL polymer with a palmitic acid substitution to target bone marrow stromal cells. A transfection efficiency similar to that of adenoviral vectors was obtained, opening the possibly to efficiently transfecting these cells without the side-effects and cell toxicity observed with viral vectors (Incani et al., 2007).
In-vivo evaluations of these modified polyplexes include use of a PEI-derived complex bearing an FGFR ligand for transfection of tumor cell lines. It demonstrated *in-vitro* and *in-vivo* specific transduction of tumor cells overexpressing the FGFR (Li & Huang, 2006), and the use of a poly[N-(2-hydroxypropyl)methacrylamide]-derived polyplex modified with an anti-P-selectin antibody. *In-vivo* specific and enhanced gene delivery to inflamed cremasteric venules was observed (Newman et al., 2009). A significant retargeting to tumor cells was also observed with a PEI polyplex carrying an antibody against a tumor-specific protein via a PEG spacer, with low expression in non-tumor cells (Duan et al., 2010).

6. Conclusions

Modification of gene therapy vectors for specific cell type gene delivery can have a significant impact on vector tropism limitations, side effects, and consolidation of gene therapy as a viable treatment. Vector modifications can be grouped in three basic strategies regardless of vector type: genetic modification (ligand insertion within the capsid), chemical modification (polymers or ligand cross-linking), or the use of adaptor molecules (bi-specific antibodies). Most studies have focused on vector design and proof-of-concept of specific gene delivery, while only few of them have evaluated the therapeutic impact of these modifications. In that sense, future studies should focus on assessing the potential of these modified vectors to improve gene therapy trials in an effort to advance from the bench science to the clinic trials. Special attention should be placed in the development of modified vectors for gene delivery to CNS and bone. Since, under normal conditions they show a limited transfection profile with the currently available vectors. Finally, parallel research should be carried out in tissue-specific promoters to design safer integrating vectors, reduce immune response, and improve the processes of vector production.

7. Acknowlegments

We are very grateful to Drs. Shunji Tomatsu and Adriana Montaño for a long time collaboration in research in this and other areas. This work was supported in part by Pontificia Universidad Javeriana (Projects ID 3763 and 4423). Rocío Cuaspa received a young researcher fellowship from the Administrative Department of Science, Technology and Innovation from Colombia (COLCIENCIAS). The authors thank María Lucía Gutiérrez and Dr. Bernd Stab for assistance with editing of the manuscript.

8. References

Alméciga-Díaz, C., Montano, A.M., Tomatsu, S. & Barrera, L. (2010). Adeno-associated virus gene transfer on Morquio A: effect of promoters and sulfatase-modifying Factor 1. *FEBS Journal*. Vol. 277, No. 17, (September 2010), pp. 3608-3619, ISSN 1742-464X.

Alméciga-Díaz, C., Rueda-Paramo, M., Espejo, A., Echeverri, O., Montano, A., Tomatsu, S. & Barrera, L. (2009). Effect of Elongation Factor 1α promoter and SUMF1 over in-vitro expression of N-acetylgalactosamine-6-sulfate sulfatase. *Molecular Biology Reports*. Vol. 36, No. 7, (September 2009), pp. 1863-1870, ISSN 0301-4851.

Arnberg, N. (2009). Adenovirus receptors: implications for tropism, treatment and targeting. *Reviews in Medical Virology*. Vol. 19, No. 3, (May 2009), pp. 165-178, ISSN 1052-9276.

Azzouz, M., Ralph, G.S., Storkebaum, E., Walmsley, L.E., Mitrophanous, K.A., Kingsman, S.M., Carmeliet, P. & Mazarakis, N.D. (2004). VEGF delivery with retrogradely transported lentivector prolongs survival in a mouse ALS model. *Nature*. Vol. 429, No. 6990, (May 2004), pp. 413-417, ISSN 0028-0836.

Bachtarzi, H., Stevenson, M. & Fisher, K. (2008). Cancer gene therapy with targeted adenoviruses. *Expert Opinion in Drug Delivery*. Vol. 5, No. 11, (November 2008), pp. 1231-1240, ISSN 1742-5247.

Bakker, A.C., Van de Loo, F.A., Joosten, L.A., Bennink, M.B., Arntz, O.J., Dmitriev, I.P., Kashentsera, E.A., Curiel, D.T. & van den Berg, W.B. (2001). A tropism-modified adenoviral vector increased the effectiveness of gene therapy for arthritis. *Gene Therapy*. Vol. 8, No. 23, (December 2001), pp. 1785-1793, ISSN 0969-7128.

Bischof, D. & Cornetta, K. (2010). Flexibility in cell targeting by pseudotyping lentiviral vectors. *Methods in Molecular Biology*. Vol. 614, (March 2010), pp. 53-68, ISSN 1940-6029.

Büning, H., Ried, M., Perabo, L., Gerner, F., Huttner, N., Enssle, J. & Hallek, M. (2003). Receptor targeting of adeno-associated virus vectors. *Gene Therapy*. Vol. 10, (July 2003), pp. 1142-1151, ISSN 0969-7128.

Campos, S.K. & Barry, M.A. (2007). Current advances and future challenges in Adenoviral vector biology and targeting. *Current Gene Therapy*. Vol. 7, No. 3, (Jun 2007), pp. 189-204, ISSN 1566-5232.

Cardoso, A.L., Simoes, S., de, A.L.P., Pelisek, J., Culmsee, C., Wagner, E. & Pedroso, d.L.M.C. (2007). siRNA delivery by a transferrin-associated lipid-based vector: a non-viral strategy to mediate gene silencing. *Journal of Gene Medicine*. Vol. 9, No. 3, (March 2007), pp. 170-183, ISSN 1099-498X.

Chen, Y.H., Chang, M. & Davidson, B.L. (2009). Molecular signatures of disease brain endothelia provide new sites for CNS-directed enzyme therapy. *Nature Medicine*. Vol. 15, No. 10, (October 2009), pp. 1215-1218, ISSN 1546-170X.

Chiu, S.J., Ueno, N.T. & Lee, R.J. (2004). Tumor-targeted gene delivery via anti-HER2 antibody (trastuzumab, Herceptin) conjugated polyethylenimine. *Journal of Controlled Release*. Vol. 97, No. 2, (June 2004), pp. 357-369, ISSN 0168-3659.

Choi, V., McCarty, D. & Samulski, R.J. (2005). AAV Hybrid Serotypes: Improved Vectors for Gene Delivery. *Current Gene Therapy*. Vol. 5, (June 2005), pp. 299-310, ISSN 1566-5232.

Cosset, F.L., Morling, F.J., Takeuchi, Y., Weiss, R.A., Collins, M.K. & Russell, S.J. (1995). Retroviral retargeting by envelopes expressing an N-terminal binding domain. *Journal of Virology*. Vol. 69, No. 10, (October 1995), pp. 6314-6322, ISSN 0022-538X.

Crompton, J., Toogood, C.I., Wallis, N. & Hay, R.T. (1994). Expression of a foreign epitope on the surface of the adenovirus hexon. *Journal of Gene Medicine*. Vol. 75 (Pt 1), (January 1994), pp. 133-139, ISSN 0022-1317.

Cronin, J., Zhang, X.Y. & Reiser, J. (2005). Altering the tropism of lentiviral vectors through pseudotyping. *Current Gene Therapy*. Vol. 5, No. 4, (August 2005), pp. 387-398, ISSN 1566-5232.

Denby, L., Work, L.M., Von Seggern, D.J., Wu, E., Mcvey, J.H., Nicklin, S.A. & Baker, A.H. (2007). Development of renal-targeted vectors through combined in vivo phage display and capsid engineering of adenoviral fibers from serotype 19p. *Molecular Therapy*. Vol. 15, No. 9, (September 2007), pp. 1647-1654, ISSN 1525-0016.

Dmitriev, I., Krasnykh, V., Miller, C.R., Wang, M., Kashentseva, E., Mikheeva, G., Belousova, N. & Curiel, D.T. (1998). An adenovirus vector with genetically modified fibers demonstrates expanded tropism via utilization of a coxsackievirus and adenovirus receptor-independent cell entry mechanism. *Journal of Virology*. Vol. 72, No. 12, (December 1998), pp. 9706-9713, ISSN 0022-538X.

Douglas, J.T. (2007). Adenoviral vectors for gene therapy. *Molecular Biotechnology*. Vol. 36, No. 1, (May 2007), pp. 71-80, ISSN 1073-6085.

Douglas, K.L. (2008). Toward development of artificial viruses for gene therapy: a comparative evaluation of viral and non-viral transfection. *Biotechnology Progress*. Vol. 24, No. 4, (July 2008), pp. 871-883, ISSN 1520-6033.

Driessen, W.H., Fujii, N., Tamamura, H. & Sullivan, S.M. (2008). Development of peptide-targeted lipoplexes to CXCR4-expressing rat glioma cells and rat proliferating endothelial cells. *Molecular Therapy*. Vol. 16, No. 3, (March 2008), pp. 516-524, ISSN 1525-0024.

Duan, Y., Yang, C., Zhang, Z., Liu, J., Zheng, J. & Kong, D. (2010). Poly(ethylene glycol)-grafted polyethylenimine modified with G250 monoclonal antibody for tumor gene therapy. *Human Gene Therapy*. Vol. 21, No. 2, (February 2010), pp. 191-198, ISSN 1557-7422.

Edelstein, M. (June 2010). Vectors used in gene therapy clinical trials, In: *Gene Therapy Clinical Trials Worldwide*, Febrary 2011, Available from: http://www.wiley.com.uk/genetherapy/clinical/.

Escors, D. & Breckpot, K. (2010). Lentiviral Vectors in Gene Therapy: Their Current Status and Future Potential. *Archivum Immunologiae et Therapiae Experimentalis*, (Feb 2010), ISSN 1661-4917.

Eto, Y., Gao, J.Q., Sekiguchi, F., Kurachi, S., Katayama, K., Maeda, M., Kawasaki, K., Mizuguchi, H., Hayakawa, T., Tsutsumi, Y., Mayumi, T. & Nakagawa, S. (2005). PEGylated adenovirus vectors containing RGD peptides on the tip of PEG show high transduction efficiency and antibody evasion ability. *Journal of Gene Medicine*. Vol. 7, No. 5, (May 2005), pp. 604-612, ISSN 1099-498X.

Fielding, A.K., Maurice, M., Morling, F.J., Cosset, F.L. & Russell, S.J. (1998). Inverse targeting of retroviral vectors: selective gene transfer in a mixed population of hematopoietic and nonhematopoietic cells. *Blood*. Vol. 91, No. 5, (March 1998), pp. 1802-1809, ISSN 0006-4971.

Fisher, K.D., Stallwood, Y., Green, N.K., Ulbrich, K., Mautner, V. & Seymour, L.W. (2001). Polymer-coated adenovirus permits efficient retargeting and evades neutralising antibodies. *Gene Therapy*. Vol. 8, No. 5, (March 2001), pp. 341-348, ISSN 0969-7128.

Flotte, T. (2004). Gene Therapy Progress and Prospects: Recombinant adeno-associated virus (rAAV) vectors. *Gene Therapy*. Vol. 11, (May 2004), pp. 805-810, ISSN 0969-7128.

Frecha, C., Szecsi, J., Cosset, F.L. & Verhoeyen, E. (2008). Strategies for targeting lentiviral vectors. *Current Gene Therapy*. Vol. 8, No. 6, (December 2008), pp. 449-460, ISSN 1566-5232.

Friedmann, T. (1992). A brief history of gene therapy. *Nature Genetics*. Vol. 2, (October 1992), pp. 93-98, ISSN 1061-4036.

Funke, S., Maisner, A., Muhlebach, M.D., Koehl, U., Grez, M., Cattaneo, R., Cichutek, K. & Buchholz, C.J. (2008). Targeted cell entry of lentiviral vectors. *Molecular Therapy*. Vol. 16, No. 8, (August 2008), pp. 1427-1436, ISSN 1525-0016.

Gigout, L., Rebollo, P., Clement, N., Jr., K.H.W., Muzyczka, N., Linden, R.M. & Weber, T. (2005). Altering AAV Tropism with Mosaic Viral Capsids. *Molecular Therapy*. Vol. 11, No. 6, (June 2005), pp. 856-865, ISSN 1525-0016.

Govindasamy, L., Padron, E., McKenna, R., Muzyczka, N., Kaludov, N., Chiorini, J.A. & Agbandje-McKenna, M. (2006). Structurally mapping the diverse phenotype of adeno-associated virus serotype 4. *Journal of Virology*. Vol. 80, No. 23, (December 2006), pp. 11556-11570, ISSN 0022-538X.

Grill, J., Van Beusechem, V.W., Van Der Valk, P., Dirven, C.M., Leonhart, A., Pherai, D.S., Haisma, H.J., Pinedo, H.M., Curiel, D.T. & Gerritsen, W.R. (2001). Combined targeting of adenoviruses to integrins and epidermal growth factor receptors increases gene transfer into primary glioma cells and spheroids. *Clinical Cancer Research*. Vol. 7, No. 3, (March 2001), pp. 641-650, ISSN 1078-0432.

Gutierrez, M., Garcia-Vallejo, F., Tomatsu, S., Ceron, F., Alméciga-Díaz, C., Domínguez, M. & Barrera, L. (2008). Construction of an Adenoassociated virus-derived vector for the treatment of Morquio A disease. *Biomedica*. Vol. 28, No. 3, (September 2008), pp. 448-459, ISSN 0120-5147.

Hauck, B., Chen, L. & Xiao, W. (2003). Generation and characterization of chimeric recombinant AAV vectors. *Molecular Therapy*. Vol. 7, No. 3, (March 2003), pp. 419-425, ISSN 1525-0016.

Heideman, D.A., Snijders, P.J., Craanen, M.E., Bloemena, E., Meijer, C.J., Meuwissen, S.G., van Beusechem, V.W., Pinedo, H.M., Curiel, D.T., Haisma, H.J. & Gerritsen, W.R.

(2001). Selective gene delivery toward gastric and esophageal adenocarcinoma cells via EpCAM-targeted adenoviral vectors. *Cancer Gene Therapy*. Vol. 8, No. 5, (May 2001), pp. 342-351, ISSN 0929-1903.

Herringson, T.P. & Altin, J.G. (2009). Convenient targeting of stealth siRNA-lipoplexes to cells with chelator lipid-anchored molecules. *Journal of Controlled Release*. Vol. 139, No. 3, (November 2009), pp. 229-238, ISSN 1873-4995.

Herringson, T.P., Patlolla, R.R. & Altin, J.G. (2009). Targeting of plasmid DNA-lipoplexes to cells with molecules anchored via a metal chelator lipid. *The Journal of Gene Medicine*. Vol. 11, No. 11, (November 2009), pp. 1048-1063, ISSN 1521-2254.

Hoare, M., Greiser, U., Schu, S., Mashayekhi, K., Aydogan, E., Murphy, M., Barry, F., Ritter, T. & O'Brien, T. (2010). Enhanced lipoplex-mediated gene expression in mesenchymal stem cells using reiterated nuclear localization sequence peptides. *Journal of Gene Medicine*. Vol. 12, No. 2, (February 2010), pp. 207-218, ISSN 1521-2254.

Horowitz, E.D., Weinberg, M.S. & Asokan, A. (2011). Glycated AAV Vectors: Chemical Redirection of Viral Tissue Tropism. *Bioconjugate Chemistry*, (March 2011), ISSN 1520-4812.

Hu, Y., Li, K., Wang, L., Yin, S., Zhang, Z. & Zhang, Y. (2010). Pegylated immuno-lipopolyplexes: A novel non-viral gene delivery system for liver cancer therapy. *Journal of Controlled Release*. Vol. 144, No. 1, (May 2010), pp. 75-81, ISSN 1873-4995.

Hu, Y., Shen, Y., Ji, B., Wang, L., Zhang, Z. & Zhang, Y. (2011). Combinational RNAi gene therapy of hepatocellular carcinoma by targeting human EGFR and TERT. *European Journal of Pharmaceutical Sciences*. Vol. 42, No. 4, (March 2011), pp. 387-391, ISSN 1879-0720.

Hughes, J.A. & Rao, G.A. (2005). Targeted polymers for gene delivery. *Expert opinion on drug delivery*. Vol. 2, No. 1, (January 2005), pp. 145-157, ISSN 1742-5247.

Incani, V., Tunis, E., Clements, B.A., Olson, C., Kucharski, C., Lavasanifar, A. & Uludag, H. (2007). Palmitic acid substitution on cationic polymers for effective delivery of plasmid DNA to bone marrow stromal cells. *Journal of Biomedical Materials Research A*. Vol. 81, No. 2, (May 2007), pp. 493-504, ISSN 1549-3296.

Jung, Y., Park, H.J., Kim, P.H., Lee, J., Hyung, W., Yang, J., Ko, H., Sohn, J.H., Kim, J.H., Huh, Y.M., Yun, C.O. & Haam, S. (2007). Retargeting of adenoviral gene delivery via Herceptin-PEG-adenovirus conjugates to breast cancer cells. *Journal of Controlled Release*. Vol. 123, No. 2, (November 2007), pp. 164-171, ISSN 1873-4995.

Kasahara, N., Dozy, A.M. & Kan, Y.W. (1994). Tissue-specific targeting of retroviral vectors through ligand-receptor interactions. *Science*. Vol. 266, No. 5189, (November 1994), pp. 1373-1376, ISSN 0036-8075.

Katane, M., Takao, E., Kubo, Y., Fujita, R. & Amanuma, H. (2002). Factors affecting the direct targeting of murine leukemia virus vectors containing peptide ligands in the envelope protein. *EMBO Reports*. Vol. 3, No. 9, (September 2002), pp. 899-904, ISSN 1469-221X.

Kayman, S.C., Park, H., Saxon, M. & Pinter, A. (1999). The hypervariable domain of the murine leukemia virus surface protein tolerates large insertions and deletions, enabling development of a retroviral particle display system. *Journal of Virology*. Vol. 73, No. 3, (March 1999), pp. 1802-1808, ISSN 0022-538X.

Khondee, S., Baoum, A., Siahaan, T.J. & Berkland, C.J. (2011). Calcium-crosslinked LABL-TAT complexes effectively target gene delivery to ICAM-1 expressing cells. *Molecular Pharmaceutics*. Vol. In Press, (April 2011), ISSN 1543-8392.

Kim, K.S., Lee, Y.K., Kim, J.S., Koo, K.H., Hong, H.J. & Park, Y.S. (2008). Targeted gene therapy of LS174 T human colon carcinoma by anti-TAG-72 immunoliposomes. *Cancer Gene Therapy*. Vol. 15, No. 5, (May 2008), pp. 331-340, ISSN 1476-5500.

Kim, N.Y., Choi, Y.B., Kang, C.I., Kim, H.H., Yang, J.M. & Shin, S. (2010). An hydrophobically modified arginine peptide vector system effectively delivers DNA into human mesenchymal stem cells and maintains transgene expression with differentiation. *Journal of Gene Medicine*. Vol. 12, No. 9, (September 2010), pp. 779-789, ISSN 1521-2254.

Kim, P.H., Sohn, J.H., Choi, J.W., Jung, Y., Kim, S.W., Haam, S. & Yun, C.O. (2011). Active targeting and safety profile of PEG-modified adenovirus conjugated with herceptin. *Biomaterials*. Vol. 32, No. 9, (March 2011), pp. 2314-2326, ISSN 1878-5905

Kim, S.H., Lee, S.H., Tian, H., Chen, X. & Park, T.G. (2009). Prostate cancer cell-specific VEGF siRNA delivery system using cell targeting peptide conjugated polyplexes. *Journal of Drug Targeting*. Vol. 17, No. 4, (May 2009), pp. 311-317, ISSN 1029-2330.

Klutz, K., Schaffert, D., Willhauck, M.J., Grunwald, G.K., Haase, R., Wunderlich, N., Zach, C., Gildehaus, F.J., Senekowitsch-Schmidtke, R., Goke, B., Wagner, E., Ogris, M. & Spitzweg, C. (2011). Epidermal Growth Factor Receptor-targeted (131)I-therapy of Liver Cancer Following Systemic Delivery of the Sodium Iodide Symporter Gene. *Molecular Therapy*. Vol. 19, No. 4, (April 2011), pp. 676-685, ISSN 1525-0024.

Kobinger, G.P., Weiner, D.J., Yu, Q.C. & Wilson, J.M. (2001). Filovirus-pseudotyped lentiviral vector can efficiently and stably transduce airway epithelia in vivo. *Nature Biotechnology*. Vol. 19, No. 3, (March 2001), pp. 225-230, ISSN 1087-0156.

Krasnykh, V., Dmitriev, I., Mikheeva, G., Miller, C.R., Belousova, N. & Curiel, D.T. (1998). Characterization of an adenovirus vector containing a heterologous peptide epitope in the HI loop of the fiber knob. *Journal of Virology*. Vol. 72, No. 3, (March 1998), pp. 1844-1852, ISSN 0022-538X.

Kwon, I. & Schaffer, D.V. (2008). Designer gene delivery vectors: molecular engineering and evolution of adeno-associated viral vectors for enhanced gene transfer. *Pharmaceutical Research*. Vol. 25, No. 3, (March 2008), pp. 489-499, ISSN 0724-8741.

Lam, J.K., Armes, S.P., Lewis, A.L. & Stolnik, S. (2009). Folate conjugated phosphorylcholine-based polycations for specific targeting in nucleic acids delivery. *Journal of Drug Targeting*. Vol. 17, No. 7, (August 2009), pp. 512-523, ISSN 1029-2330.

Lavillette, D., Russell, S.J. & Cosset, F.L. (2001). Retargeting gene delivery using surface-engineered retroviral vector particles. *Current Opinion in Biotechnology*. Vol. 12, No. 5, (October 2001), pp. 461-466, ISSN 0958-1669.

Leissner, P., Legrand, V., Schlesinger, Y., Hadji, D.A., van Raaij, M., Cusack, S., Pavirani, A. & Mehtali, M. (2001). Influence of adenoviral fiber mutations on viral encapsidation, infectivity and in vivo tropism. *Gene Therapy*. Vol. 8, No. 1, (Jannuary 2001), pp. 49-57, ISSN 0969-7128.

Lerch, T.F., Xie, Q. & Chapman, M.S. (2010). The structure of adeno-associated virus serotype 3B (AAV-3B): Insights into receptor binding and immune evasion. *Virology*. Vol. 03, No. 1, (July 2010), pp. 26-36, ISSN 1096-0341.

Li, H.J., Everts, M., Pereboeva, L., Komarova, S., Idan, A., Curiel, D.T. & Herschman, H.R. (2007). Adenovirus tumor targeting and hepatic untargeting by a coxsackie/adenovirus receptor ectodomain anti-carcinoembryonic antigen bispecific adapter. *Cancer Research*. Vol. 67, No. 11, (Jun 2007), pp. 5354-5361, ISSN 0008-5472.

Li, S.D. & Huang, L. (2006). Gene therapy progress and prospects: non-viral gene therapy by systemic delivery. *Gene Therapy*. Vol. 13, No. 18, (September 2006), pp. 1313-1319, ISSN 0969-7128.

Liang, M., Morizono, K., Pariente, N., Kamata, M., Lee, B. & Chen, I.S. (2009). Targeted transduction via CD4 by a lentiviral vector uses a clathrin-mediated entry pathway. *Journal of Virology*. Vol. 83, No. 24, (December 2009), pp. 13026-13031, ISSN 1098-5514.

Loiler, S., Conlon, T., Song, S., Tang, Q., Jr, K.W., Agarwal, A., Kapturczak, M., Li, C., Ricordi, C., Atkinson, M., Muzyczka, N. & Flotte, T. (2003). Targeting recombinant adeno-associated virus vectors to enhance gene transfer to pancreatic islets and liver. *Gene Therapy*. Vol. 10, (September 2003), pp. 1551-1558, ISSN 0969-7128.

Lopez-Barcons, L.A., Polo, D., Llorens, A., Reig, F. & Fabra, A. (2005). Targeted adriamycin delivery to MXT-B2 metastatic mammary carcinoma cells by transferrin liposomes: effect of adriamycin ADR-to-lipid ratio. *Oncology Reports*. Vol. 14, No. 5, (November 2005), pp. 1337-1343, ISSN 1021-335X.

Mazarakis, N.D., Azzouz, M., Rohll, J.B., Ellard, F.M., Wilkes, F.J., Olsen, A.L., Carter, E.E., Barber, R.D., Baban, D.F., Kingsman, S.M., Kingsman, A.J., O'Malley, K. & Mitrophanous, K.A. (2001). Rabies virus glycoprotein pseudotyping of lentiviral vectors enables retrograde axonal transport and access to the nervous system after peripheral delivery. *Human Molecular Genetics*. Vol. 10, No. 19, (September 2001), pp. 2109-2121, ISSN 0964-6906.

Merten, C.A., Engelstaedter, M., Buchholz, C.J. & Cichutek, K. (2003). Displaying epidermal growth factor on spleen necrosis virus-derived targeting vectors. *Virology*. Vol. 305, No. 1, (January 2003), pp. 106-114, ISSN 0042-6822.

Michelfelder, S., Kohlschutter, J., Skorupa, A., Pfennings, S., Muller, O., Kleinschmidt, J.A. & Trepel, M. (2009). Successful expansion but not complete restriction of tropism of adeno-associated virus by in vivo biopanning of random virus display peptide libraries. *PLoS One*. Vol. 4, No. 4, (April 2009), pp. e5122, ISSN 1932-6203.

Michelfelder, S. & Trepel, M. (2009). Adeno-associated viral vectors and their redirection to cell-type specific receptors. *Advances in Genetics*. Vol. 67, No. Pt A, (November 2009), pp. 29-60, ISSN 0065-2660.

Midoux, P., Breuzard, G., Gomez, J.P. & Pichon, C. (2008). Polymer-based gene delivery: a current review on the uptake and intracellular trafficking of polyplexes. *Current Gene Therapy*. Vol. 8, No. 5, (Oct), pp. 335-352, ISSN 1566-5232.

Miletic, H., Fischer, Y.H., Neumann, H., Hans, V., Stenzel, W., Giroglou, T., Hermann, M., Deckert, M. & Von Laer, D. (2004). Selective transduction of malignant glioma by lentiviral vectors pseudotyped with lymphocytic choriomeningitis virus glycoproteins. *Human Gene Therapy*. Vol. 15, No. 11, (November 2004), pp. 1091-1100, ISSN 1043-0342.

Mitchell, M., Nam, H.J., Carter, A., McCall, A., Rence, C., Bennett, A., Gurda, B., McKenna, R., Porter, M., Sakai, Y., Byrne, B.J., Muzyczka, N., Aslanidi, G., Zolotukhin, S. &

Agbandje-McKenna, M. (2009). Production, purification and preliminary X-ray crystallographic studies of adeno-associated virus serotype 9. *Acta Crystallographica Section F: Structural Biology and Crystallization Communications*. Vol. 65, No. Pt 7, (July 2009), pp. 715-718, ISSN 1744-3091.

Miura, Y., Yoshida, K., Nishimoto, T., Hatanaka, K., Ohnami, S., Asaka, M., Douglas, J.T., Curiel, D.T., Yoshida, T. & Aoki, K. (2007). Direct selection of targeted adenovirus vectors by random peptide display on the fiber knob. *Gene Therapy*. Vol. 14, No. 20, (October 2007), pp. 1448-1460, ISSN 0969-7128.

Morille, M., Passirani, C., Letrou-Bonneval, E., Benoit, J.P. & Pitard, B. (2009). Galactosylated DNA lipid nanocapsules for efficient hepatocyte targeting. *International Journal of Pharmaceutics*. Vol. 379, No. 2, (September 2009), pp. 293-300, ISSN 1873-3476.

Nam, H.-J., Douglas, M., Padron, E., Gurda, B., McKenna, R., Kohlbrenner, E., Aslanidi, G., Byrne, B., Muzyczka, N., Zolotukhin, S. & Agbandje-McKenna, M. (2007). Structure of Adeno-Associated virus serotype 8, a gene therapy vector. *Journal of Virology*. Vol. 81, No. 22, (August 2007), pp. 12260-12271, ISSN 0022-538X.

Newman, C.M., Crosdale, D.J., Fisher, K.D., Briggs, S.S., Norman, K.E., Seymour, L.W. & Hellewell, P.G. (2009). P-selectin dependent targeting to inflamed endothelium of recombinant P-selectin glycoprotein ligand-1 immunoglobulin chimera-coated poly[N-(2-hydroxypropyl) methacrylamide]-DNA polyplexes in vivo visualised by intravital microscopy. *Journal of Gene Medicine*. Vol. 11, No. 4, (April 2009), pp. 326-334, ISSN 1521-2254.

Ng, Q.K., Sutton, M.K., Soonsawad, P., Xing, L., Cheng, H. & Segura, T. (2009). Engineering clustered ligand binding into nonviral vectors: alphavbeta3 targeting as an example. *Molecular Therapy*. Vol. 17, No. 5, (May 2009), pp. 828-836, ISSN 1525-0024.

Nicklin, S.A., Buening, H., Dishart, K.L., Alwis, M.d., Girod, A., Hacker, U., Thrasher, A.J., Ali, R.R., Hallek, M. & Baker1, A.H. (2001a). Efficient and Selective AAV2-Mediated Gene Transfer Directed to Human Vascular Endothelial Cells. *Molecular Therapy*. Vol. 4, (September 2001), pp. 174-181, ISSN 1525-0016.

Nicklin, S.A., Von Seggern, D.J., Work, L.M., Pek, D.C., Dominiczak, A.F., Nemerow, G.R. & Baker, A.H. (2001b). Ablating adenovirus type 5 fiber-CAR binding and HI loop insertion of the SIGYPLP peptide generate an endothelial cell-selective adenovirus. *Molecular Therapy*. Vol. 4, No. 6, (December 2001), pp. 534-542, ISSN 1525-0016.

Nie, Y., Schaffert, D., Rodl, W., Ogris, M., Wagner, E. & Gunther, M. (2011). Dual-targeted polyplexes: One step towards a synthetic virus for cancer gene therapy. *Journal of Controlled Release*. Vol. In press, (March 2011), ISSN 1873-4995.

Niidome, T. & Huang, L. (2002). Gene therapy progress and prospects: nonviral vectors. *Gene Therapy*. Vol. 9, No. 24, (December 2002), pp. 1647-1652, ISSN 0969-7128.

Ogawara, K., Kuldo, J.M., Oosterhuis, K., Kroesen, B.J., Rots, M.G., Trautwein, C., Kimura, T., Haisma, H.J. & Molema, G. (2006). Functional inhibition of NF-kappaB signal transduction in alphavbeta3 integrin expressing endothelial cells by using RGD-PEG-modified adenovirus with a mutant IkappaB gene. *Arthritis Research & Therapy*. Vol. 8, No. 1, (January 2006), pp. R32, ISSN 1478-6362.

Ohno, K., Sawai, K., Iijima, Y., Levin, B. & Meruelo, D. (1997). Cell-specific targeting of Sindbis virus vectors displaying IgG-binding domains of protein A. *Nature Biotechnology*. Vol. 15, No. 8, (August 1997), pp. 763-767, ISSN 1087-0156.

Oishi, M., Nagasaki, Y., Nishiyama, N., Itaka, K., Takagi, M., Shimamoto, A., Furuichi, Y. & Kataoka, K. (2007). Enhanced growth inhibition of hepatic multicellular tumor spheroids by lactosylated poly(ethylene glycol)-siRNA conjugate formulated in PEGylated polyplexes. *ChemMedChem*. Vol. 2, No. 9, (September 2007), pp. 1290-1297, ISSN 1860-7187.

Park, J.W., Mok, H. & Park, T.G. (2010). Physical adsorption of PEG grafted and blocked poly-L-lysine copolymers on adenovirus surface for enhanced gene transduction. *Journal of Controlled Release*. Vol. 142, No. 2, (March 2010), pp. 238-244, ISSN 1873-4995.

Peng, K.W., Morling, F.J., Cosset, F.L., Murphy, G. & Russell, S.J. (1997). A gene delivery system activatable by disease-associated matrix metalloproteinases. *Human Gene Therapy*. Vol. 8, No. 6, (April 1997), pp. 729-738, ISSN 1043-0342.

Peng, K.W., Pham, L., Ye, H., Zufferey, R., Trono, D., Cosset, F.L. & Russell, S.J. (2001). Organ distribution of gene expression after intravenous infusion of targeted and untargeted lentiviral vectors. *Gene Therapy*. Vol. 8, No. 19, (October 2001), pp. 1456-1463, ISSN 0969-7128.

Peng, Z. (2005). Current status of gendicine in China: recombinant human Ad-p53 agent for treatment of cancers. *Human Gene Therapy*. Vol. 16, No. 9, (September 2005), pp. 1016-1027, ISSN 1043-0342.

Perabo, L., Goldnau, D., White, K., Endell, J., Boucas, J., Humme, S., Work, L.M., Janicki, H., Hallek, M., Baker, A.H. & Büning, H. (2006). Heparan Sulfate Proteoglycan Binding Properties of Adeno-Associated Virus Retargeting Mutants and Consequences for Their In Vivo Tropism. *Journal of Virology*. Vol. 80, No. 14, (July 2006), pp. 7265-7269, ISSN 0022-538X.

Pizzato, M., Blair, E.D., Fling, M., Kopf, J., Tomassetti, A., Weiss, R.A. & Takeuchi, Y. (2001). Evidence for nonspecific adsorption of targeted retrovirus vector particles to cells. *Gene Therapy*. Vol. 8, No. 14, (July 2001), pp. 1088-1096, ISSN 0969-7128.

Ponnazhagan, S., Mahendra, G., Kumar, S., Thompson, J.A. & Castillas, M. (2002). Conjugate-based targeting of recombinant adeno-associated virus type 2 vectors by using avidin-linked ligands. *Journal of Virology*. Vol. 76, No. 24, (December 2002), pp. 12900-12907, ISSN 0022-538X.

Ponnazhagan, S., Wang, X.S., Woody, M.J., Luo, F., Kang, L.Y., Nallari, M.L., Munshi, N.C., Zhou, S.Z. & Srivastava, A. (1996). Differential expression in human cells from the p6 promoter of human parvovirus B19 following plasmid transfection and recombinant adeno-associated virus 2 (AAV) infection: human megakaryocytic leukaemia cells are non-permissive for AAV infection. *The Journal of general virology*. Vol. 77 (Pt 6), (Jun 1996), pp. 1111-1122, ISSN 0022-1317.

Poulin, K.L., Lanthier, R.M., Smith, A.C., Christou, C., Risco Quiroz, M., Powell, K.L., O'Meara, R.W., Kothary, R., Lorimer, I.A. & Parks, R.J. (2010). Retargeting of adenovirus vectors through genetic fusion of a single-chain or single-domain antibody to capsid protein IX. *Journal of Virology*. Vol. 84, No. 19, (October 2010), pp. 10074-10086, ISSN 1098-5514.

Prill, J.M., Espenlaub, S., Samen, U., Engler, T., Schmidt, E., Vetrini, F., Rosewell, A., Grove, N., Palmer, D., Ng, P., Kochanek, S. & Kreppel, F. (2010). Modifications of Adenovirus Hexon Allow for Either Hepatocyte Detargeting or Targeting With

Potential Evasion From Kupffer Cells. *Molecular Therapy*, (October 2010), ISSN 1525-0024.

Rabinowitz, J.E., Bowles, D.E., Faust, S.M., Ledford, J.G., Cunningham, S.E. & Samulski, R.J. (2004). Cross-dressing the virion: the transcapsidation of adeno-associated virus serotypes functionally defines subgroups. *Journal of Virology*. Vol. 78, No. 9, (May 2004), pp. 4421-4432, ISSN 0022-538X.

Ranki, T., Kanerva, A., Ristimaki, A., Hakkarainen, T., Sarkioja, M., Kangasniemi, L., Raki, M., Laakkonen, P., Goodison, S. & Hemminki, A. (2007). A heparan sulfate-targeted conditionally replicative adenovirus, Ad5.pk7-Delta24, for the treatment of advanced breast cancer. *Gene Therapy*. Vol. 14, No. 1, (January 2006), pp. 58-67, ISSN 0969-7128.

Reddy, J.A., Clapp, D.W. & Low, P.S. (2001). Retargeting of viral vectors to the folate receptor endocytic pathway. *Journal of Controlled Release*. Vol. 74, No. 1-3, (July 2001), pp. 77-82, ISSN 0168-3659.

Rittner, K., Schreiber, V., Erbs, P. & Lusky, M. (2007). Targeting of adenovirus vectors carrying a tumor cell-specific peptide: in vitro and in vivo studies. *Cancer Gene Therapy*. Vol. 14, No. 5, (May 2007), pp. 509-518, ISSN 0929-1903.

Roux, P., Jeanteur, P. & Piechaczyk, M. (1989). A versatile and potentially general approach to the targeting of specific cell types by retroviruses: application to the infection of human cells by means of major histocompatibility complex class I and class II antigens by mouse ecotropic murine leukemia virus-derived viruses. *Proceedings of the National Academy of Sciences of the United States of America*. Vol. 86, No. 23, (December 1989), pp. 9079-9083, ISSN 0027-8424.

Russell, S.J., Hawkins, R.E. & Winter, G. (1993). Retroviral vectors displaying functional antibody fragments. *Nucleic Acids Research*. Vol. 21, No. 5, (March 1993), pp. 1081-1085, ISSN 0305-1048.

Schmidt, A., Haas, S.J., Hildebrandt, S., Scheibe, J., Eckhoff, B., Racek, T., Kempermann, G., Wree, A. & Putzer, B.M. (2007). Selective targeting of adenoviral vectors to neural precursor cells in the hippocampus of adult mice: new prospects for in situ gene therapy. *Stem Cells*. Vol. 25, No. 11, (November 2007), pp. 2910-2918, ISSN 1549-4918.

Sharma, A., Li, X.X., Bangari, D.S. & Mittal, S.K. (2009). Adenovirus receptors and their implications in gene delivery. *Virus Research*. Vol. 143, No. 2, (August 2009), pp. 184-194, ISSN 0168-1702.

Shi, W., Arnold, G. & Bartlett, J. (2001). Insertional Mutagenesis of the Adeno-Associated Virus Type 2 (AAV2) Capsid Gene and Generation of AAV2 Vectors Targeted to Alternative Cell-Surface Receptors. *Human Gene Therapy*. Vol. 12, (September 2001), pp. 1697-1711, ISSN 1043-0342.

Stachler, M.D. & Bartlett, J.S. (2006). Mosaic vectors comprised of modified AAV1 capsid proteins for efficient vector purification and targeting to vascular endothelial cells. *Gene Therapy*. Vol. 13, No. 11, (June 2006), pp. 926-931, ISSN 0969-7128.

Summerford, C. & Samulski, R.J. (1998). Membrane-associated heparan sulfate proteoglycan is a receptor for adeno-associated virus type 2 virions. *Journal of Virology*. Vol. 72, No. 2, (Febrary 1998), pp. 1438-1445, ISSN 0022-538X.

Surace, C., Arpicco, S., Dufay-Wojcicki, A., Marsaud, V., Bouclier, C., Clay, D., Cattel, L., Renoir, J.M. & Fattal, E. (2009). Lipoplexes targeting the CD44 hyaluronic acid receptor for efficient transfection of breast cancer cells. *Molecular Pharmaceutics*. Vol. 6, No. 4, (July 2009), pp. 1062-1073, ISSN 1543-8384.

Tomatsu, S., Montano, A.M., Alméciga-Díaz, C. & Barrera, L. (2010). Delivery of therapeutic agents to the bone. US20100008979. USA

Tros, d.I.C., Sun, Y. & Duzgunes, N. (2010). Gene delivery by lipoplexes and polyplexes. *European Journal of Pharmaceutical Sciences*. Vol. 40, No. 3, (June 2010), pp. 159-170, ISSN 1879-0720.

Verhoeyen, E. & Cosset, F.L. (2004). Surface-engineering of lentiviral vectors. *Journal of Gene Medicine*. Vol. 6 (Suppl 1), (Febrary 2004), pp. S83-94, ISSN 1099-498X.

Verma, I.M. & Weitzman, M.D. (2005). Gene Therapy: Twenty-First Century Medicine. *Annual Reviews in Biochemistry*. Vol. 74, (July 2005), pp. 711-738, ISSN 1545-4509.

Volpers, C. & Kochanek, S. (2004). Adenoviral vectors for gene transfer and therapy. *Journal of Gene Medicine*. Vol. 6 (Suppl 1), (Febrary 2004), pp. S164-171, ISSN 1099-498X.

Wagner, E., Culmsee, C. & Boeckle, S. (2005). Targeting of polyplexes: toward synthetic virus vector systems. *Advances in Genetics*. Vol. 53, pp. 333-354, ISSN 0065-2660.

Warrington, K. & Herzog, R. (2006). Treatmeant of human disease by adeno-associated viral gene transfer. *Human Genetics*. Vol. 119, (April 2006), pp. 571-603, ISSN 0340-6717.

Warrington, K.H., Gorbatyuk, O.S., Harrison, J.K., Opie, S.R., Zolotukhin, S. & Muzyczka, N. (2004). Adeno-Associated Virus Type 2 VP2 Capsid Protein Is Nonessential and Can Tolerate Large Peptide Insertions at Its N Terminus. *Journal of Virology*. Vol. 78, No. 12, (January 2004), pp. 6595-6609, ISSN 0022-538X.

Wesseling, J.G., Bosma, P.J., Krasnykh, V., Kashentseva, E.A., Blackwell, J.L., Reynolds, P.N., Li, H., Parameshwar, M., Vickers, S.M., Jaffee, E.M., Huibregtse, K., Curiel, D.T. & Dmitriev, I. (2001). Improved gene transfer efficiency to primary and established human pancreatic carcinoma target cells via epidermal growth factor receptor and integrin-targeted adenoviral vectors. *Gene Therapy*. Vol. 8, No. 13, (July 2001), pp. 969-976, ISSN 0969-7128.

White, K., Büning, H., Kritz, A., Janicki, H., McVey, J., Perabo, L., Murphy, G., Odenthal, M., Work, L., Hallek, M., Nicklin, S. & Baker, A. (2007). Engineering adeno-associated viures 2 vectors for targeted gene delivery to atherosclerotic lessions. *Gene Therapy*. Vol. 15, No. 6, (April 2007), pp. 443-451, ISSN 0969-7128.

White, S.J., Nicklin, S.A., Büning, H., Brosnan, M.J., Leike, K., Papadakis, E.D., Hallek, M. & Baker, A.H. (2004). Targeted Gene Delivery to Vascular Tissue In Vivo by Tropism-Modified Adeno-Associated Virus Vectors. *Circulation*. Vol. 109, (January 2004), pp. 513-519, ISSN 0009-7322.

Wickham, T.J., Roelvink, P.W., Brough, D.E. & Kovesdi, I. (1996). Adenovirus targeted to heparan-containing receptors increases its gene delivery efficiency to multiple cell types. *Nature Biotechnology*. Vol. 14, No. 11, (November 1996), pp. 1570-1573, ISSN 1087-0156.

Wu, B.W., Lu, J., Gallaher, T.K., Anderson, W.F. & Cannon, P.M. (2000a). Identification of regions in the Moloney murine leukemia virus SU protein that tolerate the insertion of an integrin-binding peptide. *Virology*. Vol. 269, No. 1, (March 2000), pp. 7-17, ISSN 0042-6822.

Wu, H., Han, T., Belousova, N., Krasnykh, V., Kashentseva, E., Dmitriev, I., Kataram, M., Mahasreshti, P.J. & Curiel, D.T. (2005). Identification of sites in adenovirus hexon for foreign peptide incorporation. *Journal of Virology*. Vol. 79, No. 6, (March 2005), pp. 3382-3390, ISSN 0022-538X.

Wu, P., Kudrolli, T.A., Chowdhury, W.H., Liu, M.M., Rodriguez, R. & Lupold, S.E. (2010). Adenovirus Targeting to Prostate-specific Membrane Antigen through Virus-displayed Semi-random Peptide Library Screening. *Cancer Research*, (July 2010), ISSN 1538-7445.

Wu, P., Xiao, W., Conlon, T., Hughes, J., Agbandje-McKenna, M., Ferkol, T., Flotte, T. & Muzyczka, N. (2000b). Mutational Analysis of the Adeno-Associated Virus Type 2 (AAV2) Capsid Gene and Construction of AAV2 Vectors with Altered Tropism. *Journal of Virology*. Vol. 74, No. 18, (September 2000), pp. 8635-8647, ISSN 0022-538X.

Wu, Z., Asokan, A. & Samulski, R. (2006). Adeno-associated virus serotypes: vector toolkit for human gene therapy. *Molecular Therapy*. Vol. 14, No. 3, (September 2006), pp. 316-327, ISSN 1525-0016.

Xie, Q., Bu, W., Bhatia, S., Hare, J., Somasundaram, T., Azzi, A. & Chapman, M.S. (2002). The atomic structure of adeno-associated virus (AAV-2), a vector for human gene therapy. *Proceedings of the National Academy of Sciences of the United States of America*. Vol. 99, No. 16, (August 2002), pp. 10405-10410, ISSN 0027-8424.

Yang, L., Jiang, J., Drouin, L.M., Agbandje-McKenna, M., Chen, C., Qiao, C., Pu, D., Hu, X., Wang, D.Z., Li, J. & Xiao, X. (2009). A myocardium tropic adeno-associated virus (AAV) evolved by DNA shuffling and in vivo selection. *Proceedings of the National Academy of Sciences of the United States of America*. Vol. 106, No. 10, (March 2009), pp. 3946-3951, ISSN 1091-6490.

Young, J.A., Bates, P., Willert, K. & Varmus, H.E. (1990). Efficient incorporation of human CD4 protein into avian leukosis virus particles. *Science*. Vol. 250, No. 4986, (December 1990), pp. 1421-1423, ISSN 0036-8075.

Yu, C.Y., Yuan, Z., Cao, Z., Wang, B., Qiao, C., Li, J. & Xiao, X. (2009). A muscle-targeting peptide displayed on AAV2 improves muscle tropism on systemic delivery. *Gene Therapy*. Vol. 16, No. 8, (August 2009), pp. 953-962, ISSN 1476-5462.

Yu, J.H. & Schaffer, D.V. (2005). Advanced targeting strategies for murine retroviral and adeno-associated viral vectors, In: *Advances in Biochemical Engineering/Biotechnology*, Scheper, T. (ed). 147-167, Springer, ISBN 103-540-28404-4, Berlin.

Williams, D. (2007). RAC Reviews Serious Adverse Event Associated with AAV Therapy Trial. *Molecular Therapy*, Vol. 15, No. 12, (December 2007), pp. 2053-2054, ISSN 1525-0016.

Zhang, H., Mitin, A. & Vinogradov, S.V. (2009). Efficient transfection of blood-brain barrier endothelial cells by lipoplexes and polyplexes in the presence of nuclear targeting NLS-PEG-acridine conjugates. *Bioconjugate Chemistry*. Vol. 20, No. 1, (January 2009), pp. 120-128, ISSN 1520-4812.

4

Investigation of Transfection Barriers Involved in Non-Viral Nanoparticulate Gene Delivery in Different Cell Lines

Stefanie Häfele and Regine Süss
Department of Pharmaceutical Technology and Biopharmacy, Freiburg
Germany

1. Introduction

In order to improve the delivery efficiency of genetic material into cells both *in vitro* and *in vivo*, the development of effective non viral vectors for optimized gene transfer into target cells has become an important objective. Non-viral vector systems in particular, such as cationic lipids and polymers, have been widely investigated as to their suitability as a delivery system [1-4]. In cell lines, non-viral gene transfer mediated by cationic lipid/DNA aggregates has been accomplished efficiently showing no immunogenicity and low cytotoxicity [5]. Unfortunately, non-viral gene transfer into primary cells is still inefficient and results in low transgene expression *in vivo* [6]. In contrast to the transfection of most cell lines, which can be successfully performed using a variety of methods, the introduction of foreign DNA into primary cells requires careful selection of the gene transfer technique. Whereas viral strategies are involved in immunogenic risks, non-viral methods have proved to be inefficient for most primary cell types. This might be due to the fact that biological barriers have to be overcome in order to achieve successful gene delivery.

Therefore, knowledge about the uptake mechanism and the subsequent intracellular processing of non-viral gene delivery systems is important for the development of efficient gene delivery systems. Moreover, in understanding the internalization of particles into cells, distinct pathways might be targeted.

Multiple processes are thought to be involved in the cellular internalization of particles [7], whereas clathrin-dependent uptake is the one which has been investigated the most. However, other internalization pathways such as the caveolae-dependent pathway, macro-pinocytosis, phagocytosis and the non-clathrin-non-caveolae dependent pathway are possible ways for gene delivery and further processing in the cells as well [8].

The mode of internalization may affect the kinetics of intracellular processing as well as transfection efficiency. Depending on the uptake mechanism a variety of obstacles could be the reason for low transfection efficiency. Also depending on the mode of cellular uptake, internalization may lead to either lysosomal degradation and digestion, recycling back to the membrane, transcytotic transport across the epithelial barrier or delivery to other compartments.

Once having been released into the cytosol, additional barriers such as insufficient desaggregation of the complex, poor cytoplasmic transport, cytosolic digestion by means of nucleases and finally low intra-nuclear DNA delivery have to be overcome. A promising strategy for increasing the efficiency of non-viral vectors is to target certain uptake pathways that improve the efficient delivery of particles. Such a strategy requires thorough investigation of the different internalization pathways and the subsequent intracellular events involved in each case.

In this work we concentrate on the first and second major barrier to improved transfection efficiency in human primary cells. Two different cell types were chosen because of their relevance in cardiovascular diseases: human aortic endothelial cells (HAEC) and human aortic smooth muscle cells (HASMC). Both cells are involved in the unwanted re-narrowing (restenosis) of cardiac vessels after angioplasty and therefore are the primary targets in a strategy for cardiovascular gene-therapy.

The distinct uptake mechanism of cationic lipid/DNA aggregates had to be clarified in order to gain knowledge about further intracellular processing and other barriers which still had to be overcome. To distinguish between the different endocytic pathways involved in lipoplex internalization of the Rhodamine-labeled DC-30 lipoplexes (Rh-DC-30), both general and specific inhibitors of endocytic routes were monitored in the presence of lipoplexes and analyzed by means of flow cytometry. Table 1 represents an overview of the inhibitors used. To gain more insight into the intracellular fate of lipoplexes, investigation of their co-localization with a variety of molecules was carried out using spectral bio-imaging. Transferrin alexa fluor 488 (tf) was used as a marker for clathrin-mediated uptake [9-16], cholera toxin B alexa fluor 488 (chltx-B) was used as marker for internalization via caveolae and related membrane structures [8, 17], and FITC-dextran was used as a marker for macropinocytosis.

It was subsequently investigated whether the failure of the endosomal release of the lipoplex or the desaggregation of the complex was responsible for the low transfection efficiency. Therefore, plasmid DNA was additionally introduced into the cytosol by electroporation.

Inhibitor	Uptake route	Reference
Chlorpromazine (chlp)	Clathrin	[11]
Methyl-ß-cyclodextrin (mbCD)	Clathrin and caveolae	[22-24]
Filipin (fil)	Caveolae	[25-27]
Genistein (gen)	Caveolae	[28]
LY 29004 (Ly)	Macropinocytosis	[29, 30]
Wortmannin (wm)	Macropinocytosis	[29, 30]
Nocodazole (noco)	Microtubule depolymerization	[31]
Cytochalasin-D (cch-D)	Actin skeleton disruptor	[8]

Table 1. Inhibitors for the specific endocytic routes

2. Materials

DC-30 was purchased from Avanti Polar Lipids (Birmingham, AL, USA). The Cy-5- and Rh-DNA Labeling Kits, Transferrin Alexa Fluor conjugate 488, Cholera Toxin Subunit B Alexa Fluor conjugate 488 and DAPI were purchased from Molecular Probes (Leiden, The Netherlands). Cells were purchased from ATCC (American Type Culture Collection),

Manassas, USA and pEGFP from BD Clontech Germany, Heidelberg. Unless otherwise stated, all other chemicals were purchased from Sigma/Fluka (Deisenhofen, Germany) and were of analytical grade. Additional material is described in the appropriate method section.

3. Methods

3.1 Cell culture

Human vascular smooth muscle cells (HASMC) were cultivated in smooth muscle cell medium 2 (Promocell, Heidelberg, Germany) supplemented with 5 % (v/v) FCS and human aortic endothelial (HAEC) were maintained in endothelial cell medium MV (Promocell, Heidelberg, Germany) on 100 mm culture plates. For HAEC, tissue culture plates were first coated with sterile-filtered 2 % gelatine solution for 10 min and washed twice with PBS w/o calcium and magnesium before seeding. Cells were cultivated at 37 °C in a humidified atmosphere with 5 % (v/v) CO_2.

3.2 Plasmid preparation

The plasmid pEGFP carries the green fluorescent protein coding region under the control of the cytomegalovirus immediate-early promoter region. It was isolated from Escherichia coli (Stratagene, Amsterdam, NL) with the Maxi-Prep Kit from Qiagen (Hilden, Germany). Isolated DNA was stored in TE buffer (100 mM NaCl, 10 mM Tris-HCl) at a concentration of 1 mg/mL at -20 °C after its purity was verified by determining the ratio of absorbance at 260/280 nm and by gel electrophoresis.

3.3 DNA labeling

Cy-5-labeled and Rh-labeled DNA was prepared as described for the Mirus Labeling Kit (Molecular Probes, Leiden, Netherlands).

3.4 Lipoplex formation

Enhanced green fluorescent plasmid pEGFP (either labeled for uptake studies or unlabeled for transfection studies) was mixed with DC-30® in a lipid/DNA ratio (w/w) of 5:1 according to the following protocol: lyophilized DC-30® was redispersed in sterile transfection medium (TM; 250 mM saCcharose, 25 mM NaCl) at a concentration of 1 mg/ml and incubated for 30 min at room temperature. Plasmid DNA and the respective amount of DC-30®-dispersion were diluted separately into equal volumes of TM in order to achieve the desired lipoplex concentration in 200 µL of lipoplex preparation. The dilutions were combined discontinuously by pipetting the plasmid into the liposome solution, gently mixing and incubating for at least 30 min at room temperature to allow the formation of the lipoplexes.

3.5 In vitro transfection assay

Cells were seeded in a 24-well cluster dish at a density of 10^4 cells per well 24 h prior to the experiments and cultivated in the appropriate growth medium with serum. After 24 h in culture the cells were washed with 1 ml PBS and then 400 µL growth medium containing serum was added to the cells. 200 µL of freshly prepared lipoplexes were added to the cells. After incubating for 5 h at 37 °C (5 % (v/v) CO_2) the supernatants were removed and 1 ml of the appropriate growth medium was added to each well. Thereafter, the cells were cultured further for a total of 48 h at 37 °C, 5 % (v/v) CO_2. In the control experiments cells were incubated with 200 µL culture medium or 200 µL TM and treated the same way as the lipoplex samples. Analysis was carried out by means of flow cytometry (see uptake and FACS analysis).

3.6 Electroporation experiments

Cells were cultivated to 80 % confluency as described above. Every 100 mm plate was trypsinated with 1 mL Trypsin/EDTA for 30 s (HAEC), and 90 s (HASMC) to detach the cells. Trypsinization was stopped by adding 3 ml culture medium with serum. After washing twice with ice-cold PBS, cells were redispersed in ice-cold electroporation buffer (100 mM Hepes, 137 mM NaCl, 4 mM Na_2HPO_4, 6 mM Dextrose) at a concentration of 10^7 cells/ ml. Electroporation experiments were carried out using a Gene Pulser II (BioRad Laboratories, Muenchen, Germany). 500 µL of cell suspension was poured in a chilled 0,4 cm gap cuvette. After adding 20 µg DNA (1 mg/mL TE-buffer pH 7,0; Tris 10 mM, EDTA 1 mM) the cuvette was placed on ice and electroporated with the following settings: for HAEC: 350 V, 750 µF; for HASMC: 500 V, 950 µF. After the shock, the cuvette stayed on ice for 10 min. Then, cells were transferred into a 100 mm culture plate, (gelatine-coated plates for HAEC, see section "cell culture") and incubated for 48 h at 37 °C and 5 % CO_2. Fluorescent pictures were taken with an Axiovert S 20 (Zeiss, Jena Germany, 20x).
As a positive control experiment, C3-Toxin plasmid was electroporated into the cells to see if DNA was delivered into the nucleus. Effective delivery was achieved when cells were rounded up and dead.
As cells were not vital enough for FACS analysis, fluorescent and non-fluorescent cells were counted via "Neubauer Zählkammer". Counting was repeated twice for every culture plate for at least 3 independent experiments.

3.7 Uptake studies and FACS analysis

Two days before the uptake experiment 10 000 HAEC and HASMC respectively were seeded onto a 24-well tissue culture plate. One hour before the experiment the culture medium was refreshed with 400 µL of cell specific medium containing 5 % FCS. Prior to the inhibition experiments the cells were incubated with the inhibitors (cytochalasin D (Cch-D, 10 µM) for 120 min, chlorpromazine (chlp, 56 µM), LY29004 (ly, 50 µM), wortmannin (wm, 50 nM) genistein (gen, 200 µM) and nocodazole (noco, 10 µM) for 60 min, filipin (fil, 5 µg/ml for HASMC, 10 µg/mL for HAEC) for 30 min and methyl-β-cyclodextrin (mbCD, 164 µM) for 15 min). Subsequently, the DC-30 based lipoplexes containing Cy5-labeled plasmid DNA were added and the cells were incubated at 37 °C for another 60 min. Then, cells were washed with PBS and detached with 200 µL trypsin/EDTA (0,5 mg/mL trypsin, 0,2 mg/mL EDTA) for 30 s (HAEC) or 90 s (HASMC) and harvested by centrifugation. The cell pellet was washed in one ml ice-cold PBS and resuspended again in 200 µL ice-cold PBS. Cell toxicity was measured by adding 2 µL 7-AAD (BD Biosciences), a fluorescent DNA-binding dye which only penetrates dead cells. Fluorescent positive cells were analyzed with a FACS Calibur using Cell Quest Pro software (BD Biosciences). 10 000 cells were measured for each sample. GFP was measured using fluorescence channel 1 (530+/-15 nm), Rh in fluorescence channel 2 (585+/-21 nm), 7-AAD in fluorescence channel 3 (661+/-8 nm) and Cy5 in fluorescence channel 4 (> 670 nm).
In order to determine the amount of lipoplex absorbed to the outside of the cell membrane, experiments were also performed at 4 °C. Furthermore, control experiments such as incubation only with Cy5-labeled DNA with buffer alone were performed.

3.8 Spectral bio-imaging

Cells were seeded onto 12-mm coverslips in 24-well plates 2 days prior to the experiment. Lipoplexes were prepared using DC-30® and Rh-labeled plasmid. Cells were then washed twice with PBS w/o calcium and magnesium and then incubated with 400 µL medium containing the lipoplexes. Cells were incubated simultaneously with the markers for the different pathways for 30 min to 2 h (tf alexa fluor 488 (10 µg/mL), chltx-B alexa fluor 488 (2 µg/mL) and FITC dextran 70 000, (1 µg/mL)). The amount of DNA was the same as that used in the uptake experiments. Prior to microscopic examination, the cells were fixed with 4 % paraformaldehyde (500 µL, 10 min, RT) and the coverslips were mounted on glass slides with 3 µL MobiGlow (MoBiTec, Goettingen, Germany), an antifading substance to reduce photobleaching effects.

Spectral bio-imaging was performed as described previously by Huth et al. [8] with a SpectraCube SD-200H system (Applied Spectral Imaging, Migdal HaEmek, Israel). An inverted fluorescence microscope (Axiovert S 100, Zeiss, Jena Germany) equipped with a high-pressure mercury lamp (HBO 100) for excitation and a triple bandpass filter set was used. All images were taken using a 100x/1.3 oil-immersion objective lens (Plan Neofluar, Zeiss, Jena, Germany). In the spectral range from 400 to 700 nm the objective lens shows only minimal fluctuations of transmission (85-90 %). The optical head attached to the microscope is composed of a Sagnac common-path interferometer and imaging optics including a cooled CCD camera (Hamamatsu C4880-85, Japan). Microscopic images were obtained with spectral bio-imaging 2.5 software (Applied Spectral Imaging). The acquisition time of a desired image varied from 30 to 90 s depending on the brightness of the fluorescence and the image size. Cells were first incubated with only one dye to get single-colored images. For further analysis images were then transferred to the SpectraView 1.6 software (Applied Spectral Imaging).

4. Results

4.1 Uptake experiments with inhibitors

For uptake experiments studied by means of flow cytometry, DNA was labeled with Cy-5. Cell experiments were performed at both 37 °C and 4 °C in order to distinguish cellular uptake from adsorption of lipoplexes to the outside of the cell membrane or their fusion with the cell membrane. It has been described that no energy dependent internalization process can take place at 4 °C [18]. As the size of the DC-30® lipoplexes was determined to be in the range of 300 and 500 nm [5], we assumed internalization to be an active process. The detection of positive fluorescent signal at 4 °C therefore refers to fusion or adsorption of lipoplex with the cell membrane. Fig. 1 represents the amount of fluorescent positive cells after one hour of incubation with lipoplexes at 37 °C.

The corresponding transfection efficiency is listed in Table 2 and shows that despite the fact that uptake of lipoplexes was successful in 24 % of HAEC, less than 1 % of HAEC were transfected. In HASMC, uptake reached as high as 80 %, whereas transfection was only 2 %.

Only 1 % of fluorescent cells were detected after incubation at 4 °C and therefore adsorption to the outside of the cell membrane or fusion with the cell membrane is negligible and the fluorescent positive cells as seen in Fig. 1 can be considered as resulting from cellular uptake (internalization) of the lipoplexes. Analysis of cytotoxicity confirmed results which were published previously [5].

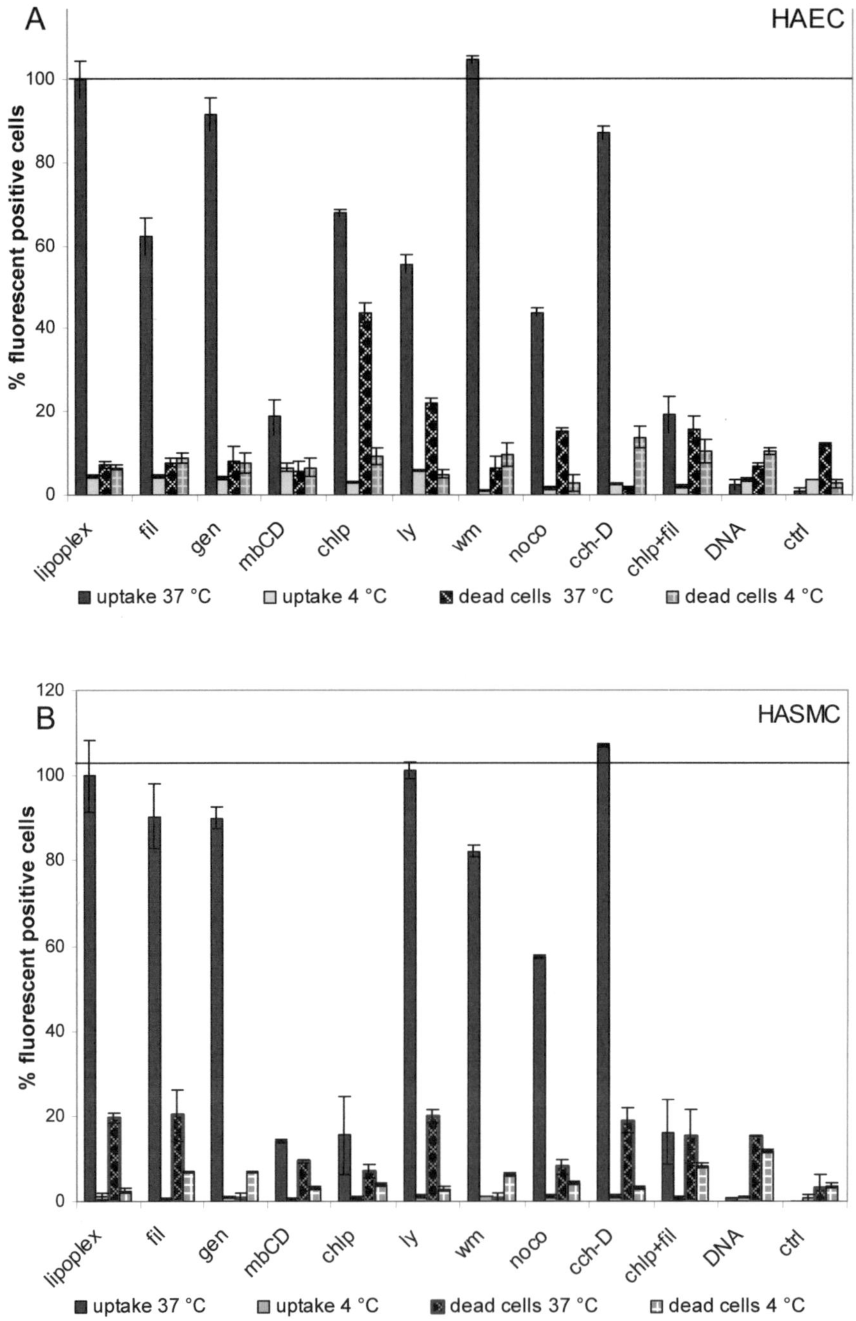

Fig. 1. Cells were incubated for one hour with Cy-5 labeled lipoplexes and analyzed by means of flow cytometry (Fl-4 channel). Prior to the measurement, every sample was additionally incubated with 7-AAD to determine the amount of dead cells (Fl-3 channel). Error bars indicate standard deviation (n=3 in 3 independent experiments).

Transfection method	Transfection agent	Transfection efficiency [%]	
		HAEC	HASMC
Non-viral cationic lipid-mediated DNA-delivery	DC-30 lipoplex	0,40 ± 0,02	2,01 ± 0,08
	DC-30 lipoplex + 100μM Chloroquine	0,70 ± 0,02	2,74 ± 0,14
	DC-30 lipoplex + 100 μM Chloroquine	0,11 ± 0,03	2,47 ± 0,22
Electroporation	DNA	43 ± 7	51 ± 8

Table 2. Influence of transfection method on transfection efficiency

Fig. 2 and Fig. 3 show the internalization of DC-30 lipoplexes by HAEC and HASMC in the presence of inhibitors of different uptake pathways. Again the incubation at 4 °C did not show any passive adsorption or fusion of DC-30® lipoplexes with the membrane in both cell types.

As depicted in Fig. 2 A the uptake of DC-30® lipoplexes by HAEC pretreated with filipin (fil) was reduced by about 40 % to 60 % relative to control values. However, another caveolae-inhibitor, genistein (gen), did not reduce lipoplex uptake significantly. Genistein affects tyrosine kinase [19], which associates with caveolae. In contrast, filipin affects 3-ß-hydroxycholesterols [20] and avoids the formation of caveolin coats ab initio. Filipin seems to intervene at the origin of internalization whereas genistein seems to inhibit further processing of caveosomes after budding out of the membrane.

The inhibitor methyl-ß-cyclodextrin (mbCD) is involved in cholesterol depletion of the plasma membrane and therefore influencing both cholesterol-rich domains (caveolae and clathrin-mediated endocytosis) and was shown to reduce lipoplex uptake significantly by 80 %.

Clathrin-dependent endocytosis was analyzed with chlorpromazine (chlp) which interacts with clathrin-coated pits and causes their loss from the surface membrane. Uptake was reduced by about 25 %. Combining the clathrin and caveolae-mediated endocytosis inhibitors chlorpromazine and filipin leads to a comparable reduction of lipoplex uptake with that achieved with mbCD.

Macropinocytosis is possibly involved in the uptake mechanism of DC-30® lipoplexes in HAEC. Pre-incubation with the macropinocytosis inhibitors LY29004 (Ly) and wortmannin (wm) only led to a significant reduction of uptake using Ly but not wortmannin.

Nocodazol (noco) acts as an inhibitor by depolymerizing microtubules and therefore prevents the transport vesicle (early endosome) from fusing with the late endosome in order to protect the early endosome´s content from digestion and degradation in the lysosomal compartment. Applying this inhibitor showed a 50 % reduction in fluorescent signal.

Incubation with cytochalasin D (Cch-D), a disrupter of the actin cytoskeleton, resulted in a reduction of about 10 % and did not seem to be strongly involved in the uptake or processing of DC-30® lipoplexes. In this context, the involvement of macropinocytosis, which is strongly actin dependent, and the different inhibition rates caused by LY and wortmannin does not clarify whether or not lipoplexes are internalized via macropinocytosis.

Fig. 2 B presents data on the internalization of DC-30® lipoplexes by HASMC. Cells pretreated with the caveolae-blocking reagents filipin and genistein showed only a slightly decreased uptake of lipoplexes. In contrast, upon incubation with the clathrin inhibitor

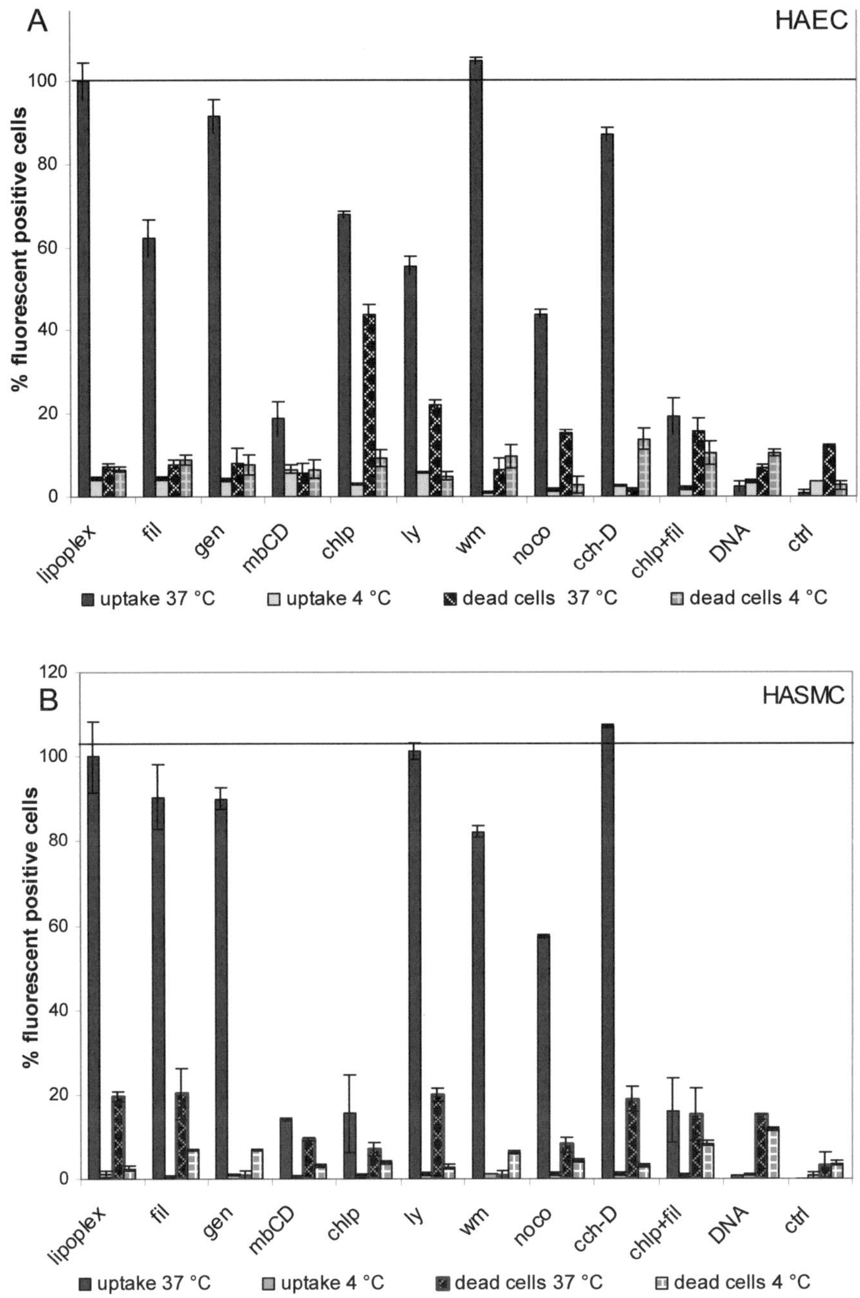

Fig. 2. After pre-incubation with different inhibitors (see Table 1) (x-range), HAEC (A) and HASMC (B) were incubated for one hour with Cy-5 labeled DC-30® lipoplexes and analyzed by means of flow cytometry (Fl-4 channel). Prior to measurement, every sample was also incubated with 7-AAD to determine the amount of dead cells (Fl-3 channel). The fluorescence intensity of lipoplexes without inhibitors was set to 100%. Error bars indicate standard deviation (n=3 in 3 independent experiments).

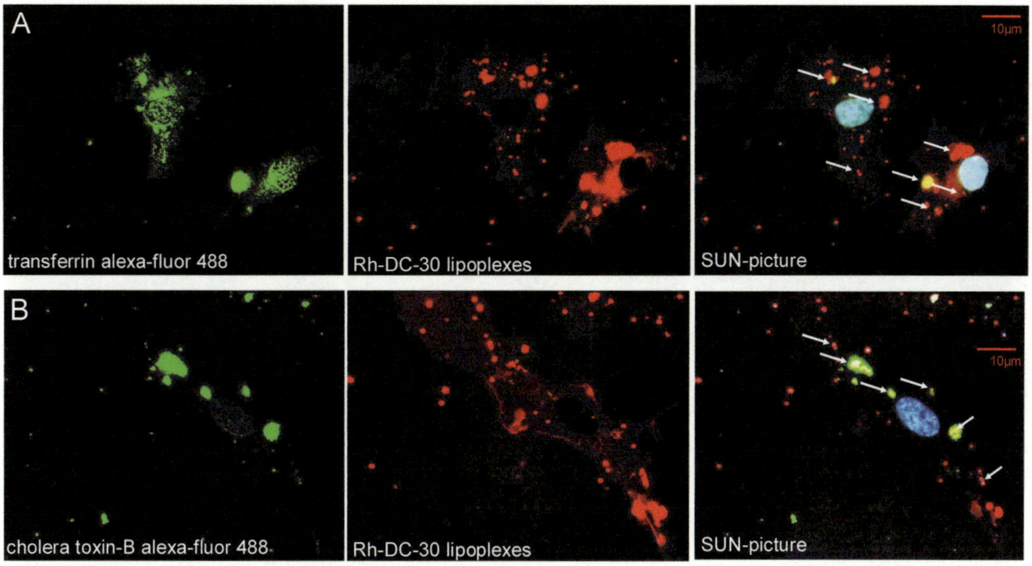

Fig. 3. HAEC were incubated for one hour with either (A) clathrin marker tf alexa-fluor 488 and Rh-lipoplexes or (B) caveolae marker choleratoxin-subunit B alexa-fluor 488 and Rh-lipoplexes. After subsequent DAPI staining of the nucleus, pictures were taken by spectral bio-imaging. I: localization of Rho-lipoplexes; II: localization of markers; III: overlay of single colour images.

chlorpromazine the highest reduction of uptake was observed (about 85 %). The same result could be achieved with mbCD, which is involved in both clathrin and caveolae-mediated pathways. Again, when combining the specific caveolae and clathrin inhibitors (chlp and fil), lipoplex uptake could not be further reduced. Macropinocytosis is also supposed to be involved in lipoplex uptake in these cells, but pre-treatment with wortmannin alone caused only a minor reduction (about 10 %) whereas Ly did not seem to effect the uptake mechanism.

On the other hand, uptake of DC-30® lipoplexes by HASMC pre-treated with nocodazole was diminished by about 45 %, which shows a correlation to the clathrin-blocking reagents. The actin-disrupting agent Cch-D did not cause a reduction of lipoplex uptake at all.

4.2 Microscopic uptake studies

The results obtained with uptake studies were confirmed using spectral-bio-imaging. Cells were first pre-incubated with the inhibitors chlormpromazine or filipin. Therefore, the internalization routes were examined via co-localization studies with markers for the clathrin- or caveolae-dependent pathways. The DNA of the lipoplex was labeled with Rhodamine (Rh). Transferrin alexa-fluor 488 was used as a clathrin marker, Choleratoxin-subunit B-Alexa Fluor 488 was a marker for internalization via caveolae-dependent endocytosis and FITC-dextran a marker for macropinocytosis. During preparation for the microscopic experiments, cells were additionally incubated with DAPI (nucleus staining) as a control. Co-localization of the lipoplex and pathway markers was determined by bio-spectral-imaging.

In HAEC after one h incubation time, co-localization of lipoplexes with tf-488 (Fig. 3A) as well as with chltx-B-488 (Fig. 3B) was detected which indicates uptake via clathrin- and caveolae-dependent pathways. No co-localization with the macropinocytosis marker FITC-dextran 70,000 could be shown.

In HASMC, Rh-labeled lipoplexes only showed co-localization with tf-488 (Fig. 4), the marker for clathrin-dependent uptake.

In both cases, spectral bio-imaging studies confirmed the results achieved by flow cytometry.

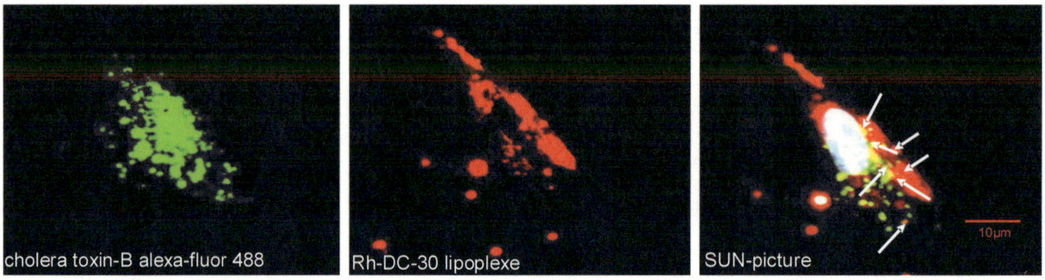

Fig. 4. HASMC were incubated for one hour with clathrin marker tf alexa-fluor 488 and Rh-lipoplexes. After subsequent DAPI staining of the nucleus pictures were taken by spectral bio-imaging. I: localization of Rh-lipoplexes; II: localization of tf alexa-fluor 488; III: overlay of single colour images.

4.3 Effects on transfection efficiency

As cellular internalization of lipoplexes was successfully achieved in both HAEC and HASMC by clathrin-dependent endocytosis, which results in the transport of lipoplexes via endosomes (Fig. 5), further investigations examined possible barriers after uptake.

For these experiments DNA was introduced into the cell by electroporation. With this method, endosomal release and disintegration of the DNA from the lipoplex are no longer involved. Basically, it can be determined that the introduced DNA is not degraded in the cytosol and is able to cross the nuclear membrane to enter the nucleus. Indeed, electroporation resulted in transfection efficiencies of 43 % in HAEC and 51 % in HASMC (Table 2, Fig. 6), indicating that transfection is restricted either by insufficient endosomal release or insufficient release of DNA from the lipoplex.

To investigate insufficient endosomal release, transfection experiments with DC-30® lipoplexes were accomplished with HAEC and HASMC as described before [5]. Additionally, prior to lipoplex incubation the cells were incubated with different concentrations of chloroquine, which represses lysosomal degradation by increasing the pH [21] to facilitate endosomal escape and therefore improve transfection efficiency. Addition of chloroquine did not lead to an increase in transfection efficiency (Table 2). This shows no insufficient endosomal escape of lipoplex.

5. Discussion

This study demonstrates, that the development of efficient non-viral gene delivery systems requires better understanding of the mechanism of the delivery and of the intracellular processing. Endocytosis is the major pathway of entry, but the involvement of specific endocytic pathways is still poorly defined. This study contributes to further clarify uptake mechanisms and barriers in gene delivery in primary cells.

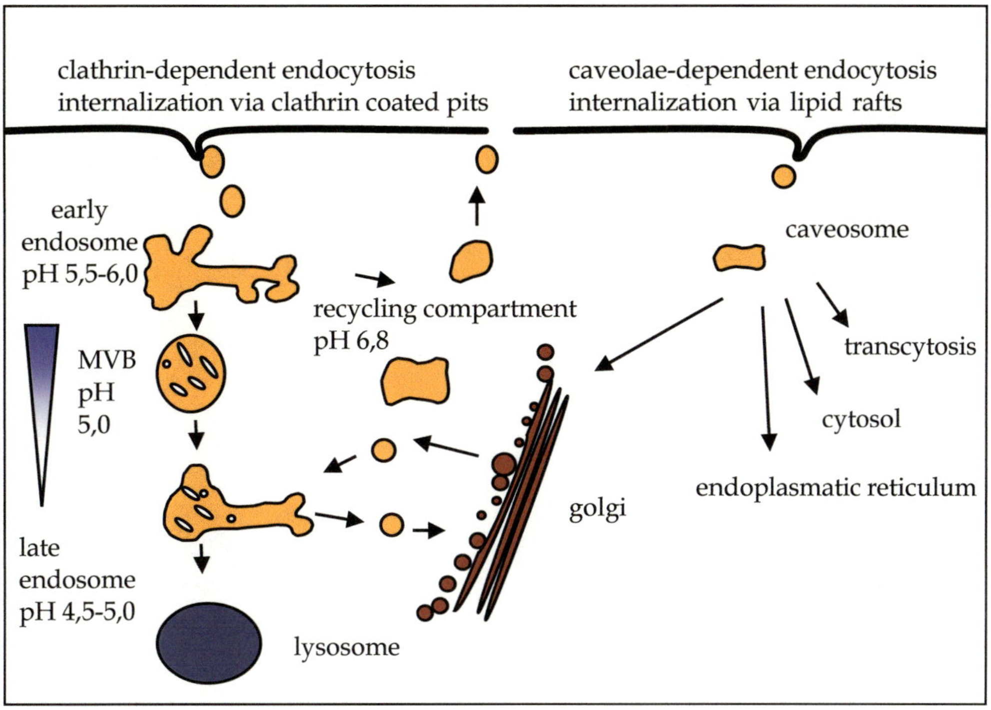

Fig. 5. Cartoon of the main cellular internalization routes of lipoplexes. On the left hand the clathrin-dependent pathway and on the right hand the caveolae-mediated uptake mechanisms are shown. Whereas the first pathway has been well investigated, caveolin-mediated internalization has not been examined in detail to date. The first step in the clathrin-dependent pathway is the budding of clathrin-coated vesicles resulting in early or sorting endosomes. Recycling back to the membrane happens in recycling endosomes. Early endosomes transform in MVB and subsequently late endosomes are formed which end up as lysosomes. Active exchange between the golgi apparatus and late endosomes is known. Particles, internalized via caveolae from so-called caveosomes offering various processing possibilities such as transcytosis, cytosolic release, delivery to the ER or transport to the golgi apparatus.

It showed, that poor transfection efficiency of primary human aorta and smooth muscle cells (HAEC and HASMC) is not due to insufficient delivery into the cell. Uptake of lipoplex reached 20 % in HAEC and 80 % in HASMC whereas transfection was less than 3 % in both cases. Furthermore, it was shown, that plasmid DNA, transferred directly into the cytosol of the cell by electroporation effectively transfected 40 to 50% of the cells. These data suggest, that DNA, once being present in the cytosol, is able to cross the nucleolae membrane and to show activity.

In the present study it was shown, that lipoplexes are partly internalized in HAEC via caveolae mediated endocytosis. The caveolae route is known to enable transport of nanoparticulate drug delivery systems into and/or through the cell without involvement of lysosomal compartments. In case of drugs being sensitive to acidic hydrolysis or enzymatic degradation, e.g., biomacromolecules such as polypetides or nucleic acids, it is important to avoid cellular routes that transport material to lysosomes. On the other side, uptake via

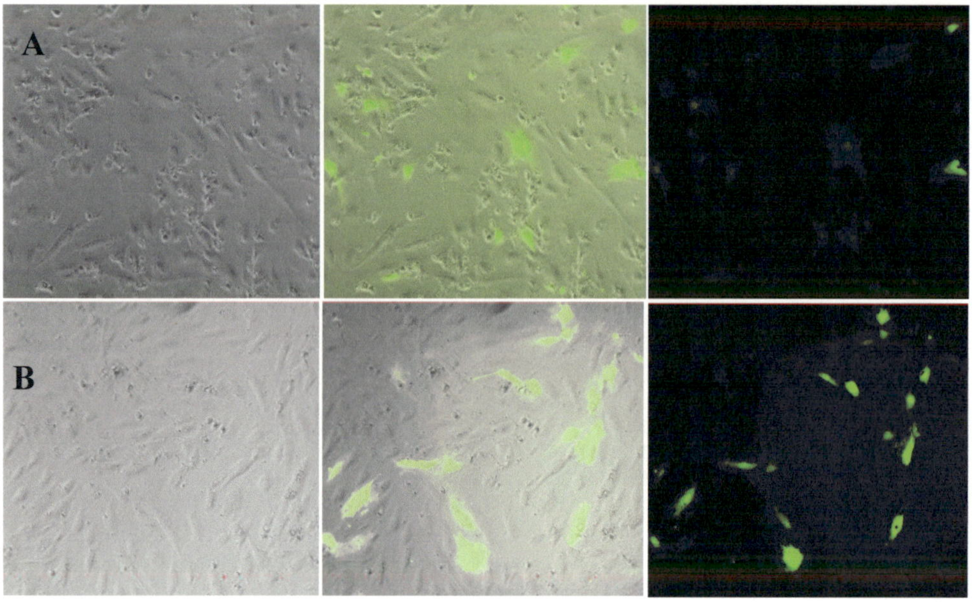

Fig. 6. HAEC (A) and HASMC (B) after electroporation of pEGFP and 48 h incubation. Left-handed: brightfield; Right handed: fluorescent picture (GFP), middle position: overlay of pictures.

caveolae does not automatically result in effective transfection as shown in this study. Although uptake in HAEC was partly achieved by the caveolae route, no transfection occurred. This is important to consider, because obviously it is not enough to focus the research on modifying particulate drug carriers, e.g., by attaching specific ligands, introducing surface charge or pH-sensitivity, or changing the particle size or elasticity in order to trigger the caveolae mediated endocytosis.
The use of different methods (flow cytometry, spectral bio-imaging, electroporation) and materials (markers and inhibitors of endocytosis pathways) contributed to the evidence that transfection of primary human aorta endothelium and smooth muscle cells was not effective due to insufficient dissociation of plasmid DNA from the lipid/DNA delivery system. This finding is of great importance for future drug deliver development in the field of gene therapy.

6. Acknowledgments

The authors thank J. Clement, F. Lewrick, U. Huth and R. Schubert for helpful discussions, B. Erhard.and Z. Khalil for technical support, K. Aktories for supply of C-3 Toxin and M. Follo for proof-reading the manuscript.

7. Abbreviations

DC-30 (DC-Chol, 3ß-[(N´,N´-Dimethylaminoethane)-carbamoyl]-cholesterol-HCl and DOPE, Dioleoylphosphatidylethanolamine 3/7 (w/w); EGFP, enhanced green fluorescent protein; HASMC, human aorta smooth muscle cells; HAEC, human aorta endothelial cells; TM, transfection medium; DAPI, 4',6-Diamino-2-phenylindol-dihydrochlorid; mbCD, methyl-beta-cyclodextrine; chlp, chlorpromazine; chtx-B, cholera toxin subunit B; tf, human transferrin; wm, wortmannin; gen, genistein; fil, filipin; noco, nocodazole; Ly, Ly294002 ; Rh, Rhodamine; cch-D, cytochalasin-D; ctrl, control; 7-AAD, 7-Amino-actinomycin

8. References

[1] K. Lundstrom, T. Boulikas, Viral and non-viral vectors in gene therapy: technology development and clinical trials, Technol Cancer Res Treat 2 (2003) 471-486.

[2] M. Thomas, A.M. Klibanov, Non-viral gene therapy: polycation-mediated DNA delivery, Appl Microbiol Biotechnol 62 (2003) 27-34.

[3] R.I. Zhdanov, O.V. Podobed, V.V. Vlassov, Cationic lipid-DNA complexes (lipoplexes) for gene transfer and therapy, Bioelectrochemistry 58 (2002) 53-64.

[4] H. Boulaiz, J.A. Marchal, J. Prados, C. Melguizo, A. Aranega, Non-viral and viral vectors for gene therapy, Cell Mol Biol (Noisy-le-grand) 51 (2005) 3-22.

[5] K. Kiefer, J. Clement, P. Garidel, R. Peschka-Süss, Transfection efficiency and cytotoxicity of nonviral gene transfer reagents in human smooth muscle and endothelial cells, Pharm Res 21 (2004) 1009-1017.

[6] O. Gresch, F.B. Engel, D. Nesic, T.T. Tran, H.M. England, E.S. Hickman, I. Korner, L. Gan, S. Chen, S. Castro-Obregon, R. Hammermann, J. Wolf, H. Muller-Hartmann, M. Nix, G. Siebenkotten, G. Kraus, K. Lun, New non-viral method for gene transfer into primary cells, Methods 33 (2004) 151-163.

[7] M.B. Bally, P. Harvie, F.M. Wong, S. Kong, E.K. Wasan, D.L. Reimer, Biological barriers to cellular delivery of lipid-based DNA carriers, Adv Drug Deliv Rev 38 (1999) 291-315.

[8] U.S. Huth, R. Schubert, R. Peschka-Süss, Investigating the uptake and intracellular fate of pH-sensitive liposomes by flow cytometry and spectral bio-imaging, J Control Release 110 (2006) 490-504.

[9] S. Rothenberger, B.J. Iacopetta, L.C. Kuhn, Endocytosis of the transferrin receptor requires the cytoplasmic domain but not its phosphorylation site, Cell 49 (1987) 423-431.

[10] I. Killisch, P. Steinlein, K. Romisch, R. Hollinshead, H. Beug, G. Griffiths, Characterization of early and late endocytic compartments of the transferrin cycle. Transferrin receptor antibody blocks erythroid differentiation by trapping the receptor in the early endosome, J Cell Sci 103 (1992) 211-232.

[11] L.H. Wang, K.G. Rothberg, R.G. Anderson, Mis-assembly of clathrin lattices on endosomes reveals a regulatory switch for coated pit formation, J Cell Biol 123 (1993) 1107-1117.

[12] Y. Shitara, Y. Kato, Y. Sugiyama, Effect of brefeldin A and lysosomotropic reagents on intracellular trafficking of epidermal growth factor and transferrin in Madin-Darby canine kidney epithelial cells, J Control Release 55 (1998) 35-43.

[13] L. Pelkmans, J. Kartenbeck, A. Helenius, Caveolar endocytosis of simian virus 40 reveals a new two-step vesicular-transport pathway to the ER, Nat Cell Biol 3 (2001) 473-483.

[14] A. Lakkaraju, Y.E. Rahman, J.M. Dubinsky, Low-density lipoprotein receptor-related protein mediates the endocytosis of anionic liposomes in neurons, J Biol Chem 277 (2002) 15085-15092.

[15] M. Karin, B. Mintz, Receptor-mediated endocytosis of transferrin in developmentally totipotent mouse teratocarcinoma stem cells, J Biol Chem 256 (1981) 3245-3252.

[16] I. Killisch, P. Steinlein, K. Romisch, R. Hollinshead, H. Beug, G. Griffiths, Characterization of early and late endocytic compartments of the transferrin cycle. Transferrin receptor antibody blocks erythroid differentiation by trapping the receptor in the early endosome, J Cell Sci 103 (Pt 1) (1992) 211-232.

[17] K. Sandvig, B. van Deurs, Membrane traffic exploited by protein toxins, Annu Rev Cell Dev Biol 18 (2002) 1-24.

[18] S. Kessner, A. Krause, U. Rothe, G. Bendas, Investigation of the cellular uptake of E-Selectin-targeted immunoliposomes by activated human endothelial cells, Biochim Biophys Acta 1514 (2001) 177-190.

[19] R.G. Parton, B. Joggerst, K. Simons, Regulated internalization of caveolae, J Cell Biol 127 (1994) 1199-1215.

[20] K. Simons, E. Ikonen, Functional rafts in cell membranes, Nature 434 (1997) 569-572.

[21] W.T. Godbey, K.K. Wu, A.G. Mikos, Tracking the intracellular path of poly(ethylenimine)/DNA complexes for gene delivery, Proc Natl Acad Sci U S A 96 (1999) 5177-5181.

[22] S.K. Rodal, G. Skretting, O. Garred, F. Vilhardt, B. van Deurs, K. Sandvig, Extraction of cholesterol with methyl-beta-cyclodextrin perturbs formation of clathrin-coated endocytic vesicles, Mol Biol Cell 10 (1999) 961-974.

[23] A. Subtil, I. Gaidarov, K. Kobylarz, M.A. Lampson, J.H. Keen, T.E. McGraw, Acute cholesterol depletion inhibits clathrin-coated pit budding, Proc Natl Acad Sci U S A 96 (1999) 6775-6780.

[24] P. Thomsen, K. Roepstorff, M. Stahlhut, B. van Deurs, Caveolae are highly immobile plasma membrane microdomains, which are not involved in constitutive endocytic trafficking, Mol Biol Cell 13 (2002) 238-250.

[25] R.M. Pelletier, M.L. Vitale, Filipin vs enzymatic localization of cholesterol in guinea pig, mink, and mallard duck testicular cells, J Histochem Cytochem 42 (1994) 1539-1554.

[26] P.A. Orlandi, P.H. Fishman, Filipin-dependent inhibition of cholera toxin: evidence for toxin internalization and activation through caveolae-like domains, J Cell Biol 141 (1998) 905-915.

[27] J.E. Schnitzer, P. Oh, E. Pinney, J. Allard, Filipin-sensitive caveolae-mediated transport in endothelium: reduced transcytosis, scavenger endocytosis, and capillary permeability of select macromolecules, J Cell Biol 127 (1994) 1217-1232.

[28] L. Pelkmans, D. Puntener, A. Helenius, Local actin polymerization and dynamin recruitment in SV40-induced internalization of caveolae, Science 296 (2002) 535-539.

[29] U. Huth, A. Wieschollek, Y. Garini, R. Schubert, R. Peschka-Süss, Fourier transformed spectral bio-imaging for studying the intracellular fate of liposomes, Cytometry A 57 (2004) 10-21.

[30] N. Araki, M.T. Johnson, J.A. Swanson, A role for phosphoinositide 3-kinase in the completion of macropinocytosis and phagocytosis by macrophages, J Cell Biol 135 (1996) 1249-1260.

[31] R.B. Kelly, Microtubules, membrane traffic, and cell organization, Cell 61 (1990) 5-7.

5

The Mechanical Agitation Method of Gene Transfer for *Ex-Vivo* Gene Therapy

Hea-Jong Chung[1], Hyun-Seo Lee[1],
Hyeon-Jin Kim[2] and Seong-Tshool Hong[1]
[1]*Laboratory of Genetics and Department of Microbiology*
Chonbuk National University Medical School
[2]*Jinis Biopharmaceuticals Co.*
Republic of Korea

1. Introduction

Gene therapy is a therapeutic method used to treat diseases by altering genes within a patient's cells. The concept of gene therapy emerged as molecular biology evolved from the mere discipline of studying DNA molecules to the scientific art of virtually manipulating the genes of cells. Explosive worldwide research was conducted after the first introduction of the concept of gene therapy into the scientific community. The original aim was to directly modify patient genes through *in vivo* gene therapeutic approaches. However, DNA molecules introduced into the body by *in vivo* gene therapy are delivered at a very low frequency into terminally differentiated tissue cells, which typically do not have the capability of self-renewal (Tenenbaum et al., 2003). Because of the short-lived nature of *in vivo* gene therapy, a defective gene in patients is only temporarily corrected by *in vivo* gene therapy (Kaloss et al., 1999). The development of gene therapeutic methods in which the corrected patient gene remains permanently has been actively pursued.

Ex vivo gene therapeutic methods have been considered as alternative options to gene therapy to overcome the short-lived nature of the corrected genes of *in vivo* gene therapy. In *ex vivo* gene therapy, the surgically removed adult stem cells, such as mesenchymal stem cells or hematopoietic stem cells, are typically cultured in a laboratory apparatus. The therapeutic DNA molecules are introduced into the isolated cells, and these transfected cells are then introduced into the patients. By using adult stem cells in *ex vivo* gene therapeutic methods, the corrected genes that are introduced are, in most cases, expressed permanently once they are corrected properly because the adult stem cells have the capability of self-renewal (Dube & Denis, 1995; Muller-Sieburg & Sieburg, 2006; Tseng et al., 2006; Nehlin & Barington 2009). In *ex vivo* gene therapy, genetic manipulation is conducted in a lab outside of the body. However, normal somatic cells, including adult stem cells, do not propagate indefinitely and are vulnerable to epigenetic modification. Therefore, long-term cultures of somatic cells isolated from the body are very difficult to sustain (Beyer & Da sliva, 2006; Tonti & Mannello, 2008). This means that the long-term culture of adult stem cells in *ex vivo* gene therapy should be avoided as much as possible. Therefore, it is absolutely necessary to deliver therapeutic DNA molecules into isolated cells immediately with high efficiency.

In current gene transfer protocols, gene delivery vehicles containing therapeutic DNA molecules make only limited contacts with their target cells by passive diffusion, thereby limiting the chances of gene delivery. In our lab, we developed a very efficient method to deliver therapeutic genes to adult stem cells based on mechanical agitation (Park et al., 2009).

In this method, mechanical agitation of the gene delivery vehicles containing cell suspensions increases the movement of gene delivery vehicles and target cells, resulting in an increase in contact between them. The application of our mechanical agitation method to the gene delivery process of *ex vivo* gene therapy, both in transfection and transduction, has increased the gene transfer efficiency more than that of any other previously known gene transfer protocol.

2. Basic principles of current gene therapeutic approaches

Gene therapy is classified as somatic gene therapy or germ line gene therapy. The application of current molecular genetic techniques used during the manipulation of transgenic or knock-out animals would definitely make gene therapy possible in virtually any type of germ line. However, all civilized societies in the world currently legally prohibit any attempts to genetically modify embryos. Thus far, gene therapy essentially implies somatic gene therapy. Compared to the easy genetic manipulation of embryonic stem cells, the genetic manipulation of somatic cells, including adult stem cells, is limited such that none of the somatic gene therapies are used practically thus far. Therefore, it is not surprising that the main quest of current gene therapy is to improve the efficiency of genetic manipulation in gene therapy, and the future success of gene therapy depends on the efficiency of genetic manipulation.

Genetic manipulation in gene therapy can be achieved by two different approaches: direct genetic manipulation of somatic cells in the body and genetic manipulation of autologous cells outside of the body. These two different strategies for gene delivery are termed *in vivo* and *ex vivo*, respectively. In the *in vivo* strategy, therapeutic genes are delivered into cells *in situ* using a variety of vectors to produce therapeutic proteins in specific sites in the body. In *ex vivo* gene therapy, genetically modified autologous cells are surgically implemented into the body. The *ex vivo* and *in vivo* gene therapies both have positive and negative aspects. Although gene therapy has been a very hot topic in biomedical science for several decades, it is still in its infancy, and a number of hurdles must be overcome to achieve the practical application of gene therapy to patients.

2.1 *In vivo* gene therapy

In vivo gene therapy is a process in which a therapeutic gene is delivered through a vector directly into the target cells of patients to produce a therapeutic effect that prevents or treats diseases (Fig. 1). Theoretically, once an ideal gene delivery vehicle for a therapeutic gene transfer is developed, the *in vivo* gene therapy should involve a very simple procedure: the injection of a solution containing the gene delivery vehicle into the body. Because of this potentially easy treatment procedure in clinics, *in vivo* gene therapy is considered the preferred gene therapeutic method than *ex vivo* gene therapy. However, *in vivo* gene therapy has a basic and fundamental problem in the delivery of therapeutic genes to target cells: the low efficiency of gene transfer.

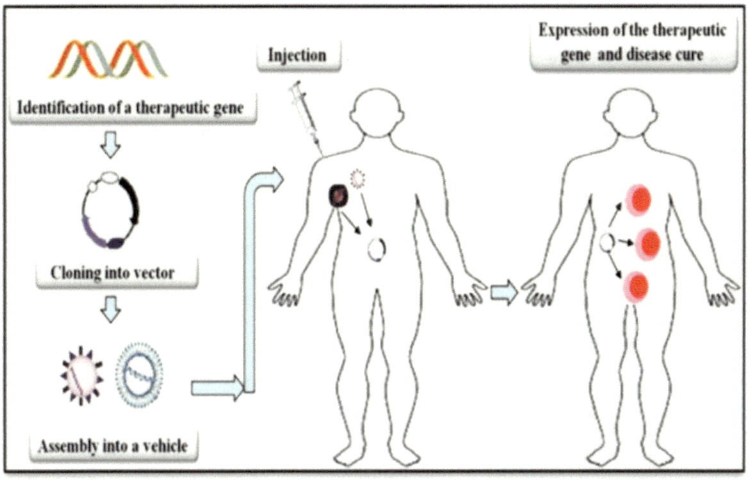

Fig. 1. Strategies for *in vivo* gene therapy. *In Vivo* gene therapy involves introduction of therapeutic DNA directly into the patient body. The DNA is introduced by cell-specific direct injection into tissue in need. Once inside the body and in contact with the specifically targeted cells, the inserted DNA is incorporated into the tissue cells where it encodes the production of the needed protein.

The bottleneck in development of *in vivo* gene therapeutic methods has been the development of an efficient method for delivery of a therapeutic gene into the target cells of the body. The main reason for poor gene delivery efficiency in *in vivo* gene therapy is rooted to the nature of the body. The cells in the body are typically surrounded by an extracellular matrix that usually provides structural support to the cells in addition to performing various other important functions (Fig. 2). The main constituent of the body is the extracellular matrix, not cells (Suki & Jason, 2008). For example, collagen proteins, which are one of the components of the extracellular matrix, constitute approximately 25-35% of the protein content of the entire body, implying that the extracellular matrix occupies the main volume of the body (Khan et al., 2009). The injected gene delivery vehicles must pass through the extracellular matrix to deliver therapeutic proteins into target cells in *in vivo* gene therapy. However, because the extracellular matrix spatially occupies such a large portion of the body, there is an unsolvable limitation for efficient gene transfer in *in vivo* gene therapy.

In addition to the low efficiency of gene delivery, *in vivo* gene therapy has another problem. The gene transfer vector is obligatorily exposed to the immune system of the body. This exposure causes an immune response that blocks gene delivery entirely. Overall, the potential immune response is another factor contributing to the low efficiency of gene delivery in *in vivo* gene therapy. Therefore, development of an ideal gene delivery vehicle for *in vivo* gene therapy is so extremely challenging that, until now, none of the *in vivo* gene therapeutic methods have not a satisfactory result.

2.2 *Ex vivo* gene therapy

In *ex vivo* gene therapy, cells are removed from a patient, maintained in culture to introduce a therapeutic gene into the cells, and then transplanted into the patient (Fig. 3). The role of the transplanted cells, which are genetically modified, is to deliver a recombinant gene

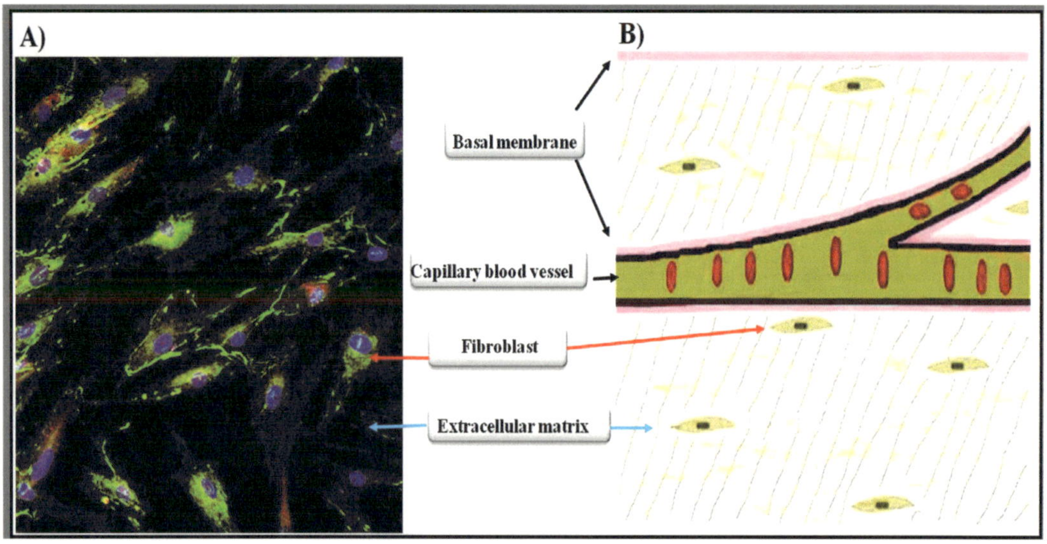

Fig. 2. Typical Anatomical Structure of Connective Tissue. A) The Confocal Microscopic Image of a Mouse Connective Tissue. B) Schematic Illustration Depicting Extracellular Matrix. The extracellular matrix (ECM) is the extracellular part of animal tissue that usually provides structural support to the animal cells in addition to performing various other important functions. The extracellular matrix is the defining feature of connective tissue in animals.

product into the patient's body. The genetically modified cells are not required to reconstitute a particular organ or tissue for the purpose of reimplementation of the cells in a location where the cells were originally obtained. For example, genetically modified hepatocytes harvested from one liver lobe may be re-infused throughout any part of the liver of patients in *ex vivo* gene therapy.

The main disadvantage of *ex vivo* gene therapy is that it requires the surgical removal of cells from the body and transplantation of the cells back to the body. These surgical steps are very painful. However, *ex vivo* therapy has several advantages over *in vivo* gene therapy. First, the efficiency of gene transfer into the targeted cells is very high compared to *in vivo* gene therapy because gene delivery is performed under controlled, optimized conditions. Second, the transduced cells can be enriched if the vector has a selectable gene marker. Third, the immunological side effects that are caused by gene delivery vehicles in *in vivo* gene therapy are usually minimized in *ex vivo* gene therapy.

2.3 *Ex-vivo* gene therapy as a practical option to correct a defective gene permanently

In vivo gene therapy introduces the therapeutic genes directly into the patient by intravascular injection. Because this approach is much simpler and less technically demanding than *ex vivo* gene therapy, which requires two surgical steps, the science of *in vivo* gene therapy has been preferentially developed. However, as discussed above, the nature of the mammalian body imposes innate, unsolved problems for *in vivo* gene therapy to achieve gene expression at therapeutically effective levels. The limitation of *in vivo* gene therapy for practical application is mainly due to low efficiency gene transfer. Because genetic manipulations are conducted in a lab in *ex vivo* gene therapy, the application of

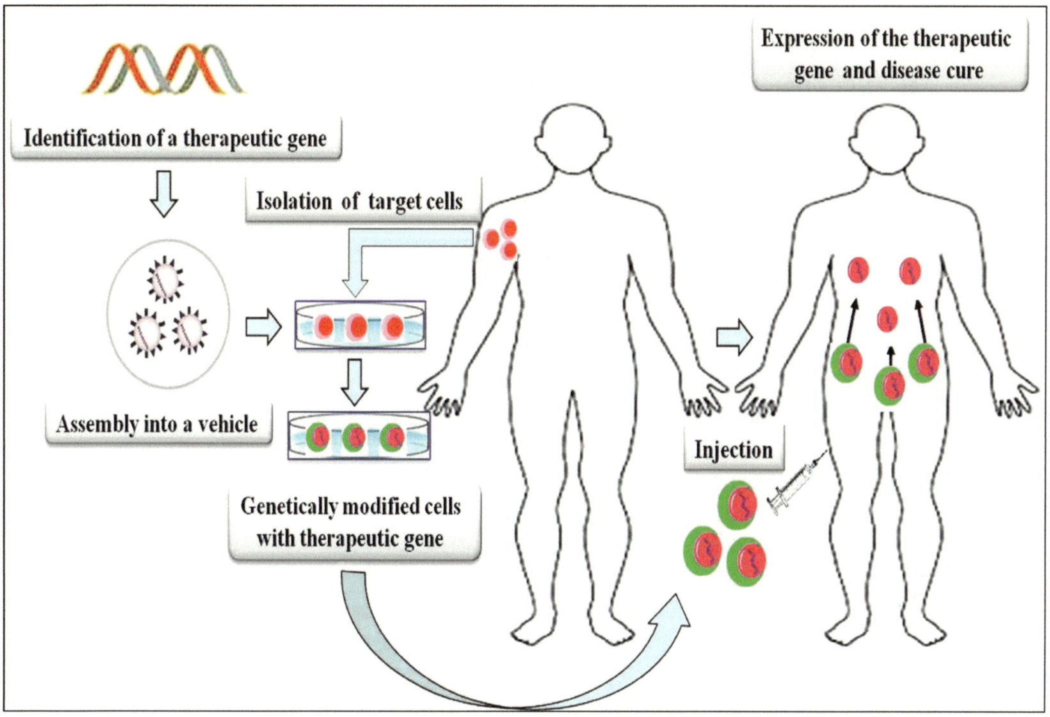

Fig. 3. Strategies for *Ex Vivo* Gene Therapy. *Ex vivo* gene therapy is performed with the genetic alterations of patients target cells happening outside of the body in as culture. Target cells from the patient are infected with a recombinant virus containing the desired therapeutic gene. These modified cells are then reintroduced into the patient body, where they produce the needed proteins that correspond to the inserted gene.

current molecular biological techniques can solve the low efficiency of gene transfer. *Ex vivo* gene therapy has the potential to ultimately solve this major problem of gene therapy, and it could be practically used in clinics. However, normal somatic cells, including adult stem cells, do not only propagate well in a typical cell culture environment and are also vulnerable to epigenetic modification (Islam et al., 2007; Martinez-Climent et al., 2006), requiring that the transfer of therapeutic genes to the isolated cells be performed as soon as possible. Therefore, one of the key factors for the success of *ex vivo* gene therapy is to deliver therapeutic DNA molecules into isolated cells promptly with high efficiency. If these problems could be solved successfully, the *ex vivo* technique could be practically applied to patients in the near future.

3. Current methods for gene delivery in *ex vivo* gene therapy

As the name implies, the success of gene therapy depends on introducing therapeutic genes into target cells with high efficiency. Since Friedmann and Roblin formulated the concept of gene therapy in 1972 (Friedmann & Roblin, 1972), the biggest challenge in gene therapy has been the development of a method to deliver therapeutic genes to target cells with high efficiency. Although gene delivery in *in vivo* gene therapy is much easier than in *ex vivo* gene therapy, gene delivery into primary cells of *in vitro* cell cultures is also quite difficult.

Typical efficiencies of gene delivery to primary cells are 5-10% in most current methods (Cai et al., 2002; Ding et al., 1999; Eiges et al., 2001; Lakshmipathy et al., 2004; Peister et al., 2004), which is not high enough for satisfactory *ex vivo* gene therapy. Because of this, many different methods of gene delivery have been developed using primary cells for *ex vivo* gene therapy. Generally, gene delivery methods can be divided into two categories, viral and non-viral.

3.1 Viral methods for gene delivery in *ex vivo* gene therapy

Viruses have evolved specialized molecular mechanisms to efficiently transport their genomes into cells. Viral vectors have developed by taking advantage of the molecular mechanisms of the virus to deliver exogenous DNA into target cells. Currently, viral vectors are frequently used molecular biology tools for delivery of genetic material into cells of a living organism (*in vivo*) or in cell culture (*in vitro*). Viral vectors are tailored to their specific applications but share a key property. Because viral vectors are essentially created from pathogenic viruses, they are modified to minimize the pathogenic properties of the original viruses. This usually involves the deletion of a portion of the viral genome that is critical for viral replication. Such viral vectors can efficiently infect cells but once the infection has taken place, they cannot replicate. The viral vectors require helper genes to provide the missing proteins for production of new virions. Replication of viral vectors is usually conducted in packaging cells that were engineered with helper genes. Therefore, viral vectors can only replicate in packaging cells and exist solely to deliver exogenous DNA to target cells where the viral vector cannot replicate.

Table 1 summarizes the types of viral vectors currently developed. In general, viral vectors are very efficient in terms of gene delivery into target cells. However, viral vectors have common problems including the following: (i) a limited DNA capacity, (ii) expression of viral genes, (iii) initiation of the antiviral immune response, (iv) reversion to a replication competent state and (v) decreasing expression over time.

Viral vectors can be classified as DNA or RNA viral vectors. DNA viral vectors are derived from viruses such as adenovirus or herpes virus, which carry their genetic material in the form of DNA. Because these viral vectors persist as an extrachromosomal element after delivery into target cells, the viral vectors remain only temporarily. One advantage of the episomal presence of the vectors is that the gene expression level is high. Because exogenous genes cannot stay indefinitely, these vectors are not suitable for *ex vivo* gene therapy. Currently, these vectors are mostly used for *in vivo* gene therapy.

Retroviral and lentiviral vectors are examples of RNA viral vectors that are replicated in target cells via reverse transcriptase to produce DNA from their RNA genomes. The DNA is then incorporated into the host's genome by an integrase. Thereafter, the virus replicates as part of the host cell's DNA, permitting long-term expression of the exogenous gene and ensuring transmission of the exogenous gene to the progeny of transduced cells. Therefore, these vectors are suitable for *ex vivo* gene therapy in which permanent gene expression is required in *in vitro* cell culture. These vectors are also widely used for *in vivo* gene therapy.

3.2 Non-viral methods for gene delivery in *ex vivo* gene therapy

Gene therapy was originally devised for the treatment of inherited genetic diseases, such as hemophilia and cystic fibrosis. However, the realm of gene therapy has been expanding to develop strategies for cancer, infectious diseases like HIV, and various complex diseases,

Vector	Genetic material	Packaging capacity	Tropism	Inflammatory potential	Vector genome forms	Main Advantages
Retrovirus	RNA	8 kb	Dividing cells	Low	Integrated	Persistent gene transfer in dividing cells
Adenovirus	dsDNA	7.5 kb	Dividing and non-dividing cells	High	Non-integrated	Extremely efficient transduction of most tissues
Adeno-associated virus	ssDNA	< 5kb	Dividing and non-dividing cells	Low	Non-integrated (90%) Integrated (>10%)	Non-inflammatory; non-pathogenic
Lentivirus	RNA	8 kb	Dividing and non-dividing cells	Low	Integrated	Persistent gene transfer in most tissues
Herpes virus	dsDNA	> 30 kb	Dividing and non-dividing cells	High	Non-integrated	Large packaging capacity; strong tropism for neurons

Table 1. A comparison of different viral vectors used for gene therapy

such as diabetes, dementia and hypertension. Genetic manipulations for these diseases are more complicated than genetic manipulations for the treatment of inherited genetic diseases. This means that current gene therapies need to deliver DNA, RNA, siRNA, or antisense sequences that alter gene expression within a specific cell population to manipulate cellular processes and responses. Viral vector-mediated gene deliveries are by far the most effective means of DNA delivery. However, the recombinant vector containing the therapeutic gene has to be packaged with viral coat proteins to make gene delivery possible, meaning that viral vector-mediated gene deliveries are limited to a DNA molecule of a certain size because the viral coat proteins have a limited DNA carrying capacity. Other than the physical limitation of viral vector-mediated gene deliveries, there are more limitations, such as immunotoxicity caused by viral coat proteins, restricted targeting of specific cell types, and recombination. Therefore, non-viral gene deliveries have been a very popular research topic, and many interesting and creative methods have been developed. The efficiency of gene delivery (*i.e.* transfection efficiency) is crucial to the success of non-viral gene deliveries. Various non-viral gene delivery methods currently developed could be classified into two groups: physical gene delivery methods and chemical gene delivery methods.

3.2.1 Physical gene delivery methods

Physical gene delivery methods are methods for transferring DNA molecules from the surrounding medium into cells. Naked DNA (*i.e.,* an uncomplexed form of DNA) is used in physical gene delivery methods. The easiest method to deliver genes into cells is to draw naked DNA into a microneedle and then inject the microneedle into cells to transfer the naked DNA directly to the cells. Though gene transfer efficiency by this method is very efficient, the method is very slow and laborious. The main drawback of this method is that microinjection can be only performed on one cell at a time, which means that this approach cannot be used for typical gene therapeutic approaches. The approach is limited to use for gene delivery into germ-line cells to produce transgenic organisms.

Currently, the most popular physical methods for gene delivery into cells are electroporation and sonoporation. The cellular membrane is punctured by an electric pulse (electroporation) (Neumann et al., 1982) or ultrasonic wave (sonoporation) (Yizhi et al., 2007). The pores in the cellular membrane are only temporarily formed, and DNA molecules pass through during the short period of time when the pores open. These methods are generally efficient and work well across a broad range of cell types. However, a high rate of cell death limits their use, especially in gene therapy. These methods are widely used for gene delivery of immortal cells in which cell viability is not a critical issue during gene transfer.

Another popular method for physical gene delivery is the use of particle bombardment. In this method, gold particles (gene gun) (Gan et al., 2000) or magnetic particles (magnetofection) (Scherer et al., 2002) are coated with naked DNA. In the gene gun method, the DNA-coated gold particles are shot into the cell using high pressure gas, and the particles pass through the cellular membrane to introduce the particles inside the cells. In the magnetofection method, a magnet is placed underneath the tissue culture dish to attract DNA-coated magnetic particles. Then, the DNA-coated magnetic particles come into contact with a cell monolayer to introduce the particles inside the cells. These methods yield reasonably high efficiency gene transfers, but do not yield better efficiencies compared to other non-viral gene transfer methods, despite the requirement for expensive equipment. Also, it is quite difficult to control the DNA entry pathway, and the metal particles in the cells following gene transfer could negatively affect cells. Therefore, these methods are not widely used.

3.2.2 Chemical gene delivery methods

Because DNA cannot pass through cellular membranes alone, various chemicals have been designed to aid the transfer of therapeutic genes into cells. The chemicals used in chemical gene delivery function to enhance the stability of the DNA molecule, to increase the efficiency of cellular uptake and intracellular trafficking, or to alter the distribution of the transferred DNA in the cells. These methods are very successful in terms of transferring genes into cells and are currently the most widely used methods. Also, chemical gene delivery methods are the easiest and most effective among various non-viral gene delivery methods developed thus far.

The most well-studied and effective approach for non-viral gene delivery is the use of cationic lipids. Positively charged cationic lipids naturally bind to negatively charged DNA in solution to condense DNA so that the DNA molecules and cationic lipids form complexes called lipoplexes. After lipoplexes are formed, the positively charged cationic lipids of the lipoplexes interact with cell membranes to allow cells to take up the lipoplexes by endocytosis. In typical cell physiology, endosomes that are formed as the result of endocytosis will fuse with lysosomes to degrade the lipoplexes containing the DNA. An exogenous gene in the lipoplexes would not have a chance to be released into the cytoplasm for gene expression if the endosomes are stable. Therefore, helper lipids are added to form lipoplexes to facilitate the endosomal escape of the exogenous gene (Herringson et al., 2009a, 2009b; Savva et al., 2005). This approach is very successful because it increases the transfection efficiency dramatically. There are various combinations of cationic lipids and helper lipids available. More than 40 products are commercially available for cationic lipid-based gene delivery, including LipoTAXI (Agilent Technologies), Lipofectamin™ (Invitrogen), NanoJuice® (Merck), Transfectam® (Promega), and LipoJet ™ (SignaGen Laboratories). The cationic lipid-based gene delivery shows a very high transfection efficiency of up to 90 in *in vitro* cell culture. Because the cationic lipid-based lipoplexes are not stably maintained in the blood, these methods are best for *ex vivo* gene therapy. However, cationic lipid-based lipoplexes show a very poor transfection efficiency with primary cells, such as stem cells, indicating that new methodological developments are required for the practical application of *ex vivo* gene therapy.

Other than cationic lipids, several different positively charged materials are used as a base material for non-viral DNA delivery, such as cationic polymers (Segura & Shea, 2001), cationic peptides consisting of poly-L-Lysine (D'Haeze et al., 2007; Mullen et al., 2000; Niidome et al., 1997), or other types of cationic proteins (De Lima et al., 1999; Jean et al., 2009; Lam et al., 2004; Lee et al., 2003; Oliveira et al., 2009; Vighi et al., 2007). These approaches produce DNA carrying complexes that are more stable. However, the transfection efficiency of this method is not better than cationic lipid-based lipoplexes. Therefore, most of these methods are designed for *in vivo* gene therapy.

4. Application of the mechanical agitation method to *ex vivo* gene therapy

One of the main obstacles for the application of adult stem cells in *ex vivo* gene therapy is the low efficiency of gene transfer to these cells. For example, electroporation or transfection in mesenchymal stem cells yields 5-10% gene delivery efficiency (Cai et al., 2002; Ding et al., 1999; Eiges et al., 2001; Lakshmipathy et al., 2004; Peister et al., 2004). Therefore, improved gene delivery methods would potentially be very beneficial for the practical application of *ex vivo* gene therapy in patient care. In current gene transfer protocols, virus particles or lipoplexes passively diffuse through the liquid culture medium to reach their target cells, which are layered on the bottom of a culture dish (Chuck & Palsson, 1996). Because the virus particles or lipoplexes contact the target cells by passive diffusion, increasing the chance of contact between virus particles or lipoplexes and their target cells would increase the chance of gene transfer and to promote higher transfer efficiencies. One simple way to increase contact between viruses or lipoplexes and target cells is through mechanical agitation. Based on this hypothesis, we developed a mechanical agitation method for retroviral transduction of primary cells or transfection by lipoplexes (Park et al., 2009). In this method, we simply implemented a step in which virus-containing or lipoplexes-containing cell suspensions are agitated to increase the movement of viruses or lipoplexes and target cells with the purpose of generating more frequent contact between them. Suspended target cells have a better chance of making physical contact with virus particles or lipoplexes than adherent target cells because of the possibility for three-dimensional contact between the cells and viruses or lipoplexes. The simple addition of the mechanical agitation step to the conventional transduction or transfection protocol increased gene transfer efficiency two-fold above the current rates these protocols (Fig. 4). In the following section, we describe one example of retroviral transduction using our mechanical agitation protocol.

A

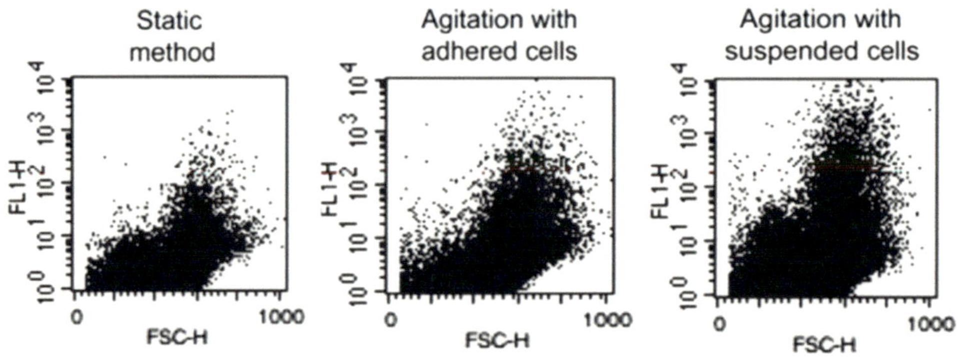

B

		Simultaneous mechanical agitation	
	Static method	Adhered cells	Suspended cells
% EGFP (+) cells	17 ± 2.7	30 ± 1.4	43 ± 2.5

Fig. 4. A Typical Example of Application of Machanical Agitation Method to Transduction of EGFP-Carrying Retrovirus (Park et al., 2009). (A) The representative FACS plots of rat mesenchymal stem cells after transduction with Retro-EGFP using the static method (left panel), mechanical agitation of viruses with adhered cells (middle panel) and simultaneous mechanical agitation of retroviruses with suspended cells (right panel). (B) Numerical representation of the transduction efficiencies of EGFP retrovirus under the static protocol versus the new agitation protocol. The transduction efficiency is defined as the percentage of cells expressing EGFP as measured using FACSCalibur. The mean percentage of GFP-positive cells is presented as the average of three independent transduction experiments (+/- SEM, n=3).

4.1 Materials

1. Packaging cell line PT67 (Clontech).
2. pCAG-EGFP expression vector (Addgene, USA) and pMSCVneo retroviral vector (Clontech, USA).
3. Lipofectamine 2,000 (Invitrogen).
4. Rat mesenchymal stem cells (isolated by flushing the femurs of two-month-old female SD rats (Damool Bioscience Co., Korea).
5. DMEM/ High glucose (Hyclone, USA) with 10% FBS (Hyclone), 2 mM L-glutamin (Invitrogen, USA), 100 µg/ml streptomycin, and 100 U/ml penicillin (Sigma, USA).
6. Selection drug, G418 (Sigma) and Polybrene (Calbiochem, USA).
7. Rat mesenchymal stem cell characterization kit (Millipore,USA).

8. TrypLE Express (Invitrogen).
9. Carl Zeiss LSM510 Meta microscope.
10. 0.45 μm cellulose acetate filter (Millipore).
11. Rocker (SLS4, Seoulin, Korea).
12. Incubator at 37°C under 5% CO_2.
13. 24-well plates and 96-well plates.
14. E-Max micro-well reader (Molecular Devices, USA).
15. Fluorescence microscope (TE2000-S, Nikon, Japan).
16. FACSCalibur instrument (Becton Dickinson, USA).

4.2 One example protocol of retroviral transduction into mesenchymal stem cells

1. Trypsinize pure rat mesenchymal stem cells (0.1 ml/cm^2) for 3 min at 37°C.
2. Adjust the cell suspension to contain 5×10^5 cells/ml.
3. Mix a 1 ml aliquot of the trypsinized rat mesenchymal stem cells directly with 1 ml virus stock in the presence of 6 μg/ml polybrene (Calbiochem, USA).
4. Seed the mixing solution in a six-well plate (Falcon, USA).
5. Mechanically agitate the plate containing the mixture of rat mesenchymal stem cells and virus on a rocker (SLS4, Seoulin, Korea) at 20 rpm for 50 min while incubating at 37°C under 5% CO_2.
6. Incubate the plate at 37°C under 5% CO_2 for 24 h.
7. Replace the supernatant containing virus particles with fresh growth medium.
8. Observe EGFP fluorescence in the transduced rat mesenchymal stem cells with a fluorescence microscope (TE2000-S, Nikon, Japan) after an 86 h incubation.

5. Conclusion and prospect

Since the first clinical trial of gene therapy in 1990, 1703 gene therapy clinical trials have been completed as of March of 2011 (http://www.wiley.com/legacy/wileychi/genmed/clinical/). However, little progress has been made since the first gene therapy clinical trial, and therefore, the Food and Drug Administration of the United States has not yet approved any human gene therapy for actual patient treatments. Although current gene therapy is still in the experimental stage, *ex vivo* gene therapeutic approaches show a great potential to treat monogenic genetic diseases as shown in the clinical trial results of adenosine deaminase deficiency and familial hypercholesterolemia (Cappelli et al., 2010 & Kassim et al., 2010). The clinical trial results of these diseases were encouraging to continually pursue *ex vivo* gene therapy.

Primary cells, including adult stem cells, have limited self-renewal ability and are vulnerable to epigenetic modification (Dube & Denis, 1995; Muller-Sieburg & Sieburg, 2006; Tseng et al., 2006; Nehlin & Barington, 2009). The long-term culture of primary cells is not possible. Therefore, it is absolutely necessary to deliver therapeutic DNA molecules into isolated cells promptly with high efficiency. However, the transfer efficiency of exogenous DNA into primary cells is very low (Beyer & Da sliva, 2006; Tonti & Mannello, 2008). The gene transfer efficiency into primary cells is several fold less than those of cell lines in current gene transfer methods. This means that improvement of the transfer efficiency of exogenous DNA into primary cells is the first obstacle for the practical use of for *ex vivo* gene therapy.

The mechanical agitation method discussed here led to a higher efficiency gene transfer, either in transfection using lipoplexes or transduction, than that of any current static transduction method. This method can potentially be applied to a variety of current transduction or transfection protocols with slight adjustments to the agitation time and speed. We believe that this protocol will contribute to various *ex vivo* gene therapies and *in vitro* gene transfer experiments for primary cells.

6. Acknowledgement

This Research was supported by the grant of Rural development administration, South Korea.

7. References

Beyer, NN., & Da Silva, ML. (2006). Mesenchynal stem cell: isolation, in vitro expansion and characterization. *Handb. Exp. Phamacol.*, Vol.174, pp.249-282.

Cai, S., Ma, Q., Yu, X., Dang, G., & Ma, D. (2002). Expression of human VEGF(121) cDNA in mouse bone marrow stromal cells. *Chin. Med. J., (Engl)* Vol.115, pp.914-918.

Cappelli, B., & Aiuti, A. (2010). Gene therapy for adenosine deaminase deficiency. *Immunol Allergy Clin. North Am.*, Vol.30, No.2, pp.249-260.

Chuck, AS., & Palsson, BO. (1996). Consistent and high rates of gene transfer can be obtained using flow-through transduction over a wide range of retroviral titers. *Hum. Gene Ther.*, Vol.7, pp.743-750.

De Lima, MC., Simões, S., Pires, P., Gaspar, R., Slepushkin, V., & Düzgüneş, N. (1999). Gene delivery mediated by cationic liposomes: from biophysical aspects to enhancement of transfection. *Mol. Membr. Biol.*, Vol.16, No.1, pp.103-109.

D'Haeze, W., Leoff, C., Freshour, G., Noel, KD., & Carlson, RW. (2007). Rhizobium etli CE3 bacteroid lipopolysaccharides are structurally similar but not identical to those produced by cultured CE3 bacteria. *J. Biol. Chem.*, Vol.282, No.23, pp.17101-17113.

Eiges, R., Schuldiner, M., Drukker, M., Yanuka, O., Itskovitz-Eldor, J., & Benvenisty, N. (2001). Establishment of human embryonic stem cell-transfected clones carrying a marker for undifferentiated cells. *Curr. Biol.*, Vol. 11, pp.514-518.

Friedmann, T., & Roblin, R. (1972). Gene Therapy for Human Genetic Disease? *Science*, Vol.175, No.25, pp.949-955.

Gan, W., Grutzendler, J., Wong, WT., Wong, ROL., & Lichtman, JW. (2000). Multicolor Diolistic Labeling of the Nervous System Using Lipophilic Dye Combinations. *Neuron*, Vol. 27, Iss. 2, pp.219-225.

Herringson, TP., Patlolla, RR., & Altin, JG. (2009). Targeting of plasmid DNA-lipoplexes to cells with molecules anchored via a metal chelator lipid. *J. Gene. Med.*, Vol.11, No.11, pp.1048-1063.

Herringson, TP., & Altin, JG. (2009). Convenient targeting of stealth siRNA-lipoplexes to cells with chelator lipid-anchored molecules. *J. Control Release.*, Vol.139, No.3, pp.229-238.

Islam, MQ., Panduri, V., & Islam, K. (2007). Generation of somatic cell hybrids for the production of biologically active factors that stimulate proliferation of other cells. *Cell Prolif.*, Vol.40, No.1, pp.91-105.

Jean, M., Smaoui, F., Lavertu, M., Méthot, S., Bouhdoud, L., Buschmann, MD., & Merzouki, A. (2009). Chitosan-plasmid nanoparticle formulations for IM and SC delivery of recombinant FGF-2 and PDGF-BB or generation of antibodies. *Gene Ther.*, Vol.16, No.9, pp.1097-1110.

Kaloss, M., Linscott, M., Wey, C., Lu, P., Long, Z., McGarrity, GJ., Otto, E., & Lyons, RM. (1999). Distribution of retroviral vectors and vector producer cells using two routes of administration in rats. *Gene therapy,* Vol.6, pp.1389-1396.

Kassim, SH., Li, H., Vandenberghe, LH., Hinderer, C., Bell, P., Marchadier, D., Wilson, A., Cromley, D., Redon, V., Yu, H., Wilson, JM., & Rader, DJ. (2010). Gene therapy in a humanized mouse model of familial hypercholesterolemia leads to marked regression of atherosclerosis. *PLoS One,* Vol.5, No.10, e13424.

Khan, T., Muise, ES., Iyengar, P., Wang, ZV., Chandalia, M., Abate, N., Zhang, BB., Bonaldo, P., Chua, S., & Scherer, PE. (2009). Metabolic Dysregulation and Adipose Tissue Fibrosis: Role of Collagen VI. *Molecular and Cellular Biology*, Vol.29, No. 6, pp.1575–1591.

Lakshmipathy, U., Pelacho, B., Sudo, K., Linehan, JL., Coucouvanis, E., Kaufman, DS., & Verfaillie, CM. (2004). Efficient transfection of embryonic and adult stem cells. *Stem Cells,* Vol. 22, pp.531-543.

Lam, JK., Ma, Y., Armes, SP., Lewis, AL., Baldwin, T., & Stolnik, S. (2004). Phosphorylcholine-polycation diblock copolymers as synthetic vectors for gene delivery. *J. Control Release.*, vol.100, No.2, pp.293-312.

Lee, LK., Siapati, EK., Jenkins, RG., McAnulty, RJ., Hart, SL., & Shamlou ,PA. (2003). Biophysical characterization of an integrin-targeted non-viral vector. *Med. Sci. Monit.*, Vol.9, No.1, pp.54-61.

Martinez-Climent , JA., Andreu, EJ., & Prosper, F. (2006). Somatic stem cells and the origin of cancer. *Clin. Transl. Oncol.*, Vol.8, No. 9, pp.647-63.

Mullen, PM., Lollo, CP., Phan, QC., Amini, A., Banaszczyk, MG., Fabrycki ,JM., Wu, D., Carlo, AT., Pezzoli , P., Coffin, CC., & Carlo, DJ. (2000). Strength of conjugate binding to plasmid DNA affects degradation rate and expression level *in vivo. Biochim. Biophys. Acta.*, Vol.1523, No. 1, pp.103-110.

Muller-Sieburg, CE., & Sieburg, HB. (2006). Clonal diversitiy of the stem cell compartment. *Cur. Opin. Hematol.*, Vol.13, No. 4, pp.243-248.

Nehlin, JO., & Barington, T. (2009). Strategies for future histocompatible stem cell therapy. *Biogerontology,* Vol.10, No.4, pp.339-376.

Neumann, E., Schaefer-Ridder, M., Wang, Y., & Hofschneider, PH. (1982). Gene transfer into mouse lyoma cells by electroporation in high electric fields. *EMBO J.,* Vol.1, No. 7, pp. 841–845.

Niidome, T., Ohmori, N., Ichinose, A., Wada, A., Mihara, H., Hirayama, T., & Aoyagi, H. (1997). Binding of cationic alpha-helical peptides to plasmid DNA and their gene transfer abilities into cells. *J. Biol. Chem.*, Vol.272, No.24, pp.15307-12.

Oliveira, AC., Ferraz, MP., Monteiro, FJ., & Simões, S. (2009). Cationic liposome-DNA complexes as gene delivery vectors: Development and behaviour towards bone-like cells. *Acta. Biomater.*, Vol.5, No.6, PP.2142-2151.

Park, JO., Park, SH. & Hong, ST. (2009). A new method for transduction of mesenchymal stem cells using mechanical agitation. *Mol. Cell,* Vol.28, No. 6, pp.515-520.

Peister, A., Mellad, JA., Wang, M., Tucker, HA., & Prockop, DJ. (2004). Stable transfection of MSCs by electroporation. *GeneTher.*, Vol. 11, pp.224-228.

Savva, M., Aljaberi, A., Feig, J., & Stolz, DB. (2005). Correlation of the physicochemical properties of symmetric 1,3-dialkoylamidopropane-based cationic lipids containing single primary and tertiary amine polar head groups with in vitro transfection activity. *Colloids Surf B Biointerfaces.*, Vol.43, No.1, pp.43-56.

Scherer, F., Anton, M., Schillinger, U., Henke, J., Bergemann, C., Krüger, A., Gänsbacher, B., & Plank, C. (2002). Magnetofection: enhancing and targeting gene delivery by magnetic force in vitro and *in vivo*. *Gene Ther.*, Vol. 9, No.2, pp. 102–109.

Segura, T., & Shea, LD. (2001). Materials for non-viral gene delivery. *Annual Review of Materials Research,* Vol. 31, pp. 25–46.

Suki, B., & Jason, HT. (2008). Bates Extracellular matrix mechanics in lung parenchymal diseases. *Respir.Physiol. Neurobiol.*, Vol.30, No.163, pp.33–43.

Tenenbaum, L., Lehtonen, E., & Monahan, PE. (2003). Evaluation of risks related to the use of adeno-associated virus-based vectors. *Curr. Gene Ther.*, Vol.3, No. 6, pp.545-565.

Tonti, GA., & Mannello, F. (2008). From bone marrow to therapeutic applications:different behaviour and genetic/epigenetic stability during mesenchymal stem cell expansion in autologous and foetal bovine sera? *Int. J. Dev. Biol.* Vol.52, pp.1023-1032.

Tseng, AS., Engel, FB., & Keating, MT. (2006). The GSK-3 inhibitor BIO promotes proliferation in mammalian cardiomyocytes. *Chem. Biol.*, Vol.13, No.9, pp.957-963.

Vighi, E., Ruozi, B., Montanari, M., Battini, R., & Leo, E. (2007). Re-dispersible cationic solid lipid nanoparticles (SLNs) freeze-dried without cryoprotectors: characterization and ability to bind the pEGFP-plasmid. *Eur. J. Pharm. Biopharm.*, Vol.67, No.2, pp.320-328.

Yizhi, Song., Garaventa, G., Bottero, S., Leprini, AE., Pallestrini, E., Castello, E., Pallestrini, EA., & Huang, WE. (2007). Ultrasound-mediated DNA transfer for bacteria. *Nucleic Acids Res.*, Vol.35, No.19, pp. 1073–1080.

6

Gene Therapy of Some Genetic Diseases by Transferring Normal Human Genomic DNA into Somatic Cells and Stem Cells from Patients

Liting Song
Hope Biomedical Research, Toronto, Ontario
Canada

1. Introduction

1.1 Viral vectors for gene therapy

Gene therapy is a way to correct mutated genes in vivo by transferring normal genes into cells of patients with genetic diseases or cancers, or to introduce new genes into cells to express therapeutic proteins. Several viruses like adenoviruses (Nayak & Herzog, 2010; Raper et al., 2003), alphaviruses (Lundstrom, 2001, 2005), retroviruses (Aiuti et al., 2009; Bordignon et al., 1989, 1995; Cavazzana-Calvo et al., 2000; Ferrari et al., 1991; Halatsch et al., 2000), lentiviruses (Dupré et al., 2004; Mortellaro et al., 2006; Nayak & Herzog, 2010), adeno-associated viruses (AAV) (Jayandharan et al., 2011; Nayak & Herzog, 2010; Terzi & Zachariou, 2008), herpes simplex viruses type 1 (HSV-I) (Epstein, 2009), have been used as vectors to deliver normal genes into cells of patients for gene therapy. However, there were limitations and hurdles in using these vectors. Some viruses like retroviruses, lentiviruses might integrate into human genomic DNA and cause cancers (Dave et al., 2004; Du et al., 2005; Hacein-Bey-Abina et al., 2003a, 2003b; Z. Li et al., 2002; Modlich et al., 2005; Seggewiss et al., 2006). Most viruses can infect both normal cells and defective/cancer cells of patients, as long as the cells have receptors of the viruses (Antar et al., 2009; K. Holmes et al., 1997; Norkin, 1995; L. Song, 2010; L. Song et al., 2009; van den Wollenberg et al., 2008; van Houdt et al., 2008), and this might lead to serious infections, inflammatory responses, and immunological reactions (Nayak & Herzog, 2010).

1.2 Highly pathogenic (virulent) viruses, moderately pathogenic viruses, and lowly or mildly pathogenic viruses

Some viruses like rabies virus, Lassa fever virus, smallpox virus, Eastern equine encephalitis virus, Ebola virus, Marburg virus, and human immunodeficiency virus are highly pathogenic and dangerous; they can cause very severe to fatal diseases in humans. For example, 399 patients had Marburg hemorrhagic fever in Angola in 2005, and 335 of them dead of the fatal disease. The human fatality rate of Ebola virus infection ranged from 50% to 89% (Balter, 2000; Peters, 2005; Rouquet et al., 2005; L. Song & Chen 1995, 1996; Virgin, 2007). Some viruses like some serotypes of seadornavirus isolated from mosquitoes in China have moderate pathogenicity, and they can cause clinical and subclinical infections.

Seadornavirus can cause mild encephalitis and fever. Multisegmented RNA viruses like influenza virus (Garten et al., 2009; E. Holmes, 2005; Karasin et al., 2000; Sun et al., 2011), rotavirus (Matthijnssens et al., 2010; Maunula & Von Bonsdorff, 2002), bluetongue virus (Batten et al., 2008), kemerovo virus (Nuttall & Moss,1989), Thogoto virus (C. Davies et al., 1987; Jones et al., 1987) are able to reassort their genomic segments in vivo, if a cell is infected by two or more different strains of a virus. This is the major reason why these viruses have multiple serotypes and subserotypes. As seadornavirus genome consists of 12 distinct segments of double-stranded RNA, it is easy to create new genotypes of seadornavirus through the reassorment event among different strains of the virus in nature. There are at least 6 different genotypes of seadornavirus in China, and there are various serotypes and subserotypes within the Chinese isolates (Q. Li et al., 1992; L. Song et al., 1995; L. Song & Chen, 1995, 1996; Tao et al., 1999; L. Xu et al., 2003; P. Xu et al., 1990; You et al., 1990). Similar seadornaviruses were isolated from mosquitoes collected in Indonesia (Brown et al., 1993) and Vietnam (Nabeshima et al., 2008). The virus was classified as a probable member of the genus Coltivirus previously, and later it was renamed as a member of a novel genus-Seadornavirus within the family of Reoviridae (Mohd Jaafar et al., 2005). Some viruses like M14-a nonpathogenic twelve-segmented double-stranded RNA virus isolated from mosquitoes in China (C. Huang et al., 1985, Liang et al., 1985) are lowly or mildly virulent viruses. The majority of viruses like hepatitis A, B, C, D, and E virus, polio virus, measles virus, mumps virus, West Nile virus, influenza virus, Coxsackie A virus, enterovirus 71, rhinoviruses, coronaviruses, norovirus, rubella virus, and the newly isolated member of bunyavirus which caused severe fever and thrombocytopenia syndrome in China (X-J. Yu et al., 2011), have moderate pathogenicity. There are very few human viruses are truly nonpathogenic viruses in nature, except some animal viruses that mainly infect animals but not humans. These mildly virulent viruses cannot cause obvious infections in humans (Csatary et al., 1985).

We should be aware that even some mild viruses which do not cause serious infections in normal people still can be dangerous to those with weakened immune systems, like late stage cancer patients, very elderly or critically ill patients, and patients with immunodeficiency disorders. Most viruses were modified and attenuated before being used as vectors for gene therapy, but in very rare situations, even those modified viral vectors can cause problems. An 18-year-old young man with partial ornithine transcarbamylase deficiency died after a clinical trial of gene therapy, even though the vector used in that trial was a modified human adenovirus type 5 virus (Raper et al., 2003).

1.3 Reovirus is not an oncolytic virus

There are Some scientists in the world have been trying to use a few so-called oncolytic viruses to cure cancers (Pennisi, 1998). One of the major problems of these therapies is that it is hard to find an ideal wild-type oncolytic virus, which only target cancer cells but not normal cells.

Normal rhesus monkey kidney LLC-MK2 cell line was established in 1955 (Evans et al., 1959; Hull et al., 1956, 1962). Normal mouse L929 cell line was first described by Stanford et al. in 1948. The L929 cell line was a cloned strain of its parental mouse cell strains L. L cell strain was made from the normal subcutaneous areolar and adipose tissue of a male mouse (Earle, 1943; Stanford et al., 1948). These two cell lines were widely used to isolate, grow, and multiplicate many types of viruses including reoviruses.

Reovirus (Respiratory Enteric Orphan Virus) is a member of the family Reoviradae. It got the name originally because it was often isolated from human respiratory and enteric systems but no obvious human disease was associated with it. Reovirus can cause cytopathic effect (CPE) in many normal cell lines like rhesus monkey kidney LLC-MK2 and MA-104E, African green embryonic monkey kidney Vero, baby hamster kidney BHK-21, Buffalo green monkey kidney BGM, African green monkey kidney BS-C-1, Madin-Darby bovine kidney (MDBK), Madin-Darby canine kidney (MDCK), human embryonic intestinal (intestinal 407), human embryonic lung (HEL), and mouse L929 cells. After a few days of cell culture, like most other viruses, reovirus will destroy and lyse the cells it infected eventually in vitro (McClain et al., 1967; Nibert et al., 1991; Ridinger et al., 1982; Rozee & Easterbrook, 1970; Schiff et al, 2007; L. Song et al., 1995, 1999b, 2000, 2009). Reovirus can infect and kill both normal cells and human tumor cells in vitro, as long as the cells have reovirus receptor-junctional adhesion molecule (Antar et al., 2009; L. Song et al., 1999b, 2000, 2009; van den Wollenberg et al., 2008; van Houdt et al., 2008). If a small number of reoviruses are injected into tumor tissues directly, the virus will infect and kill some tumor cells locally. In the meantime, the human immune system will fight with the virus, a lot of immune cells, such as T cells, B cells, natural killer cells, neutrophils, and macrophages will be recruited to the infection site, and the immune cells will produce antibodies, chemokines, and cytokines like interferons, interleukins; and after a few days, before the virus spreading to other parts of the body, the virus will be killed, and be cleared from the human body. If a large number of reoviruses are injected into the tumor body, the viruses will infect tumor cells and nearby normal cells, and spread to other organs of the body and cause systemic infection. This could be fatal for some cancer patients, as we know that many cancer patients have unbalanced, weakened, and dysfunctional immune systems. A great number of cancer patients are treated with radiation and immunosuppressive anticancer drugs, these anticancer therapies can damage immune cells further. Cancer patients with weakened immune systems have more chances to have opportunistic infections (Baggiolini et al., 1997; Bodey, 1986; Dunn et al., 2002, 2004; Locati & Murphy, 1999; Lodish et al., 2008; Luster, 1998; Murdoch & Finn, 2000; Nibert et al., 1991; Pitisuttithum et al., 2001; Schiff et al, 2007; Sutlu & Alici, 2009; Swann & Smyth, 2007; Virgin, 2007). This is the same problem we are facing when a patient has chemotherapies nowadays; there are rare drugs that only specifically and selectively target cancer cells but not normal cells. Over doses of anticancer drugs will kill both normal cells and tumor cells of patients, and lead to serious side effects and deaths; normal doses or small doses of anticancer drugs will not kill all the cancer cells, and the remained cancer cells will overexpress a membrane protein-P-glycoprotein, and be able to resistant to the cell kill effects of multi-anticancer drugs (Arkin et al., 1989; Croop et al., 1988; De Rosa et al., 2008; Debenham et al., 1982; Deuchars et al., 1987; Endicott & Ling, 1989; Goldstein et al., 1989; Juliano & Ling, 1976; Kobayashi et al., 1994, 1998; Moscow & Cowan, 1988; Pastan & Gottesman, 1987; Riordan et al., 1985; L. Song et al., 1999a).

Most people were infected by reovirus without significant symptoms, but L-H. Song et al. isolated a reovirus from the throat swabs of a patient of severe acute respiratory syndrome (SARS) in Beijing in 2003, and the virus can cause clinical symptoms similar to SARS in guinea pigs and macaques (L-H. Song et al., 2008). Antarasena et al. isolated some avian reoviruses from chickens with sudden death in Thailand (Antarasena et al., 2002). Chua et al. reported that a reovirus of bat origin could cause acute respiratory disease in humans (Chua et al., 2007). Given the fact that more than 50% of people were infected by reovirus in their lifetimes, and many of the infections occurred in the early childhood (Selb & Weber,

1994; Tai at el., 2005), and there are increasing evidences indicating that reovirus can infect normal human cells in vivo and cause some mild to serious diseases like upper respiratory illnesses, meningitis in humans (Johansson et al., 1996; Schiff et al., 2007; Tyler et al., 2004); the old concept that reoviruses were "orphan" viruses, and they were not associated with any human diseases, is not true anymore, and it should be revised.
Wild-type reovirus should not be considered as an oncolytic virus, and it is unlikely that reovirus could be an effective and practical anticancer agent (L. Song, 2010).

1.4 Non-viral vectors for gene therapy

Non-viral vectors such as peptide, polymer mediated gene therapy can only produce transient expression of genes, and the transfection efficiency is much lower compared to viral vectors (Al-Dosari & Gao, 2009; Cartier & Reszka, 2002; X. Gao et al., 2007; Niidome & Huang, 2002).

2. A possible approach for gene therapy of some genetic diseases

It is well known that a bacterium can obtain foreign DNA from another bacterium through a process of bacterial conjugation (Lederberg & Tatum, 1946). In this process, DNA is directly transferred from one cell into another cell via direct cell-to-cell contact or via a bridge-like structure between two cells. By this way, a bacteium's genomic DNA could be changed by homologous recombination with another bacterium's genomic DNA.
As above pointed out, multisegmented RNA viruses like influenza virus can reassort their genomic segments in vivo, if an animal is infected by two or more different strains of a virus in the same time period. This can create new strains of the virus, and the new strains carry the gene segments of their parental strains. There are some triple reassorted influenza virus strains in nature (V. Gregory et al., 2001; Ma et al., 2010; Octaviani et al., 2011; Rambaut et al., 2008; Smith et at., 2004; Vincent et al., 2006; Webby et al., 2000; X. Xu et al., 2002, 2004; Zhou et al., 1999).
Complementation test was used to study genetic subtypes (complementation groups) of a genetic disease like Fanconi anemia. If cells from two patients with Fanconi anemia were from two different complementation groups, the defective genes could be repaired after fusion of the two genetic complementation cells; and the hybrid cells were able to resist the attack of DNA cross-linking agents such as mitomycin C and diepoxybutane. Whereas, if the cells of two patients were from the same complementation group, the hybrid cells would still be sensitive to the attack of DNA cross-linking reagents (Buchwald, 1995; Duckworth-Rysiecki et al., 1985; Fanconi Anaemia/Breast Cancer Consortium, 1996; Giampietro et al., 1997; Joenje et al., 1995; Joenje & Patel, 2001; Levitus et al., 2004; Tischkowitz & Hodgson, 2003; Whitney et al., 1995). 14 different complementation groups of Fanconi anemia have been discovered, and 14 distinct Fanconi anemia genes have been identified (FANCA, FANCB, FANCC, FANCD1, FANCD2, FANCE, FANCF, FANCG, FNACI, FANCJ, FANCL, FANCM, FANCN, FANCP) (Alderton, 2011; Kim et al., 2011; Levitus et al., 2006; Reid et al., 2007; Smogorzewska et al., 2007; L. Song, 2009; Stoepker et al., 2011; Taniguchi & D'Andrea, 2006; Tischkowitz et al., 2008).
It is very interesting that a number of patients with some genetic diseases were cured or improved naturally later in their lives. Somatic mosaicism was involved in this form of miracle "natural gene therapy" process. Somatic mosaicism means that there are genetically different somatic cells exist in a given organism resulting from in vivo reversion of a

mutated allele to wild type. Somatic mosaicism has been found in several genetic disorders, such as hemophilia B, tyrosinemia type I, Bloom syndrome, adenosine deaminase deficiency, epidermolysis bullosa, Wiskott-Aldrich syndrome, androgen insensitivity syndrome, T-cell immunodeficiency, leukocyte adhesion deficiency type 1, Duchenne muscular dystrophy, atypical X-linked severe combined immunodeficiency, and Fanconi anemia. The mechanism of somatic mosaicism is complicated; it might be due to epigenetic alterations of DNA, copy number variations, back mutation, gene conversion, frame-restoring mutation, DNA polymerase slippage, and compensatory mutation in cis. Homologous genetic recombination between paternally and maternally derived chromosomes also plays a vital role in somatic mosaicism (Darling et al., 1999; J. Jr. Gregory et al., 2001; M. Gross et al., 2002; Hirschhorn, 2003; Lo Ten Foe et al., 1997; Mankad et al., 2006; Müller & Williams, 2009; Notini et al., 2008; Piotrowski et al., 2008; L. Song, 2009; Wada et al., 2001, 2003; Waisfisz et al., 1999; Youssoufian & Pyeritz, 2002).

Homologous genetic recombination was first discovered in bacterium *Escherichia coli* strain K-12 in 1946 by Joshua Lederberg (May 23, 1925 - February 2, 2008), winner of the 1958 Nobel Prize in Physiology or Medicine (Lederberg & Tatum, 1946; Lederberg, 1947, 1987a, 1987b; Tatum & Lederberg, 1947).

Homologous recombination happens when two homologous DNA molecules meet in vivo. They pair up and exchange some sequences. Homologous genetic recombination occurs in the processes of mitosis and meiosis. Gene recombination takes place between two nonsister chromatids of the two homologous chromosomes by crossover during meiosis. Homologous recombination happens much more often in distal regions of chromosomes and on shorter arms of chromosomes. Crossover occurs at least one time per chromosome in each of the process of meiosis. Gene sequences are exchanged during the process of meiosis by crossover (Creighton & McClintock, 1931, 1935; Holliday, 1974; International Human Genome Sequencing Consortium, 2001; Weil, 2002; Whitby, 2005).

Crossover during the process of meiosis is really a smart and fair way to let a female's eggs or a male's sperms to have genetic information from both of her/his parents; and when an egg and a sperm form a new life in the womb, the new baby carries the genetic information from both of his/her grandparents on his/her father's side and grandparents on his/her mother's side; so a baby's genetic traits are inherited from his/her four biological grandparents, this could make the baby more diversity, flexible, and fit.

Radioactive materials like radon gas in some basement rooms, ultraviolet (UV) light, toxic chemicals, reactive-oxygen compounds, polluted air, and smoking, some viral infections all can damage human genomic DNA, cause mutations, and lead to cancers. Human cells are able to cope with outside and inside challenges, and to repair the damaged DNA molecules by several ways. One of the DNA repair mechanisms is homologous recombination to repair DNA gaps, DNA double-stranded breaks, and DNA interstrand crosslinks. A damaged chromatid can be repaired by its undamaged sister chromatid or its homologous nonsister chromatid through homologous recombination during mitosis. Sister chromatids are the preferred templates over homologous or heterologous chromosomes for recombination repair in yeast and mammalian cells. Instead of crossover, gene conversion is the major result of homologous recombination. Cells seem reluctant to crossover their chromatids unnecessarily to maintain their genome's integrity and stability (Hope et al., 2007; Jackson & Bartek, 2009; Johnson & Jasin, 2001; Kadyk & Hartwell, 1992; X. Li & Heyer, 2008; Lorenz & Whitby, 2006; Willers et al., 2004).

Gene targeting (gene knockout) is a technique that a vector is used to deliver a fragment of mutated DNA into embryonic stem cells and to target its homologous DNA in the genome by homologous genetic recombination. Thousands of genes in mice were knocked out by using this method. Mario R. Capecchi, Martin J. Evans, and Oliver Smithies were awarded jointly the Nobel Prize in Physiology or Medicine in 2007 for their discoveries of principles for creating knockout mice (Bradley et al., 1984; Bronson & Smithies, 1994; Capecchi, 1989a, 1989b; Koller & Smithies, 1992; Kuehn et al., 1987; Robertson et al., 1986).
It was assumed that plant tissue grafts did not have gene exchange, but this is not true. A recent discovery found that even in plant tissue grafts, some of their genes were exchanged (Stegemann & Bock, 2009).
Based on the above observations and experiments, I proposed a possible approach for gene therapy of some genetic diseases as indicated in figure 1 (L. Song, 2009).

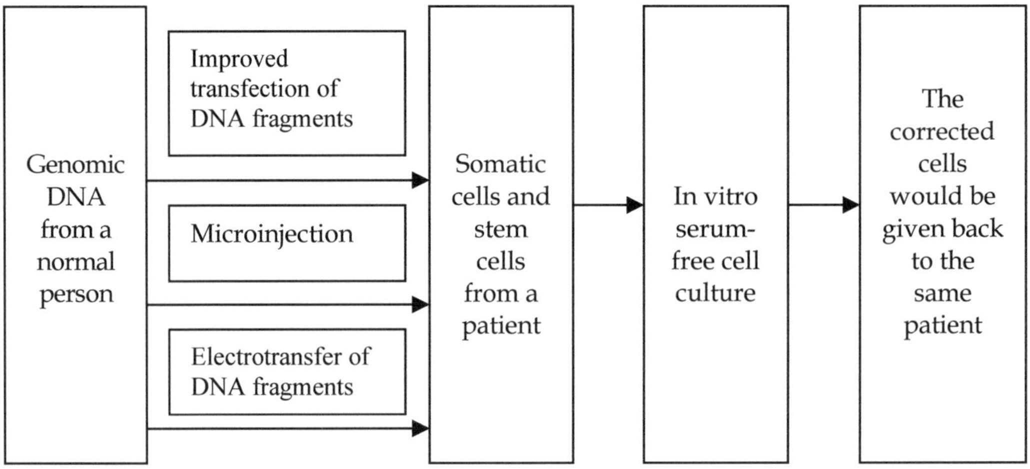

Fig. 1. Gene therapy of some genetic diseases by transferring normal human genomic DNA/DNA fragments into cells from patients.

Briefly, normal human genomic DNA or genomic DNA fragments from a healthy donor can be transferred into somatic cells and stem cells from a patient by microinjection, gene electrotransfer (electroporation), and improved transfection. After in vitro serum-free cell culture, the defective genes could be repaired by homologous genetic recombination, since the genomic DNAs of the two persons are considerably similar, although there are deletions, insertions, rearrangements, loss-of-function variants, and copy number variations (CNV) (Fujimoto et al, 2010; Levy et al., 2007; H. Park et al., 2010; The 1000 Genomes Consortium, 2010, 2011; J. Wang et al., 2008; Yim et al., 2010).

3. Discussion

3.1 Stem cells, somatic cells

Stem cells were first discovered by Ernest Armstrong McCulloch (April 27, 1926–January 20, 2011) and James Edgar Till in 1963 (Becker et al., 1963; McCulloch et al., 1964; Siminovitch et al., 1963; Till et al., 1964; Weissman & Shizuru, 2008). Stem cells have the ability to self-renew and to differentiate into different cell types. Early stage embryonic stem cells can form all types of cells. Adult stem cells only can differentiate and generate specialized cells, like bone cells, liver cells, blood cells, skin cells. The stem cells that produce all the blood cell types are called hematopoietic stem cells (Bordignon, 2006; Spangrude et al., 1988; Thomson et al., 1998; Weissman & Shizuru, 2008).

Stem cells and their differentiated cells (somatic cells) maintain a balance-homeostasis. When under stress, stem cells are activated, and start to produce more differentiated cells (Jiang et al., 2009; Martinez-Agosto et al., 2007; Till et al., 1964; Wilson et al., 2004).

Somatic cells are the end products of stem cells, they are unable to self-renew.

3.2 Induced pluripotent stem cells

In recent years, a few transcription factors (genes) were introduced into somatic cells by lentiviral or retroviral vectors, to reprogram somatic cells into pluripotent stem cells (Liao et al., 2008; I. Park et al., 2008; Takahashi et al., 2007; J. Yu et al., 2007).

Some of the genes like c-Myc that used to form induced pluripotent stem cells are oncogenes, and as above revealed, retroviral or lentiviral vectors might integrate into genome DNA randomly, these risk factors might lead to producing cancer cells. A recent study revealed that human induced stem cells were easier and faster to form tumors than human embryonic stem cells (Gutierrez-Aranda et al., 2010).

Some recently published papers disclosed that induced pluripotent stem cells could induce more immune responses and immunological rejections in the recipient mice, and had more protein-coding point mutations, more abnormal epigenomic reprogramming, and more copy number variations than normal somatic cells and normal embryonic stem cells (Gore et al., 2011; Hussein et al., 2011; Laurent et al., 2011; Lister et al., 2011; Zhao et al., 2011).

3.3 Cell membrane and nuclear envelope

Both a eukaryotic cell and a prokaryotic cell have a flexible lipid bilayer plasma membrane that controls movement of molecules in and out of the cell. A eukaryotic cell has a nucleus, while a prokaryotic cell does not have a nucleus; this is the characteristic difference between a eukaryotic cell and a prokaryotic cell.

The eukaryotic cell nucleus is surrounded by a nuclear envelope with nuclear pores. The nuclear envelope has two layers: the out nuclear membrane which faces the cytoplasm, and the inner nucleic membrane which faces the nucleoplasm. The nuclear pores are formed by nuclear pore complexes (NPCs) that span the double lipid bilayer of the nuclear envelope. The NPCs are formed by about 30 proteins. NPCs are gatekeepers of the nucleus (Alber et al., 2007; D'Angelo et al., 2006; D'Angelo & Hetzer, 2008; Devos et al., 2006; Fernandez-Martinez & Rout, 2009; Lam & Dean, 2010; Terry et al., 2007; Theerthagiri et al., 2010; E. Tran & Wente, 2006).

Ions and small molecules and DNA smaller than 200 bp can diffuse through the nuclear pore freely; while the transport of DNA molecules between 310 bp and 1500 bp from the cytosol to the nucleus is through an active transport process. DNA greater than 2 kb can rarely be seen in the nucleus (Cartier & Reszka, 2002; Hagstrom et al., 1997; Ludtke et al., 1999).

A foreign DNA molecule has to go through the human cell membrane, cytoplasm, and the nuclear envelope to reach the genomic DNA in the nucleus. This process can be performed and prompted by microinjection, electroporation, and transfection.

3.4 Microinjection

Microinjection technique has been used in transgenic animals for many years (Bishop & Smith, 1989; Chan & Yang, 2009; Charreau et al., 1996; Filipiak & Saunders, 2006; Ménoret et al., 2010; Tesson et al., 2005; Yang et al., 2008). Microinjection technique also has been used as a tool to clone animals-first, an unfertilized egg's nucleus is removed; then a nucleus of a somatic cell is microinjected into the denucleated egg; now the egg contains a whole copy of the diploid genomic DNA from the somatic cell and can be cultured in vitro to form a blastocyst; and the blastocyst is implanted into the womb of an animal; eventually a cloned animal is born (Campbell et al., 1996; Vajta & Gjerris, 2006; Willadsen, 1986; Wilmut et al., 1997).

Several different genes inserted into plasmids were microinjected into cultured mammalian somatic cells, and some genetic defective genes were corrected by homologous recombination (W. Anderson et al., 1980; Capecchi, 1980; Folger et al., 1982; Yamaizumi et al., 1983).

Feng et al. introduced a 110 kb whole human alpha globin gene cluster clone in a bacterial artificial chromosome (BAC) vector into fertilized eggs to generate transgenic mice by microinjection method. The human alpha globin gene cluster DNA was integrated into the mice genome, and human alpha globin mRNA was expressed in 3 transgenic mice (Feng et al., 2001). Similarly, Gao et al. generated transgenic mice carrying a BAC clone of a 116 kb human *apoAI/CIII/AIV/AV* gene cluster and a mutant in which the *apoCIII* enhancer was deleted from the 116 kb gene cluster by microinjection (J. Gao et al., 2005).

I assume that normal genomic DNA without a plasmid or an artificial chromosome can be directly microinjected into the nucleus of somatic cells and stem cells from a patient successfully. This method could have a higher homologous recombination rate and less immunological reactions. It is not a very convenient method, but I think it is worth the effort to try. It only needs 30 purified mouse hematopoietic stem cells to save 50% of lethally irradiated mice (Spangrude et al., 1988). Even one single stem cell transplant can significantly reconstruct the bone marrow function of some irradiated mice (Decker & Nyberg, 2001; Krause et al., 2001; Mankad et al., 2006; Osawa et al., 1996). Therefore, we might need to collect less than one hundred stem cells from a patient, and microinject normal genomic DNA into these cells. Hopefully, less than one hundred of these corrected cells are sufficient to improve a patient's physiological function significantly.

3.5 Electroporation

Electroporation or electropermeabilization has been used to transfer foreign plasmid DNA into bacteria, yeast, and mammalian cells (Escoffre et al., 2009; Favard et al., 2007; Golzio et al., 2010; Mir, 2009; Neumann et al., 1982; Somiari et al., 2000). It might be difficult to transfer large genomic DNA molecules into mammalian cells by this method. We might first digest the normal human genomic DNA by restriction enzymes, and then transfer the normal genomic DNA fragments into a patient's stem cells and somatic cells by electroporation in vitro. After a few days of in vitro cell culture in serum free media, the cells can be transplanted into the same patient. Of course, before conducting human clinical trials, this kind of experiment should be performed in animal models first.

3.6 Genomic DNA Transfection

Whole genomic DNA molecules are too big to be transfected into cells directly. Normal genomic DNA can be digested by a few restriction enzymes first, and then the purified genomic DNA fragments can be transfected into stem cells and somatic cells from patients.

Molecules commonly used for transfection are smaller than 10 kb; transfection efficiency is very low with plasmids of 12 kb or bigger (Campeau et al., 2001; Cartier & Reszka, 2002). Transfection is a relatively simple, easy, and convenient method to transfer a foreign DNA into a cell, but the current transfection methods cannot satisfy our needs when we want to transfer large DNA fragments. We have to improve the transfection efficiency, and new methods and advanced techniques are needed to transfer large genomic DNA fragments.

A cell culture medium with a little bit lower osmotic pressure can cause cell osmotic swelling, and the cells become bigger, cell membrane permeability is increased, the nuclear pores might become bigger also. Therefore, bigger size of DNA molecules might be easier to enter the swelling cells and reach the genomic DNA inside the nucleus. After transfection, the transfected cells are grown in a cell culture medium with normal osmotic pressure for a period of time, and let the cells to recover to normal. The recovered transfected cells can be transplanted into animal models of a genetic disease.

3.7 Genome sequencing and human genetic variation

Human somatic cells are diploid, each somatic cell has 23 homologous chromosome pairs (46 chromosomes), 23 of the chromosomes are from a sperm of the father and other 23 chromosomes are from an egg of the mother. The paired homologous chromosomes are similar in length, except the pair of X and Y chromosomes, an X chromosome is much longer than a Y chromosome. The human sperm cells and egg cells are haploid-each of them has 23 chromosomes.

Different species of animals or plants have different number of chromosomes. A chimpanzee has 48 chromosomes (Young et al., 1960), a dog has 78, a chicken has 78, a pig has 38, a cat has 38, a horse has 64, a cow has 60, a goat has 60, a sheep has 54, a mouse has 40, and a rat has 42 chromosomes separately (O'Brien et al., 1999); and a silkworm has 28 chromosomes (International Silkworm Genome Consortium, 2008; Xia et al., 2004). Wheat has three ploidy levels: diploid wheat (Triticum urartu, Aegilops speltoides, and Ae. tauschii) has 14 (2x), tetraploid wheat (Triticum turgidum ssp. dicoccoides) has 28 (4x), and hexaploid wheat (Triticum aestivum) has 42 (6x) chromosomes respectively; diploid wheat is the ancestor of the tetraploid and hexaploid wheat (Akhunov et al., 2005, 2010; Dvorak & Akhunov, 2005; S. Huang et al., 2002).

Each human gene has two alleles, one allele on each chromosome of the homologous pair. If the 2 alleles have the same sequence, they are called homozygotes; otherwise, they are called heterozygotes.

A specific phenotype (trait) might be determined by two alleles (recessive) or by one allele (dominant). In autosomal recessive genetic diseases like cystic fibrosis, sickle-cell anemia, and fanconi anemia (except FANCB), if a mutant gene appears on both of the paired homologous chromosomes of a person, this person has the genetic disease; if the mutant gene occurs on one of the homologous chromosomes of a person, this person is a carrier of the genetic disease. In X-linked recessive genetic diseases like Fanconi anemia subtype B, Duchenne muscular dystrophy, and Wiskott-Aldrich syndrome, if a male's X chromosome carries the mutated gene, this male has the genetic disease; if one of a female's X chromosomes carries the mutated gene, this female is a carrier; if both of a female's X chromosomes carry the mutated gene, this female has the genetic disease. On the other hand, in autosomal dominant genetic diseases like Huntington's disease, it only needs one mutated allele on any of the two homologous chromosomes to have the related genetic disease; there is no carrier of a dominant genetic disease, because every person who has the mutated allele gets the disease.

A diploid genome sequence showed that we are genetically more diverse than we have claimed before (International Human Genome Sequencing Consortium, 2001, 2004; Venter et al., 2001) based on the haploid genome sequences, and the difference between two homologous chromosomes of a pair of chromosomes inherited from one's parents is bigger than we thought before. There were more than 4.1 million DNA sequence variants in this new diploid genome. Single-base variations -single nucleotide polymorphisms (SNPs) are the major variants, small fragments insertions or deletions (indels), large fragments deletions and duplications- copy number variations also contribute to the genomic variation significantly (L. Gross, 2007; Levy et al., 2007).

J. Wang et al. sequenced a Chinese diploid genome sequence (named YH) and found about 3 million SNPs in YH's genome, of which 13.6% were new compared to the SNP database dbSNP. They compared the 3 known genome sequences and recognized that the genomes of YH, Venter, and Watson shared 1.2 million SNPs, and their unique SNPs were 31.8% (YH), 30.1% (Venter), and 33.0% (Watson) separately (J. Wang et al., 2008).

Koreans and Chinese were historically related, and they might have the same ancestors. The diploid genome sequence of a Korean male (named SJK) was significantly different from the Chinese YH; there were 1.3 million different SNPs between the two persons; even though SJK shared more SNPs with YH than with Caucasians Venter and Watson, and the Nigerian male Yoruba. 420, 083 (12.2%) SNPs of SJK were not found in the dbSNP database before, and 39.87% of the SNPs were SJK-specific (S. Ahn et al., 2009).

More than 99% of the genomic DNA sequences of a Japanese male were same to the reference human genome, but there were still 3,132,608 single nucleotide variations (SNVs) compared to other six reported human genomes (Fujimoto et al., 2010).

3.8 Copy number variations (CNV)

We are in a new era of personalized genomic medicine. With the significantly advanced and simplified new DNA sequencing tools and methods available in a few years, we would be able to know the whole genomic DNA sequence of every person in a few hours at an affordable price (less than one thousand dollars) (L. Gross, 2007).

In addition to each person has his /her unique protein-coding sequences, deletions, insertions, and inversions, copy number variations is one of the main reasons that we are different from each other genetically. Copy number variations is a hot topic of research in recent years, the aim of the studies is to disclose some possible diseases caused/or influenced by copy number variations; and how copy number variations might determine, regulate, and affect our genetic traits and social behaviours. Park et al. discovered 5,177 CNVs in 30 individuals of Korean, Chinese and Japanese, of which 3,547 were putative Asian-specific CNVs (H. Park et al., 2010). Every genome has about 40.3 CNVs averagely; the median length of CNVs is 18.9 kb. About 8% regions of the human genome are occupied by CNV regions (Yim et al., 2010).

The current research data revealed that every genetically unrelated person is significantly different from each other on protein-coding sequences, single-base variations –SNPs, small nucleotide insertions and deletions (called indels), and copy number variations.

It is time to compare genomic DNA sequences among family members, relatives, and genetically unrelated persons, to confirm that genomic DNA sequences are much more similar among family members and relatives than among genetically unrelated persons. For example, we are interested to see if a son's Y chromosome sequence is as same as his biological father's; or how many differences there are between these two if they are not the same. I assume it will be proved that genomic DNA sequences are much more similar among family members than among genetically unrelated persons. A new research showed that chromosomes with insertions or deletions could affect the process of meiosis (J. Wang et al., 2010). Therefore, if a healthy donor is a family member/relative of a patient, their genomic DNAs could be matched much better, and there should be less immunological reactions and rejections.

A gene might only be expressed from a chromosome of the paternal or maternal origin resulting from genomic imprinting effect, and some genetic diseases like Prader-Willi syndrome, Angelman syndrome, Beckwith-Wiedemann syndrome, are due to genomic imprinting (Falls et al., 1999; Hall, 1990; Tycko, 1994). Additionally, some genetic diseases such as X-linked severe combined immunodeficiency, Glucose-6-phosphate dehydrogenase deficiency, Pyruvate dehydrogenase deficiency, Wiskott-Aldrich syndrome, and Becker/Duchenne muscular dystrophy are sex linked. Hence, both genomic DNAs from a healthy male and a healthy female might be introduced into somatic cells and stem cells of a patient, to correct the mutated genes in vitro, so as to get possibly more efficient and effective gene therapy. Finally, the corrected cells would be given back to the same patient.

3.9 Human gene's exons are separated by introns

Many of the human genes have a few introns and exons, and the exons are separated by introns in the human genomic DNA. Introns in a gene can be 10 to 100 times longer than the exons. Statistically, the average exon length is about 170 bp, whereas, the average intron size is about 5419 bp; the average human gene has about 8.8 exons and 7.8 introns. The human nebulin gene has 147 introns. Some introns like the human dystrophin gene intron 44 can be more than 250,000 bp in length (Hawkins, 1988; Lodish et al., 2008; Sakharkar et al., 2004; V. Tran et al., 2005). Introns are removed from the gene to form mRNA by a process of RNA splicing (Berget et al., 1977; Chow et al., 1977) during transcription. mRNA exits the nucleus via nuclear pores, and binds to ribosomes. The ribosome moves along the mRNA, and selects the right tRNA by matching an anti-codon on a tRNA to a codon on the mRNA strand. Each tRNA can only carry a specific amino acid by the help of an enzyme called aminoacyl tRNA synthetase. This is the process of translation-an mRNA sequence is translated into a protein sequence (Goldman, 2008; Lodish et al., 2008).

The human dystrophin gene is the largest known human gene. It has more than 2, 400 kb in length, and has at least 79 exons, its intron 44 has 250 kb, its second largest intron-intron 2, is 170 kb long. 99% of the dystrophin gene sequences are present in introns. The human dystrophin gene locates at locus Xp21.2, and is mutated in patients with Duchenne and Becker muscular dystrophies (Dwi Pramono et al., 2000; Golubovsky & Manton, 2005; Koenig et al., 1987, 1988; Nishio et al., 1994; Roberts, 2001; V. Tran et al., 2005; Zhang et al., 2007).

Human hemoglobin is the protein in red blood cells responsible for transferring oxygen from the lungs to the cells of other parts of the human body . Fetal human hemoglobin has two alpha chains and 2 gamma chains; each of the polypeptide chain has a heme. After birth, the gamma globin gene expression was turned off, and two gamma chains were replaced by two β chains. Therefore, in adult human hemoglobin, there are two α chains, two β chains, and four heme groups (Feng et al., 2001; Groudine et al., 1983; Hardison, 1996; Yin et al., 2007). The human α-globin gene cluster lies on chromosome 16 (16p13.3), and is about 30 kb, it has 7 genes: zeta, pseudozeta, mu, pseudoalpha-1, alpha-2, alpha-1, theta (Barbour et al., 2000; Entrez Gene, 2011; Feng et al., 2001; Higgs et al., 1989). The human β-globin gene cluster is about 100 kb; it locates on chromosome 11 (11p15.5), and has 5 genes in the order of epsilon, gamma-G, gamma-A, delta, and beta. Both of α-globin gene and β-globin gene have three exons and two introns (Higgs et al., 1989; Yin et al., 2007).

Typically, in a viral or plasmid vector mediated gene therapy, normal mRNAs are reverse transcribed into cDNAs; and specific cDNAs are amplified by PCR method; the PCR products are purified and digested by restriction enzymes; the digested PCR products are inserted into the viral or plasmid vectors; the viral or plasmid vectors containing the normal genes are transfected/transformed into cells, in order to express normal proteins, or to correct the mutated genes in vivo.

This procedure has a problem. As the above described, the mutated genes might be separated by several introns and located in several places of the genomic DNA, the cDNA clones of the normal genes are too short to match and find the mutated genes, therefore, it is hard to correct the mutated genes in vivo, although the cloned genes might express normal proteins transiently. By transferring normal human genomic DNA into cells from patients, it can overcome this difficulty.

3.10 Non-coding sequences of genome sequences, and the miracle silkworm

We are living in an age that many important organisms have been sequenced (S. Ahn et al., 2009; Fujimoto et al., 2010; Holmes et al., 2005; International Human Genome Sequencing Consortium, 2001, 2004; International Silkworm Genome Consortium, 2008; Levy et al., 2007; O'Brien et al., 1999; Venter et al., 2001; J. Wang et al., 2008; Xia et al., 2004). We gained some valuable information from the genome sequence data of these organisms, but we are far away from knowing the secret of lives. A silkworm has a short but magical life cycle, and it proceeds in the following processes: it starts from a tiny egg; in a suitable environment, the egg turns into a small worm (larva); the small worm eats mulberry tree leaves greedily and thoroughly days and nights, and after 4 times of shedding its skin, it grows bigger and bigger; one day it starts to weave a silk house-a cocoon for itself, in about 2 days, a beautiful and perfect white colored cocoon is made by itself; the silkworm pees before weaving a cocoon, this makes its body smaller, so as to let itself be able to fit in the cocoon; inside the cocoon, the worm changes to a pupa, and before this happens, the worm poops, this makes its body further smaller; after about two weeks, the pupa becomes a moth, and it is time to get out of the cocoon; the moth is very smart, it pees inside the cocoon, the chemicals of the urine are so powerful-one of the chemicals is a special enzyme which can break down the cocoon wall, and it makes one end of the cocoon softer, so the moth can get out without trouble; the female moth comes out of the damaged cocoon, and releases sex pheromones to attract males, and mates with a few males, lays eggs after mating; and a new life cycle is started again if the environment is appropriate; or it will go through a period of hibernating.

When you think about this miracle life cycle of a silkworm, you have to believe that these abilities, talents, and skills of a silkworm are not learned from others or from the environment, because actually no one teaches it to do this step by step, especially for the first silkworm who started doing these things earlier than all the others in a group of silkworms. These natural born skills must have been inherited from its parents, and they are encoded in its genome.

It is estimated that there are only about 20,000-25,000 protein-coding genes in humans; the majority of genome sequences are non-coding sequences (International Human Genome Sequencing Consortium, 2004). We might have ignored some small protein-coding genes, and some alternatively spliced genes. The actual number of protein-coding genes might be bigger than we have claimed. (A. Ahn & Kunkel, 1993; Black, 2003; Dwi Pramono et al., 2000; Muntoni et al., 2003; Nishio et al., 1994; L. Song et al., 2003; V. Tran et al., 2005; Zhang et al., 2007). We do not know the meaning and usefulness of these non-coding sequences clearly so far, only one thing we are almost certain is that: they must have meaning and usefulness. We read many books, newspapers, and journals; we watched hundreds of movies, TV shows; we travelled numerous places, and met a lot of people. We do not know why and how we can remember all these things, and why the childhood memories can be stored in our brains for many years, and the memories can be recalled after so many years. If we can transfer the information from one person's brain to a computer, it might take up millions of gigabyte DVD space. In a human brain cell, only genomic DNA molecules could have such big storage capabilities to store such huge quantities of information. The mechanism of memory is one of the biggest challenges of our human beings; we should be able to uncover the secret of our brains with our own brains if we are on the right track. One day we might be able to know all the secrets of the silkworm and other organisms including humans.

3.11 Graft-versus-host disease (GVHD)

It is often hard to find a human leukocyte antigen (HLA)-identical sibling or a well-matched HLA unrelated donor when a patient needs hematopoietic stem cell transplant (HSCT). Sometimes, a patient had to receive a mismatched or partially matched bone marrow transplant and cord-blood transplant, when there was no HLA-matched unrelated donor available, and when a transplant was needed urgently. Acute and chronic graft-versus-host disease is the most severe and common long-term side effect of allogeneic hematopoietic stem cell transplantation (HCT). Acute GVHD was more likely to occur after mismatched marrow transplantation. Chronic GVHD was the major cause of late death of HSCT patients (Eapen et al., 2010; Laughlin et al., 2001, 2004; Mastaglio et al., 2010; Rocha et al., 2004).

Cells seem to be able to tolerate foreign DNA without immunological reactions; this is proved by the animal cloning experiments, transgenic animal models, and human and animal replication phenomena. Therefore, the possible approach I described above might have great benefits and advantages. Hopefully some genetic diseases listed below could be cured or improved by using this gene therapy method.

3.12 Fanconi anemia

Fanconi anemia (FA) is a rare chromosomal recessive genetic disease. As above cited, there are at least 14 subtypes of Fanconi anemia, and 14 genes whose mutation can cause FA are cloned. FANCB gene is on the X chromosome, and it is the only one on sex chromosomes, the other 13 FA genes are on autosomes. FA was first described by the Swiss pediatrician Guido Fanconi (1892-1979) in 1927 (Joenje & Patel, 2001; Lobitz & Velleuer, 2006; L. Song, 2009; Tischkowitz & Hodgson, 2003).

There are mouse models of Fanconi anemia available currently; FancA, FancC, FancG, FancD1, and FancD2 genes have been deleted or mutated in the mice (Parmar et al., 2009).

These 5 mouse models of Fanconi anemia will be used to prompt the research of gene therapy of these 5 subtypes of Fanconi anemia, because we can use these mouse models to do animal experiments. Normal genomic DNA or normal DNA fragments can be microinjected/electrotransfered, and transfected into stem cells and somatic cells from a mutated mouse; the corrected stem cells and somatic cells can be transplanted back to the same mouse, to see if the Fanconi anemia mouse model's physiological function is improved by this kind of gene therapy.

3.13 Sickle-cell anemia

Sickle-cell anemia is an autosomal recessive genetic disease. It results from a mutation at the sixth codon of the β hemoglobin gene on chromosome 11 (the hydrophilic amino acid glutamic acid is replaced by the hydrophobic amino acid valine). This mutation causes red blood cells to become rigid and inflexible. The patient's red blood cells are difficult to go through small capillaries, leading to stroke, chronic pain, anemia, and infection. This disease affects more than 300, 000 people worldwide (Ataga, 2009; Chang et al., 2006; Ingram, 1956, 1957; Pawliuk et al., 2001; Wu et al., 2006).

3.14 Cystic fibrosis

Cystic fibrosis is a common autosomal recessive genetic disease caused by mutations of cystic fibrosis transmembrane conductance regulator (CFTR) gene on chromosome 7 in Caucasian population (Kerem et al., 1989; Riordan et al., 1989; Rommens et al., 1989). CFTR is a cAMP-regulated chloride channel; the CFTR gene mutations lead to the cAMP-induced chloride channel dysfunction, thereby alter the transport of chloride and associated liquid, cause problems in several organ systems including respiratory system, sweat glands, pancreas, intestine, liver and gallbladder. There are more than 1800 CFTR gene mutations in the world. Cystic fibrosis affacts more than 70, 000 individuals worldwide. In 2006, the median survival age for a person with cystic fibrosis was 37 (M. Anderson et al., 1991; Collaco & Cutting, 2008; Collins, 1992; Cutting, 2010; Lee et al., 2005; Rowntree & Harris, 2003; G. Wang et al., 2005; Zielenski, 2000).

3.15 Duchenne muscular dystrophy

Duchenne muscular dystrophy (DMD) is the most common form of muscular dystrophy, it affacts about one of every 3500 males. DMD is an X-linked recessive muscle degenerative disease caused by the mutations of dystrophin. As the above stated, the DMD gene is the largest human gene (>2.4 million bp on chromosome X), its cDNA is 14 kb long. DMD gene encodes a single 427 kDa protein-dystrophin. Patient's muscle fibers do not have the 427 kDa dystrophin (Burghes et al., 1987; Campeau et al., 2001; Hoffmanet al., 1987; Koenig et al., 1987, 1988; Kunkel, 2004; Monaco et al., 1986; Nelson et al., 2009).

3.16 Huntington's disease

Huntington's disease (HD) was first described by George Huntington in 1872. HD is an autosomal dominant neurodegenerative disease caused by the mutation of the huntingtin (HTT) gene. HTT gene located at 4p16.3; it has longer CAG trinucletide repeats (more than 40 CAG repeats) in the first exon of the HTT gene than the normal gene. There are transgenic mouse, sheep and monkey models available for conducting animal experiments currently (Bates et al., 1997; Beilby, 2007; S. Davies & Ramsden, 2001; Jacobsen et al., 2010; MacDonald et al., 1993; Yang et al., 2008).

3.17 X-linked severe combined immunodeficiency (SCID-X1)

X-linked severe combined immunodeficiency (SCID-X1) is caused by the mutations of interleukin-2 receptor subunit gamma (IL2RG) gene. Patients with the disease lack of T cells and natural killer cells, their B cells are functionally impaired; therefore, they are extremely vulnerable to infections (Aiuti & Roncarolo, 2009; Cavazzana-Calvo et al., 2000; Gaspar et al., 2004; Hacein-Bey-Abina et al., 2002, 2010).

3.18 Adenosine deaminase deficiency (ADA)-SCID

ADA- SCID is a rare genetic disease caused by a mutation of a gene on chromosome 20; this gene encodes an enzyme called adenosine deaminase (ADA). The mutation can lead to lack of ADA enzyme, and the lack of ADA enzyme causes disorder of adenosine metabolism and severe combined immunodeficiency (Aiuti et al., 2002, 2009; Aiuti & Roncarolo, 2009; Bordignon et al., 1989, 1995; Ferrari et al., 1991; Gaspar et al., 2009; Mortellaro et al., 2006).

3.19 Wiskott-Aldrich syndrome (WAS)

Wiskott-Aldrich syndrome (WAS) is an X-linked recessive primary immunodeficiency disease caused by mutations of the WAS protein (WASP) gene. The WASP gene is located on chromosome Xp11.22–Xp11.23. It has 12 exons, and encodes 502 amino acids. Patients with Wiskott-Aldrich syndrome have smaller platelets and lymphocytes, and their platelet counts are decreased; they have bleeding problems, recurrent bacterial and viral infections, and higher risk of autoimmune diseases and cancers. This disease affects about 1-10 in 1 million of live births (Aiuti & Roncarolo, 2009; Bouma et al., 2009; Dupré et al., 2004; Jin et al., 2004; Qasim et al., 2009; Ramesh et al., 1997; Zhu et al., 1997).

3.20 Other diseases

This possible gene therapy method also might be used to cure other diseases such as Alzheimer's disease (Rogaev et al., 1995; Sherrington et al., 1995), Parkinson's disease (Terzi & Zachariou, 2008; Veeriah et al., 2010), X-chronic granulomatous disease (CGD) (Aiuti & Roncarolo, 2009; Kang et al., 2010), type I (insulin-dependent) (Efrat, 1998) and type II (non-insulin-dependent) (Freeman et al., 1999) diabetes.

4. Conclusion

It is possible that normal human genomic DNA to be used as materials for homologous genetic recombination to repair defective genes *in vivo*. Normal human genomic DNA or normal genomic DNA fragments can be transferred into somatic cells/stem cells from a patient by microinjection, transfection, and electroporation. The corrected cells can be transplanted back to the same patient. Cells seem to be able to tolerate foreign DNA without immunological rejections; thus, the method described above may be an effective, relatively simple gene therapy method, and it may have no or less immunological reactions and rejections. Certainly, this possible approach of gene therapy should be performed only after strict and well-designed cellular and animal experiments and human clinical trials.

5. References

Ahn, A. & Kunkel, L. (1993). The Structural and Functional Diversity of Dystrophin. *Nature Genetics*, Vol.3, No.4, (April 1993), pp. 283-291, ISSN 1061-4036

Ahn, S., Kim, T., Lee, S., Kim, D., Ghang, H., Kim, D., Kim, B., Kim, S., Kim, W., Kim, C., Park, D., Lee, Y., Kim, S., Reja, R., Jho, S., Kim, C., Cha, J., Kim, K., Lee, B., Bhak, J. & Kim, S. (2009). The First Korean Genome Sequence and Analysis: Full Genome Sequencing for a Socio-ethnic Group. *Genome Research*, Vol.19, No.9, (September 2009), pp. 1622-1629, ISSN 1088-9051

Aiuti, A., Slavin, S., Aker, M., Ficara, F., Deola, S., Mortellaro, A., Morecki, S., Andolfi, G., Tabucchi, A., Carlucci, F., Marinello, E., Cattaneo, F., Vai, S., Servida, P., Miniero, R., Roncarolo, M. & Bordignon, C. (2002). Correction of ADA-SCID by Stem Cell Gene Therapy Combined with Nonmyeloablative Conditioning. *Science*, Vol.296, No.5577, (June 2002), pp. 2410-2413, ISSN 0036-8075

Aiuti, A., Cattaneo, F., Galimberti, S., Benninghoff, U., Cassani, B., Callegaro, L., Scaramuzza, S., Andolfi, G., Mirolo, M., Brigida, I., Tabucchi, A., Carlucci, F., Eibl, M., Aker, M., Slavin, S., Al-Mousa, H., Al Ghonaium, A., Ferster, A., Duppenthaler, A., Notarangelo, L., Wintergerst, U., Buckley, R., Bregni, M., Marktel, S., Valsecchi, M., Rossi, P., Ciceri, F., Miniero, R., Bordignon, C. & Roncarolo, M. (2009). Gene Therapy for Immunodeficiency due to Adenosine Deaminase Deficiency. *The New England Journal of Medicine*, Vol.360, No.5, (January 2009), pp. 447-458, ISSN 0028-4793

Aiuti, A. & Roncarolo, M. (2009). Ten Years of Gene Therapy for Primary Immune Deficiencies. *Hematology, American Society of Hematology Education Program Book*, Vol.2009, (2009), pp. 682-689, ISSN 1520-4391

Akhunov, E., Akhunova, A. & Dvorák, J. (2005). BAC Libraries of Triticum urartu, Aegilops speltoides and Ae. tauschii, the Diploid Ancestors of Polyploid Wheat. *TAG Theoretical and Applied Genetics*, Vol.111, No.8, (November 2005), pp. 1617-1622, ISSN 0040-5752

Akhunov, E., Akhunova, A., Anderson, O., Anderson, J., Blake, N., Clegg, M., Coleman-Derr, D., Conley, E., Crossman, C., Deal, K., Dubcovsky, J., Gill, B., Gu, Y., Hadam, J., Heo, H., Huo, N., Lazo, G., Luo, M., Ma, Y., Matthews, D., McGuire, P., Morrell, P., Qualset, C., Renfro, J., Tabanao, D., Talbert, L., Tian, C., Toleno, D., Warburton, M., You, F., Zhang, W. & Dvorak, J. (2010). Nucleotide Diversity Maps Reveal Variation in Diversity among Wheat Genomes and Chromosomes. *BMC Genomics*, Vol.11, (December 2010), pp. 702. doi: 10.1186/1471-2164-11-702, ISSN 1471-2164

Alber, F., Dokudovskaya, S., Veenhoff, L., Zhang, W., Kipper, J., Devos, D., Suprapto, A., Karni-Schmidt, O., Williams, R., Chait, B., Sali, A. & Rout, M. (2007). The Molecular Architecture of the Nuclear Pore Complex. *Nature*, Vol.450, No.7170, (November 2007), pp. 695-701, ISSN 1061-4036

Alderton, G. (2011). Genomic Instability: Expanding the Reach of Fanconi Anaemia. *Nature Reviews Cancer*, Vol.11, No.3, (March 2011), pp. 158-159, ISSN 1474-175X

Al-Dosari, M. & Gao, X. (2009) Nonviral Gene Delivery: Principle, Limitations, and Recent Progress. *The AAPS Journal*, Vol.11, No.4, (December 2009), pp. 671-681, ISSN 1550-7416

Anderson, M., Gregory, R., Thompson, S., Souza, D., Paul, S., Mulligan, R., Smith, A. & Welsh, M. (1991). Demonstration that CFTR Is a Chloride Channel by Alteration of Its Anion Selectivity. *Science*, Vol.253, No.5016, (July 1991), pp. 202-205, ISSN 0036-8075

Anderson, W., Killos, L., Sanders-Haigh, L., Kretschmer, P. & Diacumakos, E. (1980). Replication and Expression of Thymidine Kinase and Human Globin Gene Microinjected into Mouse Fibroblasts. *Proceedings of the National Academy of Sciences*, Vol.77, No.9, (September 1980), pp. 5399-5403, ISSN 0027-8424

Antar, A., Konopka, J., Campbell, J., Henry, R., Perdigoto, A., Carter, B., Pozzi, A., Abel, T. & Dermody, T. (2009). Junctional Adhesion Molecule-A Is Required for Hematogenous Dissemination of Reovirus. *Cell Host & Microbe*, Vol.5, No.1, (January 2009), pp. 59-71, ISSN 1931-3128

Antarasena, C., Prommuang, Po., Promkuntod, P., Trongwongsa, L., Prommuang, Pr. & Rujikwan, S. (2002). Isolation of Avian Reoviruses Associated with Diseases of Chickens in Southern Thailand. *Songklanakarin Journal of Science and Technology*, Vol.24, No.2, (April-June 2002), pp. 329-340, ISSN 0125-3395

Arkin, H., Ohnuma, T., Kamen, B., Holland, J., & Vallabhajosula, S. (1989). Multidrug Resistance in Human Leukemia Cell Line Selected for Resistance to Trimctrexate. *Cancer Research*, Vol.49, No.23, (December 1989), pp. 6556-6561, ISSN 0008-5472

Ataga, K. (2009). Novel Therapies in Sickle Cell Disease. *Hematology, American Society of Hematology Education Program Book*, Vol.2009, (2009), pp. 54-61, ISSN 1520-4391

Baggiolini, M., Dewald, B. & Moser, B. (1997). Human Chemokines: An Update. *Annual Review of Immunology*, Vol.15, (1997), pp. 675-705, ISSN 0732-0582

Balter, M. (2000). Emerging Diseases. On the Trail of Ebola and Marburg Viruses. *Science*, Vol.290, No.5493, (November 2000), pp. 923-925, ISSN 0036-8075

Barbour, V., Tufarelli, C., Sharpe, J., Smith, Z., Ayyub, H., Heinlein, C., Sloane-Stanley, J., Indrak, K., Wood, W. & Higgs, D. (2000). α -Thalassemia Resulting from a Negative Chromosomal Position Effect. *Blood, Journal of the American Society of Hematology*, Vol.96, No.3, (August 2000), pp. 800-807, ISSN 0006-4971

Bates, G., Mangiarini, L., Mahal, A. & Davies, S. (1997). Transgenic Models of Huntington's Disease. *Human Molecular Genetics*, Vol.6, No.10, (1997), pp. 1633-1637, ISSN 0964-6906

Batten, C., Maan, S., Shaw, A., Maan, N. & Mertens, P. (2008). A European Field Strain of Bluetongue Virus Derived from Two Parental Vaccine Strains by Genome Segment Reassortment. *Virus Research*, Vol.137, No.1, (October 2008), pp. 56-63, ISSN 0168-1702

Becker, A., McCulloch E. & Till J. (1963). Cytological Demonstration of the Clonal Nature of Spleen Colonies Derived from Transplanted Mouse Marrow Cells. *Nature*, Vol.197, No.4866, (February 1963), pp. 452-454, ISSN 0028-0836

Beilby, J. (2007). DNA: Where to Now? *The Clinical Biochemist Reviews*, Vol.28, No.2, (May 2007), pp. 52-59, ISSN 0159–8090

Berget, S., Moore, C. & Sharp, P. (1977). Spliced Segments at the 5′ Terminus of Adenovirus 2 Late mRNA. *Proceedings of the National Academy of Sciences*, Vol.74, No.8, (August 1977), pp. 3171-3175, ISSN 0027-8424

Bishop, J. & Smith, P. (1989). Mechanism of Chromosomal Integration of Microinjected DNA. *Molecular Biology and Medicine*, Vol.6, No.4, (August 1989), pp. 283-298, ISSN 0735-1313

Black, D. (2003). Mechanisms of Alternative Pre-messenger RNA Splicing. *Annual Review of Biochemistry*, Vol.72, (July 2003), pp. 291-336, ISSN 0066-4154

Bodey, G. (1986). Infection in Cancer Patients. A Continuing Association. *The American Journal of Medicine*, Vol.81, No.1A, (July 1986), pp. 11-26, ISSN 0002-9343

Bordignon, C., Yu, S., Smith, C., Hantzopoulos, P., Ungers, G., Keever, C., O'Reilly, R. & Gilboa, E. (1989). Retroviral Vector-mediated High-efficiency Expression of Adenosine Deaminase (ADA) in Hematopoietic Long-term Cultures of ADA-deficient Marrow Cells. *Proceedings of the National Academy of Sciences*, Vol.86, No.17, (September 1989), pp. 6748-6752, ISSN 0027-8424

Bordignon, C., Notarangelo, L., Nobili, N., Ferrari, G., Casorati, G., Panina, P., Mazzolari, E., Maggioni, D., Rossi, C., Servida, P., Ugazio, A. & Mavilio, F. (1995). Gene Therapy in Peripheral Blood Lymphocytes and Bone Marrow for ADA- immunodeficient Patients. *Science*, Vol.270, No.5235, (October 1995), pp. 470-475, ISSN 0036-8075

Bordignon, C. (2006). Stem-cell Therapies for Blood Diseases. *Nature*, Vol.441, No.7097, (June 2006), pp. 1100-1102, ISSN 0028-0836

Bouma, G., Burns, S. & Thrasher, A. (2009). Wiskott-Aldrich Syndrome: Immunodeficiency Resulting from Defective Cell Migration and Impaired Immunostimulatory Activation. *Immunobiology*, Vol.214, No.9-10, (September 2009), pp. 778-790, ISSN 0171-2985

Bradley, A., Evans, M., Kaufman, M. & Robertson, E. (1984). Formation of Germ-line Chimaeras from Embryo-derived Teratocarcinoma Cell Lines. *Nature*, Vol.309, No.5965, (May 1984), pp. 255-256, ISSN 0028-0836

Bronson, S. & Smithies, O. (1994). Altering Mice by Homologous Recombination Using Embryonic Stem Cells. *The Journal of Biological Chemistry*, Vol.269, No.44, (November 1994), pp. 27155-27158, ISSN 0021-9258

Brown, S., Gorman, B., Tesh, R. & Knudson, D. (1993) Coltiviruses Isolated from Mosquitoes Collected in Indonesia. *Virology*, Vol.196, No.1, (September 1993), pp. 363-367, ISSN 0042-6822

Buchwald, M. (1995). Complementation Groups: One or More per Gene? *Nature Genetics*, Vol.11, No.3, (November 1995), pp. 228-230, ISSN 1061-4036

Burghes, A., Logan, C., Hu, X., Belfall, B., Worton, R. & Ray, P. (1987). A cDNA Clone from the Duchenne/Becker Muscular Dystrophy Gene. *Nature*, Vol.328, No.6129, (July-August), pp. 434-437, ISSN 0028-0836

Campbell, K., McWhir, J., Ritchie, W. & Wilmut, I. (1996). Sheep Cloned by Nuclear Transfer from a Cultured Cell Line. *Nature*, Vol.380, No.6569, (March 1996), pp. 64-66, ISSN 0028-0836

Campeau, P., Chapdelaine, P., Seigneurin-Venin, S., Massie, B. & Tremblay, J. (2001). Transfection of Large Plasmids in Primary Human Myoblasts. *Gene Therapy*, Vol.8, No.18, (September 2001), pp. 1387-1394, ISSN 0969-7128

Capecchi, M. (1980). High Efficiency Transformation by Direct Microinjection of DNA into Cultured Mammalian Cells. *Cell*, Vol.22, No.2 part 2, (November 1980), pp. 479–488, ISSN 0092-8674

Capecchi, M. (1989a). The New Mouse Genetics: Altering the Genome by Gene Targeting. *Trends in Genetics*, Vol.5, No.3, (March 1989), pp. 70-76, ISSN 0168-9479

Capecchi, M. (1989b). Altering the Genome by Homologous Recombination. *Science*, Vol.244, No.4910, (June 1989), pp. 1288-1292, ISSN 0036-8075

Cartier, R. & Reszka, R. (2002). Utilization of Synthetic Peptides Containing Nuclear Localization Signals for Nonviral Gene Transfer Systems. *Gene Therapy*, Vol.9, No.3, (February 2002), pp. 157-167, ISSN 0969-7128

Cavazzana-Calvo, M., Hacein-Bey, S., de Saint Basile, G., Gross, F., Yvon, E., Nusbaum, P., Selz, F., Hue, C., Certain, S., Casanova, J., Bousso, P., Deist, F. & Fischer, A. (2000). Gene Therapy of Human Severe Combined Immunodeficiency (SCID)-X1 Disease. *Science*, Vol.288, No.5466, (April 2000), pp. 669-672, ISSN 0036-8075

Chan, A & Yang, S. (2009). Generation of Transgenic Monkeys with Human Inherited Genetic Disease. *Methods: A Companion to Methods in Enzymology*, Vol.49, No.1, (September 2009), pp. 78-84, ISSN 1046-2023

Chang, J., Ye, L. & Kan, Y. (2006). Correction of the Sickle Cell Mutation in Embryonic Stem Cells. *Proceedings of the National Academy of Sciences*, Vol.103, No.4, (January 2006), pp. 1036-1040, ISSN 0027-8424

Charreau, B., Tesson, L., Soulillou, J., Pourcel, C. & Anegon, I. (1996). Transgenesis in Rats: Technical Aspects and Models. *Transgenic Research*, Vol.5, No.4, (July 1996), pp. 223-234, ISSN 0962-8819

Chow, L., Gelinas, R., Broker, T. & Roberts, R. (1977). An Amazing Sequence Arrangement at the 5′ Ends of Adenovirus 1 Messenger RNA. *Cell*, Vol.12, No.1, (September 1977), pp. 1-8, ISSN 0092-8674

Chua, K., Crameri, G., Hyatt, A., Yu, M., Tompang, M., Rosli, J., McEachern, J., Crameri, S., Kumarasamy, V., Eaton, B. & Wang, L. (2007). A previously Unknown Reovirus of Bat Origin Is Associated with an Acute Respiratory Disease in Humans. *Proceedings of the National Academy of Sciences*, Vol.104, No.27, (July 2007), pp. 11424-11429, ISSN 0027-8424

Collaco, J. & Cutting, G. (2008). Update on Gene Modifiers in Cystic Fibrosis. *Current Opinion in Pulmonary Medicine*, Vol.14, No.6, (November 2008), pp. 559-566, ISSN 1070-5287

Collins, F. (1992). Cystic Fibrosis: Molecular Biology and Therapeutic Implications. *Science*, Vol.256, No.5058, (May 1992), pp. 774-779, ISSN 0036-8075

Creighton, H. & McClintock, B. (1931). Correlation of Cytological and Genetical Crossing-Over in Zea Mays. *Proceedings of the National Academy of Sciences*, Vol.17, No.8, (August 1931), pp. 492-497, ISSN 0027-8424

Creighton, H. & McClintock, B. (1935). The Correlation of Cytological and Genetical Crossing-Over in Zea Mays. A Corroboration. *Proceedings of the National Academy of Sciences*, Vol.21, No.3, (March 1935), pp. 148-150, ISSN 0027-8424

Croop, J., Gros, P. & Housman, D. (1988). Genetics of Multidrug Resistance. *The Journal of Clinical Investigation*, Vol.81, No.5, (May 1988), pp. 1303-1309, ISSN 0021-9738

Csatary, L., Romvary, J., Kasza, L., Schaff, S. & Massey, R. (1985). In vivo Interference between Pathogenic and Non-pathogenic Viruses. *Journal of Medicine*, Vol.16, No.5-6, (1985), pp. 563-573, ISSN 1090-1221

Cutting, G. (2010). Modifier Genes in Mendelian Disorders: The Example of Cystic Fibrosis. *Annals of the New York Academy of Sciences*, Vol.1214, (December 2010), pp. 57-69, ISSN 0077-8923

D'Angelo, M., Anderson, D., Richard, E. & Hetzer, M. (2006). Nuclear Pores Form de novo from Both Sides of the Nuclear Envelope. *Science*, Vol.312, No.5772, (April 2006), pp. 440-443, ISSN 0036-8075

D'Angelo, M. & Hetzer, M. (2008). Structure, Dynamics and Function of Nuclear Pore Complexes. *Trends in Cell Biology*, Vol.18, No.10, (October 2008), pp. 456-466, ISSN 0962-8924

Darling, T., Yee, C., Bauer, J., Hintner, H. & Yancey, K. (1999). Revertant Mosaicism: Partial Correction of a Germ-line Mutation in COL17A1 by a Frame-restoring Mutation. *The Journal of Clinical Investigation*, Vol.103, No.10, (May 1999), pp. 1371-1377, ISSN 0021-9738

Dave, U., Jenkins, N. & Copeland, N. (2004). Gene Therapy Insertional Mutagenesis Insights. *Science*, Vol.303, No.5656, (January 2004), pp. 333, ISSN 0036-8075

Davies, C., Jones, L., Green, B. & Nuttall, P. (1987). In vivo Reassortment of Thogoto Virus (A Tick-borne Influenza-like Virus) following Oral Infection of Rhipicephalus appendiculatus Ticks. *Journal of General Virology*, Vol.68, No.part 9, (September 1987), pp. 2331-2338, ISSN 0022-1317

Davies, S. & Ramsden, D. (2001). Huntington's Disease. *Molecular Pathology*, Vol.54, No.6, (December 2001), pp. 409-413, ISSN 0021-9746

De Rosa, M., Ackerley, C., Wang, B., Ito, S., Clarke, D. & Lingwood, C. (2008). Inhibition of Multidrug Resistance by Adamantylgb3, a Globotriaosylceramide Analog. *The Journal of Biological Chemistry*, Vol.283, No.8, (February 2008), pp. 4501-4511, ISSN 0021-9258

Debenham, P., Kartner, N., Siminovitch, L., Riordan, J. & Ling, V. (1982). DNA-mediated Transfer of Multiple Drug Resistance and Plasma Membrane Glycoprotein Expression. *Molecular and Cellular Biology*, Vol.2, No.8 (August 1982), pp. 881-889, ISSN 1098-5549

Decker, G. & Nyberg, S. (2001). Evidence that a Single Stem Cell Can Lead to Multi-organ Engraftment. *Liver Transplantation,* Vol.7, No.12, (December 2001), pp. 1085-1087, ISSN 1527-6465

Deuchars, K., Du, R., Naik, M., Evernden-Porelle, D., Kartner, N., van der Bliek, A. & Ling, V. (1987). Expression of Hamster P-glycoprotein and Multidrug Resistance in DNA-mediated Transformants of Mouse LTA Cells. *Molecular and Cellular Biology*, Vol.7, No.2 (February 1987), pp. 718-724, ISSN 1098-5549

Devos, D., Dokudovskaya, S., Williams, R., Alber, F., Eswar, N., Chait, B., Rout, M. & Sali, A. (2006). Simple Fold Composition and Modular Architecture of the Nuclear Pore Complex. *Proceedings of the National Academy of Sciences*, Vol.103, No.7, (February 2006), pp. 2172-2177, ISSN 0027-8424

Du, Y., Spence, S., Jenkins, N., Copeland, N. (2005). Cooperating Cancer-gene Identification through Oncogenic-retrovirus-induced Insertional Mutagenesis. *Blood, Journal of the American Society of Hematology*, Vol.106, No.7, (October 2005), pp. 2498-2505, ISSN 0006-4971

Duckworth-Rysiecki, G., Cornish, K., Clarke, C. & Buchwald, M. (1985). Identification of Two Complementation Groups in Fanconi Anemia. *Somatic Cell and Molecular Genetics*, Vol.11, No.1, (January 1985), pp. 35-41, ISSN 0740-7750

Dunn, G., Bruce, A., Ikeda, H., Old, L. & Schreiber, R. (2002). Cancer Immunoediting: from Immunosurveillance to Tumor Escape. *Nature Immunology*, Vol.3, No.11, (November 2002), pp. 991-998, ISSN 1529-2908

Dunn, G., Old, L. & Schreiber, R. (2004). The Three Es of Cancer Immunoediting. *Annual Review of Immunology*, Vol.22, (2004), pp. 329-360, ISSN 0732-0582

Dupré, L., Trifari, S., Follenzi, A., Marangoni, F., Lain de Lera, T., Bernad, A., Martino, S., Tsuchiya, S., Bordignon, C., Naldini, L., Aiuti, A. & Roncarolo, M. (2004). Lentiviral Vector-mediated Gene Transfer in T Cells from Wiskott-Aldrich Syndrome Patients Leads to Functional Correction. *Molecular Therapy*, Vol.10, No.5, (November 2004), pp. 903-915, ISSN 1525-0016

Dvorak, J. & Akhunov, E. (2005). Tempos of Gene Locus Deletions and Duplications and Their Relationship to Recombination Rate during Diploid and Polyploid Evolution in the Aegilops-Triticum alliance. *Genetics*, Vol.171, No.1, (September 2005), pp. 323-332, ISSN 0016-6731

Dwi Pramono, Z., Takeshima, Y., Surono, A., Ishida, T. & Matsuo, M. (2000). A Novel Cryptic Exon in Intron 2 of the Human Dystrophin Gene Evolved from an Intron by Acquiring Consensus Sequences for Splicing at Different Stages of Anthropoid Evolution. *Biochemical and Biophysical Research Communications*, Vol.267, No.1, (January 2000), pp. 321-328, ISSN 0006-291X

Eapen, M., Rocha, V., Sanz, G., Scaradavou, A., Zhang, M., Arcese, W., Sirvent, A., Champlin, R., Chao, N., Gee, A., Isola, L., Laughlin, M., Marks, D., Nabhan, S., Ruggeri, A., Soiffer, R., Horowitz, M., Gluckman, E., Wagner, J., Center for International Blood and Marrow Transplant Research, Acute Leukemia Working Party Eurocord (the European Group for Blood Marrow Transplantation) & National Cord Blood Program of the New York Blood Center. (2010). Effect of Graft Source on Unrelated Donor Haemopoietic Stem-cell Transplantation in Adults with Acute Leukaemia: A Retrospective Analysis. *The Lancet Oncology*, Vol.11, No.7, (July 2010), pp. 653-660, ISSN 1470-2045

Earle, W. (1943). Production of Malignancy in vitro. IV. The Mouse Fibroblast Cultures and Changes Seen in the Living Cells. *The Journal of the National Cancer Institute*, Vol.4, (1943), pp. 165-212, ISSN 0027-8874

Efrat, S. (1998). Prospects for Gene Therapy of Insulin-dependent Diabetes Mellitus. *Diabetologia. Clinical and Experimental Diabetes and Metabolism*. Vol.41, No.12, (December 1998), pp. 1401-1409, ISSN 0012-186X

Endicott, J. & Ling, V. (1989). The Biochemistry of P-glycoprotein-mediated Multidrug Resistance. *Annual Review of Biochemistry*, Vol.58, (July 1989), pp. 137-171, ISSN 0066-4154

Entrez Gene: HBA1 Hemoglobin alpha 1. (Updated on 16-Jan-2011). *NCBI*, February 7, 2011, Available from: http://www.ncbi.nlm.nih.gov/sites/entrez?Db=gene&Cmd=ShowDetailView&TermToSearch=3039

Epstein, A. (2009). Progress and Prospects: Biological Properties and Technological Advances of Herpes Simplex Virus Type 1-based Amplicon Vectors. *Gene Therapy*, Vol.16, No.6, (June 2009), pp. 709–715, ISSN 0969-7128

Escoffre, J., Portet, T., Wasungu, L., Teissié, J., Dean, D. & Rols, M. (2009). What Is (Still Not) Known of the Mechanism by Which Electroporation Mediates Gene Transfer and Expression in Cells and Tissues. *Molecular Biotechnology*, Vol.41, No.3, (March 2009), pp. 286-295, ISSN 1073-6085

Evans, V., Kerr, H., McQuilkin, W., Earle, W. & Hull, R. (1959). Growth in vitro of a Long-term Strain of Monkey-kidney Cells in Medium NCTC 109 Free of Any Added

Protein. *The American Journal of Hygiene*, Vol.70, (November 1959), pp. 297-302, ISSN 0096-5294

Falls, J., Pulford, D., Wylie, A. & Jirtle, R. (1999). Genomic Imprinting: Implications for Human Disease. *The American Journal of Pathology*, Vol.154, No.3, (March 1999), pp. 635-647, ISSN 0002-9440

Fanconi Anaemia/Breast Cancer Consortium. (1996). Positional Cloning of the Fanconi Anaemia Group A Gene. *Nature Genetics*, Vol.14, No.3, (November 1996), pp. 324-328, ISSN 1061-4036

Favard, C., Dean, D. & Rols, M. (2007). Electrotransfer as a Non Viral Method of Gene Delivery. *Current Gene Therapy*, Vol.7, No.1, (February 2007), pp. 67-77, ISSN 1566-5232

Feng, D., Liu, D., Huang, Y., Wu, L., Li, T., Wu, M., Tang, X. & Liang, C. (2001). The Expression of Human alpha -like Globin Genes in Transgenic Mice Mediated by Bacterial Artificial Chromosome. *Proceedings of the National Academy of Sciences*, Vol.98, No.26, (December 2001), pp. 15073-15077, ISSN 0027-8424

Fernandez-Martinez, J. & Rout, M. (2009). Nuclear Pore Complex Biogenesis. *Current Opinion in Cell Biology*, Vol.21, No.4, (August 2009), pp. 603-612, ISSN 0955-0674

Ferrari, G., Rossini, S., Giavazzi, R., Maggioni, D., Nobili, N., Soldati, M., Ungers, G., Mavilio, F., Gilboa, E. & Bordignon, C. (1991). An in vivo Model of Somatic Cell Gene Therapy for Human Severe Combined Immunodeficiency. *Science*, Vol.251, No.4999, (March 1991), pp. 1363-1366, ISSN 0036-8075

Filipiak, W. & Saunders, T. (2006). Advances in Transgenic Rat Production.*Transgenic Research*, Vol.15, No.6, (December 2006), pp. 673-686, ISSN 0962-8819

Folger, K., Wong, E., Wahl, G. & Capecchi, M. (1982). Patterns of Integration of DNA Microinjected into Cultured Mammalian Cells: Evidence for Homologous Recombination between Injected Plasmid DNA Molecules. *Molecular and Cellular Biology*, Vol.2, No.11, (November 1982), pp. 1372-1387, ISSN 1098-5549

Freeman, D., Leclerc, I. & Rutter, G. (1999). Present and Potential Future Use of Gene Therapy for the Treatment of Non-insulin Dependent Diabetes Mellitus. *International Journal of Molecular Medicine*, Vol.4, No.6, (December 1999), pp. 585-592, ISSN 1107-3756

Fujimoto, A., Nakagawa, H., Hosono, N., Nakano, K., Abe, T., Boroevich, K., Nagasaki, M., Yamaguchi, R., Shibuya, T., Kubo, M., Miyano, S., Nakamura, Y. & Tsunoda, T. (2010). Whole-genome Sequencing and Comprehensive Variant Analysis of a Japanese Individual Using Massively Parallel Sequencing. *Nature Genetics*, Vol.42, No.11, (November 2010), pp. 931–936, ISSN 1061-4036

Gao, J., Wei, Y., Huang, Y., Liu, D., Liu, G., Wu, M., Wu, L., Zhang, Q., Zhang, Z., Zhang, R. & Liang, C. (2005). The Expression of Intact and Mutant Human apoAI/CIII/AIV/AV Gene Cluster in Transgenic Mice. *The Journal of Biological Chemistry*, Vol.280, No.13, (April 2005), pp. 12559-12566, ISSN 0021-9258

Gao, X., Kim, K. & Liu, D. (2007). Nonviral Gene Delivery: What We Know and What Is Next. *The AAPS Journal*, Vol.9, No.1, (March 2007), pp. E92-E104, ISSN 1550-7416

Garten, R., Davis, C., Russell, C., Shu, B., Lindstrom, S., Balish, A., Sessions, W., Xu, X., Skepner, E., Deyde, V., Okomo-Adhiambo, M., Gubareva, L., Barnes, J., Smith, C., Emery, S., Hillman, M., Rivailler, P., Smagala, J., de Graaf, M., Burke, D., Fouchier, R., Pappas, C., Alpuche-Aranda, C., López-Gatell, H., Olivera, H., López, I., Myers,

C., Faix, D., Blair, P., Yu, C., Keene, K., Dotson, P. Jr., Boxrud, D., Sambol, A., Abid, S., St George, K., Bannerman, T., Moore, A., Stringer, D., Blevins, P., Demmler-Harrison, G., Ginsberg, M., Kriner, P., Waterman, S., Smole, S., Guevara, H., Belongia, E., Clark, P., Beatrice, S., Donis, R., Katz, J., Finelli, L., Bridges, C., Shaw, M., Jernigan, D., Uyeki, T., Smith, D., Klimov, A. & Cox, N. (2009). Antigenic and Genetic Characteristics of Swine-origin 2009 A (H1N1) Influenza Viruses Circulating in Humans. *Science*, Vol.325, No.5937, (July 2009), pp. 197-201, ISSN 0036-8075

Gaspar, H., Parsley, K., Howe, S., King, D., Gilmour, K., Sinclair, J., Brouns, G., Schmidt, M., Von Kalle, C., Barington, T., Jakobsen, M., Christensen, H., Al Ghonaium, A., White, H., Smith, J., Levinsky, R., Ali, R., Kinnon, C. & Thrasher, A. (2004). Gene Therapy of X-linked Severe Combined Immunodeficiency by Use of a Pseudotyped Gammaretroviral Vector. *The Lancet*, Vol.364, No.9452, (December 2004), pp. 2181-2187, ISSN 0140-6736

Gaspar, H., Aiuti, A., Porta, F., Candotti, F., Hershfield, M. & Notarangelo, L. (2009). How I Treat ADA Deficiency. *Blood, Journal of the American Society of Hematology*, Vol.114, No.17, (October 2009), pp. 3524-3532, ISSN 0006-4971

Giampietro, P., Verlander, P., Davis, J. & Auerbach, A. (1997). Diagnosis of Fanconi Anemia in Patients without Congenital Malformations: An International Fanconi Anemia Registry Study. *The American Journal of Human Genetics*, Vol.68, No.1, (January 1997), pp. 58-61, ISSN 0148-7299

Goldman, E. (2008). Transfer RNA, In: *Encyclopedia of Life Sciences*, DOI: 10.1002/9780470015902.a0000878.pub2, John Wiley & Sons, Ltd, Retrieved from http://onlinelibrary.wiley.com/doi/10.1002/9780470015902.a0000878.pub2/full

Goldstein, L., Galski, H., Fojo, A., Willingham, M., Lai, S., Gazdar, A., Pirker, R., Green, A., Crist, W., Brodeur, G., Lieber, M., Cossman, J., Gottesman, M. & Pastan, I. (1989). Expression of a Multidrug Resistance Gene in Human Cancers. *Journal of the National Cancer Institute*, Vol.81, No.2, (January 1989), pp. 116-124, ISSN 0027-8874

Golubovsky, M. & Manton, K. (2005). Genome Organization and Three Kinds of Heritable Changes: General Description and Stochastic Factors. *Frontiers in Bioscience*, Vol.10, (January 2005), pp. 335-344, ISSN 1093-9946

Golzio, M., Escoffre, J., Portet, T., Mauroy, C., Teissié, J., Dean, D. & Rols, M. (2010). Observations of the Mechanisms of Electromediated DNA Uptake--from Vesicles to Tissues. *Current Gene Therapy*, Vol.10, No.4, (August 2010), pp. 256-266, ISSN 1566-5232

Gore, A., Li, Z., Fung, H., Young, J., Agarwal, S., Antosiewicz-Bourget, J., Canto, I., Giorgetti, A., Israel, M., Kiskinis, E., Lee, J., Loh, Y., Manos, P., Montserrat, N., Panopoulos, A., Ruiz, S., Wilbert, M., Yu, J., Kirkness, E., Izpisua Belmonte, J., Rossi, D., Thomson, J., Eggan, K., Daley, G., Goldstein, L. & Zhang K. (2011). Somatic Coding Mutations in Human Induced Pluripotent Stem Cells. *Nature*, Vol.471, No.7336, (March 2011), pp. 63-67, ISSN 0028-0836

Gregory, J. Jr., Wagner, J., Verlander, P., Levran, O., Batish, S., Eide, C., Steffenhagen, A., Hirsch, B. & Auerbach, A. (2001). Somatic Mosaicism in Fanconi Anemia: Evidence of Genotypic Reversion in Lymphohematopoietic Stem Cells. *Proceedings of the National Academy of Sciences*, Vol.98, No.5, (February 2001), pp. 2532-2537, ISSN 0027-8424

Gregory, V., Bennett, M., Orkhan, M., Al Hajjar, S., Varsano, N., Mendelson, E., Zambon, M., Ellis, J., Hay, A. & Lin, Y. (2001). Emergence of Influenza A H1N2 Reassortant Viruses in the Human Population during 2001. *Virology*, Vol.300, No.1, (August 2002), pp. 1-7, ISSN 0042-6822

Gross, L. (2007). A New Human Genome Sequence Paves the Way for Individualized Genomics. *PLoS Biol*, Vol.5, No.10, (October 2007), pp. e266. doi:10.1371/journal.pbio.0050266, ISSN 1544-9173

Gross, M., Hanenberg, H., Lobitz, S., Friedl, R., Herterich, S., Dietrich, R., Gruhn, B., Schindler, D. & Hoehn, H. (2002). Reverse Mosaicism in Fanconi Anemia: Natural Gene Therapy via Molecular Self-correction. *Cytogenetic and Genome Research*, Vol.98, No.2-3, (2002), pp. 126-135, ISSN 1424–8581

Groudine, M., Kohwi-Shigematsu, T., Gelinas, R., Stamatoyannopoulos, G. & Papayannopoulou, T. (1983). Human Fetal to Adult Hemoglobin Switching: Changes in Chromatin Structure of the beta-globin Gene Locus. *Proceedings of the National Academy of Sciences*, Vol.80, No.24, (December 1983), pp. 7551-7555, ISSN 0027-8424

Gutierrez-Aranda, I., Ramos-Mejia, V., Bueno, C., Munoz-Lopez, M., Real, P., Mácia, A., Sanchez, L., Ligero, G., Garcia-Parez, J. & Menendez, P. (2010). Human Induced Pluripotent Stem Cells Develop Teratoma More Efficiently and Faster than Human Embryonic Stem Cells Regardless the Site of Injection. *Stem Cells*, Vol.28, No.9, (September 2010), pp. 1568-1570, ISSN 1066-5099

Hacein-Bey-Abina, S., Le Deist, F., Carlier, F., Bouneaud, C., Hue, C., De Villartay, J., Thrasher, A., Wulffraat, N., Sorensen, R., Dupuis-Girod, S., Fischer, A., Davies, E., Kuis, W., Leiva, L. & Cavazzana-Calvo, M. (2002). Sustained Correction of X-linked Severe Combined Immunodeficiency by ex vivo Gene Therapy. *The New England Journal of Medicine*, Vol.346, No.16, (April 2002), pp. 1185-1193, ISSN 0028-4793

Hacein-Bey-Abina, S., von Kalle, C., Schmidt, M., Le Deist, F., Wulffraat, N., McIntyre, E., Radford, I., Villeval, J., Fraser, C., Cavazzana-Calvo, M. & Fischer, A. (2003a). A Serious Adverse Event after Successful Gene Therapy for X-linked Severe Combined Immunodeficiency. *The New England Journal of Medicine*, Vol.348, No.3, (January 2003), pp. 255–256, ISSN 0028-4793

Hacein-Bey-Abina, S., von Kalle, C., Schmidt, M., McCormack, M., Wulffraat, N., Leboulch, P., Lim, A., Osborne, C., Pawliuk, R., Morillon, E., Sorensen, R., Forster, A., Fraser, P., Cohen, J., de Saint Basile, G., Alexander, I., Wintergerst, U., Frebourg, T., Aurias, A., Stoppa-Lyonnet, D., Romana, S., Radford-Weiss, I., Gross, F., Valensi, F., Delabesse, E., Macintyre, E., Sigaux, F., Soulier, J., Leiva, L., Wissler, M., Prinz, C., Rabbitts, T., Le Deist, F., Fischer, A. & Cavazzana-Calvo, M. (2003b). LMO2-associated Clonal T Cell Proliferation in Two Patients after Gene Therapy for SCID-X1. *Science*, Vol.302, No.5644, (October 2003), pp. 415–419, ISSN 0036-8075

Hacein-Bey-Abina, S., Hauer, J., Lim, A., Picard, C., Wang, G., Berry, C., Martinache, C., Rieux-Laucat, F., Latour, S., Belohradsky, B., Leiva, L., Sorensen, R., Debré, M., Casanova, J., Blanche, S., Durandy, A., Bushman, F., Fischer, A. & Cavazzana-Calvo, M. (2010). Efficacy of Gene Therapy for X-linked Severe Combined Immunodeficiency. *The New England Journal of Medicine*, Vol.363, No.4, (July 2010), pp. 355-364, ISSN 0028-4793

Hagstrom, J., Ludtke, J., Bassik, M., Sebestyén, M., Adam, S. & Wolff, J. (1997). Nuclear Import of DNA in Digitonin-permeabilized Cells. *Journal of Cell Science*, Vol.110, No.part 18, (September 1997), pp. 2323-2331, ISSN 0021-9533

Halatsch, M., Schmidt, U., Bötefür, I., Holland, J. & Ohnuma, T. (2000). Marked Inhibition of Glioblastoma Target Cell Tumorigenicity in vitro by Retrovirus-mediated Transfer of a Hairpin Ribozyme against Deletion-mutant Epidermal Growth Factor Receptor Messenger RNA. *Journal of Neurosurgery*, Vol.92, No.2, (February 2000), pp. 297-305, ISSN 0022-3085

Hall, J. (1990). Genomic Imprinting: Review and Relevance to Human Diseases. *The American Society of Human Genetics*, Vol.46, No.5, (May 1990), pp. 857-873, ISSN 0002-9297

Hardison, R. (1996). A Brief History of Hemoglobins: Plant, Animal, Protist, and Bacteria. *Proceedings of the National Academy of Sciences*, Vol.93, No.12, (June 1996), pp. 5675-5679, ISSN 0027-8424

Hawkins, J. (1988). A Survey on Intron and Exon Lengths. *Nucleic Acids Research*, Vol.16, No.21, (November 1988), pp. 9893-9908, ISSN 0305-1048

Higgs, D., Vickers, M., Wilkie, A., Pretorius, I., Jarman, A. & Weatherall, D. (1989). A Review of the Molecular Genetics of the Human alpha-globin Gene Cluster. *Blood, Journal of the American Society of Hematology*, Vol.73, No.5, (April 1989), pp. 1081-1104, ISSN 0006-4971

Hirschhorn, R. (2003). In vivo Reversion to Normal of Inherited Mutations in Humans. *Journal of Medical Genetics*, Vol.40, No.10, (October 2003), pp. 721-728, ISSN 0022-2593

Hoffman, E., Brown, R. Jr. & Kunkel, L. (1987). Dystrophin: The Protein Product of the Duchenne Muscular Dystrophy Locus. *Cell*, Vol.51, No.6, (December 1987), pp. 919-928, ISSN 0092-8674

Holliday R. (1974). Molecular Aspects of Genetic Exchange and Gene Conversion. *Genetics*, Vol.78, No.1, (September 1974), pp. 273-287, ISSN 0016-6731

Holmes, E., Ghedin, E., Miller, N., Taylor, J., Bao, Y., St George, K., Grenfell, B., Salzberg, S., Fraser, C., Lipman, D. & Taubenberger, J. (2005). Whole-genome Analysis of Human Influenza A Virus Reveals Multiple Persistent Lineages and Reassortment among Recent H3N2 Viruses. *PLoS Biology*, Vol.3, No.9, (September 2005), pp. e300, ISSN 1544-9173

Holmes, K., Tresnan, D. & Zelus, B. (1997). Virus-receptor Interactions in the Enteric Tract. Virus-receptor Interactions. *Advances in Experimental Medicine and Biology*, Vol.412, (1997), pp. 125-133, ISSN 0065-2598

Hope, J., Cruzata, L., Duvshani, A., Mitsumoto, J., Maftahi, M. & Freyer, G. (2007). Mus81-Eme1-dependent and -independent Crossovers Form in Mitotic Cells during Double-strand Break Repair in Schizosaccharomyces pombe. *Molecular and Cellular Biology*, Vol.27, No.10, (May 2007), pp. 3828-3838, ISSN 0270-7306

Huang, C. Liang, H. & Jia, F. (1985). Beneficial Role of a Non-pathogenic Orbi-like Virus: Studies on the Interfering Effect of M14 Virus in Mice and Mosquitoes Infected with Japanese Encephalitis Virus. *Intervirology*, Vol.24, No.3, (1985), pp. 147-153, ISSN 0300-5526

Huang, S., Sirikhachornkit, A., Su, X., Faris, J., Gill, B., Haselkorn, R. & Gornicki, P. (2002). Genes Encoding Plastid Acetyl-CoA Carboxylase and 3-Phosphoglycerate Kinase of the Triticum/Aegilops Complex and the Evolutionary History of Polyploid Wheat. *Proceedings of the National Academy of Sciences*, Vol.99, No.12, (June 2002), pp. 8133-8138, ISSN 0027-8424

Hull, R., Cherry, W. & Johnson, I. (1956). The Adaptation and Maintenance of Mammalian Cells to Continuous Growth in Tissue Culture. *The Anatomical Record: Advances in Integrative Anatomy and Evolutionary Biology*, Vol.124, (1956), pp. 490–499, ISSN 0003-276X,

Hull, R., Cherry, W. & Tritch, O. (1962). Growth Characteristics of Monkey Kidney Cell Strains LLC-MK1, LLC-MK2, and LLC-MK2 (NCTC-3196) and Their Utility in Virus Research. *The Journal of Experimental Medicine*, Vol.115, (May 1962), pp. 903-918, ISSN 0022-1007

Hussein, S., Batada, N., Vuoristo, S., Ching, R., Autio, R., Närvä, E., Ng, S., Sourour, M., Hämäläinen, R., Olsson, C., Lundin, K., Mikkola, M., Trokovic, R., Peitz, M., Brüstle, O., Bazett-Jones, D., Alitalo, K., Lahesmaa, R., Nagy, A. & Otonkoski, T. (2011). Copy Number Variation and Selection during Reprogramming to Pluripotency. *Nature*, Vol.471, No.7336, (March 2011), pp. 58-62, ISSN 0028-0836

Ingram, V. (1956). A Specific Chemical Difference between the Globins of Normal Human and Sickle-cell Anaemia Haemoglobin. *Nature*, Vol.178, No.4537, (October 1956), pp. 792-794, ISSN 0028-0836

Ingram, V. (1957). Gene Mutations in Human Haemoglobin: The Chemical Difference between Normal and Sickle Cell Haemoglobin. *Nature*, Vol.180, No.4581, (August 1957), pp. 326-328, ISSN 0028-0836

International Human Genome Sequencing Consortium. (2001). Initial Sequencing and Analysis of the Human Genome. *Nature*, Vol.409, No.6822, (February 2001), pp. 860–921, ISSN 0028-0836

International Human Genome Sequencing Consortium. (2004). Finishing the Euchromatic Sequence of the Human Genome. *Nature*, Vol.431, No.7011, (October 2004), pp. 931–945, ISSN 0028-0836

International Silkworm Genome Consortium. (2008). The Genome of a Lepidopteran Model Insect, the Silkworm Bombyx mori. *Insect Biochemistry and Molecular Biology*, Vol.38, No.12, (December 2008), pp. 1036-1045, ISSN 0965-1748

Jackson, S. & Bartek, J. (2009). The DNA-damage Response in Human Biology and Disease. *Nature*, Vol.461, No.7267, (October 2009), pp. 1071-1078, ISSN 0028-0836

Jacobsen, J., Bawden, C., Rudiger, S., McLaughlan, C., Reid, S., Waldvogel, H., MacDonald, M., Gusella, J., Walker, S., Kelly, J., Webb, G., Faull, R., Rees, M. & Snell, R. (2010). An Ovine Transgenic Huntington's Disease Model. *Human Molecular Genetics*, Vol.19, No.10, (May 2010), pp. 1873-1882, ISSN 0964-6906

Jayandharan, G., Aslanidi, G., Martino, A., Jahn, S., Perrin, G., Herzog, R. & Srivastava, A. (2011). Activation of the NF-{kappa}B Pathway by Adeno-associated Virus (AAV) Vectors and Its Implications in Immune Response and Gene Therapy. *Proceedings of the National Academy of Sciences*, Vol.108, No.9, (March 2011), pp. 3743-3748, ISSN 0027-8424

Jiang, H., Patel, P., Kohlmaier, A., Grenley, M., McEwen, D. & Edgar, B. (2009). Cytokine/Jak/Stat Signaling Mediates Regeneration and Homeostasis in the Drosophila Midgut. *Cell*, Vol.137, No.7, (June 2009), pp. 1343-1355, ISSN 0092-8674

Jin, Y., Mazza, C., Christie, J., Giliani, S., Fiorini, M., Mella, P., Gandellini, F., Stewart, D., Zhu, Q., Nelson, D., Notarangelo, L. & Ochs, H. (2004). Mutations of the Wiskott-Aldrich Syndrome Protein (WASP): Hotspots, Eeffect on Transcription, and Translation and Phenotype/Genotype Correlation. *Blood, Journal of the American Society of Hematology*, Vol.104, No.13, (December 2004), pp. 4010-4019, ISSN 0006-4971

Joenje, H., Lo ten Foe, J., Oostra, A., van Berkel, C., Rooimans, M., Schroeder-Kurth, T., Wegner, R., Gille, J., Buchwald, M. & Arwert, F. (1995). Classification of Fanconi Anemia Patients by Complementation Analysis: Evidence for a Fifth Genetic Subtype. *Blood, Journal of the American Society of Hematology*, Vol.86, No.6, (September 1995), pp. 2156-2160, ISSN 0006-4971

Joenje, H. & Patel, K. (2001). The Emerging Genetic and Molecular Basis of Fanconi Anaemia. *Nature Reviews Genetics*, Vol.2, No.6, (June 2001), pp. 446-457, ISSN 1471-0056

Johansson, P., Sveger, T., Ahlfors, K., Ekstrand, J. & Svensson, L. (1996). Reovirus Type 1 Associated with Meningitis. *Scandinavian Journal of Infectious Diseases*, Vol. 28, No.2, (1996), pp. 117-120, ISSN 0036-5548

Johnson, R. & Jasin, M. (2001). Double-strand-break-induced Homologous Recombination in Mammalian Cells. *Biochemical Society Transactions*, Vol.29, No.part 2, (May 2001), pp. 196-201, ISSN 0300-5127

Jones, L., Davies, C., Green, B. & Nuttall, P. (1987). Reassortment of Thogoto Virus (A Tick-borne Influenza-like Virus) in a Vertebrate Host. *Journal of General Virology*, Vol.68, No.part 5, (May 1987), pp. 1299-1306, ISSN 0022-1317

Juliano, R. & Ling, V. (1976). A Surface Glycoprotein Modulating Drug Permeability in Chinese Hamster Ovary Cell Mutants. *Biochimica et Biophysica Acta*, Vol.455, No.1, (November 1976), pp. 152–162, ISSN 0005-2736.

Kadyk, L. & Hartwell, L. (1992). Sister Chromatids Are Preferred over Homologs as Substrates for Recombinational Repair in Saccharomyces cerevisiae. *Genetics*, Vol.132, No.2, (October 1992), pp. 387-402, ISSN 0016-6731

Kang, E., Choi, U., Theobald, N., Linton, G., Long Priel, D., Kuhns, D. & Malech, H. (2010). Retrovirus Gene Therapy for X-linked Chronic Granulomatous Disease Can Achieve Stable Long-term Correction of Oxidase Activity in Peripheral Blood Neutrophils. *Blood, Journal of the American Society of Hematology*, Vol.115, No.4, (January 2010), pp. 783-791, ISSN 0006-4971

Karasin, A., Schutten, M., Cooper, L., Smith, C., Subbarao, K., Anderson, G., Carman, S. & Olsen, C. (2000). Genetic Characterization of H3N2 Influenza Viruses Isolated from Pigs in North America, 1977-1999: Evidence for Wholly Human and Reassortant Virus Genotypes. *Virus Research*, Vol.68, No.1, (June 2000), pp. 71-85, ISSN 0168-1702

Kerem, B., Rommens, J., Buchanan, J., Markiewicz, D., Cox, T., Chakravarti, A., Buchwald, M. & Tsui, L. (1989). Identification of the Cystic Fibrosis Gene: Genetic Analysis. *Science*, Vol.245, No.4922, (September 1989), pp. 1073-1080, ISSN 0036-8075

Kim, Y., Lach, F., Desetty, R., Hanenberg, H., Auerbach, A. & Smogorzewska, A. (2011). Mutations of the SLX4 Gene in Fanconi Anemia. *Nature Genetics*, Vol.43, No.2, (February 2011), pp. 142-146, ISSN 1061-4036

Kobayashi, H., Dorai, T., Holland, J. & Ohnuma, T. (1994). Reversal of Drug Sensitivity in Multidrug-resistant Tumor Cells by an MDR1 (PGY1) Ribozyme. *Cancer Research*, Vol.54, No.5, (March 1994), PP. 1271-1275, ISSN 0008-5472

Kobayashi, H., Takemura, Y., Holland, J. & Ohnuma, T. (1998). Vincristine Saturation of Cellular Binding Sites and Its Cytotoxic Activity in Human Lymphoblastic Leukemia Cells: Mechanism of Inoculum Effect. *Biochemical Pharmacology*, Vol.55, No.8, (April 1998), pp. 1229-1234, ISSN 0006-2952

Koenig, M., Hoffman, E., Bertelson, C., Monaco, A., Feener, C. & Kunkel, L. (1987). Complete Cloning of the Duchenne Muscular Dystrophy (DMD) cDNA and Preliminary Genomic Organization of the DMD Gene in Normal and Affected Individuals. *Cell*, Vol.50, No.3, (July 1987), pp. 509-517, ISSN 0092-8674

Koenig, M., Monaco, A. & Kunkel, L. (1988). The Complete Sequence of Dystrophin Predicts a Rod-shaped Cytoskeletal Protein. *Cell*, Vol.53, No.2, (April 1988), pp. 219-228, ISSN 0092-8674

Koller, B. & Smithies, O. (1992). Altering Genes in Animals by Gene Targeting. *Annual Review of Immunology*, Vol.10, (1992), pp. 705-730, ISSN 0732-0582

Krause, D., Theise, N., Collector, M., Henegariu, O., Hwang, S., Gardner, R., Neutzel, S. & Sharkis, S. (2001). Multi-organ, Multi-lineage Engraftment by a Single Bone Marrow-derived Stem Cell. *Cell*, Vol.105, No.3, (May 2001), pp. 369-377, ISSN 0092-8674

Kuehn, M., Bradley, A., Robertson, E. & Evans, M. (1987). A Potential Animal Model for Lesch-Nyhan Syndrome through Introduction of HPRT Mutations into Mice. *Nature*, Vol.326, No.6110, (March 1987), pp. 295-298, ISSN 0028-0836

Kunkel, L. (2004). William Allan Award Address. Cloning of the DMD Gene. *The American Journal of Human Genetics*. Vol.76, No.2, (February 2005), pp. 205-214, ISSN 0002-9297

Lam, A. & Dean, A. (2010). Progress and Prospects: Nuclear Import of Nonviral Vectors. *Gene Therapy*, Vol.17, No.4, (April 2010), pp. 439-447, ISSN 0969-7128

Laughlin, M., Barker, J., Bambach, B., Koc, O., Rizzieri, D., Wagner, J., Gerson, S., Lazarus, H., Cairo, M., Stevens, C., Rubinstein, P. & Kurtzberg, J. (2001). Hematopoietic Engraftment and Survival in Adult Recipients of Umbilical-cord Blood from Unrelated Donors. *The New England Journal of Medicine*, Vol.344, No.24, (June 2001), pp. 1815-1822, ISSN 0028-4793

Laughlin, M., Eapen, M., Rubinstein, P., Wagner, J., Zhang, M., Champlin, R., Stevens, C., Barker, J., Gale, R., Lazarus, H., Marks, D., van Rood, J., Scaradavou, A. & Horowitz, M. (2004). Outcomes after Transplantation of Cord Blood or Bone Marrow from Unrelated Donors in Adults with Leukemia. *The New England Journal of Medicine*, Vol.351, No.22, (November 2004), pp. 2265-2275, ISSN 0028-4793

Laurent, L., Ulitsky, I., Slavin, I., Tran, H., Schork, A., Morey, R., Lynch, C., Harness, J., Lee, S., Barrero, M., Ku, S., Martynova, M., Semechkin, R., Galat, V., Gottesfeld, J., Izpisua Belmonte, J., Murry, C., Keirstead, H., Park, H., Schmidt, U., Laslett, A., Muller, F., Nievergelt, C., Shamir, R. & Loring, J. (2011). Dynamic Changes in the Copy Number of Pluripotency and Cell Proliferation Genes in Human ESCs and iPSCs during Reprogramming and Time in Culture. *Cell Stem Cell*, Vol.8, No.1, (January 2011), pp. 106-118, ISSN 1934-5909

Lederberg, J. & Tatum, E. (1946). Gene Recombination in Escherichia coli. *Nature*, Vol.158, No.4016, (October 1946), pp. 558, ISSN 0028-0836

Lederberg, J. (1947). Gene Recombination and Linked Segregations in Escherichia coli. *Genetics*, Vol.32, No.5, (September 1947), pp. 505-525, ISSN 0016-6731

Lederberg, J. (1987a). Gene Recombination and Linked Segregations in Escherichia coli. *Genetics*, Vol.117, No.1, (September 1987), pp. 1-4, ISSN 0016-6731

Lederberg, J. (1987b). Genetic Recombination in Bacteria: A Discovery Account. *Annual Review of Genetics*, Vol.21, (1987), pp. 23-46, ISSN 0066-4197

Lee, T., Matthews, D. & Blair, G. (2005). Novel Molecular Approaches to Cystic Fibrosis Gene Therapy. *Biochemical Journal*, Vol.387, No.part 1, (April 2005), pp. 1-15, ISSN 0264-6021

Levitus, M., Rooimans, M., Steltenpool, J., Cool, N., Oostra, A., Mathew, C., Hoatlin, M., Waisfisz, Q., Arwert, F., de Winter, J. & Joenje, H. (2004). Heterogeneity in Fanconi Anemia: Evidence for 2 New Genetic Subtypes. *Blood, Journal of the American Society of Hematology*, Vol.103, No.7, (April 2004), pp. 2498-2503, ISSN 0006-4971

Levitus, M., Joenje, H. & de Winter J. (2006). The Fanconi Anemia Pathway of Genomic Maintenance. *Cellular Oncology*, Vol.28, No.1-2, (April 2006), pp. 3-29, ISSN 1570-5870

Levy, S., Sutton, G., Ng, P., Feuk, L., Halpern, A., Walenz, B., Axelrod, N., Huang, J., Kirkness, E., Denisov, G., Lin, Y., MacDonald, J., Pang, A., Shago, M., Stockwell, T., Tsiamouri, A., Bafna, V., Bansal, V., Kravitz, S., Busam, D., Beeson, K., Mclntosh, T., Remington, K., Abril, J., Gill, J., Borman, J., Rogers, Y-H., Frazier, M., Scherer, S., Strausberg, R. & Venter, J. (2007). The Diploid Genome Sequence of an Individual Human. *PLoS Biology*, Vol.5, No.10, (October 2007), pp. e254. doi:10.1371/journal.pbio.0050254, ISSN 1544-9173

Li., Q., Xie, X., Zhi, Q., Ma, L., Abudourexiti, A., Liu, Y., Dangzheng, W., Zhang, Y., Hashan, Y., Wang, C., Hamatai, S., Liang, G., He, Y., Zhao, Z., Chen, B., Xu, P. & Zuo, J. (1992). First Isolation of 8 Strains of New Orbivirus (BANNA) from Patients with Innominate Fever in Xinjiang. *Endemic Disease Bulletin*, Vol.7, No.1, (February 1992), pp. 77-81, ISSN 1000-3711

Li, X. & Heyer, W. (2008). Homologous Recombination in DNA Repair and DNA Damage Tolerance. *Cell Research*, Vol.18, No.1, (January 2008), pp. 99-113, ISSN 1001-0602

Li, Z., Düllmann, J., Schiedlmeier, B., Schmidt, M., von Kalle, C., Meyer, J., Forster, M., Stocking, C., Wahlers, A., Frank, O., Ostertag, W., Kühlcke, K., Eckert, H., Fehse, B. & Baum, C. (2002). Murine Leukemia Induced by Retroviral Gene Marking. *Science*, Vol.296, No.5567, (April 2002), pp. 497, ISSN 0036-8075

Liang, X., Huang, Z., Wang, Y. & Xiao, P. (1985). Studies on the Interference of a Non-pathogenic Virus with the Japanese B Encephalitis Virus. *Acta Academiae Medicinae Sinicae*, Vol.7, No.4, (August 1985), pp. 290-293, ISSN 1000-503X

Liao, J., Wu, Z., Wang, Y., Cheng, L., Cui, C., Gao, Y., Chen, T., Rao, L., Chen, S., Jia, N., Dai, H., Xin, S., Kang, J., Pei, G. & Xiao, L. (2008). Enhanced Efficiency of Generating Induced Pluripotent Stem (iPS) Cells from Human Somatic Cells by a Combination of Six Transcription Factors. *Cell Research* Vol.18, No.5, (May 2008), pp. 600-603, ISSN 1001-0602

Lister, R., Pelizzola, M., Kida, Y., Hawkins, R., Nery, J., Hon, G., Antosiewicz-Bourget, J., O'Malley, R., Castanon, R., Klugman, S., Downes, M., Yu, R., Stewart, R., Ren, B.,

Thomson, J., Evans, R. & Ecker, J. (2011). Hotspots of Aberrant Epigenomic Reprogramming in Human Induced Pluripotent Stem Cells. *Nature*, Vol.471, No.7336, (March 2011), pp. 68-73, ISSN 0028-0836

Lo Ten Foe, J., Kwee, M., Rooimans, M., Oostra, A., Veerman, A., van Weel, M., Pauli, R., Shahidi, N., Dokal, I., Roberts, I., Altay, C., Gluckman, E., Gibson, R., Mathew, C., Arwert, F. & Joenje, H. (1997). Somatic Mosaicism in Fanconi Anemia: Molecular Basis and Clinical Significance. *European Journal of Human Genetics*, Vol.5, No.3, (May-June 1997), pp. 137-148, ISSN 1018-4813

Lobitz, S. & Velleuer, E. (2006). Guido Fanconi (1892-1979): A Jack of All Trades. *Nature Reviews Cancer*, Vol.6, No.11, (November 2006), pp. 893-898, ISSN 1474-175X

Locati, M. & Murphy, P. (1999). Chemokines and Chemokine Receptors: Biology and Clinical Relevance in Inflammation and AIDS. *Annual Review of Medicine*, Vol.50, (1999), pp. 425-440, ISSN 0066-4219

Lodish, H., Berk, A., Kaiser, C., Krieger, M., Scott, M., Bretscher, A., Ploegh, H. & Matsudaira, P. (2008). *Molecular Cell Biology*, W.H. Freeman and Company, ISBN-10 0-7167-7601-4, New York, USA

Lorenz, A. & Whitby, M. (2006). Crossover Promotion and Prevention. *Biochemical Society Transactions*, Vol.34, No.part 4, (August 2006), pp. 537-541, ISSN 0300-5127

Ludtke, J., Zhang, G., Sebestyen, M. & Wolff, J. (1999). A Nuclear Localization Signal Can Enhance both the Nuclear Transport and Expression of 1 kb DNA. *Journal of Cell Science*, Vol.112, No.part 12, (June 1999), pp. 2033-2041, ISSN 0021-9533

Lundstrom, K. (2001). Alphavirus Vectors for Gene Therapy Applications. *Current Gene Therapy*, Vol.1, No.1, (May 2001), pp. 19-29, ISSN 1566-5232

Lundstrom, K. (2005). Biology and Application of Alphaviruses in Gene Therapy. *Gene Therapy*, Vol.12, No.supplement 1, (October 2005), pp. S92-S97, ISSN 0969-7128

Luster, A. (1998). Chemokines-Chemotactic Cytokines that Mediate Inflammation. *The New England Journal of Medicine*, Vol.338, No.7, (February 1998), pp. 436-445, ISSN 0028-4793

Ma, W., Lager, K., Lekcharoensuk, P., Ulery, E., Janke, B., Solórzano, A., Webby, R., García-Sastre, A. & Richt, J. (2010). Viral Reassortment and Transmission after Co-infection of Pigs with Classical H1N1 and Triple-reassortant H3N2 Swine Influenza Viruses. *Journal of General Virology*, Vol.91, No.part 9, (September 2010), pp. 2314-2321, ISSN 0022-1317

MacDonald, M., Ambrose, C., Duyao, M., Myers, R., Lin, C., Srinidhi, L., Barnes, G., Taylor, S., James, M., Groot, N., MacFarlane, H., Jenkins, B., Anderson, M., Wexler, N. & Gusella, J. (1993). A Novel Gene Containing a Trinucleotide Repeat That Is Expanded and Unstable on Huntington's Disease Chromosomes. *Cell*, Vol.72, No.6, (March 1993), pp. 971-983, ISSN 0092-8674

Mankad, A., Taniguchi, T., Cox, B., Akkari, Y., Rathbun, R., Lucas, L., Bagby, G., Olson, S., D'Andrea, A., Grompe, M. (2006). Natural Gene Therapy in Monozygotic Twins with Fanconi Anemia. *Blood, Journal of the American Society of Hematology*, Vol.107, No.8, (April 2006), pp. 3084-3090, ISSN 0006-4971

Martinez-Agosto, J., Mikkola, H., Hartenstein, V. & Banerjee, U. (2007). The Hematopoietic Stem Cell and Its Niche: A Comparative View. *Genes & Development*, Vol.21, No.23, (December 2007), pp. 3044-3060, ISSN 0890-9369

Mastaglio, S., Stanghellini, M., Bordignon, C., Bondanza, A., Ciceri, F. & Bonini, C. (2010). Progress and Prospects: Graft-versus-host Disease. *Gene Therapy*, Vol.17, No.11, (November 2010), pp. 1309–1317, ISSN 0969-7128

Matthijnssens, J., Taraporewala, Z., Yang, H., Rao, S., Yuan, L., Cao, D., Hoshino, Y., Mertens, P., Carner, G., McNeal, M., Sestak, K., Van Ranst, M. & Patton, J. (2010). Simian Rotaviruses Possess Divergent Gene Constellations that Originated from Interspecies Transmission and Reassortment. *Journal of Virology*, Vol. 84, No.4, (February 2010), pp. 2013-2026, ISSN 0022-538X

Maunula, L. & Von Bonsdorff, C. (2002). Frequent Reassortments May Explain the Genetic Heterogeneity of Rotaviruses: Analysis of Finnish Rotavirus Strains. *Journal of Virology*, Vol. 76, No.23, (December 2002), pp. 11793-11800, ISSN 0022-538X

McClain, M., Spendlove, R. & Lennette, E. (1967). Infectivity Assay of Reoviruses: Comparison with Immunofluorescent Cell Count and Plaque Methods. *The Journal of Immunology*, Vol.98, No.6, (June 1967), pp. 1301-1308, ISSN 0022-1767

McCulloch, E., Siminovitch, L. & Till J. (1964). Spleen-colony Formation in Anemic Mice of Genotype WW. *Science*, Vol.144, No.1620, (May 1964), pp. 844-846, ISSN 0036-8075

Ménoret, S., Remy, S., Usal, C., Tesson, L. & Anegon, I. (2010). Generation of Transgenic Rats by Microinjection of Short DNA Fragments. *Methods in Molecular Biology*, Vol.597, (2010), pp. 81-92, ISSN 1064-3745

Mir, L. (2009). Nucleic Aacids Electrotransfer-based Gene Therapy (Electrogenetherapy): Past, Current, and Future. *Molecular Biotechnology*, Vol.43, No.2, (October 2009), pp. 167-176, ISSN 1073-6085

Modlich, U., Kustikova, O., Schmidt, M., Rudolph, C., Meyer, J., Li, Z., Kamino, K., von Neuhoff, N., Schlegelberger, B., Kuehlcke, K., Bunting, K., Schmidt, S., Deichmann, A., von Kalle, C., Fehse, B. & Baum C. (2005). Leukemias following Retroviral Transfer of Multidrug Resistance 1 (MDR1) Are Driven by Combinatorial Insertional Mutagenesis. *Blood, Journal of the American Society of Hematology*, Vol.105, No.11, (June 2005), pp. 4235-4246, ISSN 0006-4971

Mohd Jaafar, F., Attoui, H., Mertens, P., de Micco, P. & de Lamballerie, X. (2005). Structural Organization of an Encephalitic Human Isolate of Banna Virus (Genus Seadornavirus, Family Reoviridae). *Journal of General Virology*, Vol.86, No.part 4, (April 2005), pp. 1147-1157, ISSN 0022-1317

Monaco, A., Neve, R., Colletti-Feener, C., Bertelson, C., Kurnit, D. & Kunkel, L. (1986). Isolation of Candidate cDNAs for Portions of the Duchenne Muscular Dystrophy Gene. *Nature*, Vol.323, No.6089, (October 1986), pp. 646-650, ISSN 0028-0836

Mortellaro, A., Hernandez, R., Guerrini, M., Carlucci, F., Tabucchi, A., Ponzoni, M., Sanvito, F., Doglioni, C., Di Serio, C., Biasco, L., Follenzi, A., Naldini, L., Bordignon, C., Roncarolo, M. & Aiuti, A. (2006). Ex vivo Gene Therapy with Lentiviral Vectors Rescues Adenosine Deaminase (ADA)-deficient Mice and Corrects Their Immune and Metabolic Defects. *Blood, Journal of the American Society of Hematology*, Vol.108, No.9, (November 2006), pp. 2979-2988, ISSN 0006-4971

Moscow, J. & Cowan, K. (1988). Multidrug Resistance. *Journal of the National Cancer Institute*, Vol.80, No.1, (March 1988), pp. 14-20, ISSN 0027-8874

Müller, L. & Williams, D. (2009). Finding the Needle in the Hay Stack: Hematopoietic Stem Cells in Fanconi Anemia. *Mutation Research - Fundamental and Molecular Mechanisms of Mutagenesis*, Vol.668, No.1-2, (July 2009), pp. 141-149, ISSN 0027-5107

Muntoni, F., Torelli, S. & Ferlini, A. (2003). Dystrophin and Mutations: One Gene, Several Proteins, Multiple Phenotypes. *The Lancet Neurology*, Vol.2, No.12, (December 2003), pp. 731-740, ISSN 1474-4422

Murdoch, C. & Finn, A. (2000). Chemokine Receptors and Their Role in Inflammation and Infectious Diseases. *Blood, Journal of the American Society of Hematology*, Vol.95, No.10, (May 2000), pp. 3032-3043, ISSN 0006-4971

Nabeshima, T., Thi Nga, P., Guillermo, P., Parquet Mdel, C., Yu, F., Thanh Thuy, N., Minh Trang, B., Tran Hien, N., Sinh Nam, V., Inoue, S., Hasebe, F. & Morita, K. (2008). Isolation and Molecular Characterization of Banna Virus from Mosquitoes, Vietnam. *Emerging Infectious Diseases*, Vol.14, No.8, (August 2008), pp. 1276-1279, ISSN: 1080-6059

Nayak, S. & Herzog, R. (2010). Progress and Prospects: Immune Responses to Viral Vectors. *Gene Therapy*, Vol.17, No.3, (March 2010), pp. 295-304, Erratum in: *Gene Therapy*, Vol.17, No.2, (February 2010), pp. 294, ISSN 0969-7128

Nelson, S., Crosbie, R., Miceli, M. & Spencer, M. (2009). Emerging Genetic Therapies to Treat Duchenne Muscular Dystrophy. *Current Opinion in Neurology*, Vol.22, No.5, (October 2009), pp. 532-538, ISSN 1350-7540

Neumann, E., Schaefer-Ridder, M., Wang, Y. & Hofschneider, P. (1982). Gene Transfer into Mouse Lyoma Cells by Electroporation in High Electric fields. *The EMBO Journal*, Vol.1, No.7, (1982), pp. 841-845, ISSN 0261-4189

Nibert, M., Furlong, D. & Fields, B. (1991). Mechanisms of Viral Pathogenesis. Distinct Forms of Reoviruses and Their Roles during Replication in Cells and Host. *The Journal of Clinical Investigation*, Vol.88, No.3, (September 1991), pp. 727-734, ISSN 0021-9738

Niidome, T. & Huang L. (2002). Gene Therapy Progress and Prospects: Nonviral Vectors. *Gene Therapy*, Vol.9, No.24, (December 2002), pp. 1647-1652, ISSN 0969-7128

Nishio, H., Takeshima, Y., Narita, N., Yanagawa, H., Suzuki, Y., Ishikawa, Y., Ishikawa, Y., Minami, R., Nakamura, H. & Matsuo, M. (1994). Identification of a Novel First Exon in the Human Dystrophin Gene and of a New Promoter Located More than 500 kb Upstream of the Nearest Known Promoter. *Journal of Clinical Investigation*, Vol.94, No.3, (September 1994), pp. 1037-1042, ISSN 0021-9738

Norkin, L. (1995). Virus Receptors: Implications for Pathogenesis and the Design of Antiviral Agents. *Clinical Microbiology Reviews*, Vol.8, No.2, (April 1995), pp. 293-315, ISSN 0893-8512

Notini, A., Craig, J. & White, S. (2008). Copy Number Variation and Mosaicism. *Cytogenetic and Genome Research*, Vol.123, No.1-4, (2008), pp. 270-277, ISSN 1424-8581

Nuttall, P. & Moss, S. (1989). Genetic Reassortment Indicates a New Grouping for Tick-borne Orbiviruses. *Virology*, Vol.171, No.1, (July 1989), pp. 156-161, ISSN 0042-6822

O'Brien, S., Menotti-Raymond, M., Murphy, W., Nash, W., Wienberg, J., Stanyon, R., Copeland, N., Jenkins, N., Womack, J. & Marshall Graves, J. (1999). The Promise of Comparative Genomics in Mammals. *Science*, Vol.286, No.5439, (October 1999), pp. 458-462, 479-481, ISSN 0036-8075

Octaviani, C., Li, C., Noda, T. & Kawaoka, Y. (2011). Reassortment between Seasonal and Swine-origin H1N1 Influenza Viruses Generates Viruses with Enhanced Growth Capability in Cell Culture. *Virus Research*, Vol.156, No.1-2, (March 2011), pp. 147-150, ISSN 0168-1702

Osawa, M., Hanada, K., Hamada, H. & Nakauchi, H. (1996). Long-term Lymphohematopoietic Reconstitution by a Single CD34-low/Negative Hematopoietic Stem Cell. *Science*, Vol.273, No.5272, (July 1996), pp. 242-245, ISSN 0036-8075

Park, H., Kim, J., Ju, Y., Gokcumen, O., Mills, R., Kim, S., Lee, S., Suh, D., Hong, D., Kang, H., Yoo, Y., Shin, J., Kim, H., Yavartanoo, M., Chang, Y., Ha, J., Chong, W., Hwang, G., Darvishi, K., Kim, H., Yang, S., Yang, K., Kim, H., Hurles, M., Scherer, S., Carter, N., Tyler-Smith, C., Lee, C. & Seo, J. (2010). Discovery of Common Asian Copy Number Variants Using Integrated High-resolution Array CGH and Massively Parallel DNA Sequencing. *Nature Genetics*, Vol.42, No.5, (May 2010), pp. 400-405, ISSN 1061-4036

Park, I., Zhao, R., West, J., Yabuuchi, A., Huo, H., Ince, T., Lerou, P., Lensch, M. & Daley, G. (2008). Reprogramming of Human Somatic Cells to Pluripotency with Defined Factors. *Nature*, Vol.451, No.7175, (January 2008), pp. 141-146, ISSN 0028-0836

Parmar, K., D'Andrea, A. & Niedernhofer, L. (2009). Mouse Models of Fanconi Anemia. *Mutation Research - Fundamental and Molecular Mechanisms of Mutagenesis*, Vol.668, No.1-2, (July 2009), pp. 133-140, ISSN 0027-5107

Pastan, I. & Gottesman, M. (1987). Multidrug Resistance in Human Cancer. *The New England Journal of Medicine*, Vol.316, No.22, (May 1987), pp. 1388-1393, ISSN 0028-4793

Pawliuk, R., Westerman, K., Fabry, M., Payen, E., Tighe, R., Bouhassira, E., Acharya, S., Ellis, J., London, I., Eaves, C., Humphries, R., Beuzard, Y., Nagel, R. & Leboulch, P. (2001). Correction of Sickle Cell Disease in Transgenic Mouse Models by Gene Therapy. *Science*, Vol.294, No.5550, (December 2001), pp. 2368-2371, ISSN 0036-8075

Pennisi E. (1998). Training Viruses to Attack Cancers. *Science*, Vol.282, No.5392, (November 1998), pp. 1244-1246, ISSN 0036-8075

Peters, C. (2005). Marburg and Ebola--Arming Ourselves against the Deadly Filoviruses. *The New England Journal of Medicine*, Vol.352, No.25, (June 2005), pp. 2571-2573, ISSN 0028-4793

Piotrowski, A., Bruder, C., Andersson, R., Diaz de Ståhl, T., Menzel, U., Sandgren, J., Poplawski, A., von Tell, D., Crasto, C., Bogdan, A., Bartoszewski, R., Bebok, Z., Krzyzanowski, M., Jankowski, Z., Partridge, E., Komorowski, J. & Dumanski, J. (2008). Somatic Mosaicism for Copy Number Variation in Differentiated Human Tissues. *Human Mutation*, Vol.29, No.9, (September 2008), pp. 1118-1124, ISSN 1059-7794

Pitisuttithum, P., Tansuphasawadikul, S., Simpson, A., Howe, P. & White, N. (2001). A Prospective Study of AIDS-associated Cryptococcal Meningitis in Thailand Treated with High-dose Amphotericin B. *Journal of Infection*, Vol.43, No.4, (November 2001), pp. 226-233, ISSN 0163-4453

Qasim, W., Gaspar, H. & Thrasher, A. (2009). Progress and Prospects: Gene Therapy for Inherited Immunodeficiencies. *Gene Therapy*, Vol.16, No.11, (November 2009), pp. 1285–1291, ISSN 0969-7128

Rambaut, A., Pybus, O., Nelson, M., Viboud, C., Taubenberger, J. & Holmes, E. (2008). The Genomic and Epidemiological Dynamics of Human Influenza A Virus. *Nature*, Vol.453, No.7195, (May 2008), pp. 615-619, ISSN 0028-0836

Ramesh, N., Antón, I., Hartwig, J. & Geha, R. (1997). WIP, a Protein Associated with Wiskott-Aldrich Syndrome Protein, Induces Actin Polymerization and Redistribution in Lymphoid Cells. *Proceedings of the National Academy of Sciences*, Vol.94, No.26, (December 1997), pp. 14671-14676, ISSN 0027-8424

Raper, S., Chirmule, N., Lee, F., Wivel, N., Bagg, A., Gao, G., Wilson, J. & Batshaw M. (2003). Fatal Systemic Inflammatory Response Syndrome in a Ornithine Transcarbamylase Deficient Patient following Adenoviral Gene Transfer. *Molecular Genetics and Metabolism,* Vol.80, No.1-2, (September-October 2003), pp.148-158, ISSN 1096-7192

Reid, S., Schindler, D., Hanenberg, H., Barker, K., Hanks, S., Kalb, R., Neveling, K., Kelly, P., Seal, S., Freund, M., Wurm, M., Batish, S., Lach, F., Yetgin, S., Neitzel, H., Ariffin, H., Tischkowitz, M., Mathew, C., Auerbach, A. & Rahman, N. (2007). Biallelic Mutations in PALB2 Cause Fanconi Anemia Subtype FA-N and Predispose to Childhood Cancer. *Nature Genetics,* Vol.39, No.2, (February 2007), pp. 162-164, ISSN 1061-4036

Ridinger, D., Spendlove, R., Barnett, B., George, D. & Roth, J. (1982). Evaluation of Cell Lines and Immunofluorescence and Plaque Assay Procedures for Quantifying Reoviruses in Sewage. *Applied and Environmental Microbiology,* Vol.43, No.4, (April 1982), pp. 740-746, ISSN 0099-2240

Riordan, J., Deuchars, K., Kartner, N., Alon, N., Trent, J. & Ling, V. (1985). Amplification of P-glycoprotein Genes in Multidrug-resistant Mammalian Cell Lines. *Nature,* Vol.*316,* No.6031, (August 1985). pp. 817–819, ISSN 0028-0836

Riordan, J., Rommens, J., Kerem, B-S., Alon, N., Rozmahel, R., Grzelczak, Z., Zielenski, J., Lok, S., Plavsic, N., Chou, J-L., Drumm, M., Iannuzzi, M., Collins, F. & Tsui, L-C. (1989). Identification of the Cystic Fibrosis Gene: Cloning and Characterization of Complementary DNA. *Science,* Vol.245, No.4922 (September 1989), pp. 1066-1073, Erratum in: *Science,* Vol.*245,* No.4925, (September 1989), pp. 1437, ISSN 0036-8075

Roberts R. (2001). Dystrophins and Dystrobrevins. *Genome Biology,* Vol.2, No.4, (April 2001), pp. reviews3006.1–reviews3006.7, ISSN 1465-6906

Robertson, E., Bradley, A., Kuehn, M. & Evans, M. (1986). Germ-line Transmission of Genes Introduced into Cultured Pluripotential Cells by Retroviral Vector. *Nature,* Vol.323, No.6087, (October 1986), pp. 445-448, ISSN 0028-0836

Rocha, V., Labopin, M., Sanz, G., Arcese, W., Schwerdtfeger, R., Bosi, A., Jacobsen, N., Ruutu, T., de Lima, M., Finke, J., Frassoni, F., Gluckman, E., Acute Leukemia Working Party of European Blood and Marrow Transplant Group & Eurocord-Netcord Registry. (2004). Transplants of Umbilical-cord Blood or Bone Marrow from Unrelated Donors in Adults with Acute Leukemia. *The New England Journal of Medicine,* Vol.351, No.22, (November 2004), pp. 2276-2285, ISSN 0028-4793

Rogaev, E., Sherrington, R., Rogaeva, E., Levesque, G., Ikeda, M., Liang, Y., Chi, H., Lin, C., Holman, K., Tsuda, T., Mar, L., Sorbi, S., Nacmias, B., Piacentini, S., Amaducci, L., Chumakov, I., Cohen, D., Lannfelt, L., Fraser, P., Rommens, J. & St George-Hyslop, P. (1995). Familial Alzheimer's Disease in Kindreds with Missense Mutations in a Gene on Chromosome 1 Related to the Alzheimer's Disease Type 3 Gene. *Nature,* Vol.376, No.6543, (August 1995), pp. 775-778, ISSN 1061-4036

Rommens, J., Iannuzzi, M., Kerem, B-S., Drumm, M., Melmer, G., Dean, M., Rozmahel, R., Cole, J., Kennedy, D., Hidaka, N., Zsiga, M., Buchwald, M., Riordan, J., Tsui, L-C. & Collins, F. (1989). Identification of the Cystic Fibrosis Gene: Chromosome Walking and Jumping. *Science,* Vol.245, No.4922, (September 1989), pp. 1059-1065, ISSN 0036-8075

Rouquet, P., Froment, J., Bermejo, M., Kilbourn, A., Karesh, W., Reed, P., Kumulungui, B., Yaba, P., Délicat, A., Rollin, P. & Leroy, E. (2005). Wild Animal Mortality Monitoring and Human Ebola Outbreaks, Gabon and Republic of Congo, 2001-

2003. *Emerging Infectious Diseases*, Vol.11, No.2, (February 2005), pp. 283-290, ISSN 1080-6059

Rowntree, R. & Harris, A. (2003). The Phenotypic Consequences of CFTR Mutations. *Annals of Human Genetics*, Vol.67, No.part 5, (September 2003), pp. 471-485, ISSN 0003-4800

Rozee, K. & Easterbrook, K. (1970). Application of Freeze-etching Method to the Study of Reovirus-infected LLC-MK2 Cells. *Applied Microbiology*, Vol.19, No.6, (June 1970), pp. 997-1000, ISSN 0099-2240

Sakharkar, M., Chow, V. & Kangueane, P. (2004). Distributions of Exons and Introns in the Human Genome. *In Silico Biology*, Vol.4, No.4, (June 2004), pp. 387-393, ISSN 1434-3207

Schiff, L., Nibert, M & Tyler, K. (2007). Orthoreoviruses and Their Replication, In: *Fields Virology, 5th Edition, Volume One,* David M. Knipe, Peter M. Howley, Diane E. Griffin, Robert A. Lamb, Malcolm A. Martin, Bernard Roizman, pp.2388-2471, Lippincott Williams & Wilkins, ISBN-10 0781760607, Philadelphia, USA

Seggewiss, R., Pittaluga, S., Adler, R., Guenaga, F., Ferguson, C., Pilz, I., Ryu, B., Sorrentino, B., Young, W 3rd., Donahue, R., von Kalle, C., Nienhuis, A. & Dunbar, C. (2006). Acute Myeloid Leukemia Is Associated with Retroviral Gene Transfer to Hematopoietic Progenitor Cells in a Rhesus Macaque. *Blood, Journal of the American Society of Hematology,* Vol.107, No.10, (May 2006), pp. 3865-3867, ISSN 0006-4971

Selb, B. & Weber, B. (1994). A Study of Human Reovirus IgG and IgA Antibodies by ELISA and Western Blot. *Journal of Virological Methods,* Vol.47, No.1-2, (April 1994), pp. 15–25, ISSN 0166-0934

Sherrington, R., Rogaev, E., Liang, Y., Rogaeva, E., Levesque, G., Ikeda, M., Chi, H., Lin, C., Li, G., Holman, K., Tsuda, T., Mar, L., Foncin, J., Bruni, A., Montesi, M., Sorbi, S., Rainero, I., Pinessi, L., Nee, L., Chumakov, I., Pollen, D., Brookes, A., Sanseau, P., Polinsky, R., Wasco, W., Da Silva, H., Haines, J., Perkicak-Vance, M., Tanzi, R., Roses, A., Fraser, P., Rommens, J., St George-Hyslop, P.(1995). Cloning of a Gene Bearing Missense Mutations in Early-onset Familial Alzheimer's Disease. *Nature,* Vol.375, No.6534, (June 1995), pp. 754-760, ISSN 1061-4036

Siminovitch, L., McCulloch, E. & Till, J. (1963). The Distribution of Colony-forming Cells among Spleen Colonies. *Journal of Cellular and Comparative Physiology*, Vol.62, No.3, (December 1963), pp. 327-336, ISSN 0095-9898

Smith, D., Lapedes, A., de Jong, J., Bestebroer, T., Rimmelzwaan, G., Osterhaus, A. & Fouchier, R. (2004). Mapping the Antigenic and Genetic Evolution of Influenza Virus. *Science*, Vol.305, No.5682, (July 2004), pp. 371-376, ISSN 0036-8075

Smogorzewska, A., Matsuoka, S., Vinciguerra, P., McDonald, E. 3rd., Hurov, K., Luo, J., Ballif, B., Gygi, S., Hofmann, K., D'Andrea, A. & Elledge, S. (2007). Identification of the FANCI Protein, a Monoubiquitinated FANCD2 Paralog Required for DNA Repair. *Cell*, Vol.129, No.2, (April 2007), pp. 289-301, ISSN 0092-8674

Somiari, S., Glasspool-Malone, J., Drabick, J., Gilbert, R., Heller, R., Jaroszeski, M. & Malone, R. (2000). Theory and in vivo Application of Electroporative Gene Delivery. *Molecular Therapy*, Vol.2, No.3, (September 2000), pp. 178-187, ISSN 1525-0016

Song, L., Chen, B. & Zhao Z. (1995). Isolation and Identification of New Members of Coltivirus from Mosquitoes Collected in China. *Chinese Journal of Experimental and Clinical Virology*, Vol.9, No.1, (March 1995), pp. 7-10, ISSN 1003-9279

Song, L. & Chen, B. (1995). Arboviral Encephalitides (I). *Chinese Journal of Vector Biology and Control*, Vol.6, No.6, (December 1995), pp. 477-480, ISSN 1003-4692

Song, L. & Chen, B. (1996). Arboviral Encephalitides (II). *Chinese Journal of Vector Biology and Control*, Vol.7, No.1, (February 1996), pp. 66-69, ISSN 1003-4692

Song, L., Ohnuma, T. & Holland, J. (1999a). Effect of Trehalose on Cell Kills Effects of Anticancer Agents or Hyperthermia against Human Tumor Cell Lines. *Mount Sinai Journal of Medicine*, Vol.66, No.5-6, (October/November 1999), pp. 388, ISSN 0027-2507

Song, L., Gelman, I., Holland, J. & Ohnuma, T. (1999b). Study of Reovirus-induced Cytopathic Effect (CPE) and Ras Protein in Human Tumor Cell Lines. *Mount Sinai Journal of Medicine*, Vol.66, No.5-6, (October/November 1999), pp. 388, ISSN 0027-2507

Song, L., Gelman, I., Holland, J. & Ohnuma, T. (2000). Study of Reovirus-induced Cytopathic Effect (CPE), Ras, Doublestranded RNA-activated Protein Kinase (PKR) and eIF2α in Human Tumor Cell Lines. *Proceedings of the American Association for Cancer Research*, Vol.41, (2000), pp. 350, ISSN 0569-2261

Song, L., Mandecki, W. & Goldman, E. (2003). Expression of Non-open Reading Frames Isolated from Phage Display due to Translation Reinitiation. *Journal of the Federation of American Societies for Experimental Biology*, Vol.17, No.12, (September 2003), pp. 1674-1681, ISSN 0892-6638

Song, L. (2009). A Possible Approach for Stem Cell Gene Therapy of Fanconi Anemia. *Current Gene Therapy*, Vol.9, No.1, (February 2009), pp. 26-32, ISSN 1566-5232

Song, L., Ohnuma, T., Gelman, I. & Holland, J. (2009). Reovirus Infection of Cancer Cells Is Not due to Activated Ras Pathway. *Cancer Gene Therapy*, Vol.16, No.4, (April 2009), pp. 382, ISSN 0929-1903

Song, L. (2010). Comment on the AACR News of "Reovirus May Be a Novel Approach to Prostate Cancer Treatment, March 9, 2010", In: *AACR News*, March 9, 2010, 06.06.2011, Available from: http://aacrnews.wordpress.com/2010/03/09/reovirus-may-be-a-novel-approach-to-prostate-cancer-treatment/#comments

Song, L-H., Zhou, Y., He, J., Zhu, H., Huang, R., Mao, P. & Duan, Q. (2008). Comparative Sequence Analyses of a New Mammalian Reovirus Genome and the Mammalian Reovirus S1 Genes from Six New Serotype 2 Human Isolates. *Virus Genes*, Vol.37, No.3, (December 2008), pp. 392-399, ISSN 0920-8569

Spangrude, G., Heimfeld, S. & Weissman, I. (1988). Purification and Characterization of Mouse Hematopoietic Stem Cells. *Science*, Vol.241, No.4861, (July 1988), pp. 58-62, Erratum in: *Science*, Vol.244, No.4908, (June 1989), pp. 1030, ISSN 0036-8075

Stanford, K., Etrie, W. & Likely, G. (1948). The Growth in vitro of Single Isolated Tissue Cells. *The Journal of the National Cancer Institute*, Vol.9, No.3, (December 1948), pp. 229–246, ISSN 0027-8874

Stegemann, S. & Bock, R. (2009). Exchange of Genetic Material between Cells in Plant Tissue Grafts. *Science*, Vol.324, No.5927, (May 2009), pp. 649-651, ISSN 0036-8075

Stoepker, C., Hain, K., Schuster, B., Hilhorst-Hofstee, Y., Rooimans, M., Steltenpool, J., Oostra, A., Eirich, K., Korthof, E., Nieuwint, A., Jaspers, N., Bettecken, T., Joenje, H., Schindler, D., Rouse, J. & de Winter, J. (2011). SLX4, a Coordinator of Structure-specific Endonucleases, Is Mutated in a New Fanconi Anemia Subtype. *Nature Genetics*, Vol.43, No.2, (February 2011), pp. 142-146, ISSN: 1061-4036

Sun, Y., Qin, K., Wang, J., Pu, J., Tang, Q., Hu, Y., Bi, Y., Zhao, X., Yang, H., Shu, Y. & Liu, J. (2011). High Genetic Compatibility and Increased Pathogenicity of Reassortants Derived from Avian H9N2 and Pandemic H1N1/2009 Influenza Viruses. *Proceedings of the National Academy of Sciences*, Vol.108, No.10, (March 2011), pp. 4164-4169, ISSN 0027-8424

Sutlu, T. & Alici, E. (2009). Natural Killer Cell-based Immunotherapy in Cancer: Current Insights and Future Prospects. *Journal of Internal Medicine*, Vol.266, No.2, (August 2009), pp. 154-181, ISSN 0954-6820

Swann, J. & Smyth, M. (2007). Immune Surveillance of Tumors. *The Journal of Clinical Investigation*, Vol.117, No.5, (May 2007), pp. 1137-1146, ISSN 0021-9738

Tai, J., Williams, J., Edwards, K., Wright, P., Crowe, J. Jr. & Dermody, T. (2005). Prevalence of Reovirus-specific Antibodies in Young Children in Nashville, Tennessee. *The Journal of Infectious Diseases*, Vol.191, No.8, (April 2005), pp. 1221-1224, ISSN 1537-6613

Takahashi, K., Tanabe, K., Ohnuki, M., Narita, M., Ichisaka, T., Tomoda, K. & Yamanaka, S. (2007). Induction of Pluripotent Stem Cells from Adult Human Fibroblasts by Defined Factors. *Cell*, Vol.131, No.5, (November 2007), pp. 861-872, ISSN 0092-8674

Taniguchi, T. & D'Andrea, A. (2006). Molecular Pathogenesis of Fanconi Anemia: Recent Progress. *Blood, Journal of the American Society of Hematology*, Vol.107, No.11, (June 2006), pp. 4223-4233, ISSN 0006-4971

Tao, S., Cai, Z., Yang, D., Wang, H., Liu, Q., Fan, Y., Fan, X. & Chen, B. (1999). New Subtype of Coltivirus Isolated from Mosquitoes in the Northeast Part of China. *Chinese Journal of Experimental and Clinical Virology*, Vol.13, No.3, (Septmember 1999), pp. 228-230, ISSN 1003-9279

Tatum, E. & Lederberg J. (1947). Gene Recombination in the Bacterium Escherichia coli. *Journal of Bacteriology*, Vol.53, No.6, (June 1947), pp. 673-684, ISSN 0021-9193

Terry, L., Shows, E. & Wente, S. (2007). Crossing the Nuclear Envelope: Hierarchical Regulation of Nucleocytoplasmic Transport. *Science*. Vol.318, No.5855, (November 2007), pp. 1412-1416, ISSN 0036-8075

Terzi, D. & Zachariou, V. (2008). Adeno-associated Virus-mediated Gene Delivery Approaches for the Treatment of CNS Disorders. *Biotechnology Journal*, Vol.3, No.12, (December 2008), pp. 1555-1563, ISSN 1860-7314

Tesson, L., Cozzi, J., Ménoret, S., Rémy, S., Usal, C., Fraichard, A. & Anegon, I. (2005). Transgenic Modifications of the Rat Genome. *Transgenic Research*, Vol.14, No.5, (October 2005), pp. 531-546, ISSN 0962-8819

The 1000 Genomes Project Consortium. (2010). A Map of Human Genome Variation from Population-scale Sequencing. *Nature*, Vol.467, No.7319, (October 2010), pp. 1061-1073, ISSN 0028-0836

The 1000 Genomes Consortium. (2011). Mapping Copy Number Variation by Population-scale Genome. *Nature*, Vol.470, No. 7332, (February 2011), pp. 59-65, ISSN 0028-0836

Theerthagiri, G., Eisenhardt, N., Schwarz, H. & Antonin, W. (2010). The Nucleoporin Nup188 Controls Passage of Membrane Proteins across the Nuclear Pore Complex. *The Journal of Cell Biology*, Vol.189, No.7, (June 2010), pp. 1129-1142, ISSN 0021-9525

Thomson, J., Itskovitz-Eldor, J., Shapiro, S., Waknitz, M., Swiergiel, J., Marshall, V. & Jones, J. (1998). Embryonic Stem Cell Lines Derived from Human Blastocysts. *Science*, Vol.282, No.5391, (November 1998), pp. 1145-1147, Erratum in: *Science*, Vol.282, No.5395, (December 1998), pp. 1827, ISSN 0036-8075

Till, J., McCulloch, E. & Siminovitch, L. (1964). A Stochastic Model of Stem Cell Proliferation, Based on the Growth of Spleen Colony-forming Cells. *Proceedings of the National Academy of Sciences*, Vol.51, No.1, (January 1964), pp. 29–36, ISSN 0027-8424

Tischkowitz, M. & Hodgson, S. (2003). Fanconi Anaemia. *Journal of Medical Genetics*, Vol.40, No.1, (January 2003), pp. 1-10, ISSN 0022-2593

Tischkowitz, M., Easton, D., Ball, J., Hodgson, S. & Mathew, C. (2008). Cancer Incidence in Relatives of British Fanconi Anaemia Patients. *BMC Cancer*, Vol.8, (September 2008), pp. 257, doi: 10.1186/1471-2407-8-257, ISSN 1471-2407

Tran, E. & Wente, S. (2006). Dynamic Nuclear Pore Complexes: Life on the Edge. *Cell*, Vol.125, No.6, (June 2006), pp. 1041-1053, ISSN 0092-8674

Tran, V., Zhang, Z., Yagi, M., Nishiyama, A., Habara, Y., Takeshima, Y. & Matsuo, M. (2005). A Novel Cryptic Exon Identified in the 3' Region of Intron 2 of the Human Dystrophin Gene. *Journal of Human Genetics*, Vol.50, No.8, (2005), pp. 425-433, ISSN 1434-5161

Tycko, B. (1994). Genomic Imprinting: Mechanism and Role in Human Pathology. *The American Journal of Pathology*, Vol.144, No.3, (March 1994), pp. 431-443, ISSN 0002-9440

Tyler, K., Barton, E., Ibach, M., Robinson, C., Campbell, J., O'Donnell, S., Valyi-Nagy, T., Clarke, P., Wetzel, J. & Dermody, T. (2004). Isolation and Molecular Characterization of a Novel Type 3 Reovirus from a Child with Meningitis. *The Journal of Infectious Diseases*, Vol.189, No.9, (May 2004), pp. 1664-1675, ISSN 1537-6613

Vajta, G. & Gjerris, M. (2006). Science and Technology of Farm Animal Cloning: State of the Art. *Animal Reproduction Science*, Vol.92, No.3-4, (May 2006), pp. 211-230, ISSN 0378-4320

van den Wollenberg, D., van den Hengel, S., Dautzenberg, I., Cramer, S., Kranenburg, O. & Hoeben, R. (2008). A Strategy for Genetic Modification of the Spike-encoding Segment of Human Reovirus T3D for Reovirus Targeting. *Gene Therapy*, Vol.15, No.24, (December 2008), pp. 1567-1578, ISSN 0969-7128

van Houdt, W., Smakman, N., van den Wollenberg, D., Emmink, B., Veenendaal, L., van Diest, P., Hoeben, R., Borel Rinkes, I. & Kranenburg, O. (2008). Transient Infection of Freshly Isolated Human Colorectal Tumor Cells by Reovirus T3D Intermediate Subviral Particles. *Cancer Gene Therapy*, Vol.15, No.5, (May 2008), pp. 284-292, ISSN 0929-1903

Veeriah, S., Taylor, B., Meng, S., Fang, F., Yilmaz, E., Vivanco, I., Janakiraman, M., Schultz, N., Hanrahan, A., Pao, W., Ladanyi, M., Sander, C., Heguy, A., Holland, E., Paty, P., Mischel, P., Liau, L., Cloughesy, T., Mellinghoff, I., Solit, D. & Chan, T. (2010). Somatic Mutations of the Parkinson's Disease-associated Gene PARK2 in Glioblastoma and Other Human Malignancies. *Nature Genetics*, Vol.42, No.1, (January 2010), pp. 77-82, ISSN 1061-4036

Venter, J., Adams M., Myers, E., Li, P., Mural, R., Sutton, G., Smith, H., Yandell, M., Evans, C., Holt, R., Gocayne, J., Amanatides, P., Ballew, R., Huson, D., Wortman, J., Zhang, Q., Kodira, C., Zheng, X., Chen, L., Skupski, M., Subramanian, G., Thomas, P., Zhang, J., Gabor Miklos, G., Nelson, C., Broder, S., Clark, A., Nadeau, J., McKusick, V., Zinder, N., Levine, A., Roberts, R., Simon, M., Slayman, C., Hunkapiller, M., Bolanos, R., Delcher, A., Dew, I., Fasulo, D., Flanigan, M., Florea, L., Halpern, A., Hannenhalli, S., Kravitz, S., Levy, S., Mobarry, C., Reinert, K., Remington, K., Abu-Threideh, J., Beasley, E., Biddick, K., Bonazzi, V., Brandon, R., Cargill, M., Chandramouliswaran, I., Charlab, R., Chaturvedi, K., Deng, Z., Di Francesco, V., Dunn, P., Eilbeck, K., Evangelista, C., Gabrielian, A., Gan, W., Ge, W., Gong, F., Gu,

Z., Guan, P., Heiman, T., Higgins, M., Ji, R., Ke, Z., Ketchum, K., Lai, Z., Lei, Y., Li, Z., Li, J., Liang, Y., Lin, X., Lu, F., Merkulov, G., Milshina, N., Moore, H., Naik, A., Narayan, V., Neelam, B., Nusskern, D., Rusch, D., Salzberg, S., Shao, W., Shue, B., Sun, J., Wang, Z., Wang, A., Wang, X., Wang, J., Wei, M., Wides, R., Xiao, C., Yan, C., Yao, A., Ye, J., Zhan, M., Zhang, W., Zhang, H., Zhao, Q., Zheng, L., Zhong, F., Zhong, W., Zhu, S., Zhao, S., Gilbert, D., Baumhueter, S., Spier, G., Carter, C., Cravchik, A., Woodage, T., Ali, F., An, H., Awe, A., Baldwin, D., Baden, H., Barnstead, M., Barrow, I., Beeson, K., Busam, D., Carver, A., Center, A., Cheng, M., Curry, L., Danaher, S., Davenport, L., Desilets, R., Dietz, S., Dodson, K., Doup, L., Ferriera, S., Garg, N., Gluecksmann, A., Hart, B., Haynes, J., Haynes, C., Heiner, C., Hladun, S., Hostin, D., Houck, J., Howland, T., Ibegwam, C., Johnson, J., Kalush, F., Kline, L., Koduru, S., Love, A., Mann, F., May, D., McCawley, S., McIntosh, T., McMullen, I., Moy, M., Moy, L., Murphy, B., Nelson, K., Pfannkoch, C., Pratts, E., Puri, V., Qureshi, H., Reardon, M., Rodriguez, R., Rogers, Y., Romblad, D., Ruhfel, B., Scott, R., Sitter, C., Smallwood, M., Stewart, E., Strong, R., Suh, E., Thomas, R., Tint, N., Tse, S., Vech, C., Wang, G., Wetter, J., Williams, S., Williams M., Windsor, S., Winn-Deen, E., Wolfe, K., Zaveri, J., Zaveri, K., Abril, J., Guigó, R., Campbell, M., Sjolander, K., Karlak, B., Kejariwal, A., Mi, H., Lazareva, B., Hatton, T., Narechania, A., Diemer, K., Muruganujan, A., Guo, N., Sato, S., Bafna, V., Istrail, S., Lippert, R., Schwartz, R., Walenz, B., Yooseph, S., Allen, D., Basu, A., Baxendale, J., Blick, L., Caminha, M., Carnes-Stine, J., Caulk, P., Chiang, Y., Coyne, M., Dahlke, C., Mays, A., Dombroski, M., Donnelly, M., Ely, D., Esparham, S., Fosler, C., Gire, H., Glanowski, S., Glasser, K., Glodek, A., Gorokhov, M., Graham, K., Gropman, B., Harris, M., Heil, J., Henderson, S., Hoover, J., Jennings, D., Jordan, C., Jordan, J., Kasha, J., Kagan, L., Kraft, C., Levitsky, A., Lewis, M., Liu, X., Lopez, J., Ma, D., Majoros, W., McDaniel, J., Murphy, S., Newman, M., Nguyen, T., Nguyen, N., Nodell, M., Pan, S., Peck, J., Peterson, M., Rowe, W., Sanders, R., Scott, J., Simpson, M., Smith, T., Sprague, A., Stockwell, T., Turner, R., Venter, E., Wang, M., Wen, M., Wu, D., Wu, M., Xia, A., Zandieh, A. & Zhu, X. (2001) The Sequence of the Human Genome. *Science*, Vol.291, No.5507, (February 2001), pp. 1304–1351, ISSN 0036-8075

Vincent, A., Lager, K., Ma, W., Lekcharoensuk, P., Gramer, M., Loiacono, C. & Richt, J. (2006). Evaluation of Hemagglutinin Subtype 1 Swine Influenza Viruses from the United States. *Veterinary Microbiology*, Vol.118, No.3-4, (December 2006), pp. 212-222, ISSN 0378-1135

Virgin, S. (2007). Pathogenesis of Viral Infection. In: *Fields Virology, 5th Edition, Volume One,* David M. Knipe, Peter M. Howley, Diane E. Griffin, Robert A. Lamb, Malcolm A. Martin, Bernard Roizman, pp. 414-497, Lippincott Williams & Wilkins, ISBN-10: 0781760607, Philadelphia, USA

Wada, T., Schurman, S., Otsu, M., Garabedian, E., Ochs, H., Nelson, D. & Candotti, F. (2001). Somatic Mosaicism in Wiskott--Aldrich Syndrome Suggests in vivo Reversion by a DNA Slippage Mechanism. *Proceedings of the National Academy of Sciences*, Vol.98, No.15, (July 2001), pp. 8697-8702, ISSN 0027-8424

Wada, T., Konno, A., Schurman, S., Garabedian, E., Anderson, S., Kirby, M., Nelson, D. & Candotti, F. (2003). Second-site Mutation in the Wiskott-Aldrich Syndrome (WAS) Protein Gene Causes Somatic Mosaicism in Two WAS Siblings. *The Journal of Clinical Investigation*, Vol. 111, No.9, (May 2003), pp. 1389-1397, ISSN 0021-9738

Waisfisz, Q., Morgan, N., Savino, M., de Winter, J., van Berkel, C., Hoatlin, M., Ianzano, L., Gibson, R., Arwert, F., Savoia, A., Mathew, C., Pronk, J. & Joenje, H. (1999). Spontaneous Functional Correction of Homozygous Fanconi Anaemia Alleles Reveals Novel Mechanistic Basis for Reverse Mosaicism. *Nature Genetics,* Vol.22, No.4, (August 1999), pp. 379–383, ISSN 1061-4036

Wang, G., Bunnell, B., Painter, R., Quiniones, B., Tom, S., Lanson, N. Jr., Spees, J., Bertucci, D., Peister, A., Weiss, D., Valentine, V., Prockop, D. & Kolls, J. (2005). Adult Stem Cells from Bone Marrow Stroma Differentiate into Airway Epithelial Cells: Potential Therapy for Cystic Fibrosis. *Proceedings of the National Academy of Sciences,* Vol.102, No.1, (January 2005), pp. 186-191, ISSN 0027-8424

Wang, J., Wang, W., Li, R., Li, Y., Tian, G., Goodman, L., Fan, W., Zhang, J., Li, J., Zhang, J., Guo, Y., Feng, B., Li, H., Lu, Y., Fang, X., Liang, H., Du, Z., Li, D., Zhao, Y., Hu, Y., Yang, Z., Zheng, H., Hellmann, I., Inouye, M., Pool, J., Yi, X., Zhao, J., Duan, J., Zhou, Y., Qin, J., Ma, L., Li, G., Yang, Z., Zhang, G., Yang, B., Yu, C., Liang, F., Li, W., Li, S., Li, D., Ni, P., Ruan, J., Li, Q., Zhu, H., Liu, D., Lu, Z., Li, N., Guo, G., Zhang, J., Ye, J., Fang, L., Hao, Q., Chen, Q., Liang, Y., Su, Y., San, A., Ping, C., Yang, S., Chen, F., Li, L., Zhou, K., Zheng, H., Ren, Y., Yang, L., Gao, Y., Yang, G., Li, Z., Feng, X., Kristiansen, K., Wong, G., Nielsen, R., Durbin, R., Bolund, L., Zhang, X., Li, S., Yang, H. & Wang, J. (2008). The Diploid Genome Sequence of an Asian Individual. *Nature,* Vol.456, No.7218, (November 2008), pp. 60-65, ISSN 0028-0836

Wang, J., Chen P-J., Wang G. & Keller, L. (2010). Chromosome Size Differences May Affect Meiosis and Genome Size. *Science,* Vol.329, No.5989, (July 2010), pp. 293, ISSN 0036-8075

Webby, R., Swenson, S., Krauss, S., Gerrish, P., Goyal, S. & Webster, R. (2000). Evolution of Swine H3N2 Influenza Viruses in the United States. *Journal of Virology,* Vol.74, No.18, (September 2000), pp. 8243-8251, ISSN 0022-538X

Weil, C. (2002). Finding the Crosswalks on DNA. *Proceedings of the National Academy of Sciences,* Vol.99, No.9, (April 2002), pp. 5763-5765, ISSN 0027-8424

Weissman, I. & Shizuru, J. (2008). The Origins of the Identification and Isolation of Hematopoietic Stem Cells, and Their Capability to Induce Donor-specific Transplantation Tolerance and Treat Autoimmune Diseases. *Blood, Journal of the American Society of Hematology,* Vol.112, No.1, (November 2008), pp. 3543-3553, ISSN 0006-4971

Whitby, M. (2005). Making Crossovers during Meiosis. *Biochemical Society Transactions,* Vol.33, No.part 6, (December 2005), pp. 1451-1455, ISSN 0300-5127

Whitney, M., Thayer, M., Reifsteck, C., Olson, S., Smith, L., Jakobs, P., Leach, R., Naylor, S., Joenje, H. & Grompe, M. (1995). Microcell Mediated Chromosome Transfer Maps the Fanconi Anaemia Group D Gene to Chromosome 3p. *Nature Genetics,* Vol.11, No.3, (November 1995), pp. 341-343, ISSN 1061-4036

Willadsen, S. (1986). Nuclear Transplantation in Sheep Embryos. *Nature,* Vol.320, No.6057, (March 1986), pp. 63-65, ISSN 0028-0836

Willers, H., Dahm-Daphi, J. & Powell, S. (2004). Repair of Radiation Damage to DNA. *British Journal of Cancer,* Vol.90, No.7, (April 2004), pp. 1297-1301, ISSN 0007-0920

Wilmut, I., Schnieke, A., McWhir, J., Kind, A. & Campbell, K. (1997). Viable Offspring Derived from Fetal and Adult Mammalian Cells. *Nature,* Vol.385, No.6619, (February 1997), pp. 810–813, ISSN 0028-0836

Wilson, A., Murphy, M., Oskarsson, T., Kaloulis, K., Bettess, M., Oser, G., Pasche, A., Knabenhans, C., Macdonald, H. & Trumpp, A. (2004). c-Myc Controls the Balance between Hematopoietic Stem Cell Self-renewal and Differentiation. *Genes & Development*, Vol.18, No.22, (November 2004), pp. 2747-2763, ISSN 0890-9369

Wu, L., Sun, C., Ryan, T., Pawlik, K., Ren, J. & Townes, T. (2006). Correction of Sickle Cell Disease by Homologous Recombination in Embryonic Stem Cells. *Blood, Journal of the American Society of Hematology*, Vol.108, No.4, (August 2006), pp. 1183-1188, ISSN 0006-4971

Xia, Q., Zhou, Z., Lu, C., Cheng, D., Dai, F., Li, B., Zhao, P., Zha, X., Cheng, T., Chai, C., Pan, G., Xu, J., Liu, C., Lin, Y., Qian, J., Hou, Y., Wu, Z., Li, G., Pan, M., Li, C., Shen, Y., Lan, X., Yuan, L., Li, T., Xu, H., Yang, G., Wan, Y., Zhu, Y., Yu, M., Shen, W., Wu, D., Xiang, Z., Yu, J., Wang, J., Li, R., Shi, J., Li, H., Li, G., Su, J., Wang, X., Li, G., Zhang, Z., Wu, Q., Li, J., Zhang, Q., Wei, N., Xu, J., Sun, H., Dong, L., Liu, D., Zhao, S., Zhao, X., Meng, Q., Lan, F., Huang, X., Li, Y., Fang, L., Li, C., Li, D., Sun, Y., Zhang, Z., Yang, Z., Huang, Y., Xi, Y., Qi, Q., He, D., Huang, H., Zhang, X., Wang, Z., Li, W., Cao, Y., Yu, Y., Yu, H., Li, J., Ye, J., Chen, H., Zhou, Y., Liu, B., Wang, J., Ye, J., Ji, H., Li, S., Ni, P., Zhang, J., Zhang, Y., Zheng, H., Mao, B., Wang, W., Ye, C., Li, S., Wang, J., Wong, G. & Yang, H. (2004). A Draft Sequence for the Genome of the Domesticated Silkworm (Bombyx mori). *Science*, Vol.306, No.5703, (December 2004), pp. 1937-1940, ISSN 0036-8075

Xu, L., Tao, S., Cao, Y., Wang, H., Yang, D., He, Y., Liu, Q. & Chen, B. (2003). Genotyping of the Chinese Isolates of Coltivirus. *Chinese Journal of Experimental and Clinical Virology*, Vol.17, No.4, (December 2003), pp. 346-350, ISSN 1003-9279

Xu, P., Wang, Y., Zuo, J., Lin, J. & Xu, P-M. (1990). New Arboviruses Isolated from Patients with Unknown Fever and Encephalitis in Yunnan Province. *Chinese Journal of Virology*, Vol.6, No.1, (1990), pp. 27-33, ISSN 1000-8721

Xu, X., Smith, C., Mungall, B., Lindstrom, S., Hall, H., Subbarao, K., Cox, N. & Klimov, A. (2002). Intercontinental Circulation of Human Influenza A (H1N2) Reassortant Viruses during the 2001-2002 Influenza Season. *The Journal of Infectious Diseases*, Vol.186, No.10, (November 2002), pp. 1490-1493, ISSN 0022-1899

Xu, X., Lindstrom, S., Shaw, M., Smith, C., Hall, H., Mungall, B., Subbarao, K., Cox, N. & Klimov, A. (2004). Reassortment and Evolution of Current Human Influenza A and B Viruses. *Virus Research*, Vol.103, No.1-2, (July 2004), pp. 55-60, ISSN 0168-1702

Yamaizumi, M., Horwich, A. & Ruddle, F. (1983). Expression and Stabilization of Microinjected Plasmids Containing the Herpes Simplex Virus Thymidine Kinase Gene and Polyoma Virus DNA in Mouse Cells. *Molecular and Cellular Biology*, Vol.3, No.4, (April 1983), pp. 511-522, ISSN 1098-5549

Yang, S., Cheng, P., Banta, H., Piotrowska-Nitsche, K., Yang, J., Cheng, E., Snyder, B., Larkin, K., Liu, J., Orkin, J., Fang, Z., Smith, Y., Bachevalier, J., Zola, S., Li, S., Li, X. & Chan, A. (2008). Towards a Transgenic Model of Huntington's Disease in a Non-human Primate. *Nature*, Vol.453, No.7197, (June 2008), pp. 921-924, ISSN 0028-0836

Yim, S., Kim, T., Hu, H., Kim, J., Kim, B., Lee, J., Han, B., Shin, S., Jung, S. & Chung, Y. (2010). Copy Number Variations in East-Asian Population and Their Evolutionary and Functional Implications. *Human Molecular Genetics*, Vol.19, No.6, (March 2010), pp. 1001-1008, ISSN 0964-6906

Yin, W., Barkess, G., Fang, X., Xiang, P., Cao, H., Stamatoyannopoulos, G. & Li, Q. (2007). Histone Acetylation at the Human beta-globin Locus Changes with Developmental

Age. *Blood, Journal of the American Society of Hematology,* Vo.110, No.12, (December 2007), pp. 4101-4107, ISSN 0006-4971

You, Z., Wang, Y., Zhao, Z-G., He, Y., Xu, P., Zhao, Z., Cheng, Y., Cheng, W. & Zhang, H. (1990). Isolation and Identification of Two Strains of Orbivirus in Hainan Province. *Chinese Journal of Virology,* Vol.6, No.3, (1990), pp. 272-276, ISSN 1000-8721

Young, W., Merz, T., Ferguson-Smith, M. & Johnston, A. (1960). Chromosome Number of the Chimpanzee, Pan troglodytes. *Science,* Vol.131, No.3414, (June 1960), pp. 1672-1673, ISSN 0036-8075

Youssoufian, H. & Pyeritz, R. (2002). Mechanisms and Consequences of Somatic Mosaicism in Humans. *Nature Reviews Genetics,* Vol.3, No.10, (October 2002), pp. 748-758, ISSN 1471-0056

Yu, J., Vodyanik, M., Smuga-Otto, K., Antosiewicz-Bourget, J., Frane, J., Tian, S., Nie, J., Jonsdottir, G., Ruotti, V., Stewart, R., Slukvin, I. & Thomson, J. (2007). Induced Pluripotent Stem Cell Lines Derived from Human Somatic Cells. *Science,* Vol.318, No.5858, (December 2007), pp. 1917-1920, ISSN 0036-8075

Yu, X-J., Liang, M-F., Zhang, S-Y., Liu, Y., Li, J-D., Sun, Y-L., Zhang, L., Zhang, Q-F., Popov, V., Li, C., Qu, J., Li, Q., Zhang, Y-P., Hai, R., Wu, W., Wang, Q., Zhan, F-X., Wang, X-J., Kan, B., Wang, S-W., Wan, K-L., Jing, H-Q., Lu, J-X., Yin, W-W., Zhou, H., Guan, X-H., Liu, J-F., Bi, Z-Q., Liu, G-H., Ren, J., Wang, H., Zhao, Z., Song, J-D., He, J-R., Wan, T., Zhang, J-S., Fu, X-P., Sun, L-N., Dong, X-P., Feng, Z-J., Yang, W-Z., Hong, T., Zhang, Y., Walker, D., Wang, Y. & Li, D-X. (2011). Fever with Thrombocytopenia Associated with a Novel Bunyavirus in China. *The New England Journal of Medicine,* Vol.364, No.16, (April 2011), pp. 1523-1532, ISSN 0028-4793

Zhang, Z., Habara, Y., Nishiyama, A., Oyazato, Y., Yagi, M., Takeshima, Y. & Matsuo, M. (2007). Identification of Seven Novel Cryptic Exons Embedded in the Dystrophin Gene and Characterization of 14 Cryptic Dystrophin Exons. *Journal of Human Genetics,* Vol.52, No.7, (July 2007), pp. 607-617, ISSN 1434-5161

Zhao, T., Zhang, Z., Rong, Z. & Xu, Y. (2011). Immunogenicity of Induced Pluripotent Stem Cells. *Nature,* Vol.474, No.7350, (May 2011), pp. 212-215, ISSN 0028-0836

Zhou, N., Senne, D., Landgraf, J., Swenson, S., Erickson, G., Rossow, K., Liu, L., Yoon, K., Krauss, S. & Webster, R. (1999). Genetic Reassortment of Avian, Swine, and Human Influenza A Viruses in American Pigs. *Journal of Virology,* Vol.73, No.10, (October 1999), pp. 8851-8856, ISSN 0022-538X

Zhu, Q., Watanabe, C., Liu, T., Hollenbaugh, D., Blaese, R., Kanner, S., Aruffo, A., Ochs, H. (1997). Wiskott-Aldrich Syndrome/X-linked Thrombocytopenia: WASP Gene Mutations, Protein Expression, and Phenotype. *Blood, Journal of the American Society of Hematology,* Vol.90, No.7, (October 1997), pp. 2680-2689, ISSN 0006-4971

Zielenski, J. (2000). Genotype and Phenotype in Cystic Fibrosis. *Respiration,* Vol.67, No.2, (2000), pp. 117-133, ISSN 0025-7931

7

Non Viral Gene Transfer Approaches for Lysosomal Storage Disorders

Ursula Matte, Guilherme Baldo and Roberto Giugliani
Hospital de Clinicas de Porto Alegre
Brazil

1. Introduction

The lysosomal storage disorders (LSDs) are a group of almost 50 genetic diseases, characterized by mutations and loss of activity of lysosomal enzymes or, less frequently, non-lysosomal proteins that are involved in protein maturation or lysosomal biogenesis (Meikle et al, 2004). Most LSDs have an autosomal recessive inheritance, with some exceptions as Hunter syndrome (X-linked recessive), Danon disease (X-linked dominant) and Fabry disease (X-linked with a high proportion of heterozygous affected females).

Storage of distinct undegraded or partially degraded material, usually the substrate of the defective enzyme, occurs in the lysosome. The substrate type is used to group the LSDs into general categories (table 1), including mucopolysaccharidoses (characterized by the storage of mucopolysaccharides, also called glycosaminoglycans), lipidoses (storage of lipids), glycogenoses (storage of glycogen) and oligosaccharidoses (storage of small sugar chains). Despite this categorization, many clinical similarities are observed between groups as well as within each group. Generally these diseases are multisystemic, and clinical features of many LSDs include organomegaly, central nervous system dysfunction and coarse hair and faces. Most LSDs are characterized by their progressive course with high morbidity and increased mortality, although there are significant variations between different diseases, and even among patients with the same disease (Walkley 2009). Lysosomal enzymes are ubiquitously distributed, but substrate storage is usually restricted to cells, tissues and organs with higher substrate turnover.

Recently, it has been suggested that the primary gene defect and substrate storage are triggers of a complex cascade of events that lead to many of the disease manifestations (Bellettato & Scarpa, 2010). In this context, secondary substrate storage, perturbations of Calcium homeostasis and lipid trafficking would contribute to disease pathogenesis. Other manifestations, related to the lysosome's role in vescicle trafficking, including antigen presentation, innate immunity, and signal transduction would cause inflammatory and auto-immune disturbances observed in the LSD (Parkinson-Lawrence et al., 2010). In addition, general mechanisms such as unfolded protein response, reticulum stress, oxidative stress and autophagy blockade would also play a role in the pathogenesis (Vitner et al., 2010).

The incidence and prevalence of these diseases varies from different countries and regions. For example, the overall incidence of GM1 Gangliosidosis is considered to be 1:100,000-

1:200,000, however in some countries as Malta (1:3,700) and the South of Brazil (1:13,317) it is considerably higher (Baiotto et al, 2011). Large population studies suggest that the overall incidence of the LSDs vary from 1:5,000- 1:7,700 (Fuller et al, 2006).
The treatment options available for the LSDs were restricted to support measures until a few decades ago. Nowadays, specific treatments are available for a certain number of LSDs, even though some of them are still in the experimental phase or have limited effects. Treatment options listed in table 1 consider those already approved or under clinical trial, including compassionate use. Support measures and palliative care are not considered treatment options in this context.

Disease	OMIM	Gene	Enzyme	Available Treatments
Aspartylglucosaminuria	208400	*AGA*	N-aspartyl-beta-glucosaminidase	HSCT
Canavan disease	271900	*ASPA*	Aspartocylase	None
Cystinosis	219800	*CTNS*	Cystinosin	Cysteamine (drug)
Danon disease	300257	*LAMP2*	Lysosomal-associated membrane protein 2	None
Fabry disease	301500	*GLA*	A-galactosidase A	ERT
Farber disease	228000	*ASAH1*	Ceramidase	HSCT
Fucosidosis	230000	*FUCA1*	α-L-fucosidase	HSCT
Galactosialidosis	256540	*CTSA*	Cathepsin A	None
Gaucher disease	230800	*GBA*	acid β-glucosidase	ERT, GT, HSCT, PCT, SSI
GM1 gangliosidosis	230600	*GLB1*	β-Galactosidase	HSCT
Krabbe disease	245200	*GALC*	galactocerebrosidase	HSCT
Lysosomal Acid Lipase Deficiency	278000	*LIPA*	Lysosomal acid lipase	HSCT
α- mannosidosis	248500	*MAN2B1*	α -D -mannosidase	HSCT
β- mannosidosis	248510	*MANBA*	β -D-mannosidase	None
Metachromatic leucodystrophy	250100	*ARSA*	Arylsulphatase-A	HSCT
Metachromatic leucodystrophy	249900	*ARSA*	Saposin-B	HSCT
Mucolipidosis type I	256550	*NEU1*	Sialidase	None
Mucolipidosis types II/III	252500	*GNPTAB*	N-acetylglucosamine-1-phosphotransferase	None
Mucolipidosis type IIIC	252605	*GNPTG*	N-acetylglucosamine-1-phosphotransferase γ-subunit	None
Mucolipidosis type IV	252650	*MCOLN1*	Mucolipin 1	None
Mucopolysaccharidosis type I	607014	*IDUA*	α-L-iduronidase	ERT, HSCT
Mucopolysaccharidosis type II	309900	*IDS*	Iduronate sulfatase	ERT, GT, HSCT
Mucopolysaccharidosis type IIIA	252900	*SGSH*	Heparan-N-sulfatase	None
Mucopolysaccharidosis type IIIB	252920	*NAGLU*	α- N-acetylglucosaminidase	None
Mucopolysaccharidosis	252930	*HGSNAT*	AcetylCoa-glucosamine-N-	None

type IIIC			acetyltransferase	
Mucopolysaccharidosis type IIID	252940	*GNS*	N-acetylglucosamine-6-sulfatase	None
Mucopolysaccharidosis type IVA	253000	*GALNS*	N-acetylgalactosamine-6-sulphatase	ERT
Mucopolysaccharidosis type IVB	253010	*GLB1*	β-Galactosidase	None
Mucopolysaccharidosis type VI	253200	*ARSB*	N-acetylgalactosamine-4-sulphatase	ERT
Mucopolysaccharidosis type VII	253220	*GUSB*	β-Glucuronidase	None
Mucopolysaccharidosis type IX	601492	*HYAL1*	Hyaluronidase	None
Multiple sulphatase deficiency	272200	*SUMF1*	Formylglicine-generating-enzyme	None
Neuronal ceroid lipofuscinosis 1	256730	*PPT1*	Palmitoyl protein thioesterase-1	HCST
Neuronal ceroid lipofuscinosis 2	204500	*TPP1*	Tripeptydil-peptidase I	GT
Neuronal ceroid lipofuscinosis 3	204200	*CLN3*	CLN3 protein	None
Neuronal ceroid lipofuscinosis 5	256731	*CLN5*	CLN5 protein	None
Neuronal ceroid lipofuscinosis 6	601780	*CLN6*	CLN6 protein	None
Neuronal ceroid lipofuscinosis 8	600143	*CLN8*	CLN8 protein	None
Niemann-Pick disease A/B	257200	*SMPD1*	Acid sphingomyelinidase	None
Niemann-Pick disease C1	257220	*NPC1*	NPC1 protein	SSI
Niemann-Pick disease C2	607625	*NPC2*	NPC2 protein	SSI
Pompe disease	232300	*GAA*	Alpha-glucosidase	ERT, GT
Prosaposin deficiency	176801	*PSAP*	Prosaposin	None
Pycnodysostosis	265800	*CTSK*	Cathepsin K	Hormone therapy
Sandhoff disease	268800	*HEXB*	Hexosaminidase B	PCT
Schindler disease	609241	*NAGA*	Alpha-N-acetylgalactosaminidase	None
Sialic acid storage disease	269920	*SLC17A5*	Sialin	None
Sialuria	269921	*GNE*	UDP-N-acetylglucosamine-2-epimerase	None
Tay-Sachs disease	272800	*HEXA*	Hexosaminidase A	PCT, SSI

Abbreviations: GT - Gene Therapy; HSCT - Hematopoetic Stem Cell Transplantation; PCT - Pharmacological Chaperone Therapy; OMIM - Online Mendelian Inheritance in Man; SSI - Specific Substrate Inhibition; ERT - Enzyme Replacement Therapy

Table 1. List of lysosomal storage diseases with their respective OMIM accession number, gene and enzyme deficiency and treatment options (including experimental ones).

The two most widely used treatment options are Hematopoietic Stem Cell Transplantation (HSCT) and Enzyme Replacement Therapy (ERT). HSCT has proven to be efficient to some of these diseases, especially if performed early enough to prevent irreversible lesions. Nevertheless, limitations such as the need of an early diagnosis, the difficulties to find a compatible donor in short time, and the high rates of morbidity and mortality associated with the procedure still limit this type of treatment (Malatack et al, 2003). Therefore, despite the many advances in this treatment over the last 30 years (Boelens et al 2010), its use has been deferred in favor of ERT whenever it is available. Enzyme replacement therapy is approved for a growing number of LSD, especially those without CNS involvement. It has proven to reduce some visceral symptoms as hepatosplenomegaly and improve respiratory function (Sifuentes et al, 2007), however difficult-to-reach organs such as the brain and the bones are still a major challenge. Innovative routes of enzyme delivery have been tested to achieve the CNS, such as intrathecal ERT (Munoz-Rojas et al, 2008; Munoz-Rojas et al, 2010).

Other treatment approaches already under clinical use or experimentation are Specific Substrate Inhibition (SSI) and Pharmacological Chaperone Therapy (PCT). SSI aims to decrease the storage by reducing substrate synthesis through an inhibitor. PCT uses small molecules able to stabilize the mutant enzyme and help it escape proteasomal degradation, thus restoring some residual enzyme activity. All such treatments have limitations (table 2), that justify the development of gene therapy approaches for these diseases.

Approach	Brief Description	Pros	Limitations
Intravenous enzyme replacement therapy	Intravenous injection of a recombinant version of the missing enzyme	Ameliorates several visceral symptoms	High cost Does not correct difficult-to-reach sites Need of repeated injections
Intrathecal enzyme replacememnt therapy	Intrathecal injection of a recombinant version of the missing enzyme	Reaches the CNS	High Cost Need of repeated injections Efficacy uncertain
Hematopoietic stem cell tranplantation	Non-autologous transplantation of CD 34+ cells	Able to correct visceral and CNS symptoms if performed early	Limited efficacy Relatively high morbidity and mortality rates
Specific substrate inhibition	Use of drugs that can inhibit the synthesis of the undegraded material	Orally administered Reaches the CNS	Limited efficacy High cost
Pharmacological chaperone therapy	Drugs that can stabilize the mutated protein, allowing some enzyme activity	Orally administered Reaches the CNS	Works only in patients with specific mutations
Stop-codon read-through therapy	Use of molecules that can suppress stop-codon mutations	Orally administered Reaches the CNS Low cost	Works only in stop-codon mutations Clinical trials yet to be performed
Gene Therapy	Administration of a normal copy of the mutated gene	Potentially effective with single injection	Safety concerns Efficacy uncertain

Abbreviations: CNS – Central Nervous System

Table 2. Pros and limitations of different therapeutic approaches for lysosomal storage diseases.

2. Rationale for gene therapy in LSDs

The rationale for gene therapy and other enzyme-based approaches for treatment of LSDs was first introduced almost five decades ago by Christian de Duve, and can be summarized in the following sentence from his original work "In our pathogenic speculations and in our therapeutic attempts, it may be well to keep in mind that any substance which is taken up intracellularly in an endocytic process is likely to end up within lysosomes." (de Duve, 1964). His work and other pioneer studies showing cross-correction between fibroblasts from patients with Mucopolysaccharidosis type I and type II (deficient in alpha-L-iduronidase and iduronate-sulphatase, respectively) established that the enzyme produced in one cell could be uptaken by a deficient cell, thus restoring its phenotype (Fratantoni et al, 1968). Later studies identified that this uptake was a saturable, receptor-mediated process, and the main actor of this process was the mannose-6-phosphate (M6P) receptor localized in the plasmatic membrane. The post-translational modification of addition of the M6P to the protein was discovered to be a signal not only to endocytosis but also for targeting nascent hydrolases to lysosomes (Fisher et al, 1980; Sly et al., 1981).

These pivotal discoveries in the field of endocytosis and targeting of lysosomal enzymes provided the basis for treatments like HSCT and ERT. In the same way, LSDs may be considered good targets for gene therapy, despite their multisystemic involvement. The correction of a few cells could lead to the enzyme being secreted into the circulation and uptaken by the deficient cells, resulting in widespread correction of the biochemical defect (figure 1).

Since long term gene expression is desirable, most clinical and preclinical trials used viral based vectors. Initial studies on fibroblasts showed promising data using retroviruses (Anson et al, 1992). However, when tests in animal models started, it became clear that some organs as the brain would not be easily corrected, as the enzyme could not cross the blood-brain-barrier (Elinwood et al, 2004). This is a major hurdle as most LSD shows some degree of CNS involvement. Nevertheless, CNS targeted approaches could be envisaged to overcome this obstacle. For instance, Worgall et al. (2008) showed a slowing of progression of Neuronal Ceroid Lipofuscinosis 2 in ten children treated with serotype 2 adeno-associated virus expressing *CLN2* cDNA. Another clinical trial, for Pompe disease, also used adeno-associated-based vector, but in this case serotype 1 (NCT00976352-www.clinicaltrials.gov). Other two trials performed in the late 1990s used retroviral vectors for Gaucher (Dunbar et al., 1998) and Mucopolysaccharidosis type II (NCT00004454 - www.clinicaltrials.gov).

Safety issues related to immune response of the adenoviral vectors (Wilson, 2009) and the possibility of insertional mutagenesis of the retroviral vectors (Hacein-Bey-Abina S et al., 2008) led researchers to develop a series of studies in parallel using non-viral approaches to treat lysosomal storage disorders.

3. Non-viral approaches

Non-viral vectors have important safety advantages over viral approaches, including their reduced pathogenicity and capacity for insertional mutagenesis, as well as their low cost and ease of production (Fraga et al., 2008). The application of non-viral vectors to humans has, however, been held back by the poor efficiency of their delivery to cells and the transient expression of the transgenes. As new strategies are being developed for the

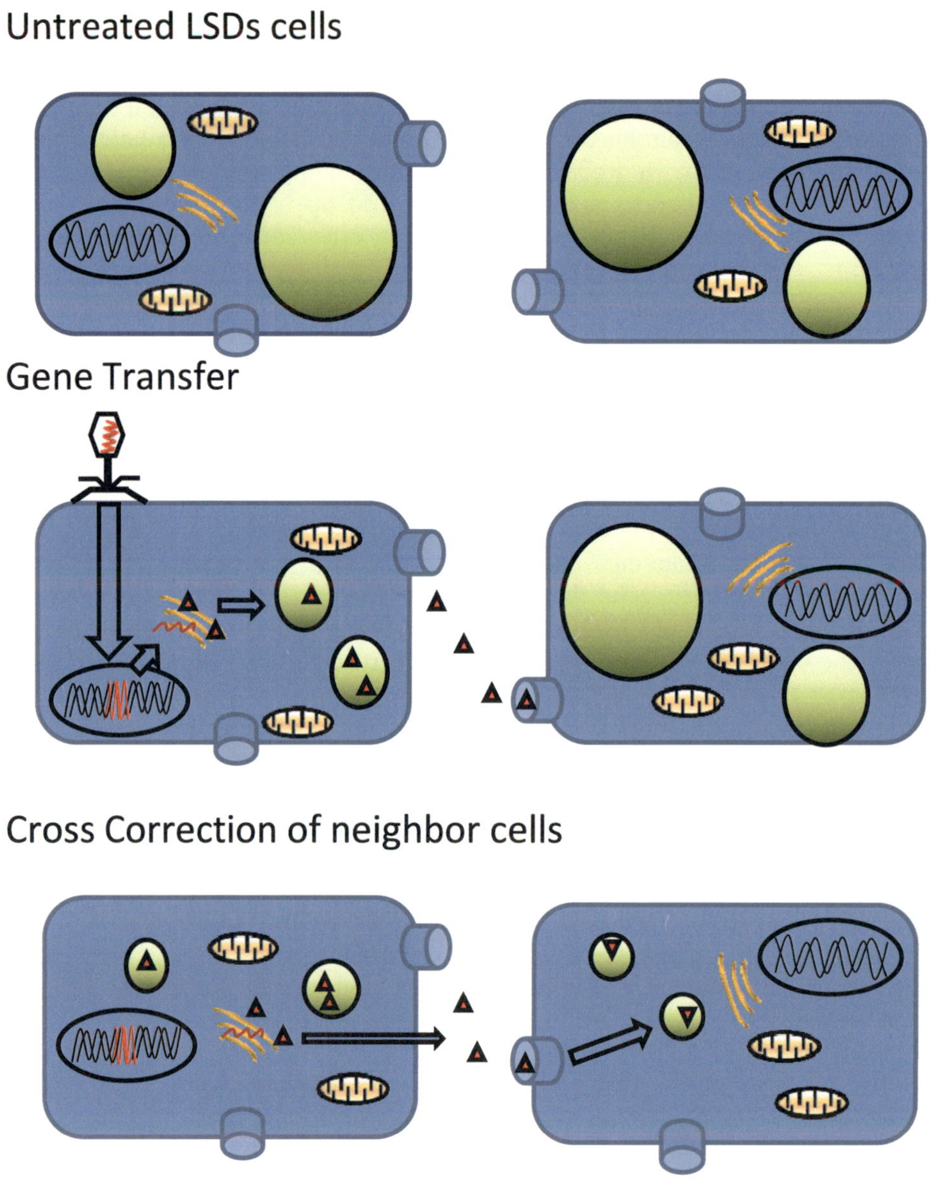

Fig. 1. Rationale for Gene Therapy in Lysosomal Storage Disorders: Cross-correction. The upper part of the figure shows two cells from a patient with LSD, with large lysosomes (green) due to accumulation of undegraded material. The gene transfer of a normal copy of the missing enzyme (red structure in the nucleus), allows the enzyme (red triangles) to be produced, and degrade the material accumulated in the lysosomes. Part of the enzyme is secreted from the recombinant cell and is captured by neighbouring cells via the mannose-6-phosphate receptors (light blue structures located on the cell membrane), reaching the lysosomes and being able to correct their phenotype, in a process called cross-correction. Note that the cell on the right was never transduced, but is able to capture the enzyme from the circulation or from the neighbouring cell.

application of non-viral vectors as nucleic acid delivery systems (Resina et al., 2009; Wasungu and Hoekstra, 2006), progress is being made in the application of this kind of therapy to LSDs.

3.1 Naked plasmid transfection

The direct injection of a plasmid containing the gene of interest and the regulatory mechanisms to ensure its expression is the simplest form of gene therapy. It has some advantages over the virus mediated gene transfer systems. First, DNA preparation is simple and can be performed at relatively low cost. In addition, the safety concerns are much lower and large amounts of DNA can be transferred. However, the major limitation of this method is that it requires a local administration and the level of transgene expression is relatively low and restricted to the injection site (Glover et al., 2005).

Hydrodynamic injection (Liu et al, 1999) is an experimental method capable to achieve efficient gene transfer and high level of transgene expression by systemic administration. In this procedure, a large volume of saline containing plasmid DNA is injected in a short period of time. The large volume and high injection rate forces the DNA solution into the liver, probably due to the permeability of liver fenestrae. A small hepatotoxicity, probably due to the large volume of saline, is observed and resolves within a few days. Even though this procedure is widely used in mice by tail vein injection, its feasibility has been demonstrated in larger animal models using a balloon occlusion catheter-based method to mimic hydrodynamic injection (Brunetti-Pierri et al, 2007; Kamimura et al, 2009).

This approach has been used in a proof-of-concept study to show the importance of coexpression of the formylglycine-generating enzyme for synthesis and secretion of functional Arylsulfatase A in a mouse model of Metachromatic Leukodystrophy (Takakusaki et al., 2005). This enzyme is a posttranslational modifying enzyme essential for activating multiple forms of sulfatases including Arylsulfatase A and therefore limits the amount of functional enzyme that can be secreted from transduced cells.

It has also been used in Mucopolysaccharidosis (MPS) type I (Camassola et al, 2005) and type VII (Richard et al, 2009). In the MPS I animals, storage content was reduced and enzyme activity was elevated in the liver and spleen. For the MPS VII model, a beneficial effect on the pathology was also observed, as liver-directed gene transfer led to the correction of secondary enzymatic elevations and to the reduction of GAGs storage in peripheral tissues and brain, as well as to histological correction in many tissues.

3.2 Liposomes and nanotechnology

Liposomes are lipid particles that resemble the cell membrane. Liposome-based gene delivery was first reported by Felgner in 1987, and is still one of the major techniques for non viral gene delivery into cells (Niidome & Huang, 2002). Lipoplexes are formed by the interaction of anionic nucleic acids binding to the surface of cationic lipids, forming multilamellar lipid–nucleic acid complexes where the negatively charged nucleic acid remains trapped inside the lipid bilayer (Dass, 2004). Since its discovery, different lipid formulations have been tested and modified. For example, stealth liposomes sterically stabilized with methoxypoly(ethylene glycol)distearoylphosphatidylethanolamine conjugates (PEG-DSPE) have long circulation half-lives following intravenous injection (Moreira et al., 2001). In addition, linear polycations such as linear, branched and dendritic vectors based on poly(ethylenimine) (PEI), poly(L-lysine) (PLL) and a range of poly(ethylene glycol) (PEG) were also developed (Hunter, 2006). Although linear PEI shows greater *in vivo* efficiency because of a dynamic structure change of the complex under high salt concentrations as found in blood (Niidome & Huang, 2002), it also possesses greater toxicity (Morille et al., 2008).

Cationic nanoemulsions have been more recently considered as potential systems for nucleic acid delivery. The interest in these systems is justified by the fact that they are biocompatible and able to form complexes with DNA protecting it from enzymatic degradation (Nam et al., 2009). Other practical advantages include ease of production and the potential for repeated administration (Al-Dorsari and Gao, 2009). We have investigated the influence of phospholipids on the properties of cationic nanoemulsions/pDNA complexes. Complexes containing the phospholipids DSPC (1,2-distearoyl-sn-glycero-3-phosphocholine) and DSPE (1,2- distearoyl-sn-glycero-3- phosphoethanolamine) were less toxic in comparison with the formulations obtained with lecithin, DOPC (1,2-dioleoyl-sn-glycero-3-phosphocholine) and DOPE (1,2-dioleoyl-sn-glycero-3-phosphoethanolamine). In addition, higher amounts of reporter DNA were detected for the formulation obtained with the DSPC phospholipid (Fraga et al., in press).

These cationic macromolecules can readily condense DNA or RNA into stable nanostructures for use in gene delivery (Hunter, 2006) but also for other nanotechnology-based approaches useful for the treatment of LSDs (Muro, 2010). Nanomaterials, as a result of their small size and their large surface area offer great promise for neuro-therapeutics (Ragnail et al., 2011) and thus may be a valid option for a large number of LSDs that affect the CNS.

Liposome-mediated gene transfer for LSD has been performed *in vitro* using patient's fibroblasts as target cells. Estruch et al. (2001) delivered therapeutic genes by integrin-mediated uptake into fibroblasts from patients with Fucosidosis and Fabry disease. The vectors consisted of a complex of lipofectin and a peptide containing an integrin-targeting domain and a poly-lysine domain to which plasmid DNA was bound. Transfected cells produced the corresponding enzyme at levels which were 10-40% of the total activity in cultures of normal fibroblasts. Although 95-98% of this activity was secreted, it did not appear to affect the viability of the cells. Our group used Lipofectamine to transduce fibroblasts from GM1 Gangliosidosis patients with the beta-galactosidase gene. Treated cells showed 33 to 100- fold increases in enzyme activity compared to untreated fibroblasts. However, after seven days enzyme activity was back to uncorrected values (Balestrin et al., 2008). When Geneticin was added to the medium (figure 2), stable expression at therapeutic levels was observed (mean 300 nmoles/h/mg prot) for 30 days, although at values lower than the normal range (mean 1,300 nmoles/h/mg prot).

In vivo, PEG-coated liposomes have been modified with monoclonal antibodies in order to reach the CNS. A liposome is coated with peptidomimetic monoclonal antibodies that undergo receptor-mediated transcytosis across the blood-brain barrier on the endogenous peptide receptor transporters (Pardridge, 2007). These Trojan horses (figure 3) may use the insulin or transferrin receptor, and since the MAb binding site is different from the binding site of the endogenous ligand, there is no interference of endogenous ligand transport (Skarlatos et al, 1995).

This approach has been used to deliver a non-viral plasmid DNA to the brain across the blood-brain-barrier after intravenous administration of liposomes coated with monoclonal antibody to the mouse transferrin receptor in a mouse model of Mucopolysaccharidosis type VII (Zhang et al, 2008). The enzyme activity was increased greater than ten-fold in brain, liver, spleen, lung, and kidney, but not in heart. A similar strategy has been used by Osborn et al (2008) for Mucopolysaccharidosis type I, although they used a plasmid bearing a fusion gene consisting of Transferrin (Tf) and α-L-iduronidase. The fusion product consisted of an enzymatically active protein that was transported into the CNS by TfR-mediated endocytosis. Short-term treatment resulted in a decrease in GAGs in the cerebellum of Mucopolysaccharidosis type I mice.

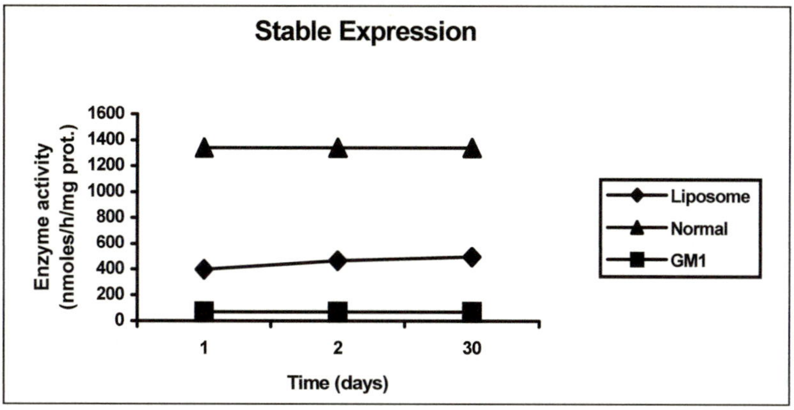

Fig. 2. Stable expression of β-Galactosidase in fibroblasts from G1 Gangliosidosis patients after *in vitro* liposome-based gene transfer. Mean values of liposome-treated cells: 300 nmoles/h/mg prot.; mean values of normal fibroblasts: 1,300 nmoles/h/mg prot.; mean values of affected fibroblasts: 68 nmoles/h/mg prot. (Balestrin et al., 2008).

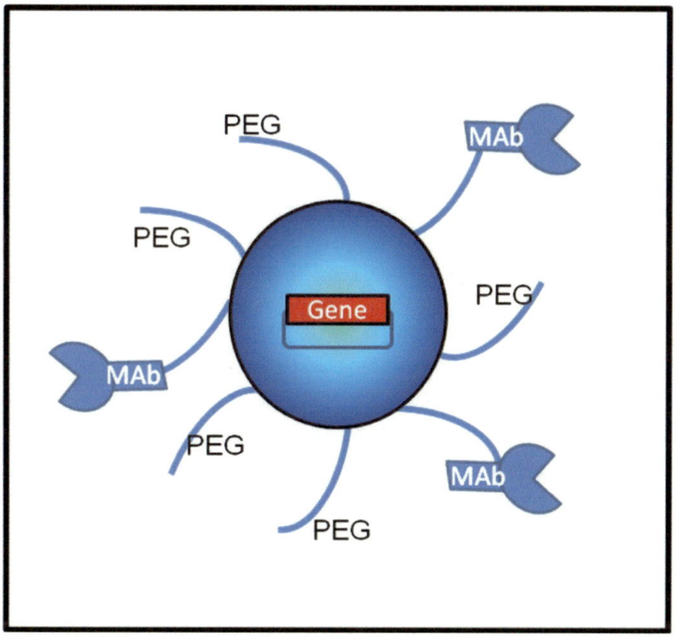

Fig. 3. Schematic view of a Trojan horse liposome. A stealth PEGylated liposome is complexed with monoclonal antibodies (MAb) that undergo receptor-mediated transcytosis across the blood-brain barrier.

3.3 Cell microencapsulation

Cell microencapsulation is an approach in which cells are trapped in a semipermeable membrane, allowing the exchange of metabolites and nutrients between them and the external environment. The membrane prevents the access of the immune system to the cells, without the need for continued immunosuppression of the host (Uludag et al., 2000). Furthermore, this technique allows the localized and controlled release, and long term duration of therapeutic products derived from the microencapsulated cells (Orive et al., 2002). Microencapsulation has become an important system for cellular preservation (Mayer et al., 2010) and a potential strategy for the controlled delivery of therapeutic products (Orive et al., 2003). Alginate has been the most important encapsulation polymer due to its abundance, easy gelling properties and biocompatibility. Agarose, chitosan, and hyaluronic acid are other polymers used for microencapsulation (Orive et al., 2003).

Cell microencapsulation presents the potential to deliver the therapeutic product of interest directly to the Central Nervous System (CNS). This has been achieved by different groups for brain tumors (Kuijlen et al 2007) and neurodegenerative diseases (Spuch et al 2010). A phase I clinical trial was conducted in Huntington's patients without signs of toxicity (Bloch et al 2004). This approach delivers the gene of interest in the spinal fluid, similar to the intrathecal enzyme replacement therapy. Thus, cell encapsulation can be suitable for the treatment of LSD, once the deficient enzyme could be released for long term directly in the CNS (Matte et al., 2011).

In order to obtain larger amounts of secreted enzyme, the encapsulated cells should be genetically modified to over-express the enzyme of interest. This enzyme would then be released to the extracapsular space (Bressel et al 2008) and uptaken by adjacent deficient cells (figure 4). This strategy has been used experimentally for different LSD, especially the Mucopolysaccharidosis (MPS).

Three *in vitro* studies were performed in LSDs other than the MPS, one in Fabry disease and the other two in Metachromatic Leukodystrophy (MLD). Naganawa et al (2002) co-cultured fibroblasts from patients with Fabry disease with microencapsulated recombinant Chinese Hamster Ovary cells (CHO) over-expressing alpha-galactosidase. The deficient cells were able to uptake the enzyme decreasing their levels of globotriaosylceramide storage. A similar approach was used by our group to test the ability of Baby Hamster Kidney (BHK) cells over-expressing ARSA to correct the deficiency of this enzyme in human skin fibroblasts from MLD patients. Fibroblasts co-cultured with the encapsulated cells for four weeks showed levels of enzyme activity higher than normal. Transmission electron microscopy showed evidence of normalization of the lysosomal ultra structure, suggesting that the secreted enzyme was able to degrade the substrate (Lagranha et al., 2008). Consiglio et al (2007) collected the conditioned media of C2C12 cells over-expressing ARSA encapsulated in polyether-sulfone polymer and used it to treat oligodendrocytes from MLD mice. The deficient cells internalized the enzyme and it was normally sorted to the lysosomal compartment, reaching 80% of physiological levels and restoring sulfatide metabolism.

Both *in vitro* and *in vivo* studies have been performed in the MPS types I, II and VII. For MPS II two studies were performed. The first was a proof of principle in which Hunter primary fibroblasts were co-cultured with alginate microcapsules containing C2C12 cell clones over-expressing IDS. After 5 days of co-culture this strategy was able to increase IDS activity inside the deficient fibroblasts to levels similar to normal (Tomanin et al 2002). The second study was a pre-clinical experiment in which APA (alginate-poli-L-lysine-alginate) microcapsules containing 1.5×10^6 allogeneic C2C12 myoblasts over-expressing IDS were implanted in the peritoneum of the MPS II mouse model. An increase in IDS activity in plasma was observed, along with a reduction on urinary GAG between the fourth and the sixth week of treatment. After 8 weeks, a reduction of 30% in the amount of GAG accumulated in the liver and 38% in the kidney were shown (Friso et al 2005).

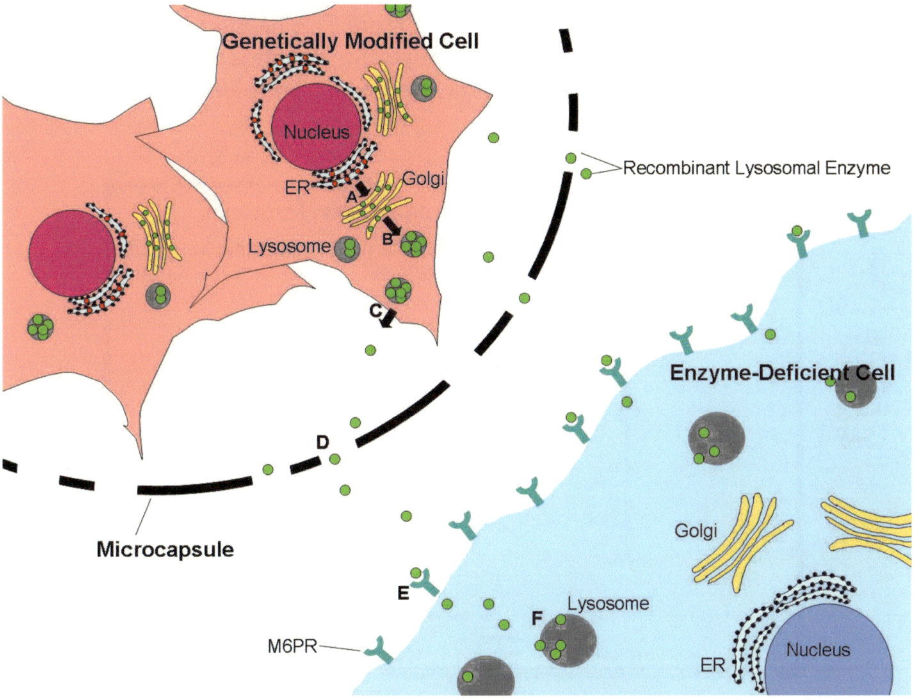

Fig. 4. Traffic of lysosomal enzymes throughout the encapsulated cells. The nascent lysosomal enzymes are glycosylated in the endoplasmic reticulum (ER) of the genetically modified cells. (A) The enzymes are phosphorylated at the residue of mannose-6 in the Golgi apparatus. (B) Most enzymes are transported to mature lysosomes. (C) Some, however, are secreted to the extracellular environment and (D) to outside of the microcapsules. (E) Phosphorylated enzymes bind to mannose-6-phosphate receptors (M6PR) of the enzyme-deficient cells (F) where they are endocyted and subsequently targeted to the lysosomes (Matte et al., 2011).

To evaluate the usefulness of this technique to treat MPS VII, Ross et al (2000a) injected APA encapsulated non-autologous cells overexpressing Gusb in the peritoneum of MPS VII mice. The results showed the presence of Gusb in the plasma 24 hours after implantation, reaching 66% of physiological levels by 2 weeks post implantation. Activity of Gusb was also detected in liver and spleen for the duration of the 8-week experiment. Accumulation of GAG was significantly reduced in liver and spleen sections and urinary GAG content reached normal levels. In another study, enzyme released by APA encapsulated 2A50 fibroblasts implanted directly into the lateral ventricles of the brain of MPS VII mice was delivered throughout most of the CNS, reversing the histological pathology (Ross et al., 2000b). *In vitro* studies were performed by Nakama et al (2006) who encapsulated immortalized recombinant human amniotic epithelial cells with MPS VII human and mouse fibroblasts and high GUSB activity was detected in the medium. Addition of mannose-6-phosphate led to decreased enzyme activity, suggesting that enzyme uptake was mediated by mannose-6-phosphate receptor.

Our group has shown that the correction of MPS I fibroblasts by recombinant encapsulated BHK cells is also mediated by mannose-6-phosphate receptor. The effect of the ratio fibroblasts:encapsulated cells was also analysed (figure 5). The amount of enzyme uptaken by the fibroblasts is essentially the same under the different ratios (5:1; 1:1; 1:5) although the enzyme activity in the medium increases, as more enzyme is released.

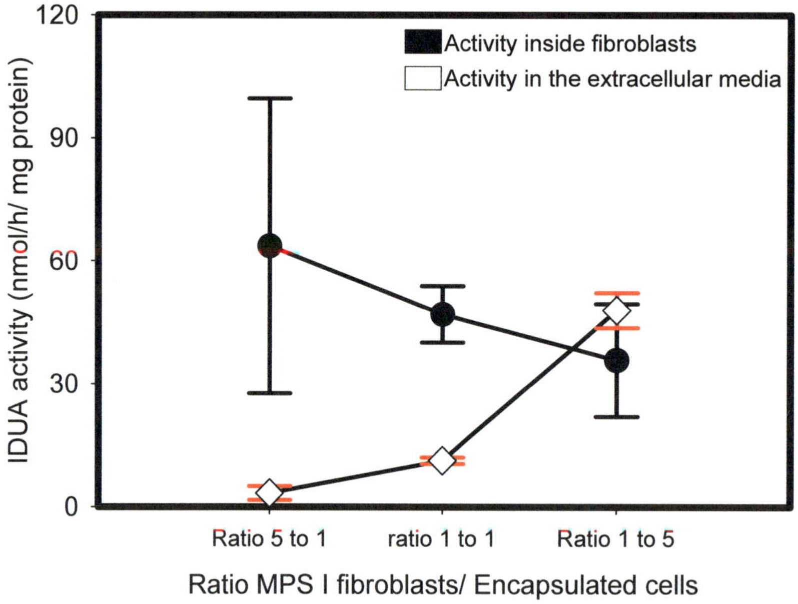

Fig. 5. IDUA enzyme activity in MPS I fibroblasts co-cultured with recombinant BHK cells overexpressing IDUA at different ratios.

Our results also showed an increase in IDUA activity in MPS I fibroblasts after 15, 30 and 45 days of co-culture with the capsules. Cytological analysis showed a marked reduction in GAG storage within MPS I cells (Baldo et al., 2011). Ongoing experiments are under way in the MPS I mouse model. The capsules were implanted in the peritoneum (figure 6) and animals were sacrificed at 4 months later. Histological analysis showed a reduction on GAG storage although plasma and tissue enzyme activity levels were not increased.

These results are quite different from those of Barsoum et al (2003) who implanted genetically modified Madin-Darby canine kidney cells (MDCK) over-expressing canine Idua in the brain parenchyma of one MPS I dog. Enzyme in plasma and cerebrospinal fluid was low but detectable for 21 days. Immunohistochemistry with anti-IDUA antibody showed the presence of the enzyme in various brain regions, however an extensive inflammatory reaction was noted, both at the sites of implantation and in the immediate vicinity. This may be the reason why histological correction of lysosomal inclusions has not been observed.

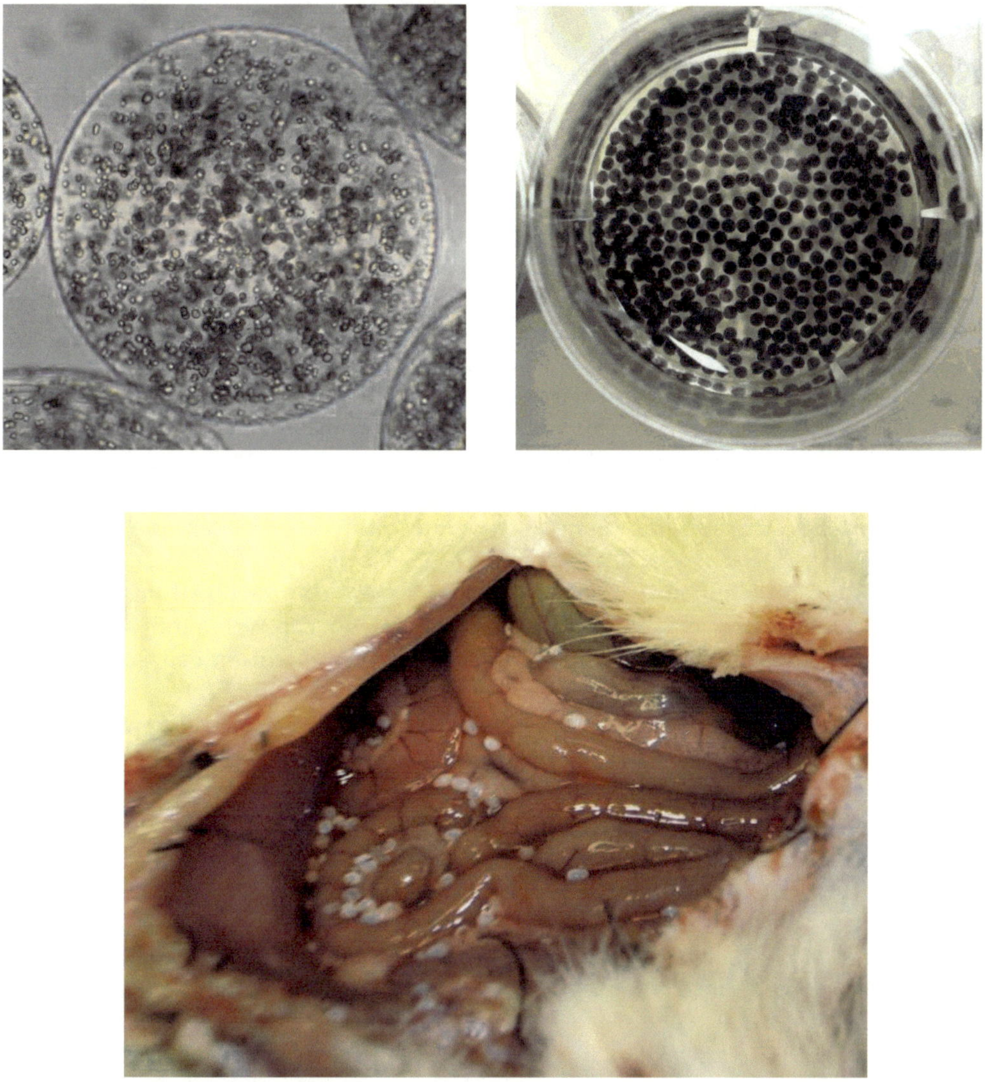

Fig. 6. Microcapsules used for the treatment of MPS I mice. Left upper panel: photomicrography of alginate beads containing recombinant BHK that overexpress IDUA (small round dots). Right upper panel: Macroscopic aspect of the microcapsules (black dots) in a 96-well plate. Capsules were ink stained to help visualization. Lower panel: Aspect of the capsules in the peritoneum ten days after implantation. Note that some capsules are attached to the intestine.

3.4 Transposon-based systems

For human gene therapy we can enumerate some important aspects of transposon systems (special emphasis in this chapter will be given to the *sleeping beauty* transposon) that make them appealing as a vector: (1) the integrated gene has stable expression, providing long-lasting expression of a therapeutic gene, which, as already mentioned, is essential for lysosomal storage diseases; (2) the transposase directs the integration of single copies of a DNA sequence into chromatin and (3) the system is binary (the transposon is not autonomous or able to transpose on its own) (Hacket et al, 2005).

The most studied transposon system, which has been used in pre-clinical studies for treatment of lysosomal disorders, is the *Sleeping beauty (SB)* system. Sleeping beauty transposon is a type of mobile element that belongs to the *Tc1/Mariner* class and that is able to transpose via movement of a DNA element in a simple cut-and-paste manner. For that, a precise piece of DNA is excised from one DNA molecule and moved to another site in the same or in a different DNA molecule (Plasterk, 1993). This reaction is catalyzed by the protein transposase, which can be supplied *in trans* by another plasmid for gene therapy purposes.

The SB transposon system consists of two components: (i) a transposon, made up of the gene of interest flanked by inverted repeats (IRs), and (ii) a source of transposase (figure 7). For Sleeping Beauty-mediated transposition, the transposase can recognize the ends of the IRs, excises the gene of interest from the delivered plasmid DNA, and then inserts it into another DNA site. Based on studies in about 2,000 integration events in either mouse or human genomes, transposons seem to integrate into random sites, including exons, introns and intergenic sequences (Carlson et al, 2003; Horie et al, 2003; Hacket et al, 2005). This is a potential problem, since it may lead to an event of insertional mutagenesis. A complete list of insertion positions of the SB tranposon can be found at the Mouse Transposon Insertion database at http://mouse.ccgb.umn.edu/transposon/ (Roberg-Perez et al, 2003).

The use of SB transposons as gene therapy approach in LSD is still recent. The first published work was conducted by Aronovich et al (2007) who studied the effects of intravenous hydrodynamic injection of the SB transposon into mice with Mucopolysaccharidosis types I or VII. Without immunomodulation, initial enzyme activities in plasma reached levels higher than 100-fold that of wild-type (WT). However, both GUSB (MPS VII) and IDUA (MPS I) levels fell to background within 4 weeks post-injection.

A second group of animals was performed with immunomodulation only in MPS I mice. Plasma IDUA persisted for over 3 months at up to 100-fold WT activity in one-third of the mice, which was sufficient to reverse lysosomal pathology in the liver and, partially, in distant organs. Histological and immunohistochemical examination of liver sections in IDUA transposon-treated WT mice revealed inflammation 10 days post-injection consisting predominantly of mononuclear cells, which can be seen as a potential side-effect.

A posterior study by the same group (Aronovich et al, 2009) was performed in another MPS I strain, which is immunodeficient (NOD/SCID mice). Using the same approach from the previous experiment, they were able to show a persistent elevation (100-fold normal) in the plasma IDUA levels for 18 weeks. Also, IDUA activity was present in all organs analyzed, including the brain. The SB transposon system proved efficacious in correcting several clinical manifestations of MPS I mice, including bone abnormalities, hepatomegaly, and accumulation of foamy macrophages in bone marrow and synovium. In 2008 the first human clinical trial using the SB transposon was approved in the USA for treatment of cancer (Williams, 2008), however although promising no clinical trials have been conducted in LSDs so far.

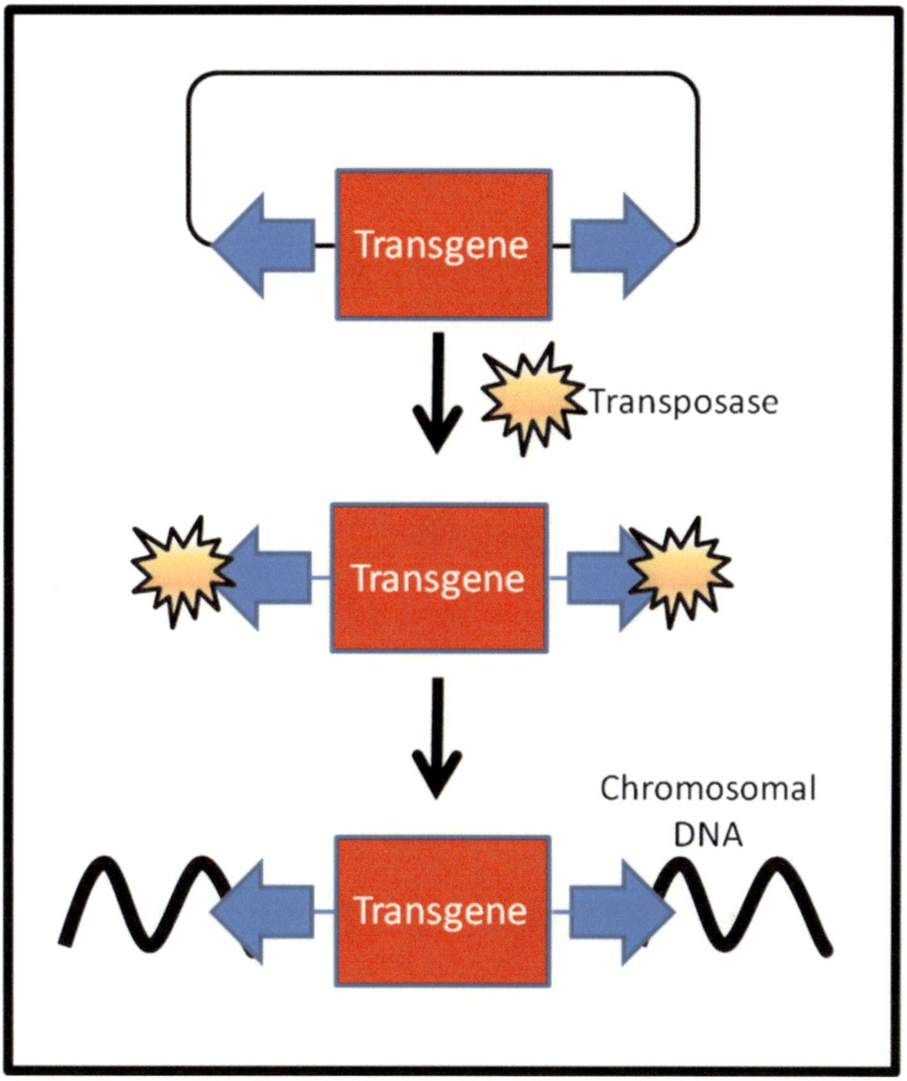

Fig. 7. SB transposon system. This simplified version of the SB transposon system shows the cut-and-paste system used by the SB transposase to insert the DNA into the host genome. The gene of interest is flanked by two inverted repeats regions (IRs, arrows) which will be recognized by the transposase (usually given in *trans* in a second plasmid) and allow the transgene to be inserted into the host genome. This way only the transgene will have prolonged expression, as transposase gene expression is transient. The SB transposon is a non-viral method of gene delivery that allows integration of the transgene in the host cell.

3.5 Minicircle gene therapy

Sustained *in vivo* transgene expression from plasmids can be difficult to achieve due to gene silencing. The mechanism by which this process occurs was postulated to be due to the deposition of repressive heterochromatin on the noncoding bacterial backbone sequences required for plasmid bacterial preparation and propagation (Chen et al, 2008; Riu et al, 2005).

Based on those findings, a new technology has emerged, known as the minicircle (MC) gene therapy. This system uses a phiC31 integrase recombination event to remove the bacterial backbone elements of the plasmid resulting in a DNA circle (the MC), encoding the mammalian expression cassette of choice and a small attR footprint (Chen et al, 2003). This has proven to be resistant to gene silencing *in vivo*, is maintained as an extrachromosomal episome, and therefore represents an interesting platform for gene replacement strategies for lysosomal storage disorders (figure 8).

This technology was recently used for treatment of MPS I mice in a proof-of-concept study (Osborn et al, 2011). In this study, the researchers performed a hydrodynamic injection of a minicircle plasmid containing the IDUA gene combined with immunomodulation, achieving stable expression of the transgene, increased IDUA tissue levels and reduction in GAG storage. As a recent technology, this is the only study performed on LSDs so far, but results are encouraging and should be tested on other diseases soon.

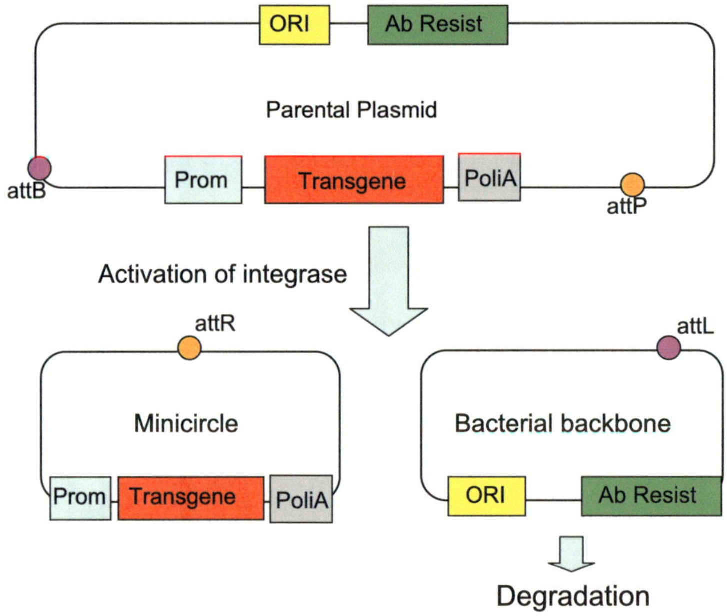

Fig. 8. Production of a minicircle plasmid. This simplified version of the process shows the parental plasmid containing both the gene of interest and the bacterial components, including origin of replication (ORI), genes that confer resistance to antibiotic (Ab resist) and sites that allow attachment of the integrase (att B and P). After activation of the integrase, a cis-recombination event occurs, separating the gene of interest and its regulatory elements from the bacterial backbone, which then is degraded.

4. Conclusions

Still nowadays most lysosomal storage disorders do not have an effective treatment. Moreover, treatments currently available are not able to correct all the manifestations of these multisystemic diseases. Despite the small number of protocols (if compared to other areas, like oncology), gene therapy approaches have shown their potential to be helpful in many of these diseases. Not only proof of concept experiments have been performed, but clinically relevant results were obtained in some cases.

The limitations of non-viral gene transfer, i.e., transient expression of the transgene and low transfection efficiency, are being slowly overcome in the last decade using improved vector design and techniques, such as nanotechnology, transposons, and minicircle approaches (to name a few) as demonstrated throughout this chapter. Novel mechanisms to help the DNA to escape endosomal degradation and pass through the nuclear envelope are also under development but were not in the scope of this chapter. Nevertheless, these improvements help non-viral gene therapy to move towards clinical trials in LSDs, which are expected to happen in the years to come. Non-viral vectors are safer than viral particles, which make them an appealing alternative for treatment of lysosomal storage disorders and even other monogenic diseases. Yet, there is a long way to clinical application but the road is paved and the scientific community advances steadily.

5. Acknowledgements

The authors are thankful to Conselho Nacional de Desenvolvimento Cientifico- CNPq and Fundacao de Amparo a Pesquisa do Rio Grande do Sul- FAPERGS.

We also would like to thank our colleagues Fabiana Quoos Mayer, Carlos Oscar Kieling, Valeska Lizzi Lagranha and Raquel Balestrin for contributing with data to this paper.

6. References

Al-Dosari, M.S., Gao X. (2009). Nonviral gene delivery: principle, limitations, and recent progress. *AAPS J*, Vol 11, No 4, pp 671-681.

Anson, D.S., Bielicki, J., Hopwood, J.J. (1992). Correction of mucopolysaccharidosis type I fibroblasts by retroviral-mediated transfer of the human alpha-L-iduronidase gene. *Hum Gene Ther*, Vol 3, No 4, pp 371-379.

Aronovich, E.L., Bell, J.B., Belur, L.R., Gunther, R., Koniar, B., Erickson, D.C., Schachern, P.A., Matise, I., McIvor, R.S., Whitley, C.B., Hackett, P.B. (2007) Prolonged expression of a lysosomal enzyme in mouse liver after Sleeping Beauty transposon-mediated gene delivery: implications for non-viral gene therapy of mucopolysaccharidoses. *J Gene Med*, Vol 9, No 5, pp 403-415.

Aronovich EL, Bell JB, Khan SA, Belur LR, Gunther R, Koniar B, Schachern PA, Parker JB, Carlson CS, Whitley CB, McIvor RS, Gupta P, Hackett PB. (2009) Systemic correction of storage disease in MPS I NOD/SCID mice using the sleeping beauty transposon system. *Mol Ther*.Vol 17, No 7, pp 1136-1144.

Baiotto, C., Sperb, F., Matte ,U., Silva, C.D., Sano, R., Coelho, J.C., Giugliani, R. (2011) Population analysis of the GLB1 gene in south Brazil. *Gen Mol Biol*, Vol 34, No 1, pp 45-48.

Baldo, G., Quoos Mayer, F., Burin, M., Carrillo-Farga, J., Matte, U., Giugliani, R. (2011) Recombinant Encapsulated Cells Overexpressing Alpha-L-Iduronidase Correct Enzyme Deficiency in Human Mucopolysaccharidosis Type I Cells. *Cells Tissues Organs*, epub.

Balestrin, R.C., Baldo, G., Vieira, M.B., Sano, R., Coelho, J.C., Giugliani, R., Matte, U. (2008) Transient high-level expression of beta-galactosidase after transfection of fibroblasts from GM1 gangliosidosis patients with plasmid DNA. *Braz J Med Biol Res*, Vol 41, No 4, PP 283-288.

Barsoum, S.C., Milgram, W., Mackay, W., Coblentz, C., Delaney, K.H., Kwiecien, J.M., Kruth, S.A., Chang P.L. (2003) Delivery of recombinant gene product to canine brain with the use of microencapsulation. *J Lab Clin Med*, Vol 142, No 6, pp 399-413.

Bellettato, C.M., Scarpa, M. (2010) Pathophysiology of neuropathic lysosomal storage disorders. *J Inherit Metab Dis,* Vol 33, No4, PP 347-362.

Bloch, J., Bachoud-Lévi, A.C., Déglon, N., Lefaucheur, J.P., Winkel, L., Palfi, S., Nguyen, J.P., Bourdet, C., Gaura, V., Remy, P., Brugières, P., Boisse, M.F., Baudic, S., Cesaro, P., Hantraye, P., Aebischer, P., Peschanski, M. (2004). Neuroprotective gene therapy for Huntington's disease, using polymer-encapsulated cells engineered to secrete human ciliary neurotrophic factor: results of a phase I study. *Hum Gene Ther,* Vol 15, No 10, pp 968-975.

Bressel, T., Paz, A.H., Baldo, G., Lima, E.O.C., Matte, U., Saraiva-Pereira, M. (2008) An effective device for generating alginate microcapsules. *Genet. Mol. Biol,* Vol 31, No 1, pp 136-140.

Brunetti-Pierri, N., Stapleton, G.E., Palmer, D.J., Zuo, Y., Mane, V.P., Finegold, M.J., Beaudet, A.L., Leland, M.M., Mullins, C.E., Ng, P. (2007) Pseudo-hydrodynamic delivery of helper-dependent adenoviral vectors into non-human primates for liver-directed gene therapy. *Mol Ther,* Vol 15, No4, pp 732- 740.

Camassola, M., Braga, L.M., Delgado-Cañedo, A., Dalberto, T.P., Matte, U., Burin, M., Giugliani, R., Nardi, N.B. (2005) Nonviral in vivo gene transfer in the mucopolysaccharidosis I murine model. *J Inherit Metab Dis,* Vol 28, No 6, pp 1035-1043.

Carlson, C.M., Dupuy, A.J., Fritz, S., Roberg-Perez, K.J., Fletcher, C.F., Largaespada, D.A. (2003) Transposon mutagenesis of the mouse germline. *Genetics* Vol 165, No 1 pp 243–256.

Chen, Z.Y., He, C.Y., Ehrhardt, A. and Kay, M.A. (2003) Minicircle DNA vectors devoid of bacterial DNA result in persistent and high-level transgene expression in vivo. *Mol Ther,* Vol 8, No 3, pp 495–500.

Chen, Z.Y., Riu, E., He, C.Y., Xu, H. and Kay, M.A. (2008) Silencing of episomal transgene expression in liver by plasmid bacterial backbone DNA is independent of CpG methylation. *Mol Ther,* Vol 16, No 3, pp 548–556.

Consiglio, A., Martino, S., Dolcetta, D. (2007) Metabolic correction in oligodendrocytes derived from metachromatic leukodystrophy mouse model by using encapsulated recombinant myoblasts. *J Neurol Sci,* Vol 255, No 1-2, pp 7-16.

Dass, C.R.(2004) Lipoplex-mediated delivery of nucleic acids: factors affecting in vivo transfection. *J Mol Med,* Vol 82, No 9, pp 579–591.

de Duve, C. (1964) From cytases to lysosomes. *Fed Proc,* Vol 23, pp 1045–1049.

Dunbar, C.E., Kohn, D.B., Schiffmann, R., Barton, N.W., Nolta, J.A., Esplin, J.A., Pensiero, M., Long, Z., Lockey, C., Emmons, R.V., Csik, S., Leitman, S., Krebs, C.B., Carter, C., Brady, R.O., Karlsson, S. (1998) Retroviral transfer of the glucocerebrosidase gene into CD34+ cells from patients with Gaucher disease: in vivo detection of transduced cells without myeloablation. *Hum Gene Ther,* Vol 9, No 17, pp 2629-2640.

Ellinwood, N.M., Vite, C.H., Haskins, M.E. (2004) Gene therapy for lysosomal storage diseases: the lessons and promise of animal models. *J Gene Med.* Vol 6, No 5, pp 481-506.

Estruch, E.J., Hart, S.L., Kinnon, C., Winchester, B.G. (2001) Non-viral, integrin-mediated gene transfer into fibroblasts from patients with lysosomal storage diseases. *J Gene Med,* Vol 3, No 5, pp 488-497.

Fischer, H.D., Gonzalez-Noriega, A., Sly, W.S., Morre, D.J. (1980) Phosphomannosyl-enzyme receptors in rat liver. Subcellular distribution and role in intracellular transport of lysosomal enzymes. J Biol Chem. Vol 255, No 20, pp 9608 - 15.

Fraga, M., Laux, M., Zandoná, B., Santos, G.R., Giuberti, C.S., Oliveira, M.C., Matte, U., Teixeira, H.F. (2008) Optimization of stearylamine-based nanoemulsions obtained by spontaneous emulsification process as nucleic acids delivery systems. *J Drug Del Sci Tech* Vol 18, No 6, pp 398-403.

Fraga, M., Bruxel, F., Lagranha, V., Teixeira, H.F., Matte, U. Influence of phospholipid composition on DNA/cationic emulsions complexes: Physicochemical properties, cytotoxicity and transfection on Hep G2 cells. *International Journal of Nanomedicine, in press.*

Fratantoni, J.C., Hall, C.W., Neufeld, E.F. (1968) Hurler and Hunter syndromes: mutual correction of the defect in cultured fibroblasts. *Science*, Vol 162, No 853, pp 570–572.

Friso, A., Tomanin, R., Alba, S. (2005) Reduction of GAG storage in MPS II mouse model following implantation of encapsulated recombinant myoblasts. *J Gene Med*, Vol 7, No 11, pp 1482-1491.

Fuller, M., Meikle, P.J., Hopwood, J.J. (2006) Epidemiology of lysosomal storage diseases: an overview. In *Fabry Disease: Perspectives from 5 Years of FOS*. Mehta A, Beck M, Sunder-Plassmann G, editors. Oxford: Oxford PharmaGenesis.

Glover D, Lipps H, Jans D (2005) Towards safe, non-viral therapeutic gene expression in humans. *Nature Reviews Genetics*, Vol 6, No 4, 299-310.

Hacein-Bey-Abina, S., Garrigue, A., Wang, G.P., Soulier, J., Lim, A., Morillon, E., Clappier, E., Caccavelli, L., Delabesse, E., Beldjord, K., Asnafi, V., MacIntyre, E., Dal Cortivo, L., Radford, I., Brousse, N., Sigaux, F., Moshous, D., Hauer, J., Borkhardt, A., Belohradsky, B.H., Wintergerst, U., Velez, M.C., Leiva, L., Sorensen, R., Wulffraat, N., Blanche, S., Bushman, F.D., Fischer, A., Cavazzana-Calvo, M. (2008) Insertional oncogenesis in 4 patients after retrovirus-mediated gene therapy of SCID-X1. *J Clin Invest*, Vol 118, No 9, pp 3132-3142.

Hackett, P.B., Ekker, S.C., Largaespada, D.A., McIvor, R.S. (2005) Sleeping beauty transposon-mediated gene therapy for prolonged expression. *Adv Genet*, Vol 54, pp 189-232.

Horie, K., Yusa, K., Yae, K., Odajima, J., Fischer, S. E., Keng, V. W., Hayakawa, T., Mizuno, S., Kondoh, G., Ijiri, T., Matsuda, Y., Plasterk, R. H., and Takeda, J. (2003) Characterization of Sleeping Beauty transposition and its application to genetic screening in mice. *Mol. Cell. Biol*, Vol 23, No 24, pp 9189–9207.

Hunter, C. (2006) Molecular hurdles in polyfectin design and mechanistic background to polycation induced cytotoxicity. *Advanced Drug Delivery Reviews*, Vol 58, pp 1523–1531.

Kamimura, K., Zhang, G., Liu, D. (2009) Image-guided, intravascular hydrodynamic gene delivery to skeletal muscle in pigs. *Mol Ther*, Vol 18, No 1, pp 93-100.

Kuijlen, J.M., de Haan, B.J., Helfrich, W., de Boer, J.F., Samplonius, D., Mooij, J.J., de Vos, P. (2006) The efficacy of alginate encapsulated CHO-K1 single chain-TRAIL producer cells in the treatment of brain tumors. *J Neurooncol* Vol 78, No 1, pp 31-39.

Lagranha, V.L., Baldo, G., de Carvalho, T.G. Burin M, Saraiva-Pereira, M.L., Matte, U., Giugliani, R. (2008) In vitro correction of ARSA deficiency in human skin fibroblasts from metachromatic leukodystrophy patients after treatment with microencapsulated recombinant cells. *Metab Brain Dis* Vol 23, No 4, pp 469-84.

Liu, F., Song, Y., Liu, D. (1999) Hydrodynamics-based transfection in animals by systemic administration of plasmid DNA. *Gene Ther*, Vol 6, No 7, pp 1258-1266.

Malatack, J.J., Consolini, D.M., Bayever, E. (2003) The status of hematopoietic stem cell transplantation in lysosomal storage disease. *Pediatr Neurol*, Vol 29, No 5, pp 391-403.

Matte U, de Carvalho T, Mayer F, Lagranha V, Giugliani R. (2011) Cell Microencapsulation: a Potential Tool for the Treatment of Neuronopathic Lysosomal Storage Diseases. *Journal of Inherited Metabolic Diseases*, epub.

Mayer, F.Q., Baldo, G., de Carvalho, T.G., Lagranha, V.L., Giugliani, R., Matte, U. (2010) Effects of cryopreservation and hypothermic storage on cell viability and enzyme activity in recombinant encapsulated cells overexpressing alpha-L-iduronidase. *Artif Organs,* Vol 34, No 5, pp 434-439.

Meikle, P.J., Fietz, M.J., Hopwood, J.J. (2004) Diagnosis of lysosomal storage disorders: current techniques and future directions. *Expert Rev Mol Diagn.* Vol 4, No 5, pp 677–691.

Moreira, J., Gaspar, R., Allen T. (2001) Targeting Stealth liposomes in a murine model of human small cell lung cancer. *Biochimica et Biophysica Acta,* Vol 1515, pp 167-176.

Morille, M., Passirani, C., Vonarbourg, A., Clavreul, A., Benoit, J.P. (2008) Progress in developing cationic vectors for non-viral systemic gene therapy against cancer. *Biomaterials,* Vol, 29, No 24-25, pp 3477-3496.

Muñoz-Rojas, M.V., Horovitz, D.D., Jardim, L.B., Raymundo, M., Llerena, J.C. Jr, de Magalhães, T.S., Vieira, T.A., Costa, R., Kakkis, E., Giugliani, R. (2010) Intrathecal administration of recombinant human N-acetylgalactosamine 4-sulfatase to a MPS VI patient with pachymeningitis cervicalis. *Mol Genet Metab,* Vol 99, No 4, pp 346-350.

Munoz-Rojas, M.V., Vieira, T., Costa, R., Fagondes, S., John, A., Jardim, L.B., Vedolin, L.M., Raymundo, M., Dickson, P.I., Kakkis, E., Giugliani, R. (2008) Intrathecal enzyme replacement therapy in a patient with mucopolysaccharidosis type I and symptomatic spinal cord compression. *Am J Med Genet A,* Vol 146A, Vol 19, pp 2538-2544.

Muro, S. (2010) New biotechnological and nanomedicine strategies for treatment of lysosomal storage disorders. *Wiley Interdiscip Rev Nanomed Nanobiotechnol,* Vol 2, No 2, pp 189-204.

Naganawa, Y., Ohsugi, K., Kase, R., Date, I., Sakuraba, H., Sakuragawa, N. (2002) In vitro study of encapsulation therapy for Fabry disease using genetically engineered CHO cell line. *Cell Transplant,* Vol 11, No 4, pp 325-329.

Nakama, H, Ohsugi, K, Otsuki, T., Date, I., Kosuga, M., Okuyama, T., Sakuragawa, N. (2006) Encapsulation cell therapy for mucopolysaccharidosis type VII using genetically engineered immortalized human amniotic epithelial cells. *Tohoku J Exp Med,* Vol 209, No 1, pp 23-32.

Nam, H.Y., Park, J.H., Kim, K., Kwon, I.C., Jeong, S.Y. (2009) Lipid-based emulsion system as non-viral gene carriers. *Arch Pharm Res* Vol 32, No 5, pp 639-646.

Niidome, T. and Huang, L. (2002) Gene Therapy Progress and Prospects: Nonviral vectors. *Gene Therapy* Vol 9, No 24, pp 1647–1652.

Orive, G., Ponce, S., Hernandez, R.M., Gascon, A.R., Igartua, M., Pedraz, J.L. (2002) Biocompatibility of microcapsules for cell imobilization alaborated with different type of alginates. *Biomaterials* Vol 23, No 18, pp 3825-3831.

Orive, G., Gascon, R.A., Hernandez, R.M., Igartua, M., Pedraz, J.L. (2003) Cell microencapsulation technology for biomedical purposes: novel insights and challenges. *Trends in Pharmacological Sciences,* Vol 24, No 5, pp 207-210.

Osborn, M.J., McElmurry, R.T., Peacock, B., Tolar, J., Blazar, B.R. (2008) Targeting of the CNS in MPS-IH using a nonviral transferrin-alpha-L-iduronidase fusion gene product. *Mol Ther,* Vol 16, No 8, pp 1459-1466.

Osborn, M.J., McElmurry, R.T., Lees, C.J., Defeo, A.P., Chen, Z.Y., Kay, M.A., Naldini, L., Freeman, G., Tolar, J., Blazar, B.R. (2011) Minicircle DNA-based Gene Therapy Coupled With Immune Modulation Permits Long-term Expression of α-L-Iduronidase in Mice With Mucopolysaccharidosis Type I. *Mol Ther,* 2011 Vol 19, No 3, pp 450-460.

Pardridge, W.M. (2007) Blood-brain barrier delivery of protein and non-viral gene therapeutics with molecular Trojan horses. *J Control Release,* Vol 122, No 3, pp 345-348.

Parkinson-Lawrence, E.J., Shandala, T., Prodoehl, M., Plew, R., Borlace, G.N., Brooks, D.A. (2010) Lysosomal storage disease: revealing lysosomal function and physiology. *Physiology (Bethesda),* Vol 25, No 2, pp 102-115.

Plasterk, R.H. (1993) Molecular mechanisms of transposition and its control. *Cell,* Vol 74, No 5, pp 781–786.

Ragnaill, M.N., Brown, M., Ye, D., Bramini, M., Callanan, S., Lynch, I., Dawson, K.A. (2011) Internal benchmarking of a human blood-brain barrier cell model for screening of nanoparticle uptake and transcytosis. *Eur J Pharm Biopharm.* Vol 77, No 3, pp 360-367.

Resina, S., Prevot, P., Thierry, A.R. (2009) Physico-chemical characteristics of lipoplexes influence cell uptake mechanisms and transfection efficacy. *PLoS One* Vol 4, No 6, e6058.

Richard, M., Arfi, A., Seguin, J., Gandolphe, C., Scherman, D. (2009) Widespread biochemical correction of murine mucopolysaccharidosis type VII pathology by liver hydrodynamic plasmid delivery. *Gene Ther,* Vol 16, No 6, pp 746-756.

Riu, E., Grimm, D., Huang, Z. and Kay, M.A. (2005). Increased maintenance and persistence of transgenes by excision of expression cassettes from plasmid sequences in vivo. *Hum Gene Ther* Vol 16, No 5, pp 558–570.

Roberg-Perez, K., Carlson, C.M., Largaespada, D.A. (2003) MTID: a database of Sleeping Beauty transposon insertions in mice. *Nucleic Acids Res,* Vol 31, No 1, pp 78-81.

Ross, C.J., Bastedo, L., Maier, S.A., Sands, M.S., Chang, P.L. (2000a) Treatment of a lysosomal storage disease, mucopolysaccharidosis VII, with microencapsulated recombinant cells. *Hum Gene Ther,* Vol 11, No 15, pp 2117-2127.

Ross, C.J., Ralph, M., Chang, P.L. (2000b) Somatic gene therapy for a neurodegenerative disease using microencapsulated recombinant cells. *Exp Neurol,* Vol 166, No 2, pp 276-286.

Sifuentes, M., Doroshow, R., Hoft, R., Mason, G., Walot, I., Diament, M., Okazaki, S., Huff, K., Cox, G.F., Swiedler, S.J., Kakkis, E.D. (2007) A follow-up study of MPS I patients treated with laronidase enzyme replacement therapy for 6 years. *Mol Genet Metab,* Vol 90, No 2, pp 171-180.

Skarlatos, S., Yoshikawa, T., Pardridge, W.M. (1995) Transport of [125I]transferrin through the rat blood-brain barrier. *Brain Res,* Vol 683, No 2, pp 164-171.

Sly, W.S., Fischer, H.D., Gonzalez-Noriega, A., Grubb, J.H., Natowicz, M. (1981) Role of the 6-phosphomannosyl-enzyme receptor in intracellular transport and adsorptive pinocytosis of lysosomal enzymes. *Methods Cell Biol,* Vol 23, pp 191-214.

Spuch. C., Antequera, D., Portero, A., Orive, G., Hernández, R.M., Molina, J.A., Bermejo-Pareja, F., Pedraz, J.L., Carro, E. (2010) The effect of encapsulated VEGF-secreting cells on brain amyloid load and behavioral impairment in a mouse model of Alzheimer's disease. *Biomaterials,* Vol 31, No21, pp 5608-5618.

Takakusaki, Y., Hisayasu, S., Hirai, Y., Shimada, T. (2005) Coexpression of formylglycine-generating enzyme is essential for synthesis and secretion of functional arylsulfatase A in a mouse model of metachromatic leukodystrophy. *Hum Gene Ther,* Vol 16, No 8, pp 929-936.

Tomanin, R., Friso, A., Alba, S., Piller Puicher, E., Mennuni, C., La Monica, N., Hortelano, G., Zacchello, F., Scarpa M. (2002) Non-viral transfer approaches for the gene therapy of mucopolysaccharidosis type II (Hunter syndrome). *Acta Paediatr Suppl,* Vol 91, No 439, pp 100-104.

Uludag, H., Vos, P., Tresco, P. (2000) Technology of mammalian cell encapsulation. *Adv Drug Delivery Reviews,* Vol 42, No 1-2, pp 29-64.

Vitner, E.B., Platt, F.M., Futerman, A.H. (2010) Common and uncommon pathogenic cascades in lysosomal storage diseases. *J Biol Chem,* Vol 285, No 27, pp 20423-20427.

Walkley, S.U. (2009) Pathogenic cascades in lysosomal disease-Why so complex? *J Inherit Metab Dis*, Vol 32, No 2, pp 181-189.

Wasungu, L., Hoekstra, D. (2006) Cationic lipids, lipoplexes and intracellular delivery of genes. *Journal of Controlled Release*, Vol. 116, No 2, pp 255-264.

Williams, D.A. (2008). Sleeping beauty vector system moves toward human trials in the United States. *Mol Ther*, Vol 16, No 9, pp 1515-1516.

Wilson JM. (2009) Lessons learned from the gene therapy trial for ornithine transcarbamylase deficiency. *Mol Genet Metab,*Vol 96, No 4, pp 151-157.

Worgall, S., Sondhi, D., Hackett, N.R., Kosofsky, B., Kekatpure, M.V., Neyzi, N., Dyke, J.P., Ballon, D., Heier, L., Greenwald, B.M., Christos, P., Mazumdar, M., Souweidane, M.M., Kaplitt, M.G., Crystal, R.G. (2008) Treatment of late infantile neuronal ceroid lipofuscinosis by CNS administration of a serotype 2 adeno-associated virus expressing CLN2 cDNA. *Hum Gene Ther*, Vol 19, No 5, pp 463-474.

Zhang, Y., Wang, Y., Boado, R.J., Pardridge, W.M. (2007) Lysosomal enzyme replacement of the brain with intravenous non-viral gene transfer. *Pharm Res,* Vol 25, No 2, pp 400-406.

8

DNA Vaccination by Electrogene Transfer

Pieranna Chiarella[1,2], Vito Michele Fazio[1,3] and Emanuela Signori[1,2]
[1]*Laboratory of Molecular Pathology and Experimental Oncology, CNR-IFT, Rome*
[2]*Laboratory of Molecular Medicine and Biotechnology*
CIR, University Campus Bio-Medico of Rome, Rome
[3]*Laboratory of Oncology, IRCCS 'Casa Sollievo della Sofferenza'*
Italy

1. Introduction

Vaccination: Traditional and new generation vaccines

Vaccination is historically one of the most important methods for the prevention of infectious diseases in humans and animals. When Edward Jenner inoculated James Phipps with a bovine poxvirus to induce protection against the closely related human pathogen smallpox virus in 1796 and then, almost a century later, Pasteur developed a live attenuated vaccine against rabies, the basic principles for vaccine development were established (Fraser and Rappuoli 2005). Traditionally, a vaccine is known as a preparation of attenuated or killed microorganisms or of subunit vaccines (purified components of a pathogen including the protein-conjugated capsular polysaccharides, toxoids, cell-free extracts, recombinant proteins and stand-alone capsular polysaccharides) administered for inducing active immunity to a specific disease.

Two types of immunization exist with intrinsic differences between them: prophylactic vaccination initiates a response against an antigen to which the immune response is naïve, leading to a long-term memory cell maintenance and protective efficacy; therapeutic vaccination stimulates the immune system to a chronically displayed antigen, leading to a clearance of an established infection.

Several infectious diseases can be prevented by vaccines produced with conventional approaches. These methods are based on the cultivation in laboratory conditions of the microorganism from which single components are isolated individually by using biochemical, microbiological and serological techniques. Each antigen is produced in pure form either directly from the bacterium or using the DNA recombinant technology, and finally tested for its ability to induce an immune response (Serruto and Rappuoli 2006).

Conventional approaches provided the basis of vaccinology and led to great achievements such as the eradication of smallpox and the virtual disappearance of diseases like diphtheria, tetanus, poliomyelitis, pertussis, measles, mumps, rubella and invasive *Haemophilus influenzae* B, increasing the life quality and expectancy (Andre 2003). Nevertheless, they present major disadvantages such as to be time-consuming and, more important, to be impractical in some circumstances due to the difficulty in cultivating some microorganisms *in vitro* and to the fact that even attenuation may result in detrimental or unwanted immune responses (Purcell et al. 2007). Moreover, in many cases the antigens expressed during infection are not produced in laboratory conditions, as well as the proteins that are most abundant and easily purified are not necessarily protective antigens and, in any case, only few molecules can be isolated and tested simultaneously (Serruto and Rappuoli 2006).

The last decade has witnessed a revolution in the approach to vaccine design and development. These advances include new delivery technologies aimed at improving the safety and immunogenicity of traditional vaccines, new strategies to identify protective antigens, generation of improved adjuvants.

Considering that new diseases are sure to emerge through evolution by mutation and gene exchange, interspecies transfer or human exposure to novel environments, more reliable approaches must be available to promptly respond to those threats (Plotkin 2005). Thanks to sophisticated technologies such as genomics, proteomics, functional genomics and synthetic chemistry, the rational identification of antigens, the synthesis of complex glycans, the generation of engineered carrier proteins are possible. This leads to identify, generate and test new vaccines, to use not only against infectious diseases but also in the treatment of autoimmune disorders, allergies, chronic inflammatory diseases and cancer. There are several vaccine modalities currently under investigation, including subunit vaccines, syntetic peptide vaccines, ex-vivo loaded dendritic cells (DCs) and genetic vaccination, that will be here discussed.

1.1 Subunit vaccines

Subunit vaccines have improved conventional attenuated or killed vaccines in many aspects, including safety and production. The systems mostly used to produce these vaccines are based on bacteria, yeast, insect or mammalian cells. However, production of recombinant vaccine proteins in these expression systems is expensive in many cases, requiring large scale fermenters and stringent purification protocols. Worldwide, only a small number of facilities exists with capabilities to produce kilograms of a specific protein to be used as immunogen, and the construction, validation, and final approval of new production facilities take many years implying important investments in capital and human resources. Additionally, some antigens require post-translational modifications that cannot be achieved using all expression systems. In the last decade, non-fermentative alternatives based on living organisms have been developed to solve such problems and provide low-cost technologies for vaccine production. Insects and plants have been adapted for subunit vaccine production with clear advantages to conventional fermentative systems, especially in terms of time of development, scaling-up production and cost-efficiency (Brun et al. 2011). Despite the improvements in the recombinant technology, these vaccines remain hard to produce due to their inherent toxicity for the bacterial/viral expression system (e.g., Human Papilloma Virus type 16-E2, wild-type p53) (van der Burg et al. 2006).

1.2 Syntetic peptide vaccines

Identification of individual epitopes within protective proteins allows the development of peptide vaccines as alternative approach respect to using a whole protein as a vaccine. Selected peptide epitopes represent the minimal immunogenic region of a protein antigen and allow for precise direction of immune responses aiming at the induction of T-cell immunity. A peptide vaccine should ideally include epitopes recognized both by B and T cells, and take into account the MHC restriction of the T-cell response. In some cases B and

T-cell epitopes can overlap substantially within the sequence of an antigen and, in others, they might be present in separate discrete regions of the antigen or present in different antigens from the targeted pathogen. The simplicity of producing clinical grade peptides allows swift changes in the design of peptide vaccines and, therefore, rapid translation of new immunological concepts, which represent a great advantage for the development of vaccines against rapidly changing viruses such as influenza (Brun et al. 2011). Despite the potential advantages of this approach, the development of successful peptide vaccines has been limited mainly by difficulties associated with stability, poor immunogenicity of simple peptides and by the MHC polymorphism of the host species (Tam 1996).

1.3 Ex-vivo loaded dendritic cells

Antigen Presenting Cells-based vaccines represent another explored field in vaccine research. With this approach, DC are harvested from the patient, pulsed with antigens or transfected with genes encoding these antigens, and readministered to the patient. This vaccine strategy has the potential to augment presentation through the MHC-class I pathway and subsequently drive the expansion of tumour-specific CTLs. In translational studies with melanoma patients, DC vaccines have demonstrated a keen ability to elicit detectable immune responses. However, such responses often fail to elicit substantial clinical responses. As it is often difficult to discern the relative contributions of DCs and effector T cells in these situations, a thorough investigation of the *in vivo* interactions between these immune cell populations may be required before a complete understanding of DC role (Palucka et al. 2007).

1.4 Genetic vaccination

Recently, new methods of vaccination such as those based on gene transfer have emerged. Genetic vaccination originates from gene therapy. The objective of genetic vaccination is to transfer in the host a gene encoding for the disease target antigen with the aim to induce a specific immune response, whereas the goal of gene therapy is to ensure production of a protein which is lacking or defective in the host. To date, the vast majority of gene therapy clinical trials have addressed cancer (66.5%), cardiovascular diseases (9.1%) and infectious diseases (6.5%). For infectious diseases, a total of 85 gene therapy trials have been carried out, the majority of these trials being performed on human immunodeficiency virus infection, tetanus, cytomegalovirus and adenovirus infections (Chiarella et al. 2008a).
Current techniques of gene transfer in mammals include packaging the DNA into carriers for gene delivery. The ideal carriers for gene delivery should be safe and yet ensure that the DNA survives the extra and intracellular environment, efficiently transfer to the appropriate cellular compartments assuring good and long-lasting expression levels.
Presently, viral vectors are more efficient than non-viral systems, achieving high levels of efficiency, estimated around 90%, for both gene delivery and expression. However, immunogenicity, inflammatory reactions, problems associated with scale-up costs and, more important, the risk of integration in the host genome, are limiting their clinical use in preclinical and clinical protocols respect to the past: i.e. during 2000 year, around 75% of clinical protocols involving gene therapy used recombinant virus-based vectors for DNA delivery (Chiarella et al. 2008a). In the last years, lot of clinical trials pointed out that the use of viral vectors as antigen delivery systems has numerous other drawbacks such as toxicity, recombination, precedent host immunity, higher immunogenicity in comparison to the

target antigen and limited DNA carrying capacity (Harrington et al. 2002; Ramirez et al. 2000). The recent advances made on the knowledge of the immune system biology have led to consider non-viral systems as naked DNA vaccination an alternative, safer and promising approach for introducing foreign antigens into the host to induce an immune response.
At the moment, non-viral systems, especially those based on plasmid DNA delivery, have become increasingly desirable in both basic research laboratories and clinical settings.

2. DNA vaccination

2.1 DNA vaccines: An emerging field

In 1990, Wolff and collaborators found that bacterial plasmid DNA encoding a reporter gene could result in *in vivo* expression of the encoded protein after simple intramuscular injection without the need for more complex vectors (Wolff et al. 1990). Following Wolff's findings a new era of vaccination started.
Naked-DNA vaccines are for definition vectors based on bacterial plasmids engineered to express the disease-specific antigen using promoter elements active in mammalian cells, without the addition of surrounding chemicals or a viral coat. The main advantages of naked DNA vaccines are safety and production in large amount, as well as stability at different temperatures and, more important, flexibility in design, since multiple antigenic targets or multiple independent cytokines or co-stimulatory sequences can be incorporated into a single DNA vector. They are also likely to be attractive from a health economics perspective: they are relatively easy to manufacture in large quantities in contrast to the complicated processes requested for attenuated virus vaccines, and do not require any special transportation or storage conditions that could hinder their widespread distribution as it happens for live pathogens-based vaccines which need to be distributed and stored in cold conditions. The genes encoding the antigens can be chemically constructed without deriving them from live virulent organisms so avoiding for operators and patients the risks of exposure to dangerous pathogens. They are commonly delivered by a simple intramuscular injection. In mammals the skeletal muscle represents approximately the 30% of the body mass, and muscle fibres are ideal targets for DNA transfection. These are stable and large syncytial cells containing several nuclei that can actively take part in immune reactions. For the easy accessibility of the skeletal muscle and good vasculature, the delivery of DNA vaccine into this organ is highly preferable (Wiendl et al. 2005). Immunisation with DNA induces all three arms of adaptive immunity (antibodies, helper T cells, CTLs), and even innate immune responses can be easily and rapidly made while maintaining fidelity to the immunological aspects necessary for a pathogen, yet excluding other undesirable proteins or immune responses (Liu 2011).
On the other hand, a major disadvantage of plasmid DNA vaccines is their poor immunogenicity when administered as an unformulated intramuscular injection. Large quantities of DNA are required to induce only modest immunogenicity and many efforts have focussed on the development of new technologies aimed at increasing the DNA vaccine potency (Chiarella et al. 2008a). That said, better strategies are needed in designing more effective vectors and combined protocols so as to induce a strong immune response to weakly immunogenic antigens. These strategies comprise new insights in studying the mechanism of action and induction of the immune response in a host injected with a DNA-based vaccine. Recently, most relevant patented strategies have been developed to enhance the plasmid DNA vaccine immunogenicity taking into account DNA plasmid construction,

epitope and antigen choice, selection and use of new adjuvants and different delivery methods.
In table 1 the advantages and disadvantages of DNA vaccines are listed.

Characteristic	Advantage/disadvantage of plasmid DNA vaccines
Antigen	In vivo antigen synthesis with native conformation
Antigen presentation	MHC-I, MHC-II, cross-priming
Immune Response	Humoural and cytotoxic
Manufacture	Easy and fast
Stability	Stable at various temperature (RT)
Risk	Does not induce the disease related to the encoded antigen
Applicability	Prophylaxis and therapy of disease
Indication of use	Infectious disease, allergy, cancer, autoimmune disease
Safety	Low risk of recombination and inflammation
Immunogenicity	Weak

Table 1. Advantages and disadvantages of plasmid DNA vaccines.

2.2 Mechanism of action and induction of the immune response

The crucial event responsible for the initiation of an immune response against a foreign antigen is recognition by specialized cells namely the antigen presenting cells (APCs), uptake and presentation of the antigen to naïve lymphocytes and induction of effector T helper (Th), cytotoxic (CTL) and B lymphocytes.
In this context the mechanism of action of DNA vaccines looks very simple. Once the DNA vaccine is delivered into the skeletal muscle, the plasmid DNA is taken up by the resident DCs and by the muscle fibres. While transfected muscle cells behave as permanent antigen reservoir as well as target of immune effector cells (Payette et al. 2001), resident DCs have the property to leave the muscle tissue and move to the closest draining lymph nodes in order to process and present the antigen to T lymphocytes (**Fig. 1**). DCs are specialized in capturing extracellular antigens by receptor-mediated endocytosis and pinocytosis mechanisms and following antigen uptake they undergo a complex multi-step maturation process. DC maturation depends also on the microbial and pathogens-derived signals which increase their capacity to migrate towards the draining lymph node. While DCs move to the lymphoid organs, they interact with various chemokines which contribute further to their maturation process (Palucka et al. 2010). Once in the lymph nodes, DCs shift from an antigen-capturing cell to a T sensitizing cell, being capable to present antigen in association with the class I and class II MHC molecules to CTLs and Th lymphocytes. Interaction between the DC and the T lymphocyte induces formation of the immunological synapse (IS) *via* complex MHC-antigen- T cell receptor (TCR) resulting in the clonal expansion of the T lymphocyte and differentiation in T memory cell. Professional DCs can also capture antigens released in the interstitial space by skeletal muscle fibres or in form of apoptotic bodies activating the cross-presentation pathway (**Fig. 1**) (Russo et al. 2000). This route allows presentation of extracellular/exogenous antigens through the MHC-I restriction pathways (Kurts et al. 2010). Therefore, extracellular antigens which normally induce a humoural immune response can also access to the MHC-I compartment through endoplasmic reticulum, leading to simultaneous stimulation of the CTL immune response. Antigen synthesized

by DC or skeletal muscle cell can also be released in the extracellular environment and activate directly the B lymphocytes through antigen-antibody interaction (**Fig.1**).
Considering the mechanism described above, plasmid DNA vaccines are able to stimulate all the principal effector cells of the adaptive immune system but due to the presence of CpG islands intrinsic to the DNA structure they can also can mimic some aspects of live infection, activating important signals of the innate immune system (Matzinger 2007). Theoretically genetic immunisation by plasmid DNA vaccines seems to confer the same broad immunological advantages as immunisation with live, attenuated vaccines does, without the accompanying safety concerns associated with live infection, such as reversion to the virulent form and/or incomplete inactivation of live vaccines. However there are some obstacles that make naked DNA vaccination less potent than traditional vaccines.

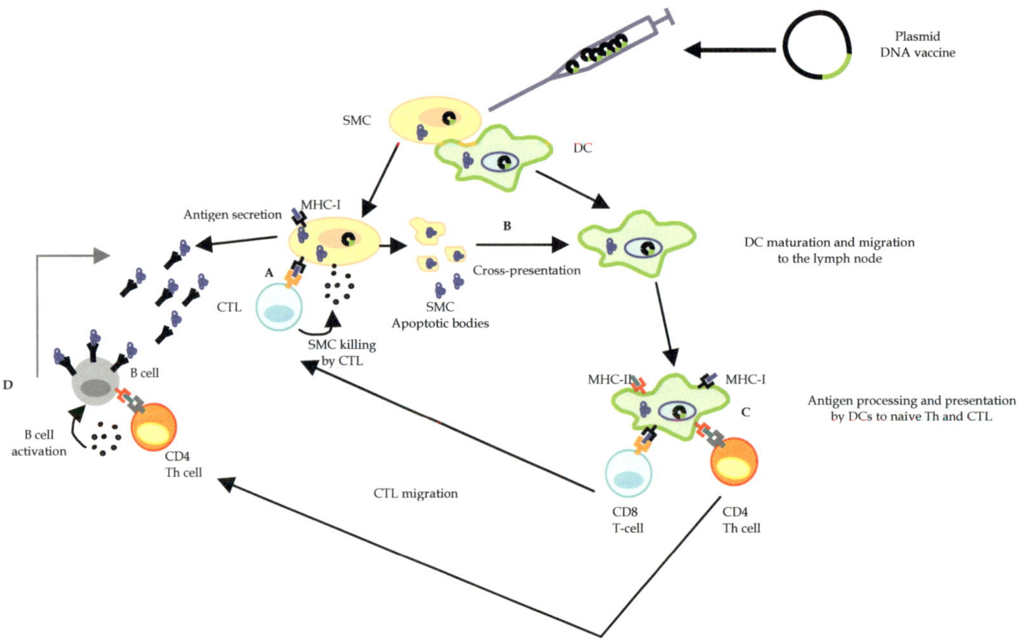

Fig. 1. Mechanism of action of plasmid DNA vaccination.

The antigen sequence is cloned into a bacterial plasmid vector specific for vaccination. The DNA vaccine is administered by intramuscular injection. After plasmid uptake by muscle cells, the gene coding for the antigen is translated into a protein. Transfected skeletal muscle cells can present the antigen to CTL through MHC-I molecules (**A**) as well as through DCs cross presentation (**B**). Plasmid is also uptaken by resident DCs which synthesize the antigen and present it in association with MHC-I molecules and MHC-II molecules to CD8+ T and CD4+ T-helper lymphocytes (**C**). Furthermore, antigen is released in the extracellular environment inducing the production of antibodies by B lymphocytes whose activation is mediated by the CD4+ T-helper cells (**D**). SMC, skeletal muscle cell; DC, dendritic cell; CTL, cytotoxic lymphocyte.CD8 T cell, CD8 T lymphocyte; CD4 Th cell, CD4 T helper lymphocyte; B cell, B lymphocyte.

2.3 DNA plasmid construction

DNA plasmid vaccines offer several advantages when compared to viral vectors or live attenuated vaccines. First of all they are easy to construct and to manipulate which is an important characteristic required to vaccines against pandemic diseases. They are also very stable at room temperature, do not require particular storage conditions which makes them ideal candidates for long-term delivery in other countries. The antigen can be chemically synthesized and cloned directly into the plasmid vaccine simplifying the operations of amplification by molecular techniques and avoiding to work with potentially dangerous live antigen source. The DNA constructs can be easily made to encode for modified proteins deprived of regions that might be dangerous or toxic to the recipient cell or that might suppress the immune response. DNA is a highly flexible molecule, the basic construct can be manipulated in several ways by genetic engineering in order to increase antigen expression, immunogenicity and uptake by recipient cells. All the modifications can affect both the vector backbone and the gene sequence incorporated into the plasmid, which can include adjuvant-like sequences with stimulating activity on the immune system (Abdulhaqq and Weiner 2008). By using this approach, enhanced antigen specific immune responses were observed, suggesting that this could be a general method for targeting antigen to selected cell types. Different strategies can be used for enhancing the plasmid DNA vaccine potency. A first strategy allows to improve the vector construct *i.e.* by working on the plasmid backbone design and construction; a second strategy allows to improve the codon usage in order to maximize the antigen synthesis.

An expression vector for genetic vaccination generally consists of the following elements: 1) a promoter/enhancer sequence; 2) the gene of interest encoding the target antigen; 3) a polyadenylation/transcriptional terminator sequence; 4) a resistance gene for plasmid selection and an origin of replication (Ori) in order to allow production of high numbers plasmid copies. The capacity of a plasmid DNA vector to drive gene expression is obtained by an optimal combination of all these requisites, and by the possibility of introducing various modifications into the plasmid backbone. The promoters mostly used for gene expression vectors are the cytomegalovirus immediately-early promoter (CMV) the simian virus SV40 early promoter (SV40) and the Rous sarcoma virus promoter (RSV). The CMV promoter is the most popular, as it drives gene expression in a wide range of cells and tissues (Lundquist et al. 1999). Plasmid DNA vectors can also contain tissue specific, synthetic and controllable promoters, whose sequences are designed for a specific use (Papadakis et al. 2004). When the expression of a gene is desired in certain tissues, promoters that control expression in a cell- tissue-specific manner are used. For instance the alpha skeletal muscle actin promoter is specifically used for selective expression in skeletal muscle cells whereas endothelial cell-specific promoters are used to drive expression in the tumour-associated endothelial cells (Dong and Nor 2009). The flexibility of DNA vector permits investigators to exploit the concept of gene expression optimisation by creating synthetic promoters, such as enhancer/promoters composed of numerous combinations of various regulatory sequences (Edelman et al. 2000; Li et al. 1999). One of these regulatory synthetic sequence, the hybrid CMV-Ub promoter, was found to have higher expression than the natural muscle promoters (Yew et al. 2001). In order to display gene expression kinetics, naturally regulated systems were developed by incorporating sequence elements that respond to the local environment of the given cell or tissue or that are regulated by small molecule drugs (Yew 2005). Thus transgene expression can be regulated by modulating expression of these transcriptional factors or by altering their activity through drug administration. However, regulation of *in vivo*

transgene expression by such approaches is unreliable, mainly due to the low levels of control associated with the complexity of these systems. Appropriate choice of regulatory elements and vector backbone can lead the gene expression kinetics from a few days to several months. Nuclear localization of plasmid DNA is another prerequisite for the effective antigen expression. To this purpose our laboratory developed a series of plasmids with a functional nuclear translocation sequence (NTS) (Ciafre et al. 1998). All the characteristics of plasmid DNA vaccines mentioned above are summarized in **Table 1**.
The codon usage is an important issue to consider in the DNA vaccine manufacture. Plasmid DNA are totally dependent on the host cell machinery for protein transcription and translation. Since codon usage of bacterial organisms is different from the codon usage of mammalian, it is mandatory to optimize codon usage in DNA vaccine to allow maximum antigen expression (Bojak et al. 2002). Various codon usage approaches are now commonly exploited in both non-human primate studies and clinical trials. This strategy has been successfully used to optimize the sequence of mycobacterial antigens (e.g., Ag85B) improving protein expression and thereby enhancing the immunogenicity of DNA vaccines against M. tuberculosis (Ko et al. 2005).

2.4 Epitope and antigen selection

The first requisite for a DNA vaccine to induce effective immune response is related to the choice of the target antigen. Sometimes the immunogenic determinant of a certain pathogen is unknown hence selection of antigen sequences has to be included as first step in the design of an epitope-based vaccine. The goal is to identify relevant T cell epitopes, able to bind to MHC class I and II molecules that are both effective and sufficient in vaccine protection against pathogen challenge or, in the case of cancer vaccines, T cell epitopes of malignant antigens that are not ignored by the immune system. In particular for tumours, highly immunogenic antigen determinants remain to be identified for most cancers types. The "direct immunological approach" which consists of deriving tumour cell lines from malignant biopsies, isolating the cancer antigens and expanding the human CTLs specific for that given antigen is now substituted by the "reverse immunological approach" (Sette and Rappuoli 2010). With this new method a candidate cancer antigen expressed on a tumour is selected by *in silico* studies. First tumour antigens are identified by exploiting immune assays based on the availability of specific polyclonal and monoclonal antibodies. Otherwise the serological analysis of recombinantly expressed clones technology (SEREX) is also supportive to identify novel tumour antigens where the blood serum of patients affected by neoplastic diseases is screened against tumour antigen cDNA expression libraries (Jager et al. 2004). Techniques employed in the molecular biology field are also helpful. The analysis of the human transcriptome based on DNA and RNA microarrays allows identification of cancer antigens in a high-throughput system. As following step, putative antigenic determinants are predicted with the aid of bioinformatics. This makes it possible to identify a variety of epitopes within an antigen sequence and to choose the best candidates for the binding to specific MHC molecules. This system works well for epitope discovery, and predictions of the MHC class I pathway is being further improved by integration with prediction tools for proteasomal cleavage and Transporter associated with Antigen Processing (TAP) binding (Larsen et al. 2007) . Furthermore, native epitopes that do not fit perfectly into the MHC groove can be modified at specific sites to increase their affinity to the MHC molecule of interest, leading to the generation of what are called "heteroclitic" epitopes (Dyall et al. 1998). The antigen determinant can be modified either by increasing the affinity of the binding to the MHC molecules or by augumenting the binding ability of the peptide–MHC complex for the TCR. The first approach is the most widely used (Dudek NL et al. 2010). This strategy is commonly exploited in the design of cancer vaccines, allowing to convert a subdominant into a dominant epitope by making it more competitive in the binding to specific MHC alleles, and thereby enhancing the potency of the vaccine. The primary and/or secondary anchor residues of an epitope can be replaced with specific aminoacids that provide much of the specificity of binding to the MHC molecule. Epitope "enhancement" is possible for both classes of human MHC resulting in priming of the $CD8^+$ cytotoxic T-lymphocytes (CTL) which can recognise the target epitope on tumour or infected cells and in activation of $CD4^+$ T helper cells whose role is crucial for promoting humoural and cytolytic responses, regardless the CTL epitope enhancement. The selection of biologically relevant epitopes within an antigen sequence is performed with different bioinformatic softwares. Several databases of MHC binding peptides now exist and a number of programs performing such predictions are available on the web. We experienced the use of SYFPEITHI, BIMAS and PROPRED I-II programs (www.syfpeithi.de; www-bimas.cit.nih.gov; www.imtech.res.in/raghava/propred)(Parker et al. 1994; Rammensee et al. 1999; Singh and Raghava 2001). They are based on different algorithms that provide estimation of the binding of a certain peptide sequence to a wide spectrum of human MHC molecules. Unfortunately, a major drawback of these programs is their intrinsic feature of being 'predictive' in estimating the binding affinity between the MHC molecule and the antigenic epitope, with approximately 70% reliability. Another limit is they cannot calculate the binding of the MHC-peptide complex to the T cell receptor, which is a crucial point to verify the immunogenicity of the tumour antigenic determinant.

Once immunogenic peptides are predicted *in silico* they need to be verified experimentally. This goal is achieved by performing *in vitro* assays to confirm their stability and binding capacity. After that, human CTL isolated from patients are assayed *in vitro* to verify their capability to recognize specifically the selected epitope on the tumour cells. This result represents the validation of the tumour antigens. Once the antigenic epitope has been validated, it can be taken in consideration for DNA vaccines manufacture and for initiating vaccination trials.

2.5 Adjuvants

It is widely accepted immunogenicity of DNA vaccines is generally weak in comparison to that of traditional vaccines. Although plasmid vaccines are capable to induce a complete immune response involving activation of CTLs, Th and B lymphocytes and a certain activation of the innate compartment of the immune system, these vaccines show low potency and efficacy when administered as unformulated injection. DNA vaccines like all the subunit vaccines, which are made of purified or recombinant antigens, require additional components to help stimulating a "comprehensive" immune reaction. Such "help" is provided by substances and components termed adjuvants.

Adjuvants of current use, either in man or in animals, have for the most part been developed empirically, without a clear understanding of their cellular and molecular mechanisms of action. Indeed adjuvants were historically defined as "the dirty little secret of the immunologist" (Janeway 1989).

The main function of an adjuvant is to create a depot of antigen at the injection site, resulting in a gradual release of small quantities of antigen over a long period of time. The adjuvant also serves as a vehicle for delivering the antigen to the lymph organs, where antigenic epitopes can be presented to T cells by professional APCs. However, recent advances in the immunological research suggest that most, if not all, adjuvants enhance T and B cell responses by engaging components of the innate immune system, rather than by exerting direct effects on the lymphocytes. In DNA vaccinations, adjuvants are used to achieve qualitative alteration of the immune response. Adjuvants confer to DNA or to subunit vaccines the ability to promote an immune response which might not occur in their absence. Here we describe certain classes of adjuvants most widely used in DNA vaccinations. A summary of the adjuvants described bellow is presented in **Table 2.**

Class of adjuvants	Adjuvant name	Nature of the adjuvant
Genetic adjuvants	Interleukin-2 Interleukin-12 Granulocyte Monocyte-Colony Stimulating Factor T-helper epitopes of toxins	Cytokine Cytokine Cytokine Peptides
Adjuvants targeting Pattern Recognition Receptors	Monophosphoryl Lipid A AS02 AS01 QS-21 CpG-DNA	Lipid derivative Oil in water emulsion Liposomal formulation Saponin Oligodeoxynucleotides
Aluminium-based compounds	Aluminium Phosphate Aluminium Hydroxide	Mineral salt Mineral salt

Table 2. Adjuvants used in vaccination with naked DNA.

2.5.1 Genetic adjuvants

Genetic adjuvants are molecules such as cytokines, chemokines and co-stimulatory factors that may be cloned into the DNA plasmid vaccine and expressed *in vivo*. These adjuvants can be encoded on the same vector expressing the antigen or inserted into a separate vector and co-injected with the vaccine. This method provides adjuvant activity at the site of antigen production, with lasting effect from transfected cells. Among various factors, cytokines are highly preferred as genetic adjuvants because they act on cells involved in the host defense and can be used to modulate immune responses. Co-delivery of cytokines in DNA vaccine formulations has been used extensively for a wide range of infectious diseases such as malaria, leishmania, schistosoma to enhance the T cell mediated responses (Ivory and Chadee 2004). One of the earliest cytokines to be incorporated into a DNA vaccine was IL-2, a well known T-cell growth factor included in several immunotherapy protocols. Addition of this cytokine to a plasmid vaccination vector resulted in enhanced antibody responses in low responder mice against malaria (Good et al. 1988) and increased production of antibodies directed against the complementary determining hypervariable region 3 of the Ig heavy chain in human B-cell lymphoma (Rinaldi et al. 2001). IL-2 contributed to increase the efficacy of a DNA vaccine against a simian immunodeficiency virus when it was fused with the immunoglobulin Fc fragment, resulting in augmentation of the cytokine half-life (Barouch et al. 2000). However, the use of IL-2 is now being limited by the emerging evidence that this cytokine can play a major role in maintaining self-tolerance and in supporting survival of $CD25^{+}$ $CD4^{+}$ regulatory T cells (T-regs) (Bayer et al. 2005; Setoguchi et al. 2005).

IL-12 is another cytokine used in DNA vaccination. It acts on T and NK cells by inducing the generation of CTLs through T-helper 1 cell activation and IFN-γ production. The beneficial effect of IL-12 in pre-clinical experimental tumour models suggested the possibility of using IL-12 as an anti-tumour agent in clinical trials. Despite some toxicity associated with certain doses of IL-12 when administered as a drug in patients affected by melanoma and colon cancer, some clinical responses were observed; this indicates that IL-12 can be used in clinical protocols of cancer therapy where a toxic effect of the cytokine could be acceptable (Atkins et al. 1997; Gollob et al. 2003). Granulocyte/macrophage colony-stimulatory factor (GM-CSF) is probably the most attractive adjuvant for DNA vaccines for its ability to recruit antigen-presenting cells to the site where antigen synthesis occurs as well as for its capacity to stimulate DC maturation. Plasmid DNA vaccines were constructed fusing GM-CSF to the S antigen of Hepatitis B Virus (HBV) to vaccinate HBV-transgenic mice. This fusion construct worked well in conferring protection from the HBV to both normal and transgenic mice (Qing et al. 2010). In another study the utility of GM-CSF as a DNA vaccine adjuvant for glycoprotein B (gB) of pseudorabies virus (PrV) was evaluated in the vaccination of a murine model. Mouse co-inoculation with a vector expressing GM-CSF enhanced the protective immunity against PrV infection. This immunity was caused by the induction of increased humoural and cellular immunity in response to PrV antigen (Yoon et al. 2006). A DNA vaccine encoding the GM-CSF gene and a DNA vaccine encoding the H1N1 influenza (A/New Caledonia/20/99) HA antigen were co-administered by particle-mediated epidermal delivery in Rhesus Macaques. After three immunizations the DNA vaccines were shown to significantly enhance both the systemic and mucosal immunogenicity of the HA influenza vaccine (Loudon et al. 2010).

Among genetic adjuvants the pathogen-derived immune-enhancing proteins are noteworthy for their ability to stimulate the immune system when they are fused with target antigens. Modified bacterial toxins, such as anthrax, diphteria and pertussis toxins, are being used in vaccination as effective carriers to deliver foreign epitopes which stimulate protective CTL responses in mammalian cells (Ballard et al. 1996; Carbonetti et al. 1999). However, the ability of modified toxins to activate the host immune system does not reside only in the delivery effect exerted on the fused antigen (Stevenson et al. 2004).

The tetanus toxin Fragment C (FrC) is one of the widely used genetic adjuvant as a fusion partner for foreign antigens. This protein was found to increase the immunogenicity of the Schistosoma mansoni glutathione S-transferase antigen when administered as genetic fusion in a live Aro-attenuated vaccine strain of Salmonella (Khan et al. 1994b) and similar results were obtained when a vaccine construct consisting of a portion of P28 glutathione S-transferase was administering intravenously as C-terminal fusion to tetanus toxin FrC in a live Aro-attenuated vaccine strain of Salmonella (Khan et al. 1994a). In cancer vaccination, a domain of the tetanus toxin FrC fused to a single antigenic determinant was demonstrated able to induce an anti-tumoural CTL mediated response in vaccinated mice (Rice et al. 2002). Likewise, in vaccination against B cell lymphoma, DNA vaccines containing the idiotypic determinants of the Ig variable region provided protective immunity against the tumour when expressed as single-chain variable fragment (sc-Fv) fused to tetanus toxin FrC (King et al. 1998). Reproducible data from several published papers, show that the high immunogenicity of the tetanus toxin FrC depends on two main attributes; 1) a conformational sequence-dependent effect ; 2) the presence of promiscuous T-helper epitopes within the protein (Umland et al. 1997). Our group has analysed the sequence of the tetanus toxin FrC, and has identified numerous T-helper epitopes in the protein domain: 1) the universal p30 T-helper epitope (FNNFTVSFWLRVPKVSASHLE aa 947-967), a strong promiscuous immunogenic T-helper epitope consisting of at least three distinct overlapping helper peptides, each of which is presented in association with multiple HLA class II alleles [42]; 2) the p21TT helper epitope (IREDNNITLKLDRCNN aa 1064-1079); 3) the p23TT epitope (VSIDKFRIFCKALNPK aa 1084-1099), 4) the pGINGKA epitope (PGINGKAIHLVNNESSE aa 916-932) [47]; 5) the p32TT epitope (LKFIIKRYTPNNEID aa 1173-1188); 6) the pGQI epitope (GQIGNDPNRDIL aa 1273-1284 (Chiarella et al. 2007). Since $CD4^{+}$ T-helper cells support both cell and humoural immunity, it seems that the antigen fusion to promiscuous T-helper peptides contributes to the activation of these lymphocytes. The result is enhancement of the immune response mediated by T-helper cells and this might explain the strong potency of the tetanus toxin FrC domain as vaccine adjuvant. Specific T-cell epitopes of FrC that are universally immunogenic, have also been widely exploited in peptide vaccination as they have been demonstrated to enhance the humoural immune response. In particular, T-helper epitopes were successfully used as vaccine carriers to induce humoural response against polysaccharide antigens when used in form of string-of-beads (Baraldo et al. 2005). This approach is based on the concept that response to the subset of antigens and epitopes, and not to the whole organism, can be sufficient for host protection. Furthermore, the availability of bioinformatic tools and softwares for prediction of the antigen binding to the human MHC molecules helps in the design of DNA vaccines. In multi-epitope vaccination, more than one CTL epitope belonging to a certain antigen of a specific disease can be linked to a series of promiscuous MHC-II binding T-helper epitope, to generate a string-of-beads vaccine, with or without intervening spacers. In several reports, vaccination with DNA constructs consisting of a single promiscuous T-helper epitope fused to antigen determinants has proved to be effective in stimulating a strong immune response when weakly immunogenic CTL epitopes are either co-injected or chemically linked to the T-helper sequence (Tymciu et al. 2004). Synthetic universal pan HLA-DR-binding T helper epitopes such as the PADRE were conceived and they were successfully used in making DNA vaccines against infectious diseases. PADRE is a synthetic universal peptide that binds to the more common HLA-DR molecules of the human population. Its efficacy in increasing immunogenicity of CTL and B epitopes was demonstrated to be higher (Alexander et al. 1994). The sequence of PADRE has been deduced from the core sequence of the ovalbumin master T-helper peptide (aa 323-339) and adapted for binding to the more representative human MHC class II molecules (del Guercio et al. 1997).

2.5.2 Adjuvants targeting pattern recognition receptors

Traditional vaccines based on live attenuated pathogens and inactivated whole pathogens have been extremely successful in preventing many common infectious diseases. The potent immunogenicity of such vaccines depends on the presence of "endogenous adjuvants" which are simply molecular portions of the pathogenic agent. *i.e.* now defined with the name of Pathogen Associated Molecular Pattern (PAMPs). These are lipopolysaccharide (LPS), CpG-containing oligonucleotides (CpG), and peptidoglycans. LPS is a Gram-negative membrane molecule consisting of a hydrophilic polysaccharide and a lipophilic phospholipid (lipid A). The lipophilic portion of LPS is such a potent stimulus on the pro-inflammatory cytokine production that it can lead to septic shock (Heine et al. 2001) whereas monophosphoryl lipid A (MPL) is a lipid A derivative included in many adjuvant formulations with good adjuvanticity and lower toxicity (Ismaili et al. 2002). MPL was the first TLR ligand approved for human use in the hepatitis B vaccine, Fendrix (GlaxoSmithKline Biologicals, Rixensart, Belgium) (Baldridge and Crane 1999). The adjuvanticity of these adjuvant molecules depends on their ability to bind and activate the TLR4. As a result, many TLR agonists or lipid A mimetics displaying TLR4-dependent immunostimulating functions, have been synthesized and proposed as new adjuvants (Johnson et al. 1999). AS02 is an oil-in-water emulsion containing MPL and QS-21, a saponin-derived immunostimulator, induces strong antibody and Th1 responses. AS02 is being evaluated in clinical trials in vaccines against malaria, human papillomavirus (HPV), HBV, tuberculosis, and HIV (Vandepapeliere et al. 2007). Smilarly to AS02, AS01 is a liposomal formulation containing MPL that induces potent humoural and cell-mediated responses, including cytotoxic T lymphocyte responses, and is being evaluated in clinical trials of vaccine against malaria.

In bacterial DNA there is a high frequency of unmethylated CpG dinucleotide sequences in comparison to the human genome which makes perception of plasmids as "foreign" elements by the human host. This is the only characteristic that confers a certain level of immunogenicity to plasmid DNA vaccines since the CpG unmethylated sequence is recognized by the Toll Like Receptor 9 preferentially expressed on the host APCs (Liu and Ulmer 2005). CpG-DNA is used as immunostimulatory potentiator in both pre-clinical peptide and DNA vaccination trials leading to activation of innate immunity and cytokine-dependent promotion of the Th-1 response. The CpG motifs, present in bacterial DNA, consist of an unmethylated CpG dinucleotide flanked by two 5′ purines and two 3′ pyrimidines. During an infection, the release of unmethylated CpG-DNA from bacteria serves as a danger signal stimulating the immune system of the host (Krieg 2002). Bacterial DNA and synthetic unmethylated CpG oligodeoxynucleotides trigger an immunostimulatory cascade that culminates in maturation, differentiation and proliferation of several immune cells creating a pro-inflammatory and Th1-biased environment. The immunostimulatory activity of this CpG-DNA is species-specific. As a result, sequences specific for the host are designed and optimized for selective TLR9 binding. In particular, *in vivo* CpG-DNA half-life has been improved by replacing phosphodiester CpG-DNA with a nuclease-resistant phosphothioate oligodeoxynucleotide although it may induce immune reaction leading to an anti-DNA immune response (Ciafre et al. 1995). Addition of the immunostimulatory CpG-DNA to peptide vaccines, tilts the balance towards a Th-1 immune response, which is often accompanied by a significant increase in IgG2a production in comparison to IgG1. The general effect of CpG-DNA addition is augmentation of the antibody serum titer against antigens and production of Th-1 cytokines such as IFN-γ (Klinman et al. 1999). By contrast, in DNA plasmid vaccination, the immunomodulating effect of bacterial CpG oligodeoxynucleotides on T-helper cell balance, shows great variability. Such variability often depends on the route of immunisation.

2.5.3 Aluminium-based compounds

Aluminium salt adjuvants (aluminium hydroxide, aluminium phosphate) are generally used in combination with protein antigens as they form a precipitated or adsorbed vaccine. An efficient, safe and well tolerated adjuvant in humans is aluminium hydroxide (Alum). It has been approved for clinical use. Although traditionally thought to function primarily by forming a long-lasting depot for antigen and by promoting their uptake by APCs, it is now clear that innate immune stimulation plays a primary role in the adjuvant activity of alum (Lambrecht et al. 2009). Aluminium hydroxide is used primarily to enhance antibody production and does not utilize TLR for its function in vivo (Gavin et al. 2006).This adjuvant induces a Th-2 biased immune response in mice whereas in humans it stimulates also a Th-1 type immunity. *In vitro* studies demonstrated that Alum can activate the inflammosome pathway to produce IL1-β (Li et al. 2007).

Recently, aluminium hydroxide has been also shown to work well in DNA vaccination in pre-clinical models (Kenney and Edelman 2003). However, the enhancing effect of aluminium hydroxide on the immune response elicited by DNA vaccines, is not related to the levels of antigen expression. Rather, it seems to affect antigen after *in vivo* expression, suggesting the adjuvanticity of this substance is strictly related to the antigen delivery mechanism (Ulmer et al. 1999).

2.6 Delivery methods

Different methods for enhancing naked DNA vaccine delivery into host cells have been studied. The best investigated strategies are based on chemical or physical devices aimed at facilitating the DNA entry into recipient cells.

2.6.1 Microparticles

Microparticle-based methods operate a DNA condensation and complexation in particles (O'Hagan et al. 2004). The encapsulation of plasmid DNA into micro- or nanospheres can provide protection from the environment prior to delivery and aid in targeting to a specific cell type for efficient delivery.

The major advantage of particulate delivery is that synthetic microparticles have excellent potential for targeting cells of the immune system stimulating antigen uptake. It has been demonstrated that particles of about 1-10 μm in diameter are preferred for their size that is readily phagocytosed by dendritic cells and other antigen-presenting cells. They are readily internalised by phagocytic cells of the immune system, leading to an enhanced antigen presentation to the immune effector cells. Furthermore, microparticulates appear to improve delivery of DNA to APCs by facilitating trafficking to the local lymphoid tissue via the afferent lymph and antigen uptake by dendritic cells (Denis-Mize et al. 2000; Denis-Mize et al. 2003; Dupuis et al. 2000). Moreover, antigen and adjuvant molecules can be delivered to the same cell at the same time being entrapped together in biodegradable microparticles such as poly-lactide-co-glycolide (PLG) or chitosan, or complexed with non-ionic block copolymers or polycations such as polyethyleneimine. Microparticulate adjuvants are currently tested in some clinical trials against human immunodeficiency virus (HIV), hepatitis B virus (HBV) and influenza (Fuller et al. 2006). DNA entrapment or encapsulation into biodegradable microspheres for DNA vaccine delivery has been illustrated in patent WO0203961 (Johnson 2003).

2.6.2 Cationic lipids/liposomes

Cationic Solid Lipid Nanoparticles (SLNs) have been recently proposed as alternative carriers for DNA delivery, due to many technological advantages such as large-scale production from substances generally recognized as safe, good storage stability and possibility of steam sterilization and lyophilisation. Cationic lipids are amphiphilic molecules composed of one or two fatty acid side chains (acyl) or alkyl, a linker and a hydrophilic amino group. The hydrophobic part can be cholesterol-derived moieties. In aqueous media, cationic lipids are assembled into a bilayer vesicular-like structure (liposomes). Liposomes/DNA complex is usually termed a lipoplex (Bolhassani et al. 2011). The future success of cationic SLNs for administration of genetic material will depend on their ability to efficiently cross the physiological barriers, selectively targeting a specific cell type in vivo and expressing therapeutic genes (Bondi and Craparo 2010).

2.6.3 Biolistic particle delivery

In order to address accelerating micro-projectiles into intact cells or tissues, is generally used a biolistic apparatus described in patent US6004287 (Loomis 1999). Application of this strategy to DNA vaccines resulted in the invention of a new DNA delivery technology that made it possible to move naked DNA plasmid into target cells on an accelerated particle carrier. This specific delivery system is based on the use of the gene gun device that, under pressurized helium, is capable of delivering plasmid DNA-coated gold beads to the epidermal layer of skin as described in patent US6436709 (Lin 2002). Because the DNA carrier is introduced directly into the skin cells, delivery of plasmid DNA vaccines using this strategy reduces the amount of DNA needed to induce immune responses. Robust immunogenicity has been shown in many different preclinical models and in clinical trials predominantly for infectious diseases (Fuller et al. 2006). In contrast to intramuscular or intradermal injection by needle, the gene gun delivery system releases plasmid DNA directly into the cells of the epidermis (Yang et al. 1990). Intradermal injection is becoming increasingly popular, as the dense network of antigen-presenting cells in the skin, absent in muscle, provides a favourable environment for induction of antigen uptake. This network of Langerhans cells (LCs) can help in the priming of both cellular and humoural immune responses. Importantly, direct transfection of Langerhans cells is carried out with very small doses of plasmid DNA (i.e. 1-10 μg), suggesting that minimum amounts of vector are required to induce the immune response. The advantage of using low doses of plasmid DNA is particularly attractive for prophylactic vaccines against infectious diseases, where a simple and rapid delivery is the main pre-requisite. Gene gun delivery has recently been used with success in a trial against the influenza virus, inducing sero-protective levels of antibody and it has been used in trials against HBV and HIV infections (Fuller et al. 2006). A further implementation of the biolistic delivery was obtained also by creating improved injection device suitable for application in human tissues. Patent US6730663 describes a flexible multi-needle injector device with a wide surface area as well as a modified injector device to be used for injection through an endoscopic device. Such a method leads to a deep injection of DNA within tissues (Hennighausen 2004).

2.6.4 Electropermeabilization

The use of electric pulses as a safe tool to deliver therapeutic molecules to tissues and organs has been rapidly developed over the last decade. This technology leads to a transient increase in the permeability of cell membranes when exposed to electric field pulses. This

process is commonly known as electropermeabilization or electroporation (EP) (Chiarella et al 2010; Favard et al. 2007; Mir et al. 1999). The simultaneous publications in 1998 by Aihara and Miyazaki and Harrison and co-workers, demonstrated EP as being a more efficient method for gene transfer into muscle than the simple i.m. injection of DNA (Aihara and Miyazaki 1998; Harrison et al. 1998). The strategy is not only promising for enhancing the gene delivery of therapeutic proteins and drugs. Infectious disease, cancer gene therapy and chemotherapy are other fields of application, making electrochemogenetherapy relevant in a variety of research branches and promising in the gene therapy field (Mir 2008; Wells 2004).
The advantage of DNA electrotransfer is dual. On the one hand, a high number of muscle cells are transfected with the DNA vaccine; on the other hand the damaged muscle cells release danger signals that favour antigen presenting cell recruitment, thus enhancing the immune response (Chiarella et al. 2008b). For this reason we consider the electropermeabilization such an important and very promising tool in the future of DNA vaccination therapy that it deserves a dedicated section of this book chapter.

3. Electrogene transfer

3.1 Mechanisms and application of gene transfer by electric fields

Naked DNA vaccination emerged as a promising approach for introducing foreign antigens into the host to induce protective immunity. The delivery of DNA vaccine into skeletal muscle is highly preferable as this organ is not only a passive site but can actively take part in immune reactions. However, one important limitation of intramuscular (i.m.) genetic vaccines is their weak performance in large animals as regards the low DNA transfection efficiency of the tissue (Escoffre et al. 2010). For this reason, novel and safe delivery systems have been developed to further improve the vaccine efficiency and immunogenicity. In several reports, electroporation-mediated DNA delivery was described as an effective tool in eliciting immune response in small and large animal models (Babiuk et al. 2002; Otten et al. 2004; Peng et al. 2007), with numerous studies proving that this technique is effective in the stimulation of humoural and cellular immunity (Dupuis et al. 2000; Tollefsen et al. 2002; Widera et al. 2000). Interest in the application of EP to DNA vaccination protocols is greatly growing in these last years for several considerations. It has been demonstrated that EP allows an augmented uptake of DNA in tissue cells especially if used in combination with hyaluronidase (McMahon et al. 2001). A higher DNA uptake *in vivo* is possible thanks to the enhancement of cell membrane permeabilization and electrophoretic movement of DNA molecules into the target cells. Moreover, if EP is applied in muscle cells, these work as a platform for antigen production within the skeletal muscle (Shirota et al. 2007). A combination of both these events facilitates target cell transfection, this resulting in a higher synthesis of the gene of interest and in an intensification of the immune response to the encoded protein.
Many studies have reported the beneficial effect of EP on the activated response by the immune system against the transferred antigen in several animal models (Tsang et al. 2007). Respect to a simple administration of DNA vaccines through i.m. injection, EP is responsible for a significant increase in antibody titre (Buchan et al. 2005), antigen-specific T-cell frequency and induction of several T-cell effector functions (Bachy et al. 2001; Capone et al. 2006). In particular, a study performed on DNA vaccination mediated by EP demonstrated that the concomitant injection of plasmid DNA and EP is crucial for the adjuvant effect exerted by EP, which is responsible for eliciting antigen-specific IgG2a antibody production

and Th-1 biased immune responses (Gronevik et al. 2005). Another study demonstrated that a single i.m. DNA vaccination in combination with EP enhanced significantly the onset and the duration of the primary antibody response affecting immune memory (Tsang et al. 2007). The use of EP for delivering a DNA vaccine encoding anthrax toxin protective agent has been demonstrated able in a rapid induction of antibodies against the antigen in 2 weeks following a single immunization in several experimental animals (Luxembourg et al. 2008).
Despite these evidences, details on possible mechanisms responsible for the positive effect of EP on the immune response to DNA vaccines were not completely characterised (Escoffre et al. 2009).
Recently EP has been reported as crucial event through which, inducing transient morphological changes and a local moderate damage in the treated muscle, is possible to generate an early production of endogenous cytokines responsible for signalling danger at the local level. The activation of a danger pro-inflammatory pathway and the recruitment of inflammatory cells result in T lymphocyte migration, indicating electropermeabilization *per se* is able to recruit and trigger cells involved in antigen presentation (Chiarella et al. 2008b). Due to these immunostimulating effects, EP is now recognised as a good adjuvant (Chiarella et al. 2007), helpful in DNA vaccination for increasing the potency and safety of this therapeutic approach due to its property to induce a higher DNA uptake and its ability to stimulate both humoural and cellular immunity. At present, numerous findings are clarifying EP mechanism (Golzio et al. 2010), also showing the easy applicability of EP to large animals. In this view, many studies are concentrated to find the most appropriate and tolerable parameters that will make EP suitable for humans (Tjelle et al. 2008; Tjelle et al. 2006). To this purpose, various electroporating devices have been developed for animal and human use (**Fig. 2**).
Because these initial results seem promising, several clinical trials based on DNA vaccination assisted by electropermeabilization are under investigation and the efficacy and tolerability of EP will be deeply studied in the near future both in preclinical and clinical gene therapy protocols.

3.2 Application of electrogene transfer in DNA vaccination protocols

The use of EP technology for DNA vaccination in the clinical settings takes advantage from the development of new protocols, which are effective in administrating the vaccine with the minimum discomfort and maximum tolerability for the patient.
The type of EP device, intensity of electrical stimulations, number of electrical pulses and administrations, and choice of the target organ, are important parameters taken into consideration for the design of clinical protocols.
Because the need to develop non-invasive or minimally invasive genetic vaccination methods has become an important issue, several studies have been focussed on the needle-free injection of DNA vaccines. A recent patent, issued in 2007, reports the combination of needle-free injection and electroporation, demonstrating that this non-invasive strategy is sufficient to introduce the DNA vaccine in a form suitable for electrotransfer into a region of the host tissue. This needle-free injection may be used in combination with suitable non invasive electrode configurations (Hofmann 2007). Safe EP protocols for human disease therapies are under investigation and many preclinical studies are described in numerous works investigating the potential of EP in both infectious and tumour diseases.

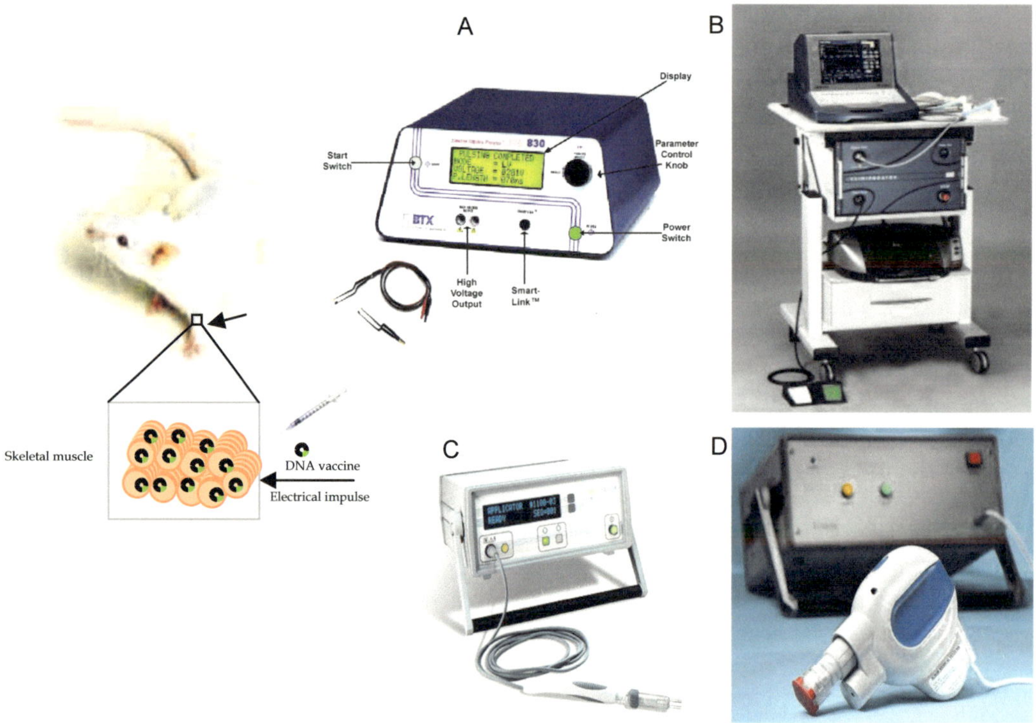

The DNA vaccine is injected into the skeletal muscle of the mouse limb and penetration into the target tissue is achieved by electropermeabilization of the muscle after DNA is injected with a syringe. The electrical impulse is applied by electrodes in contact with the skeletal muscle. Different electroporator devices are shown in the figure. A) BTX ECM 830 Harvard Apparatus; B) IGEA Cliniporator; C) Inovio MedPulser® EPT; D) Ichor TriGridTM.

Fig. 2. Administration of DNA vaccine by electropermeabilization of the muscle

HIV vaccine administration has been conducted in several animal models. Electrically-mediated delivery technology has been applied to DNA vaccines against HIV virus, and substantially higher immune responses have been achieved in mice and rabbits following vaccination with DNA encoding HIV genes. Vaccines were administered with constant electric current or constant electric voltage, causing up to 20-fold higher immune responses in comparison to the application of DNA vaccines alone (Selby 2000). In another study in mice, *in vivo* EP amplified cellular and humoural immune responses to a HIV type 1 Env DNA vaccine, enabled a 10- fold reduction in vaccine dose, and resulted in increased recruitment of inflammatory cells (Liu et al. 2008). Another study on the development of plasmid DNA vaccine able in eliciting robust cell-mediated immune response to multiple HIV type 1 (HIV-1)-derived antigens has been conducted in Rhesus macaques. Vaccination in combination with *in vivo* EP led to a more rapid onset and enhanced vaccine-specific immune responses (Luckay et al. 2007).

Also the hepatitis C virus disease is object of investigation. It was demonstrated that gene electrotransfer of a novel candidate DNA vaccine encoding an optimised version of the non structural region of HCV (from NS3 to NS5B) induces substantially more potent, broad, and long-lasting $CD4^+$ and $CD8^+$ cellular immunity than a simple naked DNA injection in mice and in Rhesus macaques. As already discussed, the T-cell responses elicited by the DNA-based electroporation strategy can be useful in prophylactic vaccine approaches against HCV and this work supports this hypothesis (Capone et al. 2006). Because the administration of a plasmid cocktail, encoding antigen and adjuvants in combination with EP, is proposed as an efficient genetic immunisation strategy, the same group designed a protocol in which Hepatitis C virus (HCV) E2 and cytokine encoding plasmids have been co-injected in the mouse quadriceps with or without EP. The vaccination outcome has been evaluated by analysis of antigen-specific cellular- mediated or antibody-mediated immunity. The co-injection of cytokine and HCV E2-encoding plasmids followed by EP, strongly enhanced T- or B-cell responses to various levels, depending on the particular combination used (Arcuri et al. 2008).

Respect to cancer, strong cellular immune responses can be induced in both mice and non-human primates, following the administration with EP of a novel HPV18 DNA vaccine encoding an E6/E7 fusion consensus protein (Yan et al. 2008).

Improvement in the efficacy of a cancer vaccine administered by electroporation, could increase its chances for clinical success. A demonstration of the inhibition of tumour growth has been reported by Curcio and collaborators. They demonstrated that a vaccination protocol using a plasmid encoding the extracellular and transmembrane domains of the Neu oncogene delivered by electroporation, prevents longterm tumour formation in cancer-prone transgenic mice (Curcio et al. 2008).

Since electropermeabilization is considered a promising delivery system for plasmid DNA vaccination, several clinical trials are now experimenting EP as a medical technology in human patients affected by infectious as well as cancer diseases (Bodles-Brakhop et al. 2009).

A summary of the clinical trials performed by DNA vaccination and EP are shown in the following tables.

Clinical trial	Condition	Pathogen	Intervention	Phase
NCT01169077	**Malaria**	Plasmodium falciparum	EP-1300	I
NCT00685412	**Human Papillomavirus infection**	HPV (E6-E7)	VGX-3100 CELLECTRA	I
NCT00563173	**Chronic Hepatitis C Virus Infection**	HCV	CHRONVAC-C®	I/IIa
NCT00545987	**AIDS (prophylactic)**	HIV	ADVAX TriGrid™	I
NCT01082692	**AIDS (therapeutic)**	HIV-1	PENNVAX-B CELLECTRA	I

Table 3. Clinical trials in infectious diseases.

Clinical trial	Condition	Antigen	Intervention	Phase
NCT01064375	**Colorectal Cancer**	CEA	tetwtCEA DNA wt CEA with tetanus toxoid Th epitope Derma Vax (electroporation device)	I/II
NCT00471133	**Intraocular Melanoma**	Tyrosinase	TriGrid	I
NCT01138410	**Melanoma**	Antibody (SCIB-1)	EP device	I/II
NCT00859729	**Prostate cancer**	PSA	pVAXrcPSAv531 DERMA VAX™	I/II
GTAC No 89	**Prostate cancer**	PSMA	EP device (Tjelle 2006)	I/II (Closed 1.4.2008)
NCT00753415	**Colon cancer Breast Cancer Melanoma**	V934/V935 hTERT	V934/V935 DNA	I

Table 4. Clinical trials in cancer diseases.

The results seem to be promising and applicable to a large cohort of diseases in the next future. Therefore electroporation would appear to be the more efficient technology for local injection of plasmid DNA vaccine into the tissue (Kato and Nakamua 1965; Wells 2010).

4. Conclusions

The last decade has witnessed a revolution in the approach to vaccine design and development. Despite considerable success in the prevention field, vaccinations against intracellular organisms, which require a cell-mediated immunity, are not yet available, while infectious diseases such as tuberculosis and malaria remain a serious problem in the Third World. Following the studies of Wolff and colleagues, in recent years immunisation with naked plasmid DNA encoding antigens has revealed a number of advantages, making DNA vaccination a promising therapeutic approach against infectious diseases and cancer. Of course improvement of vaccine efficacy has become a goal in the development of DNA vaccination protocols. Electropermeabilization has been shown to increase both the number of transfected cells and also the number of plasmids that permeate into each cell, therefore, electropermeabilization is now regarded as a promising delivery system for plasmid DNA vaccination. Intramuscular DNA vaccination combined with electropermeabilization has been described as effective in activating both humoural and cellular immune response in the host as well as in enhancing expression of the encoded antigen. Several reports showed that EP has adjuvant-like properties when combined with plasmid DNA injection. This approach is currently used not only in preclinical protocols in animals but also in humans, and studies for evaluating pain and stress induced by the treatment are currently under investigation indicating this approach as applicable and promising. Because this procedure is used safely without serious adverse effects related to the administration procedure, we strongly support improvements addressed to the efficacy of DNA vaccines administered by electropermeabilization in clinical protocols. This new approach could successfully increase chances for clinical success in humans.

5. References

Abdulhaqq, S. A., and Weiner, D. B. (2008). "DNA vaccines: developing new strategies to enhance immune responses." *Immunol Res*, 42(1-3), 219-32.

Aihara, H., and Miyazaki, J. (1998). "Gene transfer into muscle by electroporation in vivo." *Nat Biotechnol*, 16(9), 867-70.

Alexander, J., Sidney, J., Southwood, S., Ruppert, J., Oseroff, C., Maewal, A., Snoke, K., Serra, H. M., Kubo, R. T., Sette, A., and et al. (1994). "Development of high potency universal DR-restricted helper epitopes by modification of high affinity DR-blocking peptides." *Immunity*, 1(9), 751-61.

Andre, F. E. (2003). "Vaccinology: past achievements, present roadblocks and future promises." *Vaccine*, 21(7-8), 593-5.

Arcuri, M., Cappelletti, M., Zampaglione, I., Aurisicchio, L., Nicosia, A., Ciliberto, G., and Fattori, E. (2008). "Synergistic effect of gene-electro transfer and adjuvant cytokines in increasing the potency of hepatitis C virus genetic vaccination." *J Gene Med*, 10(9), 1048-54.

Atkins, M. B., Robertson, M. J., Gordon, M., Lotze, M. T., DeCoste, M., DuBois, J. S., Ritz, J., Sandler, A. B., Edington, H. D., Garzone, P. D., Mier, J. W., Canning, C. M., Battiato, L., Tahara, H., and Sherman, M. L. (1997). "Phase I evaluation of intravenous recombinant human interleukin 12 in patients with advanced malignancies." *Clin Cancer Res*, 3(3), 409-17.

Babiuk, S., Baca-Estrada, M. E., Foldvari, M., Storms, M., Rabussay, D., Widera, G., and Babiuk, L. A. (2002). "Electroporation improves the efficacy of DNA vaccines in large animals." *Vaccine*, 20(27-28), 3399-3408.

Bachy, M., Boudet, F., Bureau, M., Girerd-Chambaz, Y., Wils, P., Scherman, D., and Meric, C. (2001). "Electric pulses increase the immunogenicity of an influenza DNA vaccine injected intramuscularly in the mouse." *Vaccine*, 19(13-14), 1688-93.

Baldridge, J. R., and Crane, R. T. (1999). "Monophosphoryl lipid A (MPL) formulations for the next generation of vaccines." *Methods*, 19(1), 103-7.

Ballard, J. D., Collier, R. J., and Starnbach, M. N. (1996). "Anthrax toxin-mediated delivery of a cytotoxic T-cell epitope in vivo." *Proc Natl Acad Sci U S A*, 93(22), 12531-4.

Baraldo, K., Mori, E., Bartoloni, A., Norelli, F., Grandi, G., Rappuoli, R., Finco, O., and Del Giudice, G. (2005). "Combined conjugate vaccines: enhanced immunogenicity with the N19 polyepitope as a carrier protein." *Infect Immun*, 73(9), 5835-41.

Barouch, D. H., Craiu, A., Kuroda, M. J., Schmitz, J. E., Zheng, X. X., Santra, S., Frost, J. D., Krivulka, G. R., Lifton, M. A., Crabbs, C. L., Heidecker, G., Perry, H. C., Davies, M. E., Xie, H., Nickerson, C. E., Steenbeke, T. D., Lord, C. I., Montefiori, D. C., Strom, T. B., Shiver, J. W., Lewis, M. G., and Letvin, N. L. (2000). "Augmentation of immune responses to HIV-1 and simian immunodeficiency virus DNA vaccines by IL-2/Ig plasmid administration in rhesus monkeys." *Proc Natl Acad Sci U S A*, 97(8), 4192-7.

Bayer, A. L., Yu, A., Adeegbe, D., and Malek, T. R. (2005). "Essential role for interleukin-2 for CD4(+)CD25(+) T regulatory cell development during the neonatal period." *J Exp Med*, 201(5), 769-77.

Bodles-Brakhop, A. M., Heller, R., and Draghia-Akli, R. (2009). "Electroporation for the delivery of DNA-based vaccines and immunotherapeutics: current clinical developments." *Mol Ther*, 17(4), 585-92.

Bojak, A., Wild, J., Deml, L., and Wagner, R. (2002). "Impact of codon usage modification on T cell immunogenicity and longevity of HIV-1 gag-specific DNA vaccines." *Intervirology*, 45(4-6), 275-86.

Bolhassani, A., Safaiyan, S., and Rafati, S. (2011). "Improvement of different vaccine delivery systems for cancer therapy." *Mol Cancer*, 10, 3.

Bondi, M. L., and Craparo, E. F. (2010). "Solid lipid nanoparticles for applications in gene therapy: a review of the state of the art." *Expert Opin Drug Deliv*, 7(1), 7-18.

Brun, A., Barcena, J., Blanco, E., Borrego, B., Dory, D., Escribano, J. M., Le Gall-Recule, G., Ortego, J., and Dixon, L. K. (2011). "Current strategies for subunit and genetic viral veterinary vaccine development." *Virus Res*, 157(1), 1-12.

Buchan, S., Gronevik, E., Mathiesen, I., King, C. A., Stevenson, F. K., and Rice, J. (2005). "Electroporation as a "prime/boost" strategy for naked DNA vaccination against a tumor antigen." *J Immunol*, 174(10), 6292-8.

Capone, S., Zampaglione, I., Vitelli, A., Pezzanera, M., Kierstead, L., Burns, J., Ruggeri, L., Arcuri, M., Cappelletti, M., Meola, A., Ercole, B. B., Tafi, R., Santini, C., Luzzago, A., Fu, T. M., Colloca, S., Ciliberto, G., Cortese, R., Nicosia, A., Fattori, E., and Folgori, A. (2006). "Modulation of the immune response induced by gene electrotransfer of a hepatitis C virus DNA vaccine in nonhuman primates." *J Immunol*, 177(10), 7462-71.

Carbonetti, N. H., Irish, T. J., Chen, C. H., O'Connell, C. B., Hadley, G. A., McNamara, U., Tuskan, R. G., and Lewis, G. K. (1999). "Intracellular delivery of a cytolytic T-lymphocyte epitope peptide by pertussis toxin to major histocompatibility complex class I without involvement of the cytosolic class I antigen processing pathway." *Infect Immun*, 67(2), 602-7.

Chiarella, P., Fazio, V.M., and Signori, E. (2010). "Application of electroporation in DNA vaccination protocols." *Curr Gene Ther*,10 (4), 281-6.

Chiarella, P., Massi, E., De Robertis, M., Fazio, V. M., and Signori, E. (2008a). "Strategies for effective naked-DNA vaccination against infectious diseases." *Recent Pat Antiinfect Drug Discov*, 3(2), 93-101.

Chiarella, P., Massi, E., De Robertis, M., Sibilio, A., Parrella, P., Fazio, V. M., and Signori, E. (2008b). "Electroporation of skeletal muscle induces danger signal release and antigen-presenting cell recruitment independently of DNA vaccine administration." *Expert Opin Biol Ther*, 8(11), 1645-57.

Chiarella, P., Massi, E., De Robertis, M., Signori, E., and Fazio, V. M. (2007). "Adjuvants in vaccines and for immunisation: current trends." *Expert Opin Biol Ther*, 7(10), 1551-62.

Chu, C., Parker, R., Highlands, L., and Morales J. (2010). "Phase I of Human Papillomavirus (HPV) DNA Plasmid (VGX-3100) + Electroporation for CIN 2 or 3." *Date of access: 04/04/2011. Available from: Clinical Trials.gov.*

Ciafre, S. A., Rinaldi, M., Gasparini, P., Seripa, D., Bisceglia, L., Zelante, L., Farace, M. G., and Fazio, V. M. (1995). "Stability and functional effectiveness of phosphorothioate modified duplex DNA and synthetic 'mini-genes'." *Nucleic Acids Res*, 23(20), 4134-42.

Ciafre, S. A., Rinaldi, M., Vespignani, I., Parrella, P., Seripa, D., Signori, E., Ria, F., Farace, M. G., and Fazio, V. M. (1998). "A plasmid family containing two different expression cassettes suitable for immunomodulation and genetic immunization." *Plasmid*, 40(1), 84-9.

Curcio, C., Khan, A. S., Amici, A., Spadaro, M., Quaglino, E., Cavallo, F., Forni, G., and Draghia-Akli, R. (2008). "DNA immunization using constant-current electroporation affords long-term protection from autochthonous mammary carcinomas in cancer-prone transgenic mice." *Cancer Gene Ther*, 15(2), 108-14.

del Guercio, M. F., Alexander, J., Kubo, R. T., Arrhenius, T., Maewal, A., Appella, E., Hoffman, S. L., Jones, T., Valmori, D., Sakaguchi, K., Grey, H. M., and Sette, A. (1997). "Potent immunogenic short linear peptide constructs composed of B cell epitopes and Pan DR T helper epitopes (PADRE) for antibody responses in vivo." *Vaccine*, 15(4), 441-8.

Denis-Mize, K. S., Dupuis, M., MacKichan, M. L., Singh, M., Doe, B., O'Hagan, D., Ulmer, J. B., Donnelly, J. J., McDonald, D. M., and Ott, G. (2000). "Plasmid DNA adsorbed onto cationic microparticles mediates target gene expression and antigen presentation by dendritic cells." *Gene Ther*, 7(24), 2105-12.

Denis-Mize, K. S., Dupuis, M., Singh, M., Woo, C., Ugozzoli, M., O'Hagan, D. T., Donnelly, J. J., 3rd, Ott, G., and McDonald, D. M. (2003). "Mechanisms of increased immunogenicity for DNA-based vaccines adsorbed onto cationic microparticles." *Cell Immunol*, 225(1), 12-20.

Dong, Z., and Nor, J. E. (2009). "Transcriptional targeting of tumor endothelial cells for gene therapy." *Adv Drug Deliv Rev*, 61(7-8), 542-53.

Dudek, N.L., Perlmutter, P., Aguilar, M.I., Croft, N.P., and Purcell, A.W. (2010). "Epitope discovery and their use in peptide based vaccines." Curr Pharm Des, 16(28), 3149-57.

Dupuis, M., Denis-Mize, K., Woo, C., Goldbeck, C., Selby, M. J., Chen, M., Otten, G. R., Ulmer, J. B., Donnelly, J. J., Ott, G., and McDonald, D. M. (2000). "Distribution of DNA vaccines determines their immunogenicity after intramuscular injection in mice." *J Immunol*, 165(5), 2850-8.

Dyall, R., Bowne, W. B., Weber, L. W., LeMaoult, J., Szabo, P., Moroi, Y., Piskun, G., Lewis, J. J., Houghton, A. N., and Nikolic-Zugic, J. (1998). "Heteroclitic immunization induces tumor immunity." *J Exp Med*, 188(9), 1553-61.

Edelman, G. M., Meech, R., Owens, G. C., and Jones, F. S. (2000). "Synthetic promoter elements obtained by nucleotide sequence variation and selection for activity." *Proc Natl Acad Sci U S A*, 97(7), 3038-43.

Ertl, P. F. (2007). *Patent No. US2007248679*.

Escoffre, J. M., Portet, T., Wasungu, L., Teissie, J., Dean, D., and Rols, M. P. (2009). "What is (still not) known of the mechanism by which electroporation mediates gene transfer and expression in cells and tissues." *Mol Biotechnol*, 41(3), 286-95.

Escoffre, J. M., Teissie, J., and Rols, M. P. (2010). "Gene transfer: how can the biological barriers be overcome?" *J Membr Biol*, 236(1), 61-74.

Favard, C., Dean, D. S., and Rols, M. P. (2007). "Electrotransfer as a non viral method of gene delivery." *Curr Gene Ther*, 7(1), 67-77.

Fraser, C. M., and Rappuoli, R. (2005). "Application of microbial genomic science to advanced therapeutics." *Annu Rev Med*, 56, 459-74.

Fuller, D. H., Loudon, P., and Schmaljohn, C. (2006). "Preclinical and clinical progress of particle-mediated DNA vaccines for infectious diseases." *Methods*, 40(1), 86-97.

Gavin, A. L., Hoebe, K., Duong, B., Ota, T., Martin, C., Beutler, B., and Nemazee, D. (2006). "Adjuvant-enhanced antibody responses in the absence of toll-like receptor signaling." *Science*, 314(5807), 1936-8.

Gollob, J. A., Veenstra, K. G., Parker, R. A., Mier, J. W., McDermott, D. F., Clancy, D., Tutin, L., Koon, H., and Atkins, M. B. (2003). "Phase I trial of concurrent twice-weekly recombinant human interleukin-12 plus low-dose IL-2 in patients with melanoma or renal cell carcinoma." *J Clin Oncol*, 21(13), 2564-73.

Golzio, M., Escoffre, J. M., Portet, T., Mauroy, C., Teissie, J., Dean, D. S., and Rols, M. P. (2010) "Observations of the mechanisms of electromediated DNA uptake--from vesicles to tissues." *Curr Gene Ther*, 10(4), 256-66.

Good, M. F., Pombo, D., Lunde, M. N., Maloy, W. L., Halenbeck, R., Koths, K., Miller, L. H., and Berzofsky, J. A. (1988). "Recombinant human IL-2 overcomes genetic nonresponsiveness to malaria sporozoite peptides. Correlation of effect with biologic activity of IL-2." *J Immunol*, 141(3), 972-7.

Gothelf, A., Mir, L. M., and Gehl, J. (2003). "Electrochemotherapy: results of cancer treatment using enhanced delivery of bleomycin by electroporation." *Cancer Treat Rev*, 29(5), 371-87.

Gronevik, E., Mathiesen, I., and Lomo, T. (2005). "Early events of electroporation-mediated intramuscular DNA vaccination potentiate Th1-directed immune responses." *J Gene Med*, 7(9), 1246-54.

Harrington, L. E., Most Rv, R., Whitton, J. L., and Ahmed, R. (2002). "Recombinant vaccinia virus-induced T-cell immunity: quantitation of the response to the virus vector and the foreign epitope." *J Virol*, 76(7), 3329-37.

Harrison, R. L., Byrne, B. J., and Tung, L. (1998). "Electroporation-mediated gene transfer in cardiac tissue." *FEBS Lett*, 435(1), 1-5.

Heine, H., Rietschel, E. T., and Ulmer, A. J. (2001). "The biology of endotoxin." *Mol Biotechnol*, 19(3), 279-96.

Hennighausen, L., and Furth, P.A. (2004). "Targeting gene expression to living tissue using jet injection." *Patent No. US 6730663.*

Hofmann, G. A., Rabussay, D.P., and Zhang L. (2007). "Intradermal delivery of active agents by needle-free injection and electroporation." *Patent No. US 7171264.*

Ismaili, J., Rennesson, J., Aksoy, E., Vekemans, J., Vincart, B., Amraoui, Z., Van Laethem, F., Goldman, M., and Dubois, P. M. (2002). "Monophosphoryl lipid A activates both human dendritic cells and T cells." *J Immunol*, 168(2), 926-32.

Ivory, C., and Chadee, K. (2004). "DNA vaccines: designing strategies against parasitic infections." *Genet Vaccines Ther*, 2(1), 17.

Jager, D., Taverna, C., Zippelius, A., and Knuth, A. (2004). "Identification of tumor antigens as potential target antigens for immunotherapy by serological expression cloning." *Cancer Immunol Immunother*, 53(3), 144-7.

Janeway, C. A., Jr. (1989). "Approaching the asymptote? Evolution and revolution in immunology." *Cold Spring Harb Symp Quant Biol*, 54 Pt 1, 1-13.

Johnson, D. A., Keegan, D. S., Sowell, C. G., Livesay, M. T., Johnson, C. L., Taubner, L. M., Harris, A., Myers, K. R., Thompson, J. D., Gustafson, G. L., Rhodes, M. J., Ulrich, J. T., Ward, J. R., Yorgensen, Y. M., Cantrell, J. L., and Brookshire, V. G. (1999). "3-O-Desacyl monophosphoryl lipid A derivatives: synthesis and immunostimulant activities." *J Med Chem*, 42(22), 4640-9.

Johnson, M. E., Mossman, S., Evans, L., and Cecil T. (2003). "Microspheres and adjuvants for DNA vaccine delivery." *Patent No. WO 0203961.*

Kenney, R. T., and Edelman, R. (2003). "Survey of human-use adjuvants." *Expert Rev Vaccines*, 2(2), 167-88.

Khan, C. M., Villarreal-Ramos, B., Pierce, R. J., Demarco de Hormaeche, R., McNeill, H., Ali, T., Chatfield, S., Capron, A., Dougan, G., and Hormaeche, C. E. (1994a). "Construction, expression, and immunogenicity of multiple tandem copies of the Schistosoma mansoni peptide 115-131 of the P28 glutathione S-transferase expressed as C-terminal fusions to tetanus toxin fragment C in a live aro-attenuated vaccine strain of Salmonella." *J Immunol*, 153(12), 5634-42.

Khan, C. M., Villarreal-Ramos, B., Pierce, R. J., Riveau, G., Demarco de Hormaeche, R., McNeill, H., Ali, T., Fairweather, N., Chatfield, S., Capron, A., and et al. (1994b). "Construction, expression, and immunogenicity of the Schistosoma mansoni P28 glutathione S-transferase as a genetic fusion to tetanus toxin fragment C in a live Aro attenuated vaccine strain of Salmonella." *Proc Natl Acad Sci U S A*, 91(23), 11261-5.

King, C. A., Spellerberg, M. B., Zhu, D., Rice, J., Sahota, S. S., Thompsett, A. R., Hamblin, T. J., Radl, J., and Stevenson, F. K. (1998). "DNA vaccines with single-chain Fv fused to fragment C of tetanus toxin induce protective immunity against lymphoma and myeloma." *Nat Med*, 4(11), 1281-6.

Klinman, D. M., Barnhart, K. M., and Conover, J. (1999). "CpG motifs as immune adjuvants." *Vaccine*, 17(1), 19-25.

Ko, H. J., Ko, S. Y., Kim, Y. J., Lee, E. G., Cho, S. N., and Kang, C. Y. (2005). "Optimization of codon usage enhances the immunogenicity of a DNA vaccine encoding mycobacterial antigen Ag85B." *Infect Immun*, 73(9), 5666-74.

Krieg, A. M. (2002). "CpG motifs in bacterial DNA and their immune effects." *Annu Rev Immunol*, 20, 709-60.

Kurts, C., Robinson, B. W., and Knolle, P. A. (2010). "Cross-priming in health and disease." *Nat Rev Immunol*, 10(6), 403-14.

Lambrecht, B. N., Kool, M., Willart, M. A., and Hammad, H. (2009). "Mechanism of action of clinically approved adjuvants." *Curr Opin Immunol*, 21(1), 23-9.

Larsen, M. V., Lundegaard, C., Lamberth, K., Buus, S., Lund, O., and Nielsen, M. (2007). "Large-scale validation of methods for cytotoxic T-lymphocyte epitope prediction." *BMC Bioinformatics*, 8, 424.

Li, H., Nookala, S., and Re, F. (2007). "Aluminum hydroxide adjuvants activate caspase-1 and induce IL-1beta and IL-18 release." *J Immunol*, 178(8), 5271-6.

Li, X., Eastman, E. M., Schwartz, R. J., and Draghia-Akli, R. (1999). "Synthetic muscle promoters: activities exceeding naturally occurring regulatory sequences." *Nat Biotechnol*, 17(3), 241-5.

Lin, H. J., Huang, K.J., Yang, H.T., and Chen W.C. (2002). "Low-pressure accelerated particle gene gun." *Patent No US 6436709.*

Liu, J., Kjeken, R., Mathiesen, I., and Barouch, D. H. (2008). "Recruitment of antigen-presenting cells to the site of inoculation and augmentation of human immunodeficiency virus type 1 DNA vaccine immunogenicity by in vivo electroporation." *J Virol*, 82(11), 5643-9.

Liu, M. A. (2011). "DNA vaccines: an historical perspective and view to the future." *Immunol Rev*, 239(1), 62-84.

Liu, M. A., and Ulmer, J. B. (2005). "Human clinical trials of plasmid DNA vaccines." *Adv Genet*, 55, 25-40.

Loomis, D. J., Celeste, J., and Sanford, J. (1999). "Biolistic apparatus for delivering substances into cells and tissues." *Patent of USA, No US 6004287.*

Loudon, P. T., Yager, E. J., Lynch, D. T., Narendran, A., Stagnar, C., Franchini, A. M., Fuller, J. T., White, P. A., Nyuandi, J., Wiley, C. A., Murphey-Corb, M., and Fuller, D. H. (2010). "GM-CSF increases mucosal and systemic immunogenicity of an H1N1 influenza DNA vaccine administered into the epidermis of non-human primates." *PLoS One*, 5(6), e11021.

Luckay, A., Sidhu, M. K., Kjeken, R., Megati, S., Chong, S. Y., Roopchand, V., Garcia-Hand, D., Abdullah, R., Braun, R., Montefiori, D. C., Rosati, M., Felber, B. K., Pavlakis, G. N., Mathiesen, I., Israel, Z. R., Eldridge, J. H., and Egan, M. A. (2007). "Effect of plasmid DNA vaccine design and in vivo electroporation on the resulting vaccine-specific immune responses in rhesus macaques." *J Virol*, 81(10), 5257-69.

Lundquist, C. A., Meier, J. L., and Stinski, M. F. (1999). "A strong negative transcriptional regulatory region between the human cytomegalovirus UL127 gene and the major immediate-early enhancer." *J Virol*, 73(11), 9039-52.

Luxembourg, A., Hannaman, D., Nolan, E., Ellefsen, B., Nakamura, G., Chau, L., Tellez, O., Little, S., and Bernard, R. (2008). "Potentiation of an anthrax DNA vaccine with electroporation." *Vaccine*, 26(40), 5216-22.

Matzinger, P. (2007). "Friendly and dangerous signals: is the tissue in control?" *Nat Immunol*, 8(1), 11-3.

McMahon, J. M., Signori, E., Wells, K. E., Fazio, V. M., and Wells, D. J. (2001). "Optimisation of electrotransfer of plasmid into skeletal muscle by pretreatment with hyaluronidase -- increased expression with reduced muscle damage." *Gene Ther*, 8(16), 1264-70.

Miller, A. M., Ozenci, V., Kiessling, R., and Pisa, P. (2005). "Immune monitoring in a phase 1 trial of a PSA DNA vaccine in patients with hormone-refractory prostate cancer." *J Immunother*, 28(4), 389-95.

Mir, L. M. (2008). "Application of electroporation gene therapy: past, current, and future." *Methods Mol Biol*, 423, 3-17.

Mir, L. M., Bureau, M. F., Gehl, J., Rangara, R., Rouy, D., Caillaud, J. M., Delaere, P., Branellec, D., Schwartz, B., and Scherman, D. (1999). "High-efficiency gene transfer into skeletal muscle mediated by electric pulses." *Proc Natl Acad Sci U S A*, 96(8), 4262-7.

O'Hagan, D. T., Singh, M., and Ulmer, J. B. (2004). "Microparticles for the delivery of DNA vaccines." *Immunol Rev*, 199, 191-200.

Otten, G., Schaefer, M., Doe, B., Liu, H., Srivastava, I., zur Megede, J., O'Hagan, D., Donnelly, J., Widera, G., Rabussay, D., Lewis, M. G., Barnett, S., and Ulmer, J. B. (2004). "Enhancement of DNA vaccine potency in rhesus macaques by electroporation." *Vaccine*, 22(19), 2489-93.

Palucka, A. K., Ueno, H., Fay, J. W., and Banchereau, J. (2007). "Taming cancer by inducing immunity via dendritic cells." *Immunol Rev*, 220, 129-50.

Palucka, K., Banchereau, J., and Mellman, I. (2010). "Designing vaccines based on biology of human dendritic cell subsets." *Immunity*, 33(4), 464-78.

Papadakis, E. D., Nicklin, S. A., Baker, A. H., and White, S. J. (2004). "Promoters and control elements: designing expression cassettes for gene therapy." *Curr Gene Ther*, 4(1), 89-113.

Parker, K. C., Bednarek, M. A., and Coligan, J. E. (1994). "Scheme for ranking potential HLA-A2 binding peptides based on independent binding of individual peptide side-chains." *J Immunol*, 152(1), 163-75.

Pavlenko, M., Roos, A. K., Lundqvist, A., Palmborg, A., Miller, A. M., Ozenci, V., Bergman, B., Egevad, L., Hellstrom, M., Kiessling, R., Masucci, G., Wersall, P., Nilsson, S., and Pisa, P. (2004). "A phase I trial of DNA vaccination with a plasmid expressing prostate-specific antigen in patients with hormone-refractory prostate cancer." *Br J Cancer*, 91(4), 688-94.

Payette, P. J., Weeratna, R. D., McCluskie, M. J., and Davis, H. L. (2001). "Immune-mediated destruction of transfected myocytes following DNA vaccination occurs via multiple mechanisms." *Gene Ther*, 8(18), 1395-400.

Peng, B., Zhao, Y., Xu, L., and Xu, Y. (2007). "Electric pulses applied prior to intramuscular DNA vaccination greatly improve the vaccine immunogenicity." *Vaccine*, 25(11), 2064-73.

Plotkin, S. A. (2005). "Vaccines: past, present and future." *Nat Med*, 11(4 Suppl), S5-11.

Purcell, A. W., McCluskey, J., and Rossjohn, J. (2007). "More than one reason to rethink the use of peptides in vaccine design." *Nat Rev Drug Discov*, 6(5), 404-14.

Qing, Y., Chen, M., Zhao, J., Hu, H., Xu, H., Ling, N., Peng, M., and Ren, H. (2010). "Construction of an HBV DNA vaccine by fusion of the GM-CSF gene to the HBV-S gene and examination of its immune effects in normal and HBV-transgenic mice." *Vaccine*, 28(26), 4301-7.

Ramirez, J. C., Gherardi, M. M., Rodriguez, D., and Esteban, M. (2000). "Attenuated modified vaccinia virus Ankara can be used as an immunizing agent under conditions of preexisting immunity to the vector." *J Virol*, 74(16), 7651-5.

Rammensee, H., Bachmann, J., Emmerich, N. P., Bachor, O. A., and Stevanovic, S. (1999). "SYFPEITHI: database for MHC ligands and peptide motifs." *Immunogenetics*, 50(3-4), 213-9.

Rice, J., Buchan, S., and Stevenson, F. K. (2002). "Critical components of a DNA fusion vaccine able to induce protective cytotoxic T cells against a single epitope of a tumor antigen." *J Immunol*, 169(7), 3908-13.

Rinaldi, M., Ria, F., Parrella, P., Signori, E., Serra, A., Ciafre, S. A., Vespignani, I., Lazzari, M., Farace, M. G., Saglio, G., and Fazio, V. M. (2001). "Antibodies elicited by naked DNA vaccination against the complementary-determining region 3 hypervariable region of immunoglobulin heavy chain idiotypic determinants of B-lymphoproliferative disorders specifically react with patients' tumor cells." *Cancer Res*, 61(4), 1555-62.

Roos, A. K., King, A., and Pisa, P. (2008). "DNA vaccination for prostate cancer." *Methods Mol Biol*, 423, 463-72.

Russo, V., Tanzarella, S., Dalerba, P., Rigatti, D., Rovere, P., Villa, A., Bordignon, C., and Traversari, C. (2000). "Dendritic cells acquire the MAGE-3 human tumor antigen from apoptotic cells and induce a class I-restricted T cell response." *Proc Natl Acad Sci U S A*, 97(5), 2185-90.

Selby, M., Walsh, R., Pertile, T., Goldbeck, C., Ulmer, J., and Liu MA. (2000). "Electrically-mediated enhancement of DNA vaccine immunity and efficacy *in vivo*." *Patent No. WO/2000/045823*.

Seo, S. H., Jin, H. T., Park, S. H., Youn, J. I., and Sung, Y. C. (2009). "Optimal induction of HPV DNA vaccine-induced CD8+ T cell responses and therapeutic antitumor effect by antigen engineering and electroporation." *Vaccine*, 27(42), 5906-12.

Serruto, D., and Rappuoli, R. (2006). "Post-genomic vaccine development." *FEBS Lett*, 580(12), 2985-92.

Setoguchi, R., Hori, S., Takahashi, T., and Sakaguchi, S. (2005). "Homeostatic maintenance of natural Foxp3(+) CD25(+) CD4(+) regulatory T cells by interleukin (IL)-2 and induction of autoimmune disease by IL-2 neutralization." *J Exp Med*, 201(5), 723-35.

Sette, A., and Rappuoli, R. (2010). "Reverse vaccinology: developing vaccines in the era of genomics." *Immunity*, 33(4), 530-41.

Shirota, H., Petrenko, L., Hong, C., and Klinman, D. M. (2007). "Potential of transfected muscle cells to contribute to DNA vaccine immunogenicity." *J Immunol*, 179(1), 329-36.

Singh, H., and Raghava, G. P. (2001). "ProPred: prediction of HLA-DR binding sites." *Bioinformatics*, 17(12), 1236-7.

Stevenson, F. K., Rice, J., Ottensmeier, C. H., Thirdborough, S. M., and Zhu, D. (2004). "DNA fusion gene vaccines against cancer: from the laboratory to the clinic." *Immunol Rev*, 199, 156-80.

Tam, J. P. (1996). "Recent advances in multiple antigen peptides." *J Immunol Methods*, 196(1), 17-32.

Tjelle, T. E., Rabussay, D., Ottensmeier, C., Mathiesen, I., and Kjeken, R. (2008). "Taking electroporation-based delivery of DNA vaccination into humans: a generic clinical protocol." *Methods Mol Biol*, 423, 497-507.

Tjelle, T. E., Salte, R., Mathiesen, I., and Kjeken, R. (2006). "A novel electroporation device for gene delivery in large animals and humans." *Vaccine*, 24(21), 4667-70.

Tollefsen, S., Tjelle, T., Schneider, J., Harboe, M., Wiker, H., Hewinson, G., Huygen, K., and Mathiesen, I. (2002). "Improved cellular and humoral immune responses against Mycobacterium tuberculosis antigens after intramuscular DNA immunisation combined with muscle electroporation." *Vaccine*, 20(27-28), 3370-8.

Tsang, C., Babiuk, S., van Drunen Littel-van den Hurk, S., Babiuk, L. A., and Griebel, P. (2007). "A single DNA immunization in combination with electroporation prolongs the primary immune response and maintains immune memory for six months." *Vaccine*, 25(30), 5485-94.

Tymciu, S., Durieux-Alexandrenne, C., Wijkhuisen, A., Creminon, C., Frobert, Y., Grassi, J., Couraud, J. Y., and Boquet, D. (2004). "Enhancement of antibody responses in DNA vaccination using a vector encoding a universal T-helper cell epitope." *DNA Cell Biol*, 23(6), 395-402.

Ulmer, J. B., DeWitt, C. M., Chastain, M., Friedman, A., Donnelly, J. J., McClements, W. L., Caulfield, M. J., Bohannon, K. E., Volkin, D. B., and Evans, R. K. (1999). "Enhancement of DNA vaccine potency using conventional aluminum adjuvants." *Vaccine*, 18(1-2), 18-28.

Umland, T. C., Wingert, L. M., Swaminathan, S., Furey, W. F., Schmidt, J. J., and Sax, M. (1997). "Structure of the receptor binding fragment HC of tetanus neurotoxin." *Nat Struct Biol*, 4(10), 788-92.

van der Burg, S. H., Bijker, M. S., Welters, M. J., Offringa, R., and Melief, C. J. (2006). "Improved peptide vaccine strategies, creating synthetic artificial infections to maximize immune efficacy." *Adv Drug Deliv Rev*, 58(8), 916-30.

Vandepapeliere, P., Lau, G. K., Leroux-Roels, G., Horsmans, Y., Gane, E., Tawandee, T., Merican, M. I., Win, K. M., Trepo, C., Cooksley, G., Wettendorff, M., and Ferrari, C. (2007). "Therapeutic vaccination of chronic hepatitis B patients with virus suppression by antiviral therapy: a randomized, controlled study of co-administration of HBsAg/AS02 candidate vaccine and lamivudine." *Vaccine*, 25(51), 8585-97.

Wells, D. J. (2004). "Gene therapy progress and prospects: electroporation and other physical methods." *Gene Ther*, 11(18), 1363-9.

Wells, D. J. (2010). "Electroporation and ultrasound enhanced non-viral gene delivery in vitro and in vivo." *Cell Biol Toxicol*, 26(1), 21-8.

Widera, G., Austin, M., Rabussay, D., Goldbeck, C., Barnett, S. W., Chen, M., Leung, L., Otten, G. R., Thudium, K., Selby, M. J., and Ulmer, J. B. (2000). "Increased DNA vaccine delivery and immunogenicity by electroporation in vivo." *J Immunol*, 164(9), 4635-40.

Wiendl, H., Hohlfeld, R., and Kieseier, B. C. (2005). "Immunobiology of muscle: advances in understanding an immunological microenvironment." *Trends Immunol*, 26(7), 373-80.

Wolff, J. A., Malone, R. W., Williams, P., Chong, W., Acsadi, G., Jani, A., and Felgner, P. L. (1990). "Direct gene transfer into mouse muscle in vivo." *Science*, 247(4949 Pt 1), 1465-8.

Yan, J., Harris, K., Khan, A. S., Draghia-Akli, R., Sewell, D., and Weiner, D. B. (2008). "Cellular immunity induced by a novel HPV18 DNA vaccine encoding an E6/E7 fusion consensus protein in mice and rhesus macaques." *Vaccine*, 26(40), 5210-5.

Yang, N. S., Burkholder, J., Roberts, B., Martinell, B., and McCabe, D. (1990). "In vivo and in vitro gene transfer to mammalian somatic cells by particle bombardment." *Proc Natl Acad Sci U S A*, 87(24), 9568-72.

Yew, N. S. (2005). "Controlling the kinetics of transgene expression by plasmid design." *Adv Drug Deliv Rev*, 57(5), 769-80.

Yew, N. S., Przybylska, M., Ziegler, R. J., Liu, D., and Cheng, S. H. (2001). "High and sustained transgene expression in vivo from plasmid vectors containing a hybrid ubiquitin promoter." *Mol Ther*, 4(1), 75-82.

Yoon, H. A., Aleyas, A. G., George, J. A., Park, S. O., Han, Y. W., Lee, J. H., Cho, J. G., and Eo, S. K. (2006). "Cytokine GM-CSF genetic adjuvant facilitates prophylactic DNA vaccine against pseudorabies virus through enhanced immune responses." *Microbiol Immunol*, 50(2), 83-92.

9

Gene Delivery with Ultrasound and Microbubbles

Evan Unger and Terry Matsunaga
University of Arizona
USA

1. Introduction

Gene therapy and treatment with siRNA hold potential to treat a wide variety of different diseases. Genetic material is not usually stable and is generally hydrolyzed following intravascular administration. This makes the delivery of genes somewhat problematic since intact genetic material must usually be delivered intracellularly for therapeutic effect. For gene therapy, in most cases the gene construct must reach the cellular intranuclear sub-compartment in order to elicit the desired biological effect. Viruses have evolved to deliver DNA and RNA to cells but viral vector-based gene therapy has been associated with effects inherent in biological systems (Marshall, Muruve, Thomas). Non-viral based systems afford the potential to deliver genetic materials without the adverse biological effects of viral-based systems. In most cases, however, non-viral based gene delivery systems have been less effective than viral based systems, yielding lower levels of gene expression (Litzinger). Microbubbles, e.g. acoustically active carriers, in concert with ultrasound (Unger, Zhou) may afford potential for highly effective site directed gene therapy and delivery of other genetic materials such as siRNA (Zhigang).

2. Summary of gene delivery with microbubbles and ultrasound

The basic outline of a microbubble is shown in Figure 1. Microbubbles are composed of gas with a stabilizing shell material oftentimes consisting of lipids, albumin, or biocompatible polymers. For biomedical application they range in size from several microns in diameter to several hundred nanometers in diameter. The original biomedical application was as ultrasound contrast agents for echocardiography. Two agents, Definity®, phospholipid-coated perfluoropropane microbubbles (Lantheus, Billerica, MA) and Optison®, albumin-coated perfluoropropane microbubbles, are approved by the FDA in the US and are sold as contrast agents with approved claims for echocardiography.

Because of the large impedance mismatch between liquid and gas, when sound waves strike a microbubble, the waves are efficiently scattered back (microbubbles are excellent acoustic reflectors) and this is the basis for the use of microbubbles as ultrasound contrast agents. They are excellent reflectors of sound energy and hence are outstanding contrast agents for biomedical ultrasound imaging. Furthermore, the design of special ultrasound pulse sequences as 2nd harmonic imaging and phase inversion harmonic imaging has helped to increase ultrasound imaging by eliminating significant amounts of noise from tissue reflection.

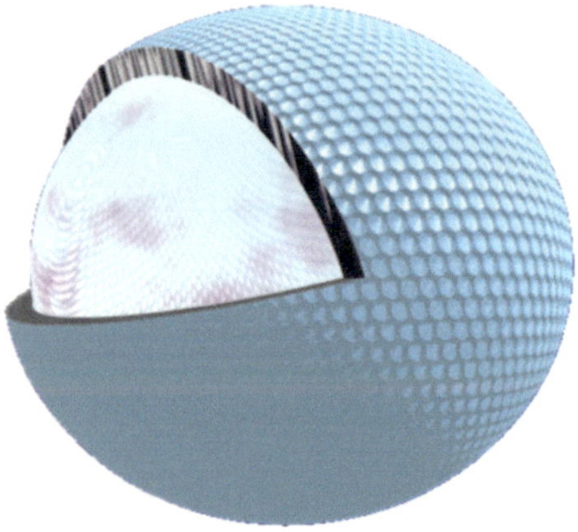

Fig. 1. Depicts a microbubble coated with a film of stabilizing material.

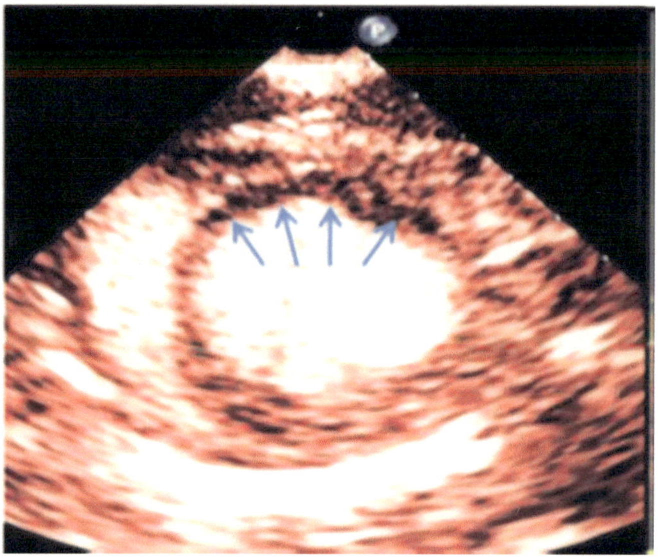

Fig. 2. Shows a contrast-enhanced echocardiogram image of a porcine heart after occlusion of the left anterior descending coronary artery (model of acute myocardial infarction). The area of decreased perfusion in the left ventricular wall is clearly seen on the post contrast images but was not detectable without contrast.

When ultrasound encounters the acoustic interface of a microbubble not only may the ultrasound be scattered, but also, because of their size and the fortuitous insonation frequencies used clinically, the microbubbles also can oscillate (stable cavitation). Depending upon the acoustic pressure, oscillating microbubbles may rupture (cavitate – described further in section 4, inertial cavitation). On the basis of cavitation it was discovered that microbubbles had therapeutic applications for gene and drug delivery and treatment of vascular thrombosis. Ultrasound effects on cell membranes may be two-fold; 1) ultrasound itself can enhance membrane permeability, thereby allowing more diffusion from the extracellular milieu (sonoporation); or, 2) can be used in conjunction with microbubbles to enhance localized delivery via microbubble bursting and subsequent radiation force induced particle penetration through the membrane surface. Cavitation can be used to increase cell permeability and local delivery of materials such as DNA for gene therapy.

A number of preclinical studies have been performed for gene (described further below) and drug delivery, but phospholipid-coated microbubbles have entered human clinical trials for treatment of vascular thrombosis. In these studies microbubbles have been administered intravenously and been shown to permeate a thrombus. Ultrasound energy has then been applied to the site of the clot to cavitate the microbubbles and dissolve the thrombus.

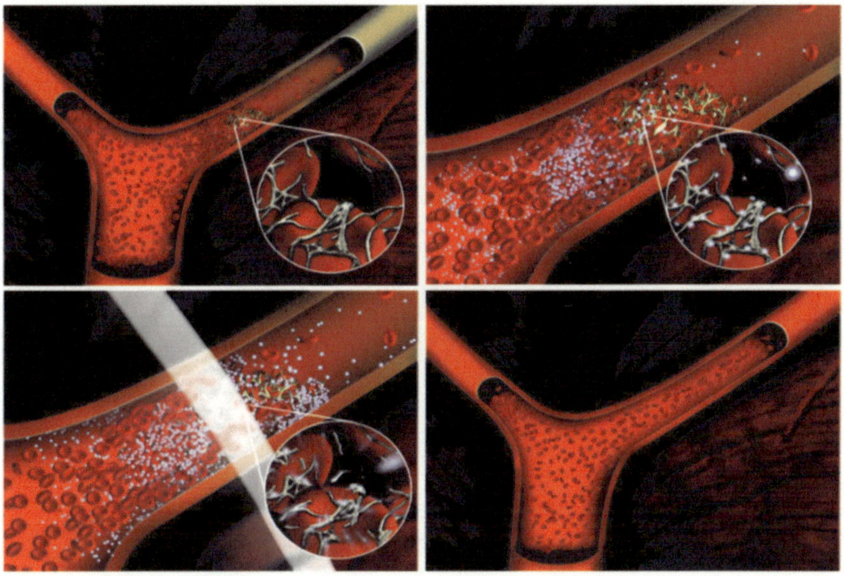

Fig. 3. Depicts and occlusive thrombus in an arterial blood vessel (upper left). Microbubbles are infused IV and permeate the clot (upper right). This can be seen on ultrasound imaging. High energy ultrasound is focused on the site of thrombus (lower left) and the microbubbles cavitate, dissolving the clot and restoring blood flow.

3. Details of microbubbles for gene delivery

Microbubbles are mainly composed of fluorinated gases. Air and nitrogen are relatively water-soluble and hence will diffuse into the blood and the bubbles will then rapidly shrink and eventually collapse from Laplace pressures. This is not to say that air and nitrogen cannot be used to make microbubbles for biomedical ultrasound applications, but that stabilizing materials will need to be more robust to preserve the microbubbles.

As opposed to oxygen and nitrogen being relatively soluble in water, perfluorocarbons are virtually insoluble in the aqueous milieu. In fact perfluorocarbons are amphiphobic. The higher the molecular weight of the fluorinated compound the less water soluble and we would predict that microbubbles prepared from that gas should be correspondingly more stable in the blood stream (all else equal). Note that perfluoropentane has a boiling point of 29°C and that perfluorohexane volatilizes at 56.6°C and therefore will be a liquid at biological temperature (presumably due to van der Waal's attractions).

Compound	Molecular Weight	Aqueous Solubility (Ostwald's Coefficient)	Boiling Point °C
Nitrogen	28	18071	-196
Oxygen	32	4865	-183
Sulfur Hexafluoride	146	5950	-64
Perfluoropropane	188	583	-36.7
Perfluorobutane	238	<500	-1.7
Perfluoropentane	288	>24 and <500	29
Perfluorohexane	338	24	56.6

Table 1. Potential Compounds for Making Gaseous Cores of Microbubbles

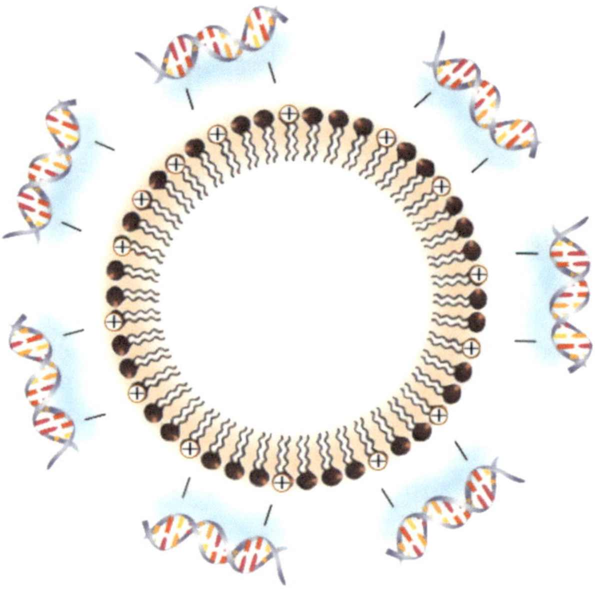

Fig. 4. Depicts a microbubble for gene delivery. The gaseous core is coated by a monolayer of phospholipid containing cationic lipid imparting a net positive charge to the microbubble. DNA, as a polyanion, is adsorbed electrostatically to the exterior surface of the microbubble.

With respect to the microbubble membrane, the above design demonstrates how DNA is adsorbed to the surface via electrostatic adhesion with cationic lipids inserted in the membrane. However, note also that there is no steric protection of the DNA, making it susceptible to biodegradation/hydrolysis. As shown below in Figure 5, microbubbles can be designed to incorporate PEG'ylated lipid (e.g. 8-10 mole percent PEG'ylated lipid) and we have still found that cationic PEG'ylated microbubbles will still adsorb useful payloads of DNA.

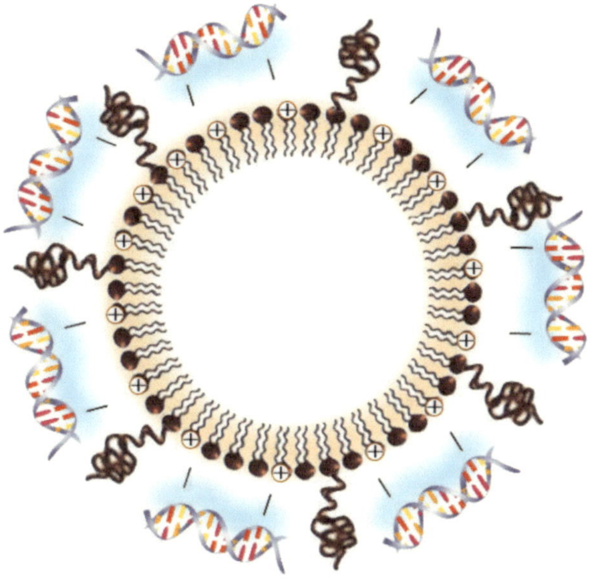

Fig. 5. Depicts a PEG'ylated cationic microbubble binding DNA.

In vivo studies with plasmid DNA using the construct depicted in Figure 5 have shown high levels of gene expression in the zones of insonation.

We predict, however, that targeted constucts that would bind to cellular targets should be more effective for gene delivery. Since microbubbles are micron-sized structures, they are not expected to extravasate from the intravscular space. However, for the purposes of delivering genes to regions in close proximity to targeted tissues, they can be targeted to eptitopes expressed on endothelial cells. Because they can also be engulfed by phagocytic cells, such as immune cells, and targeted as intracellular passengers, the nanoparticles fused to microbubble surfaces as described below (Figure 8) can also be decorated with cell surface identifiers/targets, uptake enhancers, and even intracellular targets in order to provide additional selectivity. We have prepared targeted microbubbles to a variety of different targets. Depicted below is the design for a targeted microbubble to the integrin $\alpha_v\beta_{III}$, Expressed on the endothelial surface in angiogenesis.

The microbubble construct depicted above combines several features of nanotechnology. The parent microbubble is PEG'ylated to impart stealth properties in order to prevent reticuloendothelial system elimination and includes targeting ligands directed to epitopes expressed on endothelial cells. It could be monitored as an ultrasound contrast agent and then activated with higher energy ultrasound using low MI ultrasound for imaging to monitor delivery to the target site and high MI ultrasound energy for cavitation. Upon activation the nanoparticles containing DNA would be expected to extravasate from the vasculature into the interstitial tissues. The nanoparticles could be constructed to contain targeting ligands and/or cell penetration-enhancing agents to facilitate uptake by target cells. A challenge is to design linkers to attach the nanoparticles to the surface of the parent microbubbles. One approach would be to biotinylate the nanoparticles and to have avidin tethers attached to the parent microbubbles taking advantage of the avidin/biotin interaction. This approach could be utilized in proof-of-principle studies but would not be

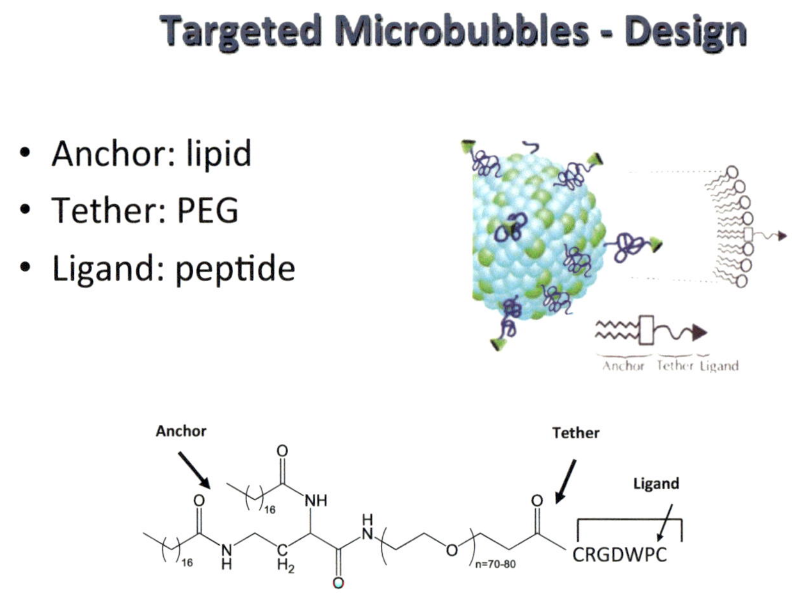

Fig. 6. Depicts a targeted microbubble. The cyclo-CRGDC analog is attached to a lipid anchor via a PEG spacer to form a bioconjugate. The bioconjugate comprises about from about 0.1 to 5 mole percent of the lipid coating the microbubble. There is additional PEG'ylated lipid from about 5-10 mole percent in the lipid coating the microbubble.

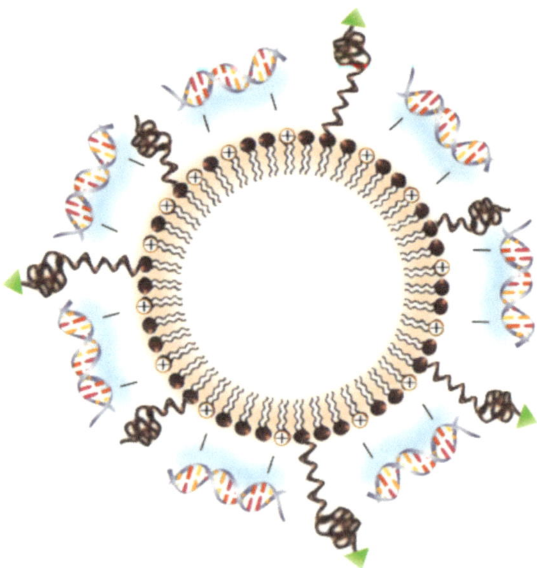

Fig. 7. Depicts a targeted cationic microbubble binding DNA. The bioconjugates are designed to bind to endothelial epitopes upregulated in disease. The microbubble can be followed and monitored by ultrasound imaging and activated with ultrasound energy for local delivery.

clinically translatable. A maleimide labeled spacer might be affixed to the microbubble and the nanoparticles might be thiolated to covalently bind the nanoparticle to the surface of the microbubbles in a potentially biocompatible manner. Another approach would be to use electrostatic interaction between the nanoparticle and the surface of the microbubbles but this must be optimized to ensure that the DNA is bound until it reaches the target site. Note also that if the bubble has excess cationic charge this may adversely affect biodistribution. Note also that it is more difficult to bind low molecular weight genetic material such as siRNA using merely electrostatic interaction.

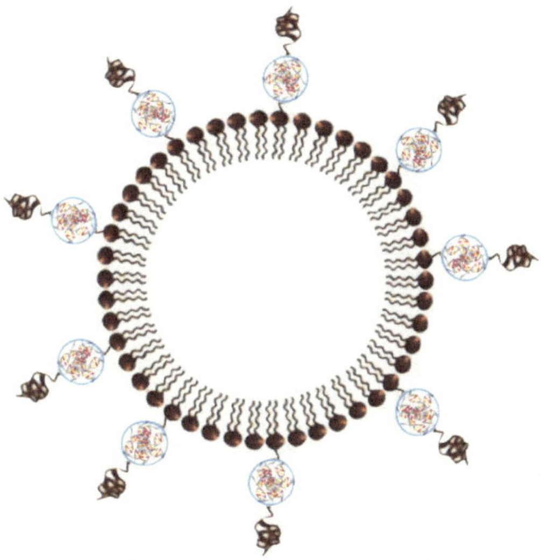

Fig. 8. Depicts a unique microbubble construct for gene delivery. The parent microbubble is PEG'ylated but the DNA (or siRNA) is condensed into nanoparticles that are bound to the surface of the microbubble. The nanoparticles have targeting ligands to bind to cell specific epitopes. Note also that the construct could be modified to comprise endothelial targeting moieties on the microbubble so that the microbubble could bind to endothelial epitopes.

4. Ultrasound – parameters and bioeffects

Ultrasound is a commonly used modality for biomedical imaging, only exceeded by X-rays in overall worldwide use. For medical imaging the power or intensity of ultrasound that can be used is limited by regulatory guidelines. The intensity of the ultrasound can be described by the mechanical index (MI) which is related to the peak negative pressure of the ultrasound wave divided by the square root of the center frequency of the ultrasound. The FDA-approved mechanical index for most body imaging ultrasound (e.g. cardiac and abdominal) is limited to an MI < 1.9. For neurovascular imaging it is limited to MI < 1.0 and for ophthalmic ultrasound to MI < 0.8.

Cavitation is a phenomenon in which ultrasound exposure at the resonance frequency of the microbubble will induce expansion and collapse of microbubbles (Apfel, Hallow). This can occur spontaneously at high acoustic pressure in the absence of exogenous microbubbles. Sufficiently high acoustic power is sufficient to create a microbubble nidus in situ and cause expansion and collapse, i.e. cavitation (Marmottant). Cavitation causes acoustic streaming and local shock waves that may radiate on the order of microns or larger depending upon the acoustic intensity and other factors (Mehier-Humbert). Cavitation can be used to increase cell permeability (i.e. sonoporation)(Deng), open the blood brain barrier or destroy tissues (i.e. sonoablation)(Conger, Feril). The acoustic pressure can be controlled to create the desired effects (Forsberg). Within the ranges of allowable acoustic pressures, in the absence of exogenous microbubbles, biomedical ultrasound imaging does not generally cause violent cavitation and ultrasound imaging is generally quite safe, particularly compared to other technologies such as X-ray imaging that uses ionizing radiation.

As shown below in Figure 9, microbubbles lower the threshold of ultrasound energy necessary for cavitation to occur. The effect is frequency dependent with a greater proportional effect at 1 MHz than at 10 MHz. Note that at 1 MHz, cavitation occurs at MI < 0.5 within the allowable ultrasound power limits for biomedical imaging. Note that microbubbles in the size range of 0.5 to 2.0 microns are quite effective in lowering the thresh-hold of energy for cavitation. Stable microbubbles for gene delivery can certainly be made in this size range. If necessary, for therapeutic applications, higher levels of ultrasound energy can be employed. Higher levels of ultrasound energy are used therapeutically for hyperthermia and focused ultrasound surgery (Brujan).

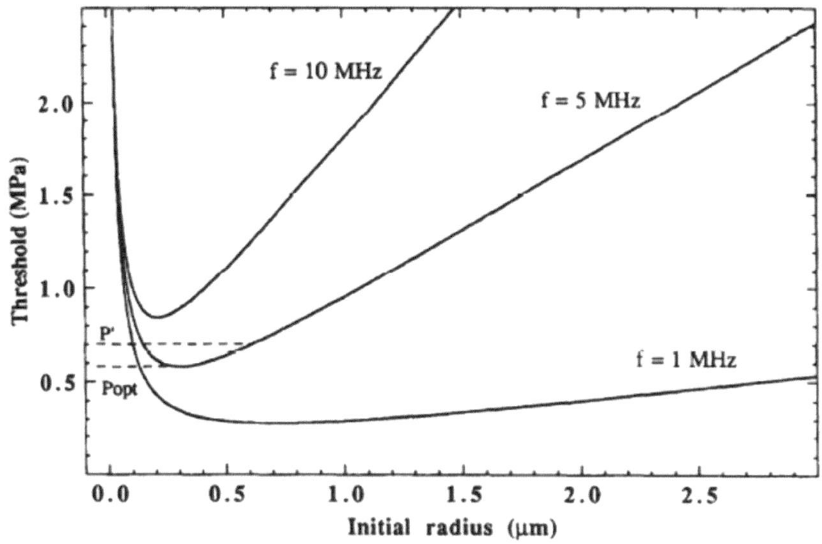

Fig. 9. Microbubbles Lower Thresh-hold of Ultrasound Energy for Cavitation (Apfel).

Figure 10, below, shows images from ultra-high speed videomicroscopy of a single bubble in response to a single high MI pulse of ultrasound energy. The microbubble expands, collapses, and fragments. The daughter fragments then undergo one additional cycle of expansion, collapse and disappear. In this process genetic materials might be released from a gene-carrying microbubble. The cavitation process will also create acoustic jets and streaming which might be used for delivering the genetic material to the target tissue or cells.

Figure 11 depicts a gene carrying microbubble in response to cavitation. The stabilizing wall material of the microbubble fragments and the genetic material is ejected with the cavitation ballistically, thereby extravasating from the vasculature to the target tissue.

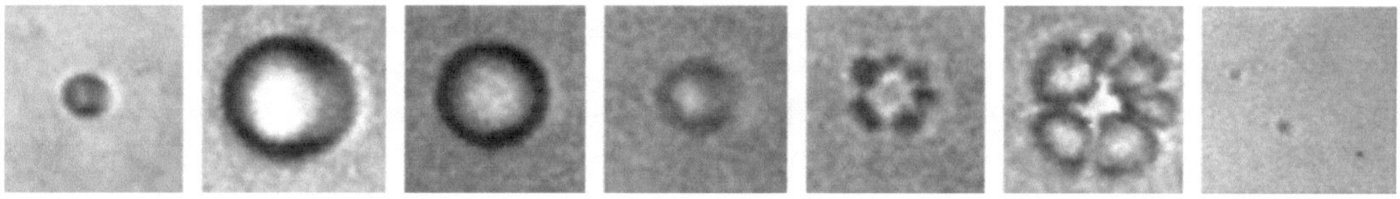

Fig. 10. Videomicroscopy images of a single bubble in response to a single ultrasonic wave.

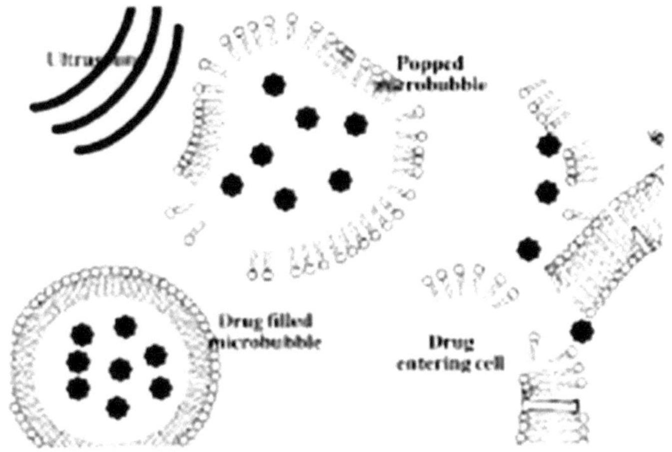

Fig. 11. A drug carrying-microbubble cavitating in response to ultrasound.

Another major mechanism in ultrasound that may be useful for drug and gene delivery is the mechanical force of microbubbles. Ultrasound exerts a radiation (pushing) force that can move microparticles and improve cellular delivery of biomaterials. Figure 12 below shows avidin-coated microbubbles flowing in blood over a biotinylated plate. The microbubbles flow and do not appear to bind but after application of relatively low MI ultrasound the microbubbles are pushed by the acoustic waves and bind to the surface of the plate. The same process can be used to improve cellular uptake of biomaterials such as DNA. The (pushing) radiation force of ultrasound occurs at lower energies than necessary for cavitation and can be used to increase efficacy from gene delivery.

An acoustic transducer that generally uses a piezoelectric material to convert electrical energy into ultrasound waves creates ultrasound waves. The transducer design varies depending upon the biomedical application. Figure 13 (below) shows the design of a three dimensional transducer for imaging and treating the heart. This transducer can be used to image the heart and visualize microbubble as they enter the myocardial circulation. Ultrasound energy can be applied to the heart to cavitate the microbubbles or for the radiation force to improve myocardial delivery. The transducer is currently being used in pre-clinical studies for microbubble enhanced sonothrombolysis to treat myocardial infarction and planned for use in clinical studies. The same transducer design could potentially be used in clinical studies for microbubble-mediated gene delivery to treat the heart.

Despite its ease of use, unwanted bioeffects can be experienced using ultrasound at high acoustic outputs. High levels of ultrasound energy with cavitation may cause cell damage, cell death and apoptosis (Miller). Ultrasound may also heat tissues and cause coagulative necrosis at high temperatures (Ter Haar). We emphasize, however, that ultrasound power levels within the limits for diagnostic ultrasound are generally safe. Ultrasound power levels can be optimized for gene therapy to maximize gene expression while minimizing unwanted bioeffects (Chen, Rahim).

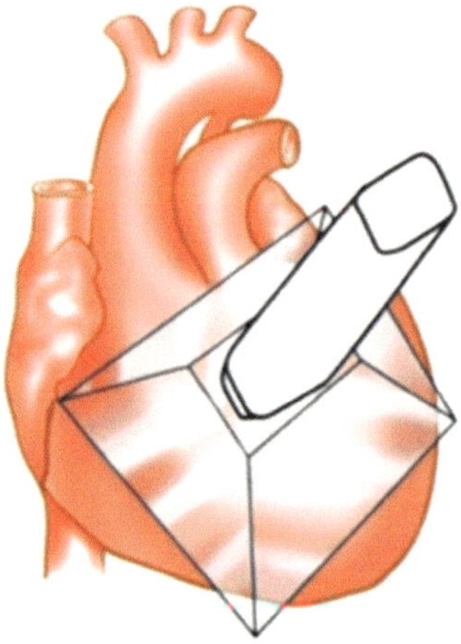

Fig. 12. Drawing of three-dimensional transducer for imaging and treating the heart.

5. Studies using microbubbles and ultrasound for gene delivery

In this section we summarize studies that have been performed using microbubbles and ultrasound for gene delivery (Klibanov, Liu, Newman).

Over the period of more that a decade a number of different studies have been performed, in vitro and in vivo. In vitro studies showed that ultrasound increased the efficacy of transfection with cationic liposomes in cell culture studies to express reporter genes. Saphenous vein grafts have been transfected with ultrasound and MBs (Kodama) to enhance graft survival after implantation (Akowuah). In vivo studies have been performed with reporter genes showing increased expression of the reporter gene after IV administration of microbubbles either binding or in association with the reporter genes. The zones of highest expression have been in the regions of tissues of insonation (except that cationic microbubbles have also been accumulated by liver, lungs, spleen and phagocytic organs). Most of the in vivo studies Have been performed with reporter genes. A few studies have performed with therapeutic genes. A wide variety of different tissues (Hauff) and cells have shown enhanced transfection with ultrasound including neuronal cells (Fischer) and skeletal muscle (Liang).

A number of groups have studied ultrasound and microbubbles to transfect tumors (Michel, Anwer). With collaborators we performed a study assessing tumor regression with transfection of the IL-12 gene with ultrasound and cationic liposomes (Anwer). In this study the liposomes were lyophilized and may have contained nitrogen gas. The tumors were insonated with 1 MHz ultrasound. Increased expression of IL-2 was observed in the insonated tumors and statistically significant tumor regression.

In addition to phospholipid coated microbubbles, MBs can be stabilizes with denatured serum albumin (e.g. Optison®, GE Healthcare Medical Diagnostics, Princeton, NJ). Albumin binds a variety of molecules and also appears to bind DNA. In one study the plasmid of AdCMV-b-Gal was attached to the microbubbles (Shohet). In these studies the solution of AdCMV-b-Gal was added to the microbubble suspension and mixed for 2 hours at 4°C. The mixture was separated into 2 distinct layers. The upper layer consisted of microbubbles with attached virus; the bottom layer, which contained unattached virus, was discarded. The concentration of microbubbles with attached AdCMV-β-Gal was $1.2x10^9$ bubbles/mL; the mean diameter was 3.5 um. The viral titer of these microbubbles was determined. Rats were anesthetized, and MBs were administered IV. Echocardiography was performed at 1.3 MHz with a mechanical index of 1.5. Images were ECG-triggered to deliver a burst of 3 frames of ultrasound every 4 to 6 cardiac cycles. The hearts of all 6 rats in the experimental group showed blue staining with 5-bromo-4-chloro-3-indolyl-β-D-galactopyranoside. None of the control rats showed myocardial staining, which confirmed that the destruction of the microbubbles containing the virus was responsible for the observed β-galactosidase expression in the rat myocardium.

Initiated in 2001, researchers began using gas-filled, albumin-shelled MBs (Optison) and non-viral carriers to increase nascent serum HDL cholesterol in mice and Sprague-Dawley rats. Initial feasibility studies were performed using reporter genes, 5-bromo-4-chloro-3-indolyl-β-D-galactopyranoside and GFP. Subsequent studies now use ApoA-I DNA plasmids in combination with Optison. In a series of rat studies performed with partial support from an NIH SBIR award (44HL095238-01), the results revealed that an average peak response of HDL-C elevation occurred within 24 hours of treatment and 88% of the responses occurred within 48 hours. The control animal group included ultrasound only, apoA-I DNA only, and microbubble only rats. These data demonstrated a rapid incorporation of the plasmid into the cell and efficient ApoA-I protein production that was later incorporated into serum HDL-C.

Summarized data revealed an average increase of 16.8% on day one post treatment. Due to wide normal variation in individual rat HDL cholesterol values, all data is plotted as a percentage from an individual animal's baseline. When examining the overall response to treatment in mg/dL, the average peak response to treatment was 14.0% (p-value <0.0001) as seen in Figure 1 (below). This response was observed uniformly across different animals and ranged from 40mg/dL HDL-C baseline to 100mg/dL HDL-C baseline.

Ongoing studies include additional design of experiments for the following: (1) optimization of sonoporation utility for raising HDL cholesterol, (2) efficient energy delivery algorithms, (3) modes and methods of delivery, and (4) mechanistic analyses of the intra-cellular plasmid location.

Ongoing studies have been performed with lipid coated MBs binding plasmid DNA with genes to treat diabetes. In vivo studies in rats have shown long-term normalization of blood glucose levels in diabetic rats. Studies are planned to test this system in primates.

Encouraging work has been performed in models of hypercholesterolemia showing the potential to perform gene therapy for H1Alpha to improve the capacity of the liver to produce HDL as treatment for atherosclerosis. Promising work continues to progress in the use of MBs binding genes to treat hemophilia. Cationic MBs binding DNA (similar to Figure 7) have been tested with ultrasound and compared to Definity^R MBs which do not bind DNA. Expression of Factor IX transgenes is more robust with the cationic MBs binding DNA than with MBs not binding DNA. In both the HI1Alpha/HDL and hemophilia treatment applications the target organ is the liver. The goal in both of these programs and in many others is to generate sustained transgene expression in the liver (Guo). Catheter mediated administration may prove attractive to maximize efficiency of delivery to hepatocytes and catheters can be deployed for delivery to other organs such as the kidneys, heart and blood vessels.

Ultrasound can be targeted to any organ for which it is possible to create an acoustic window. Most tissues are readily accessible to ultrasound. Ultrasound can be applied across

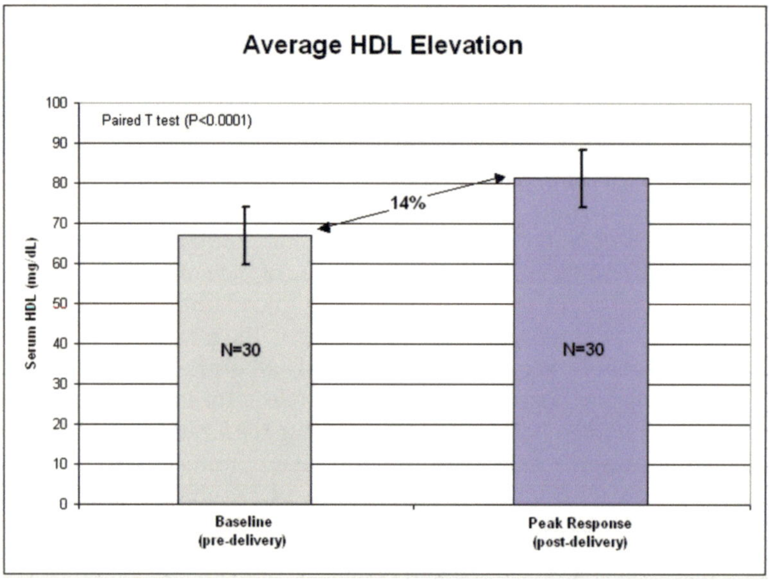

Fig. 13. Baseline to peak response measurement in 30 treated rats recorded in raw data values of mg/dL. A statically significant 14% increase was measured (p-value= 0.0001).

the intact skin or, if need be, via specialized probes. While ultrasound is blocked by air/tissue or air/fluid interfaces, even in the lung, it is possible to create acoustic windows to the bronchi with bronchoscopes and water filled balloons. Ultrasound can be targeted precisely to tissues to treat volumes of tissues ranging to more than 500 ml to less than a ml. Most studies have shown relatively low toxicity due to ultrasound and MBs. It also is possible to repeat treatment, potentially indefinitely.

Despite early studies in ultrasound and gene delivery with MBs being performed more than a decade ago, none of the ultrasound gene delivery programs with MBs, at the time of preparation of this chapter, have advanced to clinical trials. The field is still early in its development, but the tolerability, ease of use and high degrees of expression in the target tissue indicate that this technology merits serious consideration for clinical translation.

6. Conclusions

Ultrasound mediated gene delivery with acoustically active carriers (e.g. microbubbles) is a promising field that affords the potential for high levels of expression in the target tissue without the adverse bioeffects of viral-based carriers. The field is early in its development however as no clinical studies have yet been performed as of the time of preparation of this manuscript. Clinical development of this promising field will require identification of biological targets in areas of medical need and multi-disciplinary collaborations between material scientists, biologists and biopharma.

7. Acknowledgements

The Authors thank Dr. Steven Feinstein and GE Global Research, for their contributions for the ApoA-I-DNA experiments.

8. References

Akowuah EF, Gray C, Lawrie A, Sheridan PJ, Su CH, Bettinger T et al. Ultrasound-mediated delivery of TIMP-3 plasmid DNA into saphenous vein leads to increased lumen size in a porcine interposition graft model. Gene Therapy 2005; 12: 1154–1157.

Anwer K, Kao G, Proctor B, Anscombe I, Florack V, Earls R, Wilson E, McCreery T, Unger E, Rolland A, Sullivan SM. Ultrasound enhancement of cationic lipid-mediated gene transfer to primary tumors following systemic administration. Gene Ther. 2000;7 (21):1833-9.

Apfel, RE, Holland, CK. Microbubbles Lower Thresh-hold of Ultrasound Energy for Cavitation. Ultrasound Med Biol. 1991;17(2):179-85.

Brujan EA, Ikeda T, Matsumoto Y. Jet formation and shock wave emission during collapse of ultrasound-induced cavitation bubbles and their role in the therapeutic applications of high-intensity focused ultrasound. Phys Med Biol 2005; 50: 4797–4809.

Chen S, Shohet RV, Bekeredjian R, Frenkel P, Grayburn PA. Optimization of ultrasound parameters for cardiac gene delivery of adenoviral or plasmid deoxyribonucleic acid by ultrasound targeted microbubble destruction. J Am Coll Cardiol 2003; 42: 301–308.

Conger AD, Ziskin MC, Wittels H. Ultrasonic effects on mammalian multicellular tumor spheroids. .I Clin Ultrasound 1981;9:167-174.

Deng CX, Sieling F, Pan H, Cui J. Ultrasound-induced cell membrane porosity. Ultrasound Med Biol 2004; 30: 519–526. 15 Zarnitsyn VG, Prausnitz MR. Physical parameters influencing optimization of ultrasound-mediated DNA transfection. Ultrasound Med Biol 2004; 30: 527–538.

Feril LB, Kondo T, Zhao QL, Ogawa R, Tachibana K, Kudo N et al. Enhancement of ultrasound-induced apoptosis and cell lysis by echo-contrast agents. Ultrasound Med Biol 2003; 29: 331–337.

Forsberg F, Merton DA, Goldberg BB. In vivo destruction of ultrasound contrast microbubbles is independent of the mechanical index. J Ultrasound Med 2006; 25: 143–144

Guo DP, Li XY, Sun P, Tang YB, Chen XY, Chen Q et al. Ultrasound-targeted microbubble destruction improves the low density lipoprotein receptor gene expression in HepG2 cells. Biochem Biophys Res Commun 2006; 343: 470–474.

FischerAJ,StankeJJ,OmarG,AskwithCC,BurryRW.Ultrasound- mediated gene transfer into neuronal cells. J Biotechnol 2006; 122: 393–411.

Hallow DM, Mahajan AD, McCutchen TE, Prausnitz MR. Measurement and correlation of acoustic cavitation with cellular bioeffects. Ultrasound Med Biol 2006; 32: 1111–1122.

Hauff P, Seemann S, Reszka R, Schultze-Mosgau M, Reinhardt M, Buzasi T et al. Evaluation of gas-filled microparticles and sonoporation as gene delivery system: feasibility study in rodent tumor models. Radiology 2005; 236: 572–578.

Klibanov AL. Microbubble contrast agents: targeted ultrasound imaging and ultrasound-assisted drug-delivery applications. Invest Radiol 2006; 41: 354–362.

Kodama T, Tan PH, Offiah I, Partridge T, Cook T, George AJ et al. Delivery of oligodeoxynucleotides into human saphenous veins and the adjunct effect of ultrasound and microbubbles. Ultrasound Med Biol 2005; 31: 1683–1691.

Liang HD, Lu QL, Xue SA, Halliwell M, Kodama T, Cosgrove DO et al. Optimisation of ultrasound-mediated gene transfer (sonoporation) in skeletal muscle cells. Ultrasound Med Biol 2004; 30: 1523–1529.

Liu Y, Miyoshi H, Nakamura M. Encapsulated ultrasound microbubbles: therapeutic application in drug/gene delivery. J Control Release 2006; 114: 89–99.

Litzinger DC, Brown JM, Walal, Kaufman SA, et al. Fate of cationic liposomes and their complex with oligonucleotive in vivo. Biochimica et Biophysica Acta (BBA) - Biomembranes. 1996;1281(2):2139-149.

Marmottant P, Hilgenfeldt S. Controlled vesicle deformation and lysis by single oscillating bubbles. Nature 2003; 423: 153–156. 12 Sundaram J, Mellein BR, Mitragotri S. An experimental and theoretical analysis of ultrasound-induced permeabilization of cell membranes. Biophys J 2003; 84: 3087–3101. 13 Brujan EA. The role of cavitation microjets in the therapeutic applications of ultrasound. Ultrasound Med Biol 2004; 30:381–387.

Marshall E. Gene Therapy Death Prompts Review of Adenovirus Vector. Science.1999;286(5448):2244-2245.

Mehier-Humbert S, Bettinger T, Yan F, Guy RH. Ultrasound- mediated gene delivery: kinetics of plasmid internalization and gene expression. J Control Release 2005; 104: 203–211.

Michel MS, Erben P, Trojan L, Schaaf A, Kiknavelidze K, Knoll T et al. Acoustic energy: a new transfection method for cancer of the prostate, cancer of the bladder and benign kidney cells. Anticancer Res 2004; 24: 2303–2308.

Miller MW, Miller DL , Brayman AB. A review of in vitro bioeffects of inertial ultrasonic cavitation from a mechanistic perspective. Ultrasound in Med. & Biol.. Vol. 22. No. 9, pp. 1131-l 154,

Muruve DA, Barnes MJ, Stillman IE, Libermann TA. Adenoviral gene therapy leads to rapid induction of multiple chemokines and acute neutrophil dependent hepatic injury in vivo. Hum Gene Ther.1999;(10): 965–976.

Newman CMH, Bettinger T. Gene therapy progress and prospects: Ultrasound for gene transfer Gene Therapy. 2007;14 ; 465–475.

Rahim AA, Taylor SL, Bush NL, TerHaar GR, Bamber JC, Porter CD. Spatial and acoustic pressure dependence of microbubble- mediated gene delivery targeted using focused ultrasound. J Gene Med 2006; 8: 1347–1357.

Shohet RV, Chen S, Zhou Y-T, Wang Z, Meidell RS, Unger RH, Grayburn PA. Echocardiographic Destruction of Albumin Microbubbles Directs Gene Delivery to the Myocardium. Circulation 2000;101:2554-2556.

TerHaar G. Therapeutic applications of ultrasound . Prog Biophys Mol Biol 2007; 93: 111–129.

Thomas CE, EhrhardtA, Kay MA. progress and problems withthe use of viral vectors for gene therapy. 2003;4: www.nature.com/reviews/genetics p346-358.

Unger, E C, Mccreery Tp, Sweitzer Rh. Ultrasound Enhances Gene Expression of Liposomal Transfection Investigative Radiology.1997;32:723-727.

Zhigang W, Zhiyu L, Haitao R, Hong R, Qunxia Z, Ailong H et al. Ultrasound-mediated microbubble destruction enhances VEGF gene delivery to the infarcted myocardium in rats. Clin Imaging 2004; 28: 395–398.

Zhou QH, Miller DL, Carlisle RC, Seymour LW, Oupicky D. Ultrasound-enhanced transfection activity of HPMA-stabilized DNA polyplexes with prolonged plasma circulation. J Control Release 2005; 106: 416–427.

10

Ultrasound-Mediated Gene Delivery

Carol H. Miao and Andrew A. Brayman
Seattle Children's Research Institute & University of Washington, Seattle WA
United States of America

1. Introduction

Human gene therapy holds great promise in treating not only hereditary genetic disorders, but also disease states such as cancer and viral infections, and contingencies such as stroke or myocardial infarctions. It can be achieved by delivery of a correct gene into target cells with genetic deficiency or mutations, or by transfer of a therapeutic agent such as agents targeting a cancer-causing oncogene, growth factor gene, antisense oligonucleotides (ODN), or small interfering RNA (siRNA) to correct the disease state using either viral or nonviral vectors. Viral gene therapy has succeeded in many animal disease models {Snyder 1999}, and has progressed to clinical trials {Hacein-Bey-Abina *et al.* 2002; Kay *et al.* 2000}. However, significant obstacles remain, including immune responses {Manno *et al.* 2006} or tumor genesis {Hacein-Bey-Abina *et al.* 2003}. A nonviral approach would provide a safer strategy. The potential for therapeutic ultrasound (US) to effect minimally invasive nonviral gene transfer has long been recognized, and a growing body of evidence indicates that significant enhancement of transgene expression can be achieved by using high frequency acoustic energy. In addition to its well-known role in providing inexpensive, real-time imaging capability, US has been used therapeutically for years {Herzog *et al.* 1999}. The most common therapeutic application involves low acoustic intensities and is intended to heat deep tissues; *e.g.*, as used in sports medicine. At the other 'end' of the acoustic intensity spectrum is HIFU (high intensity focused ultrasound), which can be used to ablate {Fischer *et al.* 2010} or to liquefy tissues {Hall *et al.* 2009}. US of intermediate intensities has been applied to many systems, together with exogenous microbubbles [MBs], to use the acoustically-forced behavior of the MBs to generate desired bioeffects. The latter usually involves changing the permeability of endogenous barriers to otherwise impermeable materials (*e.g.*, drugs or macromolecules). Many gene therapies have been attempted by direct intramuscular or intraparenchymal injection of gene vectors; these vectors gain immediate access to the interstitial space and must then traverse the plasma membrane of the targeted cells. US contrast agents are almost always administered intravascularly. When accompanied by a gene vector, the first barrier encountered is the vascular endothelium. The next are other vascular anatomical features (*e.g.*, the basement membrane, smooth muscle layer, *etc.*) and then the outer cell membrane of the cells one hopes to target. Finally, DNA needs to be transferred across the nuclear membrane to enter the nucleus for efficient gene expression.

This review will focus almost entirely on the use of ultrasound targeted microbubble destruction (UTMD) as a means by which to deliver foreign DNA (or drugs or photo reactive nanoparticles, as other examples for which there are numerous publications) into targeted host tissues and cells. The literature on this topic is growing at an incredible rate, because almost immediately following the commercial availability of microbubble-based US contrast agents in the 1980s, it was recognized that acoustic cavitation could cause potentially undesirable bioeffects, desirable ones, or both.

Exploitation of acoustically-activated MBs for therapeutic effect remains an exciting topic. Indeed, harnessing the dynamical behavior of acoustic MBs is somewhat of the 'holy grail' of acoustically-targeted gene (or drug) delivery {Lindner 2009}. However, a healthy skepticism has been (see, *e.g.*, {Villanueva 2009} and should continue to be, applied to claims of great successes achieved using UTMD, as replication studies are few, and contradictory findings not unusual. Skepticism should obtain especially when considering 'black box' US studies.

A reasonably coherent picture of US-mediated gene therapy is emerging. With UTMD techniques, the issue ultimately reduces to the fact that US can force dynamic behaviors of MBs. Endogenous MBs are absent in most tissues of the body {Carstensen *et al.* 2000; Gross *et al.* 1985}. Exogenously-administered MBs are generally inert without acoustic exposure, but can be made to pulsate gently, or to undergo violent but highly localized dynamic behavior when driven by acoustic fields. Targeting can thus be achieved by methods as simple as co-administering MBs and gene vectors and exposing the targeted tissue to US, which will thus be the only site where bubble activation occurs. As we shall see, bioeffects typically arise when MBs are driven at pressure amplitudes sufficient to produce nonlinear bubble oscillations.

Here we will discuss the issues broadly, in the hope that the reader will gain a general understanding of the techniques, applications, apparent mechanisms, and some insights into what has been achieved. We focus most of our discussion on *in vivo* studies, as US-assisted gene therapy *in vivo* continues to be a more challenging problem than US-enhanced cell permeabilization *in vitro* or even in intact *ex vivo* tissues (see; *e.g.* {Kodama *et al.* 2005}). We have striven to be as jargon-free as possible, and have neglected mathematical treatments of the topics discussed here, as these can be found elsewhere. A few simple **abbreviations** are used: **US** (ultrasound); **MB** (microbubble); $\mathbf{P_a}$ or $\mathbf{P_r}$ (acoustic pressure amplitude or rarefaction pressure, respectively); and **pDNA** (plasmid DNA). Some words on US exposure metrics are also necessary. In some applications of therapeutic US (*e.g.*, tissue heating), the acoustic intensity in dimensions of W/cm^2 is the parameter of interest. In contrast, the occurrence and character of acoustic cavitation *in vivo* is largely determined by the presence or absence of exogenous MBs and by *peak acoustic intensity, or more properly, by the peak acoustic pressures*. These are expressed in units of mega- (MPa) or kiloPascals (kPa), where 1 MPa = 10 atm. Acoustic intensity scales as the square of the pressure amplitude. The quality of acoustic reporting in the US-mediated gene therapy literature varies widely. We will describe most acoustic exposures in terms of the pressure amplitude (P_a) or the peak rarefactional acoustic pressure (P_r), sometimes inferred by us. In any case, it is not our purpose here to be rigorously quantitative.

2. Ultrasound-targeted microbubble destruction: Physics & technology

There are many potential applications for UTMD gene delivery; a large body of work has been conducted using both *in vitro* and *in vivo* model systems to understand if, and how, UTMD 'works' to produce therapeutic effects. Most studies have as their ultimate goal the application of the technology to effect minimally-invasive treatment of disease or contingency, although *in vitro* UTMD transfection techniques are being used for cell-based therapies {Otani *et al.* 2009}. Specific applications to various organs or for various clinical conditions will be discussed in **§5**. Here it is sufficient to note that in UTMD-based gene delivery studies, much of the work has focused on model or surrogate systems; *e.g.*, the delivery of reporter genes rather than therapeutic ones. However, therapeutic gene transfer effects such as tumor volume reduction have been reported in some model systems.

Therapeutic US has the potential for enhancing minimally invasive gene therapies. For gene therapies involving naked DNA vectors in particular, UTMD techniques have many desired characteristics. These include (1) low toxicity of all components of the treatment, (2) low immunogenicity of the vectors, (3) low invasiveness (*e.g.*, the vector and gas bodies can be administered intravascularly, and for sonographically-accessible organs, the therapeutic US can be applied through the skin), (4) there is good potential for repeated application, (5) organs can be targeted with high specificity, and (6) the technique has broad applicability (again related to sonographic accessibility). However, low efficiencies remain a problem.

2.1 What is ultrasound targeted microbubble destruction?

Here we hope to provide a sense of the types of MBs often used in US-mediated gene therapies, the ways in which US can cause these MBs to be destroyed (either gradually or abruptly) and/or otherwise activated, and the mechanisms by which UTMD-induced microvascular damage, extravasation, and target cell uptake of gene vectors may occur. A more comprehensive discussion of the physics can be found in {Wu & Nyborg 2008}.

In broad terms, the targeting 'part' of UTMD therapies is based *principally* on the fact that MBs present in tissues respond dynamically only if the area is exposed to US. Ligands incorporated into the MB shell may enhance accumulation of the MBs and any vector load they carry in a region of interest, but it is the selective acoustic exposure which 'activates' the MBs. As mentioned, site-specific ligands can be added to MB shells to improve retention in regions of interest. This field has received considerable attention {Ferrara *et al.* 2009}. Some degree of targeting can also be achieved by acoustically 'pushing' bubbles to a region of interest. A propagating acoustic field exerts a radiation force on MBs {Sarvazyan *et al.* 2010}, and this force can propel them in the direction of wave propagation. If the MB is undergoing radial oscillations {Emmer *et al.* 2007}, the bubble lurches forward, slowing as it expands and accelerating as it collapses. Radiation force can be used to concentrate MBs along a specific wall of an intracavitary space {Horie *et al.* 2010}, or blood vessel.

The MB destruction 'part' of UTMD occurs in response to the acoustic exposure, and may result in release of lipid or aqueous-phase drugs {Smith *et al.* 2010} or produce small-scale damage to microvessels which allows normally impermeable materials (drugs, plasmids, even objects as large as cells or MB fragments) to escape the vascular lumen and enter the interstitial space. Cellular permeabilization is also associated with MB activation.

2.2 Ultrasound contrast agents and other stabilized gas bodies

Microbubble US contrast agent evolution from early, agitated saline or sugar solutions to protein-shelled agents containing air to lipid- or polymer-shelled agents using relatively insoluble gases was rapid. The evolution of these agents continues {Qin *et al.* 2009}, as do new applications for them {Cosgrove & Harvey 2009}. US contrast agents are typically micron-sized gas bodies which are stabilized against diffusion by a shell {Overvelde *et al.* 2010; Sarkar *et al.* 2009}; most contrast agent MBs have mean diameters of ~2 μm. New agents currently under development for imaging or therapy are smaller still, and are considered to be nanobubbles {Krupka *et al.* 2009}. Multi-layered structures in which a gas body stabilized by a lipid monolayer is contained in an aqueous compartment bounded by a lipid bilayer (echogenic liposomes) are also under development. *When used for imaging, US contrast agents are unique amongst contrast agents in that they respond dynamically to the signal used to interrogate tissues for their presence.* It is this same property that is exploited for UTMD therapies or therapy models.

2.3 Microbubble destruction: Shell disruption and shell/gas body fragmentation

There are three principal mechanisms by which US or time can destroy a shelled MB {Chomas *et al.* 2001}. In increasing order of 'violence' to the MBs, these are: (1) static diffusion, in which gas dissolves into the surrounding host fluid. This may be rapid if the bubble is 'free' (without stabilizing shell) or very slow if a stabilizing shell is present; (2) acoustically-forced shell disruption, which leads to accelerated diffusive loss of gas relative to unperturbed shelled bubbles; and (3) shell fragmentation and rapid loss of gas.

A micron-sized free air bubble can be expected to dissolve in water in ~30 ms {Sarkar *et al.* 2009}, which is why relatively insoluble gases such as perfluorocarbons are now used in modern contrast agents, and a stabilizing shell is employed. The principal mechanism by which bubble shell materials stabilize MBs against diffusion is by reducing the surface tension at the bubble surface. Shell properties also affect the dynamic responses and stability of MBs at P_a below the shell fragmentation threshold {Emmer *et al.* 2007; Ferrara *et al.* 2009}.

Acoustically-forced MB dissolution can occur when the P_a is sufficient to drive MB oscillations which stretch and compress the shell sufficiently to produce relatively small defects in the shell, which may re-seal {Huang 2008}. Very high physical stresses develop in the shells as the MB oscillates, even when the driving pressures are only a few hundred kPa {Stride & Saffari 2003}. Small shell defects lead to more rapid dissolution of the gas body than would otherwise occur, but complete gas dissolution may require many acoustic cycles {Smith *et al.* 2010}. For examples, Optison MBs exposed to 3.5 MHz US of P_a > 0.15 MPa undergo accelerated loss of gas, indicating shell compromise {Porter *et al.* 2006}. Shell disruption P_a thresholds for albumin-stabilized Optison and surfactant stabilized Sonazoid are similar; at 1.1 MHz, these are 0.13 MPa or 0.15 MPa, respectively. At 3.5 MHz, these thresholds are somewhat higher (Optison: 0.48 MPa; Sonazoid: 0.58 MPa) {Chen *et al.* 2003}. Others have reported a somewhat lower threshold (0.15 MPa) for Optison shell disruption at 3.5 MHz {Porter *et al.* 2006}. Likewise, {Borden *et al.* 2005} studied the behavior of lipid monolayer-encapsulated MBs at 2.25 MHz using single-cycle pulses, and found that the P_r threshold for slow MB dissolution to be in the range of 0.4 – 0.6 MPa, and the P_r threshold for MB fragmentation to be 0.8 MPa. A P_a of around 0.3 MPa was also found to be the threshold for soft-shelled contrast agent MB disruption {de Jong *et al.* 2009}. Echogenic liposomes also appear to have two pressure thresholds; one associated with compromise of the shell of the interior gas body, and a higher one associated with disruption of the outer lipid bilayer {Smith *et al.* 2010}. Rapid fragmentation occurs on a time scale of microseconds when P_a is sufficient to buckle and completely rupture the shell {Marmottant *et al.* 2005}, creating free gas bodies which may then dissolve, grow by rectified diffusion, coalesce into larger bubbles, or dissolve, depending stochastically on exposure conditions.

2.4 Microbubble dynamics: An overview of how gas bodies respond to ultrasound

At very low P_a, MB volume oscillations are related linearly to P_a. At modest P_as of a few hundred kPa (or less), MB volume oscillations become non-linearly related to P_a, with bubble expansion being relatively slow and bubble collapse much faster, being governed by the inertia of the in-rushing surrounding fluid to a greater extent than by the compressive phase of the applied pressure field; hence the phenomenon of bubbles undergoing acoustically-driven expansions followed by rapid, inertially-dominated collapse is termed 'inertial cavitation'. This typically occurs when a MB has been driven by the rarefaction phase of the acoustic wave to a diameter roughly 2 - 3 times the initial diameter {Chomas *et al.* 2001}. At very modest P_as, inertial cavitation can be stable and sustained for an almost indefinite number of acoustic cycles. For example, {Church & Carstensen 2001} found that surfactant-coated Sonazoid MBs could undergo repetitive inertial collapses and rebounds when driven by 2.5 MHz US at acoustic pressures greater than about 0.3 - 0.4 MPa; for this agent, irreversible post-collapse fragmentation occurred at a P_a of ~ 1.5 MPa. Others have reported that a 3 μm bubble exposed to 2.25 MHz US can be expected to undergo expansion, inertial collapse, and fragmentation at a P_a just over 0.3 MPa {Chomas *et al.* 2001}. The albumin-shelled, first-generation US contrast agent Albunex began to emit acoustic signatures characteristic of nonlinear oscillations at acoustic pressures as low as 0.005 - 0.010 MPa {Krishna & Newhouse 1997}. At even modest P_a (*e.g.*, 0.6 MPa at 1 MHz), some contrast agent bubbles can expand to 10 times or larger than their equilibrium radius; under such conditions, inertial collapse is expected. Fragmentation of the inertially-collapsing bubble occurs at some instant near the time of minimum bubble radius {Postema & Schmitz 2007}. Inertial bubble collapse is so rapid and the gas so compressed that the maximum temperature inside the bubble can reach more than 5000 K {Apfel & Holland 1991}. Light emissions {Matula 2003} and reactive free radicals may be produced {Okada *et al.* 2009}. MB rebound and fragmentation can re-emit acoustic energy at many times the excitation pressures. These emissions also contain higher frequency spectral components which can produce local heating. In the present context, however, it appears that the most important determinant of UTMD gene delivery methods is that *bubble expansion and collapse can produce local tissue distortions or damage which are presumed to be the principal mechanism by which microvascular bioeffects become manifest, and target cell permeabilization occurs.*

Cavitation bubbles can interact with nearby boundaries; these interactions can produce high velocity fluid jets and induce bubble translation, with the directions of fluid jets and translation depending on the boundary's properties. For rigid boundaries, bubbles closer to the boundary than about twice the fully-expanded radius of the bubble {Kodama & Tomita 2000} may collapse asymmetrically, with a high velocity water jet 'punching through' the bubble and impinging on the rigid boundary. Near rigid, planar boundaries, an oscillating MB translates toward the boundary and if collapse jetting occurs, the jet is directed toward the rigid surface {Plesset & Chapman 1971} with sufficient water hammer pressure to damage the surface {Blake & Gibson 1987}. *In vivo,* however, this condition would seem rare.

MBs driven to oscillate near pressure release boundaries (an air-water interface, for example), collapse jets which occur are directed away from the boundary, as is the direction of bubble translation {Chahine 1977; Robinson *et al.* 2001}.

Oscillating MBs collapsing near a 'soft', planar boundary (*e.g.*, gels or large vessel walls) also undergo translation and jetting, but the directions of jetting and translation can be either toward or away from the boundary, being determined by bubble size, bubble distance from the boundary, and the mechanical properties of the boundary (see. *e.g.*, {Kodama & Tomita 2000; Shima *et al.* 1989}. Deformation of the elastic boundary stores energy which is 'returned' as the bubble collapses; this creates a hydrodynamic pressure gradient which in turn produces fluid flow away from the elastic boundary. If the pressure gradient is large enough, bubble collapse jets directed away from the boundary, and bubble translation away from the boundary, can result {Blake & Gibson 1987}. Liquid jets were observed in an early experimental study of acoustically forced MB behavior in a 200 µm diameter cellulose tube {Postema *et al.* 2004}. In vessel-simulating gel tunnels, at 1.7 MHz, the P_a at which Optison MBs began to emit broadband noise characteristic of inertial collapse and rebound was weakly dependent on tunnel diameter (~0.8 MPa in 90 µm diameter tunnels *vs.* ~0.6 MPa in 800 µm tunnels) {Sassaroli & Hynynen 2007}. Single-MB dynamics observations in actual microvessels were acquired using a rat cecum model; MBs translated toward the vessel walls and a toroidal bubble morphology consistent with the formation of a microjet was observed {Caskey *et al.* 2007}.

Where bioeffects attributable to inertial cavitation occur, cavitation jets directed toward cells or tissues have long been assumed to be causative. Vessel 'stretching' during bubble expansion has also been proposed as a mechanism of vessel damage {Miao *et al.* 2008}. Very high speed imaging of MBs driven to growth and inertial collapse in microvessels of rat mesentery {Chen *et al.* 2010; Chen *et al.* 2011} indicate that (1) MB collapse jets form frequently in the intravascular environment, (2) jets are typically directed *away* from the nearest blood vessel wall, (3) blood vessel expansion in response to bubble growth is minimal, and (4) tissues 'follow' the collapsing bubbles such that inward vessel distortions are much greater than outward distortions, with inward vessel wall motion having speeds of 5 - 10 m/s and the events occurring on microsecond time scales. This is perhaps one mechanism by which vessel permeabilization occurs. In any case, permeabilization of biological transport barriers is associated with some cell killing, both *in vitro* {Brayman *et al.* 1999} and *in vivo* {Ferrara 2008; Miller *et al.* 2011; Price *et al.* 1998; Skyba *et al.* 1998}

Finally, it is worth mentioning that MB-excitation techniques for cellular permeabilization need not use US to achieve MB activation or cell permeabilization; targeted laser illumination can also be used effectively. For a recent research paper on this topic, using a liposome MB contrast agent, see {Zhou *et al.* 2010}.

2.5 Effect of different shell compositions or agents on gene delivery

It is difficult to compare the efficacy of different contrast agents in US-mediated gene delivery between different studies, because MB type, concentration as injected, rate of injection, total dose, animal model, US exposure source, exposure conditions, and even the way the MBs are handled vary widely and can influence outcome. MB concentration is a determinant of UTMD-mediated pDNA expression in mouse liver {Miao *et al.* 2005; Shen *et al.* 2008}. Different agents have different 'native' concentrations, and agents with similar gas content but dissimilar shells can have different efficacies in enhancing gene delivery under otherwise comparable conditions (*cf.* effects of Optison and PESDA MBs; {Pislaru *et al.* 2003}). Relatively large differences between contrast agent types in UTMD gene delivery have been observed, but the reasons are not always clear. With equalized MB concentrations and either Optison, SonoVue or Sonazoid contrast agents, UTMD-mediated transfer of phosphorodiamidate morpholino oligomer to a dystrophin-deficient murine heart model induced dystrophin-positive cells in the hearts when harvested 7 days after treatment.

Optison and Sonazoid were equivalent in effectiveness, producing about four times greater expression than did SonoVue {Alter *et al.* 2009}.

2.6 Sensitivity of stabilized gas bodies to technique

Bubbles are buoyant, fragile, can coalesce into larger bubbles, or 'disappear' as gas is lost to diffusion. In many *in vivo* studies of UTMD, the MBs and gene vectors are infused slowly; this prolongs the time window in which acoustic treatments can occur, but aggravates the problem of time-dependent changes in MB distribution and delivery {Kaya *et al.* 2009}. It is worth noting that MBs can be destroyed by static pressure or tension; an over-pressure of only ~0.3 MPa can destroy them {Stringham *et al.* 2009}. MBs can also be destroyed by drawing up or injecting an MB suspension *too rapidly* when using a small gauge needle {Talu *et al.* 2008}; thus one can unwittingly alter experimental outcome by 'over-enthusiasm'.

3. Breaching the physical barriers to gene delivery using ultrasound

In order to achieve efficient gene expression following ultrasound-mediated gene delivery, multiple barriers need to be overcome to allow pDNA to enter into the nucleus of target cells including penetrating vascular and cellular membranes as well as trafficking through different intracellular compartments.

US contrast agents are intended to be intravascular agents. Whether the gene vector is administered as a simple mixture with the gas body suspension, or is in some way linked to the gas bodies, they are also intravascular agents in vascular UTMD methods. The first barrier encountered is the vascular endothelium. The next are other vascular anatomical features (*e.g.*, the basement membrane, smooth muscle layer, *etc.*) and then the outer cell membrane of the cells one hopes to target. Some intracellular membranous compartments must also be traversed. However, MBs have been used with intramuscular or intraparenchymal injections of vectors, and some successes reported. In UTMD-based gene transfer methods using vascular approaches, to mediate gene therapy *via* acoustic excitation, gas bodies must first exert their influence from within the vascular lumen.

Most of the available evidence from *in vivo* studies indicate that vessel permeabilization effects occur principally in the microcirculation; larger vessels are too robust to be penetrated by cavitation events, even if their vascular endothelium can be effectively destroyed by intraluminal inertial cavitation {Hwang *et al.* 2005}. Extravasation of dyes, nanoparticles or macromolecules through microvessels is almost always accompanied by extravasation of red cells (see below); since these have diameters on the order of 6 μm, breaches in the endothelial wall can be quite large. However, there is also some evidence that more subtle effects, such as partial opening of the tight junctions between endothelial cells, can also contribute. Assuming that the gene vector escapes the intravascular compartment and enters the interstitium, it must then enter the surrounding cells; thus the plasma membrane is the second major barrier encountered by the vectors. Lethal effects of cavitation occurring in the cardiac microcirculation can extend outward into the myocardium {Miller *et al.* 2011}; there is good reason to expect that sub lethal poration of cells located within a few cell diameters of the intravascular cavitation event(s) also occurs.

3.1 Extravasation of dyes, nanoparticles and cells

Evans blue [EB] is an azo dye which binds serum albumin with high affinity, and is normally unable to pass through the endothelium. Extravasation of EB through reversible or

irreversible capillary modification has been observed in small animal (rat) hearts exposed to low-MHz frequency US with the use of various contrast agent MBs, accompanied by premature ventricular contractions {Li *et al.* 2004}. The effect was sensitive to P_a (apparent threshold somewhat less than 1.6 MPa at 1.5 MHz) and to the concentration of the injected MBs {Miller et al. 2004}. The effect appears to be of mechanical origin {Miller *et al.* 2004} With injection of dilute Definity suspensions, extravasation of EB from canine hearts, and cell killing of cardiomycetes within the ultrasonically-interrogated area also occurs under diagnostically realistic exposure conditions {Miller *et al.* 2006}.
Erythrocyte extravasation has been observed in rat kidney glomerular capillaries exposed to diagnostic US with contrast agent MBs in the circulation {Miller et al. 2010a, Miller et al., 2010b}; such damage was associated with tissue inflammation at 1 week and fibrosis at 4 weeks {Miller *et al.* 2009}. A threshold P_a of ~0.8 MPa was indicated {Miller *et al.* 2007}. Glomerular capillary hemorrhage with contrast-enhanced diagnostic US also occurs in large animals (pigs) exposed to 1.5 MHz, 1.7 MPa US {Miller *et al.* 2010}. Petechial hemorrhage on intestinal blood vessels in an *in vivo* murine model was observed with the contrast agent Albunex, with apparent P_a thresholds of 0.4 MPa at 0.4 MHz, 0.8 MPa at 1.1 MHz, or 2.3 MPa at 2.3 MHz; the thresholds were lower with the agent Levovist than with Albunex {Miller & Gies 1998a, Miller & Gies 1998b}. At 2.25 MHz, a threshold P_a of between 0.85 and 1.0 MPa was indicated for vessel damage in exteriorized rat cremaster muscle containing Definity MBs {Samuel *et al.* 2009}. Similarly, intravital observation of red cell extravasation from rat cremaster muscle capillaries containing MB contrast agent was observed more than a decade ago {Price *et al.* 1998; Skyba *et al.* 1998}. Microscopic observations of US and MB-induced red cell extravasation have been reported in glass catfish {Maruvada & Hynynen 2004}. In exteriorized rat spinotrapezius muscle, 1 MHz US at a P_a of 0.75 MPa was shown to result in extravasation of 100 nm diameter microspheres co-injected with contrast agent MBs {Song *et al.* 2002}. In rats, *in vivo* exposure of the kidneys following injection of MBs resulted in red cell extravasation from the glomerular capillaries into Bowman's space with an apparent threshold P_a of ~ 0.73 MPa (at ~ 1 MHz), with nearly 40% of histological sections taken from the focal plane showing extravasation at a P_a of 1.8 MPa {Miller *et al.* 2007}. Intravital microscopy and concurrent cavitation detection was used to study the relationship between bubble dynamics and extravasation of red cells from rat cremaster muscle using 2.25 MHz US, and Definity contrast agent infused *via* the tail vein. Vascular damage and acoustic emissions from the MBs were correlated. The greatest amount of red cell extravasation and the greatest cumulated bubble acoustic emissions occurred at 10 Hz pulse repetition frequency **[PRF]**, indicating that the time for tissue refill with bubbles following each pulse was ~100 ms. In experiments in which pulses were applied at 100 Hz PRF and the P_a varied from 0 - 2.0 MPa, there was no vascular damage at $P_r \leq 0.85$ MPa, but unambiguous damage occurred at $P_r \geq 1.0$ MPa {Samuel *et al.* 2009}. Finally, there is evidence that low amplitude US induced MB oscillations (1 MHz, P_r = 0.1 MPa, SonoVue bubbles) can increase the permeability of primary endothelial monolayer cultures *in vitro*. Insonation produced immediate influx of Ca^{2+} ions into the cells, indicating poration of the endothelial plasma membranes. The effect was essentially abolished by application of catalase, strongly suggesting a role for extracellularly-produced H_2O_2 associated with nonlinear bubble oscillations. Moreover, histochemical staining for a protein associated with gap junctions showed an approximately 50% increase immediately after insonation, but returned to control levels within 30 minutes of insonation {Juffermans *et al.* 2009}.

3.2 Transient poration of the cell membrane

Two mechanisms by which US and MBs facilitate poration of cell membranes are prominent; these are: (1) cavitational; *e.g.*, the opening of transient holes in membranes in consequence to local shear forces exerted on membranes by fluid flow ('micro streaming') around oscillating bubbles, local shock waves (which produce large pressure gradients across a cell), or cavitation microjets, or (2) endocytosis {Doinikov & Bouakaz 2010; Walton & Shohet 2009}. Other mechanisms have been proposed, of course. However, it appears that shear stresses associated with bubble activation is probably the principal mechanism. A third mechanism by which normally 'tight' physiological barriers may be permeabilized is by sonochemical stimulation.

Transient pores of a few hundred nanometers in diameter and lifetimes of several seconds can be formed in cell membranes by acoustically-driven, single MB oscillations {Deng *et al.* 2004; Han *et al.* 2007; Zhou *et al.* 2008; Zhou *et al.* 2009}. Voltage clamp studies of *Xenopus* oocytes exposed to 1 MHz US showed that without MBs, there was no change in current at P_r as high as 1.2 MPa. With Optison MBs, opening and resealing of individual pores was observable even at P_r as low as 0.2 MPa. The transmembrane current was carried by influx of Ca^{2+} ions. The transmembrane current was greater at 0.4 MPa than at 0.2 MPa; in both cases, pore lifetime was ~2 s. More generally, the effect was P_a dependent, increasing slowly with increasing P_a over the range of 0.3 - 0.55 MPa, and then inflecting sharply upward at higher P_a {Deng *et al.* 2004}. Pore opening showed a high level of temporal correlation with inertial cavitation noise {Zhou *et al.* 2008}. Pore size was estimated as 220 ± 80 (mean ± SD) nanometers, and refined estimates of pore resealing times indicated closure in 3 - 5 s {Zhou *et al.* 2009}. *In vitro* studies of cells in contact with SonoVue MBs excited by 1 MHz US at P_a of 0.05 - 2.50 MPa have shown Ca^{2+} influx associated with poration {Juffermans *et al.* 2008}. Sonoporation to naked DNA *in vitro* is correlated with inertial cavitation activity {Qiu *et al.* 2010}, and depends in part on the fluidity of the membrane at the time of UTMD treatment {Zarnitsyn & Prausnitz 2004}, with higher reporter gene transfection rates at 37 °C than at 21 °C. This is consistent with the need for porated membranes to reseal rapidly in order to maintain viability. Still others have shown that 1 MHz US at P_a as low as 0.1 MPa can permeabilize cells *in vitro* to pDNA {Rahim *et al.* 2006}. In cell suspensions containing Definity MBs, the P_a thresholds for cell permeabilization to 70 kDa FITC-dextran, propidium iodide (indicating cell death) and MB destruction were 75 kPa at 0.5 MHz, 200 kPa at 2.5 MHz, and 600 kPa at 5 MHz {Karshafian *et al.* 2009}. However, the idea that cellular poration results from inertial cavitation has been challenged on the basis of observations of cavitation noise and permeabilization of *in vitro* cell monolayers to 500 kDa FITC dextran; the supporting data indicate that permeabilization precedes the occurrence of broadband noise associated with inertial collapse and rebound cavitation. The authors conclude that the forces associated with microstreaming around activated bubbles is the principal mechanism of sonoporation {Forbes *et al.* 2008}. More study is clearly needed.

US and MB-induced cell lysis and reversible poration in other cell types *in vitro* are strongly correlated with inertial cavitation {Chen *et al.* 2003a; Chen *et al.* 2003b; Lai *et al.* 2006}. Cell surface antigens may be stripped off the surface of viable cells during such events {Brayman *et al.* 1999}. While *in vitro* UTMD-based transfection with naked DNA is often associated with high cell mortality, this is not always the case {Wang *et al.* 2009}.

The use of the collapse jets of MBs generated by laser pulses to selectively and directionally sonoporate individual cells has reached a high level of sophistication, producing pore sizes of ~ 200 nm {Sankin *et al.* 2010}, which may someday prove useful for cell therapies. This is very similar to pore size determined by sonoporation of *Xenopus* oocytes using 1.07 MHz US of 0.3 MPa P_a with Definity MBs; *viz.*, a mean pore size of 220 ± 80 nm diameter {Zhou Y *et al.* 2009}. Lipoplexes, which are normally taken up by cells *via* endocytosis, are taken up poorly when 'PEGylated' (coated with polyethylene glycol). However, when PEGylated pDNA/lipolexes were attached to acoustically activated MBs, large increases in PEGylated lipoplex transfection were achieved in an *in vitro* model system, relative to ether 'free' PEGylated lipolexes, or lipolexes + MB simple (un-linked) mixtures {Lentacker *et al.* 2009}. The investigators also used a number of endocytosis inhibitors; their results indicate that endocytosis was not the primary mechanism involved. They postulate that lipoplex-loaded MBs collapsing near cell monolayers in culture plates released the lipolexes, resulting in high local lipoplex concentrations, that some of the released lipolexes became entrained in MB collapse jets and were 'injected' into the cells with the fluid jet (see also {Miller 2000}). However, Meijering and colleagues, using fluorescently labeled dextrans of ~4 - 500 kDa, present data which indicate that the principal mechanism by which UTMD treatment (1 MHz US, 0.2 MPa P_r, SonoVue MBs) facilitates macromolecule delivery across the plasma membrane is *via* induction of endocytosis. Sonoporation was also observed, but did not seem to be the mechanism for macromolecular uptake {Meijering *et al.* 2009}. It is clear that the our understanding of the mechanism(s) of UTMD-enhanced uptake of macromolecules remains incomplete.

3.3 Entry of pDNA into the nucleus

Following delivery of pDNA across the plasma membrane of cells into cytoplasm, pDNA may travel through multiple cellular compartments and finally enter the nucleus *via* diffusion {Liang *et al.* 2004} or other assisted mechanism to produce efficient transgene expression. UTMD may facilitate overcoming some of these barriers most likely *via* cavitation bioeffects. It was reported that long-term exposure to therapeutic ultrasound (1 MHz, 2 W/cm^2, 30% duty cycle for 30 mins) can overcome the rate-limiting step of driving DNA into the cell nucleus {Duvshani-Eshet & Machluf 2005}. One thousand fold higher gene expression levels of luciferase was achieved with minimal loss in cell viability (<20%) in three different cell types (BHK, LNCaP, and BCE). These data implied that therapeutic US is the main driving force delivering pDNA not only to the cell cytoplasm but also to the nucleus. However, in this case, no MB was used. The same group {Duvshani-Eshet *et al.* 2006} showed that adding Optison further increased transfection levels. Confocal and atomic force microscopy studies indicated that long-term therapeutic US application localizes the pDNA in cell and nucleus regardless of Optison addition. In addition, the use Optison did not affect the kinetics of protein expression, indicating Optison did not affect DNA trafficking to the nucleus. They hypothesized that US application by itself plays a major role in delivering DNA to the nucleus.

An interesting recent report used Doxorubicin (DOX) as a molecular nanotheranostic agent to study UTMD-mediated intracellular delivery and nuclear trafficking {Mohan & Rapoport 2010}. DOX is a popular research tool due to its inherent fluorescence and was encapsulated in poly(ethylene glycol)-co-polycaprolactone (PEG-PCL) micelles or PEG-PCL stabilized perfluorocarbon nanodroplets in this study. US triggered DOX trafficking into cell nuclei; the trafficking was further enhanced in the presence of phase-transition nanodroplets which become gas MBs upon US exposure of sufficient P_r. This was believed to be due to cavitation induced transient permeabilization of both plasma and nuclear membranes, thus allowing DOX penetration into the cell nuclei. Whether MBs and/or nanodroplet emulsions can significantly augment DNA delivery to the nucleus needs further investigation.

Once pDNA enters the nucleus, some DNA can be condensed by histones and form persistent nucleosome-like structures. Persistent gene expression from these stable episomal pDNA genomes requires the introduction of specific cis-acting elements in the gene transfer constructs. We have demonstrated that incorporation of locus control region and intron elements into specific gene transfer constructs can achieve persistent expression of therapeutic-levels of coagulation proteins in the liver following nonviral gene therapy {Miao *et al.* 2001; Miao *et al.* 2003; Ye *et al.* 2003}. The locus control region {Yant *et al.* 2003} can contribute to the open chromatin structure of the pDNA genome and avoid silencing of the transgene expression cassette {Miao *et al.* 2005}. Furthermore, addition of an intron element significantly enhanced the transcription efficiency of stable mRNA {Miao *et al.* 2005}. Thus, gene transfer of episomal pDNA into slow-dividing or terminally differentiated cells facilitated by UTMD has high potential to achieve a therapeutic effect to treat specific diseases. For gene transfer into dividing cells where integration of target genes are required, incorporation of other systems such as sleeping beauty transposons {Aronovich *et al.* 2011; Yant *et al.* 2007} or PhiC31 integrase {Keravala *et al.* 2011} with UTMD-mediated nonviral gene transfer methodology can lead to long-term transgene expression.

4. The vectors: Packaging desired genes for ultrasound-mediated delivery

4.1 Naked DNA: Plasmids

Naked plasmid DNA provides many advantages as a nonviral gene transfer vector, including: (1) ease of preparation, (2) cost-effectiveness, (3) minimum toxicity, and (4) it is least immunogenic of the vectors. Indeed, the immunogenic CpG moiety can be modified easily if needed. Most importantly, quality control is quite easy compared to other pDNA complexes containing synthetic vehicles. However, it has been a very challenging problem to deliver naked pDNA into specific cells due to its large size and negative charge. *In vivo* delivery of naked pDNA is especially difficult with additional impediments of instability of pDNA in blood serum as well as in cellular sub-compartments such as cytosol, endosome, and nucleus after cell entry. Recently a hydrodynamic approach has been developed to drive efficient gene delivery into liver {Liu *et al.* 1999} and muscle {Danko *et al.* 1997} resulting in therapeutic levels of transgene expression in animal disease models, including hemophilia B {Miao *et al.* 2003} and others {Zhang *et al.* 2000}. This method in its current form is not suitable for clinical use; however, notable recent advances have been made in large animal models (*vide, e.g.*, {Fabre *et al.* 2008; Kamimura *et al.* 2009; Suda *et al.* 2008}. Alternatively, innovative US and MB technology to facilitate delivery of naked pDNA is a potential clinically feasible nonviral gene therapy approach {Miao *et al.* 2005; Shen *et al.* 2008; Song *et al.* 2011}.

The potential for sonoporation to increase pDNA loading of cells was recognized years ago {Fechheimer *et al.* 1987}. Sonoporation-enhanced transport of nanoparticles into cells is dependent on molecular size; uptake of particles ≤ 37 nm diameter was enhanced by sonoporation without gross damage, but particle uptake generally declined as particle size increased {Mehier-Humbert *et al.* 2005a}. pDNA gene expression is faster with sonoporation than with liposome-based methods which depend on endocytosis {Mehier-Humbert *et al.* 2005}, indicating that pDNA enters cells through transient pores. Moreover, due to the risk of pDNA degradation by serum nucleases and removal by phagocytes {Niidome & Huang

2002}, injection of a nonviral gene transfer vector long before US treatment occurs is unlikely to be effective. With simultaneous delivery of pDNA and US exposure, UTMD can significantly facilitate the transfer of naked pDNA up to several hundred fold *in vitro* {Miller *et al.* 2002; Newman & Bettinger 2007} and up to several thousand fold *in vivo*, depending on different US and transfection systems {Chen *et al.* 2010; Miao *et al.* 2005; Shen *et al.* 2008; Song *et al.* 2011}. Furthermore, with introduction of specific cis-acting elements in the gene transfer constructs, persistent expression of near-therapeutic levels of proteins can be achieved from episomal plasmids following UTMD-mediated gene therapy {Miao *et al.* 2005}. These results demonstrate that development of UTMD has high potential to achieve a therapeutic effect for treating specific diseases.

4.2 Encapsulated or compacted DNA

Polyanionic solutes can be complexed to phospholipid polar head groups *via* Ca^{2+} bridges {Huster *et al.* 1999}. Thus, anionic DNA molecules can be compacted onto cationic MB lipid shells. Polylysine has also been used to link naked DNA to phospholipid MB shells {Wang *et al.* 2009}. It appears to be widely believed that enhanced efficiency of gene delivery can be obtained with pDNA in close proximity to MBs and any cell membrane 'defects' they may create, thereby increasing the probability that pDNA will be available to enter through these pores prior to their closure. Thus far, however, there has been inconsistent support for this idea. For example, pDNA coupled electrostatically with cationic MBs were used for local delivery of DNA to vascular muscle cells. One percent of cells were transduced with 40% of the cells remaining viable {Phillips *et al.* 2010}. However, reporter plasmid bound to the cationic MB preparation MRX-225 was used to transfect canine myocardium which was exposed to diagnostic US. Reporter gene activity was only observed in the myocardium of those animals that received MB-linked DNA and were exposed to US but not in control untreated animals {Vannan *et al.* 2002}. It is not clear if the pDNA-MB linkage influenced the experimental outcome.

Due to large size of DNA molecules and the concerns of enzymatic degradation of the injected pDNA as well as the low pDNA concentration in the vicinity of sonoporated cell membranes, polymer-coated MBs that can bind and protect the pDNA have been developed for UTMD-mediated gene delivery. Coating albumin-shelled MBs with poly(allylamine hydrochloride) (PAH) makes the surface charge of the MBs positive, but did not affect the size distribution of the MBs. The cationic coating allowed the MBs to bind to 100 fg of pDNA per MB and protected the bound DNA against nucleases. The PAH coating also significantly increased the lifetime of MBs (half-life ~7 h), making them more convenient for *in vivo* applications {Lentacker *et al.* 2006}.

Another approach to compacting DNA onto MBs is to first incubate the pDNA with a cationic lipid such as GL67 or a cationic polymer such as polyethylenimine (PEI), followed by mixing with MBs. PEI/DNA mixed with SonoVue MBs were injected intravenously in tumor-bearing mice. Following US exposure, reporter gene expression in tumor xenografts was significantly enhanced without causing any apparently adverse effect. Furthermore, with UTMD and PEI complex, vectors carrying a short hairpin RNA (shRNA) targeting human survivin were efficiently delivered into the tumor site, leading to inhibition of surviving gene expression and apoptosis of the tumor cells {Chen *et al.* 2010}.

DNA loading of MB shells can be impressive, but may also be limiting to high yield gene therapies using UTMD. By first forming pDNA-Lipofectamine 2000 complexes, mixing these with home-made phospholipid mixtures, agitating under a perflutren atmosphere to generate MBs, and then repeatedly washing the bubbles to remove unassociated DNA, a per bubble loading of 50 x 10^{-15} gram/MB was achieved {Chen *et al.* 2006}. Similar binding rates (approximately 100 fg/MB) were reported by others {Carson *et al.* 2011}. Using a layer-by-layer approach, DNA loading of pre-existing cationic MBs was increased 10-fold by first bringing anionic DNA to the surface of the cationic bubble, followed by binding a coating of poly-cationic polylysine to the DNA, followed by more DNA, *etc.* Loading as high as ~2500 fg DNA/MB was achieved, without apparent impact on the bubbles' dynamical response to acoustic excitation {Borden *et al.* 2007}. However, others have found that *in vitro* transfection rates are not enhanced by conjugation of reporter pDNA to MB shells {Tlaxca *et al.* 2010}, as found in the *in vivo* canine myocardium example discussed earlier in this section.

4.3 Viral vectors

There have been many reports that US treatment alone, or in combination with MBs, can increase transgene uptake by cells {Miller *et al.* 2002; Newman & Bettinger 2007}. Even with the difficulty of translating UTMD-mediated results obtained under tissue culture conditions (*e.g.*, infinite media for suspended cells *vs.* nearby noncompliant boundaries for monolayers) to the fully 3-D, viscoelastic intravascular environment *in vivo*, *in vitro* experiments often have the advantage of being better controlled and the results therefore more easily understood. This is not always the case, however. Zheng and colleagues exposed two different endothelial pigment cell lines to adenoviral gene vectors in combination with US or US and MBs (1 - 3 W/cm^2; P_r appears to have been ~0.17 - 0.30 MPa at 1 MHz; SonoVue MBs were used when bubbles were employed). They found that treatment with US and MBs increased adenoviral gene transfer in human retinal pigment epithelium cells, but was without effect on rat retinal pigment epithelial cells under otherwise identical conditions {Zheng *et al.* 2009}. The differences were speculated to arise in consequence to differing ability of the two cell lines to phagocytize the SonoVue MBs, to which the adenoviral vectors were believed to be attached.

It is difficult to limit the specificity of delivery of viral vectors, which are usually delivered systemically. By using retrovirus-loaded MBs, UTMD facilitated the delivery of viral vectors in a restricted area of cells exposed to P_r of 0.4 MPa or greater, despite uniform dispersion of the vector {Taylor *et al.* 2007}. An envelope-deficient retroviral vector was combined with cationic MBs and added to target cells. Transduction efficiencies and sites can thus be controlled by means of US exposure. These results emphasize that UTMD can not only facilitate the delivery of nonviral vectors, but also has the potential to enhance efficiencies and restrict targeted sites of viral gene transfer.

4.4 Small RNAs and oligonucleotides

Small RNAs and oligonucleotides (ODN) have recently been developed as promising therapeutics to treat diseases like viral infections, cancer, and several genetic disorders. Among these, small inhibitory RNA (RNAi or siRNA) based therapeutics have been investigated for treating a number of different diseases, including viral infections (*e.g.*, hepatitis, HIV, influenza), cancer, Huntington's disease, and others. Other therapeutic agents including microRNA (miRNA), transfer RNA (tRNA), and antisense ODN are also being developed to regulate gene or cell functions as treatment regimens. Since these agents are small, it is expected that they will be good candidates for augmented delivery by UTMD.

The US contrast agent pioneer Thomas Porter recognized early that UTMD delivery of oligonucleotides had the potential to influence vascular tissue remodeling after injury. In a 2001 study, an oligonucleotide which inhibits vascular smooth muscle cell proliferation was bound to albumin-shelled MBs and UTMD effected by transcutaneous application of 20 kHz US to porcine carotid artery walls following balloon catheter injury. Thirty days after treatment, the percent area stenosis in UTMD-treated animals was half that in controls {Porter *et al.* 2001}. The uptake of ODNs into intact *ex vivo* human saphenous veins and isolated smooth muscle cells from the veins was also potentiated by US {Kodama *et al.* 2005}. In addition, UTMD facilitated the delivery of antisense ODN targeting the human androgen receptor (AR) in prostate tumor cells, resulting in 49% transfected cells, associated with a decrease in AR expression compared to untreated controls {Haag *et al.* 2006}.

UTMD-mediated sonoporation (frequency: 1 MHz; intensity: 2 W/cm^2; exposure time: 2 min) was capable of enhancing *in vivo* siRNA delivery into salivary gland of rats, leading to significant GAPDH gene silencing by 10-50% for 48 hours {Sakai *et al.* 2009}. No gene silencing was observed with exposure to US only in the absence of Optison MBs. Intraventricular co-injection of siRNA-GFP and MB BR14 with concomitant ultrasonic exposure resulted in a substantial reduction in EGFP expression in the coronary artery in EGFP transgenic mice {Tsunoda *et al.* 2005}. Liposomal MBs combined with US can efficiently delivery siRNA with only 10s of US exposure *in vitro*. siRNA was also efficiently delivered into the tibialis muscles using the same system and the gene-silencing effect could be sustained for more than 3 weeks {Negishi *et al.* 2008}. These results demonstrate that UTMD-mediated delivery of siRNA can serve as a very useful tool for loss-of-function genetic engineering both *in vitro* and *in vivo*.

4.5 Transduced cell therapy

Cell therapy is a promising strategy for many applications, including genetic diseases, cancer, regenerative medicine, and others. However, it is very difficult to transfect certain cell types and maintain their viability following transfection, including hematopoietic and mesenchymal stem cells, T cells, and others which are important targets for cell therapy using the transfection methods currently available. UTMD has been demonstrated to facilitate the delivery of siRNA into mesenchymal stem cells (MSCs) {Otani *et al.* 2009}, which knocked down mRNA expression of specific genes, leading to the improvement of cellular function and viability. The application of UTMD has high potential to facilitate the delivery of genetic materials into target cells and can be expanded for use in a variety of cell therapy protocols.

5. Selected applications of ultrasound-mediated gene delivery

5.1 Cardiovascular

Recent reviews of cardiac applications of UTMD are provided elsewhere {Laing & McPherson 2009; Porter 2009}. Desired endpoints may be improved vascular function (*e.g.*, following ischemia) or inhibition of vascularization to 'starve' tumors. The following discussion is intended only to provide an indication of some of the exciting avenues of research in the area.

Cardiovascular graft remodeling: Tissue remodeling after transplantation surgery is required for long term transplant success. It has been shown that US-mediated gene therapy can improve transplanted vessel patency after surgery. Carotid interposition saphenous vein grafts in pigs were treated *ex vivo* prior to transplantation with 1 MHz US at ~1.8 MPa P_a with both a MB contrast agent and a plasmid encoding for metalloproteinase 3 (TIMP-3; the enzyme inhibits post-graft vessel restriction) present during US exposure. At 4 weeks, luminal diameters in animals receiving the transfected grafts were significantly greater than in controls {Akowuah *et al.* 2005}. Similarly, US treatment enhanced the delivery of an adenoviral vector to the aortic root, yielding a 2.5-fold enhancement in gene delivery {Beeri *et al.* 2002}. A technical issue of note is that a balloon catheter was used to briefly occlude the aortic root above the sinuses to increase the dwell time of the injected MBs and adenoviral vectors.

Reperfusion therapies: US-mediated gene therapy to improve myocardial reperfusion following induced myocardial infarcts in mice was studied using Definity MBs, and UTMD achieved using high frequency (8 MHz), relatively high P_a (estimated ~4.5 MPa) US from a diagnostic US machine. Plasmids were either empty (controls) or encoded for Stem Cell Factor (SCF; expected to enhance reperfusion by recruitment of cells during tissue remodeling) or VEGF (expected to stimulate angiogenesis). At 21 days, UTMD with either VEGF or SCF-bearing pDNA increased the microvessel density and blood flow relative to controls {Fujii *et al.* 2009}. Similarly, reperfusion of ischemic rat hind limbs was improved by US-mediated gene therapy. Cationic lipid-shelled MBs and a pDNA encoding for VEGF-165 were used; US frequency and amplitude were 1.3 MHz and ~2 MPa, respectively {Kobulnik *et al.* 2009}. A murine cardiac infarct model treated with UTMD with pDNA encoding for either VEGF or stem cell factor (SCF) has been reported to increase reperfusion; the observation that SCF-encoding pDNA increased perfusion was interpreted as evidence for the recruitment of reparative cells into the area of infarction {Fujii *et al.* 2009}.

Expression of a reporter plasmid gene delivered to the myocardium by UTMD methods was relatively brief (4 d), but was improved by retreatment {Bekeredjian *et al.* 2003}. Under similar exposure conditions, damage to the heart was negligible {Bekeredjian *et al.* 2004}. However, UTMD-enhanced gene delivery to the heart is often attended by at least minimal damage, which can include extravasation of large molecules and red cells {Hernot *et al.* 2010}. It is noteworthy that under diagnostic US exposure conditions, premature ventricular contractions can occur with the use of US contrast agents (see, *e.g.* {Miller *et al.* 2005}), and in contrast with the results of {Hernot *et al.* 2010} these have been unambiguously correlated with cell killing of cardiomycetes. In rats, using 1.7 MHz ultrasound, premature complexes and cardiomycete death were observable at P_as of 2 MPa or greater {Miller *et al.* 2011}. Premature contraction complexes appear to be related directly to extravascular cell killing, so even absent gross side effects, some side effects can be expected in gene therapies involving UTMD. This has important implications not only for safety, but also efficacy; *i.e.*, one hopes to transfect the target cells, not kill them. It seems unlikely that transfection to meaningful extents can be achieved without some cell killing, so attempts to optimize UTMD treatments must strive to achieve an acceptable balance between desired effect (transfection) and undesired effect (killing of the target cells).

When treating the heart using reporter genes, MBs and a diagnostic scanner as the acoustic source, superior results were obtained by moving the scan head about to 'paint' a larger volume of tissue {Geis *et al.* 2009}. Another noteworthy finding was that moving the beam relative to the heart did not increase Evans blue dye extravasation, which suggests less microcirculation damage per unit transgene expression when the insonifying beam is moved relative to the target.

Inhibition of neovascularization: A substantial literature on therapies to inhibit neoangiogenesis exists. Here we mention one recent example: MBs and pDNA encoding for pigment epithelium derived factor, which inhibits neovascularization in the retina, were injected into the vitreous humor of rats having laser-induced choroidal injury, which leads to neovascularization. The eyes were treated immediately with 0.3 MHz US of P_a estimated to be in the range of 0.1 - 0.3 MPa. At 28 days post treatment, choroidal neovascularization was inhibited in the UTMD group relative to untreated controls {Zhou XY *et al.* 2009}. Similarly, pDNA carrying a silencing sequence for the gene coding for survivin were introduced into implanted murine tumors using UTMD methods. Treated tumors were sonicated with 3 MHz US at an intensity of 2 W/cm^2 (estimated P_r: 0.2 - 0.5 MPa). Transgene expression was significantly increased in tumors treated with UTMB. It was proposed that the technique could be applied therapeutically to tumors to increase in tumor cell apoptosis *via* the silencing effect on survivin expression in transfected cells {Chen *et al.* 2010}.

5.2 Skeletal muscle

Among the applications for gene therapy in skeletal muscle is the treatment of muscular dystrophy (see, e.g., {Alter *et al.* 2009} and references therein). As a specific recent example, Kodama and colleagues used various means to attempt delivery of PGL3 luciferase pDNA into murine skeletal muscle. Optison, human albumin MBs or acoustic liposomes (all formulated with C_3F_8 gas) were compared, using a 1 MHz US source; P_a was 0.2 MPa. Treatment with plasmid, US and either Optison or liposomes increased luciferase expression relative to controls. The ~200 nm diameter acoustic liposomes produced the highest expression rates, presumably because of their very high concentration {Kodama *et al.* 2010}.

5.3 Pancreas

Pancreatic gene therapies have focused principally on treatments for diabetes types I and II. The feasibility of using pDNA and UTMD methods to deliver transgenes to the pancreas has been described by Grayburn and colleagues. Following injection of reporter gene pDNA attached to the MB phospholipid shells, the reporter gene was expressed with fairly high spatial specificity, declining after 4 days, but with measurable expression persisting for as long as 21 days ({Chen *et al.* 2006}; see internal citations for a discussion of viral approaches). US of ~3 MHz was used, with an apparent P_a of ~1 MPa at the pancreas. When plasmid vectors carrying human insulin and hexokinase I gene were delivered using UTMD, transgene expression was obtained in islets and decreased circulating glucose levels were observed in treated rats. These data indicate that UTMD allows relatively noninvasive delivery of genes to pancreatic islets to modulate beta cell function. More recently, the same group reported that delivery of NeuroD1 gene driven by a rat insulin promoter (RAP3.1) into rats by UTMD-mediated gene delivery targeting pancreas *in vivo* promoted islet regeneration from surviving beta-cells, with normalization of glucose, insulin and C-peptide levels at 30 days {Chen *et al.* 2010}.

5.4 Liver

Liver is a major organ for protein synthesis, and therefore represents an important target for gene therapy. We will discuss here UTMD-mediated gene therapy targeting liver for treating non-tumoral diseases.

Our group has extensively studied gene delivery of reporter and therapeutic genes into the liver. We have demonstrated that UTMD (1 MHz US) can significantly enhance gene transfer of naked pDNA into the mouse liver in the presence of either Optison {Miao 2005} or Definity MBs {Shen *et al.* 2008}. Transgene expression was dependent exponentially on P_r, with an inflection point usually between 1 and 2.5 MPa followed by a plateau above 3 MPa {Song *et al.* 2011a}, consistent with an inertial cavitation mechanism. More than thousand-fold enhancement of gene transfer efficiencies was obtained compared to control experiments in the absence of UTMD. Recently we have gained preliminary success in scaling up pDNA delivery in larger animal models, including rats {Song *et al.* 2011b } and dogs {Noble *et al.* 2011}. Previously we have shown that near therapeutic levels of factor IX were achieved by UTMD-mediated gene delivery in mice. Technical improvements to further enhance gene transfer of factor VIII for treatment of hemophilia A and factor IX for treatment of hemophilia B are currently being pursued in small and large animal models.

5.5 Kidney

A number of kidney diseases could be potentially treated with gene therapies. Hydrodynamic approaches have met with some success. Xing *et al.* attempted to improve on these results by combining hydrodynamic and UTMD approaches to naked DNA reporter gene delivery to surgically-exposed rat kidneys. Combined US (unspecified frequency) from a Sonotron 2000 hand-held diagnostic US machine and hydrodynamic therapy together yielded better reporter gene transfection than hydrodynamic therapy alone, producing an approximately 4-fold increase in reported gene expression when the estimated P_a was in the range of 0.3 - 0.8 MPa and no MBs were used. The effect was intensity-dependent. When Optison MBs were injected with the naked DNA during hydrodynamic therapy and US exposure, the same effect (4-fold increase in gene expression) was observed at an intensity of only 1 Watt/cm^2 (estimated 0.2 - 0.5 MPa P_a) {Xing *et al.* 2009}.

5.6 Skin (DNA vaccine)

The failure of wounds to heal in diabetic patients is a significant clinical problem. Gene therapies which promote angiogenesis represent a promising approach to this problem. VEGF-encoding gene vectors (either minicircle naked DNA; a supercoiled form with a molecular weight estimated as 331 g/mol, or naked DNA borne on the gene carrier branched polyethylinimine) were tested for efficacy in inducing circulating VEGF expression and accelerating wound healing in an induced diabetic mouse model. Wounds were treated by peripheral injection of gene vectors with or without exposure to US (1 MHz, 2 W/cm^2, 20% duty cycle; estimated 0.25 - 0.5 MPa). In some treatments, SonoVue MBs were injected with the microcircle DNA prior to sonication. Markedly greater levels of circulating VEGF were observed in mice treated with [VEGF-encoding minicircle DNA + US + MBs] relative to controls, but not as high as those obtained using the polyethylinimine gene carrier. Nonetheless, the [minicircle DNA + US + MBs] treatment produced a significant improvement in healing rates of the treated skin wounds {Yoon *et al.* 2009}.

5.7 Other solid organs

Brain: Much work has been done on 'opening' (*i.e.*, making more permeable) the blood-brain barrier, which so tightly regulates traffic between the vascular space and the brain that chemotherapeutic agents often cannot cross the barrier {Meairs & Alonso 2007}. Much success with tracer molecules (*e.g.*, Evans blue dye, gadolinium MRI contrast agents, *etc.*) has been achieved using UTMD methods, principally in small animal models. However, low energy US applied through the temporal bone of swine produced short-term permeabilization of the blood-brain barrier with exogenous MBs (see {Xie *et al.* 2008} and citations within). However, we have found no reports of UTMD gene therapies attempted in the brain.

5.8 Endothelium

There are many papers which indicate that endothelial cells *in vitro* can express transgenes delivered by UTMD methods (see {Su *et al.* 2010} and internal references for recent examples). Su and colleagues found that treatment with 1 MHz US of 1 MPa P_r together with pGL3 pDNA and MBs yielded a 100-fold increase in luciferase expression relative to pDNA treatment alone. It remains to be determined if endothelial cells *in vivo* can be 'recruited' as effective synthesizers and secretors of therapeutic gene expression products.

5.9 Cell therapies: *Ex vivo* gene therapy

In this section, we discuss several examples of US-mediated gene delivery using cell cultures *in vitro*; these may have some mechanistic relevance to the *in vivo* condition. However, some of the results obtained using *in vitro* cells may have direct bearing on cell therapies.
Shock waves and MBs have been used *in vitro* to increase pDNA uptake in cultured HEK cells; the technique worked, but was associated with substantial cell killing {Bekeredjian *et al.* 2007} as might be expected (see, *e.g.*, {Brayman *et al.* 1999; Hwang *et al.* 2006; Hwang *et al.* 2003}). As a general rule, only a small fraction (~5 - 10%) of cells insonated with MBs *in vitro* undergo transient poration; these yields are often associated with cell killing rates of ~50% (see, *e.g.* {AIUM 2000; AIUM 2008} and references therein). If those cells can be sorted (*e.g.*, by flow cytometry) and cultured to increase cell numbers, this may be acceptable for cell therapies - if the gene vector is integrated into the host genome. An obvious problem for cell therapies based on this approach with naked DNA, however, is that the pDNA does not replicate with the host cell, and so there would be little to be gained by increasing cell numbers of the transfected subpopulation of cells. However, using suspended KHT-C cells, and 3 V% Definity, high levels of *in vitro* permeabilization to 70 kDa fluorescein isothiocyanate (FITC) - dextran were achieved using 0.5 MHz US at a P_a of 0.57 MPa, 16 cycle pulses repeated at 3 kHz PRF. About 30% of the cells were permeabilized, with >95% retention of viability {Karshafian *et al.* 2009}. If similar results can be obtained with naked DNA, the prospects for cell therapies using cells transfected using *in vitro* UTMD seem much brighter.

5.10 Gene therapies for tumoricidal activity

Strategies currently under investigation for treatment of cancers include anti-angiogenic therapies, the introduction of 'suicide genes' which either induce apoptosis or sensitize cells to subsequent treatment with drugs {Aoi *et al.* 2008; Azuma *et al.* 2008; Daigeler *et al.* 2010; Kirn *et al.* 2002; Zhou *et al.* 2010}, or down-regulate oncogenes {Wang *et al.* 2009}. Naked DNA bearing the Herpes-derived 'suicide gene' for thymidine kinase has been delivered to murine squamous cell carcinomas by UTMD methods (1.3 MHz, estimated P_r ~1.8 MPa). The DNA was bound to lipid shelled MBs at a rate of about 100 fg DNA/MB. With daily ganciclovir treatments beginning 3 d after UTMD and pDNA treatment, tumor doubling times were significantly reduced (by ~17%) in the UTMD-treated tumors {Carson *et al.* 2011}.

In tumors as in other systems, extravasation of gene vectors seems to be a constraint for delivery of antitumoral therapeutics which are delivered intravascularly. Here, too, UTMD appears to aid in increasing vascular permeability. For example, in implanted subcutaneous hepatomas, extravasation of Evans blue dye was 5-fold higher in the UTMD and plasmid-treated tumors than in untreated control tumors; there was no increase in Evans blue extravasation when US was applied without MBs. In this case, however, there was no significant transfection by the pDNA {Bekeredjian *et al.* 2007}. UTMD techniques have been used successfully to introduce the gene for tumor suppression protein p53 into murine retinoblastoma xenografts; when insonated in the presence of MBs or liposomes, significant expression of p53 resulted; there was no expression in the plasmid-only or plasmid + US groups {Luo *et al.* 2010}.

6. Concluding remarks

Much exciting work on ultrasound-mediated gene delivery has already been done, but the field remains young and even preclinical applications involving therapeutic genes are relatively few. A few generalities may be put forth: In most (but not all) cases, ultrasound-mediated gene delivery is dependent on, or greatly facilitated by, exogenous microbubbles. Where this is the case, the acoustic exposures are usually such that the bubbles can be expected to behave in a nonlinear way. Given the intense effort being devoted to the topic, we can anticipate with some confidence that successful gene therapies in large animals and early human trials will be achieved in the near future.

7. Acknowledgements

The authors acknowledge gratefully the support of NIH grants 5R01HL069049 (C.H.M., A.A.B), 5R21/R33HL089038 (C.H.M., A.A.B); 5R01HL082600 (C.H.M.); 1R01CA917794 (A.A.B.), and 1RO1CA109557 (A.A.B.), 5RO1EB000350 (A.A.B.) and Bayer Hemophilia Award (C.H.M.). We thank Drs. Thomas J. Matula, Wayne Kreider, Michael R. Bailey, Peter J. Kaczkowski, Mark Borden, Misty Noble, Sophia Song and Ms. Hong Chen for helpful discussions during preparation of this manuscript.

8. References

AIUM. (2000) Mechanical Bioeffects from Diagnostic Ultrasound: AIUM Consensus Statements. Section 6 - Mechanical bioeffects in the presence of gas-carrier ultrasound contrast agents. *J Ultrasound Med* 19: 120 - 142.

AIUM. (2008) American Institute of Ultrasound in Medicine Consensus Report on Potential Bioeffects of Diagnostic Ultrasound: Executive Summary. *J Ultrasound Med* 27: 503-515.

Akowuah EF, Gray C, Lawrie A, Sheridan PJ, Su CH, Bettinger T, Brisken AF, Gunn J, Crossman DC, Francis SE, Baker AH, Newman CM. (2005) Ultrasound-mediated delivery of TIMP-3 plasmid DNA into saphenous vein leads to increased lumen size in a porcine interposition graft model. *Gene Ther* 12: 1154-1157.

Alter J, Sennoga CA, Lopes DM, Eckersley RJ, Wells DJ. (2009) Microbubble stability is a major determinant of the efficiency of ultrasound and microbubble mediated in vivo gene transfer. *Ultrasound Med Biol* 35: 976-984.

Aoi A, Watanabe Y, Mori S, Takahashi M, Vassaux G, Kodama T. (2008) Herpes simplex virus thymidine kinase-mediated suicide gene therapy using nano/microbubbles and ultrasound. *Ultrasound Med Biol* 34: 425-434.

Apfel RE, Holland CK. (1991) Gauging the likelihood of cavitation from short-pulse, low duty cycle diagnostic ultrasound. *Ultrasound Med Biol* 17: 179 - 185.

Aronovich EL, McIvor RS, Hackett PB. (2011) The Sleeping Beauty transposon system - a non-viral vector for gene therapy. *Human Molec Genetics* Epub ahead of print.

Azuma H, Tomita N, Sakamoto T, Kiyama S, Inamoto T, Takahara K, Kotake Y, Segawa N, Morishita R, Takahara S, Hayasaki H, Otsuki Y, Horie S, Tanigawa N, Katsuoka Y. (2008) Marked regression of liver metastasis by combined therapy of ultrasound-mediated NF kappaB-decoy transfer and transportal injection of paclitaxel, in mouse. *Int J Cancer* 122: 1645-1656.

Beeri R, Guerrero JL, Supple G, Sullivan S, Levine RA, Hajjar RJ. (2002) New efficient catheter-based system for myocardial gene delivery. *Circulation* 106: 1756-1759.

Bekeredjian R, Bohris C, Hansen A, Katus HA, Kuecherer HF, Hardt SE. (2007) Impact of microbubbles on shock wave-mediated DNA uptake in cells in vitro. *Ultrasound Med Biol* 33: 743-750.

Bekeredjian R, Chen S, Frenkel PA, Grayburn PA, Shohet RV. (2003) Ultrasound-targeted microbubble destruction can repeatedly direct highly specific plasmid expression to the heart. *Circulation* 108: 1022-1026.

Bekeredjian R, Chen S, Pan W, Grayburn PA, Shohet RV. (2004) Effects of ultrasound-targeted microbubble destruction on cardiac gene expression. *Ultrasound Med Biol* 30: 539-543.

Bekeredjian R, Kroll RD, Fein E, Tinkov S, Coester C, Winter G, Katus HA, Kulaksiz H. (2007) Ultrasound targeted microbubble destruction increases capillary permeability in hepatomas. *Ultrasound Med Biol* 33: 1592-1598.

Blake JR, Gibson DC. (1987) Cavitation bubbles near boundaries. *Ann Rev Fluid Mechanics* 19: 99 - 123.

Borden MA, Caskey CF, Little E, Gillies RJ, Ferrara KW. (2007) DNA and polylysine adsorption and multilayer construction onto cationic lipid-coated microbubbles. *Langmuir* 23: 9401-9408.

Borden MA, Kruse DE, Caskey CF, Zhao S, Dayton PA, Ferrara KW. (2005) Influence of lipid shell physicochemical properties on ultrasound-induced microbubble destruction. *IEEE Trans UFFC* 52: 992-2002.

Brayman AA, Coppage ML, Vaidya S, Miller MW. (1999) Transient poration and cell surface receptor removal from human lymphocytes in vitro by 1 MHz ultrasound. *Ultrasound Med Biol* 25: 999-1008.

Carson AR, McTiernan CF, Lavery L, Hodnick A, Grata M, Leng X, Wang J, Chen X, Modzelewski RA, Villanueva FS. (2011) Gene therapy of carcinoma using ultrasound-targeted microbubble destruction. *Ultrasound Med Biol* 37: 393-402.

Carstensen EL, Gracewski S, Dalecki D. (2000) The search for cavitation in vivo. *Ultrasound Med Biol* 26: 1377-1385.

Caskey CF, Stieger SM, Qin S, Dayton PA, Ferrara KW. (2007) Direct observations of ultrasound microbubble contrast agent interaction with the microvessel wall. *J Acoust Soc America* 122: 1191-1200.

Chahine GL. (1977) Interaction between an oscillating bubble and a free-surface. *J Fluid Eng-T ASME* 99: 709-716.

Chen H, Brayman AA, Bailey MR, Matula TJ. (2010) Blood vessel rupture by cavitation. *Urological Res* 38: 321-326.

Chen H, Kreider W, Brayman AA, Bailey MR, Matula TJ. (2011) Blood vessel deformations on microsecond time scales by ultrasonic cavitation. *Phys Review Lett* 106: 034301-034304.

Chen S, Ding JH, Bekeredjian R, Yang BZ, Shohet RV, Johnston SA, Hohmeier HE, Newgard CB, Grayburn PA. (2006) Efficient gene delivery to pancreatic islets with ultrasonic microbubble destruction technology. *Proc Nat Acad Sci USA* 103: 8469-8474.

Chen S, Shimoda M, Wang MY, Ding J, Noguchi H, Matsumoto S, Grayburn PA. (2010) Regeneration of pancreatic islets in vivo by ultrasound-targeted gene therapy. *Gene Ther* 17: 1411-1420.

Chen W-S, Matula TJ, Brayman AA, Crum LA. (2003) A comparison of the fragmentation thresholds and inertial cavitation doses of different ultrasound contrast agents. *J Acoust Soc America* 113: 643 - 651.

Chen WS, Brayman AA, Matula TJ, Crum LA. (2003a) Inertial cavitation dose and hemolysis produced in vitro with or without Optison. *Ultrasound Med Biol* 29: 725-737.

Chen WS, Brayman AA, Matula TJ, Crum LA, Miller MW. (2003b) The pulse length-dependence of inertial cavitation dose and hemolysis. *Ultrasound Med Biol* 29: 739-748.

Chen ZY, Liang K, Qiu RX. (2010) Targeted gene delivery in tumor xenografts by the combination of ultrasound-targeted microbubble destruction and polyethylenimine to inhibit survivin gene expression and induce apoptosis. *J Exp Clin Cancer Res* 29: 152.

Chomas JE, Dayton P, Allen J, Morgan K, Ferrara KW. (2001) Mechanisms of contrast agent destruction. *IEEE Trans UFFC* 48: 232-248.

Chomas JE, Dayton P, Ferarra K. (2001) Threshold of fragmentation for ultrasonic contrast agents. *J Biomedical Optics* 6: 141 - 159.

Church CC, Carstensen EL. (2001) "Stable" inertial cavitation. *Ultrasound Med Biol* 27: 1435 - 1437.

Cosgrove D, Harvey C. (2009) Clinical uses of microbubbles in diagnosis and treatment. *Medical and Biological Engineering and Computing* 47: 813-826.

Daigeler A, Chromik AM, Haendschke K, Emmelmann S, Siepmann M, Hensel K, Schmitz G, Klein-Hitpass L, Steinau HU, Lehnhardt M, Hauser J. (2010) Synergistic effects of sonoporation and taurolidin/TRAIL on apoptosis in human fibrosarcoma. *Ultrasound Med Biol* 36: 1893-1906.

Danko I, Williams P, Herweijer H, Zhang G, Latendresse JS, Bock I, Wolff JA. (1997) High expression of naked plasmid DNA in muscles of young rodents. *Human Molec Genetics* 6: 1435-1443.

de Jong N, Emmer M, van Wamel A, Versluis M. (2009) Ultrasonic characterization of ultrasound contrast agents. *Medical and Biological Engineering and Computing* 47: 861-873.

Deng CX, Sieling F, Pan H, Cui J. (2004) Ultrasound-induced cell membrane porosity. *Ultrasound Med Biol* 30: 519-526.

Doinikov AA, Bouakaz A. (2010) Theoretical investigation of shear stress generated by a contrast microbubble on the cell membrane as a mechanism for sonoporation. *J Acoust Soc America* 128: 11-19.

Duvshani-Eshet M, Baruch L, Kesselman E, Shimoni E, Machluf M. (2006) Therapeutic ultrasound-mediated DNA to cell and nucleus: bioeffects revealed by confocal and atomic force microscopy. *Gene Ther* 13: 163-172.

Duvshani-Eshet M, Machluf M. (2005) Therapeutic ultrasound optimization for gene delivery: a key factor achieving nuclear DNA localization. *J Controlled Release* 108: 513-528.

Emmer M, van Wamel A, Goertz DE, de Jong N. (2007) The onset of microbubble vibration. *Ultrasound Med Biol* 33: 941-949.

Fabre JW, Grehan A, Whitehorne M, Sawyer GJ, Dong X, Salehi S, Eckley L, Zhang X, Seddon M, Shah AM, Davenport M, Rela M. (2008) Hydrodynamic gene delivery to the pig liver via an isolated segment of the inferior vena cava. *Gene Ther* 15: 452-462.

Fechheimer M, Boylan JF, Parker S, Sisken JE, Patel GL, Zimmer SG. (1987) Transfection of mammalian cells with plasmid DNA by scrape loading and sonication loading. *Proc Nat Acad Sci USA* 84: 8463-8467.

Ferrara KW. (2008) Driving delivery vehicles with ultrasound. *Adv Drug Deliv Rev* 60: 1097-1102.

Ferrara KW, Borden MA, Zhang H. (2009) Lipid-shelled vehicles: engineering for ultrasound molecular imaging and drug delivery. *Accounts Chem Res* 42: 881-892.

Fischer K, Gedroyc W, Jolesz FA. (2010) Focused ultrasound as a local therapy for liver cancer. *Cancer J* 16: 118-124.

Forbes MM, Steinberg RL, O'Brien WD, Jr. (2008) Examination of inertial cavitation of Optison in producing sonoporation of Chinese hamster ovary cells. *Ultrasound Med Biol* 34: 2009-2018.

Fujii H, Sun Z, Li SH, Wu J, Fazel S, Weisel RD, Rakowski H, Lindner J, Li RK. (2009) Ultrasound-targeted gene delivery induces angiogenesis after a myocardial infarction in mice. *JACC Cardiovascular Imaging* 2: 869-879.

Geis NA, Mayer CR, Kroll RD, Hardt SE, Katus HA, Bekeredjian R. (2009) Spatial distribution of ultrasound targeted microbubble destruction increases cardiac transgene expression but not capillary permeability. *Ultrasound Med Biol* 35: 1119-1126.

Gross DR, Miller DL, Williams AR. (1985) A search for ultrasonic cavitation within the canine cardiovascular system. *Ultrasound Med Biol* 11: 85-97.

Haag P, Frauscher F, Gradl J, Seitz A, Schafer G, Lindner JR, Klibanov AL, Bartsch G, Klocker H, Eder IE. (2006) Microbubble-enhanced ultrasound to deliver an antisense oligodeoxynucleotide targeting the human androgen receptor into prostate tumours. *J Steroid Biochem and Molec Biol* 102: 103-113.

Hacein-Bey-Abina S, Le Deist F, Carlier F, Bouneaud C, Hue C, De Villartay JP, Thrasher AJ, Wulffraat N, Sorensen R, Dupuis-Girod S, Fischer A, Davies EG, Kuis W, Leiva L, Cavazzana-Calvo M. (2002) Sustained correction of X-linked severe combined immunodeficiency by ex vivo gene therapy. *New England J Med* 346: 1185-1193.

Hacein-Bey-Abina S, von Kalle C, Schmidt M, Le Deist F, Wulffraat N, McIntyre E, Radford I, Villeval JL, Fraser CC, Cavazzana-Calvo M, Fischer A. (2003) A serious adverse event after successful gene therapy for X-linked severe combined immunodeficiency. *New England J Med* 2003; 348: 255-256.

Hall TL, Hempel CR, Wojno K, Xu Z, Cain CA, Roberts WW. (2009) Histotripsy of the prostate: dose effects in a chronic canine model. *Urology* 74: 932-937.

Han YW, Ikegami A, Chung P, Zhang L, Deng CX. (2007) Sonoporation is an efficient tool for intracellular fluorescent dextran delivery and one-step double-crossover mutant construction in Fusobacterium nucleatum. *Appl Environ Microbiol* 73: 3677-3683.

Hernot S, Cosyns B, Droogmans S, Garbar C, Couck P, Vanhove C, Caveliers V, van Camp G, Bossuyt A, LaHoutte T. (2010) Effect of high-intensity ultrasound-targeted microbubble destruction of perfusion and function of the rat heart assessed by pinhole-gated SPECT. *Ultrasound Med Biol* 36: 158 - 165.

Horie S, Watanabe Y, Chen R, Mori S, Matsumura Y, Kodama T. (2010) Development of localized gene delivery using dual intensity ultrasound in the bladder. *Ultrasound Med Biol* 36: 1867 - 1875.

Huang SL. (2008) Liposomes in ultrasonic drug and gene delivery. *Adv Drug Deliv Rev* 60: 1167-1176.

Huster D, Paasche G, Dietrich U, Zschornig O, Gutberlet T, Gawrisch K, Arnold K. (1999) Investigation of phospholipid area compression induced by calcium-mediated dextran sulfate interaction. *Biophys J* 77: 879-887.

Hwang JH, Brayman AA, Reidy MA, Matula TJ, Kimmey MB, Crum LA. (2005) Vascular effects induced by combined 1-MHz ultrasound and microbubble contrast agent treatments in vivo. *Ultrasound Med Biol* 31: 553-564.

Hwang JH, Tu J, Brayman AA, Matula TJ, Crum LA. (2006) Correlation between inertial cavitation dose and endothelial cell damage in vivo. *Ultrasound Med Biol* 32: 1611-1619.

Hwang JH, Vaezy S, Martin RW, Cho MY, Noble ML, Crum LA, Kimmey MB. (2003) High-intensity focused US: a potential new treatment for GI bleeding. *Gastrointest Endosc* 58: 111-115.

Juffermans LJ, Kamp O, Dijkmans PA, Visser CA, Musters RJ. (2008) Low-intensity ultrasound-exposed microbubbles provoke local hyperpolarization of the cell membrane via activation of BK(Ca) channels. *Ultrasound Med Biol* 34: 502-508.

Juffermans LJ, van Dijk A, Jongenelen CAM, Drukarch B, Reijerkerk AR, de Vries HE, Kamp O, Musters RJ. (2009) Ultrasound and microbubble-induced intra- and intercellular bioeffects in primary endothelial cells. *Ultrasound Med Biol* 35: 1917 - 1927.

Kamimura K, Suda T, Xu W, Zhang G, Liu D. (2009) Image-guided, lobe-specific hydrodynamic gene delivery to swine liver. *Molecular Ther* 17: 491-499.

Karshafian R, Bevan PD, Williams R, Samac S, Burns PN. (2009) Sonoporation by ultrasound-activated microbubble contrast agents: Effect of acoustic exposure parameters on cell membrane permeability and cell viability. *Ultrasound Med Biol* 35: 847 - 860.

Kay MA, Manno CS, Ragni MV, Larson PJ, Couto LB, McClelland A, Glader B, Chew AJ, Tai SJ, Herzog RW, Arruda V, Johnson F, Scallan C, Skarsgard E, Flake AW, High KA. (2000) Evidence for gene transfer and expression of factor IX in haemophilia B patients treated with an AAV vector. *Nature Genetics* 224: 257-261.

Kaya M, Gregory V TS, Dayton PA. (2009) Changes in lipid-encapsulated microbubble population during continuous infusion and methods to maintain consistency. *Ultrasound Med Biol* 35: 1748 - 1755.

Keravala A, Chavez CL, Hu G, Woodard LE, Monahan PE, Calos MP. (2011) Long-term phenotypic correction in factor IX knockout mice by using phiC31 integrase-mediated gene therapy. *Gene Ther* Epub ahead of print.

Kirn D, Niculescu-Duvaz I, Hallden G, Springer CJ. (2002) The emerging fields of suicide gene therapy and virotherapy. *Trends Molec Sci* 8: S68-73.

Kobulnik J, Kuliszewski MA, Stewart DJ, Lindner JR, Leong-Poi H. (2009) Comparison of gene delivery techniques for therapeutic angiogenesis: ultrasound-mediated destruction of carrier microbubbles versus direct intramuscular injection. *J Am Coll Cardiol* 54: 1735-1742.

Kodama T, Aoi A, Watanabe Y, Horie S, Kodama M, Li L, Chen R, Teramoto N, Morikawa H, Mori S, Fukumoto M. (2010) Evaluation of transfection efficiency in skeletal muscle using nano/microbubbles and ultrasound. *Ultrasound Med Biol* 36: 1196 - 1205.

Kodama T, Tan PH, Offiah I, Partridge T, Cook T, George AJ, Blomley MJ. (2005) Delivery of oligodeoxynucleotides into human saphenous veins and the adjunct effect of ultrasound and microbubbles. *Ultrasound Med Biol* 31: 1683-1691.

Kodama T, Tomita Y. (2000) Cavitation bubble behavior and bubble-shock wave interaction near a gelatin surface as a study of in vivo bubble dynamics. *Appl Phys B-Lasers* 70: 139-149.

Krupka TM, Solorio L, Wilson RE, Wu H, Azar N, Exner AA. (2009) Formulation and characterization of echogenic lipid-Pluronic nanobubbles. *Mol Pharm* 7: 49-59.

Lai CY, Wu CH, Chen CC, Li PC. (2006) Quantitative relations of acoustic inertial cavitation with sonoporation and cell viability. *Ultrasound Med Biol* 32: 1931-1941.

Laing ST, McPherson DD. (2009) Cardiovascular therapeutic uses of targeted ultrasound contrast agents. *Cardiovascular Res* 83: 626 - 634.

Lentacker I, De Geest BG, Vandenbroucke RE, Peeters L, Demeester J, De Smedt SC, Sanders NN. (2006) Ultrasound-responsive polymer-coated microbubbles that bind and protect DNA. *Langmuir* 22: 7273-7278.

Lentacker I, Wang N, Vandenbroucke RE, Demeester J, De Smedt SC, Sanders NN. (2009) Ultrasound exposure of lipoplex loaded microbubbles facilitates direct cytoplasmic entry of the lipoplexes. *Mol Pharmaceutics* 6: 457 - 467.

Li P, Armstrong WF, Miller DL. (2004) Impact of myocardial contrast echocardiography on vascular permeability: comparison of three different contrast agents. *Ultrasound Med Biol* 30: 83-91.

Liang HD, Lu QL, Xue SA, Halliwell M, Kodama T, Cosgrove DO, Stauss HJ, Partridge TA, Blomley MJ. (2004) Optimisation of ultrasound-mediated gene transfer (sonoporation) in skeletal muscle cells. *Ultrasound Med Biol* 30: 1523-1529.

Lindner JR. (2009) Contrast ultrasound molecular imaging: harnessing the power of bubbles. *Cardiovascular Res* 83: 615-616.

Liu F, Song Y, Liu D. (1999) Hydrodynamics-based transfection in animals by systemic administration of plasmid DNA. *Gene Ther* 6: 1258-1266.

Luo J, Zhou X, Diao L, Wang Z. (2010) Experimental research on wild-type p53 plasmid transfected into retinoblastoma cells and tissues using an ultrasound microbubble intensifier. *J Int Med Res* 38: 1005-1015.

Manno CS, Pierce GF, Arruda VR, Glader B, Ragni M, Rasko JJ, Ozelo MC, Hoots K, Blatt P, Konkle B, Dake M, Kaye R, Razavi M, Zajko A, Zehnder J, Rustagi PK, Nakai H, Chew A, Leonard D, Wright JF, Lessard RR, Sommer JM, Tigges M, Sabatino D, Luk A, Jiang H, Mingozzi F, Couto L, Ertl HC, High KA, Kay MA. (2006) Successful transduction of liver in hemophilia by AAV-Factor IX and limitations imposed by the host immune response. *Nature Med* 12: 342-347.

Marmottant P, de Jong N, Hilgenfeldt S, Lohse D. (2005) A model for large amplitude oscillations of coated bubbles accounting for buckling and rupture. *J Acoust Soc America* 118: 3499 - 3505.

Maruvada S, Hynynen K. (2004) Optical monitoring of ultrasound-induced bioeffects in glass catfish. *Ultrasound Med Biol* 30: 67-74.

Matula TJ. (2003) Bubble levitation and translation under single-bubble sonoluminescence conditions. *J Acoust Soc America* 114: 775-781.

Meairs S, Alonso A. (2007) Ultrasound, microbubbles and the blood-brain barrier. *Prog Biophys Mol Biol* 93: 354-362.

Mehier-Humbert S, Bettinger T, Yan F, Guy RH. (2005) Plasma membrane poration induced by ultrasound exposure: implication for drug delivery. *J Control Release* 104: 213-222.

Meijering BD, Juffermans LJ, van Wamel A, Henning RH, Zuhorn IS, Emmer M, Versteilen AM, Paulus WJ, van Gilst WH, Kooiman K, de Jong N, Musters RJ, Deelman LE, Kamp O. (2009) Ultrasound and microbubble-targeted delivery of macromolecules is regulated by induction of endocytosis and pore formation. *Circ Res* 104: 679-687.

Miao CH. (2005) A novel gene expression system: non-viral gene transfer for hemophilia as model systems. *Adv Genetics* 54: 143 - 177.

Miao CH, Brayman AA, Loeb KR, Ye P, Zhou L, Mourad P, Crum LA. (2005) Ultrasound enhances gene delivery of human factor IX plasmid. *Human Gene Ther* 16: 893-905.

Miao CH, Thompson AR, Loeb K, Ye X. (2001) Long-term and therapeutic-level hepatic gene expression of human factor IX after naked plasmid transfer in vivo. *Molecular Therapy* 3: 947-957.

Miao CH, Ye X, Thompson AR. (2003) High-level factor VIII gene expression in vivo achieved by nonviral liver-specific gene therapy vectors. *Human Gene Ther* 14: 1297-1305.

Miao H, Gracewski SM, Dalecki D. (2008) Ultrasonic excitation of a bubble inside a deformable tube: implications for ultrasonically induced hemorrhage. *J Acoust Soc America* 124: 2374-2384.

Miller D, Li P, Armstrong WF. (2004) The effect of time and of vasoactive drugs on capillary leakage induced during myocardial contrast echocardiography. *Echocardiography* 21: 125-132.

Miller DL, Dou C, Wiggins RC. (2009) Glomerular capillary hemorrhage induced in rats by diagnostic ultrasound with gas-body contrast agent produces intratubular obstruction. *Ultrasound Med Biol* 35: 869-877.

Miller DL, Dou C, Wiggins RC. (2010a) Contrast-enhanced diagnostic ultrasound causes renal tissue damage in a porcine model. *J Ultrasound Med* 29: 1391-1401.

Miller DL, Dou C, Wiggins RC. (2010b) In vivo gas body efficacy for glomerular capillary hemorrhage induced by diagnostic ultrasound in rats. *IEEE Trans Biomed Eng* 57: 167-174.

Miller DL, Dou C, Wiggins RC, Wharram BL, Goyal M, Williams AR. (2007) An in vivo rat model simulating imaging of human kidney by diagnostic ultrasound with gas-body contrast agent. *Ultrasound Med Biol* 33: 129-135.

Miller DL, Dou H, Lucchesi BR. (2011) Are ECG premature complexes induced by ultrasonic cavitation electrophysiological responses to irreversible cardiomycete injury? *Ultrasound Med Biol* 37: 312 - 320.

Miller DL, Driscoll EM, Dou C, Armstrong WF, Lucchesi BR. (2006) Microvascular permeabilization and cardiomyocyte injury provoked by myocardial contrast echocardiography in a canine model. *J Am Coll Cardiol* 47: 1464-1468.

Miller DL, Gies RA. (1998a) Gas-body-based contrast agent enhances vascular bioeffects of 1.09 MHz ultrasound on mouse intestine. *Ultrasound Med Biol* 24: 1201-1208.

Miller DL, Gies RA. (1998b) The interaction of ultrasonic heating and cavitation in vascular bioeffects on mouse intestine. *Ultrasound Med Biol* 24: 123-128.

Miller DL, Gies RA. (2000) The influence of ultrasound frequency and gas-body composition on the contrast agent-mediated enhancement of vascular bioeffects in mouse intestine. *Ultrasound Med Biol* 26: 307-313.

Miller DL, Li P, Dou C, Gordon D, Edwards CA, Armstrong WF. (2005) Influence of contrast agent dose and ultrasound exposure on cardiomyocyte injury induced by myocardial contrast echocardiography in rats. *Radiology* 237: 137-143.

Miller DL, Li P, Gordon D, Armstrong WF. (2005) Histological characterization of microlesions induced by myocardial contrast echocardiography. *Echocardiography* 22: 25-34.

Miller DL, Pislaru SV, Greenleaf JE. (2002) Sonoporation: mechanical DNA delivery by ultrasonic cavitation. *Somatic Cell Molec Genetics* 27: 115-134.

Miller MW. (2000) Gene transfection and drug delivery. *Ultrasound Med Biol* 26 Suppl 1: S59-62.

Mohan P, Rapoport N. (2010) Doxorubicin as a molecular nanotheranostic agent: effect of doxorubicin encapsulation in micelles or nanoemulsions on the ultrasound-mediated intracellular delivery and nuclear trafficking. *Molecular Pharmaceutics* 7: 1959-1973.

Negishi Y, Endo Y, Fukuyama T, Suzuki R, Takizawa T, Omata D, Maruyama K, Aramaki Y. (2008) Delivery of siRNA into the cytoplasm by liposomal bubbles and ultrasound. *J Control Release* 132: 124-130.

Newman CM, Bettinger T. (2007) Gene therapy progress and prospects: ultrasound for gene transfer. *Gene Ther* 14: 465-475.

Niidome T, Huang L.(2002) Gene therapy progress and prospects: nonviral vectors. *Gene Ther* 9: 1647-1652.

Noble ML, Brayman AA, Kuhr CS, Graves SS, Keilman GW, Chen L, Loeb KR, Storb RF, Miao CH. (2011) Effective gene transfer using microbubble-assisted ultrasound therapy in canine livers. *American Society of Gene and Cell Therapy 14th Annual Meeting 2011:* Oral abstract presentation.

Okada K, Kudo N, Hassan MA, Kondo T, Yamamoto K. (2009) Threshold curves obtained under various gaseous conditions for free radical generation by burst ultrasound - Effects of dissolved gas, microbubbles and gas transport from the air. *Ultrasonics Sonochem* 16: 512-518.

Otani K, Yamahara K, Ohnishi S, Obata H, Kitamura S, Nagaya N. (2009) Nonviral delivery of siRNA into mesenchymal stem cells by a combination of ultrasound and microbubbles. *J Control Release* 133: 146-153.

Overvelde M, Garbinb V, Sijl J, Dollet B, de Jong N, Lohse D, Versluis M. (2010) Nonlinear shell behavior of phospholipid-coated microbubbles. *Ultrasound Med Biol* 36: 2080 - 2092.

Phillips LC, Klibanov AL, Wamhoff BR, Hossack JA. (2010) Targeted gene transfection from microbubbles into vascular smooth muscle cells using focused, ultrasound-mediated delivery. *Ultrasound Med Biol* 36: 1470-1480.

Pislaru SV, Pislaru C, Kinnick RR, Singh R, Gulati R, Greenleaf JF, Simari RD. (2003) Optimization of ultrasound-mediated gene transfer: comparison of contrast agents and ultrasound modalities. *Eur Heart J* 24: 1690-1698.

Plesset MS, Chapman RB. (1971) Collapse of an initially spherical vapour cavity in the neighbourhood of a solid boundary. *J Fluid Mech* 47: 283-290.

Porter TM, Smith DAB, Holland CK. (2006) Acoustic techniques for assessing the Optison destruction threshold. *J Ultrasound Med* 25: 1519-1529.

Porter TR. (2009) The utilization of ultrasound and microbubbles for therapy in acute coronary syndromes. *Cardiovasc Res* 83: 636-642.

Porter TR, Hiser WL, Kricsfeld D, Deligonul U, Xie F, Iversen P, Radio S. (2001) Inhibition of carotid artery neointimal formation with intravenous microbubbles. *Ultrasound Med Biol* 27: 259-265.

Postema M, Schmitz G. (2007) Ultrasonic bubbles in medicine: influence of the shell. *Ultrasonics Sonochem* 14: 438 - 444.

Postema M, van Wamel A, Lancee CT, de Jong N. (2004) Ultrasound-induced encapsulated microbubble phenomena. *Ultrasound Med Biol* 30: 827-840.

Price RJ, Skyba DM, Kaul S, Skalak TC. (1998) Delivery of colloidal particles and red blood cells to tissue through microvessel ruptures created by targeted microbubble destruction with ultrasound. *Circulation* 98: 1264-1267.

Qin S, Caskey CF, Ferrara KW. (2009) Ultrasound contrast microbubbles in imaging and therapy: physical principles and engineering. *Phys Med Biol* 54: R27-57.

Qiu Y, Luo Y, Zhang Y, Cui W, Zhang D, Wu J, Zhang J, Tu J. (2010) The correlation between acoustic cavitation and sonoporation involved in ultrasound-mediated DNA transfection with polyethylenimine (PEI) in vitro. *J Control Release* 145: 40-48.

Rahim AA, Taylor SL, Bush NL, ter Haar GR, Bamber JC, Porter CD. (2006) Spatial and acoustic pressure dependence of microbubble-mediated gene delivery targeted using focused ultrasound. *J Gene Med* 8: 1347-1357.

Robinson PB, Blake JR, Kodama T, Shima A, Tomita Y. (2001) Interaction of cavitation bubbles with a free surface. *J Appl Phys* 89: 8225-8237.

Sakai T, Kawaguchi M, Kosuge Y. (2009) siRNA-mediated gene silencing in the salivary gland using in vivo microbubble-enhanced sonoporation. *Oral Diseases* 15: 505-511.

Samuel S, Cooper MA, Bull JL, Fowlkes JB, Miller DL. (2009) An ex vivo study of the correlation between acoustic emission and microvascular damage. *Ultrasound Med Biol* 35: 1574-1586.

Sankin GN, Yuan F, Zhong P. (2010) Pulsating tandem microbubble for localized and directional single-cell membrane poration. *Physical Rev Lett* 105: 078101.

Sarkar K, Katiyar A, Jain P. (2009) Growth and dissolution of an encapsulated contrast microbubble: effects of encapsulation permeability. *Ultrasound Med Biol* 35: 1385-1396.

Sarvazyan AP, Rudenko OV, Nyborg WL. (2010) Biomedical applications of radiation force of ultrasound: historical roots and physical basis. *Ultrasound Med Biol* 36: 1379-1394.

Sassaroli E, Hynynen K. (2007) Cavitation threshold of microbubbles in gel tunnels by focused ultrasound. *Ultrasound Med Biol* 33: 1651-1660.

Shen ZP, Brayman AA, Chen L, Miao CH. (2008) Ultrasound with microbubbles enhances gene expression of plasmid DNA in the liver via intraportal delivery. *Gene Ther* 15: 1147-1155.

Shima A, Tomita Y, Gibson DC, Blake JR. (1989) The growth and collapse of cavitation bubbles near composite surfaces. *J Fluid Mech* 203: 199 - 214.

Skyba DM, Price RJ, Linka AZ, Skalak TC, Kaul S. (1998) Direct in vivo visualization of intravascular destruction of microbubbles by ultrasound and its local effects on tissue. *Circulation* 98: 290-293.

Smith DA, Vaidya SS, Kopechek JA, Huang SL, Klegerman ME, McPherson DD, Holland CK. (2010) Ultrasound-triggered release of recombinant tissue-type plasminogen activator from echogenic liposomes. *Ultrasound Med Biol* 36: 145-157.

Snyder RO. (1999) Adeno-associated virus-mediated gene delivery. *J Gene Med* 1: 166-175.

Song J, Chappell JC, Qi M, VanGieson EJ, Kaul S, Price RJ. (2002) Influence of injection site, microvascular pressure and ultrasound variables on microbubble-mediated delivery of microspheres to muscle. *J Am Coll Cardiol* 39: 726-731.

Song S, Noble ML, Sun SX, Chen L, Brayman AA, Miao CH. (2011b) Optimization of high intensity therapeutic ultrasound and microbubbles for gene delivery into rat liver. *American Society of Gene and Cell Therapy 14th Annual Meeting:* Oral abstract presentation.

Song S, Shen Z, Chen L, Brayman AA, Miao AA. (2011a) Explorations of high-intensity therapuetic ultrasound and microbubble-mediated gene delivery in mouse liver. *Gene Therapy* Mar 31. [Epub ahead of print].

Stride E, Saffari N. (2003) On the destruction of microbubble ultrasound contrast agents. *Ultrasound Med Biol* 29: 563-573.

Stringham SB, Viskovska MA, Richardson ES, Ohmine S, Husseini GA, Murray BK, Pitt WG. (2009) Over-pressure suppresses ultrasonic-induced drug uptake. *Ultrasound Med Biol* 35: 409-415.

Su CH, Chang CY, Wang HH, Wu YJ, Bettinger T, Tsai CH, Yeh HI. (2010) Ultrasonic microbubble-mediated gene delivery causes phenotypic changes of human aortic endothelial cells. *Ultrasound Med Biol* 36: 449-458.

Suda T, Suda K, Liu D. (2008) Computer-assisted hydrodynamic gene delivery. *Molecular Therapy* 16: 1098-1104.

Talu E, Powell RL, Longo ML, Dayton PA. (2008) Needle size and injection rate impact microbubble contrast agent population. *Ultrasound Med Biol* 34: 1182-1185.

Taylor SL, Rahim AA, Bush NL, Bamber JC, Porter CD. (2007) Targeted retroviral gene delivery using ultrasound. *J Gene Med* 9: 77-87.

Tlaxca JL, Anderson CR, Klibanov AL, Lowrey B, Hossack JA, Alexander JS, Lawrence MB, Rychak JJ. (2010) Analysis of in vitro transfection by sonoporation using cationic and neutral microbubbles. *Ultrasound Med Biol* 36: 1907-1918.

Tsunoda S, Mazda O, Oda Y, Iida Y, Akabame S, Kishida T, Shin-Ya M, Asada H, Gojo S, Imanishi J, Matsubara H, Yoshikawa T. (2005) Sonoporation using microbubble BR14 promotes pDNA/siRNA transduction to murine heart. *Biochem Biophys Res Comm* 336: 118-127.

Vannan M, McCreery T, Li P, Han Z, Unger E, Kuersten B, Nabel E, Rajagopalan S. (2002) Ultrasound-mediated transfection of canine myocardium by intravenous administration of cationic microbubble-linked plasmid DNA. *J Am Soc Cardiogr* 15: 214-218.

Villanueva FS. (2009) Ultrasound mediated destruction of DNA-loaded microbubbles for enhancement of cell-based therapies: new promise amidst a confluence of uncertainties? *J Am Coll Cardiogr Cardiovasc Imaging* 2: 880-882.

Walton CB, Shohet RV. (2009) Tiny bubbles and endocytosis? *Circ Res* 104: 563-565.

Wang JF, Wu CJ, Zhang CM, Qiu QY, Zheng M. (2009) Ultrasound-mediated microbubble destruction facilitates gene transfection in rat C6 glioma cells. *Mol Biol Rep* 36: 1263-1267.

Wang ZX, Wang ZG, Ran HT, Ren JL, Zhang Y, Li Q, Zhu YF, Ao M. (2009) The treatment of liver fibrosis induced by hepatocyte growth factor-directed, ultrasound-targeted microbubble destruction in rats. *Clin Imaging* 33: 454-461.

Wu J, Nyborg WL. (2008) Ultrasound, cavitation bubbles and their interaction with cells. *Advanced Drug Delivery Reviews* 60: 1103-1116.

Xie F, Boska MD, Lof J, Uberti MG, Tsutsui JM, Porter TR. (2008) Effects of transcranial ultrasound and intravenous microbubbles on blood brain barrier permeability in a large animal model. *Ultrasound Med Biol* 34: 2028-2034.

Xing Y, Pua EC, Lu X, Zhong P. (2009) Low-amplitude ultrasound enhances hydrodynamic-based gene delivery to rat kidney. *Biochem Biophys Res Commun* 386: 217-222.

Yant SR, Huang Y, Akache B, Kay MA. (2007) Site-directed transposon integration in human cells. *Nucleic Acids Res* 35: e50.

Ye X, Loeb KR, Stafford DW, Thompson AR, Miao CH. (2003) Complete and sustained phenotypic correction of hemophilia B in mice following hepatic gene transfer of a high-expressing human factor IX plasmid. *J Thrombosis Haemostasis* 1: 103-111.

Yoon CS, Jung HS, Kwon MJ, Lee SH, Kim CW, Kim MK, Lee M, Park JH. (2009) Sonoporation of the minicircle-VEGF(165) for wound healing of diabetic mice. *Pharm Res* 26: 794-801.

Zarnitsyn VG, Prausnitz MR. (2004) Physical parameters influencing optimization of ultrasound-mediated DNA transfection. *Ultrasound Med Biol* 30: 527-538.

Zhang G, Song YK, Liu D. (2000) Long-term expression of human alpha1-antitrypsin gene in mouse liver achieved by intravenous administration of plasmid DNA using a hydrodynamics-based procedure. *Gene Ther* 7: 1344-1349.

Zheng XZ, Li HL, Du LF, Wang HP, Gu Q. (2009) Comparative analysis of gene transfer to human and rat retinal pigment epithelium cell line by a combinatorial use of recombinant adeno- associated virus and ultrasound or/and microbubbles. *Bosn J Basic Med Sci* 9: 174-181.

Zhou S, Li S, Liu Z, Tang Y, Wang Z, Gong J, Liu C. (2010) Ultrasound-targeted microbubble destruction mediated herpes simplex virus-thymidine kinase gene treats hepatoma in mice. *J Exp Clin Cancer Res* 29: 170.

Zhou XY, Liao Q, Pu YM, Tang YQ, Gong X, Li J, Xu Y, Wang ZG. (2009) Ultrasound-mediated microbubble delivery of pigment epithelium-derived factor gene into retina inhibits choroidal neovascularization. *Chinese Medical J* 122: 2711-2717.

Zhou Y, Cui J, Deng CX. (2008) Dynamics of sonoporation correlated with acoustic cavitation activities. *Biophysical J* 94: L51-53.

Zhou Y, Kumon RE, Cui J, Deng CX. (2009) The size of sonoporation pores on the cell membrane. *Ultrasound Med Biol* 35: 1756 - 1760.

Zhou Y, Zhou XY, Wang ZG, Zhu YF, Li P. (2010) Elevation of plasma membrane permeability upon laser irradiation of extracellular microbubbles. *Lasers Med Sci* 25: 587-594.

11

Polyamine – Lipid Conjugates as Effective Gene Carriers: Chemical Structure, Morphology, and Gene Transfer Activity

Takehisa Dewa, Tomohiro Asai, Naoto Oku and Mamoru Nango
Graduate School of Engineering, Nagoya Institute of Technology
University of Shizuoka Graduate School of Pharmaceutical Sciences
Japan

1. Introduction

Development of more efficient and safer gene carriers using nonviral compounds is one of the most challenging aspects of gene therapy (Kay, 1997; Lasic, 1997). Compared to viral carrier systems, nonviral gene carrier systems have advantages in simplicity of use, lack of specific immune response, and ease of mass production due to the low cost of preparation; however, they have the disadvantage of low transfection efficiency, which needs to be overcome (Miller, 1998; Li & Huang, 2000). To improve the efficiency of nonviral carriers, many synthetic organic compounds, including cationic lipids (Felgner & Ringold, 1989; MacDonald et al., 1999; Felgner et al., 1987; Behr et al., 1989; Meyer et al., 1998), polycations (Boussif et al., 1995; Petersen et al., 2002; Koide et al., 2006; Russ et al., 2008; Haensler & Szoka, 1993; Shim & Kwon, 2009), and combinations thereof (Guillot-Nieckowski et al., 2007; Wu et al., 2001; Ewert et al., 2006; Takahashi et al., 2007; Matsui et al., 2006; Mustapa et al., 2009; Kogure et al., 2008), have been developed as nonviral gene carriers (Mintzer, M. A. & Simanek, E. E., 2009; also references cited therein). Substantial research has been reported on structure–activity relationships for cationic amphiphiles concerning the cationic and hydrophobic portions (Remy et al., 1994; Geall et al., 1999; Ewert et al, 2002; Byk et al., 1998; McGregor et al., 2001). Such amphiphiles form self-assembling micelles and liposomes in an aqueous phase, the structures of which have been investigated using small-angle X-ray scattering (SAXS), transmission electron microscopy (TEM), and atomic force microscopy (AFM) to gain knowledge about structure–activity relationship, particularly those involving ordered structures (lamellar, inverted hexagonal, and cubic phases) and their morphological changes (Koltover et al., 1998; Koynova, Wang & MacDonald, 2006) as well as about the size of complexes (Aoyama et al., 2003).

The mechanism of gene delivery by such cationic carriers probably involves an endosomal pathway (Wrobel & Collins (1995)): (i) cellular uptake via endocytosis, (ii) DNA release from endosome, and (iii) entry into the nucleus. Many researchers have devised cationic compounds that facilitate the process, for example, ligand-conjugated molecules targeting a receptor such as integrin (Mustapa et al., 2007; Varga, Wickham & Lauffenburger, 2000), pH-responsive or cleavable molecules that enable escape of DNA from endosome (Russ et al, 2008; Oupicky, Parker & Seymour, 2002; Dauty et al., 2001; Miyake et al., 2004; Anderson,

Lynn & Lange, 2003), and conjugation of nuclear localization signal peptides (NLS) (Zanta et al., 1999; Manickam & Oupicky, 2006) for steps (i)-(iii), respectively. For cationic lipids/DNA complexes (lipoplexes), it has been proposed that a morphological change from lamellar to inverted hexagonal phase in the acidic endosomal environment facilitates the endosomal release and escape of DNA (Bell et al., 2003; Xu & Szoka, 1996). In addition to investigation of intracellular trafficking of polycation–DNA complexes (polyplexes and lipoplexes), observation of morphology and metamorphosis of the complexes is very important to shed light on the mechanism of gene transfer and provide information for development of novel synthetic carriers (Koynova, Wang & MacDonald, 2006; Wan et al., 2008; Tarahovsky, Koynova & MacDonald, 2004).

We have reported that polycationic liposomes (PCL) containing cetylated polyethylenimine (cetyl-PEI) possess high gene transfer activity (Yamazaki et al., 2000; Oku et al., 2001; Matsuura et al., 2003). The cetyl-PEI molecule is anchored by the hydrophobic cetyl portion and is distributed over the liposomal surface. In our previous report, we proposed a possible mechanism of PCL-mediated gene transfer wherein PCL/DNA complexes are uptaken by endosomal pathway; this was based on tracking of fluorescence-labeled components, PCL lipid, cetyl-PEI, and DNA, which the release and transfer of cetyl PEI / DNA complex into the nucleus via the cytosol (Sugiyama et al., 2004). Compaction of DNA is therefore crucial, and both electrostatic and hydrophobic interactions in the cetyl PEI / DNA complex are responsible for its effective compaction.

PEI is used as a gene transfer vector by itself, however, it has inherent disadvantages, *i.e.*, cytotoxicity and polydispersity. We have previously reported successful syntheses of a series of polyamine–dicetyl phosphate (DCP) conjugates via reaction of a novel synthetic intermediate, dimerized DCP anhydride (compound **1** in Scheme 1), with various polyamines, spermidine, spermine, and PEI (Scheme 1) (Dewa et al., 2004a). Since spermidine and spermine are naturally occurring polyamines, we expected low cytotoxicity. When suspended in aqueous solution, they form micellar aggregates and exhibit moderate gene-transfer activity, the magnitude of which is relatively insensitive to the modification of the polyamine portion. We also observed the morphology of the conjugate / DNA complex by using atomic force microscopy (AFM). We discuss briefly the relation between the assembling structure of the conjugate/DNA and their transfection efficiency.

In this report, we describe (1) facile synthetic strategy of polyamine-lipid conjugates in brief and (2) evidence demonstrating that the transgene activity is dramatically enhanced when the conjugates are assembled into liposomes containing cholesterol and phospholipid and that the activity is susceptible to the chemical modification of the conjugate both in the polyamine and in the hydrophobic chain portions (Scheme 1). We show further that (3) gene transfer activity of the corresponding PCLs strongly depends on the type of polyamine in the conjugate, with notable differences between the lower molecular weight polyamines (spermidine and spermine) on one hand and the polymer type (PEI(1800)) on the other.

We also examined (4) the morphology of the lipoplexes by AFM and discuss the relationship between the structure of lipoplexes and their transfection efficiency. AFM analysis has a considerable advantage for observation of lipoplex morphology, especially for less ordered structures (Oberle et al., 2000), however, until now little clear evidence has been reported on the relationship between morphological change and DNA release. In this research, DNA release as a result of disassociation of the complex was revealed by AFM (Dewa et al., 2010). We discuss morphology–activity relationships on the basis of electrophoresis analysis, dynamic light scattering (DLS) and AFM observation. Furthermore we introduce (5) our recent effort for synthesis of cleavable polyamine-lipid conjugates under a reductive cytosolic condition.

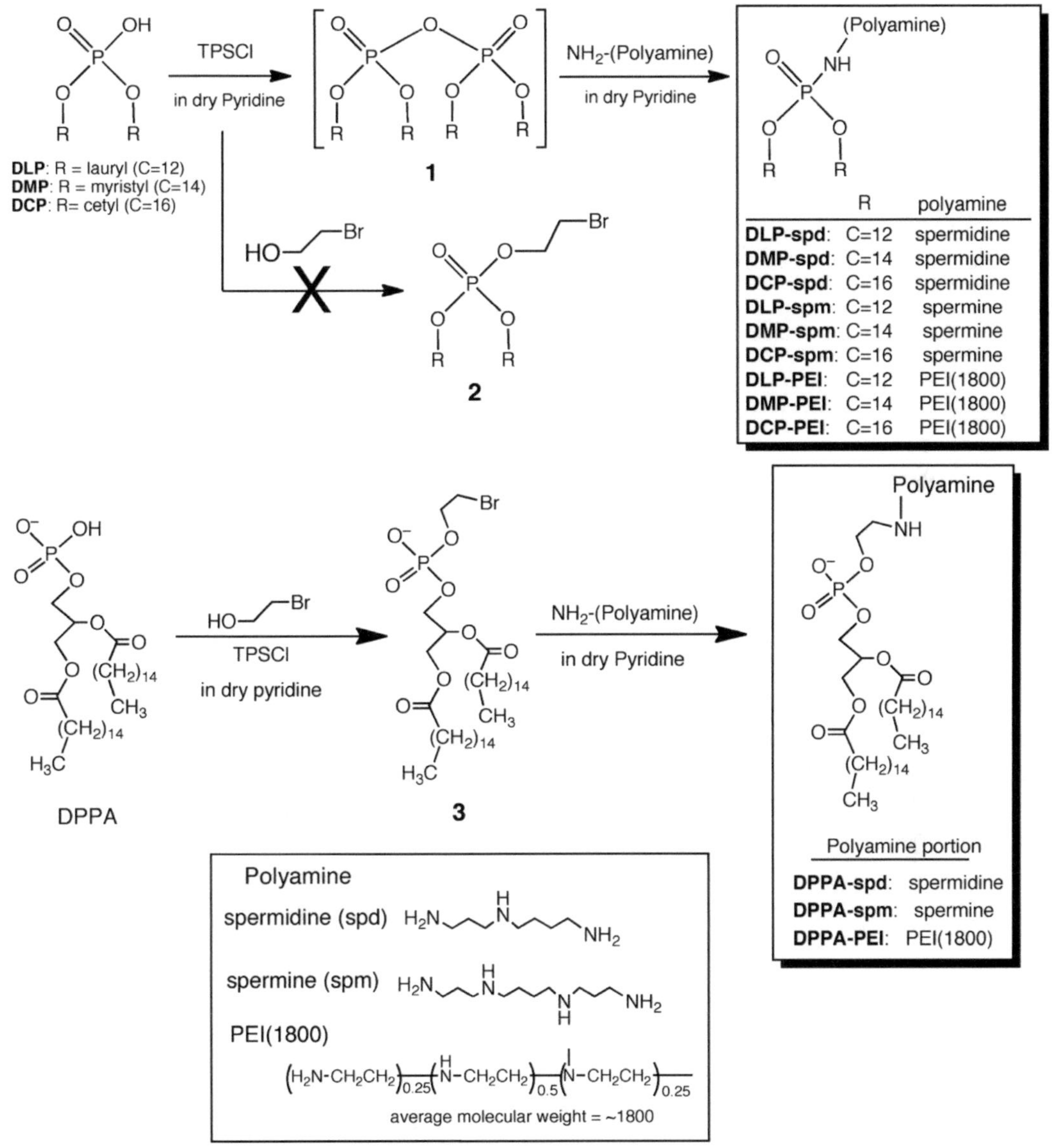

Scheme 1. Synthetic Strategy for Polyamine-lipid Conjugates.

2. Synthetic strategy of various polyamine-lipid conjugates via facile synthetic routes

In many cases, polycationic compounds have been synthesized through multi step reactions including protection/deprotection reactions on polyamine moieties. Our polyamine-lipid compounds can be prepared via two-step reactions without such protection/deprotection reactions. The synthetic schemes are shown in Scheme 1, where two types of polyamine-lipid conjugate; dialkyl phosphate- and diacylphosphatidic acid-based compounds, are described. In this section, we showed a synthetic strategy for polyamine-lipid conjugates via facile routes (Dewa et al., 2004a,b, 2010).

2.1 Polyamine-dialkyl phosphate conjugates via a synthetic intermediate 1

Our preliminary idea for the syntheses of polyamine-dicetyl phosphate (DCP) conjugates was to use the bromoethylated compound, **2**, as a synthetic intermediate via condensation of DCP and 2-bromoethanol (Scheme 1) by using 1,3,5-triisopropylbenzenesulfonyl chloride, TPSCl (Uragami, Miyake & Regen, 2000; Tanaka, et al., 1987). Instead of the expected adduct, **2**, however, we obtained another product having high R_f value, 0.97 (R_f = 0.56 for DCP by eluting $CHCl_3/MeOH/H_2O$ = 13/6/1, v/v/v). The resulting product is stable enough to be isolated by column chromatography. SIMS indicates almost double molecular mass, 1075.4 (546.9 for DCP). The observed IR absorption band at 952 cm^{-1} is assignable to the P–O–P stretching mode. The ^{31}P NMR spectrum of the product, whose signals appear at δ= -12.27 and -0.13 ppm, is clearly distinguishable from that of DCP having a signal at δ= 2.15 ppm. This evidence, taken together, leaves no doubt that the product is dimerized DCP in anhydrous form, **1**, [$(C_{64}H_{133}O_7P_2)^+$ calcd 1075.9] connected via P–O–P bonding. There are some prior examples in the synthesis of pyrophosphate derivatives bearing small alkyl moieties, methyl, ethyl, propyl, and butyl (Cullis, Kaye & Trippett, 1987), however, the dimerized anhydride, **1**, bearing phospholipid-like long alkyl chains is an unprecedented compound. This compound is a convenient synthetic intermediate for formimg phosphoramidate bonds, as described below.

The anhydride **1** readily react with amines, *e.g.*, spermidine, spermine, and even polymer, PEI(1800), to form the phosphoramidate, P–N bond, providing the corresponding adducts shown in Scheme 1. The reactivity toward these nucleophiles indicates that the anhydrous compound **1** is potentially a good synthetic intermediate for making polyamine-dialkyl phosphate conjugates via the P–N bond. When reacted with spermine, for example, the adduct **DCP-spm** readily forms, concomitantly with the loss of DCP. The ^{31}P NMR signal of compound **DCP-spm** is shifted downfield, to 9.76 ppm compared with that of DCP at 2.15 ppm, indicating the formation of the P–N bond in the compound. The down-field-shifted signal is attributed to the lower electronegativity of the nitrogen atom in spermine relative to the oxygen atom in DCP. Anhydride **1** is a useful synthetic intermediate because it is (1) stable yet reactive with amino groups, (2) very simple and easy to prepare, and (3) produced in high yield (~90 %). Furthermore, modification on the hydrophobic chain is easy when various dialkyl phosphates were used. These compounds could hence provide new category of polycationic lipids. Gall et al. have developed cationic lipid derivatives bearing P-N linkage, which possess gene transfer activity (Gall et al., 2010).

2.2 Polyamine-diacylphosphatidic acid conjugates via a synthetic intermediate 3

To diacylphosphatidic acid can be attached 2-bromoethanol with TPSCl, giving an intermediate **3**. When this reacted with an amino group of polyamine compounds via nucleophilic substitution reaction, a corresponding polyamine conjugate was formed as shown in Scheme 1 (Dewa et al., 2004b). Purified products can be afforded by column chromatography using an amino group-modified silicagel.

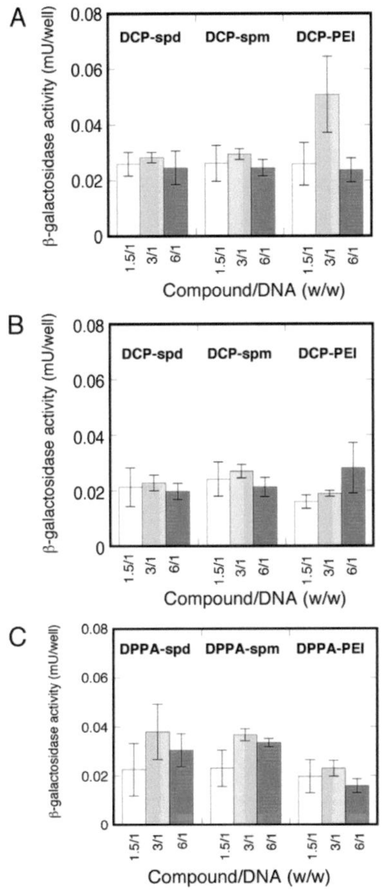

Fig. 1. Transfection efficacy of polyamine-DCP (A and B) and polyamine-DPPA conjugates (C) on VSMC, in the absence (A and C) and the presence of 20% of FBS (B). The ratios of compound/β-galactosidase plasmid DNA (w/w) were 1.5/1, 3/1, and 6/1, respectively.

3. Transfection efficacy of various polyamine-lipid conjugates as micellar carriers

First, we describes trasnsfection efficacy of these polyamine-lipid conjugates. Figure 1A shows the efficacy of these carriers using β-galactosidase activity (milli-unit/well), in the absence of FBS. Compared with the commercially available transfection reagent, *O*-ethyl DOPC (E-DOPC) (MacDonald et al., 1999), which produced 0.1 milli-unit/well transgene expression, the compounds, **DCP-spd**, **DCP-spm**, **and DCP-PEI**, exhibit moderate efficiency, ~30 to 50 % of the efficiency of E-DOPC. The transfection efficiencies of the components themselves, *i.e.*, DCP, spermidine, spermine, and PEI(1800) were almost negligible. Thus, the transfection activity results from the conjugation of two moieties, a hydrophilic polyamine and a hydrophobic DCP. Compound **DCP-PEI** shows the highest efficiency at 3/1 (w/w) of **DCP-PEI** /DNA, whereas the efficiency of the other compounds are comparable and insensitive to the compound/DNA ratio within the range of error. In

Figure 1B is shown the transfection efficiency in the presence of 20% FBS. The efficiency of these compounds was not influenced by the presence of 20% FBS, retaining 80–100 % of the activity (except compound **DCP-PEI** at 3/1 (w/w)). Such serum-resistant activity was also observed for the PCL gene transfection system previously reported (Matsuura et al., 2003). It is well known that serum often inhibits transfection; such inhibition is due to binding of negatively charged serum proteins to the cationic transfection reagents resulting in forming aggregates ineffective to the transfection. Although it is not clear why the polyamine-DCP conjugates are not influenced by the presence of the serum, the polyamine part may be assumed to efficiently interact with DNA via electrostatic interactions.

Polyamine-DPPA derivatives also exhibited transfection activity, whose extent is almost comparable to the polyamine-DCP derivatives (Figure 1C). The tendency of the activity is **DPPA-spd** ≥ **DPPA-spm** > **DPPA-PEI**. In the following section, we will discuss on the relationship between gene transfer activity and morphology of polyamine-lipid complexes.

4. Morphology of the micellar and complexes with DNA

It was found that DNA (ColE1 plasmid DNA) complex with various polyamines and polyamine–lipid conjugates by monitoring decrease of fluorescence from EtBr initially intercalated into DNA. With an increase in the cation (N) /anion (P) ratio, defined as N/P, the relative fluorescence intensity decreased as a result of complexation of DNA and polyamine. The polymeric molecule, PEI(1800) (N ~ 42 per molecule) most efficiently forms a complex with DNA; the complexation was almost complete at N/P = 3. Spermidine (N = 3 per molecule) and spermine (N = 4 per molecule) are less effective than PEI(1800), however, with complexation being complete at around N/P~7. For polyamine-DCP conjugates, the tendency for the fluorescence intensity to decrease is due to the complexation with DNA in the same way as that of the free amines, that is, **DCP-spd** < **DCP-spm** < **DCP-PEI**. DPPA-polyamine conjugates exhibited similar DNA condensation manner to DCP-polyamines, however, the tendency of DNA condensation was opposite way. The EtBr replacement experiment suggested that the tendency of DNA condensation is **DPPA-spd** > **DPPA-spm** > **DPPA-PEI**; the order is opposite to that of DCP-conjugates with regard to the polyamine portions.

In Table 1, the size of the micellar and complex with DNA was summarized. The mean particle diameters of various polyamine-DCP conjugates in an aqueous suspension, as given by dynamic light scattering is summarized in Table 1: 155 ± 54 nm for **DCP-spd**, 173 ± 46 nm for **DCP-spm**, 128 ± 38 nm for **DCP-PEI**, 90 ± 8 nm for **DPPA-spd**, 106 ± 41 nm for **DPPA-spm**, and 218 ± 35 nm for **DPPA-PEI**. AFM images for the suspension of these compounds exhibited spherical or ellipsoidal particles, whose sizes, defined according to diameter for the spheres and major × minor axes for the ellipsoid, were 132 nm for **DCP-spd**, 156 nm for **DCP-spm**, 209 × 145 nm for **DCP-PEI**, 96 nm for **DPPA-spd**, 111 nm for **DPPA-spm**, and 201 nm for **DPPA-PEI** (Figures 2A, B, C, D, E, and F, respectively). The particle sizes for these compounds as observed by AFM show good agreement with those obtained by DLS. The molecular shapes of these compounds are regarded to be the "cone" type, due to the attachment of the large polyamine moiety. We have endeavored to make liposome from these compounds, however, entrapment of a fluorescence probe, calcein, was impossible. Therefore, we assume that the particle consisting of polyamine-DCP conjugates is a micelle-like aggregate.

Compound	DLS (nm)		AFM / shape (size (nm)) and height (nm) [b)]			
	Micellar aggregate	Complex with DNA	Micelle aggregate		Complex with DNA	
DCP-spd	155 ± 54	409 ± 115	sphere (132)	21	aggregate (~1000 × 437)	16
DCP-spm	173 ± 46	237 ± 127	sphere (156)	24	aggregate (569 × 317)	20
DCP-PEI	128 ± 38	115 ± 40	ellipsoid (209 × 145)	12	sphere (120)	20
DPPA-spd	90 ± 8	140 ± 40	sphere (96)	24	sphere (129)	21
DPPA-spm	106 ± 41	109 ± 40	sphere (112)	16	sphere (172)	37
DPPA-PEI	218 ± 35	205 ± 39	aggregate (201)	12	aggregate (201)	17

a) The ratio of polyamine conjugate / DNA was 3/1 (w/w). Complexation of polyamine conjugate with DNA was carried out in water.
b) Sample solution was spread on a mica surface and dried. AFM images were obtained under dry condition. Width and height of the complexes were estimated from the AFM images in Figs 2 and 3.

Table 1. Estimated size and shape of polyamine-lipid micelles and complexes with ColE1 DNA suspended in aqueous solution [a)]

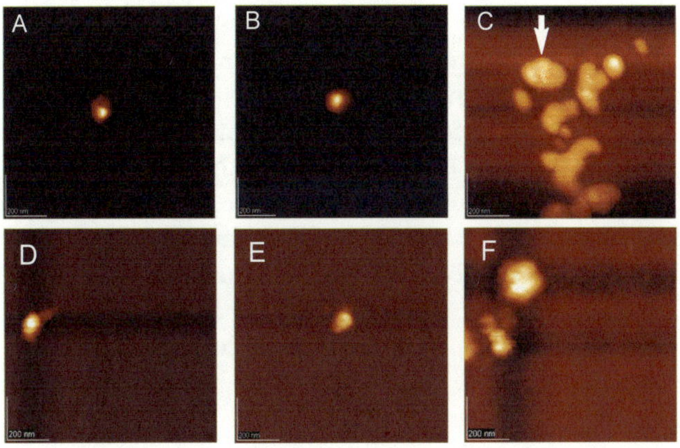

Fig. 2. AFM images of arrays of compounds, **DCP-spd** (A), **DCP-spm** (B), **DCP-PEI** (C), **DPPA-spd** (D), **DPPA-spm** (E), and **DPPA-PEI** (F). The compound was suspended in distilled water then dropped onto a mica surface by spin coating. All scale bars represent 200 nm. The object indicated by the arrow is discussed in the text.

Particle sizes of the conjugate/DNA (3/1: w/w) complex evaluated by DLS is 409 ± 115 nm for **DCP-spd**, 237 ± 127 nm for **DCP-spm**, 115 ± 40 nm for **DCP-PEI**, 140 ± 40 nm for **DPPA-spd**, 109 ± 40 nm for **DPPA-spm**, and 205 ± 39 nm for **DPPA-PEI**, respectively (Table 1). With increase in the size of polyamine portion in DCP-conjugates, the particle size significantly decreases, whereas opposite tendency was observed in DPPA-conjugates. AFM images support the tendency. Figure 3 shows an AFM image of DNA (A) and of the complexes it forms with various polyamines (B – I). Figure 3A reveals a clear image of partially-coiled ColE1 plasmid DNA (6646 bp), whose size is estimated to be 300~ 400 nm.

The height is ~ 2 nm, corresponding to the diameter of B-form DNA, ca. 2.4 nm. When DNA was complexed with compound **DCP-spd**, a "spider nest"-like structure was observed (Figure 3D). The size of the "quasi-ellipsoidal core region" is ~1000 × 437 nm and the height is ~16 nm. The height of the radiating peripheral "nest" region is ~ 2 nm, suggesting the nest region consists of free DNA. The height of the core region (~16 nm) is clearly larger than that of the DNA part, therefore, the core region of the structure must consist of the **DCP-spd**/DNA complex. Thus, complexation of compound **DCP-spd** and DNA gives rise to a segregated array, having complex and free DNA portions. The compound **DCP-spm** forms a similar but distinguishably different complex structure with DNA (Figure 3E), which resembles a "pearl necklace-like" aggregate (Yoshikawa et al., 1996), 569 × 317 nm in the plane of the substrate and 4~20 nm in height. The size of the pearl parts is 120 ~ 170 nm in diameter and 11 ~ 20 nm in height. These parts are connected by a region that is 4 ~ 5 nm in height. It appears from the image that the assembly consists of a tightly packed **DCP-spm**/DNA complex and regions of partially compacted DNA parts. Pronounced compaction of the complex was observed for the **DCP-PEI**/DNA, which formed a spherical cluster (120 nm in width and ~20 nm in height) (Figure 3F). The order of increasing compaction of DNA, **DCP-spd < DCP-spm < DCP-PEI**, is consistent with the extent of intercalation of EtBr as mentioned above, that is, the more tightly packed was the DNA complex, the lower was the extent of intercalation of EtBr. The tendency of size of the complex and the DNA condensation for DPPA-polyamine conjugates, that is, **DPPA-spd** (G) > **DPPA-spm** (H) > **DPPA-PEI** (I). One may wonder why the morphologies of the complexes, DCP- and DPPA-based conjugates, as well as **DCP-spd** and **DCP-spm** with DNA are so different despite the structural difference in cationic portion seems very little. It might come from the difference in delicate balance of hydrophilic/hydrophobic factor and/or molecular shapes which reflect a packing parameter.

Upon comparison, of the observed DNA complex with free polyamines, spermine (Figure 3B) and PEI (Figure 3C), the complex size and shape are obviously distinguishable from the corresponding conjugate forms; much larger complexes form with these free polyamines. The dimension of the spermine/DNA complex (Figure 3B) is ~3 μm; the compaction of DNA is obviously incomplete, judging from the presence of the "nest" portion of DNA that are similar to peripheral part of the **DCP-spd**/DNA complex (Figure 3D). The PEI/DNA complex is smaller (416 × 218 nm by 22 nm high) than the former complex, suggesting that the greater cationic charge makes the complex smaller. When one considers the effect of the hydrophobic portion in the polyamine compound on the size of the complex, it is clear that hydrophobic alkyl parts in the conjugates play an important role in the compaction of DNA, which is most prominently observed in conjugate **DCP-PEI** (Figure 3C vs 3F). From these results, the prominent transfection efficiency of **DCP-PEI** likely results from the more efficient compaction of DNA in the complex **DCP-PEI**/DNA, whereas the lower activity of **DCP-spd** and **DCP-spm** is likely due to their much weaker compaction.

Although the precise mechanism remains to be clarified, the compaction by these polyamine compounds probably plays an important role because entry into the nucleus is thought to be a key step and a smaller complex is likely to be associated with more efficient transfection. The conjugates in this study possibly decompose into separate polyamine and DCP portions in endosome. We assume that two critically important factors are involved in the present transfection system; compaction of DNA by polyamine part and with hydrophobic dialkyl portion and decomposition of the complex in endosome so as to liberate the

DNA/polyamine complex to be transported into nucleous. As previous report, DNA accompanied with cetyl-PEI enters into nucleus.

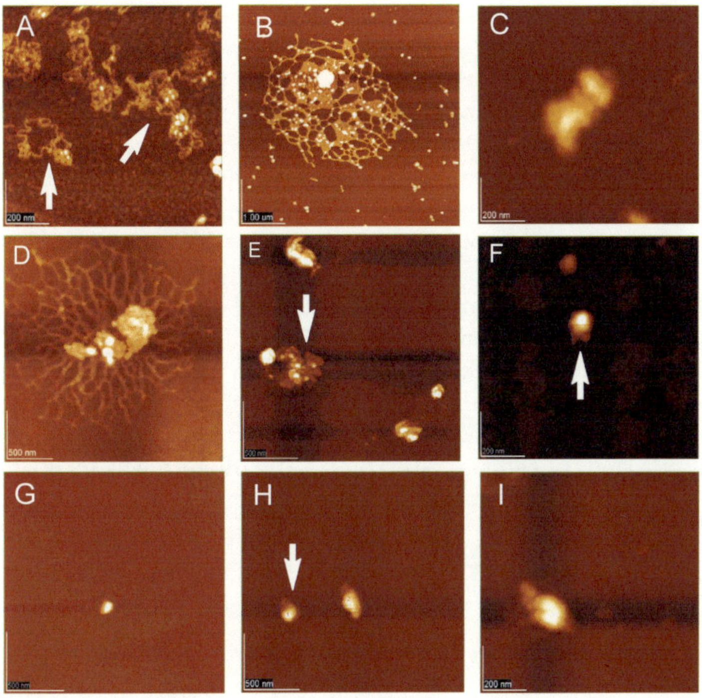

Fig. 3. AFM images of polyamine-ColE1 plasmid DNA complexes: (A), ColE1 plasmid DNA alone on polylysine-treated mica; (B), spermine/DNA; (C), PEI(1800)/DNA; (D), **DCP-spd**/DNA; (E), **DCP-spm**/DNA; (F), **DCP-PEI**/DNA; (G), **DPPA-spd**/DNA; (H), **DPPA-spm**/DNA; (I), **DPPA-PEI**/DNA. The polyamine/DNA ratio was 3/1 (w/w). Scale bars inserted in these images represent (A) 200, (B) 1000, (C) 200, (D) 500, (E) 500, (F) 200, (G) 500, (H) 500, and (I) 200 nm, respectively. The objects indicated by arrow(s) are discussed in the text.

In this section, we described novel types of polyamine-dialkyl phosphate conjugates that have moderate gene transfection activity for β-galactosidase assay. These conjugates are easy to prepare via a novel synthetic intermediate, dimerized DCP anhydride, **1**. The synthetic approaches described herein are flexible and possess potential for the rationale design of highly efficient gene carriers with single or narrow ranges of molecular weight.

5. Morphological effect of polyamine-lipid/DNA complexes on their transfection activity

As described above, when the polyamine-lipid conjugates were suspended in aqueous solution, they form micellar aggregates and exhibit moderate gene-transfer activity, the magnitude of which is relatively insensitive to the modification of the polyamine portion. Here we describe that preformed bilayer structure (as polycation liposomes, PCLs) significantly improves transfection efficacy compared with micellar aggregate form.

5.1 Preparation of Micellar Aggregates, PCL Vectors, and their complexes with DNA

Polycation liposome suspensions were typically prepared as follows: polyamine conjugate, phospholipid, 1,2-dioleoyl-*sn*-glycero-3-phosphoethanolamine (DOPE), and cholesterol (1/1/1 as a molar ratio) were dissolved in t-butyl alcohol. After removal of the solvent under reduced pressure, the residual solvent was removed by freeze-drying overnight. The lyophilized powder was hydrated with Tris-HCl buffer (20 mM, pH 8.0) followed by three freeze–thaw cycles and the resultant suspension was then subsequently extruded through polycarbonate membranes of 0.4, 0.2, and 0.1-µm pore diameter at room temperature. A suspension of the polyamine conjugate alone was prepared in the Tris-HCl buffer (20 mM, pH 8.0) by ultrasonication for 3 min. For convenience, particles so prepared are termed "micellar aggregates". Hereafter, polycationic liposomes (PCL) composed of the conjugates are described as "**conjugate**(PCL)", such as **DCP-spd**(PCL). Otherwise, micellar aggregates are described as just the name of conjugate, such as **DCP-spd**.

A plasmid encoding luciferase gene, pCAG-luc3 (6480 bp, a gift of DNAVEC Institute, Tsukuba, Japan), was amplified in E. coli JM109 (Nippon Gene, Toyama, Japan) and purified as described before (Matsuura et al., 2003). One microgram of the plasmid DNA in a TE buffer was added to a suspension of PCL containing 1 mM of polyamine conjugate so as to give the desired nitrogen/phosphate ratio, N/P. The mixture was incubated for 20 min at room temperature when used for transfection.

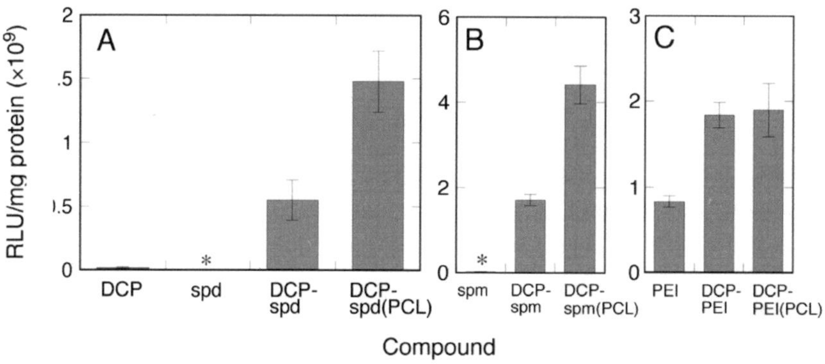

Fig. 4. Transfection efficacy of polyamine–lipid conjugates, **DCP-spd** (A), **DCP-spm** (B), and **DCP-PEI** (C), and their constituents, DCP (A) and polyamines, spermidine (spd, A), spermine (spm, B) and PEI1800 (PEI, C), on COS-1 cells. Efficacy was evaluated with the luciferase activity. The observed values for spermidine and spermine indicated by the asterisks (*) were apparently negligible on the activity scale shown. The conjugates **DCP-spd**, **DCP-spm**, and **DCP-PEI** represent their micellar aggregate forms, and **DCP-spd**(PCL), **DCP-spm**(PCL), and **DCP-PEI**(PCL) represent the conjugate-based PCLs (conjugate/DOPE/cholesterol = 1/1/1 (mol/mol/mol)). The nitrogen/phosphate (N/P) ratio was 16/1 for the polyamine conjugate/DNA complexes. For the monoanionic DCP, the molar ratio, DCP/nucleotide = 16/1, was applied as a negative control experiment. Transfection was conducted in the presence of 10% FBS.

5.2 Transfection procedure

COS-1 cells were cultured in Dulbecco's modified Eagle medium (DMEM) supplemented with 10% fetal bovine serum (FBS, Japan Bioserum Co. Ltd.) under a humidified atmosphere of 5% CO_2 in air. One day before a transfection experiment, 1×10^5 COS-1 cells were seeded onto each of several 35-mm dishes and incubated overnight in a CO_2 incubator. Then, the cells were washed twice with DMEM, and a suspension of lipoplex (1 μg DNA) was added to them in the presence of 10% FBS-DMEM. After 3 h incubation (37°C, 5% CO_2), the cells were washed twice with DMEM and cultured for another 48 h in 10% FBS-DMEM. The cells in the 35-mm dishes were washed twice with phosphate-buffered saline at 37°C, and 200 μL of cell lysis buffer (LC-β, TOYO B-Net Co. Ltd., Tokyo) were added. After 15 min incubation, the cells were collected with a cell scraper, frozen at -80 °C, and then thawed at room temperature. The lysate was centrifuged at 15,000 rpm for 5 min at 4 °C. The supernatant was subjected to the luciferase assay (Pica Gene, TOYO B-Net Co. Ltd., Tokyo) using a luminophotometer (Luminescencer-PSN AB-2200, ATTO). The observed intensity in instrument light units was normalized to the amount of protein determined by BCA protein assay Kit (PIERCE) to give a relative light unit (RLU/mg protein).

5.3 Transfection efficacy of micellar aggregates and PCL vectors: Comparison of the dicetyl phosphate derivatives of spermidine, sperimine, and polyamine

Figure 4A shows the transfection efficacy of the polyamine conjugate, **DCP-spd**, and its constituent molecules, DCP and spermidine (spd). The conjugate (in this case an aqueous micellar suspension) shows greatly increased efficacy relative to the constituent molecules, DCP and spermidine. For these polyamine/DNA complexes, the nitrogen/phosphorous ratio (N/P) was 16. The data of the figure indicate that coupling the lipophilic and cationic portions is essential to obtain gene transfer. Such an effect of conjugating these two moieties was also observed for the spermine conjugate, **DCP-spm** (Figure 4B). When the conjugates were further formulated with DOPE and cholesterol (conjugate/DOPE/cholesterol = 1/1/1 (mol/mol/mol)) to generate polycationic liposomes (PCL) (**DCP-spd**(PCL) and **DCP-spm**(PCL)), efficacies were further enhanced by a factor of 2–3 relative to the micellar aggregate suspensions (**DCP-spd** and **DCP-spm**). The polycation PEI(1800) itself showed moderate activity and the conjugate, **DCP-PEI**, exhibited even greater activity. However, in contrast to the other conjugates, the activity of the liposomal form, **DCP-PEI**(PCL), was comparable to that of the micellar version, **DCP-PEI**. The cytotoxicity of the conjugates, both as micellar aggregates and PCLs, was low; the latter vectors, which exhibited higher activity, also had slightly higher toxicity than the former.

It was found that the DOPE-based PCL exhibits significantly greater activity than the DPPC-based compound for both of the **DCP-spd**(PCL) and the **DCP-spm**(PCL). This is indicative of a lipid-mediated gene transfer mechanism; DOPE is well-known as a "helper" lipid, which is believed to facilitate membrane fusion and endosomal escape of the DNA (Felgner et al., 1994). DOPE in the present PCL systems presumably also plays a role in the mechanism to expedite membrane fusion and destabilization of the endosomal membrane. DPPC, whose T_m is 41.5 °C, renders the PCL more stable and more rigid than does DOPE. Thus, it is likely that the fusogenic property of DOPE is responsible for the enhanced transfection activity of its complexes relative to those containing DPPC.

5.4 Optimal structure of the conjugate molecules for gene transfer

The facile synthetic route provides a variety of polycationic compounds that can be exploited to examine the effect of the polycationic and hydrophobic portions on transfection efficiency. We hence examined the effect on transfection activity of different polyamine

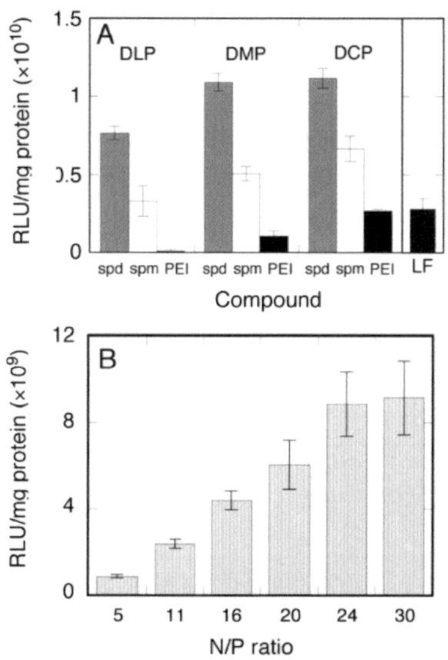

Fig. 5. (A) Effect of polyamine and hydrophobic portions on PCL-mediated gene transfer efficiency. PCL were composed of polyamine conjugate/DOPE/Cholesterol (1/1/1 mol/mol/mol). N/P ratio was 24. Transfection was done in the presence of 10% FBS. LF represents Lipofectamine™ 2000 as a positive control experiment. (B) Effect of the N/P ratio on the transfection efficacy of **DCP-spm**(PCL) (**DCP-spm**/DOPE/cholesterol = 1/1/1 (mol/mol/mol)). Transfection was in the presence of 10% FBS.

conjugates incorporated into PCLs: C12, C14, or C16 alkyl chain in the lipophilic portion and spermidine, spermine, or PEI(1800) as the polycationic head group of the conjugate. The data on these compounds are shown in Figure 5A. This result reveals clear tendencies of longer length of the alkyl group and the lower molecular weight of the polyamines (spermidine, spermine) to enhance transfection. When compared with a commercial product, Lipofectamine™ 2000, the **DCP-spd**(PCL) possessed 3.6-fold higher activity.

5.5 N/P-dependent efficacy and complexation of PCL with DNA

Figure 5B shows the dependence of **DCP-spm**(PCL) efficacy on the ratio of the number of nitrogen atoms in the conjugate to that of phosphate in the DNA (N/P). The efficacy increases with the N/P ratio essentially linearly up to 24. A similar N/P-dependence has been also observed for **DCP-spd**(PCL) (data not shown for clarity), indicating that excess polyamine relative to DNA is needed for effective gene transfer by PCLs. In contrast, the transfection activity of micellar aggregates **DCP-spd** and **DCP-spm** reaches plateau values in the N/P range of 11–16 ($1\sim2 \times 10^9$ of RLU/mg protein). This tendency is consistent with our previous data obtained with the β-galactosidase expression system (Dewa et al., 2004a).

5.6 Chemical structure of the polyamine conjugates

The polyamine-dialkyl phosphate conjugates can be readily synthesized via a two-step reaction: (i) formation of dimerized dialkyl phosphate anhydride and (ii) its nucleophilic substitution with polyamines. The synthetic strategy gives access to a wide variety of polyamine–dialkyl phosphate derivatives. Conjugation of the polyamine and hydrophobic portions is required for an effective gene carrier (Figure 4). Such amphiphilicity is essential to condense DNA molecules, which requires both electrostatic and hydrophobic interactions (Yamazaki, 2000; Dewa et al., 2004a,b). We tested a number of combinations of dialkyl and polyamine portions for their activity in gene transfection. The longer alkyl chain exhibited higher efficiency (Figure 5A). The ζ-potential of the DOPE-based PCL increased with alkyl chain length, for example, 27.6, 33.4, and 37.1 mV for **DLP-spd**(PCL), **DMP-spd**(PCL), and **DCP-spd**(PCL), respectively, showing that the conjugate with the longer chain length provides the higher positive potential. The hydrophobic interaction results in stable incorporation of the conjugate into the PCL, consistent with transfection activity in the order of C16 ≥ C14 > C12. We found that the micellar aggregate of **DCP-PEI** conjugate exhibited slightly higher transfection activity than the low-molecular weight amine conjugates, **DCP-spd** and **DCP-spm**, however, the activity of **DCP-PEI**(PCL) was marginal. The size of **DCP-PEI**(PCL)/DNA lipoplex is significantly greater than that of the other lipoplexes (Table 2, entry 14). The **DCP-PEI** conjugate is composed of DCP/PEI(1800) = ~1/1, judged by ^{1}H-NMR (Dewa et al., 2004a). As previously reported, the cetyl-PEI, whose PCL possesses high transfection activity, consists of 10 cetyl portions in the polymer (Matsuura et al., 2003). The cetyl-PEI can attach to the PCL surface via the anchoring of cetyl portions in the lipid bilayer. However, that is not the case for **DCP-PEI**(PCL); the single hydrophobic portion in the conjugate is not enough to provide adequate covering of PEI over the PCL surface. This may cause "PEI-protrusion" from the surface, which gives rise to the large and heterogeneous aggregation seen upon combination with DNA molecules. This is likely the reason for the lower activity of the **DCP-PEI**(PCL). Taken together, these considerations suggest that a homogeneous positive charge distribution on the PCL surface is important to the transfection activity.

5.7 Morphological analysis of the complexes with DNA

5.7.1 Formation of complex with DNA

To elucidate the characteristics of N/P-dependence, formation of **DCP-spd**(PCL)/DNA and **DCP-spm**(PCL)/DNA lipoplexes was analyzed by agarose gel electrophoreses and DLS analysis. Electrophoretic analysis showed N/P ratio-dependent complexation; in the lower N/P range of 5–16, the open circular DNA band vanished and the supercoiled DNA band gradually faded for both of **DCP-spd**(PCL) and **DCP-spm**(PCL) and in the higher N/P range, 20–30, the latter DNA band totally disappeared. These observations indicate that the DNA molecules are completely entrapped within the lipoplex. Ethidium bromide (EtBr) replacement experiments also reveal condensation of DNA in the N/P range of 5–30 (Dewa et al., 2010).

The particle size of lipoplexes estimated by DLS analysis is summarized in Table 2. The diameters of the **DCP-spd**(PCL) and **DCP-spm**(PCL) alone are 158 ± 56, and 159 ± 30 nm, respectively (entries 1 and 7). Lipoplexes were larger and their size increased with increasing N/P up to 5 (entries 2 and 8 at N/P = 2 and entries 3 and 9 at N/P = 5). At N/P = 5, the PCL/DNA lipoplexes became larger with a broad distribution from 650 nm to over 1 μm (entries 3 and 9). In the higher N/P range (N/P = 16–24), sizes were reduced, converging at 261 ± 114 nm (**DCP-spd**(PCL), entry 5) and 256 ± 116 nm (**DCP-spm**(PCL), entry 11). ζ-potential measurements indicated the polarity of surface charge of lipoplexes inverts from negative in the lower N/P (5–11) to positive in the higher N/P (>16) regions.

AFM images revealed characteristic morphologies of lipoplexes in the both low and high N/P ranges (Figures 6A-D). When the **DCP-spd**(PCL)/DNA and **DCP-spm**(PCL)/DNA lipoplexes at N/P = 5 were put on PLL-treated mica (positively charged surface), large aggregates in the sub-~micrometer size range (600–1200 nm, Figures 6A and B) were observed. These structures resembled by bead-like aggregates (Yoshikawa et al., 1996) composed of small particles (80–120 nm in diameter, 8–20 nm in height) connected to one another. Such aggregates were not observed on a negatively-charged bare mica. This is understandable since the lipoplex at N/P = 5 is negatively charged, and the lipoplex must be adsorbed on the PLL-mica surface through electrostatic interaction to be imaged. The outer periphery of the large aggregates is rich in DNA molecules, presumably those were so loosely attached that they were liberated from the aggregates during electrophoresis.

entry	compound	N/P ratio	pH	size (nm)	
				PCL	Micellar aggregate
1	**DCP-spd**	–	8	158 ± 56	249 ± 106
2		2	8	231 ± 89	
3		5	8	651 ± 501	1181 ± 1057
4		16	8	190 ± 83	
5		24	8	261 ± 114	1791 ± 1630
6		24	4	985 ± 1437	1624 ± 1566
7	**DCP-spm**	–	8	159 ± 30	225 ± 102
8		2	8	293 ± 112	
9		5	8	764 ± 378	321 ± 181
10		16	8	296 ± 168	
11		24	8	256 ± 116	1767 ± 1284
12		24	4	1033 ± 1060	1209 ± 949
13	**DCP-PEI**	–	8	214 ± 90	275 ± 184
14		24	8	1062 ± 783	317 ± 243

Table 2. DLS analysis of various polyamine-dicetyl phosphate conjugate/DNA complexes

At the high N/P = 24, spherical complexes were observed for **DCP-spd**(PCL) and **DCP-spm**(PCL) complexes; their diameters were 200–400 nm for **DCP-spd**(PCL)/DNA (C) and 150–250 nm for **DCP-spm**(PCL)/DNA lipoplexes (D), and their heights were 12–30 and 27–60 nm, respectively. The size of the complexes is in good agreement with the values observed by DLS. The detailed topography of these **DCP-spd**(PCL)/DNA and **DCP-spm**(PCL)/DNA lipoplexes showed flat-topped spheres and spherical structures (line profiles (i)–(iii) for (C) and (iv)–(vi) for (D)). The profiles (ii) and (iii) are characteristically "step-like" (arrows). The heights indicated in (ii) are 6, 10, and 14 nm. Considering the thickness of lipid bilayer (4 nm) and the diameter of DNA (2 nm), these three values correspond to one bilayer (4 nm) + DNA (2 nm) = 6 nm, a double bilayer (8 nm) + DNA = 10 nm, and a triple bilayer (12 nm) + DNA = 14 nm, respectively. Thus, the step-like structure is reasonably indicative of a smectic lamellar assembly, where DNA molecules are laminated between bilayers.

Compared with **DCP-spd**(PCL) and **DCP-spm**(PCL) lipoplexes, the size of the **DCP-PEI**(PCL)/DNA lipoplex (N/P = 24) is large and has a broad distribution (1062 ± 783 nm, Table 2, entry 14). AFM images of the **DCP-PEI**(PCL)/DNA lipoplex show aggregates with heterogeneous and featureless shapes (Figure 6E and F). EtBr replacement experiments revealed DNA condensation in a similar manner to that of **DCP-spd**(PCL) and **DCP-spm**(PCL).

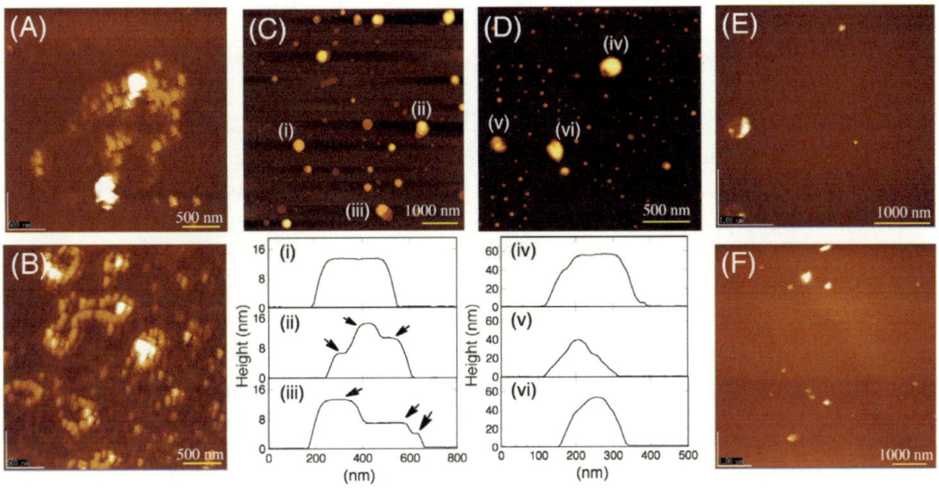

Fig. 6. AFM images of PCL/plasmid DNA (ColE1; 6646 bp) lipoplexes: (A), **DCP-spd**(PCL)/DNA (N/P = 5); (B), **DCP-spm**(PCL)/DNA (N/P = 5); (C), **DCP-spd**(PCL)/DNA (N/P = 24); (D), **DCP-spm**(PCL)/DNA (N/P = 24); (E and F), **DCP-PEI**(PCL)/DNA complex (N/P = 24). Scale bars shown in the images are 500 nm (A, B, and D) and 1000 nm (C, E, and F). The PCL/DNA complexes were applied to PLL-mica (A and B) and bare mica (C, D, E, F). All images were taken under an ambient air conditions. Height profiles of the objects (i)-(iii) in C and (iv)-(v) in D are shown below these images. Arrows in (ii) and (iii) indicate step-like profiles discussed in the text. Images E and F for **DCP-PEI**(PCL)/DNA were taken from a different area of the bare mica surface.

5.7.2 Effect of bilayer structure on the transfection activity

In the series of polyamines tested in this study, the low molecular weight polyamines were found to be more effective gene carriers when these conjugates were assembled into PCLs. The transfection activity of the PCL was ~3 times larger than as the corresponding micellar aggregate (Figure 4). The effect of the helper lipid, DOPE, was clearly substantial when compared with DPPC used instead of DOPE. DOPE, a predominantly non-lamellar lipid, is thought to facilitate fusion and destabilization of the endosomal membrane after uptake of cationic lipid/DNA complexes into a cell. In our previous report, we described intercellular trafficking of PCL (composed of cetyl-PEI and DOPE)-DNA complexes, which were taken up into cells by endosomal pathway (Sugiyama et al., 2004), followed by endosomal escape. In fact, transfection activity of the present PCLs was inhibited by nigericin, which is able to dissipate the pH gradient across the endosomal membranes, by 30-50%, suggesting that endosomal pathway is likely involved in the mechanism in the present lipoplex system. It appears therefore, that the mechanism of the lipofection by the compounds in this study may be similar to that of this and other agents known to be enhanced by DOPE. The lipoplexes made from the bilayer-structured PCLs evidently involve lamellar assemblies, given that AFM images reveal the presence of step-like profiles ((ii) and (iii) in Figure 6). The step-like profiles imply a lamellar complex, in which DNA rods (2 nm in diameter) are laminated between bilayers (4 nm thickness). Such an intrinsic bilayer structure may predispose lipoplexes to interact with cell and endosomal membranes. This is not the case for micellar aggregates, whose morphology is large spheres, in which polyamine conjugate and DNA molecules likely aggregate randomly (Table 2 entry 5). This may be one of the reasons for the higher activity of PCL-based lipoplex, whose size is more favorable to transfection.

The linear dependence of activity on N/P (Figure 5B) is related to the morphology of the lipoplex. The electrophoresis experiment and AFM images (Figures 6A-D) suggest a reasonable explanation of the dependence, namely, the following: In the low N/P range (~5), the PCLs inadequately condense DNA molecules, giving the bead-like structures (Figures 6A and B). The DNA molecules loosely packed in the complex are readily released during electrophoresis. Such a complex, whose ζ-potential is negative, is too large to be introduced into the cell membrane via endocytosis; therefore the transfection level is low. With increasing N/P ratio, the morphology of the lipoplex transforms from large bead-like structure into smaller particles, wherein DNA molecules are condensed more tightly (Figures 6C and D). The size of the lipoplexes, whose ζ-potential is positive, is 150–400 nm, is more favorable for cellular uptake via endocytosis (Koynova, Wang & MacDonald, 2006). Given that the lamellar assembly in the lipoplex is responsible for its effectiveness as a gene carrier (Koltover et al., 1998; Koynova, Wang & MacDonald, 2006), the population of active species for gene transfer would increase with increasing in the N/P. Although highly positive-charged carriers are generally toxic, the PCL described here exhibit low cytotoxicity, an advantage for in vitro and in vivo applications.

5.7.3 Disassembly of the lipoplexes and DNA release

When the **DCP-spd**(PCL)/DNA and **DCP-spm**(PCL)/DNA lipoplexes (N/P = 24) were incubated in acidic solution (down to pH 4), the particle sizes measured by DLS became significantly larger and exhibited broad distributions (Table 2, entries 6 and 12). AFM imaging revealed morphological transformation of the PCL/DNA complexes upon acidification. When the dispersion of **DCP-spd**(PCL)/DNA lipoplexes (N/P = 24) was acidified at pH 4 for 1 h by addition of acetic acid, deformed structures were observed on bare mica (Figure 7A). Relative to the original structure (Figure 6C), the complex is decisively deformed by the acid treatment. Although some of flat-topped sphere complexes remain, the predominant morphology is particles connected with strings. The height of the clusters is 25–53 nm and they are connected with string portions that are 6–10 nm high. When the acid-treated complex solution was put on PLL-mica, additional deformed objects appeared on the surface (Figure 7B). A "beads on a string" deformed structure is composed of very small particles (50~100 nm in diameter) and string parts (~70 nm in width and 2–5 nm in height). The beads on a string structure observed on the positively charged surface must consist of DNA-rich fragments associated with some lipid components. The **DCP-spm**(PCL)/DNA lipoplex maintains its spherical structure on bare mica (Figure 7C). On the PLL-mica, on the other hand, deformed structures were observed as in the case of **DCP-spd**(PCL)/DNA lipoplex (Figure 7D). Such morphological changes upon acidification result from disassembly of the lipoplexes and the accompanying DNA release. Gel electrophoretic analysis provided evidence for the DNA release; the released plasmid band increased with the acidification from pH 8 to pH 4. In sharp contrast, such a morphological change was not observed for the micellar aggregate **DCP-spd**. DLS analysis indicates an insensitivity of the micellar aggregates to acidification (Table 2, entries 6 and 12).

Facile escape from the acidic endosomal compartment is necessary for efficient gene transfer. Disassembly of the lipoplex associated with DNA release has been clearly observed by AFM imaging (Figure 7) and by electrophoretic analyses. Upon acidification (down to pH4), the extent of protonation of the polyamine portion is increased. Assuming that the lipoplex forms smectic lamella, electrostatic repulsion between layers must be increased with such protonation, resulting in the disruption of the lipoplex. For lipoplexes composed of **DCP-spd**(PCL) and **DCP-spm**(PCL), disruption accompanying DNA release has been confirmed. In sharp contrast, the size and shape of micellar aggregate/DNA complexes composed of **DCP-spd** and **DCP-spm** are insensitive to acidification (Table 2, entries 6 and 12). This would be due to their amorphous structure, which does not respond to pH change. Thus, the disassembly of the lipoplex composed of the bilayer-structured PCL is essential in effective gene transfer, especially in the process of endosomal escape, where lipid exchange and flip-flop are involved in disrupting the membrane and leading to DNA release (Xu & Szoka, 1996). Although the acidity of this experimental condition (pH4) seems higher than that in endosome (pH5.5), such a protonation process on the polyamines should be involved in the endosomal environment, because the protonation on the polyamines whose pKa values are > 8 may proceed rather gradually in the acidic region, especially in the self-assembled lamellar structure, where polyamines are densely packed. This finding suggests a strategy for molecular design—especially in the polyamine portion—in which a morphological transformation of lipoplexes is taken advantage of for new nonviral transfection strategies.

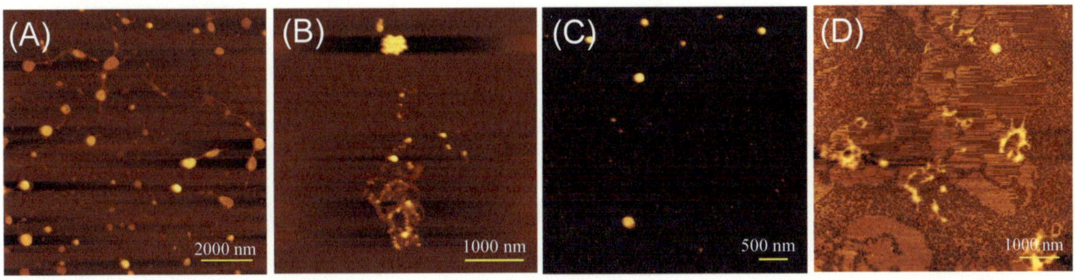

Fig. 7. AFM images of disassembled lipoplexes, **DCP-spd**(PCL)/DNA (A and B) and **DCP-spm**(PCL)/DNA (C and D) by acidification at pH 4. The acid-treated suspensions of complexes were put on bare mica (A, C) and PLL-mica (B and D). After removal of the solution the images were acquired. Scale bars: 2000 nm (A), 1000 nm (B), 500 nm (C), 1000 nm (D).

6. Cleavable peptide-phospholipid conjugates under physiological conditions

Detachable conjugates between cationic and hydrophobic lipid portions may facilitate the DNA release from complexes in intracellular reductive environment. This is a promising strategy for improvement of efficacy of non-viral gene delivery. Such approaches have been reported using disulfide-linked polymer (Oba et al., 2008) and gemini lipids (Behr). Recently, we have successfully synthesized oligo-arginine bearing phospholipids via disulfide linkage, DPPE-SS-R_n (Scheme 2). Oligo-arginines, e.g., TAT peptide, are well known for effective carriers across cell membranes (Futaki et al., 2001). The reaction scheme is shown in Scheme 2. In brief, 1,2-dipalmitoyl-*sn*-glycero-3-phospho-ethanolamine (DPPE) was reacted with a heterobifunctional coupling agent, *N*-succinimidyl-3-(2-pyridyldithio)-propionate

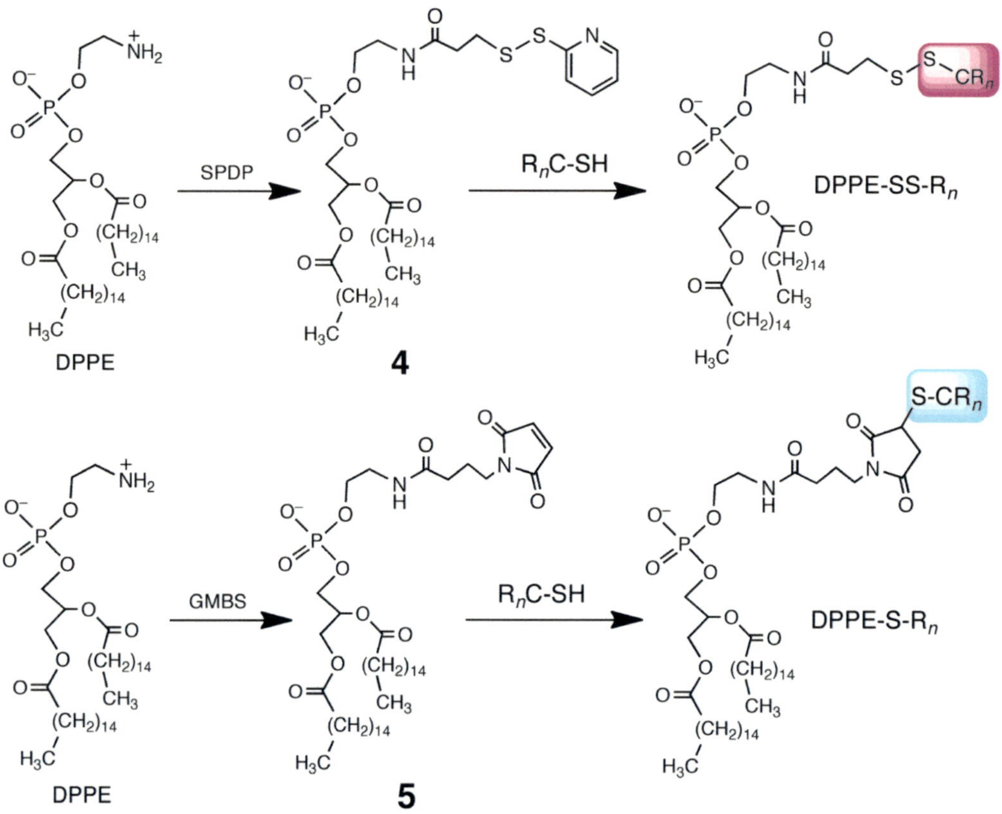

Scheme 2. Synthetic strategy for peptide-phospholipid conjugates

(SPDP) to form compound **4**, followed by coupling with oligopeptides, $(Arg)_nCys$ (R_nC; n = 5, 8). Undetachable type of analogous conjugates (DPPE-S-R_n) were also synthesized with a coupling agent, *N*-(4-maleimidobutyroxy)succinimide (GMBS) and DPPE to form compound **5**, followed by coupling with $(Arg)_nCys$. When the disulfide-type conjugates were applied to gene delivery assay in vitro, 3-5 times higher trasnfection activity was observed compared with the corresponding undetachable conjugates. This result suggests that such a cleavable type of peptide-phospholipid conjugate is one of promising components to assemble effective non-viral vectors.

7. Conclusions

We described herein that PCL composed of the low-molecular-weight polyamine conjugates, DCP-spermidine (**DCP-spd**) and DCP-spermine (**DCP-spm**), exhibit much higher gene transfer activity than PEI(1800) conjugate-based **DCP-PEI**(PCL). The former compounds generate 150–400 nm diameter lipoplexes whereas the latter gives rise to large aggregates. In the case of the former compounds, AFM images clearly reveal a morphological change upon acidification, indicating DNA release from the lipoplexes, whereas, in contrast, the morphology of micellar aggregates is insensitive to pH change. A pH-dependent transformation is crucial in gene transfer; and the chemical structure of the polyamine portion may therefore play an important role in the acidification-induced transformation. We have also described the relation between the N/P-dependence of transfection activity and the morphology of the lipoplexes as revealed by AFM. Morphological study with AFM provided useful information for understanding the basis of lipoplexes with superior activity and for design strategies leading to optimally efficient gene carriers. Our recent efforts have demonstrated that such a DCP-polyaimie-based liposomes are effective for systemic siRNA delivery (Asai et al., 2001).

8. Acknowledgments

The authors thank Dr. Robert C. MacDonald for helpful comments and discussion. The present work was supported by "Grant-in-Aid for Scientific Research on Innovative Areas 2006 (Molecular Science of Fluctuations towards Biological Functions)" (201107510, 23107713) from the Ministry of Education, Culture, Sports, Science and Technology (MEXT) of the Japanese Government.

9. References

Anderson, D. G., Lynn, D. M. & Lange, R. (2003) Semi-automated synthesis and screening of a large library of degradable cationic polymers for gene delivery. *Angew. Chem. Int. Ed.* 42, 3153–3158.

Aoyama, Y., Kanamori, T., Nakai, T., Sasaki, T., Horiuchi, S., Sando, S. & Niidome, T. (2003) Artificial viruses and their application to gene delivery. Size-controlled gene coating with glycocluster nanoparticles. *J. Am. Chem. Soc.* 125, 3455–3457.

Asai, T., Matsushita, S., Kenjo, E., Tsuzuku, T., Yonenaga, N., Koide, H., Hatanaka, K., Dewa, T., Nango, M., Maeda, N., Kikuchi, H. & Oku, N. (2011). Dicetyl Phosphate-Tetraethylenepentamine-Based Liposomes for Systemic siRNA Delivery. *Bioconjugate Chem.* 22, 429–435.

Behr, J.-P., Demeneix, B., Loeffler, J. P. & Perez-Mutul, J. (1989) Efficient gene transfer into mammalian primary endocrine cells with lipopolyamine-coated DNA. *Proc. Natl. Acad. Sci. U.S.A.* 86, 6982–6986.

Bell, P. C., Bergsma, M., Dolbnya, I. P., Bras, W., Stuart, M. C. A., Rowan, A. E., Feiters, M. C. & Engberts, J. B. F. N. (2003) Transfection mediated by gemini surfactants: Engineered escape from the endosomal compartment. *J. Am. Chem. Soc.* 125, 1551–1558.

Boussif, O., Lezoulch, F., Zanta, M. A., Mergny, M. D., Scherman, D., Demeneix, B. & Behr, J.-P. (1995) A Versatile vector for gene and oligonucleotide transfer into cells in culture and in vivo: Polyethylenimine. *Proc. Natl. Acad. Sci. U.S.A.* 92, 7297–7301.

Byk, G., Dubertret, C., Escriou, V., Frederic, M., Jaslin, G., Rangara, R., Pitard, B., Crouzet, J., Wils, P., Schwartz, B. & Scherman, D. (1998) Synthesis, activity, and structure-activity relationship studies of novel cationic lipids for DNA transfer. *J. Med. Chem.* 41, 224–235.

Chittimalla, C., Zammut-Italiano, L., Zuber, G. & Jean-Paul Behr, J.-P. (2005). Monomolecular DNA Nanoparticles for Intravenous Delivery of Genes. *J. Am. Chem. Soc.*, 127, 11436-11441.

Cullis, P. M., Kaye, A. D. & Trippett, S. (1987). On the mechanism of reaction of activated phospholyl compounds with phosphoryl anions: a reassessment of the role of dioxadiphosphetanes. *J. Chem. Soc., Chem. Commun.* 1464 - 1466.

Ewert, K., Ahmad, A., Evans, H. M., Schmidt, H.-W., and Safinya, C. R. (2002) Efficient synthesis and cell-transfection properties of a new multivalent cationic lipid for nonviral gene delivery. *J. Med. Chem. 45*, 5023–5029.

Ewert, K. K., Evans, H. M., Zidovska, A., Bouxsein, N. F., Ahmad, A. & Safinya, C. R. (2006) A columnar phase of dendritic lipid-based cationic liposome-DNA complexes for gene delivery: Hexagonally ordered cylindrical micelles embedded in a DNA honeycomb lattice. *J. Am. Chem. Soc.* 128, 3998–4006.

Dauty, E., Remy, J.-S., Blessing, T. & Behr, J.-P. (2001) Dimerizable cationic detergents with a low cmc condense plasmid DNA into nanometric particles and transfect cells in culture. *J. Am. Chem. Soc.* 123, 9227–9234.

Dewa, T., Ieda, Y., Morita, K., Wang, L., MacDonald, R. C., Iida, K., Yamashita, K., Oku, N. & Nango, M. (2004a). Novel polyamine–dialkyl phosphate conjugates for gene carriers. Facile synthetic route via an unprecedented dialkyl phosphate. *Bioconjugate Chem.* 15, 824–830.

Dewa, T., Ieda, Y., Morita, K., Yoshida, K., Wang, L., MacDonald, R. C., Iida, K., Yamashita, K., Oku, N. & Nango, M. (2004b). Novel Polycationic phospholipid Conjugates for Gene Carriers. *Kobunshi Ronbunshu*, 61, 634-639.

Dewa, T., Asai, T., Tsunoda, Y., Kato, K., Baba, D., Uchida, M., Sumino, A., Niwata, K., Umemoto, T., Iida, K., Oku, N. & Nango, M. (2010). Liposomal Polyamine-Dialkyl Phosphate Conjugates as Effective Gene Carriers: Chemical Structure, Morphology, and Gene Transfer Activity. *Bioconjugate Chem.* 21, 844–852.

Felgner, P. L., Gadek, T. R., Holm, M., Roman, R., Chan, H. W., Wenz, M., Northrop, J. P., Ringold, G. M. & Danielsen, M. (1987) Lipofection: A highly efficient, lipid-mediated DNA-transfection procedure. *Proc. Natl. Acad. Sci. U.S.A.* 84, 7413–7417.

Felgner, P. L. & Ringold, G. M. (1989) Cationic liposome-mediated transfection. *Nature* 337, 387–388.

Felgner, J. H., Kumar, R., Sridhar, C. N., Wheeler, C. J., Tsai, Y. J., Border, R., Ramsey, P., Martin, M. & Felgner, P. L. (1994). Enhanced gene delivery and mechanism studies with a novel series of cationic lipid formulations. *J. Biol. Chem.* 269, 2550–2561.

Futaki, S., Suzuki, T., Ohashi, W., Yagami, T.,Tanaka, S., Ueda, K. & Sugiura, Y. (2001). Arginine-rich Peptides. An Abundant Source of Membrane-permeable Peptides Having Potential as Carriers for Intracellular Protein delivery. *J. Biol. Chem.* 276, 5836–5840.

Gall, T. L., Loizeau, D., Picquet, E., Carmoy, N., Yaouanc, J.-J., Burel-Deschamps, L., Delépine, P., Giamarchi, P., Paul-Alain Jaffrées, P.-A., Lehn, P. & Montier, T. (2010). A Novel Cationic Lipophosphoramide with Diunsaturated Lipid Chains:

Synthesis, Physicochemical Properties, and Transfection Activities. *J. Med. Chem.* 53, 1496–1508.

Geall, A. J., Eaton, M. A. W., Baker, T., Catterall, C. & Blagbrough, I. S. (1999) The regiochemical distribution of positive charges along cholesterol polyamine carbamates plays significant roles in modulating DNA binding affinity and lipofection. *FEBS Lett.* 459, 337–342.

Guillot-Nieckowski, M., Joester, D., Stöhr, M., Losson, M., Adrian, M., Wagner, B., Kansy, M., Heinzelmann, H., Pugin, R., Diederich, F. & Gallani, J.-L. (2007) Self-assembly, DNA complexation, and pH response of amphiphilic dendrimers for gene transfection. *Langmuir* 23, 737–746.

Haensler, J.& Szoka, Jr. F. C. (1993) Polyamidoamine cascade polymers mediate efficient transfection of cells in culture. *Bioconjugate Chem.* 4, 372–379.

Kay, M. A., Liu, D. & Hoogerbrugge, P. M. (1997). Gene Therapy. *Proc. Natl. Acad. Sci. U.S.A.* 94, 12744–12746.

Kogure, K., Akita, H., Yamada, Y., and Harashima, H. (2008) Multifunctional envelope-type nano device (MEND) as a non-viral gene delivery system. *Adv. Drug Deliv. Rev.* 60, 559–571.

Koide, A., Kishimura, A., Osada, K., Jang, W.-D., Yamasaki, Y., Kataoka, K., Harada, A. & Nagasaki, Y. (2006) Semipermeable polymer vesicle (PICsome) self-assembled in aqueous medium from a pair of oppositely charged block copolymers: Physiologically stable micro-/nanocontainers of water-soluble macromolecules. *J. Am. Chem. Soc.* 128, 5988–5989.

Koltover, I., Salditt, T., Rädler, J. O. & Safinya, C. R. (1998) An inverted hexagonal phase of cationic liposome-DNA complexes related to DNA release and delivery. *Science, 281,* 78–81.

Koynova, R., Wang, L. & MacDonald, R. C. (2006) An intracellular lamellar-nonlamellar phase transition rationalizes the superior performance of some cationic lipid transfection agents. *Proc. Natl. Acad. Sci. U.S.A.* 103, 14373–14378.

Lasic, D. D. (1997) *Liposomes in Gene Derivary,* CRC Press, New York.

Li, S. & Huang, L. (2000) Nonviral gene therapy: promises and challenges, *Gene Therapy* 7, 31–34.

MacDonald, R.C., Ashley, G. W., Shida, M. M., Rakhmanova, V. A., Tarahovsky, Y. S., Pantazatos, D. P., Kennedy, M. T., Pozharski, E. V., Baker, K. A., Jones, R. D., Rosenzweig, H. S., Choi, K. L., Qiu, R. & McIntosh, T. J. (1999). Physical and biological properties of cationic triesters of phosphatidylcholine. *Biophys. J.* 77, 2612 - 2629.

Manickam D. S. & Oupicky, D. (2006) Multiblock reducible copolypeptides containing histidine-rich and nuclear localization sequences for gene delivery. *Bioconjugate Chem.* 17, 1395–1403.

Matsui, K., Sando, S., Sera, T., Aoyama, Y., Sasaki, Y., Komatsu, T., Terashima, T. & Kikuchi, J. (2006) Cerasome as an Infusible, cell-friendly, and serum-compatible transfection agent in a viral size. *J. Am. Chem. Soc.* 128, 3114–3115.

Matsuura, M., Yamazaki, Y., Sugiyama, M., Kondo, M., Ori, H., Nango, M. & Oku, N. (2003) Polycation liposome-mediated gene transfer in vivo. *Biochim. Biophys. Acta* 1612, 136 - 143.

McGregor, C., Perrin, C., Monck, M., Camilleri, P. & Kirby, A. J. (2001) Rational approaches to the design of cationic gemini surfactants for gene delivery. *J. Am. Chem. Soc.* 123, 6215–6220.

Meyer, O., Kirpotin, D., Hong, K., Sternberg, B., Park, J. W., Woodle, M. C. & Papahadjopoulos, D. (1998) Cationic liposomes coated with polyethylene glycol as carriers for oligonucleotides. *J. Biol. Chem.* 273, 15621–15627.

Miller, A. D. (1998) Cationic liposomes for gene therapy. *Angew. Chem. Int. Ed.* 37, 1768–1785.

Mintzer, M. A. & Simanek, E. E. (2009) Nonviral vectors for gene delivery. *Chem. Rev. 109,* 259–302.

Miyata, K., Kakizawa, Y., Nishiyama, N., Harada, A., Yamasaki, Y., Koyama, H. & Kataoka, K. (2004) Block catiomer polyplexes with regulated densities of charge and disulfide cross-linking directed to enhance gene expression. *J. Am. Chem. Soc.* 126, 2355–2361.

Mustapa, M. F. M., Bell, P. C., Hurley, C. A., Nicol, A., Guénin, E., Sarkar, S., Writer, M. J., Barker, S. E., Wong, J. B., Pilkington-Miksa, M. A., Papahadjopoulos-Sternberg, B., Shamlou, P. A., Hailes, H. C., Hart, S. L., Zicha, D. & Tabor, A. B. (2007) Biophysical characterization of an integrin-targeted lipopolyplex gene delivery vector. *Biochemistry* 46, 12930–12944.

Mustapa, M. F. M., Grosse, S., M., Kudsiova, L., Elbs, M., Raiber, E.-A., Wong, J. B., Brain, A. P. R., Armer, H. E. J., Warley, A., Keppler, M., Ng, T., Lawrence, M. J., Hart, S. L., Hailes, H. C., and Tabor, A. B. (2009) Stabilized integrin-targeting ternary LPD (Lipopolyplex) vectors for gene delivery designed to disassemble within the target cell. *Bioconjugate Chem. 20,* 518–532.

Oba, M., Aoyagi, K., Miyata, K., Matsumoto, Y., Itaka, K., Nishiyama, N., Yamasaki, Y., Koyama, H. & Kataoka, K. (2008). Polyplex Micelles with Cyclic RGD Peptide Ligands and Disulfide Cross-Links Directing to the Enhanced Transfection via Controlled Intracellular Trafficking *Mol. Pharmacuetics* 5, 1080–1092.

Oberle, V., Bakowsky, U., Zuhorn, I. S. & Hoekstra, D. (2000). Lipoplex formation under equilibrium conditions reveals a three-step mechanism. *Biophys. J. 79,* 1447–1454.

Oku, N., Yamazaki, M., Matsuura, M., Sugiyama, M., Hasegawa, M. & Nango, M. (2001) A novel non-viral gene transfer system, polycation liposomes. *Adv. Drug Deliv. Rev.* 52, 209 - 218.

Oupicky, D., Parker, A. L. & Seymour, L. W. (2002) Laterally stabilized complexes of DNA with linear reducible polycations: Strategy for triggered intracellular activation of DNA delivery vectors. *J. Am. Chem. Soc.* 124, 8–9.

Petersen, H., Fechner, P. M., Martin, A. L., Kunath, K., Stolnik, S., Roberts, C. J., Fischer, D., Davies, M. C. & Kissel, T. (2002) Polyethylenimine-graft-poly(ethylene glycol) copolymers: influence of copolymer block structure on DNA complexation and biological activities as gene delivery system. *Bioconjugate Chem.* 13, 845–854.

Remy, J.-S., Sirlin, C., Vierling, P. & Behr, J.-P. (1994) Gene transfer with a series of lipophilic DNA-binding molecules. *Bioconjugate Chem.* 5, 647–654.

Russ, V., Elfberg, H., Thoma, C., Kloeckner, J., Ogris, M. & Wagner, E. (2008) Novel degradable oligoethylenimine acrylate ester-based pseudodendrimers for in vitro and in vivo gene transfer. *Gene Therapy* 15, 18–29.

Shim, M. S. & Kwon, Y. J. (2009) Acid-responsive linear polyethylenimine for efficient, specific, and biocompatible siRNA delivery. *Bioconjugate Chem.* 20, 488–499.

Sugiyama, M., Matsuura, M., Takeuchi, Y., Kosaka, J., Nango, M. & Oku N. (2004) Possible mechanism of polycation liposome (PCL)-mediated gene transfer. *Biochim. Biophys. Acta* 1660, 24 - 30.

Takahashi, T., Hirose, J., Kojima, C., Harada, A. & Kono, K. (2007) Synthesis of poly(amidoamine) dendron-bearing lipids with poly(ethylene glycol) grafts and their use for stabilization of nonviral gene vectors. *Bioconjugate Chem.* 18, 1163–1169.

Tanaka, T., Sakata, T., Fujimoto, K. & Ikehara, M. (1987). Synthesis of oligonucleotide with aliphatic amino or phosphate group at the 5′ end by the phosphotriester method on a polystyrene support. *Nucleic Acids Res.* 15, 6209 - 6224.

Tarahovsky, Y. S., Koynova, R. & MacDonald, R. C. (2004) DNA release from lipoplexes by anionic lipids: Correlation with lipid mesomorphism, interfacial curvature, and membrane fusion. *Biophys. J.* 87, 1054–1064.

Uragami, M., Miyake, Y. & Regen, S. L. (2000). Influence of headgroup chirality on the mixing behavior of phosphatidylglycerol mimics in fluid bilayers. *Langmuir* 16, 3491 - 3496.

Varga, C. M., Wickham, T. J. & Lauffenburger, D. A. (2000) Receptor-mediated targeting of gene delivery vectors: Insights from molecular mechanisms for improved vehicle design. *Biotechnol. Bioeng.* 70, 593–605.

Wan, L., Manickam, D. S., Oupicky, D. & Mao, G. (2008) DNA release dynamics from reducible polyplexes by atomic force microscopy. *Langmuir* 24, 12474–12482.

Wrobel, I. & Collins, D. (1995) Fusion of cationic liposomes with mammalian cells occurs after endocytosis. *Biochim. Biophys. Acta* 1235, 296 - 304.

Wu, J., Lizarzaburu, M. E., Kurth, M. J., Liu, L., Wege, H., Zern, M. A. & Nantz, M. H. (2001) Cationic lipid polymerization as a novel approach for constructing new DNA delivery agents. *Bioconjugate Chem. 12*, 251–257.

Xu, Y. & Szoka, Jr. F. C. (1996) Mechanism of DNA release from cationic liposome/DNA complexes used in cell transfection. *Biochemistry* 35, 5616–5623.

Yamazaki, Y., Nango, M., Matsuura, M., Hasegawa, Y., Hasegawa, M. & Oku, N. (2000) Polyamine liposomes, a novel nonviral gene transfer system, constructed drom cetylated polyethyleninine. *Gene Therapy,* 7, 1148 - 1155.

Yoshikawa, Y., Emi, N., Kanbe, T., Yoshikawa, K. & Saito, H. (1996). Folding and aggregation of DNA chains induced by complexation with lipospermine: formation of a nucleosome-like structure and network assembly. *FEBS Lett.* 396, 71 - 76.

Zanta, M. A., Beleguise-Valladier, P. & Behr, J.-P. (1999) Gene delivery: A single nuclear localization signal peptide is sufficient to carry DNA to the cell nucleus. *Proc. Natl. Acad. Sci. U.S.A.* 96, 91–96.

12

Technological Aspects of Scalable Processes for the Production of Functional Liposomes for Gene Therapy

Julia E. Trevisan[1], Leide P. Cavalcanti[2], Cristiano L. P. Oliveira[3], Lucimara G. de La Torre[1] and Maria Helena A. Santana[1]

[1]*University of Campinas*
[2]*Brazilian Synchrotron Light National Lab*
[3]*University of São Paulo*
Brazil

1. Introduction

The success of gene delivery systems in *in vivo* or *in vitro* applications depends on efficient transfection. Cationic liposomes remain a promising alternative for nonviral DNA carriers, mainly because they protect DNA from interstitial fluids and easily interact with cells (Gregoriadis, 1993; Lasic, 1997). However, in order to be effective in the immunological response, cationic liposomes must be functional and reach their specific target. Stability, reduced toxicity, efficiency in delivering genes to cells, and specific targeting to the nucleus are essential requirements for prophylactic and/or therapeutic performance. In order to achieve these standards, important physico-chemical parameters in liposomes must be controlled, such as the functionality of the lipids, the concentration of the cationic lipid, DNA loading (reflected by the $R_{+/-}$ molar charge ratio), the zeta potential, size, and polydispersity.

Several laboratory experiments have already explored DNA vaccines using cationic lipids. A classical investigation of lipid functionality and composition, as well as the efficiency of cationic liposomes as DNA carriers, was performed by Perrie and colleagues (Perrie & Gregoriadis, 2000; Perrie et al., 2001). The plasmid pRc/CMV HBS encoding the S (small) region of hepatitis B surface antigen was encapsulated in dehydrated-hydrated liposomes composed of egg phosphatidylcholine (EPC, bilayer-forming lipid), 1,2-dioleoyl-3-trimethylammonium-propane (DOTAP, cationic lipid), 1,2-dioleoyl-*sn*-glycero-3-phosphoethanolamine (DOPE, helper lipid) in a 50:25:25 percent molar ratio. The authors demonstrated that the encapsulation process protects the DNA vaccine against incubation with sodium dodecyl sulfate (SDS) due to DNA incorporation inside the liposome lamella (Perrie & Gregoriadis, 2000), and a better immunological response was obtained with cationic liposomes compared to naked DNA.

Concerning size and polydispersity, different authors have reported that nanoparticle size is an important parameter for transfection success (Ma et al., 2007; Ogris et al., 1998; Rejman et al., 2004; Ross & Hui, 1999; Wiewrodt et al., 2002). Indeed, most of the variability in transfection procedures is a consequence of non-viral gene delivery systems with high polydispersity index values. The polydispersity index is related to the width of the particle size distribution. High polydispersity indicates that greater population fractions are out of the optimum size range for cell transfection (Hsieh et al., 2009).

In this sense, a rational design associated with a technological process able to construct functional liposomes efficiently is needed. Otherwise, the technological processes must be scalable in order to guarantee the reproducibility of the formulation when more liposomes have to be produced for pre-clinical and clinical assays before industrial production. In addition, deep understanding of the phenomena involved, as well as the correlation among operational variables and the physico-chemical parameters, allows more precise control of the quality of the final product and a rational optimization of the process. Therefore, process and product must be strongly linked to assure the desired biological performance.

The literature reports valuable results regarding the biological performance of cationic liposomes in vaccination and gene therapy. However, to the best of our knowledge, no study has yet focused on the approach connecting design, product, and production process. We obtained promising immunological responses and a prophylactic effect against tuberculosis (TB) using cationic dehydrated-hydrated liposomes (DRV) complexed to DNA containing the hsp65 gene on the external surface (Rosada et al., 2008). Hsp65 is a heat shock protein from *M. leprae*. The hsp65 gene has been extensively studied and its biological effects evaluated for protection against and the treatment of tuberculosis (de Paula et al., 2007; Silva et al., 2005). Formulations based on the hsp65 gene have been used in different immunization strategies and the evaluation of protection against *M. tuberculosis* challenge (Souza et al., 2008).

We developed a novel and non-toxic formulation of cationic liposomes in which the hsp65 DNA vaccine was entrapped or complexed on the external surface of the cationic DRV. The formulation was used to immunize mice by intramuscular or intranasal routes. A single intranasal dose of the formulation elicited humoral and cellular immune responses that were as strong as those induced by four intramuscular doses of naked DNA in the mouse model of TB. The formulation also allowed a 16-fold reduction in the amount of DNA administered. Moreover, this formulation was demonstrated to be safe, biocompatible, stable, and easy to manufacture at low cost. We think that this strategy can be applied to human vaccination against TB in a single dose or in prime-boost protocols with a tremendous impact on controlling this neglected disease (Rosada et al., 2008).

The net positive surface charge imparted by DOTAP drives electrostatic binding to the cell membrane. The fusogenic properties of phosphatidylethanolamine promote the exchange of lipids with the endosomal membrane and delivery of DNA into the cytoplasm (Xu and Szoka, 1996). Finally, the presence of EPC provides stability to the liposomes, reduces the cytotoxicity of the cationic lipids, and delimits the diameter of liposome construction, which influences macrophage phagocytosis. For the same lipid composition, the complexation of DNA on the surface of liposomes generated more cell accessibility (non-electrostatically bound DNA) to DNA in relation to encapsulated DNA, and controlled antibody production related to DOTAP/DOPE lipoplexes (de la Torre et al., 2009). The liposomes were prepared using Bangham's method (Bangham et al., 1965) and characterized according to size, polydispersity, and zeta potential. DNA loading and availability on the external surface of liposomes were also determined (Rosada et al., 2008).

For the next pre-clinical and clinical assays, a scalable process had to be established in order to evaluate the capability of the system in scale transposition, reproducing the physico-chemical and biological properties of the previously prepared liposomes on a laboratory scale.

In this chapter, we review the top-down and bottom-up approaches for liposome production and DNA complexation aiming at gene vaccines. The technological processes are classified into strategies and the feasibility to scale transposition envisaged. The physico-chemical aspects of the processes and properties of the produced liposomes are correlated, connecting product and process. In addition, we report our experience with a scalable production of previously designed cationic DNA-EPC/DOPE/DOTAP liposomes in a top-down process involving ultra-turrax and microchannel microfluidizer devices for the homogenation and reduction of liposome size.

2. Liposomes: Structure, formation, and characterization

In general, amphiphile molecules, when dispersed in a liquid medium, undergo internal self-organization, generating colloidal aggregates. Liposomes are formed through the aggregation of phospholipid molecules in an aqueous medium. Initially, a plain bilayer structure is formed when the relative volumes between the non-polar and polar parts of the phospholipid molecules are favorable (packing factor is close to 1) for vesiculation in closed structures. The timing of spontaneous self-aggregation is long, and in technological processes this time is reduced by promoting vesiculation via the addition of energy to the system and remotion of the organic solvent or detergent in which the lipids were initially dispersed (Gregoriadis, 1990; Lasic, 1993). Primary aggregation generates unilamellar liposomes, which undergo secondary aggregation, forming multilamellar liposomes (Figure 1).

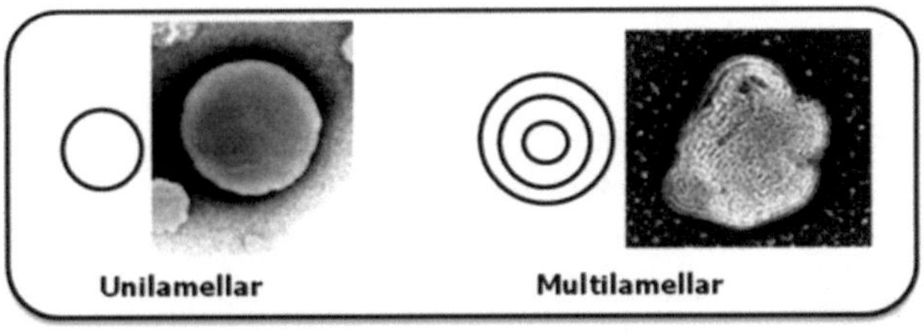

Fig. 1. Unilamellar and multilamellar liposomes.

The main physico-chemical characterization of cationic liposomes for gene vaccines includes average hydrodynamic diameter and size distribution, zeta potential, and morphology. These characterizations have been well described in the modern literature, including techniques, equipment, and the software used for analyzing data.
Regarding the average hydrodynamic diameter and size distribution, photon correlation spectroscopy (PCS) and dynamic laser light scattering using a Ne-He laser are generally used for measurements at various incidence angles. Particle diameter is calculated from the translational diffusion coefficient using the Stokes-Einstein equation:

$$d(H) = (kT)/(3\pi\eta D) \qquad (1)$$

Where d(H) is the hydrodynamic diameter, D is the translational diffusion coefficient, k is Boltzmann's constant, T is the absolute temperature, and η is the viscosity. The mean diameter and size distribution are estimated by an adequate algorithm analysis. The results of the population distributions are expressed as the intensity of scattered light and automatically converted to number-weighted mean diameter and size distribution by adequate software. For more accurate size characterization, intensity and number-weighted

mean diameters are considered. Although the whole range of diameters is shown in the intensity-weighted distribution, the proportionality to the sixth power of particle diameter underestimates small particles, which are only very weakly weighted (Egelhaaf et al., 1996). The corresponding number-weighted distribution converted using the Mie theory is in equivalent proportion to the first power of the diameter and determines the actual number of particles yielding the observed intensity in each size class (Hulst, 1969).
Several structural parameters involved in the process of liposome preparation can be studied and controlled using X-ray techniques. The simple piling of several polar lipid bilayers produces an X-ray diffraction pattern from which one can determine the periodicity, the type of lattice, and an estimate of water molecules in the interface. The colloidal size of self aggregates, such as the dispersion of liposomes, can be characterized by small angle X-ray scattering techniques directly in the liquid buffer media, complementing some indirect microscopy methods (Kratky 1988). Structural phase transition, swelling, crystallization, permeation, nucleation, and other properties will be reflected in a change in the scattering pattern. More than a few dimensions in polar lipid/water systems, such as, lattice periodicity and arrangement, aggregate size, and defects, are on the order of magnitude of the X-ray wavelength, a few Angstroms. The bigger the particle (up to a few hundred Angstroms), the smaller the scattering angle. The terms small angle X-ray scattering (SAXS) and wide angle X-ray scattering (WAXS) are applied. X-ray diffraction is a particular case of scattering for ordered systems.

2.1 Small angle X-ray scattering (SAXS)

Here, we present an outline of the main features of the general X-ray techniques applied specifically to the case of liposome characterization. For better comprehension of the theory of X-ray scattering, the reader may like to consult the works of Glatter (Glatter & Kratky 1982, Glatter 1991) and Kratky (Kratky & Laggner 2001). For the notation, as a convention in the literature, and in order to avoid dependence on wavelength values, the scattering angle is normalized using the following equation:

$$q = |\mathbf{q}| = \frac{4\pi}{\lambda}\sin\theta \qquad (2)$$

Where q is the wave vector, 2θ the scattering angle, and λ the incident wavelength. By using the wave vector instead of angles, one can directly compare experiments performed with different X-ray wavelengths. SAXS is the elastic scattering that occurs when X-rays strike a sample of given material. The electrons of each atom in the sample will re-emit the same energy isotropically. The total scattering amplitude, or amplitude "form factor" F(q), is a sum of all scattered waves in all directions as defined in Equation 3,

$$F(\vec{q}) = \int \rho(\vec{r}) e^{-i\vec{q}\cdot\vec{r}} d\vec{r} \qquad (3)$$

Where $\rho(\vec{r}) e^{-i\vec{q}\cdot\vec{r}}$ is the amplitude of the wave scattered by an atom located at position r. The result is a maximum intensity in the direction of the incident beam decreasing smoothly as a function of the scattering angle. The intensity of the scattering will depend directly on the electronic density $\rho(\vec{r})$ of the sample, i.e., the number of electrons per unit of volume. More specifically, for our case, the higher the difference between the electronic densities of the scattering centers of the sample (e.g., liposomes) and the media (e.g., buffer solution), the

higher the total scattering intensity. Lipid/water systems generally contain light atoms (low atomic number) and, consequently, very low electronic density contrast. A way to increase the scattering intensity is to use high flux X-ray sources, such as synchrotrons. The SAXS experiment will give information on the particle/system structure. Usually, the main goal of the SAXS analysis is the determination of the electron density $\rho(\vec{r})$. This is the so called inverse scattering problem since the information is given in reciprocal space. There are several procedures that can be applied to determine $\rho(\vec{r})$. One possible approach is the calculation of a theoretical intensity obtained for an assumed model object and the comparison to the experimental data. The more information one has about the sample, the more consistent the model will be and, consequently, the simpler the SAXS analysis. Nevertheless, some parameters can be determined directly from the scattering curve, for instance, the radius of gyration of a particle, Rg, which is the root mean square of the distances of all electrons from the center of gravity of the particle. The Rg is determined using the Guinier method, which approximates the scattering function to a simple distribution in the limit of very small angles (q~0.01Å^{-1}). A graph plotting ln I(q) versus q^2 in the limit for very low angles might be characterized by a straight line with an angular coefficient proportional to Rg^2.
Considering that the particles are spheres with radius r, it yields:

$$R_g{}^2 = \frac{3}{5} r^2 \tag{4}$$

The two requirements for using Guinier approximation are: the sample should be a monodisperse colloidal system, which implies no interaction between the scattering centers, and the experimental data must have a minimum q such that d<π/q, where d is the maximum particle dimension that can be studied (Glatter 1982). For systems of large unilamellar vesicles in which the dimensions of the particles are not inside the limit of SAXS experiments, other methods, such as visible light scattering, can be used (Glatter 2002). In some cases, determining the cross section distance would be interesting, such as in large unilamellar vesicle systems, where the thickness of the lamellae is inside the limits of the Guinier approximation. In this case, the graph of I(q)q^2 versus q, called the "thickness Guinier plot", is used to determine the radius of gyration of the thickness RT com $RT = T / \sqrt{12}$, were T is the bilayer thickness). Another approach is to obtain the electron density across the thickness of the vesicle, $\rho_t(x)$. The latter approach can be applied both for unilamellar of multilamellar vesicles as will be discussed next.

2.2 X ray diffraction (XRD)

Diffraction can be viewed as a particular case of scattering: Due to the periodicity, d, of the system, the sum or integration of all scattered intensities turns into an interference pattern. In analogy, the function S(q) which is the result of the integration, is called the "structure factor". The scattering curve, or diffraction pattern, presents peaks for certain scattering angles, θ, which can satisfy Bragg's condition (Azaroff 1968):

$$n\lambda = 2d \sin\theta \tag{5}$$

Where λ is the wavelength of the incident X-ray beam and n is the order of diffraction. We can observe a diffraction pattern, for example, in multilamellar lipid vesicles, which have a lipid bilayer periodicity on the order of 50 Å. The determination of the period of the bilayer is useful for characterizing the structural phase of the system and its transitions. If several orders of diffraction are observed, the structure factor function can be reconstructed and the electronic density profile of the lipid bilayer determined (Pachence & Blasie 1991). The incorporation of compounds inside the lipid bilayer can alter the density profile and be controlled (Sato et al. 2009). Also the matrix of acyl chains is a periodic arrangement with distances between chains on the order of 5 Å. The determination of this parameter is helpful for controlling the stability of the liposome. Any change in these distances will be followed by a dislocation of the diffraction peak.

2.3 Simultaneous determination of form factor and structure factor

Some systems present both form factor and structure factor. The scattering intensity from such a system can be written by the following expression:

$$I(q) = c\langle P(q)S(q)\rangle \tag{6}$$

Where c is related to the concentration of particles in the system, $P(q)=|F(q)|^2$ is the intensity form factor of the particles and carries information about particle shape and contrast and S(q) is the system structure factor, which carries information about possible interparticle interactions or arrangements. The brackets "⟨ ⟩" indicate that in the general case these two contributions have to be averaged together in the calculation. For highly anisotropic systems, like vesicles for example, where the transversal dimensions are much larger than the perpendicular dimension, the form factor can be considered as only corresponding to the perpendicular direction (1D function) and equation 6 can be rewritten as,

$$I(q) = \frac{c}{q^2}\langle P(q)S(q)\rangle \tag{7}$$

One usual approach is to use the decoupling approximation and treat the form factor and structure factor separately. For a lamellar system, the structure factor is well described by the MCT theory (Zhang et al. 1994)

$$S(q) = 1 + 2\sum_{n=1}^{N-1}\left(1-\frac{n}{N}\right)\cos(nqd)\; e^{-(d/2\pi)^2 q^2 \eta\gamma}(\pi q)^{-(d/2\pi)^2 q^2 \eta} \tag{8}$$

The average number of coherent scattering bilayers in the stack is denoted as N, γ is Eulers' constant and d the separation between layers. The Caillé parameter η involves both the bending modulus K of lipid bilayers and the bulk modulus B for compression (Caille 1972, Zhang et al. 1994).

$$\eta = \frac{\pi\, k\, T}{2d^2\sqrt{BK}} \tag{9}$$

The description of the form factor can be done in several levels of detail. One of the simplest approximations is to consider a two step model given by (Nallet et al. 1993),

$$P(q) = \frac{4}{q^2}\left\{\Delta\rho_H \sin\left[q(\delta_H+\delta_T)\right] - \Delta\rho_H \sin(q\delta_T) + \Delta\rho_T \sin(q\delta_T)\right\}^2 \tag{10}$$

Where $\Delta\rho_H$ and $\Delta\rho_T$ are respectively the head group and tail group electron density contrasts and δ_H and δ_T are the sizes of the head group and tail group. Following the step model strategy, Glatter and co-workers developed the deconvolution square root method (Glatter & Kratky 1982, Fritz & Glatter 2006) where the electron density is described by several step functions and it is applied a constrained least squares fitting routine to obtain the step heights. Another strategy was proposed by Pabst et.al (Pabst et al. 2000), which models the bilayer using a two Gaussian system: a central Gaussian placed at the origin, which can model the central part of the tail groups, and is known to have negative contrast with respect to a water buffer (when using X-Rays), and a second Gaussian placed at a certain distance Z in such a way that it can model the position of the head group region. This approach and the two step model cannot describe high quality data, principally for high q values (Oliveira et al. Unpublished work). In a recent development, Oliveira and co-workers combined the advantages of the Gaussian description with the stability introduced by the Glatter method, enabling a more flexible and stable model procedure.

In this approach the profile is described by a symmetric sum of several equally spaced Gaussian functions. The amplitude of each Gaussian is smoothened by extra constraints. The constraints are used to ensure the numerical stability of the nonlinear least-square fit. By proper choice of the amplitude of each Gaussian it is possible to build a smooth profile that can describe more accurately the electron density of the bilayer. Usually, 4 Gaussians function are sufficient to describe a bilayer profile satisfactorily. The electron density is defined as

$$\rho(z) = \sum_{n=1}^{4} a_n \left[G_s(z, z_n, \sigma_n) + G_s(z, -z_n, \sigma_n) \right] / (1 + \delta_{i1}) \qquad \begin{matrix} \delta_{i1} = 1, i = 1 \\ \delta_{i1} = 0, i = 2,3,4 \end{matrix} \tag{11}$$

$$G_s(z, z_n, \sigma) = \frac{1}{\sigma\sqrt{2\pi}} \exp\left[-(z - z_n)^2 / 2\sigma^2 \right] \tag{12}$$

and the Kroninger delta function δ_{i1} is used to avoid double counting for the central Gaussian. n is the order of Gaussian used. The profile is defined by the values of the amplitude factors a_n. Given a half bilayer thickness Z the centers of the Gaussians and the standard deviations (σ values) are defined as follows:

$$z_n = (n-1)2\sigma, \qquad \sigma = \frac{Z}{2n_{\max}\sqrt{2\ln 2}} \tag{13}$$

This choice of the centers and standard deviations gives a reasonable overlap between the Gaussian functions enabling the construction of smooth profiles. A typical profile built using equation 11 is shown in the figure 2 (left). One of the advantages of using a Gaussian set of functions for the representation of the profile is that, for the one-dimensional case of centro-symmetric bilayers, the integral in equation 3 has one analytical solution, given by:

$$F(q,n) = \sqrt{2\pi}\sigma \exp\left(-\frac{\sigma^2 q^2}{2} \right) \cos(q\, z_n) \tag{14}$$

The final scattering amplitude is just the addition of all the F(q,n) terms:

$$F(q) = \sum_{n=1}^{4} a_n F(q,n) \tag{15}$$

Regardless the methodology to calculate the form factor, this procedure gives the scattering contribution from the built shape of the electron density profile. For the multilamelar vesicles this profile will be a repeating unit for each vesicle layer. By using the structure factor given from the modified Caillé theory (equation 8), the final scattering intensity is then given by:

$$I_{MLV}(q) = \left(\left|F(q)\right|^2 S_{MCT}(q) + N_{diff} \left|F(q)\right|^2 \right) \tag{16}$$

Where the second term gives rise to a diffusive scattering which might appear from the presence of single bilayers in the sample. Smearing effects, which are a consequence of the collimation of the camera pinholes, wavelength bandwidth, detector resolution, etc, can be taken into account by the use of the resolution function R(⟨q⟩,q), as described in the work of Pedersen (Pedersen et al. 1990). The final expression used to describe the data from multilamellar vesicles is given by:

$$I(q)_{FIT} = Sc_1 \frac{I_{MLV}(\langle q \rangle)}{q^2} + BG \tag{17}$$

Sc_1 is an overall scale factor and BG is a constant background. Both are optimized during data fitting. Using the above mentioned procedure it is possible to perform a full curve fitting, retrieving simultaneously information about the form factor and structure factor. A simulated example and an application to real experimental data are shown in Figure 2(right).

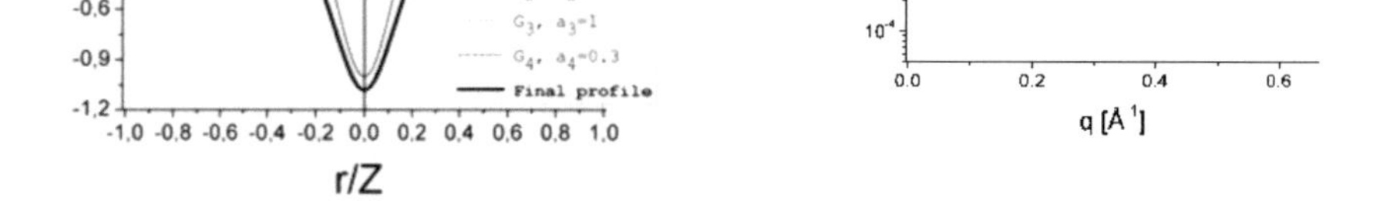

Fig. 2. Left: Construction of the electron density profile using four Gaussians (G1, G2, G3 and G4) with four different amplitudes (-1, -0.3, 1, 0.3). They are shown in four different lines. The final resultant electron density profile from the Gaussian model is shown in solid thick line. Right: Fitting of experimental data using the 4-Gaussians approach. Open circles: experimental data for Egg phosphatidylcholine (EPC) liposome system. Solid curve: Theoretical intensity I(q). Dotted line: structure factors S(q). Dashed line: intensity form factor P(q). The obtained number of layers was N=50, Interplanar distance d=73.5±0.2Å, Caillé parameter of η=0.13±0.01 and bilayer half size of Z=30.00±0.06Å. The obtained electron density profile is shown in the inset.

3. Top-down and bottom-up approaches in processes

In general, the processes for producing nanomaterials can be characterized as two main approaches, top-down or bottom-up. The top-down approach starts with large particles that are comminuted to a nanometric size through the application of high-energy forces. This is the classical approach for the majority of nanoparticle production processes. Top-down approaches require highly precise control of the variables of the process in order to obtain the narrow particle size (Mijatovic et al., 2005). Lithography is the classical example. Other high-energy processes include grinding, high impact homogenization, ultrasound waves, and extrusion through nanoporous membranes (Sanguansri & Augustin, 2006).

Bottom-up approaches are based on the self-organization of molecules under thermodynamic control, generating nanostructures from atoms and molecules as a result of the effects of the chemical, physical, and process interventions on the balance of the intermolecular and intramolecular forces of the system components (Sanguansri & Augustin, 2006). Bottom-up approaches focus on the construction of functional materials, mimetizing the hierarchic organization of the molecules in live organisms, though the science still does not dominate the complex auto-aggregate structures in nature.

Regarding liposome production, top-down approaches comprise the high-energy comminution of a polydispersed population of multilamellar liposomes formed under non-controlled aggregation. The bottom-up approach manipulates the phospholipid molecules in controlled local aggregation in space and time, generating a monodispersed population of nano-sized unilamellar liposomes. Figure 3 illustrates top-down and bottom-up approaches for liposome production.

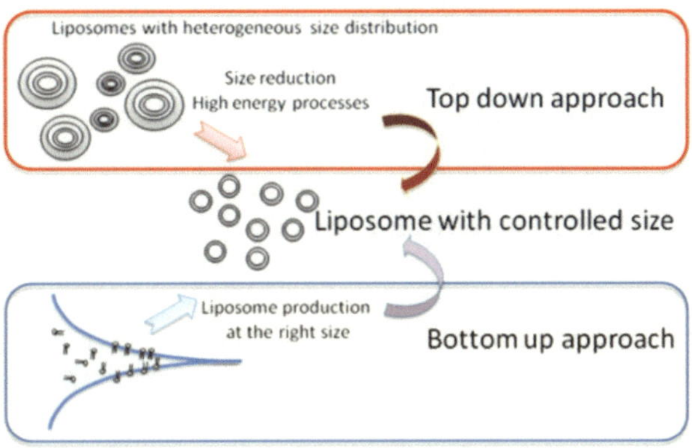

Fig. 3. Scheme of top-down and bottom-up approaches for liposome production.

4. Technological processes

Most of the conventional methods for liposome production require an additional unit operation for size reduction and polydispersity, as they are top-down approaches. In this approach, liposomes are produced from the hydration of a thin film of lipids using Bangham's method (Bangham et al., 1965), multitubular system (Torre et al., 2007; Tournier et al., 1999), detergent depletion or emulsion methods, ether/ethanol injection, and reverse phase evaporation (Lasic, 1993; New, 1990). All of these processes are discontinuous and only the ether/ethanol injection and multitubular system are scalable. Shearing or impact strategies are

the general key for homogenation and reducing liposome size. Mechanical stirring, extrusion through orifices (French press), extrusion through membranes, high-pressure impactor, and microchannel microfluidizer are equipment used in high-energy processes.
Bottom-up processes are low energy processes inspired by biological systems and used for the development of functional nanomaterials, such as supramolecular structures, self-aggregated monolayers, Langmuir-Blodgett films, aggregated peptide nanotubes, and deposited polyelectrolites or proteins in multilayers (Mijatovic et al., 2005; Shimomura & Sawadaishi, 2001).
Microfluidic systems have been the main representatives of bottom-up processing for liposome production in continuous and scaled up processes. Different microfluidic systems can be applied to the production of liposomes and giant liposomes (Ota et al., 2009; Shum et al., 2008; Wagner et al., 2002). DNA complexation on the external surface of liposomes also constitute a promising technology for the production of gene vaccines.

4.1 Microfluidic systems for the production of cationic liposomes

Among different microfluidic geometries, hydrodynamic focusing (HF) is a promising technology and liposomes can be produced in sizes ranging from 50 to 500 nm (Jahn et al., 2004, 2007; Wagner et al., 2002). The HF consists of a device with four-microchannel intersection geometry (Figure 4A). The organic solvent, miscible in water (isopropanol, ethanol), containing dispersed lipids are injected in the middle stream and hydrodynamically compressed by two aqueous (or buffered) streams. The precise upstream flow rates are achieved using syringe pumps that control the position of the focused stream in the downstream channel and, consequently, the process quality parameters (Baldas & Caen, 2010). The use of stereo microscopy is recommended to monitor the process as presented in the schematic representation of the experimental apparatus in Figure 4B. The laminar flow rate allows the formation of a well defined region between the two miscible fluids. The interfacial forces between two miscible solvents (for example, water and isopropanol or water and ethanol) control the convective-diffusive process and liposome self-assembly (Jahn et al., 2010). From the phenomenological point of view, the continuous flow mode allows the continuous diffusion of water and alcohol, reducing lipid solubility, which causes thermodynamic instability and generates liposomes (Jahn et al., 2008). The continuous flow mode also increases productivity.
The HF geometry for liposome production is based on the conventional method of ethanol injection (bulk) adapted for microfluidic systems. Conventional ethanol injection consists of the controlled addition of an ethanol/lipid stream in a tank reactor containing buffered water under controlled agitation. The advantage is the use of ethanol; compared to other organic solvents (e.g., chloroform and methanol), it is less harmful and, depending on the lipid concentration, there may be no need for post-treatment size reduction (Kremer & Esker, 1977). Some of the disadvantages are low lipid concentration in ethanol (higher concentrations require post-treatment for size reduction) and a difficulty achieving reproducibility (Wagner et al., 2002).
The representative parameters for liposome size and polydispersity control in HF are channel geometry (deep and width), volumetric flow buffer/alcohol rate-ratio (FRR), and total volumetric flow rate (buffer+alcohol flow rates). Solvent diffusivity in water is another important parameter (Jahn et al., 2004, 2007, 2010). Basically, the narrower the microchannel width, the smaller the liposome size. For total volumetric flow rate, which promotes flow velocity at the channel, higher FRRs (which corresponds to an increased proportion of buffer

to lipid/solvent flow) correspond to smaller liposome diameter (Janh et al., 2010). However, caution is required in this flow rate analysis as the final alcohol content in the liposome colloidal dispersion can change with FRR and as a consequence of particle size. Alcohol can be used to disrupt liposomes and, at low concentrations, liposome size can be increased due to alcohol incorporation into the bilayer. Precise analysis can be performed if the alcohol is removed after liposome processing. By decreasing the total volumetric flow rate, the residence time can be increased and a lower average vesicle diameter and narrower size distribution obtained. This behavior indicates that if increasing the total volumetric flow rate, the microchannel length must be longer to complete the alcohol diffusion, otherwise large particles will be obtained due to bulk mixing downstream of the channel (Janh et al., 2010).

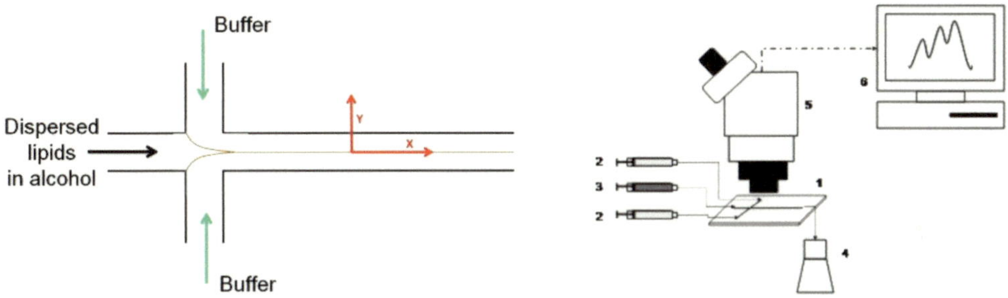

A B

Fig. 4. (A) Schematic representation of hydrodynamic focusing (HF) in a microfluidic device with four-channel intersection geometry. The organic solvent (miscible in water) containing the dispersed lipids is injected in the middle stream and hydrodynamically compressed by two aqueous (or buffered) streams. The flow is in the x direction and alcohol diffusion is in the y direction. (B) Schematic representation of the experimental apparatus for liposome production using HF: (1) microfluidic device; (2) water syringe pumps; (3) syringe pump for lipids/ethanol stream; (4) collector flask; (5) stereo microscopy; (6) computer data acquisition (adapted from Zhang et al., 2008).

The lipid concentration in alcohol is also another important parameter for controlling size. The development of vaccines for *in vivo* applications requires the highest drug-loading capacity. In terms of gene vaccines, the DNA-loading capacity correlates with the cationic lipid content, defined by the molar charge rate ($R_{+/-}$) between the cationic charges (from the cationic lipid) and negative charges (from the DNA). The $R_{+/-}$ and total lipid content are project parameters for scaling up (or scaling out) processes. As an example, the $R_{+/-}$ of the tuberculosis gene vaccine is 10 and the total lipid concentration 64 mM (Rosada et al., 2008). These parameters require cationic liposome production in a high lipid concentration under unusual microfluidic conditions. Aiming to explore the effect of lipid concentration on microfluidic HF processes, we investigated the influence of high lipid content (100 mM) and lipid composition in ethanol (EPC or EPC/DOTAP/DOPE) as a function of average size. We understand that the studied molar concentration is greater than the lipid solubility in ethanol (approximately 4 mM for EPC) (New, 1990) and, in this case, the lipid dispersion offers an additional barrier to ethanol diffusion into water. Based on this assumption, we simulated the required microchannel length for complete ethanol diffusion from a central stream (after HF) as a function of the lipid concentration in the ethanol stream considering the mass continuity equation (according to Figure 4A), without a chemical reaction (Equation 18). This simulation was performed based on a microfluidic glass device produced by the wet photolithographic process. The microchannels were etched with HF solution; upstream channels measured 140 ± 1 μm in width and downstream channels 200 ± 1 μm after the T junction. The microchannel was 50 ± 2 μm deep and the diffusion length 5 cm.

$$\frac{\partial C_E}{\partial t}+\left(v_x\frac{\partial C_E}{\partial x}+v_y\frac{\partial C_E}{\partial y}+v_z\frac{\partial C_E}{\partial z}\right)=D_{EW}\left(\frac{\partial^2 C_E}{\partial x^2}+\frac{\partial^2 C_E}{\partial y^2}+\frac{\partial^2 C_E}{\partial z^2}\right) \quad (18)$$

Where D_{EW} is the ethanol diffusion coefficient in water and C_E is the ethanol concentration. The Cartesian coordinates are used because the microchannel area presents rectangular geometry. Considering laminar flow in x direction and mass transfer along the y direction (Figure 4A), Equation 18 can be adapted for short times according to the Higbie penetration model (Higbie, 1935):

$$N_E=\sqrt{\frac{4.D_{EA}}{\pi.t}}.(C_{E_0}-C_{E\infty}) \quad (19)$$

Where *t* is the quotient between the difference in flow rates (water and ethanol) and distance x. The influence of lipid concentration was considered an additional barrier for ethanol diffusion due to the presence of lipid aggregates dispersed in the ethanol stream. In this case, the ethanol diffusion depends on the concentration gradient through ethanol/water streams, as well as its hydrophobic characteristics, with similar behavior as ethanol diffusion from aqueous solution to a phospholipid bilayer (Galindo-Rodriguez et al., 2004). The hydrophobic characteristics of the lipid can be expressed as the partition coefficient octanol/water ($P_{o/w}$= 0,478). In this context, D_{EW} was corrected by the partition coefficient according to Equation 20.

$$D_{EW}'=0,478*D_{EW} \quad (20)$$

Where D_{EW}' is the effective diffusion coefficient.
Figure 5 presents the simulation of the distance (x) for total ethanol diffusion as a function of ethanol flow rate (at a fixed FRR of 6.26 and 20). Increasing the lipid concentration in the ethanol stream, the distance x to complete ethanol diffusion will increase.

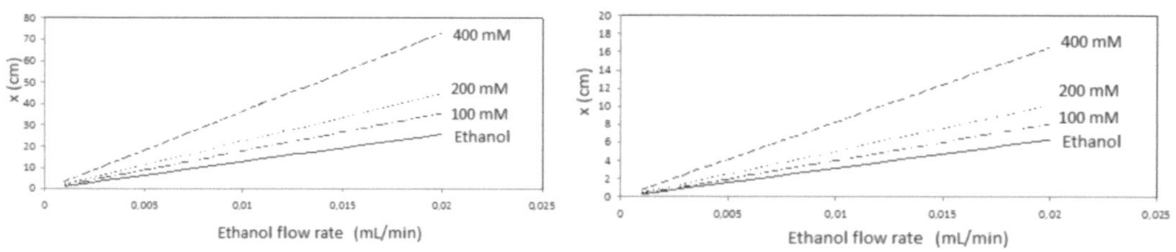

Fig. 5. Simulation of the distance for total ethanol diffusion into the water stream. The lipid (EPC) concentration was considered as an additional barrier to ethanol diffusion. (A) FRR = 6.26. (B) FRR = 20.

According to the simulation, ethanol dispersion requires the lowest length for ethanol diffusion for a lipid concentration of 100 mM (among the simulated concentrations). Experimental evaluations with this lipid concentration were performed at different total flow velocities (total flow rate) and lipid compositions (EPC and EPC/DOTAP/DOPE - cationic liposomes) as presented in Table 1. The average diameter is strongly influenced by the total flow velocity and lipid composition. Decreasing the flow velocity decreases the average size, and this behavior is not dependent on the FRR. This parameter is associated with the residence time inside the microchannel, suggesting that higher residence time is required to control liposome size. Another interesting parameter is the lipid composition. The viscosity of the ethanol dispersion was 1.07 and 1.21 cP for EPC/DOTAP/DOPE and EPC, respectively. Lower viscosity probably offers lower mass transfer resistence, reflecting smaller diameters (and standard deviations) and polydispersity index values. This difference reflected in HF is confirmed by stereomicroscopic observation along the microchannel. A high polydispersity index (Table 1) can also indicate the possibility for further process optimization in terms of flow velocity, FRR, and lipid concentration.

Lipid composition	Total flow velocity (cm/min)	FRR	Z-average (nm)	Polidispersity index
EPC	5.6	6	342.8 ± 134.5	0.427 ± 0.140
	4	7	271.6 ± 37.5	0.408 ± 0.145
EPC/DOTAP/DOPE	8.1	10.6	162.1 ± 88.13	0.606 ± 0.157
	6.1	7.7	92.92 ± 10.14	0.441 ± 0.028

FRR: volumetric flow buffer/alcohol rate-ratio.
Total lipid concentration of 100 mM in ethanol stream.

Table 1. Average liposome size (Z-average) obtained at different lipid compositions and flow rates.

4.2 Microfluidic systems for electrostatic complexation of DNA

The electrostatic interactions between DNA and cationic liposomes produce particles with different sizes and morphology (Mannisto et al., 2002; Oberle et al., 2000) that depend on $R_{+/-}$, buffer ionic strength, order of component addition, reaction conditions, and the type of lipids (Mount et al., 2003; Zelphati et al., 1998). In this context, HF can also be used to control the diffusion process for DNA compaction, producing well organized aggregates. The flow velocity is the major parameter controlling the aggregation process (Dootz et al., 2006).
Otten et al. (2005) investigated the HF microfluidic device to produce cationic liposome-DNA complexes. The DNA solution is introduced in the central stream and the cationic liposome stream introduced at a lateral position. The average liposome size was 200 nm (composed of 1:1 DOTAP and DOPC with a lipid concentration of 25 mg.mL^{-1}), and the DNA was calf thymus (5 mg.mL^{-1}). The flow velocity was 100 mm.s^{-1}, varying with $v_{Liposome} = 13v_{DNA}$ and $v_{Lipossomas} = 130v_{DNA}$, where v is the flow velocity. The authors concluded that the complex is formed in two steps. The first step relates to the formation of a multilamellar complex, followed by the second step in which DNA is organized inside the lamellae. The central stream can be focused according the FRR, and reducing the diffusional length allows faster mixing (Knight et al., 1998).

A micromixer (Jellema et al., 2010) and multi-inlet microfluidic HF (MF) system (Koh et al., 2010) were recently investigated as alternatives for producing the liposome-DNA complexes. These studies point out new and promising alternatives aiming to control the aggregation process between DNA and cationic liposomes.

5. Physico-chemical aspects

The processes that use top-down strategies for liposome production differ according to the remotion of solvent and/or application of shear. The remotion of solvent is carried out by evaporation (Bangham´s method or multitubular system), spray drying or evaporation in reverse phase, sublimation (dehydration–hydration), or solubilization in water by ether/ethanol injection in diluted or concentrated phases. The incomplete remotion of solvent has a direct impact on liposome size.

We have observed that the presence of organic solvent in spray-dried lipid structures generates more amorphous or more crystalline domains due to the packing of lipids in the bilayers (Alves and Santana, 2004). The operational conditions interfere with the drying rate, and mass transfer limitations result in the complete evaporation of ethanol. The higher the evaporation rate, the higher the amount of ethanol remaining inside the particles because a shield of packed lipids close to the surface and more amorphous structures are formed. At a slower rate of evaporation, it is more controlled, generating more crystalline structures. The subsequent hydration of the solid particles with different levels of crystallinity influences the size and polydispersity of the generated liposomes.

Similar mass transfer limitations are present when the organic solvent is removed by diffusion in water. A compromise between the diffusion and vesiculation rates controls particle size. The opposite rates of diffusion and hydration depend on the barrier created by the phospholipids, which is a function of its concentration and depends on the interaction among lipids. In previous studies, we characterized the packing of pseudo-ternary mixed Langmuir monolayers of EPC/DOTAP/DOPE using surface–molecular area curves. The interactions and miscibility behavior were inferred from the curves by calculating the excess free energy of the mixture (ΔG_{Exc}). The deviation from ideal showed dependence on the lipid polar head type and monolayer composition (Rigoletto et al., 2011).

The rates of vesiculation and solvent diffusion are comparable in magnitude only at very low lipid concentrations, generating small liposomes in an excess of water. Under other conditions, the barrier created by the extension of the primary aggregation of lipids delays solvent remotion, generating large multilamellar liposomes. Otherwise, the rate of vesiculation is associated with the hydrophobicity of the non-polar groups. Therefore, the vesiculation rate in the primary aggregate controls liposome size. When cationic lipids are used, such as in the DOTAP/DOPE/EPC system, the electrostatic repulsion among the molecules benefits solvent diffusion and hydration, generating smaller liposomes.

Because of the softness of the primary aggregate and the bilayer fluidity imparted by the phase transition temperature, liposomes are prone to fusion due to the non-ordered Brownian movement of the colloids in the medium, and multilamellar vesicles are generated in a broad range of sizes. The remaining solvent generates polydispersed liposomes, which are more favorable for fusion. However, charged lipids stabilize liposomes. Therefore, mass transfer is critical in discontinuous processing, controlling liposome size and polydispersity.

Despite limitations in mass transfer and interactions, discontinuous processes are still preferable due to the simplicity in carrying out massive liposome production and scaling up

processes. In this context, the development of technologies that promote the production of cationic liposomes with controlled size and low polydispersity index, with low energy consumption and the elimination of organic solvents, is still a challenge.
Continuous processes in microchannels with HF reduce the limitations due to mass transfer in the interface of the primary aggregate, and the continuous operation decreases interactions among particles due to Brownian movement. Therefore, particle size is controlled by the relative flow rates between the phases and by microchannel length.

6. A case study of the production of cationic liposomes and gene vaccines in scalable top-down processing

Although top-down strategies are important and high shear processing has various uses, no systematic studies have been carried out on the effects of liposome comminution on the physico-chemical and surface properties of liposomes. The data in the literature are sparse in regards to the kind of impellers, comminution equipment, or type of lipids used.
Aiming to produce the gene vaccine composed of EPC/DOTAP/DOPE liposomes with DNA complexed on their external surface, we initially studied the significance of the process variables for the properties of liposomes composed of egg lecithin. Mechanical forces were used for homogenation and comminution in Caules type stirrer, Ultra-Turrax, and microchannel microfluidizer equipment. A main variable was selected and its effects on the physico-chemical properties of the liposomes characterized. Finally, a scalable discontinuous process was established and EPC/DOTAP/DOPE liposomes produced and complexed with DNA. The physico-chemical and biological properties of the gene vaccine were compared with our previous gene vaccine prepared using Bangham's method.

6.1 Effects of the process variables on liposome properties

6.1.1 Statistical analysis

We studied the effects of the shear rate using multi-factorial statistical experimental planning (Montgomery 2008) in order to delineate the relative importance and influence of the shear rate and feed flow rate on the mean diameter, polydispersity, zeta potential, and viscosity of egg lecithin liposomes. The liposomes were prepared with high lipid concentration (300 mM), aiming for applications in scaling up processes. Food grade egg lecithin (60% phosphatidylcholine content) from Degussa (GmbH Germany) and ethanol 99-100% from Labsynth ltda. (São Paulo- Brazil) were used as the lipid and solvent, respectively.
Figure 6 shows the experimental outline for liposome preparation. The 300 mM ethanol-lipid suspension in a beacker (1) was fed at a previously defined flow rate through a peristaltic pump (2) into the bottom of a 150 mL beaker with four fins containing pure Milli Q water (3). Continuous mechanical stirring was provided by a Caules type stirrer or Ultra-Turrax® IKA T25 (Ika Works) (4). The final lipid concentration was 50 mM. After the feeding was complete, stirring was maintained for an additional 15 min. Comminution was also carried out in a microchannel microfluidizer (Microfluidizer® M-110P) with 100 mL of a liposome dispersion pre-processed through an Ultra-Turrax® at 5000 to 21000 s^{-1} shear rate and 0.09 to 0.96 $mL.s^{-1}$. The microfluidizer worked in the pressure range of 200 to 1500 bar and for various passages. All liposome dispersions were stored at 8°C for 12 hours before characterization.

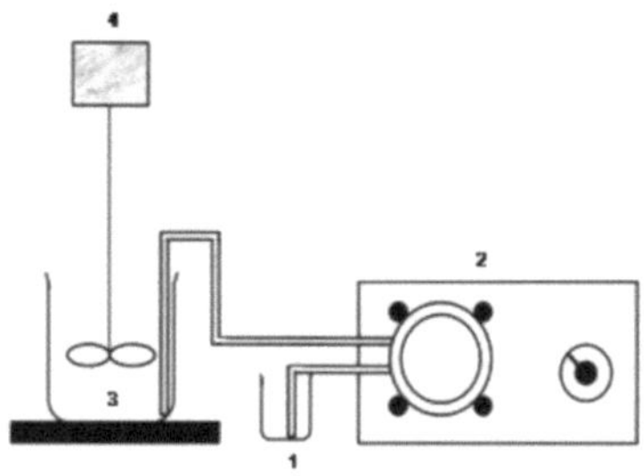

Fig. 6. Scheme of the experimental set-up used for liposome preparation using (A) Ultra-Turrax® or Caules mechanical stirrer. 1) Tank containing the lipid dispersion in ethanol; 2) peristaltic pump; 3) tank with four fins containing (150 mL) water; 4) Ultra-Turrax® or Caules mechanical stirrer. (B) Microchannel microfluidizer system processed the samples from the Ultra-Turrax®.

6.1.2 Significance of shear and feed flow rates

The effects of the shear rate and feed flow rate on the mean diameter, polydispersity, and zeta potential are presented in Table 2 and in terms of the significance of the independent variables and their interaction in the Pareto graphics in Figure 8. For the Caules type stirrer, the effects of shear rate and feed flow rate on the mean diameter of liposomes were not significant (Figure 7A1). The shear rate was significant for polydispersity (Figure 7A2), and both variables were significant for zeta potential (Figure 7A3). The interactions between the variables were not significant for the three response variables.

Table A

Factors	-	0	+
1: Shear rate (s^{-1})	2,860	12,140	21,430
2: Inlet lipid solution flow rate (mL/s)	0.09	0.54	0.96

Experiment	1	2	Diameter (nm)	Polydispersity	Zeta Potential (mV)
1	-1	-1	386.10	0.37	-53.73
2	1	-1	254.73	0.31	-56.33
3	-1	1	550.20	0.58	-53.73
4	1	1	246.50	0.35	-48.57
5	0	0	374.83	0.47	-55.90
6	0	0	359.00	0.36	-54.60
7	0	0	358.90	0.45	-54.40

Table B

Factors	-	0	+
1: Shear rate (s^{-1})	1,000	1,750	2,530
2: Inlet lipid solution flow rate (mL/s)	0.09	0.54	0.96

Experiment	1	2	Diameter (nm)	Polydispersity	Zeta Potential (mV)
1	-1	-1	626.17	0.65	-55.00
2	1	-1	414.87	0.51	-71.27
3	-1	1	616.47	0.68	-57.50
4	1	1	446.77	0.51	-52.60
5	0	0	582.77	0.65	-57.27
6	0	0	642.67	0.58	-55.80
7	0	0	567.40	0.62	-56.00

Table 2. (A,B) Physico-chemical properties of liposomes as a function of the operational variables.

Data obtained using ultra-turrax showed a significant influence of the shear and feed flow rates, as well as their interactions, on the mean diameter and polydispersity (Figure 7B1,B2). However, these variables had no significant effect on the zeta potential (Figure 7B3). The mean diameter was influenced more by shear rate, whereas both shear rate and feed flow rate were significant for polydispersity.

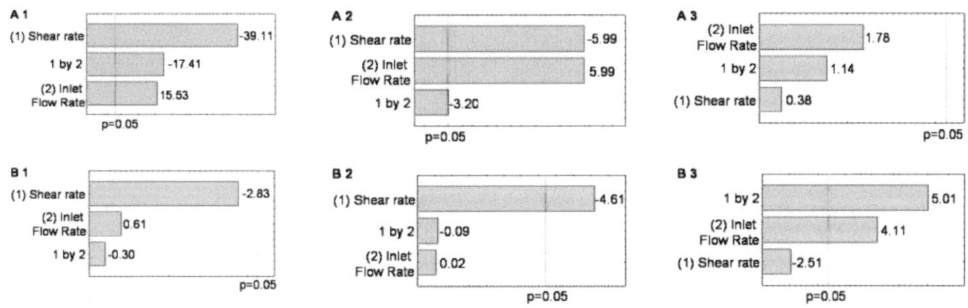

Fig. 7. Pareto´s graphic for liposome production using (A) Caules and (B) Ultra-Turrax® stirrers. (A1,B1) mean diameter hidrodinâmico médio cumulativo, (A2,B2) polydispersity, (A3,B3) zeta potential.

The results show that the shear rate range of the Caules stirrer did not comminute the aggregates less than 600 nm in size, but it destroyed the progressive aggregations, influencing the polydispersity and zeta potential. However, the higher shear rates provided by the ultra-turrax better control phospholipid aggregation, generating smaller liposomes. Control is strongly dependent on the intensity of shear, and sizes in the range of 200 nm were obtained at the superior shear rate limit (21530 s^{-1}) provided by the equipment. Feed flow rate influence mainly occurs at the inferior shear rate limit (2860 s^{-1}). Though the shear rate range for ultra-turrax interferes with primary liposome aggregation, the zeta potential is not influenced. Therefore, for egg lecithin (300 mM concentration) liposomes, the shear rate range between 1000 and 21430 s^{-1} delimits the liposome size from approximately 600 to 200 nm.

6.1.3 Effects of the shear rate on the liposome properties

Mean diameter - Additional data allowed the construction of the curve presented in Figure 8A. The curve shows a clear relationship between liposome comminution and shear rate, with the mean diameter exponentially decaying with applied shear rate. The error bars are higher at lower shear rates due to the poor homogenization of liposomes provided by the lower pumping capabilities of the mechanical systems.

The microchannel microfluidizer, working in the pressure range of 200 to 1500 bars, provided shear rates in the range of 2×10^5 to 6×10^5 s^{-1} .The data from the microchannel microfluidizer were obtained for pre-treated liposomes using Ultra-Turrax at shear and feed flow rates of 5600 to 24000 s^{-1} and 0.09 to 0.96 $mL.s^{-1}$, respectively. The results show that the pre-formed liposomes reached the nanometric range (100 nm) in only one passage using Ultra-Turrax and the high shear rate range of the microchannel microfluidizer.

This comminution behavior agrees with the results reported by Diat et al. (1993a). Through a balance between elastic and viscous forces in the liposomes, the mean diameter is reduced according to the square root of the applied shear rate (Equation 21).

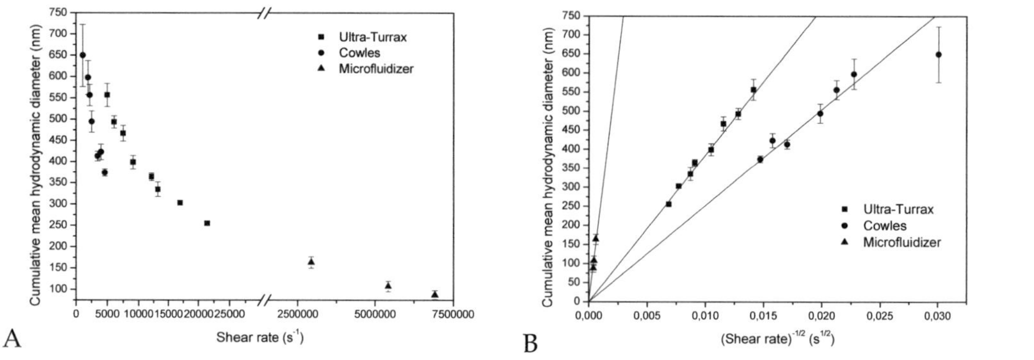

Fig. 8. Cumulative hydrodynamic mean diameter as a function of the shear rate provided by Caules stirrer, Ultra-Turrax®, or microchannel microfluidizer. (A) Z-average values obtained from light scattering measurements. (B) Linear relationship from Equation 21 proposed by Diat et al. (1993a).

$$R = \sqrt{\frac{4.\pi.\left(2.k + \bar{k}\right)}{\mu.d.\dot{\gamma}}} \tag{21}$$

Where R is the liposome radius at equilibrium, k and k are the average and Gaussian elastic constant of the membrane, respectively, μ is the viscosity of the liposome dispersion, $\dot{\gamma}$ is the shear rate, and d is the interlamellar distance. The different slopes for the straight lines in Figure 9B were obtained for the shear rate ranges of the devices used, agreeing with the mass balance between elastic and viscous forces in the liposomes described by Diat et al. (1993b). Higher shear rates produce higher slopes, indicating the presence of liposomes with higher elastic constant, lower viscosity, and shorter interlamellar distance.

6.1.3.1 Viscosity, surface tension, and zeta potential

The shear rate also reduced the viscosity of the liposome dispersion from 5 to 2 mPa, but no significant changes were observed in the surface tension as a consequence of the reduction in size. However, the reduction in size also resulted in rearrangement of the lipids in the external layer, changing the zeta potential from -50 to -40 mV.

6.1.3.2 Lamellar packing

Small angle X-ray scattering (SAXS) characterization showed changes in the interlamellar distances for the applied shear rate ranges (Figure 9). The distance decreased with higher shear rates. The decreasing interlamellar distance was a consequence of the loss of interlamellar water, calculated to be up to 12% for the highest level of shear rate, as well as of lipid packing in the liposome, found to be less than 2%. The water layer is calculated as the difference between the full period and the bilayer thickness (see Table 4). These factors may explain the observed changes in zeta potential and the different slopes of the straight lines obtained for the studied shear rate ranges. In addition to the interlamellar distance and packing, the elasticity of the bilayer may also be influenced by the shear rate and changes in the elastic constants determined. In general, elastic modulus is not the same as stiffness. Elastic modulus is a property of the constituent material, whereas stiffness is a property of the structure. In the case of liposomes, the elastic modulus is an intensive property of the lipids, and stiffness is an extensive property dependent on the structure and packing of the aggregate. Therefore, we associated the changes in the slope of the straight lines in Figure 8B with changes in the elastic constants as a consequence of the changes in packing in the liposomes.

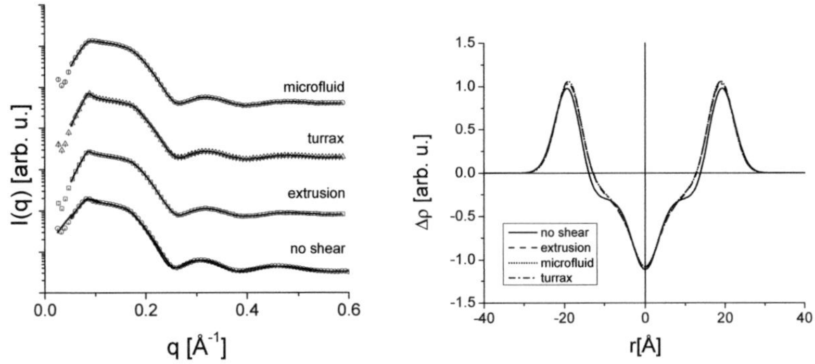

Fig. 9. Left: Small angle X-ray scattering (SAXS) profiles determined for the liposomes treated under moderate shear (extruded through polycarbonate membranes) and high shear produced by Ultra-Turrax® (21430 s^{-1}) and microchannel microfluidizer devices (6 961 000 s^{-1}). Right: Electron density profile across the bilayer obtained from the fitting (see Table 3).

Sample	Period[Å]	Bilayer thickness[Å]	N	η
no shear	76.7±0.2	59,9±0.1	3.2±0.1	0.18±0.02
Extrusion	73.4±0.1	59,3±0.1	3.4±0.1	0.26±0.01
Turrax	72.5±0.2	59,1±0.1	4.1±0.1	0.26±0.01
Microfluid	72.3±0.1	59,2±0.2	2.3±0.1	0.09±0.01

N is the average number of bilayers and η is the Caillé parameter.

Table 3. Structural parameters obtained from full curve modeling of SAXS data.

6.1.3.3 Morphology

Figure 10 presents transmission electronic microscope images of the liposomes under various shear treatments compared to control (Bangham's method).

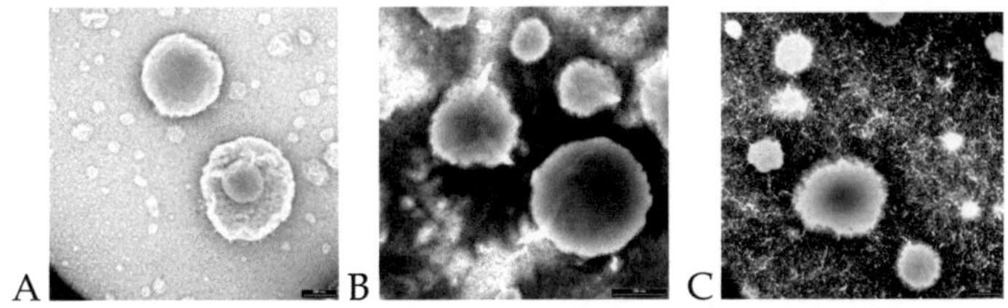

Fig. 10. Transmission electronic microscopy of liposomes obtained using (A) Bangham's method followed by extrusion in membranes, (B) ultra-turrax under a shear rate of 21430 s^{-1}, (C) microchannel microfluidizer under a shear rate 6 961 000 s^{-1}. Bars :200nm

Under low shear, the liposome surface looks thicker (Figure 10A), whereas it looks more packed with ultra-turrax treatment (Figure 10B). However, in both cases the liposome morphology is spherical. Under the highest shear, the morphology of the liposomes was not spherical, and irregularities in the surface reflect stretching of the aggregated structure (Figure 8C). These results reflect the observed change in packing and zeta potential as a consequence of the shear rate.

6.1.4 Scalable top-down process for liposome production

The scalable process described in Figure 11 was established based on these results and validated for the production of EPC/DOPE/DOTAP liposomes. Previous assays (data not shown) validated the changes in the purity of EPC from 99-100% (analytical grade) to 96-98% (commercial grade) and the lipid concentration from 16 mM (used in the Bangham's method) to 64 mM.

The injection of ethanol was used modified for the higher lipid concentration. Lipid concentration in the ethanol phase was previously optimized with an aim to minimize the concentration of ethanol in the liposome formulation, as well as prevent obstructions of the microchannels in the microfluidizer.

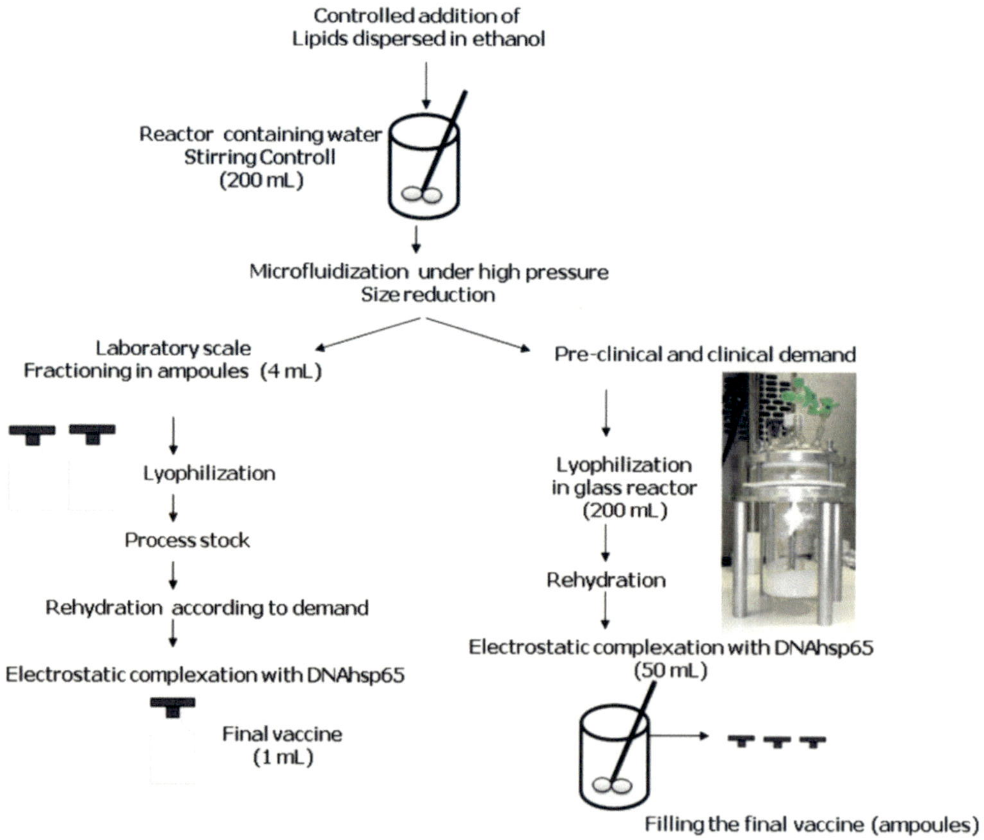

Fig. 11. Schematic diagram of the scalable process for cationic liposome production.

7. Conclusions

The top-down and bottom-up approaches are valuable for liposome production. By understanding the physico-chemical aspects and behavior of variables involved in the process, we can establish a conscious scalable process for liposome production and connect functional liposomes, the performance of the production process, and the final properties of the gene vaccine as a product. The results presented in this chapter open opportunities for the development of new gene or non-gene vaccines in future research using scalable top-down and bottom-up processes.

8. Acknowledgment

The authors acknowledge the University of Campinas, the Brazilian Synchrotron Light National Laboratory, and the financial agencies FAPESP and CNPq in Brazil.

9. References

Alves, G. P., and Santana, M. H. A. (2004) Phospholipid dry powders produced by spray drying processing: Structural, thermodynamic and physical properties, *Powder Technology*, Vol. 145, pp 139-148, ISSN 0032-5910.

Azaroff, L. V. (1968) *Elements of x-ray crystallography*, McGraw Hill Book, New York.

Baldas, L., and Caen, R. (2010) Experimental methods *in: Microfluidics*, Vol. Edited by Stéphane Colin, pp 330-348.

Bangham, A. D., Standish, M. M., and Watkins, J. C. (1965) Diffusion of univalent ions across lamellae of swollen phospholipids, *Journal of Molecular Biology*, Vol. 13, p 238, ISSN 0022-2836.

Caille, A. (1972) *C. R. Seances Acad. Sci. B*, Vol. 274, p 891, ISSN 0249-6313.

Ciccariello, S., and Sobry, R. (1999) Small-angle scattering intensity behaviours of cylindrical, spherical and planar lamellae, *Journal of Applied Crystallography*, Vol. 32, pp 892-901, ISSN 0021-8898.

Cullity, B. D. (1978) *Elements of x ray diffraction*, 2nd ed., Addison Wesley, USA.

de Paula, L., Silva, C. L., Carlos, D., Matias-Peres, C., Sorgi, C. A., Soares, E. G., Souza, P. R., Blades, C. R., Galleti, F. C., Bonato, V. L., Goncalves, E. D., Silva, E. V., and Faccioli, L. H. (2007) Comparison of different delivery systems of DNA vaccination for the induction of protection against tuberculosis in mice and guinea pigs, *Genet Vaccines Ther*, Vol. 5, p 2, ISSN 1479-0556.

Diat, O., and Roux, D. (1993a) Preparation of monodisperse multilayer vesicles of controlled size and high encapsulation ratio, *Journal De Physique II*, Vol. 3, pp 9-14, ISSN 1155-4312.

Diat, O.; Roux, D.; Nallet, F. (1993b) Effect of Shear on a Lyotropic Lamellar Phase. *Journal de Physique II*, Vol.3, pp. 1427-1452.

Dootz, R., Otten, A., Koster, S., Struth, B., and Pfohl, T. (2006) Evolution of DNA compaction in microchannels, *Journal of Physics-Condensed Matter*, Vol. 18, pp S639-S652, ISSN 0953-8984.

Egelhaaf, S. U., Wehrli, E., Muller, M., Adrian, M., and Schurtenberger, P. (1996) Determination of the size distribution of lecithin liposomes: A comparative study using freeze fracture, cryoelectron microscopy and dynamic light scattering, *Journal of Microscopy-Oxford*, Vol. 184, pp 214-228, ISSN 0022-2720.

Fritz, G., and Glatter, O. (2006) Structure and interaction in dense colloidal systems: Evaluation of scattering data by the generalized indirect fourier transformation method, *Journal of Physics: Condensed Matter*, Vol. 18, pp S2403-S2419, ISSN 0953-8984.

Galindo-Rodriguez, S., Allemann, E., Fessi, H., and Doelker, E. (2004) Physicochemical parameters associated with nanoparticle formation in the salting-out, emulsification-diffusion, and nanoprecipitation methods, *Pharmaceutical Research*, Vol. 21, pp 1428-1439, ISSN 0724-8741.

Glatter, O. (1982) Data treatment, In *Small angle x ray scattering* (Glatter, O. & Kratky, O., Eds.), p 137, Academic Press, London.

Glatter, O. (1991) Scattering studies on colloids of biological interest (amphiphilic systems), In *Trends in colloid and interface science v* (Corti, M. & Mallamace, F., Eds.), pp 46-54, Springer Berlin / Heidelberg.

Glatter, O. (2002) Neutrons, x-rays and light: Scattering methods applied to soft condensed matter, In *Static light scattering of large systems* (Lindner, P. & Zemb, T., Eds.), pp 171-201, Elsevier, ISBN 0-444-51122-9, Amsterdam.

Glatter, O., and Kratky, O., (Eds.) (1982) *Small angle x ray scattering*, Academic Press, London.

Gregoriadis, G. (1993) *Liposome technology*, CRC Press, Inc, ISBN 0-8493-6709-3.

Higbie, R. (1935) The rate of absorption of a pure gas into a still liquid during short periods of exposure, *Transactions of the American Institute of Chemical Engineers*, Vol. 31, pp 365-389, ISSN 0096-7408.

Hsieh, A. T. H., Hori, N., Massoudi, R., Pan, P. J. H., Sasaki, H., Lin, Y. A., and Lee, A. P. (2009) Nonviral gene vector formation in monodispersed picolitre incubator for consistent gene delivery, *Lab on a Chip*, Vol. 9, pp 2638-2643, ISSN 1473-0197.

Hulst, H. C. v. d. (1957) *Light scattering by small particles*, Wiley, New York.

Jahn, A., Reiner, J. E., Vreeland, W. N., DeVoe, D. L., Locascio, L. E., and Gaitan, M. (2008) Preparation of nanoparticles by continuous-flow microfluidics, *Journal of Nanoparticle Research*, Vol. 10, pp 925-934, ISSN 1388-0764.

Jahn, A., Stavis, S. M., Hong, J. S., Vreeland, W. N., Devoe, D. L., and Gaitan, M. (2010) Microfluidic mixing and the formation of nanoscale lipid vesicles, *Acs Nano*, Vol. 4, pp 2077-2087, ISSN 1936-0851.

Jahn, A., Vreeland, W. N., DeVoe, D. L., Locascio, L. E., and Gaitan, M. (2007) Microfluidic directed formation of liposomes of controlled size, *Langmuir*, Vol. 23, pp 6289-6293, ISSN 0743-7463.

Jahn, A., Vreeland, W. N., Gaitan, M., and Locascio, L. E. (2004) Controlled vesicle self-assembly in microfluidic channels with hydrodynamic focusing, *Journal of the American Chemical Society*, Vol. 126, pp 2674-2675, ISSN 0002-7863.

Jellema, R. K., Bomans, P., Deckers, N., Ungethum, L., Reutelingsperger, C. P. M., Hofstra, L., and Frederik, P. M. (2010) Transfection efficiency of lipoplexes for site-directed delivery, *Journal of Liposome Research*, Vol. 20, pp 258-267, ISSN 0898-2104.

Knight, J. B., Vishwanath, A., Brody, J. P., and Austin, R. H. (1998) Hydrodynamic focusing on a silicon chip: Mixing nanoliters in microseconds, *Physical Review Letters*, Vol. 80, pp 3863-3866, ISSN 0031-9007.

Koh, C. G., Zhang, X. L., Liu, S. J., Golan, S., Yu, B., Yang, X. J., Guan, J. J., Jin, Y., Talmon, Y., Muthusamy, N., Chan, K. K., Byrd, J. C., Lee, R. J., Marcucci, G., and Lee, L. J. (2010) Delivery of antisense oligodeoxyribonucleotide lipopolyplex nanoparticles assembled by microfluidic hydrodynamic focusing, *J. Control. Release*, Vol. 141, pp 62-69, ISSN 0168-3659.

Kratky, O. (1988) The importance of x-ray small-angle scattering in colloid research, In *Dispersed systems* (Hummel, K. & Schurz, J., Eds.), pp 1-14, Springer Berlin / Heidelberg.

Kratky, O., and Laggner, P. (2001) X-ray small-angle scattering, In *Encyclopedia of physical science and technology* (Robert, A. M., Ed.), pp 939-988, Academic Press, ISBN 978-0-12-227410-7, New York.

Kremer, J. M. H., Esker, M. W. J., Pathmamanoharan, C., and Wiersema, P. H. (1977) Vesicles of variable diameter prepared by a modified injection method, *Biochemistry*, Vol. 16, pp 3932-3935, ISSN 0006-2960.

Lasic, D. D. (1993) *Liposomes: From physics to applications*, Amsterdam:Elsevier Science Publishers B.V.

Mannisto, M., Vanderkerken, S., Toncheva, V., Elomaa, M., Ruponen, M., Schacht, E., and Urtti, A. (2002) Structure-activity relationships of poly(l-lysines): Effects of pegylation and molecular shape on physicochemical and biological properties in gene delivery, *J. Control. Release*, Vol. 83, pp 169-182, ISSN 0168-3659.

Mijatovic, D., Eijkel, J. C. T., and van den Berg, A. (2005) Technologies for nanofluidic systems: Top-down vs. Bottom-up - a review, *Lab on a Chip*, Vol. 5, pp 492-500, ISSN 1473-0189.

Montgomery, D. C. (2008) *Design and analysis of experiments*, John Wiley & Sons.

Mount, C. N., Lee, L. K., Yasin, A., Scott, A., Fearn, T., and Shamlou, P. A. (2003) The influence of physico-chemical and process conditions on the physical stability of plasmid DNA complexes using response surface methodology, *Biotechnology and Applied Biochemistry*, Vol. 37, pp 225-234, ISSN 0885-4513.

Nagle, J. F., Zhang, R., Tristram-Nagle, S., Sun, W., Petrache, H. I., and Suter, R. M. (1996) X-ray structure determination of fully hydrated l alpha phase dipalmitoylphosphatidylcholine bilayers, *Biophys J*, Vol. 70, pp 1419-1431, ISSN 0006-3495.

Nallet, F., Laversanne, R., and Roux, D. (1993) Modelling x-ray or neutron scattering spectra of lyotropic lamellar phases : Interplay between form and structure factors, *J. Phys. II France*, Vol. 3, pp 487-502.

New, R. R. C. (1990) *Liposomes: A practical approach (the practical approach series)*.

Oberle, V., Bakowsky, U., Zuhorn, I. S., and Hoekstra, D. (2000) Lipoplex formation under equilibrium conditions reveals a three-step mechanism, *Biophysical Journal*, Vol. 79, pp 1447-1454, ISSN 0006-3495.

Ogris, M., Steinlein, P., Kursa, M., Mechtler, K., Kircheis, R., and Wagner, E. (1998) The size of DNA/transferrin-pei complexes is an important factor for gene expression in cultured cells, *Gene Therapy*, Vol. 5, pp 1425-1433, ISSN 0969-7128.

Oliveira, C. L. P., Sankar R., Kloesgen, M. B., and Pedersen, J. S. (Unpublished work).

Ota, S., Yoshizawa, S., and Takeuchi, S. (2009) Microfluidic formation of monodisperse, cell-sized, and unilamellar vesicles, *Angewandte Chemie-International Edition*, Vol. 48, pp 6533-6537, ISSN 1433-7851.

Otten, A., Koster, S., Struth, B., Snigirev, A., and Pfohl, T. (2005) Microfluidics of soft matter investigated by small-angle x-ray scattering, *Journal of Synchrotron Radiation*, Vol. 12, pp 745-750, ISSN 0909-0495.

Pabst, G., Rappolt, M., Amenitsch, H., and Laggner, P. (2000) Structural information from multilamellar liposomes at full hydration: Full q-range fitting with high quality x-ray data, *Physical Review E*, Vol. 62, p 4000.

Pachence, J. M., and Blasie, J. K. (1991) Structural investigation of the covalent and electrostatic binding of yeast cytochrome c to the surface of various ultrathin lipid multilayers using x-ray diffraction, *Biophysical journal*, Vol. 59, pp 894-900, ISSN 0006-3495.

Pedersen, J. S., Posselt, D., and Mortensen, K. (1990) Analytical treatment of the resolution function for small-angle scattering, *Journal of Applied Crystallography*, Vol. 23, pp 321-333, ISSN 0021-8898.

Perrie, Y., Frederik, P. M., and Gregoriadis, G. (2001) Liposome-mediated DNA vaccination: The effect of vesicle composition, *Vaccine*, Vol. 19, pp 3301-3310, ISSN 0264-410X.

Perrie, Y., and Gregoriadis, G. (2000) Liposome-entrapped plasmid DNA: Characterisation studies, *Biochimica Et Biophysica Acta-General Subjects*, Vol. 1475, pp 125-132, ISSN 0304-4165.

Rejman, J., Oberle, V., Zuhorn, I. S., and Hoekstra, D. (2004) Size-dependent internalization of particles via the pathways of clathrin-and caveolae-mediated endocytosis, *Biochemical Journal*, Vol. 377, pp 159-169, ISSN 0264-6021.

Rigoletto, T. D., Zaniquelli, M. E. D., Santana, M. H. A., and de la Torre, L. G. (2011) Surface miscibility of epc/dotap/dope in binary and ternary mixed monolayers, *Colloids and Surfaces B-Biointerfaces*, Vol. 83, pp 260-269, ISSN 0927-7765.

Rosada, R. S., de la Torre, L. G., Frantz, F. G., Trombone, A. P. F., Zarate-Blades, C. R., Fonseca, D. M., Souza, P. R. M., Brandao, I. T., Masson, A. P., Soares, E. G., Ramos, S. G., Faccioli, L. H., Silva, C. L., Santana, M. H. A., and Coelho-Castelo, A. A. M. (2008) Protection against tuberculosis by a single intranasal administration of DNA-hsp65 vaccine complexed with cationic liposomes, *BMC Immunol.*, Vol. 9, p 13, ISSN 1471-2172.

Ross, P. C., and Hui, S. W. (1999) Lipoplex size is a major determinant of in vitro lipofection efficiency, *Gene Therapy*, Vol. 6, pp 651-659, ISSN 0969-7128.

Sato, T., Sakai, H., Sou, K., Medebach, M., Glatter, O., and Tsuchida, E. (2009) Static structures and dynamics of hemoglobin vesicle (hbv) developed as a transfusion alternative, *J Phys Chem B*, Vol. 113, pp 8418-8428, ISSN 1520-6106.

Shimomura, M., and Sawadaishi, T. (2001) Bottom-up strategy of materials fabrication: A new trend in nanotechnology of soft materials, *Current Opinion in Colloid & Interface Science*, Vol. 6, pp 11-16, ISSN 1359-0294.

Shum, H. C., Lee, D., Yoon, I., Kodger, T., and Weitz, D. A. (2008) Double emulsion templated monodisperse phospholipid vesicles, *Langmuir*, Vol. 24, pp 7651-7653, ISSN 0743-7463.

Silva, C. L., Bonato, V. L. D., Coelho-Castelo, A. A. M., De Souza, A. O., Santos, S. A., Lima, K. M., Faccioli, L. H., and Rodrigues, J. M. (2005) Immunotherapy with plasmid DNA encoding mycobacterial hsp65 in association with chemotherapy is a more rapid and efficient form of treatment for tuberculosis in mice, *Gene Therapy*, Vol. 12, pp 281-287, ISSN 0969-7128.

Torre, L. G., Carneiro, A. L., Rosada, R. S., Silva, C. L., and Santana, M. H. A. (2007) A mathematical model describing the kinetic of cationic liposome production from dried lipid films adsorbed in a multitubular system, *Brazilian Journal of Chemical Engineering*, Vol. 24, pp 477-486, ISSN 0104-6632.

Tournier, V. H., Trionex, M. S., and Chable-Beaumont, C. G. L. (1999) Liposomes with enhanced entrapment capacity and their use in imaging, In *US Patent* (Bracco Reserach S.A, Ed.).

Wagner, A., Vorauer-Uhl, K., Kreismayr, G., and Katinger, H. (2002) The crossflow injection technique: An improvement of the ethanol injection method, *Journal of Liposome Research*, Vol. 12, pp 259-270, ISSN 0898-2104.

Wiewrodt, R., Thomas, A. P., Cipelletti, L., Christofidou-Solomidou, M., Weitz, D. A., Feinstein, S. I., Schaffer, D., Albelda, S. M., Koval, M., and Muzykantov, V. R. (2002) Size-dependent intracellular immunotargeting of therapeutic cargoes into endothelial cells, *Blood*, Vol. 99, pp 912-922, ISSN 0006-4971.

Xu, Y., Szoka, F.C.J. (1996) Mechanism of DNA release from cationic liposome/DNA complexes used in cell transfection, *Biochemistry*, Vol. 35, pp. 5616-5623, ISSN: 0006-2960.

Zelphati, O., Nguyen, C., Ferrari, M., Felgner, J., Tsai, Y., and Felgner, P. L. (1998) Stable and monodisperse lipoplex formulations for gene delivery, *Gene Therapy*, Vol. 5, pp 1272-1282, ISSN 0969-7128.

Zhang, R., Suter, R. M., and Nagle, J. F. (1994) Theory of the structure factor of lipid bilayers, *Phys Rev E Stat Phys Plasmas Fluids Relat Interdiscip Topics*, Vol. 50, pp 5047-5060, ISSN 1063-651X.

Zhang, R., Tristram-Nagle, S., Sun, W., Headrick, R. L., Irving, T. C., Suter, R. M., and Nagle, J. F. (1996) Small-angle x-ray scattering from lipid bilayers is well described by modified caille theory but not by paracrystalline theory, *Biophys J*, Vol. 70, pp 349-357, ISSN 0006-3495.

Zhang, S. B., Zhao, B., Jiang, H. M., Wang, B., and Ma, B. C. (2007) Cationic lipids and polymers mediated vectors for delivery of sirna, *J. Control. Release*, Vol. 123, pp 1-10, ISSN 0168-3659.

Zhang, S. H., Shen, S. C., Chen, Z., Yun, J. X., Yao, K. J., Chen, B. B., and Chen, J. Z. (2008) Preparation of solid lipid nanoparticles in co-flowing microchannels, *Chemical Engineering Journal*, Vol. 144, pp 324-328, ISSN 1385-8947.

13

Cationic Liposomes in Different Structural Levels for Gene Delivery

Yinan Zhao, Defu Zhi and Shubiao Zhang
SEAC-ME Key Laboratory of Biochemical Engineering
College of Life Science, Dalian Nationalities University
China

1. Introduction

Over the last few decades, as a promising strategy for the treatment of many refractory diseases, such as inherited diseases (Martin-Rendon & Blake, 2003) and acquired immuno-deficiency syndrome (AIDS) (Fanning et al., 2003), gene therapy, the objective to allow a gene to express the protein coded in the target cells and consequently to treat disease by the protein secreted from cells transfected, has become an invaluable experimental tool to study gene function and its regulation (El-Aneed, 2004). The success of gene therapy critically depends on suitable transfection vectors, which have the high efficiency transfer of genes to target cells as well as a favorable safety profile. Broadly, these vectors are mainly classified into two categories: viral and non-viral (Liu & Huang, 2002). Currently, viral vectors based on many different viruses such as adenovirus and retrovirus have achieved some success particularly in cancer gene therapy (Williams et al., 2010), and their performance and pathogenicity have been evaluated in animal models. However, several issues including difficulty in production, limited opportunity for repeated administrations due to acute inflammatory response, and delayed humeral or cellular immune responses need to be addressed, so that their clinical potential can be fully realized (Love et al., 2010). Thus it is necessary to develop more efficient and flexible security system in the category of vectors for gene delivery. Synthetic non-viral vectors are potential alternatives to viral vectors, and may help to overcome some of these problems (Zhang et al., 2010). Among these, cationic compounds (mainly including cationic lipids and cationic polymers) are believed to cause less safety problems due to their relative simplicity, and have been the most extensively studied.

Since the first description of successful *in vitro* transfection with cationic lipid by Felgner et al. in 1987 (Felgner et al., 1987), numerous cationic lipids have been synthesised and used for delivery of nucleic acids into cells during the last 20 years. Cationic liposomes are composed of lipid constituents, and have improved the gene delivery efficacy owing to their typical bilayer structure. Some helper lipids such as dioleylphosphatidyl choline (DOPC) or dioleylphosphatidyl ethanolamine (DOPE), typically neutrally lipids (Zuhorn et al., 2005), are often employed with cationic lipids, and play very important role during the formation of lipoplexes by combining cationic liposomes and genes, as they could determine the morphologies of lipoplexes.

Cationic polymer, which condenses DNA by ionic interaction (at physiological pH), form a particulate complex, polyplex, capable of gene transfer into the targeted cells (El-Aneed, 2004). They can condense the negatively charged DNA to a relatively small size and reduce its susceptibility to nucleases so that they may be favorable for improving transfection efficacy. The introduction of polycations (such as poly-L-lysine and protamine) in cationic liposomes, as co-polymer may provide a synergistic effect on the transfection efficiency and a promising solution to the problem frustrating us (Gao & Huang, 1996; Li & Huang, 1997).

In this chapter, we review the effect of cationic liposomes in different structural levels for gene delivery, and help furthering the understanding of the mechanism governing the formation and behaviour of cationic liposomes in gene delivery. The first level for studying on the structure-activity relationship of cationic lipids is the synthesis of new vectors, as well as attempts to improve transfection efficiencies and decrease cytotoxicity, through hydrophilic, hydrophobic and linker domain modifications. The second one is the study on morphologies of lipoplexes through the effects of helper lipids and particle sizes. The last one is the hybridized utilization of non-viral vectors including the complexes of cationic lipsomes and polymers, conjugates of lipids and peptides and of targeting moieties and lipids.

2. Chemical structure of cationic compounds

To understand the relationship between chemical structure and gene delivery, a large series of cationic lipids have been developed. In general, a cationic lipid used for gene therapy is constituted of three basic domains: a hydrophilic cationic headgroup, a hydrophobic domain, and a linker bond which joins the hydrophilic and hydrophobic regions (Fig. 1.) (Gao & Hui, 2001). The chemical structure of cationic lipids determines the physical parameters of the liposome and is an essential factor in both transfection activity and cytotoxicity levels. The effect of chemical structure modifications on gene delivery is discussed in detail through analyzing the large amount of literatures and exemplified thereinafter.

2.1 Headgroup domain

Since the first description of successful *in vitro* transfection with cationic lipid—DOTMA (Fig. 1.) by Felgner et al. in 1987 (Felgner et al., 1987), progress has been made in the design and analysis of each domain. The effect of transfection efficiency and cytotoxicity is associated with the cationic nature of the vectors, which is mainly determined by the structure of its hydrophilic headgroup. In general, the different types of headgroups fall into the following categories: primary, secondary, tertiary amines or quaternary ammonium salts (of which polyamines have often seen the most success) and guanidinium, amidine, as well as heterocyclic ring (Heyes et al., 2002). In addition, other charged groups that have been shown capable of binding plasmids have since been employed. For example, Floch et al. (Floch et al., 2000) showed that cationic lipids (Fig. 2.) characterized by a cationic charge carried by a phosphorus or arsenic atom instead of a nitrogen atom, led to an increased transfection efficiency (up to 7 times according to the cell lines tested) and reduced toxicity.

In hydrophilic headgroup, tertiary amine or quaternary ammonium groups are the most frequently used in many of the established cationic lipids (Felgner et al., 1987; Gao & Huang, 1991; Leventis & Silvius, 1990). A typical example that modified to the chemical structure of headgroup was described by Felgner et al. (Felgner et al., 1994). They synthesized a series of 2,3-dialkyloxy quaternary ammonium compounds containing a hydroxyl moiety (Fig. 3.), which were more efficient in transfection compared with DOTMA that lacks a hydroxyl group on the quaternary amine. In our previous work, we also synthesized a series of cationic lipids containing a hydroxyl moiety on the quaternary amine for liposome-mediated gene delivery (Fig. 4.). Several cationic liposomes with relatively higher transfection efficiency were selected after *in vitro* transfection studies of the prepared cationic liposomes, whose biological performance was superior or parallel to that of the commercial transfection agents, Lipofectamine2000 and DOTAP. It is suggested that the headgroup hydration can be decreased by the incorporation of a hydroxyalkyl chain capable of hydrogen bonding to neighbouring headgroups while it improves the compaction of DNA by several mechanisms, for example, DNA can form hydrogen bonds with the lipid, and the hydroxyl group can enhance the membrane hydration. Accordingly, several groups have synthesised cationic lipids that varied the chain length of the hydroxyalkyl moiety, while keeping the remaining structure unchanged, and observed that the activity of lipid increased with the decrease in the hydroxyalkyl chain length. It shows that a decrease in the number of carbon atoms in the hydroxyalkyl chain, providing more rigidity to the terminal hydroxyl group, are very efficient in compacting DNA, which is responsible for the more observed transfection activity (Felgner et al., 1994; Bennett et al.,1997).

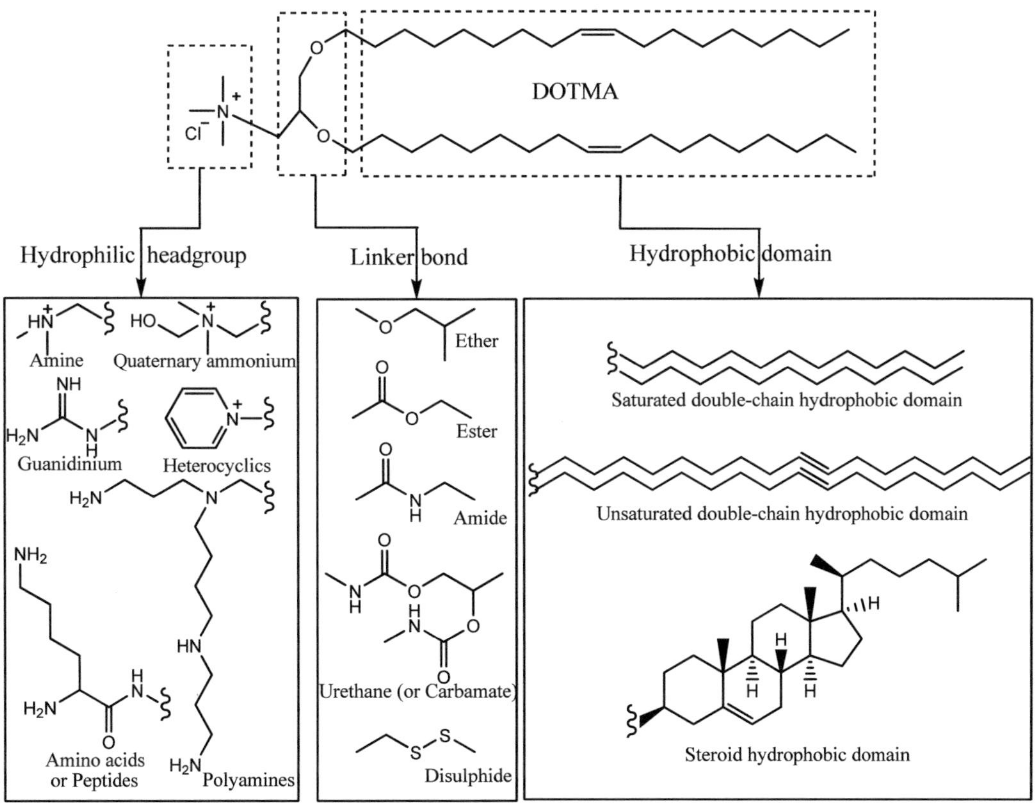

Fig. 1. Representative structure of the cationic lipid DOTMA. Examples of cationic lipid structural components: hydrophilic headgroup, linker bond, and hydrophobic domain.

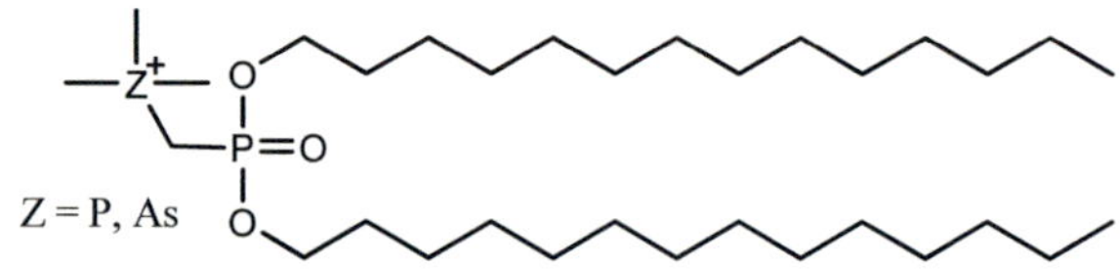

Fig. 2. Alternative cations in the lipid headgroup.

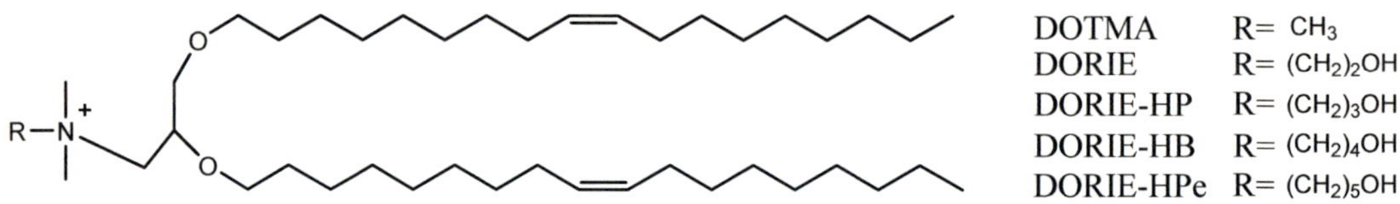

Fig. 3. Double-chain cationic lipids containing a hydroxyl moiety on the quaternary amine.

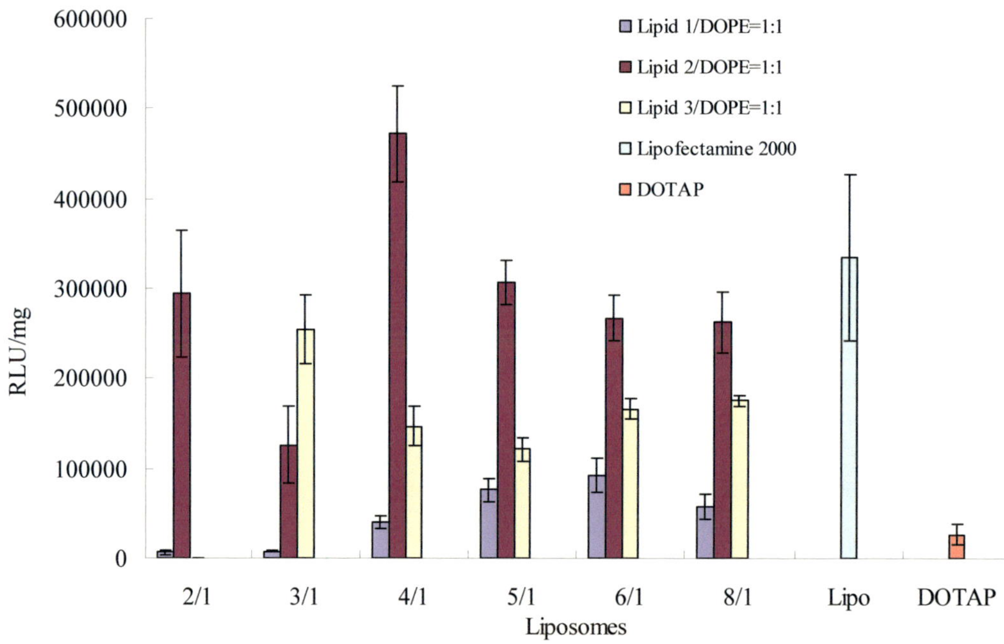

Fig. 4. Transfection comparisons of lipids synthesized and commercial reagents.

A number of cationic lipids that spread the positive charge of the cationic head by delocalizing it into a heterocyclic ring have been designed in an attempt to improve transfection efficacy and to lower toxicity. Heterocyclic cationic lipids with morpholine or piperazine polar heads conjugated to cholesterol directly or via a spacer (Fig. 5.) have been reported to compare favourably with linear polyamine head groups with similar or greater number of charges (Gao & Hui, 2001). And then, the use of imidazole or pyridine rings have been also reported to display higher transfection efficiency and reduced cytotoxicity when compared with classical transfection systems (Ilies et al., 2003; Medvedeva et al., 2009).

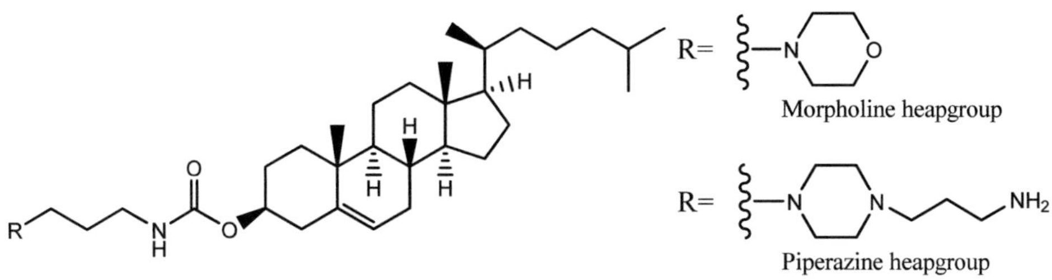

Fig. 5. Heterocyclic cationic lipids with morpholine or piperazine polar heads.

Guanidine and its salts are important intermediates for organic synthesis and medicine; they have also been proposed for making cationic lipids for gene delivery. Yingyongnarongkul et al. (Yingyongnarongkul et al., 2004) studied a library of aminoglycerol–diamine conjugate-based cationic lipids with urea linkage between varying length of diamines and hydrophobic chains, and found two compounds with bis-guanidinium and one tail had transfection activity superior to that of the commercial lipid transfection reagent effective and merit further investigation. In addition, several cationic lipids containing guanidine (Floch et al., 2000), amidine (Lensink et al., 2009), or cyclic guanidine (Frederic at al., 2000) in the head group have been studied.

As a way to not only bind DNA but to compact DNA, polyvalent cationic lipids known as lipopolyamines and lipospermine were synthesized, e.g., DOSPA, DOGS (Behr et al., 1989), are claimed to be more efficient than single-charged lipids such as DOTMA, DOTAP, DC-Chol, DMRIE (Ferrari et al., 1998). The choice of headgroup may depend on the desired and specific function of the cationic lipid, but for gene transfection it is essential that the headgroups of cationic lipid interact strongly with the minor groove of DNA via its multivalent headgroup, and has the ability to efficiently condense DNA. In addition, a few parameters, such as the shape (linear, T-shaped, globular, branched) and the length of the multivalent headgroup, and the distance between two consecutive nitrogen atoms in the polyamine, are also important in transfection efficiency and cytotoxicity (Byk et al., 1998; Fujiwara et al., 2000).

In summary, the choice of cationic headgroups has expanded into the use of natural architectures and functional groups with recognized DNA binding modes. Multivalent cationic lipids are more likely to be the most efficient in compacting DNA; however, they are prone to formation of micelles typically contributing to increased toxicity (Pedroso de Lima et al., 2003). The incorporation of a heteroatomic group as the substitution of the liner amine headgroup, such as pyridinium and guanidine, can improve the compaction of DNA by the positive charge of the cationic head, and then transfection efficiency is increased and toxicity is decreased significantly.

2.2 Hydrophobic domain

The hydrophobic domains represent the non-polar hydrocarbon moieties of cationic lipids and are usually made of two types of hydrophobic moieties—aliphatic chains, steroid domain. Transfection efficiency and toxicity of cationic lipids can be affected by structural variations in the hydrophobic domain such as length, the specific type of chemical bonds, and the relative position of the hydrocarbon chains (Zhi at al., 2010).

Cationic lipids with aliphatic chains have been very thoroughly researched. The chains are either linear and saturated or linear and mono-unsaturated and used in liposomal vectors ranging from C5:0 to C18:1, but oleyl, lauryl, myristyl, palmityl and stearyl, have been the most researched ones (Niculescu-Duvaz et al., 2003). A common variation is the use of branched (Ferrari et al., 2002), acetylenic (Fletcher et al., 2006) chains and *cis*-monounsaturated alkyl chains (Bennett at al., 1997).

It is commonly believed that cationic lipids have one to four hydrocarbon chains. Several studies have also shown that incorporating aliphatic chains with different numbers can improve transfection efficiency potentially by promoting endosomal escape (Felgner et al., 1987; Tang & Hughes, 1999a; Gaucheron at al., 2002; Zhi et al., 2010). Cationic lipids with double-chain hydrocarbons in the hydrophobic domain represent the majority of cationic lipids synthesized so far. Cationic lipids containing two aliphatic chains such as DOTMA and DOTAP, are among the most active lipids for systemic gene delivery. However, Tang et al. (Tang & Hughes, 1999a) demonstrated that 6-lauroxyhexyl ornithinate (LHON) with one tail was more efficient and of lower cytotoxicity compared to DOTAP. Generally speaking, for aliphatic chains, single-tailed and three-tailed cationic lipids are better known as surfactants because of their ability to form micelles in solution, but they are more toxic and less efficient than their double-tailed counterparts. Usually, cationic lipids with double-tailed hydrocarbons are capable of forming liposomes by themselves or with a helper phospholipid. Therefore, most of the aliphatic chains in the cationic lipids are double-tailed.

It is generally agreed that the length and saturation of the aliphatic chains incorporated into cationic lipids significantly affect their transfection efficiency. In order to gain chain length–activity correlation, Felgner et al. (Felgner et al., 1994) studied a series of hydroxyethyl quaternary ammonium lipids with myristoyl (diC14:0, DMRIE), palmitoyl (diC16:0, DPRIE), stearoyl (diC18:0, DSRIE), and oleoyl (diC18:1, DORIE) chains. They observed that a comparison of vectors based solely on the lengths of the two aliphatic chains led to identify the order C14:0 > C18:1 > C16:0 > C18:0. Our study on double-chain cationic lipids also showed increasing transfection efficiency with decrease of the chain length (Liu et al., 2008). It was therefore proposed that cationic lipids with shorter chain length (for saturated chains) were generally important for acquiring high transfection efficiency, since they are responsible for membrane fluidity and good lipid mixing within the bilayer. Beyond that, the best chains in terms of benefit to transfection are frequently the unsaturated ones. The overwhelming majority of results showed that the unsaturated C18:1 oleyl was the optimal aliphatic chain, which was frequently the best choice for good transfection (Fletcher et al., 2006).

Some new vectors were designed to covalently connect some special moieties in the hydrophobic chains, in order to get the relationship between hydrophobic chains and transfection efficiency. Jacopin et al. (Jacopin et al., 2001) synthesized a glycosylated analogue (Fig. 6.) of the dialkylamidoglycylcarboxyspermines, which formed stable particles at low charge ratio and was efficient for gene delivery. Many groups also reported a few other glycosylated cationic bolaamphiphiles similar to the compound (Fabio et al., 2003; Brunelle et al., 2009). In addition, the fluorinated part of the hydrophobic chain can also influence the transfection efficiency of cationic lipids *in vivo* and *in vitro*. Many varieties of fluorinated cationic lipids have been developed as transfecting agents, which are very efficient in compacting DNA and delivering genes into cells *in vivo* and *in vitro* (Gaucheron et al., 2001a, 2001b, 2001c, 2001d).

In the steroid groups, cholesterol is by far the most frequently encountered and used as an alternative to aliphatic chains because of its rigidity, as well as its endogenous biodegradability and fusion activity. An example is cationic lipid 'GL-67' (Fig. 7.), which has been found to be particularly efficient for gene transfer to cultured cells and in murine lungs

(Lee et al., 1996). Other steroid compounds used as hydrophobic moieties for cationic lipids include vitamin D (Ren et al., 2000), bile acids (Randazzo et al., 2009), antibiotic (Kichler et al., 2005), cholestane and litocholic acid (Fujiwara et al., 2000).

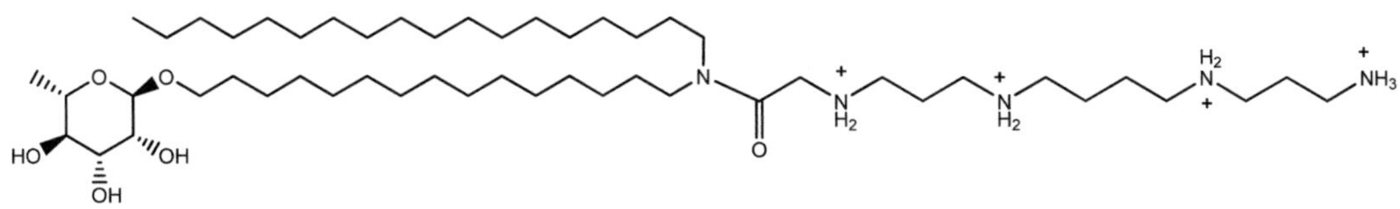

Fig. 6. Glycosylated analogue of lipopolyamines.

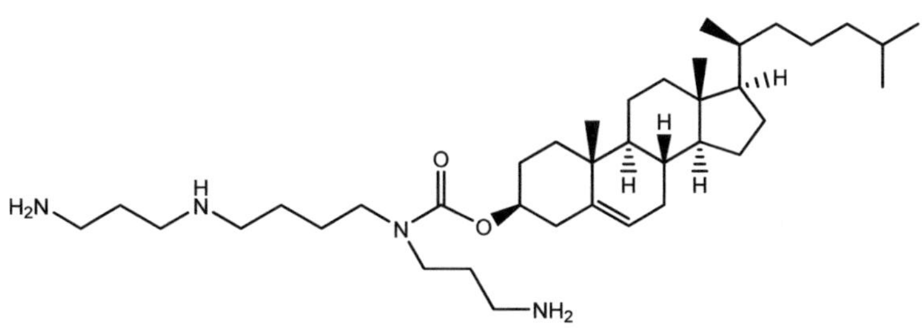

Fig. 7. Chemical structure of GL-67.

To summarise, the hydrophobic domain of cationic lipids mainly includes aliphatic chains and steroid domain, which determines the phase transition temperature and the fluidity of the bilayer, and influences the stability and toxicity of liposomes, the DNA protection from nucleases, and the DNA release from complex.

2.3 Linker bond

For lipids without a backbone, the linker bond that acts as a connector between the hydrophobic and cationic headgroup domains can affect the transfection efficiency, biodegradability and stability of cationic lipids. Linker bonds are commonly ether, ester (Leventis & Silvius, 1990), amide (Behr et al., 1989) or urethane (or carbamate) (Lee et al., 1996) groups (Koynova & Tenchov, 2010), but other groups such as redox-sensitive disulphide (Byk et al., 1998, 2000) have also been employed (Fig. 1.). Cationic lipids with ether bonds such as DOTMA in the linker domain generally render better transfection efficiency, but they are too stable to be biodegraded thus may cause higher toxicity. Compared with ether bonds, although cationic lipids with ester bonds such as DOTAP are more biodegradable and associated with less cytotoxicity in cultured cells (Leventis & Silvius, 1990; Choi et al., 2001), those with ester may also decrease the stability of liposomes in systemic circulation.

The chemistry of the linker has most often been of the carbamate or amide variety, both of which are chemically stable and biodegradable, and cationic lipids with these linkers could be used as efficient gene delivery carriers (Ren et al., 2001; Liu et al., 2005a, 2005b, 2008). A typical example of cationic lipid with carbamate linker is DC-Chol, which was the first lipid used in clinical trials because of its combined properties of transfection efficiency, stability, and low toxicity (Gao & Huang, 1995). As well known, when incorporating a carbamate group into the linker, it may therefore be hoped that the pH drop will act as a trigger, disconnecting the hydrophobic and hydrophilic portions of the lipoplex, and thereby to release DNA after entering endosomes in cell because of the pH decreasing (Liu et al., 2005a, 2008). We synthesized a series of carbamate-linked cationic lipids for liposome-mediated gene delivery, which proved to have good gene transfection properties (Fig. 4.).

It is familiar to chemists that compounds comprising redox-sensitive disulphide bonds is stable chemically as long as no reducing agents, and it is expected that these disulphide-linked lipids can keep stable in the circulation system while decomposing to release DNA after entering endosomes in cells (in a similar manner as the pH-sensitive systems) (Tang & Hughes, 1999b). Byk et al. (Byk et al., 1998, 2000) prepared a series of lipopolyamines that harbor a disulfide bridge within different positions in the backbone of the lipids as biosensitive function. They found that an early release of DNA during or after penetration into cells, probably promoted by reduction of a disulfide bridge placed between the polyamine and the lipid, implied a total loss of transfection efficiency.

In addition, structural variations at the linker region such as length, the specific type of chemical bonds and the relative position of the hydrocarbon chains can affect the transfection efficiency, biodegradability and stability of cationic lipids (Fujiwara et al., 2000). The level of hydration and toxicity of the lipid can also be determined by the length of the linker (Floch et al., 2000). In a word, the use of linkers incorporating functional groups that are cleavable on shorter time scales and under specific stimuli is however of emerging interest, as DNA release may here be facilitated by a triggered decomplexation mechanism.

From the chemistry point of view, the structure of cationic compounds is an important factor for their transfection activity and toxicity. Some common conclusions can be achieved by comparing the different structures and their transfection activity in the same family or different families of lipids. The transfection efficiency is not only determined by one domain of cationic lipids, but also depends on the combination of them (Tang & Hughes, 1999a). In general, it seems when researchers design cationic compounds for gene delivery, the balances between the opposite factors including fluidity and rigidity, symmetry and asymmetry, saturation and unsaturation, linearity and branching, short chain and long chain, hydrophilicity and lipophilicity of compounds should be taken into serious consideration.

3. Helper lipids and morphology of lipoplexes

Neutrally charged helper lipids such as DOPE, DOPC (Fig. 8.), are often employed with cationic lipids in order to gain high transfection efficiency (Felgner & Ringold, 1989). When cationic liposomes are mixed with DNA, lipoplexes are formed with heterogeneous morphologies including beads on a string structure (Felgner & Ringold, 1989), spaghettis or meatballs structure (Sternberg et al., 1994), multilamellar structure L^{C}_{α}, inverted hexagonal phase structure H^{C}_{II} (Koltover et al., 1998), a map-pin structure (Sternberg et al., 1998) and a sliding columnar phase (O'Hern & Lubensky, 1998). Helper lipids play very important role during the formation of lipoplexes by combining cationic liposomes and genes, as they could determine the morphologies of lipoplexes. It has shown lipoplex size is very important for gene transfer to actively endocytosing cells (Ross & Hui, 1999), as such the influences on transfection efficiency: DNA ratio, types of liposomes, incubation time in polyanion containing media, and time of serum addition, are channeled mostly through their influences on lipoplex size.

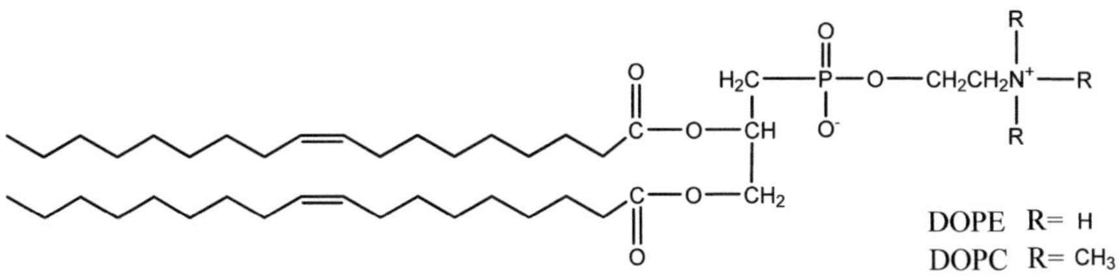

Fig. 8. Chemical structure of DOPE and DOPC.

3.1 DOPE

DOPE often presents a super synergistic effect when used in cationic liposomes, because DOPE destabilized lipid bilayers, and it was believed to be involved in endosomal disruption (Litzinger & Huang, 1992), allowing the release of DNA into the cytosol (Farhood et al., 1995) and leading to mixed bilayers (Scarzello et al., 2005). Most studies have shown that lipoplexes containing the non-bilayer-phase-preferring lipid DOPE or cholesterol would promote H^{C}_{II} organization (Zuhorn et al., 2005). A transition from the L^{C}_{α} phase to the H^{C}_{II} phase could be expected by increasing weight fraction of DOPE, via controlling the spontaneous radius of curvature "Ro" of the lipid layers, favored by the elastic free energy (Safinya, 2001). Another helper lipid, cholesterol, could also promote $H_{II}{}^{C}$ organization as DOPE. It has been proved that *in vivo* applications cholesterol was a more effective helper lipid than DOPE (Lasic, 1997).

Koltover et al. (Koltover et al., 1998) disclosed the reason in the level of phase transition through synchrotron small-angle X-ray scattering (SAXS) and optical microscopy to show the phase transition from $L_{\alpha}{}^{C}$ to $H_{II}{}^{C}$ induced by DOPE via controlling the spontaneous curvature $C_o = 1/R_o$ of the lipid monolayer. It has been concluded that DOPE facilitates endosomal escape by forming an unstable inverted hexagonal phase at the endosomal pH that destabilizes both the complex and the endosomal membrane. But in a recent study (Leal et al., 2010), they developed CL-siRNA complexes with a novel cubic phase nanostructure exhibiting efficient silencing at low toxicity by using glycerol monooleate other than DOPE as the helper lipid. The inverse bicontinuous gyroid cubic nanostructure was unequivocally established from synchrotron X-ray scattering data, while fluorescence microscopy revealed colocalization of lipid and siRNA in complexes.

Tubes of lipoplexes containing DOTAP/MOG, DOTAP or DOTAP/PC, and DOTAP/DOPE were observed in freeze-fracture electron micrographs. The tubes were extremely short and appeared bead-like in lipoplexes containing DOTAP/MOG, slightly longer in those containing DOTAP or DOTAP/PC, and extensively elongated in DOTAP/DOPE lipoplexes (Xu et al., 1999). The spaghetti-like structures, occurring at DNA: lipid concentrations which were used during transfection and their diameter came closest to the diameter of the nuclear pores, may be the active cationic lipoplexes (Zhdanov et al., 2002). In the study of the structure and morphology of DC-Chol–DOPE/DNA complexes it was found the existence of cluster-like aggregates made of multilamellar DNA/lipid domains coexisting with other multilamellar lipoplexes or, alternatively, with DNA-coated vesicles (Amenitsch et al., 2010). The further study showed that DC-Chol-DOPE/DNA lipoplexes preferentially used a raft mediated endocytosis, while DOTAP-DOPC/DNA systems were mainly internalized by not specific fluid phase macropinocitosys. Most efficient multicomponent lipoplexes, incorporating different lipid species in their lipid bilayer, can use multiple endocytic pathways to enter cells. Their data demonstrated that efficiency of endocytosis was regulated by shape coupling between lipoplex and membrane lipids to suggest that such a shape-dependent coupling regulated efficient formation of endocytic vesicles thus determining the success of internalization (Marchini et al., 2010).

Kato et al. (Kato et al., 2010) observed the effect of phase separation of the membrane by changing PE from DOPE to dipalmitoylethanolamine (DPPE), which corresponded to a change from a homogeneous single phase to two segregated phases of liquid-ordered and liquid-disordered states on the membrane. This study further proved that helper lipids could change the morphologies of lipoplexes through the mutual interaction with DNA based on their chemical structures. Several helper lipids such as dilauroylphosphatidylethanolamine (C12:0), dimiristoylphosphatidylethanolamine (C14:0), dipalmitoylphosphatidylethanolamine (C16:0), diphytanoylphosphatidylethanolamine (C16:0, branched), distearoylphosphatidylethanolamine (DSPE, C18:0) were compared with DOPE (C18:1) to show that the branched and unsaturated species combined with cationic lipids acted in physical synergism to increase transfection efficiency (Heinze et al., 2010).

3.2 DOPC

Ewert et al. (Ewert et al., 2004) demonstrated that σ_M, the average membrane charge density of the CL-vector, was a key universal parameter that governed the transfection behavior of L_α^C complexes in cells. DOPC favors the formation of L_α^C type of lipoplexes, in which, a system of DOPC/DOTAP-DNA lipoplex showed a strong dependence on the molar fraction of neutral lipid DOPC (ΦDOPC) and therefore membrane charge density σ_M. The transfection efficiency started low for 0.5 < ΦDOPC < 0.7 and increased dramatically to a similar value, at ΦDOPC = 0.2, with H_{II}^C lipoplex achieved by the DOPE/DOTAP-DNA. In contrast to L_α^C complexes, H_{II}^C complexes containing DOPE exhibited no dependence on σ_M. The transfection efficiency increased exponentially with a linear increase of σ_M for the MVL5/DOPC/DNA lipoplex bearing L_α^C (Ewert et al., 2002). And then, they found that the curve of transfection efficiency versus σ_M assumed a bell-shape with increasing σ_M using MVL type of cationic lipids (Ahmad et al., 2005). Ewert et al. (Ewert et al., 2006) also found that hexagonally arranged tubular lipid micelles (H_I^C) surrounded by DNA rods were formed though DOPC was used in the dendritic lipid-based cationic liposome.

Later it has been proved that the enhanced transfection efficiency was supported by a meso-scale computer modeling of cationic lipid lipoplexes in L_α^C phase at high concentrations of cationic lipid (Farago et al., 2006). Recently, a study (Kedika & Srilakshmi, 2011) showed that DOPC was a more efficacious colipid than DOPE. The difference in the transfection efficiencies of lipoplexes in the presence of colipids DOPE and DOPC was explained as the uptake of the lipoplexes in the presence of DOPE took place mainly from the fusion of the lipoplexes with the plasma membrane, whereas "endocytosis" facilitated uptake in the presence of DOPC. Many researchers have agreed membrane charge density σ_M is a universal parameter governing the transfection efficiency of L^C_α lipoplexs (Ewert et al., 2005a, 2005b; Lin, 2003). But for the question, which morphology among L_α^C governed main by DOPC and H_{II}^C governed mainly by DOPE is favored in terms of transfection efficiency, we still need to carry out more research.

3.3 Lipoplex sizes

Another parameter of morphologies affecting transfection efficiency is lipoplex sizes, for the important role of lipoplex sizes in determining the nature of the entry pathway by endocytosis (Wasungu & Hoekstra, 2006). Though it is difficult to unify the size effect of lipoplexs on the transfection activity so far, most transfection complexes fall within an average size range of 100-300nm. The lipoplex particles can be categorized as small (≤100nm), medium (100-200nm), large (200-1000nm) or giant (≥1000nm). (Donkuru et al., 2010).

Some times large lipoplexes sizes could be more efficient to transfer genes because large particles lead to maximum contact with cells (Kennedy et al., 2000), the formation of large intracellular vesicles which are more easily disrupted, thus releasing DNA into the cytoplasm (Escriou et al., 1998), phagocytic activity accompanied by endosomal escape (Xu et al., 1999) and faster sedimentation and better cellular trafficking (Lee et al., 2003). At the same time, some reports supported that particles with smaller size would gain high transfection efficiency (Pitard et al., 1997; Kneuer et al., 2006). The requirement for efficient transfection may be different *in vivo* and *in vitro*. Compared with *in vitro* delivery, small particles tend to have high transfection efficiency *in vivo* because of the ability of small particles to traverse narrow capillary networks. Large particles typically have low *in vivo* transfection efficiencies, while 200-400nm is the optimal size for lipoplexes *in vitro* (Zhdanov et al., 2002; Kennedy et al., 2000). Measurement of the endosomal uptake of fluorescent dextran beads of various sizes clarified that particles smaller than 200 nm were predominantly taken up by means of clathrin mediated endocytosis; with increasing the size, a shift to another mechanism occurred, so that particles larger than 500 nm were taken up predominantly by caveolae mediated pathways (Rejman et al., 2004).

Carriere et al. (Carriere et al., 2002) have proved that lipofection inhibition by serum was largely due to the serum inhibition of lipoplex size growth, and may be overcome by using large, stable lipoplexes. Lipoplexes of over 700 nm mean diameter induced efficient transfection in the presence or absence of serum (Turek et al., 2000), but lipoplexes of less than 250 nm in size showed efficient transfection only in the absence of serum. It was reported that the particle sizes may be one of the factors that were contributed to serum resistance of EDL (ethanol-dried lipid-DNA) lipoplexes, and the large cationic lipoplexes may delay the dissociation of DNA with lipid, thereby enhancing DNA transfection efficiency (Lian & Ho, 2003).

Although a general rule is not obtained until now, there is no doubt that high transfection would be gained from large lipoplexes when endocytosis is dominant, because large particles facilitate membrane contact and fusion. When cells are not actively endocytosing, either small particles may have high transfection efficiency, or lipoplex sizes don't correlate with lipofection efficiency. The possibility of a final agreement on the lipoplexes size effect may be very small, as the other conditions of every transfection case could be different. The controllable assembly of lipoplexes may provide a solution to this problem.

4. Hybrid vectors based on cationic lipids

The hybridized utilization of non-viral vectors also provides an alternative solution to the delivery of genes. We could hybridize cationic lipsomes and polymers; introduce peptides and targeting moieties into lipids for approaching the requirements of gene therapy (Zhang et al., 2010).

4.1 Hybrids of cationic liposomes and polymers

Cationic polymers could combine with DNA to form a particulate complex, polyplex, capable of gene transfer into the targeted cells (El-Aneed, 2004), because most of them are completely soluble in water. Therefore, they have the obvious advantage of compressing DNA molecules to a relatively small size (Gershon et al., 1993; Ruponen et al., 1999). But they do not contain a hydrophobic moiety (Elouahabi & Ruysschaert, 2005), this may hinder the transfection efficiency and cause cytotoxicity to some degree.

Liposome-mediated gene transfer could be improved by natural polycations such as protamine sulfate (PS), poly(L-lysine) (PLL), and spermine (Li & Huang, 1997; Cheng et al., 2009). The addition of poly(L-lysine) and protamine dramatically reduced the particle size of the complex formed between DNA and cationic liposomes and rendered DNA resistant to the nucleases (Gao & Huang, 1996). These polycations could form a complex with DNA and condense DNA from extended conformation to highly compact structure into 30-100 nm in size. A type of hybrid vectors were developed by Huang et al. (Gao & Huang, 1996; Lee & Huang, 1996) in which poly(lysine)-condensed DNA was entrapped into folate-targeted cationic liposomes (LPD). They found LPD vectors to be more efficient and less cytotoxic compared to conventional cationic liposomal vectors. Later, they modified LPDs through different cationic liposomes wherein LPDs were used to deliver antisense oligodeoxynucleotide and siRNA (Li & Huang, 2006; Chen et al., 2009; Gao & Huang, 2009).

As a cationic polymer, PEI is commonly used for the delivery of genes. The hybrid usage with cationic liposomes provides a promising way to the field of gene transfer. In a study, the combination of PEI and DOTAP-Chol caused more than 10-fold increase in the transfection efficiency and less toxicity in many cells compared with using polymer or liposome alone(Lee et al., 2003). Nearly at the same time, PEI2K-DNA-Dosper complexes showed much more cellular uptake of DNA than PEI2K-DNA complexes and two times higher transfection than Dosper-DNA complexes. It has been hypothesized that Dosper improved the cellular uptake of PEI2K-DNA complexes and PEI2K improved a transfer of the complexes from lysosomes to nucleus (Lampela et al., 2003).

In recent years, chitosan-based carriers have become one of the non-viral vectors that have gained increasing interest as a safer and cost-effective delivery system for gene materials, as they have beneficial qualities such as low toxicity, low immunogenicity, excellent biocompatibility as well as a high positive charge density (Zhang et al., 2007; Mao et al., 2010). Katas et al. (Katas & Alpar, 2006) may be the first group to investigate the use of chitosan to deliver siRNA *in vitro*. Two types of cell lines, CHO K1 and HEK 293 were used to reveal that preparation method of siRNA association to the chitosan played an important role on the silencing effect. Chitosan-TPP nanoparticles with entrapped siRNA were shown to be better vectors as siRNA delivery vehicles compared to chitosan-siRNA complexes possibly due to their high binding capacity and loading efficiency. We have combined chitosans and cationic liposomes to form a ternary lipopolyplex which could facilitate the delivery of genes into cells more efficiently than the utilization of a lipoplex or a polyplex alone (Fig. 9.). The confocal microscopy method proved that exogenous DNA molecules entered the nucleus through the nuclear membrane other than via the NPC. The results explored novel ways based on the hybrid vectors to enhance the pDNA delivery with chitosans and with further suitable intracellular mechanism, allowing the development of nonviral gene delivery and may provide the most exciting solution for hybrid biomaterials design used for beneficial candidates for gene therapy.

4.2 Conjugates of peptides and lipids

One of the most challenge things for gene delivery by cationic liposome method is the toxicity of cationic lipids originated in the cationic nature. The replacement of cationic head

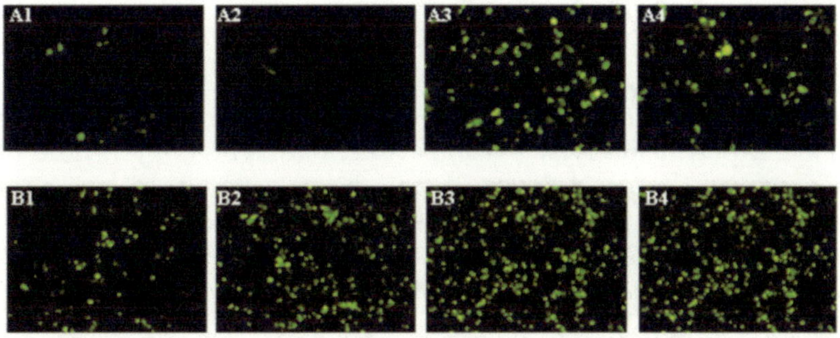

Fig. 9. The role of chitosans on transfection efficiency of cationic liposomes. (A in Hela cells, A1: lipoplex, A2: polyplex, A3: lipopolyplex 1, A4: lipopolyplex 2; B in Hep2 cells, B1: lipoplex, B2: lipopolyplex 1, B3: lipopolyplex 2, B4: lipopolyplex 3)

groups has been a major trend with other more biocompatible groups, such as peptides, in recent years, as the cationic lipids with quaternary ammonium head groups can become cytotoxic by interacting with critical enzymes such as PKC (Bottega & Epand, 1992). The commonly used headgroups are peptides consisting of amino acids, such as lysine, arginine, histine, ornigine and tryptophan. Therefore, the conjugates of peptides and lipids are much less toxic, whilst keeping the same transfection efficiency (Behr et al., 1989; Ahn et al., 2004). The first polypeptide cationic liposome prepared by a polycondensation reaction was described by Folda et al. (Folda et al., 1982). A subset of lipitoids with a repeated side chain trimer motif conjugated with dimyristoyl phosphatidyl-ethanolamine (DMPE) mediated DNA were also found to transfer cells with high efficiency (Huang et al., 1998). A compound which contained cholesterol and a dipeptide consisting of glycine and sterically protected arginine has been proved to be suitable for *in vitro* transfection in the presence of 10% sera more efficiently than other cholesterol derivatives (Sochanik et al., 2000). Peptide-based gemini surfactants GS could lead to an increase in levels of gene expression *in vitro* compared to well-established non-viral reagents (McGregor et al., 2001).

Obata et al. (Obata et al., 2008) have proved that the lysine- or arginine-type lipids exhibited higher gene expression efficiencies than that of Lipofectamine2000, with COS-7 cells. A series of new lipophilic peptides possessing a cationic tripeptide headgroup were effective non-viral vectors for gene delivery. Then, they also synthesized a series of cationic amino acid-based lipids having a spacer between the cationic head group and hydrophobic moieties and examined the influence of the spacer on a liposome gene delivery system. (Obata et al., 2009). At present, they are investigating the ability of cationic liposomes composed of 1,5-dihexadecyl *N*-arginyl-L-glutamate (Arg-Glu2C_{16}) to carry nucleic acids into neuronal cells. Arg-Glu2C_{16}, as a model cationic amino acid-based lipid, had a high capability as a gene carrier, even for neuronal transfection (Obata et al., 2010). Coles et al. (Coles et al., 2010) has synthesized positively charged peptide-based carriers which could interact with DNA improved by performing isothermal titration calorimetry and particle size and zeta potential experiments. The particle sizes of the carrier/DNA complexes varied over the different charge ratios from 200-800nm. The utilization of lipophilic carriers is a promising approach to improve the bioavailability of gene delivery.

Some peptide head groups could endow additional functions to the lipids, such as membrane-disturbing ability. In a hybrid molecule, the covalent coupling of an amphipathic and membrane-disturbing peptide to a lipid moiety might create a stable and efficient peptide-based gene transfer system. The luciferase activity induced by the dioleoylmelittin/DNA complex was 5-500-fold higher than that induced by a cationic lipid/DNA complex, depending on the cationic lipid and the cell-line (Legendre et al., 1997). Later, a membrane-disrupting peptide derived from the influenza virus was covalently linked to different polymethacrylates using N-succinimidyl 3-(2-pyridyldithio)propionate (SPDP) as a coupling agent to increase the transfection efficiency of polyplexes based on these polymers. *In vitro* transfection and toxicity were tested in COS-7 cells, and these experiments showed that the polyplexes with grafted peptides had a substantially higher transfection activity than the control polyplexes, while the toxicity remained unchanged (Funhoff et al., 2005).

4.3 Conjugates of targeting moieties and lipids

For a number of gene therapy applications, targeted gene delivery systems have attracted great attention due to their potential in directing the therapeutic genes to the target cells, and it may help minimize adverse effects such as cytotoxicity or immune reactions, as well as maximizing the efficacy of the therapeutic response. The targeted delivery of the lipoplexes may be achieved through the addition of targeting moieties (e.g., ligands) into liposomes by direct formulation, with no covalent bond to any lipid (Seol et al., 2000); conjugated to helper lipid (Dauty et al., 2002), or connected directly to the cationic lipids (Kawakami et al., 2000a; Gaucheron et al., 2001c). For targeted lipoplexes, modified with a targeting moiety such as folate (Dauty et al., 2002), galactose(Kawakami et al., 2000a; Gaucheron et al., 2001c), mannose (Kawakami et al., 2000b), antibodies (Duan et al., 2008) and transferrin (Seol et al., 2000; Sakaguchi et al., 2008), the uptake can be receptor mediated and enhanced (Zhang et al., 2010).

Targeting of the folate receptor (FR) had received much attention in recent years, since the folate receptor is a tumor marker over expressed in large numbers of cancer cells, including cancers of the ovary, kidney, uterus, testis, brain, colon, and in addition, folic acid is a relatively small molecule (MW 441 Da), therefore, it has the advantages of being stable and nonimmunogenic compared to monoclonal antibodies (Kane et al., 1986), and still having a relatively high receptor affinity. In a study, the folate moiety was attached to a lipid membrane anchor via a cysteinyl-PEG_{3400} spacer, which greatly increased specific cellular uptake to FR overexpressing cancer cells in comparison with unmodified cationic liposome and can significantly improve the transfection efficiency of a cationic liposomal formulation (Reddy et al., 2002). Recently, Yoshizawa et al. (Yoshizawa et al., 2008) developed a folate-linked nanoparticle (NP-F), which was composed of cholesteryl-3β-carboxyamidoethylene-N-hydroxyethylamine, Tween 80 and folate-poly(ethylene glycol)-distearoyl-phosphatidylethanolamine conjugate (f-PEG2000-DSPE), and was delivered synthetic siRNA with high transfection efficiency and selectivity into nasopharyngeal tumor KB cells.

The asialoglycoprotein receptor (ASPGR), present at the surface of hepatocytes, could recognize and bind to β-D-galactoside terminated glycoproteins for the targeting of cationic vector-based gene delivery systems (Ashwell & Harford, 1982). Kawakami et al. (Kawakami et al., 1998) have studied liposomal with asialoglycoprotein receptor gene carrier systems for gene delivery to hepatocytes, which was a novel galactosylated cholesterol derivatives, cholesten-5-yloxy-N-(4-((1-imino-2-β-D-thiogalactosylethyl)amino)alkyl) formamide. In human hepatoma cells (HepG2), the liposomes containing this galactolipid showed higher transfection activities than DC-Chol liposomes based on a receptor-mediated mechanism.

Later, they used galactosylated cationic liposomes to target liver cell asialoglycoprotein receptors *in vivo* (Kawakami et al., 2000a). Many groups also reported a few other glycosylated cationic bolaamphiphiles similar to the compound (Letrou-Bonneval et al., 2008). Brunelle et al. (Brunelle et al., 2009) synthesized a new series of dissymmetric hemifluorocarbon bolaamphiphiles (Fig. 10.), and the dissymmetric functionalization of diiodoperfluorooctane led to bolaamphiphile molecules composed of a partially fluorocarbon core end-capped with a glycoside and an ammonium salt. They found that the incorporation of two fluorinated segments in the molecular structure of the bolaamphiphiles is detrimental for an efficient DNA condensation.

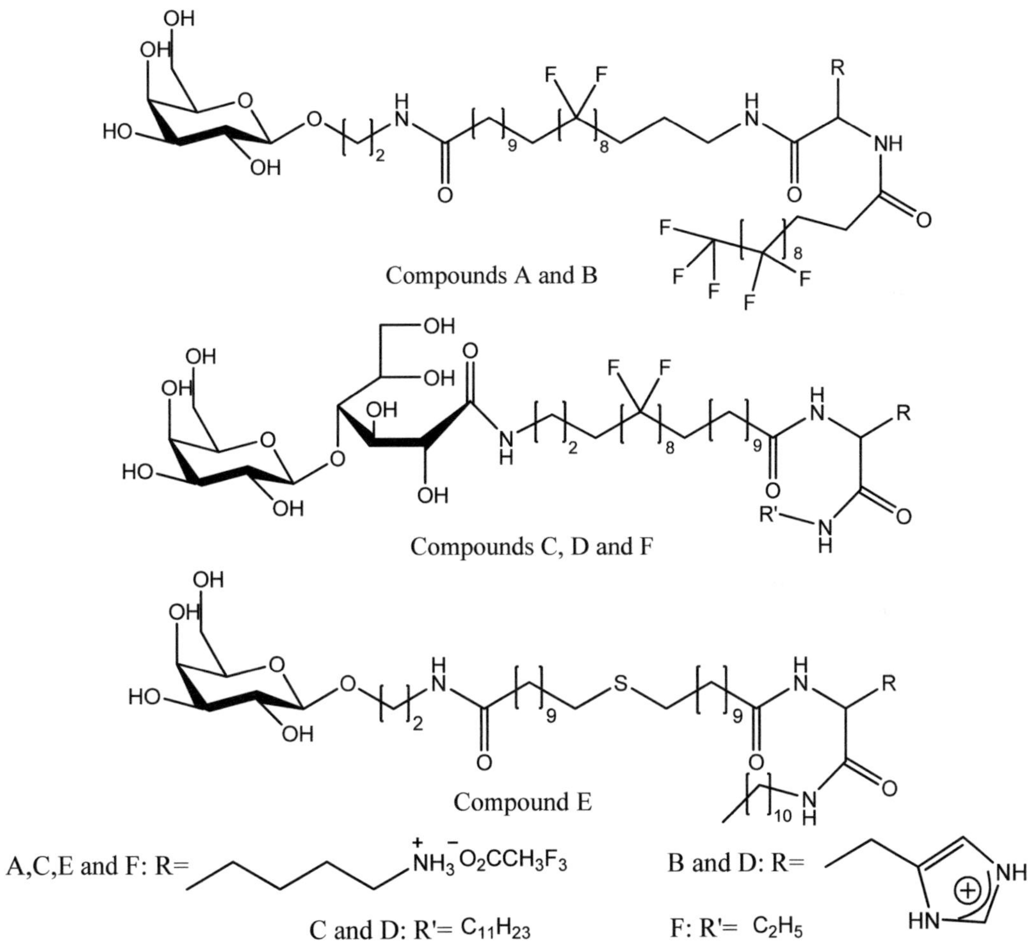

Fig. 10. A set of dissymmetric hemifluorocarbon bolaamphiphiles.

The mannose receptor (MR) is found on the surface of macrophages and dendritic cells can recognize complex carbohydrates that are located on glycoproteins that are a part of many different biological processes, and bind terminal mannoses found on vector. Kawakami et al. (Kawakami et al., 2000b) have developed a novel mannosylated cholesterol derivative, Man-C4-Chol, consisting of modified cationic liposomes with mannose moieties for NPC-selective gene delivery via mannose receptors on NPC. The mannosylated cationic

liposomes can deliver pDNA to liver nonparenchymal cells (Kawakami et al., 2000b) and splenic DCs and improve immune activation in DNA vaccines (Hattori et al., 2004).
Since theirs early use for the targeting to erythroblasts (Zhang et al., 2010), targeting proteins such as antibodies or transferrin have become one of the most widely used ligands for targeting of synthetic vectors, and been used in conjunction with cationic lipoplexes (Rao, 2010) to mediate uptake of plasmid DNA and antisense oligonucleotides. Another important class of cell proteins with promise for targeted gene delivery is growth factor receptor, which is a most commonly single pass transmembrane protein with an extracellular ligand binding domain and an intracellular region with enzymatic activity, usually a tyrosine kinase domain, which transmits a growth factor signal from the cell's environment to its interior. It has been used to target polylysine complexes (Cristiano & Roth, 1996), liposomes (Kikuchi, 1996), PEI polyplexes (Cristiano & Roth, 1996), and adenovirus-derived peptides (Medina-Kauwe et al., 2001) to receptor-positive cells.
Targeting provides a generic strategy to improve the specificity of a pharmaceutical formulation independently of the specificity of the drug or gene itself, primarily through a modulation of the carriers' biodistribution, so that a dose differential is created between healthy and diseased tissue.

5. Conclusion

Cationic lipisomes-mediated gene transfer has shown to be a safe and effective way to transfer genes for gene therapy, and will gain clinical application in the near future. Some traditional cationic lipids have been used in gene transfer for a long time; many of them have trademarks such as lipofectin, lipofectamine and transfectam. These cationic lipids, however, may not be enough for the application in clinical trials; on the other hand, they have some shortcomings for a special application field. Therefore, many novel cationic lipids in chemical structure nature have been researching to meet the requirements with respect to gene therapy. Besides the lipid structure the next level should be the formulations of cationic liposomes, as in order to increase transfection efficiency and to decrease cytotoxicity other ingredients such as heper lipids could be chosen. Different formulations may cause various morphologies of lipoplexes formed by the combination between cationic liposomes and genes. It shows that the purposeful design of morphologies could increase transfection efficiency. The hybrid utilization of non-viral vectors based on cationic liposomes provides another solution to gene delivery. Much research has shown the promising combination between cationic lipsomes and polymers, the favorable conjugation between lipids and peptides and between targeting moieties and lipids.

6. Acknowledgement

The study was supported by the National Natural Science Foundation of China (20876027 and 21046008) and Program for New Century Excellent Talents in University (NCET-08-0654) and the Fundamental Research Funds for the Central Universities (DC10020103).

7. References

Ahmad, A.; Evans, H.M.; Ewert, K.; George, C.X.; Samuel, C.E. & Safinya1, C.R. (2005). New Multivalent Cationic Lipids Reveal Bell Curve for Transfection Efficiency Versus

Membrane Charge Density: Lipid–DNA Complexes for Gene Delivery. *J. Gene. Med.*, Vol.7, No.6, pp. 739-748, ISSN 1099-498X

Ahn, C.H.; Chae, S.Y.; Bae, Y.H. & Kim, S.W. (2004). Synthesis of Biodegradable Multi-block Copolymers of Poly(L-lysine) and Poly(ethylene glycol) As a Non-viral Gene Carrier. *J. Controlled Release*, Vol.97, No.3, pp. 567–574, ISSN 0168-3659

Amenitsch, H.; Caracciolo, G.; Foglia, P.; Fuscoletti, V.; Giansanti, P.; Marianecci, C.; Pozzi, D. & Laganà, A. (2011). Existence of Hybrid Structures in Cationic Liposome/DNA Complexes Revealed by Their Interaction with Plasma Proteins. *Colloids Surf., B*, Vol.82, No.1, pp. 141-146, ISSN 0927-7765

Ashwell, G. & Harford, J. (1982). Carbohydrate-specific Receptors of the Liver. *Annu. ReV. Biochem.*, Vol.51, pp. 531–554, ISSN 0066-4154

Behr, J.P.; Demeneix, B.; Loeffler, J.P. & Perez-Mutul, J. (1989). Efficient Gene-transfer into Mammalian Primary Endocrine-cells with Lipopolyamine-coated DNA. *Proc. Natl. Acad. Sci. U.S.A.*, Vol.86, No.18, pp. 6982–6986, ISSN 0027-8424

Bennett, M.J.; Aberle, A.M.; Balasubramaniam, R.P.; Malone, J.G.; Malone, R.W. & Nantz, M.H. (1997). Cationic Lipid-mediated Gene Delivery to Murine Lung: Correlation of Lipid Hydration with in Vivo Transfection Activity. *J. Med. Chem.*, Vol.40, No.25, pp. 4069-4078, ISSN 0022-2623

Bottega, R. & Epand, R.M. (1992). Inhibition of Protein Kinase C by Cationic Amphiphiles. *Biochemistry*, Vol.31, No.37, pp. 9025-9030, ISSN 0006-2960

Brunelle, M.; Polidori, A.; Denoyelle, S.; Fabiano, A.S.; Vuillaume, P.Y.; Laurent-Lewandowski, S. & Pucci, B. (2009). A Structure-activity Investigation of Hemifluorinated Bifunctional Bolaamphiphiles Designed for Gene Delivery. *C. R. Chimie.*, Vol.12, No.1-2, pp. 188-208, ISSN 1631-0748

Byk, G.; Dubertret, C.; Escriou, V.; Frederic, M.; Jaslin, G.; Rangara, R.; Pitard, B.; Crouzet, J.; Wils, P.; Schwartz, B. & Scherman, D. (1998). Synthesis, Activity, and Structure-Activity Relationship Studies of Novel Cationic Lipids for DNA Transfer. *J. Med. Chem.*, Vol.41, No.2, pp. 224-235, ISSN 0022-2623

Byk, G.; Wetzer, B.; Frederic, M.; Dubertret, C.; Pitard, B.; Jaslin, G. & Scherman, D. (2000). Reduction-sensitive Lipopolyamines as a Novel Nonviral Gene Delivery System for Modulated Release of DNA with Improved Transgene Expression. *J. Med. Chem.*, Vol.43, No.23, pp. 4377-4387, ISSN 0022-2623

Carriere, M.; Tranchant, I.; Niore, P.A.; Byk, G.; Mignet, N.; Escriou, V.; Scherman, D. & Herscovici, J. (2002). Optimization of Cationic Lipid Mediated Gene Transfer: Structure-function, Physico-chemical, and Cellular Studies. *J. Liposome. Res.*, Vol.12, No.1-2, pp. 95-106, ISSN 0898-2104

Chen, Y.C.; Sen, J.; Bathula, S.R.; Yang, Q.; Fittipaldi, R. & Huang, L. (2009). Novel Cationic Lipid That Delivers siRNA and Enhances Therapeutic Effect in Lung Cancer Cells. *Mol. Pharm.*, Vol.6, No.3, pp. 696-705, ISSN 1543-8384

Cheng, H.; Zhu, J.L.; Zeng, X.; Jing, Y.; Zhang, X.Z. & Zhuo, R.X. (2009). Targeted Gene Delivery Dediated by Folate-polyethylenimine-block-poly(ethylene glycol) with Receptor Selectivity. *Bioconjugate Chem.*, Vol.20, No.3, pp. 481-487, ISSN 1043-1082

Choi, J.S.; Lee, E.J.; Jang, H.S. & Park, J.S. (2001). New Cationic Liposomes for Gene Transfer into Mammalian Cells with High Efficiency and Low Toxicity. *Bioconjugate Chem.*, Vol.12, No.1, pp. 108-113, ISSN 1043-1082

Coles, D.J.; Esposito, A.; Chuah, H.T. & Toth, I. (2010). The Synthesis and Characterization of Lipophilic Peptide-based Carriers for Gene Delivery.*Tetrahedron*, Vol.66, No.29, pp. 5435-5441, ISSN 0040-4020

Cristiano, R.J. & Roth, J.A. (1996). Epidermal Growth Factor Mediated DNA Delivery into Lung Cancer Cells via the Epidermal Growth Factor Receptor. *Cancer Gene Ther.*, Vol.3, No.1, pp. 4-10, ISSN 0929-1903

Dauty, E.; Remy, J. S.; Zuber, G. & Behr, J.-P. (2002). Intracellular Delivery of Nanometric DNA Particles via the Folate Receptor. *Bioconjugate Chem.*, Vol.13, No.4, pp. 831–839, ISSN 1043-1082

Donkuru, M.D.; Badea, I.; Wettig, S.; Verrall, R.; Elsabahy, M. & Foldvari, M. (2010). Advancing Nonviral Gene Delivery: Lipid- and Surfactant-based Nanoparticle Design Strategies. *Nanomedicine (Lond)*, Vol.5, No.7, pp. 1103-1127, ISSN 1743-5889

Duan, Y.J.; Zheng, J.N.; Han, S.F.; Wu, Y.; Wang, Y.M.; Li, D.J.; Kong, D.L. & Yu, Y.T. (2008). A Tumor Targeted Gene Vector Modified with G250 Monoclonal Antibody for Gene Therapy. *J. Controlled Release*, Vol.127, No.2, pp. 173-179, ISSN 0168-3659

El-Aneed, A. (2004). An Overview of Current Delivery Systems in Cancer Gene Therapy. *J. Controlled Release*, Vol.94, No.1, pp. 1-14, ISSN 0168-3659

Elouahabi, A. & Ruysschaert, J.M. (2005). Formation and Intracellular Trafficking of Lipoplexes and Polyplexes. *Mol. Ther.*, Vol.11, No.3, pp. 336–347, ISSN 1525-0016

Escriou, V.; Ciolina, C.; Lacroix, F.; Byk, G.; Scherman, D. & Wils, P. (1998). Cationic Lipid-mediated Gene Transfer: Effect of Serum on Cellular Uptake and Intracellular Fate of Lipopolyamine/DNA Complexes. *Biochim. Biophys. Acta.*, Vol.1368, No.2, pp. 276-288, ISSN 0005-2736

Ewert, K.; Ahmad, A.; Evans, H.M. & Safinya, C.R. (2005a). Cationic Lipid-DNA Complexes for Non-viral Gene Therapy: Relating Supramolecular Structures to Cellular Pathways. *Expert Opin. Biol. Ther.*, Vol.5, No.1, pp. 33-53, ISSN 1471-2598

Ewert, K.; Ahmad, A.; Evans, H.M.; Schmidt, H.W. & Safinya, C.R. (2002). Efficient Synthesis and Cell-transfection Properties of a New Nultivalent Cationic Lipid for Nonviral Gene Delivery. *J. Med. Chem.*, Vol.45, No.23, pp. 5023-5029, ISSN 0022-2623

Ewert, K.; Evans, H.M.; Ahmad, A.N.; Slack, L.; Lin, A.J.; Martin-Herranz, A. & Safinya, C.R. (2005b). Lipoplex Structures and Their Distinct Cellular Pathways. *Adv. Genet.*, Vol.53, No.8, pp. 119-155, ISBN 13:978-0-12-374621-4

Ewert, K.; Evans, H.M.; Zidovska, A.; Bouxsein, N.F.; Ahmad, A. & Safinya, C.R. (2006). A Columnar Phase of Dendritic Lipid-based Cationic Liposome-DNA Complexes for Gene Delivery: Hexagonally Ordered Cylindrical Micelles Embedded in A DNA Honeycomb Lattice. *J. Am. Chem. Soc.*, Vol.128, No.12, pp. 3998-4006, ISSN 0002-7863

Ewert, K.; Slack, N.L.; Ahmad, A.; Evans, H.M.; Lin, A.J.; Samuel, C.E. & Safinya, C.R. (2004). Cationic Lipid-DNA Complexes for Gene Therapy: Understanding the Relationship Between Complex Structure and Gene Delivery Pathways at The Molecular Level. *Curr. Med. Chem.*, Vol.11, No.2, pp. 133-149, ISSN 1568-0118

Fabio, K.; Gaucheron, J.; Giorgio, C.D. & Vierling P. (2003). Novel Galactosylated Polyamine Bolaamphiphiles for Gene Delivery. *Bioconjugate Chem.*, Vol.14, No.2, pp. 358-367, ISSN 1043-1082

Fanning, G.; Amado, R. & Symonds, G.J. (2003). Gene Therapy for HIV/AIDS: The Potential for a New Therapeutic Regimen. *J Gene Med*, Vol.5, No.8, pp. 645-653, ISSN 1521-2254

Farago, O.; Gronbech-Jensen, N. & Pincus, P. (2006). Mesoscale Computer Modeling of Lipid-DNA Complexes for Gene Therapy. *Phys. Rev. Lett.*, Vol.96, No.4, pp. 018102-018106, ISSN 0031-9007

Farhood, H.; Serbina, N. & Huang, L. (1995). The Role of Dioleoyl Phosphatidylethanolamine in Cationic Liposome Mediated Gene Transfer. *Biochim. Biophys. Act.*, Vol.1235, No.2, pp. 289-295, ISSN 0005-2736

Felgner, J.H.; Kumar, R.; Sridhar, C.N.; Wheeler, C.J.; Tsai, Y.J.; Border, R.; Ramsey, P.; Martin, M. & Felgner, P.L. (1994). Enhanced Gene Delivery and Mechanism Studies with a Novel Series of Cationic Lipid Formulations. *J. Biol. Chem.*, Vol.269, No.4, pp. 2550-2561, ISSN 0021-9258

Felgner, P.L.; Gadek, T.R.; Holm, M.; Roman, R.; Chan, H.S.; Wenz, M.; Northrop, J.P.; Ringgold, G.M. & Danielson, M. (1987). Lipofection: A Highly Efficient, Lipid-Mediated DNA-transfection Procedure. *Proc. Natl. Acad. Sci. U.S.A.*, Vol.84, No.21, pp. 7413-7417, ISSN 0027-8424

Felgner, P.L. & Ringold, G.M. (1989). Cationic Liposome-mediated Transfection. *Nature*, Vol.11, No.2, pp. 387-388, ISSN 0028-0836

Ferrari, M.E.; Nguyen, C.M.; Zelphati, O.; Tsai, Y. & Felgner, P.L. (1998). Analytical Methods for the Characterization of Cationic Lipid Nucleic Acid Complexes. *Hum. Gene Ther.*, Vol.9, No.3, pp. 341-351, ISSN 1043-0342

Ferrari, M.E.; Rusalov, D.; Enas, J. & Wheeler, C.J. (2002). Synergy between Cationic Lipid and Co-lipid Determines the Macroscopic Structure and Transfection Activity of Lipoplexes. *Nucleic Acids Res.*, Vol.30, No.8, pp. 1808-1816, ISSN 0305-1048

Fletcher, S.; Ahmad, A.; Perouzel, E.; Heron, A.; Miller, A.D. & Jorgensen, M.R. (2006). In Vivo Studies of Dialkynoyl Analogues of DOTAP Demonstrate Improved Gene Transfer Efficiency of Cationic Liposomes in Mouse Lung. *J. Med. Chem.*, Vol.49, No.1, pp. 349-357, ISSN 0022-2623

Floch, V.; Loisel, S.; Guénin, E.; Hervé, A.C.; Yaouanc, J.J.; Clément, J.C.; Férec, C. & Des Abbayes, H. (2000). Cation Substitution in Cationic Phosphonolipids: A New Concept to Improve Transfection Activity and Decrease Cellular Toxicity. *J. Med. Chem.*, Vol.43, No.23, pp. 4617-4628, ISSN 0022-2623

Folda, T.; Gros, L. & Ringsdorf, H. (1982). Polyreactions in Oriented Systems, 29[a]). Formation of Oriented Polypeptides and Polyamides in Monolayers and Liposomes. *Makromol Chem Rapid Commun*, Vol.3, No.3, pp. 167–174, ISSN 0173-2803

Frederic, M.; Scherman, D. & Byk, G. (2000). Introduction of Cyclic Guanidines into Cationic Lipids for Non-viral Gene Delivery. *Tetrahedron Lett.*, Vol.41, No.5, pp. 675-679, ISSN 0040-4039

Fujiwara, T.; Hasegawa, S.; Hirashima, N.; Nakanishi, M. & Ohwada, T. (2000). Gene Transfection Activities of Amphiphilic Steroid–polyamine Conjugates. *Biochim. Biophys. Acta, Biomembr.*, Vol.1468, No.1-2, pp. 396-402, ISSN 0005-2736

Funhoff, A.M.; van Nostrum, C.F.; Lok, M.C.; Kruijtzer, J.A.; Crommelin, D.J. & Hennink, W.E. (2005). Cationic Polymethacrylates with Covalently Linked Membrane Destabilizing Peptides as Gene Delivery Vectors. *J. Controlled Release*, Vol.101, No.1-3, pp. 233–246, ISSN 0168-3659

Gao, H. & Hui, K.M. (2001). Synthesis of a Novel Series of Cationic Lipids that Can Act As Efficient Gene Delivery Vehicles Through Systematic Heterocyclic Substitution of Cholesterol Derivatives. *Gene Ther*, Vol.8, No.11, pp. 855-863, ISSN 0969-7128

Gao, K. & Huang, L. (2009). Nonviral Methods for siRNA Delivery. *Mol. Pharm.*, Vol.6, No.3, pp. 651-658, ISSN 1543-8384

Gao, X. & Huang, L. (1991). A Novel Cationic Liposome Reagent for Efficient Transfection of Mammalian Cells. *Biochem. Biophys. Res. Commun.*, Vol.179, No.1, pp. 280-285, ISSN 0006-291X

Gao, X. & Huang, L. (1995). Cationic Liposome-mediated Gene Transfer. *Gene Ther*, Vol.2, No.10, pp. 710-722, ISSN 0969-7128

Gao, X. & Huang, L. (1996). Potentiation of Cationic Liposomemediated Gene Delivery by Polycations. *Biochemistry*, Vol.35, No.3, pp. 1027-1036, ISSN 0006-2960

Gaucheron, J.; Boulanger, C.; Santaella, C.; Sbirrazzuoli, N.; Boussif, O. & Vierling, P. (2001a). In Vitro Cationic Lipid-mediated Gene Delivery with Fluorinated Glycerophosphoethanolamine Helper Lipids. *Bioconjugate Chem.*, Vol.12, No.6, pp. 949-963, ISSN 1043-1082

Gaucheron, J.; Santaella, C. & Vierling, P. (2001b). Highly Fluorinated Lipospermines for Gene Transfer: Synthesis and Evaluation of Their in Vitro Transfection Efficiency. *Bioconjugate Chem.*, Vol.12, No.1, pp. 114-128, ISSN 1043-1082

Gaucheron, J.; Santaella, C. & Vierling, P. (2001c). In Vitro Gene Transfer with a Novel Galactosylated Spermine Bolaamphiphile. *Bioconjugate Chem.*, Vol.12, No.4, pp. 569-575, ISSN 1043-1082

Gaucheron, J.; Santaella, C. & Vierling, P. (2001d). Improved in Vitro Gene Transfer Mediated by Fluorinated Lipoplexes in the Presence of a Bile Salt Surfactant. *J. Med. Chem.*, Vol.3, No.4, pp. 338-344, ISSN 0022-2623

Gaucheron, J.; Wong, T.; Wong, K.F.; Maurer, N. & Cullis, P.R. (2002). Synthesis and Properties of Novel Tetraalkyl Cationic Lipids. *Bioconjugate Chem.*, Vol.13, No.3, pp. 671-675, ISSN 1043-1082

Gershon, H.; Ghirlando, R.; Guttman, S.B. & Minsky, A. (1993). Mode of Formation and Structural Features of DNA-Cationic Liposome Complexes Used for Transfection. *Biochemistry*, Vol.32, No.28, pp. 7143–7151, ISSN 0006-2960

Hattori, Y.; Kawakami, S.; Suzuki, S.; Yamashita, F. & Hashida, M. (2004). Enhancement of Immune Responses by DNA Vaccination Through Targeted Gene Delivery Using Mannosylated Cationic Liposome Formulations Following Intravenous Administration in Mice. *Biochem. Biophys. Res. Commun.*, Vol.317, No.4, pp. 992–999, ISSN 0006-291X

Heinze, M.; Brezesinski, G. & Dobner, B. (2010). LangnerA: Novel Cationic Lipids Based on Malonic Acid Amides Backbone: Transfection Efficacy and Cell Toxicity Properties. *Bioconjugate Chem.*, Vol.21, No. 4, pp. 696-708, ISSN 1043-1802

Heyes, J.A.; Niculescu-Duvaz, D.; Cooper, R.G. & Springer, C.J. (2002). Synthesis of Novel Cationic Lipids: Effect of Structural Modification on the Efficiency of Gene Transfer. *J. Med. Chem.*, Vol.45, No.1, pp. 99–114, ISSN 0022-2623

Huang, C.Y.; Uno, T.; Murphy, J.E.; Lee, S.; Hamer, J.D.; Escobedo, J.A.; Cohen, F.E.; Radhakrishnan, R.; Dwarki, V. & Zuckermann R.N. (1998). Lipitoids-novel Cationic Lipids for Cellular Delivery of Plasmid DNA in Vitro. *Chem Biol.*, Vol.5, No.6, pp. 345–354, ISSN 1074-5521

Legendre, J.Y.; Trzeciak, A.; Bohrmann, B.; Deuschle, U.; Kitas, E. & Supersaxo, A. (1997). Dioleoylmelittin as a Novel Serum-Insensitive Reagent for Efficient Transfection of Mammalian Cells. *Bioconjugate Chem.*, Vol.8, No.1, pp. 57–63, ISSN 1043-1082

Ilies, M.A.; Seitz, W.A.; Caproiu, M.T.; Wentz, M.; Garfield, R.E. & Balaban, A.T. (2003). Pyridinium-based Cationic Lipids As Gene-transfer Agents. *Eur. J. Org. Chem.*, Vol.2003, No.14, pp. 2645–2655, ISSN 1099-0690

Jacopin, C.; Hofland, H.; Scherman, D. & Herscovici, J. (2001). Synthesis and Transfecting Properties of a Glycosylated Polycationic DNA Vector. *Bioorg. Med. Chem. Lett.*, Vol.11, No.3, pp. 419-422, ISSN 0960-894X

Kane, M.A.; Elwood, P.C.; Portillo, R.M.; Antony, A.C. & Kolhouse, J.F. (1986). The Interrelationship of the Soluble and Membrane-associated Folate-binding Proteins in Human KB cells. *J. Biol. Chem.*, Vol.261, No.33, pp. 15625–15631, ISSN 0021-9258

Katas, H. & Alpar, H.O. (2006). Development and Characterisation of Chitosan Nanoparticles for siRNA Delivery. *J. Controlled Release*, Vol.115, No.2, pp. 216-225, ISSN 0168-3659

Kato, A.; Tsuji, A.; Yanagisawa, M.; Saeki, D.; Juni, K.; Morimoto, Y. & Yoshikawa, K. (2010). Phase Separation on a Phospholipid Membrane Inducing a Characteristic Localization of DNA Accompanied by Its Structural Transition. *J. Phys. Chem. Lett.*, Vol.1, No. 23, pp. 3391-3395, ISSN 1948-7185

Kawakami, S.; Fumoto, S.; Nishikawa, M.; Yamashita, F. & Hashida, M. (2000a). In Vivo Gene Delivery to the Liver Using Novel Galactosylated Cationic Liposomes. *Pharm. Res.*, Vol.17, No.3, pp. 306–313, ISSN 0724-8741

Kawakami, S.; Sato, A.; Nishikawa, M.; Yamashita, F. & Hashida, M. (2000b). Mannose Receptor-mediated Gene Transfer into Macrophages Using Novel Mannosylated Cationic Liposomes. *Gene Ther*, Vol.7, No.4, pp. 292–299, ISSN 0969-7128

Kawakami, S.; Yamashita, F.; Nishikawa, M.; Takakura, Y. & Hashida, M. (1998). Asialoglycoprotein Receptor-mediated Gene Transfer Using Novel Galactosylated Cationic Liposomes. *Biochem. Biophys. Res. Commun.*, Vol.252, No.1, pp. 78-83, ISSN 0006-291X

Kedika, B. & Patri, S.V. (2011). Design, Synthesis, and in Vitro Transfection Biology of Novel Tocopherol Based Monocationic Lipids: A Structure-Activity Investigation. *J. Med. Chem.*, Vol.54, No.2, pp. 548–561, ISSN 0022-2623

Kennedy, M.T.; Pozharski, E.V.; Rakhmanova, V.A. & MacDonald, R.C. (2000). Factors Governing the Assembly of Cationic Phospholipid-DNA Complexes. *Biophys. J.*, Vol.78, No.3, pp. 1620-1633, ISSN 0006-3495

Kichler, A.; Leborgne, C.; Savage, P.B. & Danos, O. (2005). Cationic Steroid Antibiotics Demonstrate DNA Delivery Properties. *J. Controlled Release*, Vol.107, No.1, pp. 174-182, ISSN 0168-3659

Kikuchi, A.; Sugaya, S.; Ueda, H.; Tanaka, K.; Aramaki, Y.; Hara, T.; Arima, H.; Tsuchiya, S. & Fuwa, T. (1996). Efficient Gene Transfer to EGF Receptor Overexpressing Cancer Cells by Means of EGF-labeled Cationic Liposomes. *Biochem. Biophys. Res. Commun.*, Vol.227, No.3, pp. 666–671, ISSN 0006-291X

Kneuer, C.; Ehrhardt, C.; Bakowsky, H.; Kumar, M.N.; Oberle, V.; Lehr, C.M.; Hoekstra, D. & Bakowsky, U. (2006). The Influence of Physicochemical Parameters on the Efficacy of Non-viral DNA Transfection Complexes: a Comparative Study. *J. Nanosci Nanotechnol.*, Vol.6, No.9-10, pp. 2776-2782, ISSN 1550-7033

Koltover, I.; Salditt, T.; Radler, J.O. & Safinya, C.R. (1998). An Inverted Hexagonal Phase of Cationic Liposome-DNA Complexes Related to DNA Release and Delivery. *Science*, Vol.281, No.5373, pp. 78-81, ISSN 0036-8075

Koynova, R. & Tenchov, B. (2010). Cationic Lipids: Nolecular Structure/Transfection Activity Relationships and Interactions with Biomembranes. *Top Curr Chem*, Vol.296, No.2010, pp. 51-93, ISSN 0340-1022

Lampela, P.; Elomaa, M.; Ruponen, M.; Urtti, A.; Mannisto, P.T. & Raasmaja, A. (2003). Different Synergistic Roles of Small Polyethylenimine and Dosper in Gene Delivery. *J. Controlled Release*, Vol.88, No.1, pp. 173-183, ISSN 0168-3659

Lasic, D.D. (1997). Recent Developments in Medical Applications of Liposomes: Sterically Stabilized Liposomes in Cancer Therapy and Gene Delivery in Vivo. *J. Controlled Release*, Vol.48, No.2-3, pp. 203-222, ISSN 0168-3659

Leal, C.; Bouxsein, N. F.; Ewert, K.K. & Safinya C.R. (2010). Highly Efficient Gene Silencing Activity of siRNA Embedded in a Nanostructured Gyroid Cubic Lipid Matrix. *J. Am. Chem. Soc.*, Vol.132, No.47, pp. 16841-16847, ISSN 0002-7863

Lee, C.H.; Ni, Y.H.; Chen, C.C.; Chou, C.K. & Chang, F.H. (2003). Synergistic Effect of Polyethylenimine and Cationic Liposomes in Nucleic acid Delivery to Human Cancer Cells. *Biochim. Biophys. Acta, Biomembr.*, Vol.1611, No.1-2, pp. 55-62, ISSN 0005-2736

Lee, E.R.; Marshall, J.; Siegel, C.S.; Jiang, C.; Yew, N.S.; Nichols, M.R.; Nietupski, J.B.; Ziegler, R.J.; Lane, M.B.; Wang, K.X.; Wan, N.C.; Scheule, R.K.; Harris, D.J.; Smith, A.E. & Cheng, S.H. (1996). Detailed Analysis of Structures and Formulations of Cationic Lipids for Efficient Gene Transfer to the Lung. *Hum. Gene Ther.*, Vol.7, No.14, pp. 1701-1717, ISSN 1043-0342

Lee, L.K.; Siapati, E.K.; Jenkins, R.G.; McAnulty, R.J.; Hart, S.L. & Shamlou, P.A. (2003). Biophysical Characterization of an Integrin-targeted Non-viral Vector. *Med. Sci. Monit.*, Vol.9, No.1, pp. 54-61, ISSN 1234-1010

Lee, R.J. & Huang, L. (1996). Folate-targeted, Anionic Liposome-entrapped Polylysine-condensed DNA for Tumor Cell-specific Gene Transfer. *J. Biol. Chem.*, Vol.271, No.14, pp. 8481-8487, ISSN 0021-9258

Letrou-Bonneval, E.; Chèvre, R.; Lambert, O.; Costet, P.; André, C.; Tellier, C. & Pitard, B. (2008). Galactosylated Multimodular Lipoplexes for Specific Gene Transfer into Primary Hepatocytes. *J Gene Med*, Vol.10, No.11, pp. 1198-1209, ISSN 1521-2254

Lensink, M.F.; Lonez, C.; Ruysschaert, J.M. & Vandenbranden, M. (2009). Characterization of the Cationic DiC_{14}-amidine Bilayer by Mixed DMPC/DiC_{14}-amidine Molecular Dynamics Simulations Shows an Interdigitated Nonlamellar Bilayer Phase. *Langmuir*, Vol.25, No.9, pp. 5230-5238, ISSN 0743-7463

Leventis, R. & Silvius, J.R. (1990). Interactions of Mammalian Cells with Lipid Dispersions Containing Novel Metabolizable Cationic Amphiphiles. *Biochim. Biophys. Acta, Biomembr.*, Vol.1023, No.1, pp. 124-132, ISSN 0005-2736

Lian, T. & Ho, R.J. (2003). Design and Characterization of a Novel Lipid-DNA Complex That Resists serum-induced Destabilization. *J. Pharm. Sci.*, Vol.92, No.12, pp. 2373-2385, ISSN 0022-3549

Lin, A.J.; Slack, N.L.; Ahmad, A.C.; George, X.; Samuel, C.E. & Safinya, C.R. (2003). Three-dimensional Imaging of Lipid Gene-carriers: Membrane Charge Density Controls

Universal Transfection Behavior in Lamellar Cationic Liposome-DNA Complexes. *Biophys. J.*, Vol.84, No. 5, pp. 3307-3316, ISSN 0006-3495

Litzinger, D. & Huang, L. (1992). Phosphatidylethanolamine Liposomes: Drug Delivery, Gene Transfer and Immunodiagnostic Applications. *Biochim.Biophys.Act.*, Vol.1113, No.2, pp. 201-227, ISSN 0005-2736

Liu, D.L.; Hu, J.J.; Qiao, W.H.; Li, Z.S.; Zhang, S.B.; Cheng, L.B. (2005a). Synthesis of Carbamate-linked Lipids for Gene Delivery. *Bioorg. Med. Chem. Lett.*, Vol.15, No.12, pp. 3147–3150, ISSN 0960-894X

Liu, D.L.; Hu, J.J.; Qiao, W.H.; Li, Z.S.; Zhang, S.B.; Cheng, L.B. (2005b). Synthesis and Characterization of a Series of Carbamate-linked Cationic Lipids for Gene Delivery. *Lipids*, Vol.40, No.8, pp. 839–848, ISSN 0024-4201

Liu, D.L.; Qiao, W.H.; Li, Z.S.; Chen, Y.; Cui, X.; Li, K.; Yu, L.; Yan, K.; Zhu, L.; Guo, Y. & Cheng, L.B. (2008). Structure–function Relationship Research of Glycerol Backbone-based Cationic Lipids for Gene Delivery. *Chem. Biol. Drug Des.*, Vol.71, No.4, pp. 336–344, ISSN 1747-0277

Liu, F. & Huang, L. (2002). Development of Non-viral Vectors for Systemic Gene Delivery. *J. Controlled Release*, Vol.78, No.1-3, pp. 259-266, ISSN 0168-3659

Li, S. & Huang, L. (1997). In Vivo Gene Transfer via Intravenous Administration of Cationic Lipid-protamine-DNA (LPD) Complexes. *Gene Ther*, Vol.4, No.9, pp. 891-900, ISSN 0969-7128

Li, S.D. & Huang, L. (2006). Targeted Delivery of Antisense Oligodeoxynucleotide and Small Interference RNA into Lung Cancer Cells. *Mol. Pharm.*, Vol.3, No.5, pp. 579–588, ISSN 1543-8384

Love, K.T.; Mahon, K.P.; Levins, C.G.; Whitehead, K.A.; Querbes, W.; Dorkin, J.R.; Qin, J. & Anderson, D.G. (2010). Lipid-like Materials for Low-dose, in Vivo Gene Silencing. *Proc. Natl. Acad. Sci. U.S.A.*, Vol.107, No.5, pp. 1864–1869, ISSN 0027-8424

Mao, S.; Sun, W. & Kissel, T. (2010). Chitosan-based Formulations for Delivery of DNA and siRNA. *Adv Drug Deliv Rev.*, Vol.62, No.1, pp. 12-27, ISSN 0169-409X

Marchini, C.; Pozzi, D.; Montani, M.; Alfonsi, C.; Amici, A.; Amenitsch, H.; Sanctis, S.C.D. & Caracciolo, G. (2010). Tailoring Lipoplex Composition to the Lipid Composition of Plasma Membrane: A Trojan Horse for Cell Entry. *Langmuir*, Vol.26, No.17, pp. 13867-13873, ISSN 0743-7463

Martin-Rendon, E. & Blake, D.J. (2003). Protein Glycosylation in Disease: New Insights into the Congenital Muscular Dystrophies. *Trends Pharmacol Sci*, Vol.24, No.4, pp. 178-183, ISSN 0165-6147

McGregor, C.; Perrin, C.; Monck, M.; Camilleri, P. & Kirby, A.J. (2001). Rational Approaches to the Design of Cationic Gemini Surfactants for Gene Delivery. *J. Am. Chem. Soc.*, Vol.123, No.26, pp. 6215-6220, ISSN 0002-7863

Medina-Kauwe, L.K.; Maguire, M.; Kasahara, N. & Kedes, L. (2001). Nonviral Gene Delivery to Human Breast Cancer Cells by Targeted Ad5 Penton Proteins. *Gene Ther*, Vol.8, No.23, pp. 1753–1761, ISSN 0969-7128

Medvedeva, D.A.; Maslov, M.A.; Serikov, R.N.; Morozova, N.G.; Serebrenikova, G.A.; Sheglov, D.V.; Latyshev, A.V.; Vlassov, V.V.; Zenkova, M.A. (2009). Novel Cholesterol-Based Cationic Lipids for Gene Delivery. *J. Med. Chem.*, Vol.52, No.21, pp. 6558-6568, ISSN 0022-2623

Niculescu-Duvaz, D.; Heyes, J. & Springer, C. J. (2003). Structure-activity Relationship in Cationic Lipid Mediated Gene Transfection. *Curr. Med. Chem.*, Vol.10, No.14, pp. 1233-1261, ISSN 0929-8673

Obata, Y.; Ciofani, G.; Raffa, V.; Cuschieri, A. & Takeoka. S. (2010). Evaluation of Cationic Liposomes Composed of an Amino Acid-based Lipid for Neuronal Transfection. *Nanomed: Nanotech, Biol. Med.*, Vol.6, No.1, pp. 70-77, ISSN 1549-9634

Obata, Y.; Saito, S.; Takeda, N. & Takeoka, S. (2009). Plasmid DNA-encapsulating Liposomes: Effect of a Spacer between the Cationic Head Group and Hydrophobic Moieties of the Lipids on Gene Expression Efficiency. *Biochim. Biophys. Acta, Biomembr.*, Vol.1788, No.5, pp. 1148-1158, ISSN 0005-2736

Obata, Y.; Suzuki, D. & Takeoka, S. (2008). Evaluation of Cationic Assemblies Constructed with Amino Acid Based Lipids for Plasmid DNA Delivery. *Bioconjugate Chem.*, Vol.19, No.5, pp. 1055–1063, ISSN 1043-1082

O'Hern, C.S. & Lubensky, T.C. (1998). Sliding Columnar Phase of DNA-Lipid Complexes. *Phys. Rev. Lett.*, Vol.80, No.19, pp. 4345-4348, ISSN 0031-9007

Randazzo, R.A.S.; Bucki , R.; Janmey, P.A. & Diamond, S.L. (2009). A Series of Cationic Sterol Lipids with Gene Transfer and Bactericidal Activity. *Bioorg Med Chem.*, Vol.17, No.9, pp. 3257-3265, ISSN 0968-0896

Rao, N.M. (2010). Cationic Lipid-mediated Nucleic Acid Delivery: Beyond Being Cationic. *Chem* Phys Lipids, Vol.163, No.3, pp. 245-252, ISSN 0009-3084

Reddy, J.A.; Abburi, C.; Hofland. H.; Howard, S.J.; Vlahov, I.; Wils, P. & Leamon C.P. (2002). Folate-targeted, Cationic Liposome-mediated Gene Transfer into Disseminated Peritoneal Tumors. *Gene Ther*, Vol.9, No.22, pp. 1542–1550, ISSN 0969-7128

Pedroso de Lima, M.C.; Neves, S.; Filipe, A; Düzgünes, N. & Simoes, S. (2003). Cationic Liposomes for Gene Delivery: From Biophysics to Biological Applications. *Curr. Med. Chem.*, Vol.10, No.14, pp. 1221-1231, ISSN 0929-8673

Pitard, B.; Aguerre, O.; Airiau, M.; Lachagès, A.M.; Boukhnikachvili, T.; Byk, G.; Dubertret, C.; Herviou, C.; Scherman, D.; Mayaux, J.F. & Crouzet, J. (1997). Virus-sized Self-assembling Lamellar Complexes between Plasmid DNA and Cationic Micelles Promote Gene Transfer. *Proc. Natl. Acad. Sci. U. S. A.*, Vol.94, No.26, pp. 14412-14417, ISSN 0027-8424

Rejman, J.; Oberle, V.; & Zuhorn, I.S. (2004). Size-dependent Internalization of Particles via the Pathways of Clathrin-and Caveolae-mediated Endocytosis. *Biochem. J.*, Vol.377, No.1, pp. 159-169, ISSN 0264-6021

Ren, T.; Zhang, G.; Liu, F. & Liu, D. (2000). Synthesis and Evaluation of Vitamin D-based Cationic Lipids for Gene Delivery in Vitro. *Bioorg. Med. Chem. Lett.*, Vol.10, No.9, pp. 891-894, ISSN 0960-894X

Ren, T.; Zhang, G.S. & Liu, D.X. (2001). Synthesis of Bifunctional Cationic Compound for Gene Delivery. *Tetrahedron Lett.*, Vol.42, No.6, pp. 1007–1010, ISSN 0040-4039

Ross, P.C. & Hui, S.W. (1999). Lipoplex Size Is a Major Determinant of in Vitro Lipofection Efficiency. *Gene. Ther.*, Vol.6, No.4, pp. 651-659, ISSN 0969-7128

Ruponen, M.; Ylä-Herttuala, S. & Urtti, A. (1999). Interactions of Polymeric and Liposomal Gene Delivery Systems with Extracellular Glycosaminoglycans: Physicochemical and Transfection Studies. *Biochim. Biophys. Acta, Biomembr.*, Vol.1415, No.2, pp. 331-341, ISSN 0005-2736

Safinya, C.R. (2001). Structures of Lipid–DNA Complexes: Supramolecular Assembly and Gene Delivery. *Curr. Opin. Struct. Biol.* Vol.11, No.4, pp. 440- 448 ISSN 0959-440X

Sakaguchi, N.; Kojima, C.; Harada, A.; Koiwai, K.; Shimizu, K.; Emi, N. & Kono, K. (2008). Generation of Highly Potent Nonviral Gene Vectors by Complexation of Lipoplexes and Transferrin-bearing Fusogenic Polymer-modified Liposomes in Aqueous Glucose Solution. *Biomaterials,* Vol.29, No.9, pp. 1262-1272, ISSN 0142-9612

Scarzello, M.J.; Smisterova, A.; Wagenaar, M.C.; Stuart, D.; Hoekstra,□J.B. & Engberts, R. (2005). Sunfish Cationic Amphiphiles: Toward an Adaptative Lipoplex Morphology. *J. Am. Chem. Soc.* Vol.127, No.29, pp. 10420-10429, ISSN 0002-7863

Seol, J.G., Heo, D.S., Kim, H.K., Yoon, J.-H., Choi, B.I., Lee, H.-S., Kim, N.K. & Kim, C.Y. (2000). Selective Gene Expression in Hepatic Tumor with Trans-arterial Delivery of DNA/Liposome/Transferrin Complex. *In Vivo,* Vol.14, No.3, pp. 513–518, ISSN 0258-851X

Sochanik, A.; Kaida, I.; Mitrus, I.; Rajca, A. & Szala, S. (2000). A New Cholesterol Derivative Suitable for Transfecting Certain Type of Cells in the Presence of 10% Serum. *Cancer Gene Ther.,* Vol.7, No.4, pp. 513–520, ISSN 0929-1903

Sternberg, B.; Sorgib, F.L. & Huang, L. (1994). New Structures in Complex Formation between DNA and Cationic Liposomes Visualized by Freeze-fracture Electron Microscopy. *FEBS. Lett.,* Vol.356, No.2-3, pp. 361-366, ISSN 0014-5793

Sternberg, B.; Hong, K.; Zheng, W. & Papahadjopoulos, D. (1998). Ultrastructural Characterization of Cationic Liposome-DNA Complexes Showing Enhanced Stability in Serum and High Transfection Activity in Vivo. *Biochim. Biophys. Act.,* Vol.1375, No.1-2, pp. 23-35, ISSN 0005-2736

Tang, F. & Hughes, J.A. (1999a). Synthesis of a Single-tailed Cationic Lipid and Investigation of Its Transfection. *J. Controlled Release,* Vol.62, No.3, pp. 345-358, ISSN 0168-3659

Tang, F. & Hughes, J.A. (1999b). Use of Dithiodiglycolic Acid As a Tether for Cationic Lipids Decreases the Cytotoxicity and Increases Transgene Expression of Plasmid DNA in Vitro. *Bioconjugate Chem.,* Vol.10, No.5, pp. 791–796, ISSN 1043-1082

Turek, J.; Dubertret, C.; Jaslin, G.; Antonakis, K.; Scherman, D. & Pitard, B. (2000). Formulations Which Increase the Size of Lipoplexes Prevent Serum-associated Inhibition of Transfection. *J. Gene. Med.,* Vol.2, No.1, pp. 32-40, ISSN 1099-498X

Wasungu, L. & Hoekstra, D. (2006). Cationic Lipids, Lipoplexes and Intracellular Delivery of Genes. *J. Controlled Release,* Vol.116, No.2, pp. 255-264, ISSN 0168-3659

Williams, P.D.; Ranjzad, P.; Kakar, S.J. & Kingston, P.A. (2010). Development of Viral Vectors for Use in Cardiovascular Gene Therapy. *Viruses,* Vol.2, No.2, pp. 334-371, ISSN 1999-4915

Xu, Y.; Hui, S.W.; Frederik, P. & Szoka, F.C.J. (1999). Physicochemical Characterization and Purification of Cationic Lipoplexes. *Biophys. J.,* Vol.77, No.1, pp. 341-353, ISSN 0006-3495

Yingyongnarongkul, B.E.; Howarth, M.; Elliott, T. & Bradley, M. (2004). Solid Phase Synthesis of 89 Polyamine-based Cationic Lipids for DNA Delivery to Mammalian Cells. *Chem. Eur. J.,* Vol.10, No.2, pp. 463–473, ISSN 1521-3765

Yoshizawa, T.; Hattori, Y.; Hakoshima, M.; Koga, K. & Maitani, Y. (2008). Folate-linked Lipid-based Nanoparticles for Synthetic siRNA Delivery in KB Tumor xenografts. *Eur J Pharm Biopharm.,* Vol.70, No.3, pp. 718-725, ISSN 0939-6411

Zuhorn, I.S.; Bakowsky, U.; Polushkin, E.; Visser, W.H.; Stuart, M.C.; Engberts, J.B. & Hoekstra, D. (2005). Nonbilayer Phase of Lipoplex-membrane Mixture Determines Endosomal Escape of Genetic Cargo and Transfection Efficiency. *Mol. Ther.*, Vol.11, No.5, pp. 801-810, ISSN 1525-0016

Zhang, Z.; Yang, C.; Duan, Y.; Wang, Y.; Liu, J.; Wang, L. & Kong, D. (2010). Poly(ethylene glycol) Analogs Grafted with Low Molecular Weight Poly(ethylene imine) As Non-viral Gene Vectors. *Acta Biomater.*, Vol.6, No.7, pp. 2650-2657, ISSN 1742-7061

Zhang, S.B.; Zhao, B.D.; Jiang, H.M.; Wang, B. & Ma, B.C. (2007). Cationic Lipids and Polymers Mediated Vectors for Delivery of siRNA. *J. Controlled Release*, Vol.123, No.1, pp. 1-10, ISSN 0168-3659

Zhang, S.B.; Zhao, Y.N.; Zhao, B.D. & Wang, B. (2010). Hybrids of Nonviral Vectors for Gene Delivery. *Bioconjugate Chem.*, Vol.21, No.6, pp. 1003-1009, ISSN 1043-1082

Zhdanov, R.I.; Podobed, O.V. & Vlassov, V.V. (2002). Cationic Lipid–DNA Complexes-lipoplexes-for Gene Transfer and Therapy. *Bioelectrochemistry.* Vol.58, No.1, pp. 53-64, ISSN 1567-5394

Zhi, D.F.; Zhang, S.B.; Wang, B., Zhao, Y.N., Yang B.L. & Yu S.J. (2010). Transfection Efficiency of Cationic Lipids with Different Hydrophobic Domains in Gene Delivery. *Bioconjugate Chem.*, Vol.21, No.4, pp. 563-577, ISSN 1043-1082

14

Neutral Liposomes and DNA Transfection

Michela Pisani, Giovanna Mobbili and Paolo Bruni
Marche Polytechnic University
Italy

1. Introduction

Non viral gene transfer vectors for human gene therapy (HGT) applications represent today one of the widest fields of chemical, biological and medical research. Some authors (Kostaleros & Miller, 2005) have expressed the opinion that the future of a safe and efficient gene therapy will depend on suitable synthetic vectors of genetic material, rather than on viruses. The reason for this preference is based on the consideration that viruses, although characterized by high transfection efficiency of genetic material, may suffer from some serious disadvantages such as immune response (Marshall, 2000) and potential oncogenic activity (Hacein-Bey-Abina et al., 2003), as well as a high cost of preparation of the transferring system. On the contrary, synthetic vectors have many potential advantages, such as lack of immunogenicity and oncogenicity, no limits to the size of nucleic acids to be carried inside the cells (Harrington et al., 1997; Roush, 1997; Willard, 2000) and finally preparation procedures cheap and easy to perform. Nevertheless an awkward problem that accompanies their use is the low efficiency of the transfections *in vivo*. Among the synthetic vectors, the most explored by the researchers are the cationic liposomes (CLs), after Felgner and collaborators (Felgner et al., 1997) described the synthesis of the first cation lipid, *N*-[1-(2,3-dioleoyloxy)propyl]-*N,N,N*-trimethylammonium chloride (DOTMA) and demonstrated that it was able to bind DNA and transfect it both *in vitro* and *in vivo* experiments. Other cationic lipids followed and became popular, such as the commercially widely used N-[1-(2,3-dioleoyloxy)propyl]-N,N,N-trimethylammonium methylsulfate (DOTAP), 1,2-dioleoyl-3-dimethylammonium-propane (DODAP), dimethyldioctadecylammonium bromide (DDAB) and 3β-[N-(N',N'-dimethylaminoethane)-carbamoyl]cholesterol hydrochloride (DC-Chol); many others were synthesized during the past years and are still being synthesized. A few years after the Felgner's discovery scientists' interest was focused also on cationic polymers (Wu, G.Y. & Wu; C.H., 1987), that became popular after the discovery of polyethylenimines (Boussif, 1995) and are still the object of great interest. Both classes of cationic compounds owe their interest to the formation of stable complexes with DNA, called lipoplexes and polyplexes respectively, formed through an electrostatic interaction between the cationic head of lipids and the negative phosphates of DNA. The great amount of data and experiments reported in the literature with cationic vectors and some encouraging results in *in vivo* transfection experiments have led to the significant milestone of 20% of the ongoing clinical trials run with synthetic vectors (Edelstein et al., 2004): however the goal of a higher efficiency is still a problem to be solved. As recently stated (Safinya et al., 2006), the long-term target of research in this area is to develop a general fundamental theory, that may help to design and implement the synthesis of specialized vectors able to offer the highest efficiency in the various *in vivo* applications. Accordingly, the prevailing opinion is that more exhaustive research and development will be required before such efficiency becomes competitive with viral vectors. As a matter of fact the experience shows that also the cationic carriers suffer from some serious drawbacks, affecting more or less negatively their efficiency of transfection: namely some inherent cytotoxicity (Filion & Phillips, 1998; Lv et al., 2006) that causes negative effects on cells, such as shrinking and inhibition of the protein kinase C (PKC) and a limited stability of their complexes with plasmid DNA in serum (Foradada et al., 2000), responsible for the current restriction of a generalized and extensive use. In this situation the idea of using neutral liposomes as carriers of DNA seems to be interesting and can offer good prospects. It is well known that neutral liposomes are generally non toxic (Koiv et al., 1995) and relatively stable in serum (Tardi et al., 1996), which makes them potentially interesting gene transfer vectors. Despite these strategic features, neutral liposomes (NLs) have not yet received wide attention in the context of the HGT, even though the researchers' initial interest for DNA entrapment was turned to neutral liposomes (Budker et al., 1978). Likely, there are two causes for this situation: the first, and more important, is the lack of positive charge that makes virtually impossible to realize an interaction stable enough between NLs and DNA; the second is the great leading role assumed by the cationic carriers, which have polarized the researchers' interest, leaving other alternatives aside.

In this chapter we will deal with NLs following two separate paths, according to different functions they exert in HGT applications. The former will deal with their role of helpers of DNA transfection when used in mixture with cationic liposomes; the latter with their achievements and perspectives as autonomous and independent carriers of DNA. A survey of the literature published so far, though not too extensive, enables to foresee interesting prospects for NLs as promising synthetic vectors of genetic material. Perhaps they will be considered in a near future as an alternative to cationic vectors, rather than a provocative challenge. This forecast is supported by the results of several studies: of course deeper investigation is necessary in order to define a frame appropriate to treat correctly the many aspects of the transfection process and find better experimental conditions to warrant high transfection efficiency, particularly *in vivo*. The large number of studies carried on so far and the very large number of data collected in the field of cationic liposomes will help in building this frame and exploring the different aspects of the specific transfection with NLs.

2. Neutral lipids as helpers of cationic liposomes in DNA transfection

Since the discovery of the cationic liposomes as DNA carriers for gene transfer applications it has been clear that higher efficiencies could be obtained by adding a neutral lipid to the lipoplexes with the role of transfection helper. The approach followed in this section is not to evaluate all the issues related to DNA transfection with lipoplexes mediated by neutral lipids, but rather discuss the specific role of neutral lipids in determining the lipoplex transfection efficiency. The ultimate purpose is to highlight the factors that cause such increase of efficiency and check how they may help in designing the best experimental conditions for the transfections procedures with independent NLs.

Cationic systems for gene therapy are generally prepared by mixing a cationic lipid with DNA and a neutral helper co-lipid; such non toxic helper induces the dual result to reduce the amount of the toxic cationic component and, more important, to alter the physical properties of the delivery vehicle, in a way that favours some of the most complex steps of the whole mechanism of transfection: the consequence is that both actions affect the quality of the transfection. The most widely used neutral helpers in DNA transfection experiments are the 1,2-dioleoyl-*sn*-glycero-3-phosphocholine (DOPC) and the 1,2-dioleoyl-*sn*-glycero-3-phosphoethanolamine (DOPE), sometimes in combination with cholesterol: the main difference between the two phospholipids is that DOPC induces a lamellar L_{α}^{C} phase in the lipoplexes, while DOPE induces an inverted hexagonal H_{II}^{C} phase. Earlier studies led to propose that DOPE is responsible for more efficient transfections because its hexagonal phase is able to fuse readily with anionic vesicles (Koltover et al., 1998) and destabilize the bilayer membranes, making easier the DNA escape from the endosomes, once the lipoplex has entered the cells. Therefore it was believed that DOPE was more useful than DOPC to realize the most efficient transfections. In support of this claim it was also suggested (Mui et al., 2000) that the inverted hexagonal phase promoted by DOPE has a higher ability to disrupt the membrane integrity than the lamellar one induced by DOPC. It turned soon evident that the situation was not so simple and the interpretation was not unambiguous: indeed, if it is verified that the DNA complex with cationic DOTAP, in which DOPE is present as helper in an amount of 70%, transfects better than the corresponding complex including the same amount of DOPC (Koltover et al., 1998), lamellar L_{α}^{C} complexes, showing similar transfection efficiency, were also synthesized (Lin et al., 2003). More generally, many literature data show the difficulty in finding a general correlation between vector formulations and transfection efficiency. Trying to explain these apparently contradictory results, some researchers have recently suggested the opportunity to consider the possibility that complexes can bear a structural modification within the phase of the interaction of the systems DNA-carrier with each individual cell, the transition L_{α}^{C} to H_{II}^{C} phase being an example among others (Safinya, 2001). Starting from the observation that a large number of efficient complexes are assembled in the L_{α}^{C} phase, it was suggested (Caracciolo & Caminiti, 2005) that perhaps a compelling correlation between the structure of a complex and its transfection efficiency does not simply exist and that the lower transfection efficiency of the synthetic carriers of DNA with respect to virus depends on a poor understanding of the supramolecular structures of the complexes, on the mechanism of their interaction with cells and of the release of DNA within the nucleus. If these statements are true, and there are reasons to confirm them, a more exhaustive knowledge of the subject is particularly important also with reference to the use of NLs as independent carriers of DNA, because it is likely that similar problems will arise and the need to overcome them will be even more important. Of course, understanding the mechanism is crucial for any successful design of a non viral gene delivery, whatever path has been chosen. Besides some early studies, that assumed a fusion between liposomes and cell membranes as the initial step of the process, it is today recognized that the uptake into an endocytic pathway is required for fusion to occur (Wrobel & Collins, 1995) and the whole aspect has been the object of deep attention (Liu & Huang, 2002) leading to suggest some main steps, namely non specific interaction with the cell surface, endocytosis into endocytic vesicles, trafficking and release of the DNA from endosomal compartment, nuclear uptake and transgene expression.

Special attention was also devoted to the intracellular trafficking of cationic vectors and the role of neutral helpers (Elouahabi & Ruysschaert, 2005): six steps of the whole transfection process were identified and analyzed, namely (i) interaction between vectors and nucleic acids with formation of complexes, (ii) binding of a complex to the cell, (iii) effect of serum, (iv) uptake of the complex by the cell, (v) escape from endosomes and dissociation of the complex and finally (vi) nuclear entry of DNA.

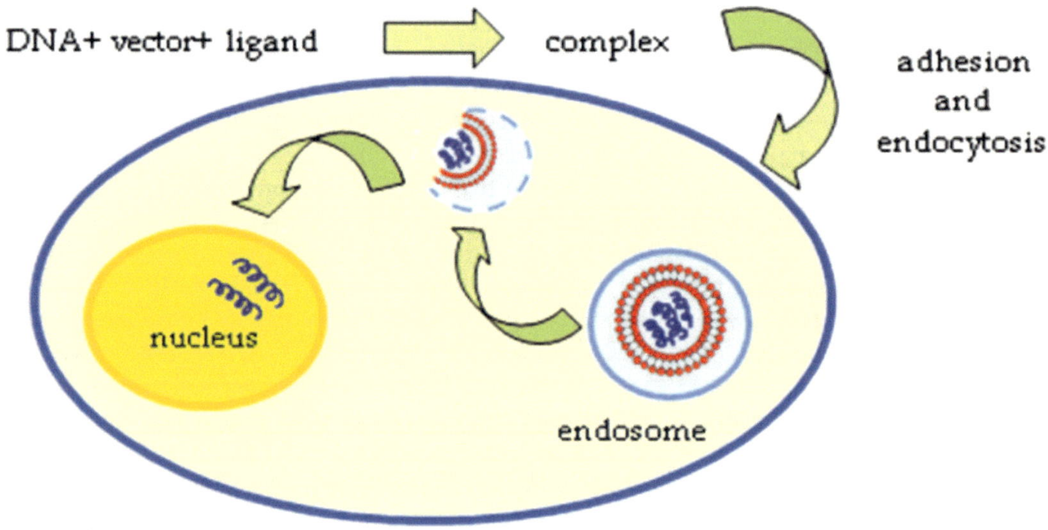

Fig. 1. A schematic representation of the steps involved in the liposome mediated DNA transfection.

We will consider here only the aspects likely to have significant involvements on the transfection process operated by NLs as unique carriers of genetic material. Neutral helpers play a not marginal role in the formation of the complexes: meaningful, though in some way contradictory, is the role of the helpers in determining the effect of serum on the uptake of lipoplexes, an issue that has implications in the *in vivo* transfections. No significant inhibition of serum was observed in transfecting COS-7 cells with cationic pyridinium-derived lipids (SAINT) in DOPE/DNA lipoplexes (Zuhorn et al., 2002), while a strong inhibitory effect operates in lipoplexes obtained by polycationic lipids like DOGS. However this negative effect may be avoided if one operates at slight alkaline pH that favours a lamellar organisation of the lipoplexes (Boukhnikachvili et al., 1997). Likewise DOTAP/DOPE and DC-Chol/DOPE prepared at high +/- charge ratio are not sensitive to the inhibitory effect of serum and indeed, at some ratios, are even more efficient (Yang & Huang, 1997). A different perspective on the role of helpers is offered by other researchers: it was observed (Fasbender & al., 1997) that when DOPE is incorporated into the complexes of DNA with three different cationics, its effect on the gene expression in COS-1 cells is different, depending on each cationic lipid. When the cationic lipids and DOPE were formulated separately and then complexed with DNA, no difference in activity was observed over that obtained with cationic lipids alone. Finally (Felgner et al., 1994) unsaturated PE co-lipids enhance lipoplexes activity while saturated PE and PC have no enhancing effect or even have an inhibitory effect.

CATIONIC LIPIDS

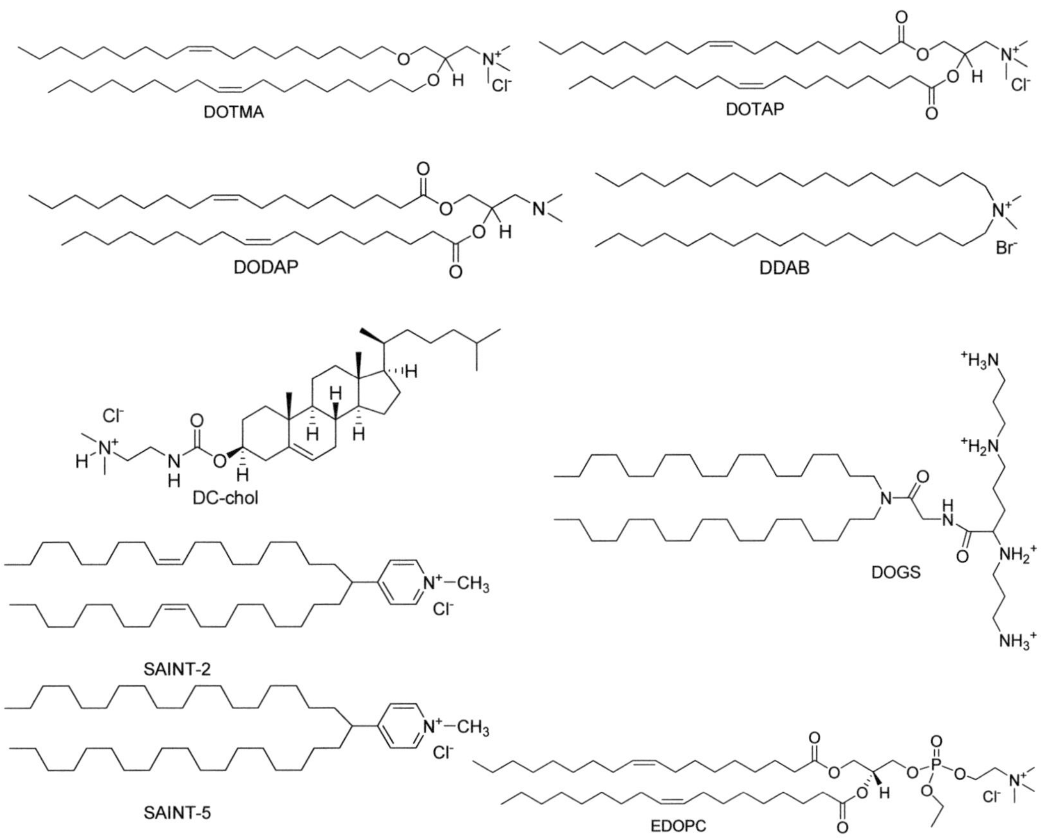

The escape of DNA from the endosomes is strictly depending on the nature of the neutral co-lipid: it was found that the fusion with endosomes is likely the way for the release of DNA into the cytoplasm. This mechanism was supported by the finding that efficient transfections require the fusogenic lipid DOPE, which is able to promote a transition from bilayers to hexagonal structures, the latter being known to catalyze the fusion process (Koltover et al., 1998; Mok & Cullis, 1997). The ability of liposomes to fuse with endosomal membranes was also proved by several studies (Koltover et al., 1998; Farhood et al., 1995; Mok & Cullis, 1997) and some evidence was found that the helper lipids can adapt their actions depending on the cationic lipid and the target cells (Fasbender et al., 1997).

In order to better clear up the situation, an interesting study was made a few years ago (Zuhorn et al., 2005). It provides deeper insight into the involvement of helper lipids in the liposomes mediated gene delivery. Two different helpers, DOPE, which has a propensity to adopt an inverted hexagonal phase, and the lamellar phase forming dipalmitoylphosphatidylethanolamine (DPPE), have been compared as neutral co-lipids in lipoplexes formed with SAINT-2 and plasmid DNA, with the specific aim of studying the endosomal escape of the genetic cargo in the cytosol for transport to the nucleus. As usual, it was found that the helper determines the *in vitro* transfection efficiency (COS-7 cells were used), DPPE inducing a significantly lower efficiency (≅ 25% of cell transfected) than DOPE

(≅ 75%), despite an equal interaction of both SAINT-2/DNA/DOPE and SAINT-2/DNA/DPPE with cells. Assuming that the translocation of the nucleic acids through the endosomal membrane is the crucial step of the overall process, a mimic membrane consisting of phosphatidylserine (PS): phosphatidylcholine (PC): phosphatidylethanolamine (PE) anionic vesicle was used to simulate this step. Without helper lipids, a limited fraction of DNA was released from SAINT-2 lipoplex and no effect was promoted by the inclusion of DOPC. On the contrary, inclusion of DOPE significantly enhanced the amount of DNA released and, more interesting, a comparable effect was induced by DPPE (40% release for DPPE versus 50% for DOPE). This result can find an explanation since the *x*-ray diffraction analysis after incubation of SAINT-2/DPPE with the anionic PS:PC:PE (1:1:2) revealed the presence of a mixed lamellar-hexagonal phase. The lower efficiency of the DPPE containing complex is consistent with this partial transition from the lamellar to the hexagonal phase. These results confirm that the limiting step in the overall transfection pathway depends on the level of DNA translocation through the endosomal membrane. The results obtained in the transfections with two different lipoplexes containing SAINT with different tails, namely SAINT-2 (C18:1) and SAINT-5 (C18:0) lead (Zuhorn et al., 2002) to analogous conclusions. Both amphiphiles may make transfection and DOPE strongly promotes the SAINT-2 mediated one, but not the SAINT-5. The relatively rigid SAINT-5 membrane forms structurally deformed lipoplexes hampering the plasmid translocation through endosomal and/or nuclear membranes.

What it has been said so far makes clear that there are still many aspects concerning the DNA transfection process that require a better investigation: among them, the need of a comprehensive knowledge of what really happens when a lipid-DNA complex interacts with a cell, an issue extremely important also in the neutral lipid mediated DNA transfections. In this connection a new perspective has gained recently ground: it identifies as one of the most critical factors of the transfection process the evolution of the structure of the lipoplexes that occurs when they interact with cells. That means to introduce the idea that the differences in the transfection efficiency, often observed and not always unambiguously interpreted, may depend on each particular cellular variety and emphasize the importance to consider both lipid composition of lipoplexes and target membranes (Koynova et al., 2005). Ancestors of this new perspective are some studies that demonstrated the ability of anionic lipids to promote the release of DNA from lipoplexes, by neutralizing their positive charge (Szoka et al. 1996; Zelphati & Szoka, 1996; McDonald et al., 1999). It was observed that the DNA release from complexes with the cationic lipids o-ethyldioleoylphosphatidylcholinium (EDOPC) or DOTAP, after mixing them with some different negatively charged lipids, depends on both lipoplexes and negative lipids. Most significant, the transfection efficiencies of DNA complexes with two very similar cationic phospholipids, bearing only a minimal structural difference in one of the two hydrocarbon tails, the carbon-carbon double bond bearing oleoyldecanoyl-ethylphosphatidylcholine (C18:1/C10-EPC) and the completely saturated stearoyldecanoyl-ethylphosphatidylcholine (C18:0/C10-EPC) were compared (Koynova et al., 2006). The former complex shows a 50-fold higher transfection efficiency than the latter in human umbilical artery endothelial cells. A reasonable explanation of this different behaviour lies in the great difference of these lipids in the phase evolution found in mixing with biomembrane mimicking lipid mixtures (DOPC/DOPE/DOPS/chol). The C18:1 lipoplex underwent a transition to the fusogenic non lamellar cubic phase, whereas the C18:0 did not. All these new perspectives must be seriously considered by all aiming at studying the DNA transfection with NLs, since an analogous behaviour will be probably characterize those experimental setups.

Before ending these considerations on the role of the helper co-lipids in the processes of non viral DNA transfection, it is advisable to say something about a neglected aspect of the topic. As a matter of fact it is surprising that the continuous growing of number and features of cationic lipids, in the search for most suitable vectors of genetic material, no analogous interest has been reserved, for many years, for new co-lipids. The idea that improved transfections could be realized also with the aid of new and more appropriate helpers has developed only in the last ten years. After the discovery that high transfection efficiency could be obtained with fluorinated double chain lipospermines, forming fluorinated lipoplexes (Gaucheron et al., 2001a, 2001b), a partially fluorinated analogue of DOPE, identified as [F8E11][C16]OPE from the number of fluorine atoms, was synthesized and compared with DOPE as helper of fluorinated lipoplexes (Boussif et al., 2001): this compound, inactive itself in promoting transfection, increased the *in vitro* and *in vivo* gene transfer of the lipoplex obtained from the pentacationic pcTG90 to a larger extent than DOPE. The synthesis was then extended to more fluorinated glycerophosphoethanolamines (Gaucheron et al., 2001) confirming that lipoplexes formulated with fluorinated helper lipids are attractive candidates for gene delivery both *in vitro* and *in vivo*. Several reasons were identified to explain these results: fluorinated co-lipids have a larger ability to preserve the integrity of complexed DNA in a biological environment and a larger propensity to promote fusion with endosomes and subsequent destabilisation, allowing more efficient DNA release in the cytosol; their high hydrophobic and lipophobic character can preserve the lipoplexes from the effect of the interactions with lipophilic and hydrophilic biocompounds; finally fluorinated DOPE compounds are expected to have a greater tendency to promote a lamellar to a an inverted hexagonal phase transition with the consequence of a higher effectiveness in disrupting membranes than DOPE.

It is commonly accepted that one of the main features of DOPE as helper depends on its polymorphism under various concentration and temperature conditions. Its ability to enhance transfection efficiency is related to its preference for the fusogenic H_{II} phase, which can promote fusion with cellular membranes, especially the endosomal ones, thereby facilitating the escape of the genetic material; however, the low L_{α}/H_{II} phase transition temperature (T_h = 10 °C) makes cationic liposomes too unstable in the *in vivo* environment. An approach to solve the problem might be to synthesize analogues of DOPE in which the phase transition is near the physiological temperature. Some molecules having these characteristics have been synthesized (Fletcher et al., 2006) and correspond to a series of dialkynoyl analogues of DOPE where the cis-double bond in the two oleoyl fatty acid chains is replaced by a triple bond located in different positions of the hydrocarbon tails. With this modified geometry a new intermolecular packing is realized, able to induce an increase of the phase transition at the physiological conditions.

The achievements just shown were based on the concept to modify DOPE: a different approach to the search for more efficient helpers has been realized by synthesizing completely new lipids characterized by the presence of an imidazole polar head (Mével et al., 2008). These lipophosphoramides are neutral at physiological pH: the protonation occurring in the acidic compartments of the cell, namely the endosomes, induces fusion of liposomes with endosomes and structural changes that favour the release of DNA in the cytosol. Three phosphoramidates with a cationic polar head derived from natural aminoesters or a methylimidazolium salt were also synthesized and these cationic lipids were formulated with each one of the two new helpers and with cholesterol or DOPE for a comparison of transfections; it is worth noticing that the new helper lipids can improve the transfection by a factor of 100 compared with DOPE.

3. Liposomes and membrane fusion mimicking

A remote introduction to the processes of gene transfer is represented by a series of studies aiming at mimicking the process of cell fusion by using model membranes mainly composed of phosphatidylcholine (PC) and phosphatidylserine (PS). It was demonstrated that addition of liposomes containing these lipids fuse with plasma membranes in the presence of Ca^{2+} and Mg^{2+} (Papahadjopoulos et al., 1976). Considering that cellular fusion is one of the most fundamental processes in life and that its role has been recognized in the interaction of liposomes with endosomes within the processes of DNA transfection, such studies are highly significant for the knowledge of this particular step of the non viral GT and in designing lipids with the highest characteristics of fusion. The study of the effect of divalent metal cations in the interaction and mixing of membrane components in vesicles prepared from phospholipids led to find that low amounts of Ca^{2+} and Mg^{2+} induce extensive mixing of vesicle membrane components and important structural rearrangements to form new membrane structures. The result is a true fusion rather than a simple mixing of vesicles that occurs in the absence of cations. Some evidence was found that fusion of vesicle membranes by Ca^{2+} and Mg^{2+} is not simply due to electrostatic charge neutralization, but rather to changes in molecular packing. It is possible to see here an anticipation of the phase transitions that many years after was demonstrated to occur in DNA transfection with co-lipid added lipoplexes, as reported in the previous section. These results have been confirmed by finding that Ca^{2+} and Mg^{2+} produce structurally different complexes with PE (Newton et al., 1978). A different behaviour in fusion induced by these two cations was found in mixture of PS/PC, PS/PE and PS/PC/PE (Düzgünes et al. 1981). The extent of fusion by Ca^{2+} in mixed PE/PC was lower compared to that of pure PS vesicles and was completely inhibited when PC reached 50% in the mixture; rapid fusion was instead obtained in mixtures PS/PE. Mg^{2+} can fuse PS only in the presence of PE. The fusogenic capacity of Mg^{2+} was instead completely absent in mixtures PS/PC/PE with 10% of PC. These results show clearly a marked difference between Ca^{2+} and Mg^{2+} against fusion: as we will see later, this difference will appear also in some processes concerning the formation of complexes of DNA with neutral liposomes.

A rational mechanism to interpret these results was tried out: kinetics of the interaction between PS vesicles in the presence of Ca^{2+} (Portis et al., 1979) show the formation of two different complexes: the former develops when the cations bind only to individual vesicles, the latter, which seems correlated with the beginning of membrane fusion, when the vesicles come to close apposition; the former complex is obtained also with Mg^{2+}. Its characteristics led to suggest that this complex is formed when the divalent cations bind to PS head groups on one bilayer only (cis complex). The latter, obtained only with Ca^{2+}, shows different characteristics and seems to involve a polydentate chelation of Ca^{2+} with the head groups of PS from apposed membranes (trans complex). The formation of this PS/Ca^{2+} complex is of crucial importance for the fusion of the vesicles. Apart from the names used to identify these complexes, it is worth noting that the structure suggested for the latter complex agrees with the one found in the complex between the neutral lipid DPPC and DNA, promoted by divalent metal cations, showing a L_{α}^{C} phase. A more detailed study (Wilschut et al., 1980) allowed to obtain further information about the process: it was demonstrated that fusion is one of the earliest events during the Ca^{2+}-induced aggregation of SUVs (small unilamellar vesicles) of PS and occurs at a similar time scale, which means that fusion doesn't require initial rupture of the vesicles. The close contact between the vesicles induced by Ca^{2+} is sufficient to trigger the immediate fusion of the two membranes and the mixing of the internal volumes with a relative low leakiness of their content: which makes the Ca^{2+}/PS system an almost ideal model for membrane fusion. This model has been later deeply developed and is the basis to explain the processes which occur in the cytosol when the complexes liposomes/DNA encounter the endosomes and release the DNA. With these last findings the route to the DNA delivery to cells by means of liposomes was opened.

4. The neutral liposomes as independent DNA transfection agents

After the Bangham's work (Bangham et al., 1965) liposomes were extensively used as models of biological membranes (Sessa & Weissmann, 1968) on the basis of their lamellar structure. It was seen that they are able to discriminate ions as natural membranes do, and that it is easy to vary their surface charge, in order to modulate the diffusion of a large amount of cations and anions. It was proved that it is possible to incorporate proteins in their lamellar structure and that their composition can be modified to mimic the properties of a large variety of natural membranes. Basically, it was recognized that liposomes are a valuable instrument to study many problems concerning natural membrane structure and function. What's more, it was assumed that, if liposomes were able to incorporate proteins, enzymes, drugs or nucleic acids, an important step towards a true *in vitro* replica of the membranes of living systems would be obtained.

4.1 Liposomes and polynucleotide entrapment

Soon these foreseen opportunities began to turn into actual tasks: liposomes started being applied as carriers of different molecules into target cells (Dimitriadis, 1979; Tyrrell et al., 1976; Finkelstein & Weissmann, 1978) or of enzymes in enzyme replaced therapy (Gregoriadis & Buckland, 1973). It was in those years that the entrapment of synthetic polynucleotides (Magee et al., 1976), as well as natural ones (Hoffman et al., 1978; Lurquin, 1979), was undertaken. Large unilamellar liposomes were obtained (Dimitriadis, 1978) by adding ribonucleic acid (globin mRNA) to PS and it was demonstrated that mRNA is really entrapped and not simply adhering to the surface. A different experiment was realized with the aim of clearing up the mechanism of crossing the hydrophobic barriers formed by protein-lipid membranes and the nature of bonds, providing adsorption of polynucleotides in the membranes (a mechanism unknown at that time). It was demonstrated (Budker et al., 1978) that polynucleotides are adsorbed by liposomes of PC forming stable complexes in the presence of Mg^{2+} or Ca^{2+} ions, but not in the absence of these ions. This result suggested that this interaction is due to the action of bivalent cations, which crosslink phosphate groups of polynucleotides with the ones of PC. It was also found that the complexes obtained are stable, but that the addition of monovalent cations reduces the extent of complexation.

It has been said already that one of the main reasons of the success of cationic liposomes resides in their positive charge that enables attractive interactions both with the negative phosphate groups of the polynucleotides and the negatively charged cell wall. Encapsulation of DNA into a vector is of course the first and irreplaceable step to realize a synthetic vector driven gene therapy and must be solved within neutral liposomes, where the absence of charge does not allow the formation of a stable aggregation with negative DNA. However gene transfer and gene therapy need an efficient encapsulation of plasmid DNA into neutral liposomes and an attractive interaction with the negative cell wall which is the necessary step for the endocytic internalisation of the construct. The methods generally used to realize a stable entrapment can be schematically indicated in three main classes: reverse phase evaporation, dehydration-rehydration and freeze-thawing. According to the first method the nucleic acids are dissolved in water and the solution is added to lipids dispersed in an organic solvent, then evaporated to induce vesiculation (Szoka & Papahadjopoulos, 1978). In the second procedure the nucleic acids are added to a dispersion of SULs (small unilamellar liposomes) and the mixture is dehydrated until almost dryness; afterwards the material is rehydrated and vortexed to induce the formation of liposomal aggregates (Deamer & Barchfeld, 1982). The third method involves the addition of nucleic acids to a dispersion of SULs followed by numerous freeze-thawing operations and by a final extrusion to obtain homogeneously sized vesicles (Chapman et al., 1990). The last method was applied to encapsulate a 3368 base pair DNA (Monnard et al., 1997), using liposomes prepared with 1-palmitoyl-2-oleoyl-*sn*-glycero-3-phosphocholine (POPC) mixed with a little amount of the negative PS or the cationic didodecyl-methylammonium bromide (DDAB) as cosurfatants. The yields of entrapment calculated over the amount of the initial material were 27% in pure POPC, 26% in POPC/PS 9:1 and 50% in POPC/DDAB 99:1. While the addition of PS has evidently no influence on the entrapment, the one of traces of the positive DDAB, doubles the percentage of entrapped DNA. An important contribute to the entrapment of nucleic acids in neutral liposomes was done some years later (Bayley & Sullivan, 2000). Plasmid DNAs (pDNA) were trapped into pure DOPC, DOPC/DOPE 1:1 and DOPC/DOPE/Chol 1:1:1 by simply adding $CaCl_2$ and ethanol to the initial mixture DNA/lipids. With optimized amounts of ethanol and calcium the entrapment percentages were 65-70% for DOPC, 70-80% for DOPC/DOPE 1:1 and only 35-40% for DOPC/DOPE/Chol 1:1:1. Most important the neutral liposome complexes obtained from DOPC and DOPC/DOPE are stable for at least two weeks in PBS (phosphate buffered saline) at 4 °C.

4.2 Some early experiments of DNA delivery to cells by means of liposomes

The need of modifying the expression of the eukaryotic genome to study the protein synthesis led to encapsulate a functional rabbit globin mRNA in lecithin liposomes, made by neutral PC and PE, to realize its selective insertion into differentiated eukaryotic cells in vitro and express a globin-like protein (Ostro et al., 1978). The authors claimed this result as the first successful attempt to entrap and deliver high molecular weight RNA with a liposome. New applications followed and led to improve the technique. Poliovirus RNA was encapsulated in liposomes of PS and delivered efficiently to cells in an infectious form

(Wilson et al., 1979). A comparison between large unilamellar vesicles (LUVs) and multilamellar vesicles (MLVs) of PS indicates that LUVs deliver their content to cell cytoplasm much more efficiently than MLVs and that LUV-entrapped poliovirus RNA produces infection titers 10 to 100 fold higher than when delivered with other techniques. Likewise, DNA isolated from simian virus 40 (SV40) was encapsulated in LUVs of PS and delivered to a monkey cell line (Fraley et al., 1980). The infectivity realized with this method was enhanced at least 100 fold over that of free naked DNA. This process was then used as a probe to study liposome-cell interactions and determine conditions favouring the intracellular delivery of liposome content to cells (Fraley et al., 1981). The efficiency of DNA delivery was found dependent both on size of vesicles and the resistance of liposomes to cell induced leakage of content. Acidic phospholipids are much more effective in both binding and delivery, and PS was found to be the best in both events. Inclusion of cholesterol in liposomes reduces the cell-induced leakage of vesicle content and enhances the delivery of DNA to cells. A brief exposure of cells to glycerol solutions enhances infectivity of the SV40 DNA when encapsulated into the negatively charged liposome of PS, but not in neutral and positively charged liposomes. Morphological studies indicate that the glycerol treatment stimulates membrane vacuolisation and suggest that the enhanced uptake of liposomes occurs by an endocytic-like process. As it was said in a previous paragraph, endocytosis is the mechanism followed in the phase of the internalisation of the complexes liposome/DNA into cells. Additional attempts to transfect DNA to cells by means of bivalent cations mediated complexes of neutral liposomes are reported by the literature (Kovalenko et al., 1996).

4.3 The problem of the uptake of liposomes by the reticuloendothelial system

It is known that many liposomes are removed in liver and spleen from the blood circulation within minutes: this property, beneficial when they are employed to carry drugs for treating intracellular infections of the reticuloendothelial system (RES), has limited their use as delivery carriers of material to sites beyond the RES. Designing liposomes with prolonged circulation time requires a reduction of the rate of their clearance by the RES and of the leakage of liposome cargo in blood stream. The search for a solution of the problem has led to the discovery of the so called stealth liposomes, sterically stabilized by the presence of bulky groups: the so-called PEG-liposomes, namely polyethyleneglycol functionalized liposomes, are the most important tools in ensuring a prolonged circulation time in blood. The incorporation of PEG into conventional liposomes provides a steric barrier at the liposome surface that inhibits opsonisation, therefore extending the persistence time of liposomes in the blood. Positive effects are a prolonged circulation lifetime of lipoplexes and a reduced formation of aggregates (Klibanov et al., 1990; Papahadjopoulos et al., 1991). The incorporation of 1,2-dioleoyl-N-(methoxy-polyethyleneglycol-succinyl-)phosphatidylethanolamine (PEG-PE) in liposomes composed of egg phosphatidylcholine-cholesterol, exposed to human serum at 37 °C increases the blood circulation half-life ten times the one of simple phosphatidylcholine-cholesterol liposome (Klibanov et al., 1990). While PEG-lipids play an active role in limiting excessive inhibition and fusion during the self-assembling phase when cationic lipids associate with anionic DNA protecting DNA from nuclease degradation in plasma, the steric barrier introduced by PEG is expected to inhibit also the process of fusion with the endosomes and by consequence reduce the transfection activity. Conflicting results have been obtained so far. It has been found (Song et al., 2002) that, owing to the presence of PEG lipids with long acyl chains (< 14 carbons), the contact between complexes and endosomal membranes doesn't allow membrane disruption. In general it seems that the biological and physicochemical characteristics of the DNA/copolymer complexes, including PEG, are influenced by the copolymer architecture (Deshpande et al., 2004) and that the transfection efficiency is strongly correlated with the level of cellular association and uptake of the DNA/copolymer complexes.

4.4 The structure of the complexes of DNA with zwitterionic liposomes

In previous paragraphs we pointed out that the structure of the lipoplexes represents a fundamental tool in understanding and planning DNA transfection systems. The same remarks are valid for complexes of DNA with neutral (zwitterionic) liposomes in order to evaluate correctly their behaviour and, in case, design the necessary developments to achieve better results in DNA transfection experiments both *in vitro* and *in vivo*. These complexes were initially studied in order to understand the influence of DNA structural transition of neutral lipids: DSC thermograms of the DPPC/DNA/Ca^{2+} complex (Tarahovsky et al., 1996) reveal a distinct maximum at the temperature of 316.3 K in addition to the main maximum at 314.6 K. Since a direct relationship was observed between the molar proportion of DNA in samples and the value of the height of the second peak, it was hence assumed that the higher temperature transition corresponds to the formation of the complex. In another work (Kharakoz et al., 1999) it was demonstrated that DPPC/DNA complexes could be obtained by simply mixing the DNA solutions with an aqueous lipid dispersion in the presence of Ca^{2+} and that their formation could be obtained with both MLVs and ULVs. The stoichiometry was determined in 4.5 to 5 strongly bound lipid molecules per molecule of nucleotide, depending on the method used in a temperature-scanning ultrasonic study. From this result and the ones obtained in a small angle x-ray scattering experiment (SAXS), a model was proposed (McManus et al., 2003) for the interaction of DNA and DPPC in the presence of $CaCl_2$. The lamellar repeat distance in complexes with MLVs at 298 K increases slightly as Ca^{2+} concentration increases, but it drops to a minimum at a Ca^{2+} concentration equal to 5 mM. At this concentration a special compact structural arrangement is observed, indicative of increased order. Combining this finding with the above result on the ratio of 4.5 to 5 lipid molecules per molecule of nucleotide, it was inferred that roughly one $CaCl_2$ binds two DPPC molecules and a model was proposed where every Ca^{2+} bridges two adjacent DPPC molecules through their phosphate groups. A different possibility was formerly considered (Bruni et al., 1997) in a study on the interactions of bivalent metal cations with double-stranded polynucleotides or DNA and egg yolk PC. Scatchard plots of PC/DNA/Mn^{2+} and DNA/Mn^{2+} complexes, combined with data of elemental analysis, support an arrangement where each Mn^{2+} bridges two DNA phosphates with three PC molecules. One more schematic model for interpreting the DNA-lipid interaction mediated by Ca^{2+} and Mg^{2+} has been working on the zwitterionic 1,2-dimyristoylphopsphoetyhanolamine (DMPE). Following this suggestion (Gromelski & Brezesinski, 2006) the divalent cations bridge the negative part of the zwitterionic phospholipid headgroups, thereby making the lipid monolayers positive. Divalent cations also interact with the negative DNA phosphate moieties, condensing the DNA and leading to an ordered alignment of the DNA strands. If not all charges are screened by the divalent cations, the DNA aggregate remains partially negative and can interact either via divalent cations with the lipid phosphate groups or directly with the positively charged ethanolamine groups of DMPE when the lipid phosphate groups are bridged by divalent cations.

NEUTRAL LIPIDS

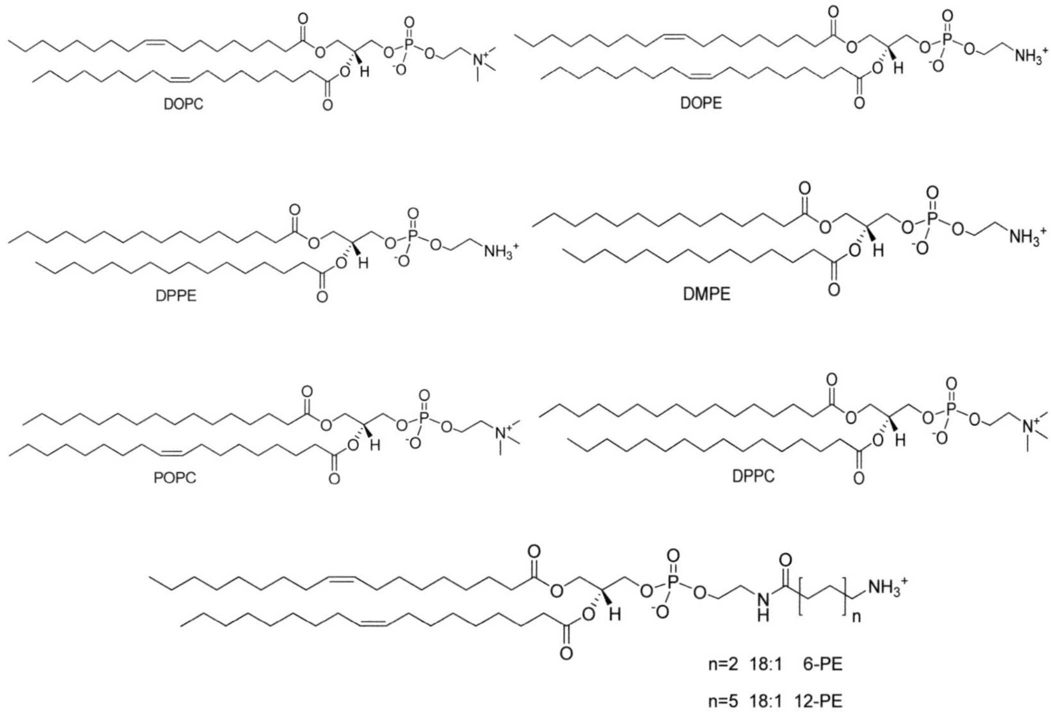

This new class of complexes consists of ternary systems NLs/DNA/M^{2+} where M refers mostly to Ca, Mg, a choice consistent with the previously reported experiments of membrane fusion, and sometimes Mn. The formation of the ternary complexes is the result of a self assembling process in which the driving force is represented by the release of the counter-ion entropy upon neutralization of DNA phosphate groups by metal cations (Cl^- in the examples discussed). Studies on the structure of these ternary complexes were undertaken mainly by means of x-ray diffraction technique.

In all the experiments performed by the authors of this review, XRD measurements were carried out at the high brilliance beamline ID02 of the European Synchrotron Radiation Facility (Grenoble, France). The energy of the incident beam was 12.5 keV (λ= 0.995 Å), the beam size 100x100 μm^2, and the sample-to-detector distance 1.2 m. The 2D diffraction patterns were collected by a CCD detector. The small angle q range from q_{min} = 0.1 nm^{-1} to q_{max} = 4 nm^{-1} with a resolution of 5 x 10^{-3} nm^{-1} (fwhm) was investigated: the samples were held in a 1 mm-sized glass capillary. To avoid radiation damage, each sample was exposed to radiation for 3 sec/frame. To calculate the electron density maps, the integrated intensities of the diffraction peaks were determined by fitting the data with series of Lorentz functions, using a nonlinear baseline. The Lorentz correction was performed multiplying each integrated intensity by sin θ and the intensities were then calibrated dividing by the multiplicity of the reflection (Harper et al., 2001; Francescangeli et al., 1996). The square root of the corrected peak was finally used to determine the modulus of the form factor F of each respective reflection. The electron density profile $\Delta\rho$ along the normal to the bilayers was calculated by Fourier sum,

$$\Delta\rho = \frac{\rho(z) - \langle\rho\rangle}{\left[\langle\rho^2(z)\rangle - \langle\rho\rangle^2\right]^{1/2}} = \sum_{l=1}^{N} F_l \cos\left(2\pi\, l \frac{z}{d}\right)$$

where $\rho(z)$ is the electron density, $\langle\rho\rangle$ its average value, N the highest order of fundamental reflection observed in the SAXS pattern; F_l is the form factor of the $(00l)$ reflection, d the thickness of the repeating unit and the origin of the z axis is chosen in the middle of the lipid bilayers. The phase problem was solved by means of a pattern recognition approach based on the histogram of the electron density map (Tristram-Nagle et al., 1998) and the results were found to be in agreement with those obtained with different approaches.

In a first example (Francescangeli et al., 2003), a DOPC liposome was mixed with calf thymus DNA in hepes buffered aqueous solutions of divalent cations and simultaneous small (SAXS) and wide (WAXS) angle x-ray scattering measurements were carried out.

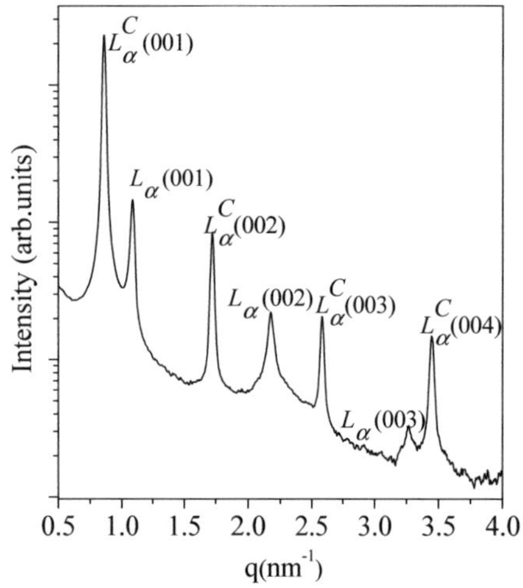

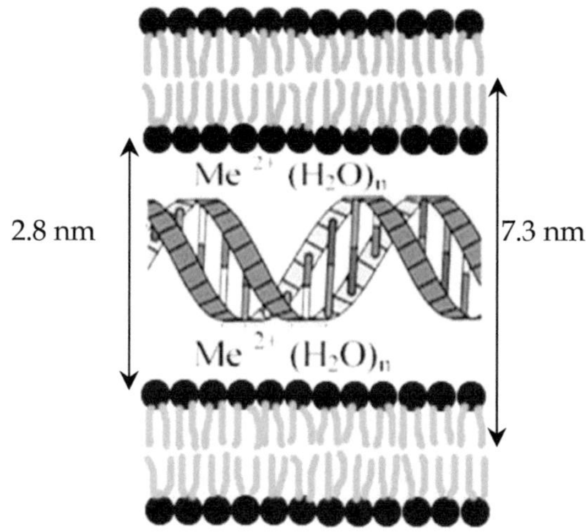

Fig. 2. Left: synchrotron SAXS pattern of DOPC/DNA/Mn^{2+} complex at molar ratio 3:4:12. (Reprinted from MROC, 2011, 8, 38) Right: the model proposed for the L_α^C phase of the ternary complex, reporting the main structural parameters.

In a typical experiment the mole ratio DOPC:DNA:Mn^{2+} was 3:4:12 and the corresponding synchrotron x-ray diffraction (XRD) pattern (Figure 2, left) at 298 K is reported. Two series of spacings are present in the x-ray pattern: the one indicated with the symbol L_α^C (d= 7.34 nm), independent of the concentration of the cation, has been attributed to the ternary complex and the one indicated with the symbol L_α (d= 5.88 nm) to the complex DOPC/Mn^{2+}. The ternary complex is characterized by the lamellar symmetry of the L_α^C (Luzzati, 1968), consisting of an ordered multilamellar assembly where the hydrated DNA helices are sandwiched between the liposome bilayers. This structure is similar to that found in CLs/DNA complexes (Rädler et al., 1997; Podgornik et al. 1989). A pictorial representation (Figure 3, left) of the ternary complex DOPC/DNA/Mn^{2+} has been proposed:

the DNA strands are sandwiched between the lipid bilayers and bound together through the hydrated metal ions: the value of 2.8 nm between two lipid bilayers is sufficient to accommodate a hydrated double strand of DNA (Figure 2, right).

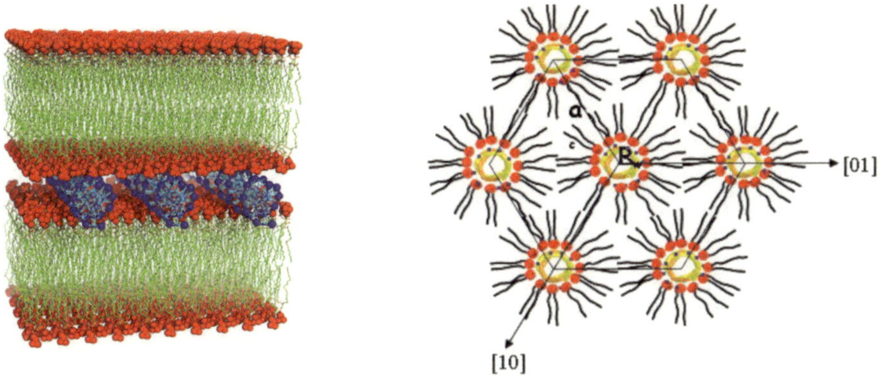

Fig. 3. A pictorial image of the DOPC/DNA/Mn^{2+} (left) and of the DOPE/DNA/M^{2+} (right) ternary complexes.

The simultaneous presence of two lamellar structures, confirmed by an analogous XRD study (Uhrikova et al., 2005), was interpreted by plotting (Figure 4, left) the integrated intensities of the first order diffraction peaks of the DNA complex and of the DOPC liposome as a function of the ratio of the metal ion concentration versus the one of the DNA phosphate groups.

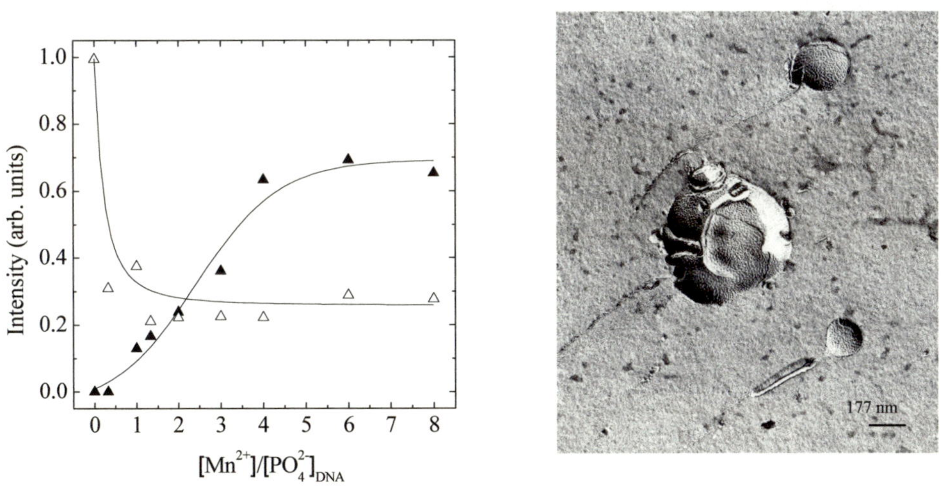

Fig. 4. Left: integrated intensities of the first order diffraction peak of the ternary complex (▲) and of DOPC liposome (△) as a function of the ratio of the metal ion concentration to the concentration of DNA phosphate groups. (Reprinted from Phys. Rev. E, 2003, 67, 11904). Right: freeze-fracture EM micrograph of the DOPC/DNA/Mn^{2+} complex.

An increase of the Mn^{2+} concentration favours the formation of the ternary complex accompanied to a complementary reduction of the DOPC: the saturation is reached at a ratio $[Mn^{2+}]:[PO_4^{2-}] \cong 6$, corresponding to a constant volume fraction of the two structures (~ 70% to ~ 30% respectively). A freeze-fracture EM micrograph of the ternary complex has also been made and reported in figure 4 (right). An analogous study was made with the neutral liposome 1,2-dipalmitoylphosphatidylcholine (DPPC), bearing completely saturated hydrocarbon tails (McManus et al., 2003) : as for DOPC two coexisting phases are present and the ternary complex shows a lamellar structure, the DNA layers being embedded in the DPPC layers. The repeat distance is 7.84 nm at 298 K. At this temperature the DPPC/DNA/Ca^{2+} complex is in the gel thermotropic phase ($L_{\beta'}$).
These works have been followed by an extended approach to ternary complexes based on NLs, bearing unsaturated (DOPC, DLPC and DOPE) or saturated (DPPC) hydrocarbon tails. A twofold goal has been pursued when investigating the microscopic structures of lipids and their corresponding ternary complexes: to test whether different metal cations are equally active in promoting the DNA condensation with different lipids and ascertain to what extent structure and phase symmetry of the lipids affect the structure of the complexes; two aspects that have fundamental implications in view of an approach to gene delivery based application of these complexes. Different varieties of DNA (calf-thymus, salmon sperm and plasmid) complexed with DOPC and DLPC (Pisani et al., 2005) or DPPC (Pisani et al. 2006), in the presence of different cations (Ca^{2+}, Mn^{2+}, Co^{2+}, Fe^{2+}, Mg^{2+}), exhibit the already discussed multilamellar liquid-crystalline L_α^C phase, consisting of ordered assemblies, where hydrated DNA helices are sandwiched between the lipid bilayers, and the metal cations mediate the binding of the phosphate groups of DNA with the lipid polar heads. Also within these assemblies the L_α^C phase coexists with the uncomplexed L_α phase of the parent lipid. A systematic series of SAXS measurements in DOPC/DNA_{ct}/M^{2+} complexes, prepared with different metal cations, was performed as a function of the number of metal ion moles (n).
The results obtained from these spectra are reported in figure 5: a remarkable constancy of the lamellar spacings of the L_α^C accompanied by a slight decrease of the lamellar repeat distance of the uncomplexed L_α, reported in the figure agrees with the model proposed in figure 3. As an example we report (Figure 6) the analysis of the ternary complex with Mg^{2+}: again two sets of peaks (each one including fundamental and high-order harmonics) related to distinct lamellar structures L_α^C and L_α, with layer spacings d_1= 7.52 nm and d_2= 5.9 nm respectively, are present. The SAXS pattern (A), and the relative electron density profile (B) are shown: in the latter, the two peaks with the maximum of electron density correspond to phospholipids' polar headgroups, while the minimum correlates with the terminal hydrocarbon chain region.
The distance between the centres of the density maxima gives a good approximation of the bilayer thickness (d_{PP} = 4.51 nm): it follows that the water-layer thickness can be calculated as $d_W = d_1 - d_{PP} = 7.52 - 4.51 = 3.01$ nm sufficient to accommodate a double stranded DNA helix surrounded by one water hydration layer plus two thin layers of hydrated metal ions. Likewise, it was calculated a water layer thicknesses d_W in the range of 2.8-3.0 nm in the complexes with DLPC and in the range of 2.9-3.2 nm in the ones with DPPC, depending on metal cation.
The SAXS pattern of the DPPC/DNA/Ca^{2+} (Figure **7,** left) shows a correlation peak, marked as DNA in the figure, corresponding to the DNA-DNA interaction, indicative of a higher

organization of the DNA chains between the liposome layers. The thermotropic phase behaviour in a temperature range between 303 K and 328 K, well above the main transition temperature of the pure lipid (Tm = 314 K) was studied (Figure 7, right), leading to the important conclusion that coexistence of complexed and uncomplexed phases persists over the whole explored thermal range. A further relevant effect is observed: while the uncomplexed lipid exhibits the same thermotropic phase behaviour as pure DPPC, i.e. $L_{\beta'}$ $-P_{\beta'}$ $-L_{\alpha}$, the mesomorphic behaviour of the bound lipid in the complex is partially altered. This is highlighted by the disappearance of the ripple phase and the remarkable increase of the main transition temperature: the observed thermotropic phase sequence of the complex goes directly from $L^{c}_{\beta'}$ to L^{c}_{α}. (Pisani et al. 2006). In addition the effect of the temperature on the formation of the DOPC/DNA/Mn^{2+} complex has been determined (Francescangeli et al., 2003): figure 8 shows the temperature evolution of the XRD patterns of this complex in the range 290 to 320 K (left) and the temperature dependence (right) of the integrated intensities of the two small-angle reflections for the L^{C}_{α} phase for the ternary complex and the L_{α} phase of DOPC, respectively.

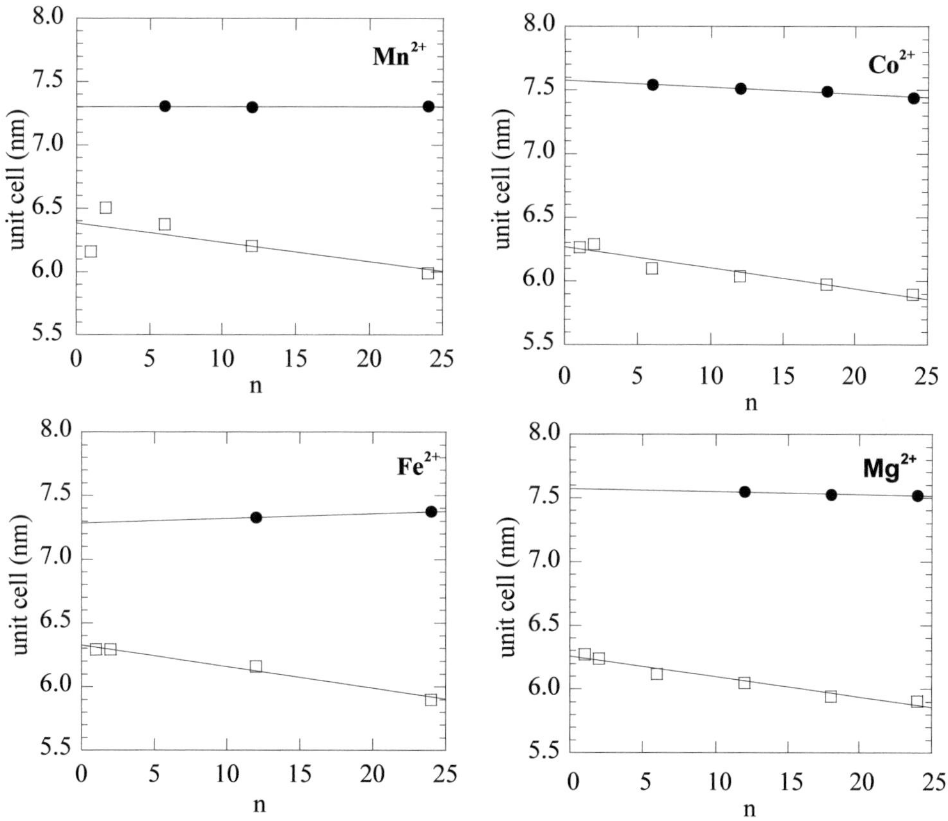

Fig. 5. Lamellar d-spacings of the L^{C}_{α} of ternary complex DOPC/DNA_{ct}/M^{2+} (•) and of the L_{α} phase of DOPC (∀) as a function of the metal mole number n in the DOPC/DNA_{ct}/M^{2+} complexes at molar ratios 3:4:n. (Reprinted from: M. Pisani, P. Bruni, C. Conti, E. Giorgini, O. Francescangeli. Self-Assembled Liposome-DNA-Metal Complexes Related to DNA Delivery. Mol. Cryst. Liq. Cryst., 2005, 434, 643).

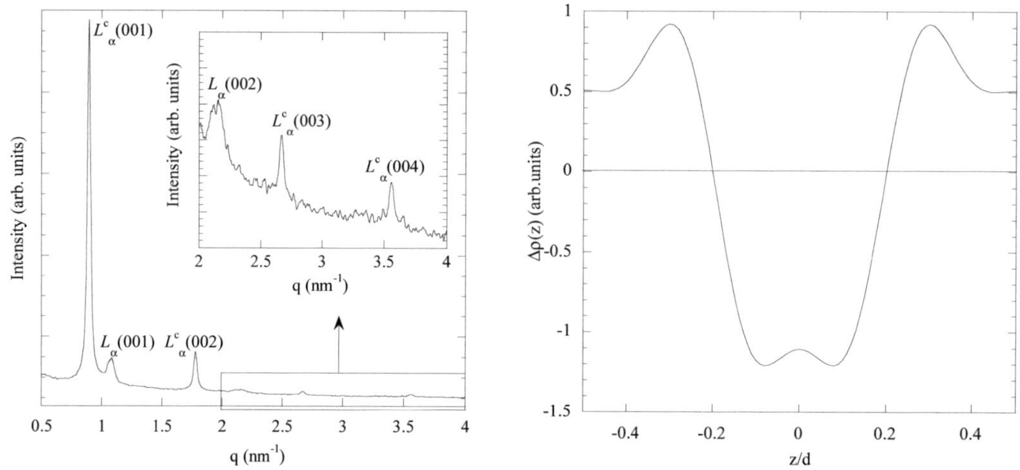

Fig. 6. Left: synchrotron SAXS pattern of the ternary complex DLPC/DNA$_{ct}$/Mn^{2+} at 3:4:12 molar ratio. Right: electron density profile along the normal to the bilayers in the L_{α}^{C} phase. (Reprinted from: M. Pisani, P. Bruni, C. Conti, E. Giorgini, O. Francescangeli. Self-Assembled Liposome-DNA-Metal Complexes Related to DNA Delivery. Mol. Cryst. Liq. Cryst., 2005, 434, 643).

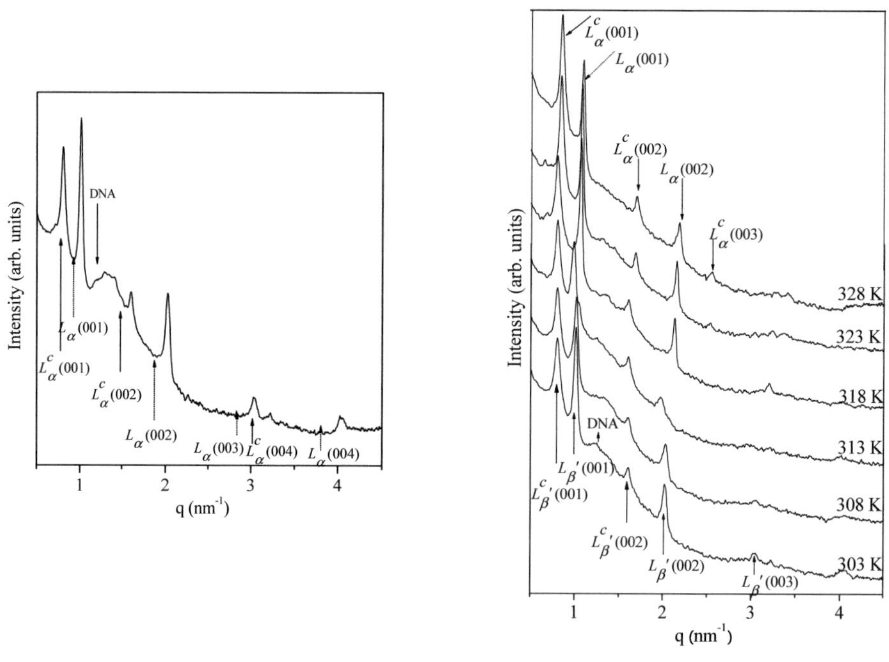

Fig. 7. Left: SAXS pattern of DPPC/DNA/Ca^{2+} complex at molar ratio 3:4:24. Right: synchrotron XRD patterns as a function of temperature.

The evolution of the equilibrium concentrations of the two phases clearly shows that the increase of the temperature favours the formation of the complex, the relative concentrations of the lamellar phases of pure lipids lowering in favour of the one of the ternary complex.

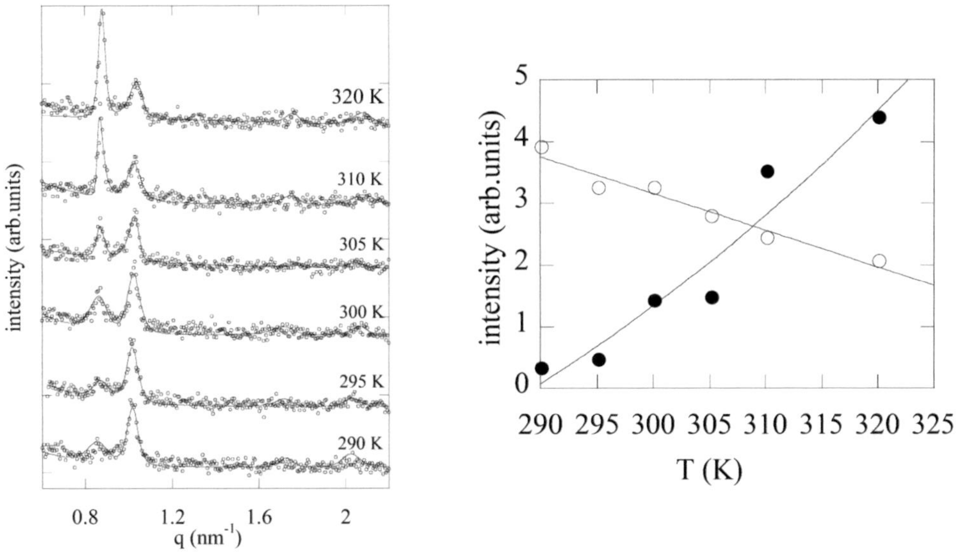

Fig. 8. Left: temperature evolution of the XRD patterns of DOPC/DNA/Mn^{2+} in the range 290 to 320 K. Right: temperature dependence of the integrated intensities of the two small-angle reflections for the L_α^C and the L_α phases. (Reprinted from Rec. Res. Devel. in Macromol., 2003, 7, 247).

The complex DOPC/DNA/Mn^{2+} has also been studied in a solid supported phase (Caracciolo et al., 2004) by Energy Dispersion X-ray Diffraction (Caminiti & Rossi Albertini, 1999; Caracciolo et al., 2002) and it has been found that its structure is essentially identical to that in aqueous solution. The effect of hydration on the structural features of these multilamellar systems has also been explored (Caminiti et al., 2005), considering that adsorbed water plays a major role in the effectiveness of lipid drug delivery systems where lipid-cell interactions are involved. The hydration kinetics of oriented DOPC shows that the long-range order in a multilamellar lipid system strictly depends on the hydration level: adsorbed water molecules first promote a spatial coherence along the normal to the lipid bilayers, then penetrate the interbilayer region and behave as bulk water, producing disorder. The existence of a correlation between the degree of hydration of lipid bilayers and the structure of interbilayer water (Ge & Freed, 2003; Zhou et al., 1999) has been confirmed.

We have already reported that DOPE induces a structural transformation of the lipoplexes when added as a co-lipid: the equilibrium phase of pure DOPE in excess water consists of an inverted hexagonal H_{II} lattice (Turner & Gruner, 1992), whose structure elements are infinitely long rigid rods, all identical and cristallographically equivalent, regularly packed in a 2D hexagonal lattice. The cylinders are filled by water and dispersed in the continuous medium of the hydrocarbon chains, whereas the polar groups are located at the water-hydrocarbon interface. The SAXS pattern of pure DOPE allows to calculate a unit cell spacing a = 7.44 nm (Francescangeli et al., 2004) and its electron density profile calculated along the [10] direction (Figure 9, left) shows an average diameter of the water core d_W = 3.02 nm. DOPE and divalent metal cations Mn^{2+}, Mg^{2+}, Co^{2+} and Fe^{2+} in water solution condense DNA into ternary complexes DOPE/DNA/M^{2+} characterized by an inverted-hexagonal phase H_{II}^{C}. Also in this case two different sets of peaks with different unit cell spacings, namely a = 7.45 nm and a_C= 6.87 nm respectively, have been observed. The former corresponds to the phase H_{II} of pure DOPE, the latter is instead consistent with the 2D columnar inverted hexagonal phase H_{II}^{C} of the DOPE/DNA/Fe^{2+} complexes.

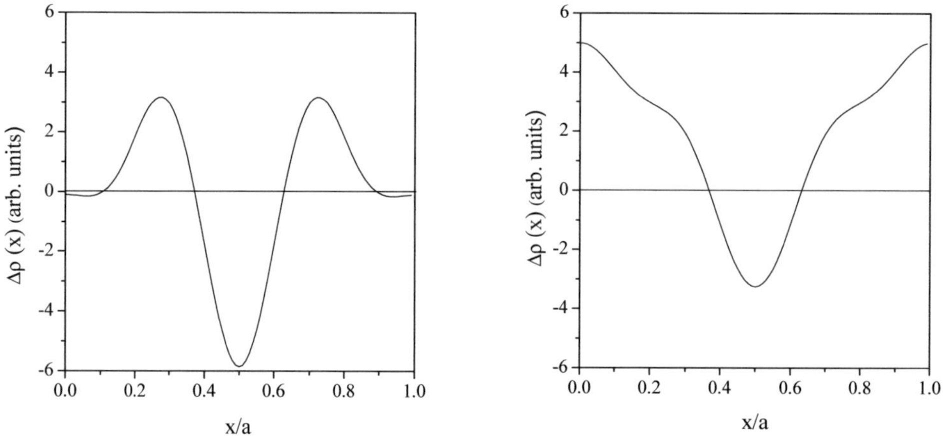

Fig. 9. Left: electron density profile of the pure DOPE along the [10] direction of the unit cell: the origin corresponds to the centre of water core. Right: electron density profile of the complex DOPE/DNA/Fe^{2+}.

In this structure DNA strands are supposed to fill the water gap inside the cylinders of pure DOPE, as it is supported by the electron density profiles (Figure 9 right) calculated along the [10] direction. The two shoulders, at z/d ~ 0.26 and 0.73 respectively, correspond to phosphate groups and are used to localize the centres of the polar head. From the structural data, values of d_{PP} = 3.26 nm and d_L = 4.36 nm were calculated, leading to a water layer thickness d_W = 2.51 nm, large enough to accommodate a double-stranded DNA molecule surrounded by a hydration layer (Podgornik et al., 1989). A pictorial representation of this structure is reported in Figure 3 (right). Unlike complexes organized in the L_α^C the ratio between H_{II} and H_{II}^{C} depends also on the incubation time: after 48 hours, phase H_{II} disappears completely and is transformed into the H_{II}^{C} of ternary complex.

The effect of pegylation on NLs has also been studied (Pisani at al., 2008, 2009) in mixed complexes DOPE/DOPE-PEG(350)/DNA/M^{2+} (M = Ca, Mg, Mn). XRD investigation on the complex with Mn^{2+} shows that with 3% of DOPE-PEG, the two phases H_{II}^{C} and H_{II} coexist as usual: the former being attributed to DOPE/DOPE-PEG(350)/DNA/Mn^{2+}, the latter to DOPE/DOPE-PEG(350)/Mn^{2+}. Interestingly a new phase, indexed in the SAXS pattern as Q (Figure 10), appears at higher concentrations of DOPE-PEG (6, 9 and 15%): the corresponding peaks are spaced in the ratios $\sqrt{2};\sqrt{3};\sqrt{4};\sqrt{6};\sqrt{8};\sqrt{9};\sqrt{10}$ consistent with a cubic Q224 phase with the space group *Pn3m*. A transition $H_{II} \rightarrow Q_{II}$ has been found in different contexts (Koynova et al., 1997) : this ability, together with the well known fusogenic property of DOPE and its destabilizing effect on targeted endosomal membranes makes the complexes DOPE/DOPE-PEG(350)/DNA/Mn^{2+} extremely interesting for application in HGT.

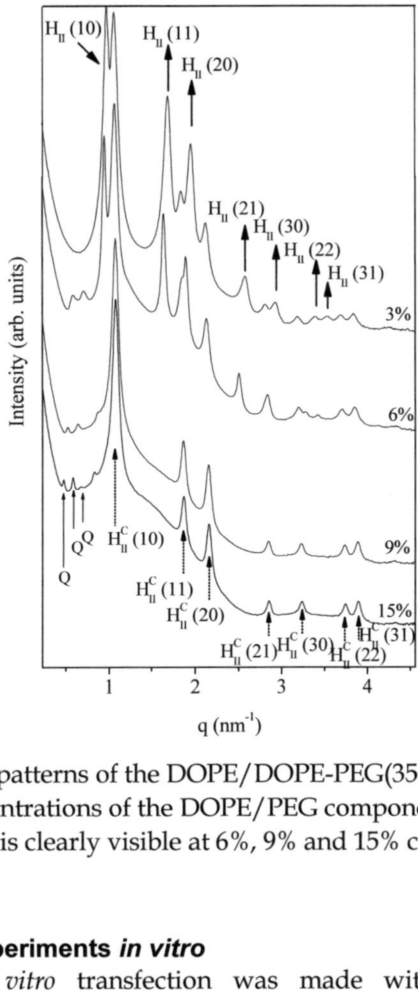

Fig. 10. Synchrotron XRD patterns of the DOPE/DOPE-PEG(350)/DNA/Mn^{2+} complex as a function of different concentrations of the DOPE/PEG component in the lipid mixture. The pattern of the cubic phase is clearly visible at 6%, 9% and 15% concentration of the pegilated DOPE.

4.5 DNA transfection experiments *in vitro*

A first attempt of *in vitro* transfection was made with a couple of complexes DOPC/pDNA/M^{2+}, with M = Ca or Mn, on a mouse fibroplast NIH 3T3 cell line (Bruni et al., 2006): using standard methods the green fluorescent protein was expressed by both complexes. Figure 11 reports an improved result obtained later, using a 15 mM concentration of Ca^{2+} in the complex.

Other attempts of *in vitro* transfections made in our laboratories are compared in a series of histograms (Figure 12) which show that the low efficiency of pure DOPC can be increased by addition of both 1, 2-dioleoyl-*sn*-glycero-3-phosphoethanolamine-N-hexanoylamine (6PE) or 1,2-dioleoyl-*sn*-glycero-3-phosphoethanolamine-N-dodecanoylamine (12PE) to DOPC/DNA/M^{2+}. This result confirms that the transfection efficiency is strongly dependent on an appropriate mixutures of liposomes as DNA carriers.

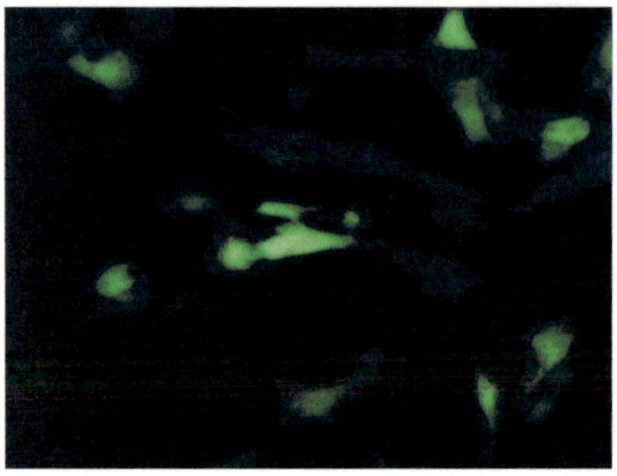

Fig. 11. Fluorescence micrograph of mouse fibroplast NIH 3T3 cells transfected with pGreen Lantern complexed with DOPC liposome in presence of Ca^{2+}.

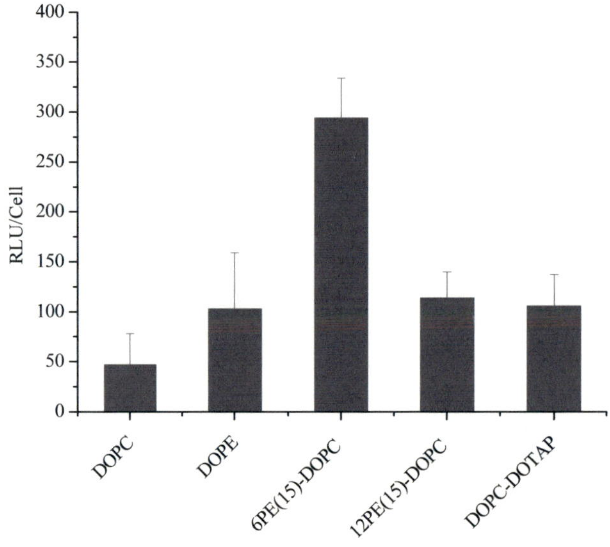

Fig. 12. Luciferase expression following 6hrs transfection with different complexes in NIH3T3 cell line. Expression efficiency is expressed as Relative Luminometric Units per cell (RLU/cell).

An interesting comparison among in vitro transfection efficiencies by DOPE/DNA complexes mediated by cations bearing different charges such as K^+, Mg^{2+}, Ca^{2+}, La^{3+} has been proposed (Tresset et al., 2007). At physiological pH pure DOPE has a slightly negative charge which is not altered by K^+ owing to its low density of binding sites. On the contrary high charge density has been measured for Mg^{2+} and Ca^{2+} and particularly for La^{3+} (100-fold higher than the two bivalent cations). SAXS of the corresponding ternary complexes show the absence of any ordered structure induced by K^+, whereas the usual presence of the two H_{II} and H_{II}^{C} phases has been confirmed with the other cations. Transfection efficiency has been measured on the two cell lines U87 and hepG2: due to the absence of a complexation by K^+, as revealed by x-rays, no transfection has been observed in this case. Instead the efficiency increases in the order $Mg^{2+} < Ca^{2+} < La^{3+}$, the last being 2.6-fold higher than the lipoplex DNA/DOTAP/DOPE. It is also of great importance that the highest efficiency measured with La^{3+} complex has been obtained with ion concentration of three orders of magnitude lower than that of Ca^{2+}: a result extremely favourable in relation to toxicity, as it has been proved.

5. Conclusions and perspectives

At present the use of NLs as autonomous carriers of genetic material in human gene therapy can be considered an opportunity that needs extensive exploration to become a real alternative to CLs. Considering the many limits the latter still meet, particularly in the *in vivo* applications, and their slow progress, it seems important to take also the parallel way of NLs as possible autonomous carriers: lack of toxicity and high stability in serum are important characteristics in their favour. Some of the results outlined here are worth interesting developments. It has been found that complexes reflect the structure and symmetry of the parent lipids and that the different bivalent metal cations are equally active in promoting the DNA condensation into the ternary complexes; these achievements will provide structure-composition correlation, that may be used in designing at the best these materials as non-viral DNA carriers in HGT. Additional developments of the research in this field, currently investigated in our laboratories, concern the use of pegylated NLs in the management of brain related diseases, where CLs have started being experimented (Zhang et al., 2002; Pardridge, 2007; Boardo, 2007). Better results could be perhaps obtained with NLs, thanks to their ability to reduce opsonisation. The recent interest in the so-called intelligent carriers which is developing on CLs (Voinea & Simionescu, 2002; Shi et al., 2002; Alvarez-Lorenzo et al., 2009) could also represent an interesting opportunity for NLs. The structural knowledge of complexes of DNA with NLs is only one of the aspects which will presumably affect the transfection: many other aspects, such as Z-potential values, complex size, and efficient DNA entrapment are all very important acquisitions to be obtained. The entry of NLs in the world of HGT and the consequent opportunity to compare properties and activity with the ones of cationic and anionic liposomes will lead to a better understanding of that processes. In this connection is encouraging to quote the opinion of Rädler, one of the most outstanding experts in cationic lipids: "the resources devoted to creating less toxic cationic-DNA complexes, may perhaps, in the future be balanced by research exploiting the possibility of creating comparable complexes from entirely non toxic components such as the NLs/DNA/M^{2+} complexes".

6. References

Alvarez-Lorenzo, C.; Bromberg, L. & Concheiro, A. (2009). Light-sensitive intelligent drug delivery systems. *Photochem. Photobiol.*, 85, 848–860, 0031-8655.

Bailay, A.L. & Sullivan, S.M. (2000). Efficient encapsulation of DNA plasmids in small neutral liposomes induced by ethanol and calcium. *Biochim. Biophys. Acta*, 1468, 239-252, 005-2736.

Bangham, A.D., Standish, M.M. & Weissmann, G. (1965). The action of steroids and streptolysin S on the permeability of phospholipids structures to cations. *J. Mol. Biol.*, 13, 253-259, 0022-2836.

Boado R.J. (2007). Blood-brain barrier transport of non-viral gene and RNAi therapeutics. *Pharm. Res.*, 24, 1772-1787, 0724-8741.

Boukhnikachvili. T., Aguerre-Chariol, O., Airlau, M., Lesieur, S., Ollivon, M: & Vacus, J. (1997). Structure of in-serum transfecting DNA-cationic lipid complexes. *FEBS Lett.*, 409, 188-194, 0014-5793.

Boussif, O., Lezoualch, F., Zanta, M. A.,. Mergny, M. D., Scherman, D., Demeneix, B.J. & Behr P. (1995). A versatile vector for gene and oligonucleotide transfer into cells in culture and in vivo: polyethylenimine *Proc. Natl. Acad. Sci. USA, 92,* 7297-7301, 0027-8424.

Boussif, O., Gaucheron, J., Boulanger, C., Santaella, C., Kolbe, H.V.J. & Vierling, P. (2001). Enhanced in vitro and in vivo cationic lipid-mediated gene delivery with a fluorinated glycerophospho-ethanolamine. *J.Gen. Med.*, 3, 109-114, 1099-498X.

Bruni, P., Gobbi, G., Morgganti, G., Iacussi, M. &Maurelli E. (1997). Use and activity of metals in biological systems. The interaction of bivalent metal cations with double-stranded polynucleotides and phospholipids. *Gazz. Chim. Ital.*, 127, 513-517, 0016-5603.

Bruni, P.; Pisani, M.; Amici, A.; Marchini, C.; Montani, M. & Francescangeli, O. (2006). Self-assembled ternary complexes of neutral liposomes, deoxyribonucleic acid and bivalent metal cations. Promising vectors for gene transfer? *Applied Physics Letters,* 88, 73901, 1-3, 0003-6951.

Budker, V. G., Kazatchkov, Y. A. & Naumova, L. P. (1978). Polynucleotides adsorb on mitochondrial and model lipid membranes in the presence of bivalent cations. *FEBS Lett.*, 95, 143-146, 0014-5793.

Caminiti, R. & Rossi Albertini, V. (1999). The kinetics of phase transitions observed by energy-dispersive X-ray diffraction. *Int. Rev. Phys. Chem.*, 18, 263-299, 0144-235X.

Caminiti, R.; Caracciolo, G.; Pisani, M. & Bruni, P. (2005). Effect of hydration on the long-range order of lipid multilayers investigated by in situ time-resolved energy dispersive X-ray diffraction. *Chem. Phys. Lett.*, 409, 331-336, 0009-2614.

Caracciolo, G.; Caminiti, R.; Pozzi, D.; Friello, M.; Boffi, F. & Congiu Castellano A. (2002). Self-assembly of cationic liposomes-DNA complexes: a structural and thermodynamic study by EDXD. *Chem. Phys. Lett.*, 351, 222-228, 0009-2614.

Caracciolo, G.; Sadun, C.; Caminiti, R.; Pisani, M.; Bruni, P. & Francescangeli, O. (2004). Structure of solid-supported lipid-DNA-metal complexes investigated by energy dispersive X-ray diffraction. *Chem. Phys. Lett.*, 397, 138-143, 0009-2614.

Caracciolo, G. & Caminiti, R. (2005). Do DC-Chol/DOPE-DNA complexes really form an inverted hexagonal phase? *Chem. Phys. Lett.*, 411, 327-332, 0009-2614.

Chapman, C.J., Erdahl, W.L., Taylor, R.W. & Pfeiffer, D.R. (1990). Factors affecting solute entrapment in phospholipid vesicles prepared by the freeze-thaw extrusion method: a possible general method for improving the efficiency of entrapment. *Chem. Phys. Lipids,* 55, 73-83, 0009-3084.

Deamer, D.W. & Barchfield, G.L. (1982). Encapsulation of macromolecules by lipid vesicles under simulated prebiotic conditions. *J.Mol. Evol.*, 18, 203-206, 0022-2844.

Deshpande, M.C.; Davies, M.C.; Garnett, M.C.; Williams, P.M.; Armitage, D.; Bailey, L.; Vamvakaki, M.; Armes, S.P. & Stolnik, S. (2004): The effect of poly(ethylene glycol) molecular architecture on cellular interaction and uptake of DNA complexes. *J. Control. Release,* 97, 143–156, 0168-3659.

Dimitriadis, G.J. (1978). Entrapment of ribonucleic acid in liposomes. *FEBS Lett.*, 86, 289-293, 0014-5793.

Dimitriadis, G.J. & Butters, T.D. (1979). Liposome-mediated ricin toxicity in ricin-resistant cells. *FEBS Lett.*, 98, 33-36, 0014-5793.

Düzgünes, N., Wilschut, J., Fraley, R. & Papahadjopoulos, D. 1981. Studies on the mechanism of membrane fusion. Role of head-group composition in calcium- and magnesium-induced fusion of mixed phospholipid vesicles. *Biochim. Biophys. Acta*, 642, 182-195, 0005-2736.

Edelstein, M.J., Abedi, M.R., Wicson, J. & Edelstein, M.R. (2004): Gene therapy clinical trials worldwide 1989-2004. *J. Genet. Med.*, 6, 597-602, 1226-1769.

Elouahabi, A. & Ruysschaert, J.M. (2005). Formation and intracellular trafficking of lipoplexes and polyplexes. *Mol. Ther.*, 11, 336-347, 1525-0016.

Farhood, H., Serbina, N. & Huang, L. (1995), The role of dioleyl phosphatidylethaloamine in cationic liposome- mediated gene transfer. *Biochim. Biophys. Acta*, 1235, 289-295, 0005-2736.

Fasbender, A., Marshall, J., Moninger, T.O., Grust, T., Cheng, S. & Welsh, M.J. (1997). Effect of co-lipids in enhancing cationic-lipid mediated gene transfer in vitro and in vivo. *Gen. Ther.*, 4, 716-725, 0969-7128.

Felgner, P.L., Gadek,T.R., Holm, M., Roman, R., Chan, H.W., Wenz, M., Northrop, J.P., Ringold, G.M. & Danielsen, M. (1987). Lipofection: A highly efficient, lipid-mediated DNA-transfection procedure. *Proc. Natl. Acad. Sci. USA*, 84, 7413-7417, 0027-8424.

Felgner, J.H., R Kumar, C N Sridhar, C J Wheeler, Y J Tsai, R Border, P Ramsey, M Martin, & P L Felgner. (1994). Enhanced gene delivery and mechanism studies with a novel series of cationic lipid formulations. *J. Biol. Chem.*, 269, 2550-2561, 0021-9258.

Filion, M.C., Phillips, N.C. (1998). Major limitations in the use of cationic liposomes for DANN delivery. *Int. J. Pharm.*, 162, 159-170, 0378-5143.

Finkelstein, M. & Weissmann, G. (1978). The introduction of enzymes into cells by means of liposomes. *J. Lip. Res.*, 19, 289-303, 0022-2275.

Fletcher S., Ahmad, A., Perouzel, E., Jorgensen & M.R., Miller, A.D. (2006). A dialkynoyl analog of DOPE improves gene transfer of lower-charged cationic lipoplexes. *Org. Biomol. Chem.*, 4, 196-199, 1477-0520.

Foradada, M.; Pujol, M.D.; Bermudez, J. & Esterlich, J. (2000). Chemical degradation of liposomes by serum components detected by NMR. *Chem. Phys. Lipids*, 104, 133-148, 0009-3084.

Fraley, R., Subramani, S., Berg, P. & Papahadjopoulos, D. (1980). Introduction of liposome-encapsulated SV40 DNA into cells. *J. Biol. Chem.*, 255, 10431-10435, 0021-9258.

Fraley, R., Straubinger, R.M., Rule, G., Springer, A.L. & Papahadjopoulos, D. (1981). Liposome-mediated delivery of deoxyribonucleic acid to cells: enhanced efficiency of delivery related to lipid composition and incubation conditions. *Biochemistry*, 20, 6978-6987, 0006-2960.

Francescangeli, O.; Rinaldi, D.; Laus, M.; Galli, G. & Gallot, B.J. (1996). An X-ray study of a smectic C and smectic A liquid crystal polyacrylate. *J. Phys. II*, 6, 77-89.

Francescangeli, O., Pisani, M., Stanic, V., Bruni, P. & Iacussi, M. (2003). Supramolecular ordering of self-assembled liposome-DNA- metal complexes. *Recent Res. Dev. Macromol. Res.*, 7, 247-263, 81-271-0025-0.

Francescangeli, O., Stanic, V., Gobbi, L., Bruni, P., Iacussi, M., Tosi, G. & Bernstorff, S. (2003). Structure of self-assembled liposome-DNA-metal complexes. *Phys. Rev. E*, 67, 11904 (1-11), 1539-3755.

Francescangeli, O.; Pisani, M.; Stanic, V.; Bruni, P. & Weiss, T.M. (2004). Evidence of an inverted hexagonal phase in self-assembled phospholipid-DNA-metal complexes. *Europhysics Letters*, 67, 669-675, 0295-5075.

Gaucheron, J., Santaella, C. & Vierling, P. (2001a). Higly fluorinated lipospermines fo gene transfer: synthesis and evaluation of their in vitro transfection efficiency. *Bioconj. Chem.*, 12, 114-128, 1043-1802.

Gaucheron, J., Santaella, C. & Vierling, P. (2001b). Improved in vitro gene transfer mediated by fluorinated lipoplexes in the presence of a bile salt surfactant. *J.Gene Med.*, 3, 338-344, 1029-498X..

Gaucheron, J., Boulanger, C., Santaella, C., Sbirrazzuoli, N., Boussif. O. & Vierling, P. (2001c). In vitro cationic lipid-mediated gene delivery with fluorinated glycerophosphoethanolamine helper lipids. *Bioconj. Chem.*, 12, 949-963, 1043-1802.

Ge, M. & Freed J.H. (2003). Hydration, structure and molecular interactions in the headgroup region of dioleoylphosphatidylcholine bilayers: an electron spin resonance study. *Biophys. J.*, 85, 4023-4040, 006-3495.

Gregoriadis, G. & Buckland R. A. (1973). Enzyme-containing Liposomes alleviate a Model for Storage Disease. *Nature,* 244, 170-172, 0038-0836.

Gromelski, S. & Brezezinski, G. (2006). DNA condensation and interaction with zwittrionic phospolipids mediated by divalent cations. *Langmuir*, 22, 6293-6301, 0743-7463.

Hacein-Bey-Abina, S. et al. (2003). LMO2-Associated clonal T cell proliferation in two patients after gene therapy for SCID-X1. *Science*, 302, 415-419, 0036-8075.

Harper, P. E.; Mannock, D.A.; Lewis, R.N.A.H.; McElhaney, R.N. & Gruner, S.M. (2001). X-Ray diffraction structures of some phosphatidylethanolamine lamellar and inverted hexagonal phases. *Biophys. J.*, 81, 2693-2706, 0006-3495.

Harrington, J.J., Van Bokkelen, G., Mays, R.W., Gustashaw, K. & Williard, H.F. (1997). Formation of *de novo* centromeres and construction of first-generation human artificial microchromosome. *Nat. Genet.*, 15, 345-355, 1061-4036.

Hoffman, R.M., Margolis, R.B. & Bergelson, L.D. (1978). Binding and entrapment of high molecular weight DNA by lecithin liposomes. *FEBS Lett.*, 93, 365-368, 0014-5793.

Kharakoz, D.P., Khusainova, R.S., Gorelov, A.V. & Dawson, K.A. (1999). Stoichiometry of dipalmitoylphosphatidylcholine-DNA interaction in the presence of Ca^{2+}: a temperature-scanning ultrasonic study. *FEBS Lett.*, 466, 27-29, 0014-5793.

Klibanov, A.L., Maruyama, K:, Torchilin, V.P. & Huang, L. (1990). Amphipatic polyethylenglycos effectively prolong the
circulation time of liposomes. *FEBS,* 268, 235-237, 0014-5793.

Koiv, A., Palvimo, J. & Kinnunen, P.K. (1995). Evidence for ternary complex by histone H1, DNA and liposomes. *Biochemistry*, 34, 8018-8027, 0006-2960.

Koltover, L., Salditt, T., Rädler, J.O. & Safinya, C.R. (1998). An inverted hexagonal phase of cationic liposome-DNA complexes related to DNA release and delivery. *Science,* 281, 78-81, 0036-8075.

Kostarelos, K. & Miller, A.D. (2005). Synthetic, self-assembly ABCD nanoparticles; a structural paradigm for synthetic non-viral vectors. *Chem. Soc. Rev.*, 34, 970-994, 0306-0012.

Kovalenko D.V.; Shafei, R.A.; Zelenina, I.A.; Semenova, M.L.; Samuilova, O.V. & Zhdanov, R.I. (1996). Metallo nucleoliposome complexes as a vehicle for gene delivery to mouse skeletal muscles in vivo. *Genetika, 32*, 1299-1301, 1022-7954.

Koynova, R.; Tenchov, B. & Rapp, G. (1997). Low amounts of PEG-lipid induce cubic phase in phosphatidylethanolamine dispersions. *Biochim. Biophys. Acta*, 1326, 167-170, 0005-2736.

Koynova, R., Wang, L., Tarahovsky, W. & McDonald, R.C. (2005). Lipid phase control of DNA delivery. *Bioconj. Chem.*, 16, 1335-1339, 1043-1802.

Koynova, R., Wang, Li. & MacDonald, R.C. (2006). An intracellular lamellar-non lamellar phase transition rationalizes the superior performance of some cationic lipid transfection agents. *Proc. Natl. Acad. Sci. USA*, 103, 14373-14378, 0027-8424.

Lin, A.J., Slack, N.L., Ahmad, A., George, C.X., Samuel, C.E. & Safinya, C.R. (2003). Three-dimensional imaging of lipid gene-carriers: membrane charge density controls universal transfection behavior in lamellar cationic liposome-DNA complexes *Biophys. J.*, 84, 3307-3316, 0006-3495.

Liu, F. & Huang, L. (2002). Development of non-viral vectors for systemic gene delivery. *J. Control. Rel.*, 78, 259-266, 0168-3659.

Lurquin, P.F. (1979). Entrapment of plasmid DNA by liposomes and their interactions with plant protoplast. *Nucleic Acid Res.*, 6, 3773-3784, 0305-1048.

Luzzati, V. (1968). *Biological Membranes*, Academic Press, New York, London.

Lv, H., Zhang, S., Wang,B., Cui, S. & Yan, J. (2006). Toxicity of cationic lipids and cationic polymers in gene delivery. *J.Control. Rel.*, 114, 100-109, 0168-5659.

Magee, W., Talcott, M., Straub, S. & Vriend, D. (1976). A comparison of negatively and positively charged liposomes containing entrapped polynosinic polycytidylic acid for interferon induction in mice. *Biochim. Biophys. Acta*, 451,610-618, 0304-4165.

Marshall, E. (2000). Gene Therapy on Trial. *Science*, 288, 951-957, 0036-8075.

McDonald, R.C., Ashley, G.W., Shida M.M., Rakhmanova, V.A., Tarahovsky, Y.S., Pantazatos, P.P., Kennedy, M.T., Pozharski, E.V., Baker, K.A., Jones, R.D., Rosenzweig, H.S., Choi, K.L., Qiu, R.Z. & McIntosh T. J. (1999). Physical and Biological Properties of cationic triesters of phosphatidylcholine. *Biophys. J.*, 77, 2612-2629, 0006-3495.

McManus, J.J., Rädler, J.O. & Dawson, K.A. (2003). Does calcium turn a zwitterionic lipid cationic? *J. Phys. Chem. B*, 107,
9869-9875, 1520-6106.

McManus, J.J., Rädler, J.O. & Dawson, K.A. (2003). Phase behavior of DPPC in a DNA-calcium-zwitterionic lipid complex studied by small-angle x-ray scattering. *Langmuir*, 19, 9630-9637, 0743-7463.

Mével, M., Neveu, C., Goncalves, C., Yaouanc, J.J., Pichon, C., Jaffrès, P.A. & Midoux, P. (2008). Novel neutral imidazole-lipophosphoramides for transfection assays. *Chem Comm.*, 3124-3126, 1359-7345.

Mok, K.W. & Cullis, P.R. (1997). Structural and fusogenic properties of cationic liposomes in the presence of plasmid DNA. *Biophys. J.*, 73, 2534-2545, 0006-3495.

Monnard, P.A., Oberholzer, T. & Luisi, P.L. (1997). Entrapment of nucleic acids in liposomes. *Biochim. Biophys. Acta*, 1329, 39-50, 0005-2736.

Mui, H., Ahkong, Q.F., Chow, L. & Hope, M.J. (2000). Membrane perturbation and the mechanism of lipid-mediated transfer of DNA into cells. *Biochim. Biophys. Acta,* 1467, 281-292, 0005-2736.

Newton, C., Pangborn, W, Nir, S. & Papahadjopoulos, D. (1978). Specificity of Ca^{2+} and Mg^{2+} binding to phsphatidylserine vesicles and resultant phase changes of bilayer membrane structure. *Biochim. Biphys. Acta,* 506, 281-287, 0005-2736.

Ostro, M.J., Giacomini, D., Lavelle, D., Paxton, W. & Dray, S. (1978). Evidence for traslation of rabbit globin mRNA after liposome mediated insertion into a human cell line. *Nature,* 274, 921-923, 0028-0836.

Papahadjopoulos, D., Vail, W.J., Pangborn, W. & Poste, G. (1976). Studies on membrane fusion. II. Induction in fusion in pure phospholipid membranes by calcium ions an other divalent metals. *Biochim. Biophys. Acta,* 448, 265-283, 0005-2736.

Papahadjopoulos, D.; Allen, T.M.; Gabizon, A.; Mayhew, E.; Matthay, K.; Huang, S.K.; Lee, K.D.; Woodle, M.C.; Lasic, D.D.; Redemann, C. & Martin, F.J. (1991). Sterically stabilized liposomes: improvements in pharmacokinetics and antitumor therapeutic efficacy. *Proc. Natl. Acad. Sci. USA,* 88, 11460-11464, 0027-8424.

Pardridge, W.M. (2007). shRNA and siRNA delivery to the brain. *Adv. Drug Del. Reviews,* 59, 141–152, 0169-409X..

Pisani, M., Bruni, P., Conti, C., Giorgini, E. & Francescangeli, O. (2005). Self.-asembled liposome-DNA metal complexes related to DNA delivery. *Mol. Cryst. Liq. Cryst.,* 434, 315-323, 1542-1406.

Pisani, M., Bruni, P., Caracciolo, G., Caminiti, R. & Francescangeli, O. (2006). Structure and phase behavior of self-assembled DOPC-DNA-Metal Cation complexes. *J. Phys. Chem. B,* 110, 13203-13211, 1520-6106.

Pisani, M., Fino, V., Bruni, P., Di Cola, E. & Francescangeli, O. (2008). Metal induced cubic phase in poly(ethyleneglycol)-functionalized dioleoylphosphatidylethanolamine aqueous dispersions. *J. Phys. Chem. Letters B,* 112, 5276-5278, 1520-6106.

Pisani, M., Fino, V., Bruni, P. & Francescangeli, O. (2009). DNA condensation into inverted hexagonal phase in aqueous dispersion of poly(ethylene)-functionalized dioleoylphosphatidylethanolamine and metal cations. *Mol. Cryst. Liq. Cryst.,* 500, 132-143, 1542-1406.

Podgornik, R., Rau, D.C. & Parsegian, V.A. (1989). The action of interhelical forces on the organisation of DNA double helices: fluctuation-enhanced decay of electrostatic double-layer and hydration forces. *Macromolecules,* 22, 1780-1786, 0024-9297.

Portis, A., Newton, C., Pangborn, W. & Papahadjopoulos, D. (1979). Studies on the mechanism of membrane fusion: Evidence for an intermembrane Ca^{2+}-phospholipid complex, synergism with Mg^{2+} and inhibition by spectrin. *Biochemistry,* 18, 780-790, 0006-2960.

Rädler, J.O., Koltover, I., Salditt, T. & Safinya, C.R. (1997). Structure of DNA-Cationic liposome complexes: DNA intercalation in multilateral membranes in distinct interhelical packing regimes. *Science,* 275, 810-814, 0036-8075.

Roush, W. (1997). Molecular biology: counterfeit chromosomes for humans. *Science,* 276, 38-39, 0036-8075.

Safinya, C.R., (2001). Structures of lipid-DNA complexes: supramolecular assembly and gene delivery. *Curr. Opin. Struct. Biol.,* 11, 440-448, 0959-440X.

Safinya, C.R., Ewert, K., Ahmad, A., Evans, H.M., Raviv, U., Needleman, D.J., Lin, A.J., Slack, N.L., George, C. & Samuel, C.E. (2006). Cationic liposome-DNA complexes: from liquid crystal science to gene delivery applications. *Phil. Trans. R. Soc. A*, 364, 2573-2596, 1364-503X

Sessa, G. & Weissmann, G. (1968). Phospholipid spherules (liposomes) a model for biological membranes. *J. Lipid Res.*, 9, 310-318, 0022-2275.

Shi, G., Guo, W., Stephenson, S.M. & Lee, R.J. (2002). Efficient intracellular drug and gene delivery using folate receptor-targeted pH-sensitive liposomes composed of cationic/anionic lipid combinations. *J. Control Rel.*, 80, 309–319, 0168-3659.

Song, L.Y., Ahkong, Q.F.; Rong, Q., Wang, Z., Ansell, S., Hope, M.J. & Mui, B. (2002). Characterization of the inhibitory effect of PEG-lipid conjugates on the intracellular delivery of plasmid and antisense DNA mediated by cationic lipid liposomes. *Biochim. Biophys. Acta,* 1558, 1–13, 005-2736.

Szoka, F. & Papahadjopoulos, D. (1978). Procedure for preparation of liposomes with large internal aqueous space and high capture by reverse-phase evaporation. *Proc. Natl. Acad. Sci. USA*, 75, 4194-4198, 0027-8424.

Szoka, F.C.,Jr., Xu, Y. & Zelphati, O. (1996). How are nucleic acids released in the cell from cationic-nucleic acid complexes. *J. Liposome Res.*, 6, 567-587, 0898-2104.

Tarahowsky, Y.S., Khusainova, R.S., Gorelov, A.V., Nicolaeva, T.I., Deev, A.A., Dawson, A.K. & Ivanitsky, G.R. (1996).

DNA initiates polymorphic structural transitions in lecithin. *FEBS Lett.*, 390, 133-136, 0014-5793.

Tardi, P.G., Boman, N.L. & Cullis, P.R. (1996). Liposomal doxorubicin. *J. Drug Target.*, 4, 129-140, 1061-186X.

Tresset, G., Cheong, W.C.D., Tan, Y.L.S., Boulaire, J. & Lam, Y.M. (2007). Phospholipid based artificial viruses assembled by multivalent cations. *Biophys. J.*, 93, 637-644, 0006-3495.

Tristram-Nagle, S.; Peytrache, H.I. & Nagle, J.F. (1998). Structure and interactions of fully hydrated dioleoylphosphatidylcholine bilayers. *Biophys. J.*, 75, 917-925, 0006-3495.

Turner, D.C. & Gruner, S.M. (1992). X-ray diffraction reconstruction of the inverted hexagonal (H_{II}) phase in lipid-water systems. *Biochemistry*, 31, 1340-1355, 0006-2960.

Tyrrell, D.A., Heath, T.D., Colley, C.M. & Ryman, B.E. (1976). New aspects of liposomes. *Biochim. Biophys. Acta*, 457, 259-302, 0005-2736.

Uhrikova, D., Hanulova, M.; Funari, S.S., Khusainova, R.S., Sersen, F., Balgavy, P. (2005). The structure of DNA-DOPC aggregates formed in presence of calcium and magnesium ions: a small-angle synchrotron X-ray diffraction study. *Biochim: Biophys. Acta*, , 1713, 15-28, 005-2736.

Voinea, M. & Simionescu, M. (2002). Designing of intelligent liposomes for efficient delivery of drugs. *J. Cell. Mol. Med.*, 6, 465-474, 1582-1838.

Willard, H.F. (2000). Artificial Chromosomes Coming to Life. *Science*, 290, 1308-1309, 0036-8075.

Wilschut, J., Düzgünes, N., Fraley, R. & Papahadiopoulos, D. (1980). Studies on the mechanism of membrane fusion: kinetics of calcium ion induced fusion of phosphatidylserine vesicles followed by a new assay for mixing of aqueous vesicle contents. *Biochemistry*, 19, 6011-6021, 0006-2960.

Wilson, T., Papahadjopoulos, D. & Taber, R. (1979). The introduction of poliovirus DNA into cells via lipid vesicles (lipoosmes). *Cell*, 17, 77-84, 0092-8674.

Worthington, C.R. & Khare, R.S. (1978). Structure determination of lipid bilayers. *Biophys. J.*, 23, 407-425, 0006-3495.

Wrobel, I. & Collins, D. (1995). Fusion of cationic liposomes with mammalian cells occurs after endocytosis. *Biochim. Biophys. Acta*, 1235, 296-304, 0005-2736.

Wu, G.Y. & Wu; C.H. (1987). Receptor-mediated in vitro gene transformation by a soluble DNA carrier system.. *J. Biol. Chem.*, 262, 4429-4432, 0021-9258.

Yang, J.P. & Huang, L. (1997). Overcoming the inhibitory effect of serum on lipofection by increasing the charge ratio of cationic liposome to DNA. *Gen. Ther.*, 4, 950-960, 0969-7128.

Zelphati, O. & Szoka F.C. (1996). Liposomes as a carrier for intracellular delivery of antisense olinucleotides: a real or magic bullet? *J. Control. Rel.*, 41, 99-119, 0168-3659.

Zhang, Y., Zhu, C. & Pardridge W.M. (2002). Antisense gene therapy of brain cancer with an artificial virus gene delivery system. *Mol. Ther.*, 6, 67-72, 1525-0016.

Zhou, Z., Sayer, B.G., Hughes, D.W., Stark, R.E. & Epand, R.M. (1999). Studies of phospholipid hydration by high-resolution magic-angle spinning nuclear magnetic resonance. *Biophys. J.*, 76, 387-399, 0006-3495.

Zuhorn, I.S., Oberle,V., Wisser, W.H., Engberts, J.B.F.N., Bakowski, U., Polushkin, E. & Hoekstra, D. (2002). Phase behaviour of cationic amphiphiles and their mixtures with helper lipids influences lipoplex shape, DNA traslocation and transfection efficiency. *Biophys. J.*, 83, 2096-2108, 0006-3495.

Zuhorn, I.S., Visser, W.H., Bakowsky, U., Engberts, J.B. & Hoekxtra, D. (2002). Interference of serum with lipoplex-cell intraction: modulation of intracellular processing. *Biochim. Biophys. Acta*, 1560, 25-36, 005-2736.

Zuhorn, I.S., Bakowski, U., Polushkin, E., Wisser, W.H., Stuart, M.C.A., Engberts, J.B.F.N. & Hoekstra, D. (2005). Nonbilayer Phase of Lipoplex-Membrane mIxture Determines Endosomal Escape of Genetic Cargo and Transfection Efficiency. *Mol. Ther.*, 11, 801-810, 1525-0016.

15

Non-Viral Gene Delivery Systems Based on Cholesterol Cationic Lipids: Structure-Activity Relationships

Michael A. Maslov[1] and Marina A. Zenkova[2]
[1]*Moscow State Academy of Fine Chemical Technologies, Moscow*
[2]*Institute of Chemical Biology and Fundamental Medicine SB RAS, Novosibirsk*
Russia

1. Introduction

Gene therapy as an alternative to conventional medicine implies the elimination of the cause of a disease via the introduction of therapeutic nucleic acids (antisense oligonucleotide, or siRNA, or transgene expressing plasmid DNA, or aptamers, etc) into the cells of the organism (Blau & Springer, 1995; Lv et al., 2006; Karmali & Chaudhuri, 2007; Rayburn & Zhang R., 2008; and references in it). However, efficient delivery of genes at the physiological level into cells of living organism (''transfection'') is always more simple in theory than in practice. Both the therapeutic nucleic acids and cell membrane are negatively charged and therefore the spontaneous entry of naked nucleic acid inside cells is unlikely to be an efficient process. In other words, the development of clinically viable gene-targeted therapeutics and the design of safe and efficient gene delivery reagents (''transfection vectors'') are inseparable problems. (Templeton, Ed. 2010).

Prior to reaching the nucleus, the therapeutic nucleic acids must overcome a number of biological barriers, in particular, the cellular, endosomal, and nuclear membranes. This process is achieved by the utilization of appropriate delivery systems, that protect the genetic material from the destructive action of enzymes and encourage their penetration into the intracellular space, transfer through the nuclear membrane, and further expression in the nucleus (Eliyahu et al., 2005). In addition, these delivery systems should be nontoxic, non-immunogenic and biocompatible.

The administration of genes for therapeutic purposes can be achieved using one of three different approaches. The first approach consists of a direct injection of naked non-protected DNA into the cell resulting in a high level of transgene expression. The simplicity of this approach ensures it can be reasonably applied in a number of experimental protocols (Huang et al., Eds.; 2005). However, therapeutic application of unprotected naked nucleic acids is limited by the easily accessible organs (skin or muscles) for direct injection and is not applicable for systemic delivery due to a number of factors, the most important of which being extracellular nucleases. Gene-modified viruses and virus like particles represent the second approach for the cellular delivery of therapeutic nucleic acids. Viruses are efficient in transducing cells. However, the safety concerns regarding the use of viruses in humans make non-viral delivery systems an attractive alternative.

The third approached is focused upon the use of non-viral vectors. Non-viral vectors are particularly suitable with respect to their simplicity of use, large-scale production and lack of specific immune response. Non-viral vectors can be grouped into three main categories: cationic lipids, cationic polymers, and peptides. In comparison with their viral counterparts, these vectors are currently considerably less efficient, but their well-defined physical and chemical composition coupled with their reduced immunogenicity and toxicity make them promising candidates for gene delivery (El-Aneed, 2004; Dass, 2002; Verma & Weitzman, 2005).

Another important method of gene delivery is lipofection, a method based on the use of cationic lipids/cationic liposomes for gene transfer (Templeton, Ed. 2010; Huang, et al., Eds.; 2005; Karmali & Chaudhuri, 2007; Tseng et al., 2009). Cationic lipids have many potential advantages and have thus been viewed favorably in comparison with other non-viral vectors, including the significant simplicity and ease of production, good repeatability and biodegradability, potential commercial value, and their wide range of clinical application and safety.

The cationic liposomes are formed using cationic lipids, comprising a wide range of chemical compounds with a common structural feature, namely, the presence of both positively charged hydrophilic and hydrophobic domains. Of the most significant interest are biodegradable cationic lipids of natural origin (Lv et al., 2006). Long-chain hydrocarbons, steroids, and diglycerides are used as the hydrophobic domains (Zhi et al., 2010). The cationic hydrophilic domain can be represented by one (monocationic lipids) or more (polycationic lipids) positively charged groups. Monocationic lipids are most often secondary, tertiary or quaternary derivatives of aliphatic or heterocyclic nitrogen bases. In polycationic lipids, natural or synthetic polyamines or amino acids are used as the hydrophilic domains. The stability and toxicity of cationic lipids in biological systems, are determined by the type of bond connecting hydrophobic and hydrophilic domains.

In addition to cationic lipids, the zwitterionic helper lipid has a major impact upon the structure and activity of lipoplexes. A helper lipid can improve the ability of cationic liposomes to transfect cells. *In vitro* studies show that liposomes composed of an equimolar mixture of dioleoylphosphatidylethanolamine (DOPE) and cationic lipids (DOTMA, DOTAP) can mediate higher levels of transfection than those containing only the cationic lipid (Hui et al., 1996; Mok et al, 1997; Kerner et al., 2001). This fact has been attributed to the ability of DOPE tendency to undergo a transition from a bilayer to a hexagonal configuration under acidic pH, possibly facilitating fusion with, or destabilization of target membranes, in particular endosomal membranes (Zuidam & Barenholz, 1998; Zuidam et al., 1999).

Cholesterol initially used as a helper lipid form more stable but less efficient complexes than those containing DOPE *in vitro*. However, cholesterol containing lipoplexes have shown a higher rate of biological activity when compared to lipoplexes with DOPE, when these complexes were utilized *in vivo* (Liu et al., 1997; Sternberg et al., 1998; Smith et al., 1998; Simberg et al., 2003). The significant transfection activity attained was attributed to an improved cell binding and uptake of the lipoplexes promoted by the presence of cholesterol (Crook et al., 1998) and/or better stability of the lipoplex in serum (Simberg et al., 2003).

In 1991, Gao et al. reported the synthesis and application of the cholesterol-based cationic lipid 3-β-[*N*-(*N*′,*N*′-dimethylaminoethyl)carbamoyl]-cholesterol (DC-Chol, **1a**), which was combined with DOPE to transfect mammalian cells (Gao & Huang, 1991). Since then, considerable endeavors have been made in the synthesis of steroidal cationic lipids, due to their potential applications in gene therapy (Zhdanov et al., 1998; Gao & Hui, 2001; Choi et al., 2001; Geall et al., 2000; Percot et al., 2004; Ding et al., 2008; Medvedeva et al., 2009; Maslov et al., 2010). The cationic amphiphiles containing cholesterol as a hydrophobic residue possess a high transfection activity and a low toxicity, finding use in the studies of both the structure-activity relationships and membrane fusion mechanisms (Noguchi et al, 1998; Kearns et al., 2008). Found within the synthesized cholesterol derivatives are commercially available lipids, (DC-Chol) and N^1-cholesteryloxycarbonyl-3,7-diazanonane-1,9-diamine (CDAN). The liposomes prepared with DC-Chol or CDAN and DOPE lipids are widely used to deliver the plasmid DNA for tumor immunotherapy or artificial immunization and are under clinical trials for the therapy of mucoviscidosis.

The efficiency of liposome mediated gene delivery is ascertained not only by the structure of cationic and helper lipids, properties of the nucleic acid, but also by the size and ζ-potential of the lipoplex formed with the nucleic acid. Therefore, the efficiency of the lipid vehicles for nucleic acid delivery is dependent upon the structure of cationic amphiphile whose chemical design requires a tailored approach, taking into account the lipid composition of the membranes, the nature of cell receptors, and the chemical processes in the intracellular environment.

Thus, in this chapter we summarize recent results on the design and structure-activity relationships of cholesterol-based cationic lipids with multiple architectures. We show that some of the designed cationic lipids (liposomal formulations) mediate efficient cellular accumulation, endosomal escape and the biological activity of the delivered nucleic acids (siRNAs, transgene expressing DNA, etc).

2. Cholesterol-containing cationic lipids and polymers

2.1 DC-Chol

Cationic lipid DC-Chol (**1a**) was originally synthesized by Gao et al. (Gao & Huang, 1991) and is available commercially. The DC-Chol was formulated as a cationic liposome with the helper lipid DOPE which promotes the fusion of lipoplexes with the cell membrane resulting in an increase of the DNA transfection efficiency (Zuidam & Barenholz, 1998; Lin et al., 2003).

Cationic liposomes DC-Chol/DOPE have been used extensively both *in vitro* and *in vivo,* displaying high transfection efficiencies (TE) (Litzinger et al., 1996; Song et al., 1997; Porter et al., 1998). There are documented reports that cationic liposomes DC-Chol/DOPE work well in various cell lines e.g. A431 human epithermoid carcinoma cells, A549 human lung carcinoma cells, L929 mouse fibroblast cells, YPT minipig primary endothelial cells (Gao & Huang, 1991), COS-7 cells, CFNPE-9o and 16HBE14o epithelial cell lines (Caplen et al., 1995), SKnSH and the primary rat neuronal cells (Ajmani et al.,1999), glioma cells (Esposito et al., 2003).

An experimental study of DNA compaction with the liposomes DC-Chol/DOPE that covered the whole range of mixed lipid composition and several lipid/DNA charge ratios was published (Rodriguez-Pulido et al., 2008; Munoz-Ubeda et al., 2010). A series of experimental techniques (electrophoretic mobility, SAXS, and fluorescence anisotropy), together with a theoretical aggregation-disaggregation model, has attested to the fact that DC-Chol/ DOPE cationic liposomes, with an average hydrodynamic diameter of (120+/-10) nm, properly condense and compact DNA and the liposomes composition is a key factor pertaining to the properties and structure of the resulting lipoplex.

Commercially available, DC-Chol is widely used for the development of novel approaches for DNA delivery, i.e. as a component of cationic solid lipid nanoparticles (SLNs) (Choi et al., 2008). The SLNs for gene delivery composed of DC-Chol, DOPE, and Tween 80 with TC (tricaprin) as a core in various ratios were produced by the melt homogenization method. The SLNs were bound to the cellular membrane 10 min after transfection, and translocated to the cytosol 60 min later. After 24 h, the SLNs were detectable in the nucleus and cytosol. SLNs showed high transfection efficiency in comparison with commercially available Lipofectin. In fact, PCR analysis indicated that SLNs prolonged the mRNA expression of the plasmid in various organs for up to 5 days. The SLNs-mediated transfection of the p53 gene resulted in the efficient reestablishment of wild-type p53 function in lung cancer cells and restored the apoptotic pathway (Choi et al., 2008).

The use of the most thoroughly investigated cationic lipids DC-Chol, DOTAP, and dimethyldioctadecylammonium (DDA) as vaccine delivery systems to form an antigen depot at the site of injection (SOI) and to induce immunological responses *in vivo* was reported (Henriksen-Lacey et al., 2011). DC-Chol, DOTAP, and DDA liposomes incorporating immunomodulating trehalose dibehenate (TDB) were prepared. DC-Chol/TDB liposomes were stable under storage and were retained at a significantly better degree at the SOI, with nearly 40% of the original dose still detectable 14 days p.i, in comparison with DOTAP/TDB liposomes. With regards to the depot effect at the SOI, the formulations were able to cause antigen retention between the range of 59 and 79% of the antigen dose recovered one day p.i.

The key step in lipid-mediated DNA delivery may be the structural changes of lipid carriers resulting in DNA release (Tarahovsky et al., 2004; Koynova et al., 2006; Hoekstra et al., 2007). In recent times, it was shown that multicomponent lipoplexes are superior in transfection with respect to the binary ones usually employed for gene delivery (Caracciolo et al., 2005a; 2005b; 2006). For instance, the four-component lipid system incorporating cationic lipids DOTAP, DC-Chol and neutral helper lipids dioleoylphosphocholine (DOPC) and DOPE transfer DNA into mouse fibroblast (NIH 3T3) and tumoral myofibroblast-like (A17) cell lines more efficiently than the thoroughly studied DOTAP/DOPC and DC-Chol/DOPE cationic liposomes separately. To answer the question concerning how TE will change with an increasing number of lipid components, the multicomponent lipoplexes were studied incorporating three to six lipid species simultaneously and the TE was then evaluated with respect to mouse fibroblast (NIH 3T3), ovarian (CHO) and tumoral myofibroblast-like (A17) cell lines (Caracciolo et al., 2007). These multicomponent lipoplexes exhibited a much higher TE (about two orders of magnitude) than binary lipoplexes that are more commonly employed for gene delivery. Furthermore, a trend was discovered that the TE increases in correlation with the number of lipid components (with some exceptions as a result of lipid composition). This discovery may be related to the higher fusogenicity and compatibility of vesicles composed of several lipid components with respect to single lipids (Caracciolo et al., 2007). The existence of different regimes of stability was demonstrated for these multicomponent lipoplexes: the most efficient lipoplexes exhibited intermediate 'optimal stability'. To this end, lipoplexes DOTAP/DOPC-DNA were the least resistant mixture to disintegration; DC-Chol/DOPE/DOPC-DNA, the most resistant mixture to disintegration; and DOTAP/DC-Chol/DOPC/DOPE-DNA, the mixture exhibiting an intermediated behavior and characterized by a high TE. The extent of DNA release estimated by electrophoresis was in total concurrence with the structural stability of lipoplexes revealed by SAXS and TE (Caracciolo et al., 2007).

2.2 Monocationic lipids

The basic structure of the cholesterol-based cationic lipids used in gene therapy includes four functional domains: 1) Appositively charged headgroup capable to bind with the negatively charged phosphate group of nucleic acid; 2) a hydrophobic cholesterol anchor, which interacts with the cellular membrane; 3) a spacer group; 4) a linker group, which connects the positively charged head and the hydrophobic domain.

In order to estimate the contribution of each functional domain into the efficacy of DNA delivery and cytotoxicity, various types of cholesterol cationic lipids were synthesized. In the first investigation of the structure-activity relationship, it was revealed that in order to achieve an efficient transfection, the tertiary ammonium group must be connected to the cholesterol by a short spacer *via* the ester or urethane bond. (Farhood et al., 1992).

In further studies the 3-deoxycholesterol cationic derivatives **2a-c** were synthesized, which are shown to be more efficient than DC-Chol (**1a**) or lipid **1b** (Takeuchi et al. 1996). It was observed that introduction of the ethyl or propyl groups into the cationic head results in the decrease of the transfection efficiency (TE). The value of the surface charge (ζ-potential) for the liposomes based on lipids **1a,b, 2a-c, 3a** and their analogs was in positive correlation with TE of the HeLa, COS-7, and NIH 3T3 cells. Cationic liposomes **2a**/DOPE, having the highest ζ-potential, demonstrated the highest TE in all cell lines tested. Furthermore, the activity of the liposomes derived from the compounds **2c** and **3a** having the lowest ζ-potential, was less than 20% of the activity of lipid **2a** (Takeuchi et al., 1996). Moreover, it was found that to achieve an efficient transfection, the size of the complexes should be neither smaller (<400 nm) nor larger (>1.4 µm) (Kawaura et al., 1998).

Lipid **2d,** containing the 2-hydroxyethyl group was found to be more active than the compound **2a** with dimethylamine group, both in the presence and absence of serum (Okayama et al., 1997). Further modifications of the lipid structure by introduction of additional 2-hydroxyethyl groups (compounds **2e-i**) into the cationic head resulted in the collapse of transfection activity. Similarly, the derivative **2f** containing the primary amino group was almost not active. The TE of the lipid **2d** was 2-fold higher in comparison with the activity of lipids **2a** and **2h** (Hasegawa et al, 2002). Based on fluorescence resonance energy transfer (FRET) it was observed that DNA is released differently from the lipoplexes by means of anionic liposomes. Furthermore, both the release rate and the amount of unbound DNA have a positive correlation with the TE. The transfection efficiency of nanoparticles composed of the lipid **2d** was 11.5-fold higher than the TE of DC-Chol (**1a**) and was comparable with Lipofectamine 2000, DMRIE-C and Tfx-20 (Hattori et al., 2007). The size of the nonoplex was 290 nm, and the highest TE *in vitro* was observed for the nitrogen/phosphate (N/P) ratio of 3, when the nanoplex was positively charged. The *in vivo* delivery directly into the tumor demonstrated that the optimum TE corresponds to the N/P ratio of 1; meanwhile the size of nanocomplexes was around 145 nm, and ξ-potential was negative (-16.9 mV). After the intravenous, intramuscular and peroral administration, there was no transgene expression detected in any organ.

Lipids containing ester (**3b,c**), ether (**3d-f**) and urethane (**1b**) bonds were synthesized (Ghosh et al., 2000; Ghosh et al., 2002) in order to study the influence of linker type on the TE. It was subsequently demonstrated, that the presence of the urethane-based linkage in the compound **1b** led to the 6-fold decrease of the TE, in comparison to the ether lipid **3d**. However, in our opinion, this kind of comparison is fallacious due to presence of the different type of cationic head in the structure of the lipids **1b** and **3d**. Cholesterol lipids with the ether linkage **3d,e** were significantly more efficient than their analogues **3b,c** with ester bond. The increase of the spacer length by one oxyethylene unit (lipid **3f**) resulted in the decrease of the TE. The efficiency of the **3d**-based liposomes was comparable with the Lipofectamine. Lipid **3e** with 2-hydroxyethyl substituent efficiently transected cells without DOPE. A comparison of the liposome mediated siRNA delivery in the presence of serum was carried out for the lipids with ether (**3g**) and urethane (**1c**) linkage. (Han et al., 2008). The cellular accumulation of the fluorescein-labeled siRNA mediated by liposome **1c**/DOPE was inhibited by serum, while liposomes **3g**/DOPE had the ability to efficiently deliver siRNA into the cell in the presence of serum. Liposomes **3g**/DOPE were successfully applied for silencing survivin and green fluorescent protein (GFP).

A comparative study of the TE of DC-Chol (**1a**), and lipids **1c-e** was performed in order to estimate the effect of the cationic headgroup in the cholesterol lipids containing the urethane linker group (Kearns et al., 2008). The lipids **1c** and **1d**, containing both primary and secondary amino groups, were able to transport DNA into the melanoma B16-F10 cells. These data differ from the results received for the 3-deoxycholesterol derivatives **2a-f**, where the lipid **2f** with primary amino group display extremely low TE in comparison of the analogue **2a** with the tertiary amino group. It was observed that lipids **1c** and **1d** containing primary and secondary amino groups are less toxic, in comparison to the lipids with tertiary (**1a**) and quaternary (**1e**) amino groups. The highest TE achieved for liposomes with lipids **1c** and **1d** could be a result of the ability of these liposomes to penetrate into the cells, to interact with the endosomal membrane and to release the nucleic acid into the cytoplasm.

Cationic liposomes formed by lipid **1f** in combination with DOPE were able to deliver DNA into the cells (Reynier et al., 2002; Lesage, 2002). The TE of these liposomes was 2-fold higher in comparison with DC-Chol (**1a**)/DOPE liposomes. What is more, the TE increased in the presence of 4% PEG 8000. Using the liposomes **1e**/DOPE and **1f**/DOPE (1:1) the relocation of DNA within the lipoplexes upon the transfection was monitored in addition to the localization of the plasmid DNA inside the cell nucleus was visualized using immunogold labeling (Briane, et al., 2002).

As mentioned above, the introduction of the 2-hydroxyethyl substituent into the cationic headgroup can increase the TE (Okayama et al., 1997; Hasegawa et al, 2002). The cationic lipid **1h** was synthesized and formed stable liposomes with DOPE with the monomodal size distribution (Percot et al, 2004). *In vivo* direct injection into the tumor of the liposomes **1h**/DOPE and **1g**/DOPE demonstrated that the TE of the 2-hydroxyethyl-containing lipid **1h** was slightly lower than the TE of the lipid **1g** containing trimethylammonium headgroup. In order to study the effect of 2-hydroxyethyl group on the TE more thoroughly, the activity the lipids **1b** and **1h-k** was tested and compared with the activity of DC-Chol (**1a**) and 3-deoxycholesterol derivative **2d** (Ding, et al., 2008). It was discovered that lipids without OH-groups (DC-Chol and **1b**) had the higher TE in comparison with the 2-hydroxyethyl-containing lipids **1h-k**, excluding lipid **2d**. Liposomes **2d**/DOPE possessed the highest TE *in vitro* (comparable with Lipofectamine2000) when N/P ratio was equal to 3, and were characterized by the big sizes of both liposomes itself (400 nm) and lipoplexes. The maximal level of the luciferase gene expression *in vivo* after intratracheal administration of the lipoplexes **1k**/DOPE-pDNA was 2-fold higher than the levels for the **1h**/DOPE, **1j**/DOPE and 4-fold higher than for DC-Chol (**1a**)/DOPE. The liposomes containing lipid **2d** were the least active.

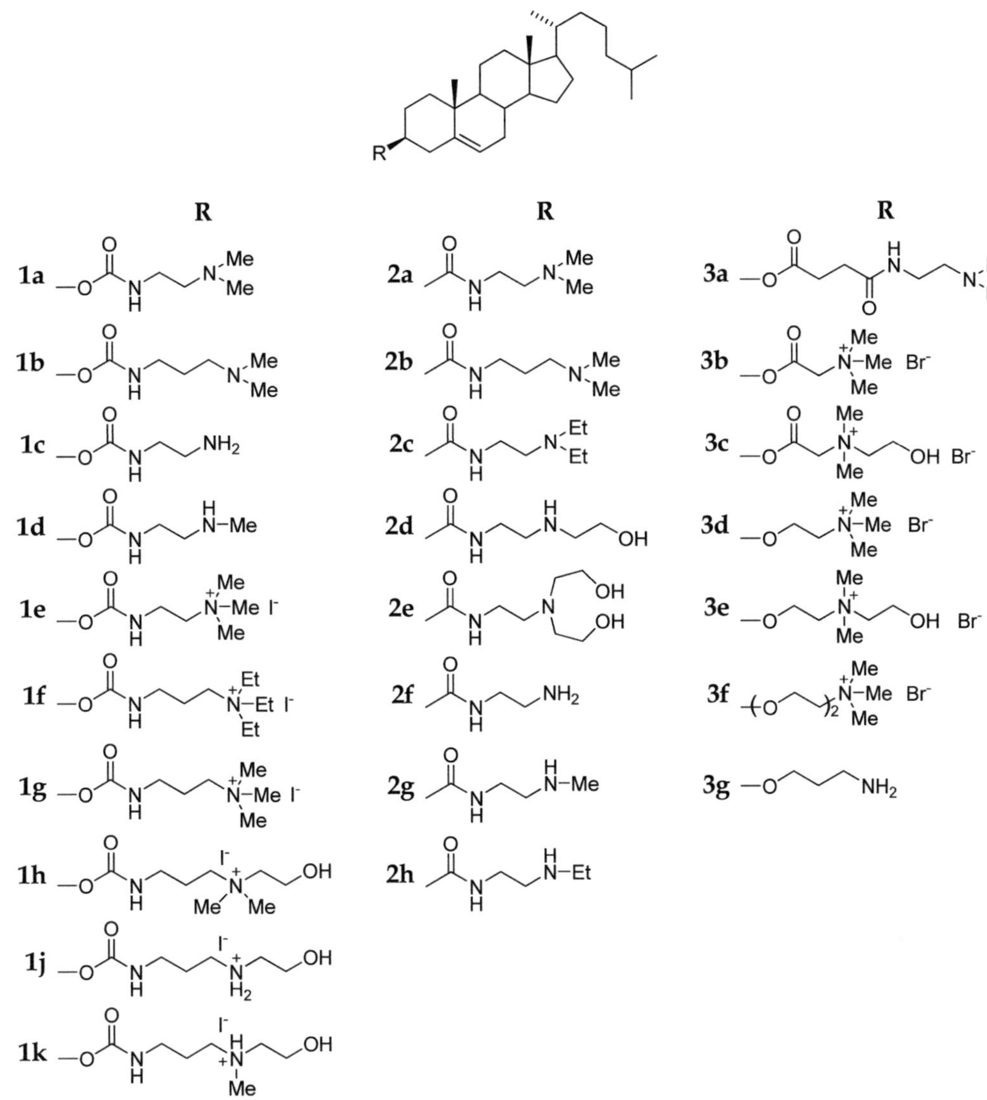

It was found that heterocyclic cationic lipids containing imidazolinium (Solodin et al., 1995) or pyridinium polar heads (Ilies et al., 2006) reveal a higher TE and a reduced level of cytotoxicity in comparison with the classical transfectants. To study the influence of this type of heterocyclic polar head on the TE, the cholesterol-based lipids containing heterocyclic amine connected to the cholesterol residue *via* urethane (**4a-f**, **6a**), ether (**5a-5h**) and ester linkers (**6b-f**) were synthesized (Gao & Hui, 2001; Bajaj et al., 2008c; Medvedeva et al., 2009).

The study of the transfection activity for the lipids **4a-f** revealed that liposomes **4c**/DOPE and **4f**/DOPE displayed the highest TE, which from 3 to 6-fold exceeded the TE of DC-Chol (**1a**)/DOPE and Lipofectamine 2000 (Gao & Hui, 2001). The serum (from 1 to 10%) have no effect on cells transfection mediated by these cationic liposomes at different N/P ratios. It was observed that these liposomes gained a negative charge in the presence of serum. *In* *vivo* DNA delivery (direct administration into the spleen) was efficient at low N/P ratios, but as yet, no reasonable explanation for this occurrence has been found.

Liposomes formed from lipids **5a-g** and DOPE were able to transfect 50-80% of cells, and the TE increased when the N/P ratio increases (Bajaj et al., 2008c). The highest TE was observed for lipid **5f** containing *N,N*-dimethylaminopyridinium headgroup. This lipid transfected cells in the presence of serum without any loss of activity. The experiments with sodium dodecylsulphate (SDS)-induced DNA release from the lipoplexes demonstrated that DNA is released from the complex with liposomes 5f/DOPE in an unhurried manner. This could possibly be a result of a more effective lipid shielding of DNA. This is probably a reason for the high TE displayed by liposomes **5f**/DOPE, even in the presence of the serum.

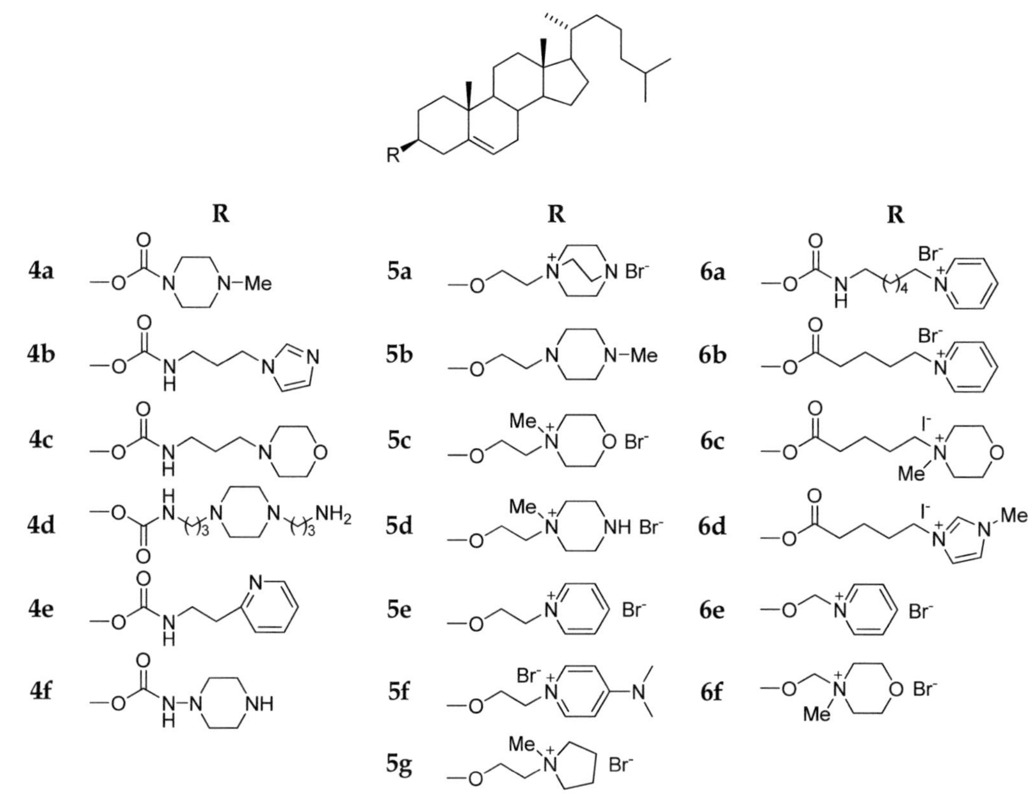

The structure-activity relationships study for the series of lipids **6a-f**, containing different heterocyclic cationic groups and linkers, permitted us to determine that lipids containing pyridinium (**6a,b**) or *N*-methylimidazium (**6d**) heads and ester or urethane linkers are the most promising in terms of transfection (Medvedeva et al., 2009). It was also revealed, that the ability of these lipids to deliver the oligodeoxyribonucleotides and pDNA into cells, correlates positively with their ability to form lipoplexes with the size not exceeding 100 nm. Cholesterol-based lipids containing heterocyclic polar heads linked *via* biodegradable β-glucosyl spacer were prepared (Maslov et al., 2010).

The study of the biological activity of the cationic glycolipids **7a-d** demonstrated that nucleic acids could be efficiently delivered only by means of cationic liposomes; however this was not possible using individual lipids. The delivery of fluorescein-labeled oligonucleotide was comparable for the liposomes **7d**/DOPE and Lipofectamine 2000. In the case of the siRNA delivery, the highest TE was observed for the liposomes **7c**/DOPE and the GFP gene-silencing was observed both in the absence and in the presence of serum in the culture media.

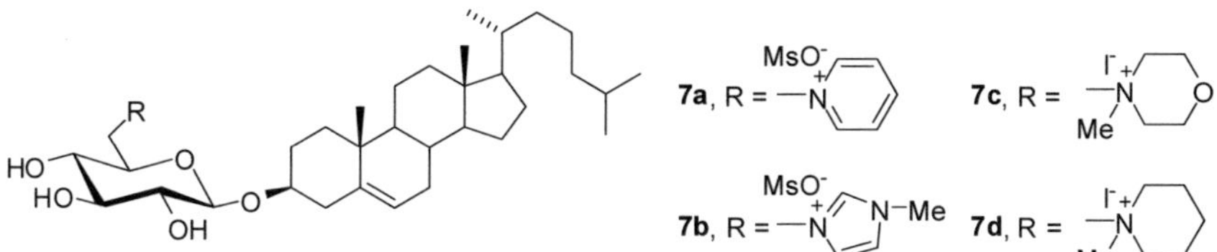

7a-d

2.3 Stimuli-responsive cationic lipids

It was revealed that lipoplexes enter the cells *via* nonspecific endocytosis, which occurs after the electrostatic binding of the positively charged lipoplexes to the negatively charged components of the cell membrane (Rejman, et al., 2006; Belting et al., 2005). There are a number of obstacles, hindering the efficient cationic liposome-mediated gene transfection: DNA release from the endosomes, DNA dissociation from the lipoplexes (Escriou et al., 1998; Rolland, 1998; Zabner et al., 1995) as well as insufficient release of DNA from endosomes. The use of stimuli-responsive delivery systems offers a new opportunity for the improvement of the delivery of nucleic acid (Ganta et al., 2008). Therefore, pH and redox microenvironment can be used as biological stimuli to improve the TE of lipoplexes. To achieve a stimuli-responsive release of DNA it is necessary to design cationic lipids containing trigger-groups, which specifically react to the alteration of the pH value, or to the presence of the intracellular reducing agents.

2.3.1 Redox-responsive disulfide cationic lipids

Thiol-disulfide exchange reactions play an important role in the biological functions of living cells; notably in the stabilization of the protein structure and redox cycles. The strong intracellular reductive micro-environment can stimulate the disintegration of the lipoplexes if these compounds contain the disulfide cationic lipids that are stable outside the cells, but could be reduced in the cells by intracellular reductive agents, *e.g.* glutathione (Tang & Hughes, 1998). The reduction of the disulfide bond will enhance the release of DNA from the DNA-liposomes complexes. Previously, it was demonstrated that the transfection of the plasmid DNA by the glycerolipids containing disulfide bonds was higher compared to the transfection activity of its non-disulfide analogue (Tang & Hughes, 1998).
Lipid **8a** containing cholesterol, was synthesized and its activity to mediate DNA transfer was compared with the activity of both non-disulfide analogue **8b** and DC-Chol (**1a**) (Tang & Hughes, 1999). In the presence of glutathione (10 mM) a 50% DNA release from the complex with liposomes **8a**/DOPE was observed, while the lipoplexes formed by lipid **8b** did not release DNA. The TE for the disulfide lipid **8a** was 100-fold higher, in comparison with the DC-Chol (**1a**) and 7-fold higher when compared to the lipid **8b,** in spite of the fact, that the amount of DNA internalized by cells was lower in the case of **8a**.
Lipids **9a-c** based on thiocholesterol (in the mixture with DOPE) were more active in comparison to PEI and DOTAP/DOPE when transfecting CV-1 cells (Huang et al., 2005).

Nanolipoparticles (NLP) were formed from lipids **9a-c** and PEG was added for the steric stabilization. The treatment of NLP with cysteine or glutathione changed the surface charge of the particles; the modification of the NLP surface with Tat-protein resulted in the increase of the TE of the neutral and negatively charged NLP.

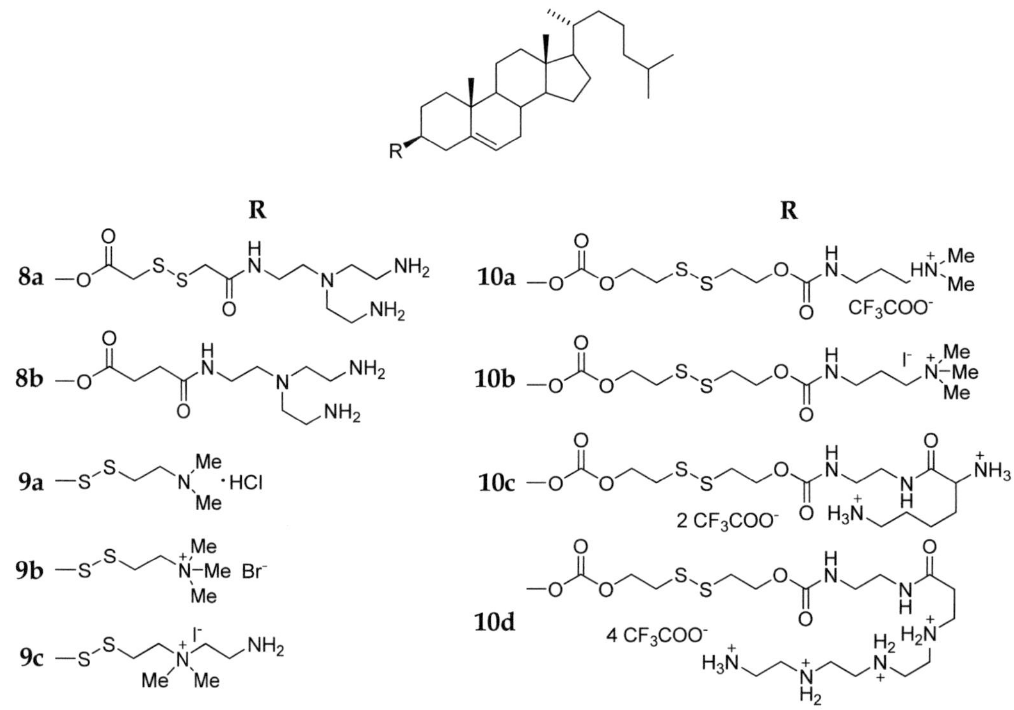

To find new efficient transfectants, the water-soluble low-toxic cholesterol-based lipids **10a-d** were synthesized. The lipids contain the positively-charged headgroups connected to the cholesterol backbone *via* the disulfide and carbonate linkers (Sheng et al., 2011). The atomic force microscopy indicated that mixing the cationic lipids and DNA gave compact, condensed lipoplexes with a size 200-300 nm. The addition of dithiotreitol (10 mM) resulted in the disassembly of these complexes into tiny, irregular-shaped fragments and small sized pieces, confirming the cleavage of disulfide bonds and distortion of the stable lipoplexes. Lipid **10c**, which contained the natural aminoacid lysine, displayed the highest TE in respect to COS-7 cells, both in the presence and absence of serum. The least active was lipid **10b** with the quaternary amino group. It is worthy of note, that lipid **10a** was almost as active as **10c** at low N/P ratio (up to 5). This ratio is characterized by the formation of the small lipoplexes (approximately 250 nm) with the negative ξ-potential.

2.3.2 pH-responsive cationic lipids

It is known that endocytosis is accompanied by a noticeable increase in the environment acidity from the physiological value of pH 7.4 to 6.5–6.0 in endosomes and to 5.0 in primary or secondary lysosomes (Mukherjee et al., 1997). Endocytosed lipoplexes may be digested by acidic hydrolases, active at the acidic pH of the lysosome. In order to protect DNA from such hydrolytic degradation and enhance the release of DNA from endosome pH-sensitive cationic lipids were synthesized (Budker et al., 1996). These lipids contain weakly basic lysosomotropic imidazole head group which acts as a proton sponge, preventing the acidification of endosomal environment and inhibiting the degradative hydrolysis. Another approach to enhance the DNA release is the incorporation of the chemical trigger-bond into lipid that could be hydrolyzed at a specific pH gradient. Therefore, incorporation of acid-labile bonds into the lipid structure favors the lipoplex destabilization and facilitates the DNA release from the endosomal compartment to the cytoplasm, thus improving the transfection efficiency (Boomer et al., 2002; Guo & Szoka, 2003). Furthermore, the use of biodegradable cationic lipids lowers the cytotoxicity of cationic liposomes, making them promising transfection agents.

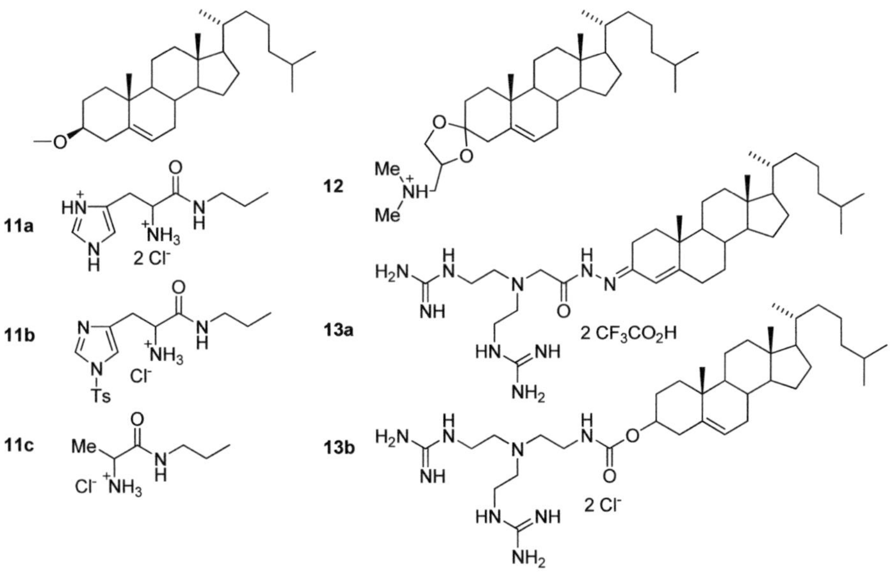

Cholesterol-based, endosomal, pH-sensitive, histidylated, cationic lipid (**11a**), its less pH-sensitive analogue with the electron-deficient head group (**11b**) and cationic lipid, which does not contain histidine headgroup (**11c**) were synthesized (Singh, et al., 2004). Lipid **11b** exhibited lower TE than lipid **11a** in relation to 293T7 cells. The activities of both lipids were inhibited in the presence of Bafilomycin A1, demonstrating the involvement of imidazole ring protonation in the endosomal escape of DNA. However, the TE of histidinylated lipid **11a** did not exceed this value for lipid **11c**. The lipid **12** with an acid-sensitive ketal bond was hydrolyzed in acidic medium where an ether analogue remained undegraded (Zhu, et al., 2002). Lipid (**12**) achieved levels of gene delivery similar to DC-Chol (**1a**), but the toxicity was correspondingly low.

In recent time a new series of cationic steroid derivatives, containing guanidinium headgroup connected with the hydrophobic cholesterol *via* the acid-sensitive acylhydrazone linker have been developed (Aissaoui et al., 2004). The lipid **13a** was found to possess a low cytotoxicity and was able to mediate the efficient gene transfection into various mammalian cell lines *in vitro*. The TE of the lipid **13a** was comparable with TE of its analogue **13b**, which did not contain the acid-labile group. Colloidally stable

13a/DOPE-DNA complexes were prepared and administered *via* nasal instillation into the mouse airways. A significant expression of the reporter protein in the lung homogenates was subsequently detected. It should be noted, the TE in the experimental groups was much higher compared to the control group of mice receiving the identical dose of "naked" DNA.

2.4 Cholesterol gemini-surfactants

Recently, a new class of surfactants was discovered. These so-called 'dimeric' or 'gemini-surfactants' attract a considerable amount of scientific attention as being of particular importance in biology. For instance, the ability to form "bilayer bridges"was demonstrated for some gemini-surfactants containing long hydrophobic spacers (Moss & Li, 1992). The structure of these gemini-surfactants resembles the structure of lipids found in the membrane of the thermophiles archaebacteria. Other gemini-surfactants were specially synthesized for the usage as nucleic acids carriers into the cells (Kirby et al., 2003;) and the effects of the nature of the spacer, hydrocarbon chains, and headgroups on the transfection activity of these compounds were studied in detail.

Dimeric lipids **14a-k**, differing in the length of the spacer and the type of the cationic headgroup, were synthesized, and the transfection activity of these compounds was compared with this parameter for the monomeric lipids **3d** and **3e** (Bajaj et al., 2007a; Biswas et al., 2011). Lipids formed different aggregates, depending on the structure of the cationic head. For instance, individual vesicles with sizes from 20 to 160 nm were formed by the compounds **14a-e**. In turn, for lipids **14f-k** formation of vesicular conglomerates of various lengths composed of the individual vesicles was observed. These conglomerates were formed due to the hydrogen bonding interactions imposed by the 2-hydroxyethylated headgroups of the lipids of each vesicle of geminies **14f-k** (Biswas et al., 2011). The maximal TE was observed for the lipid **14c**, containing pentamethylene spacer, and, on the contrary, lipid **14e** was not active in the absence of serum in the culture media. A different morphology of the lipoplexes formed by these lipids and DNA was subjected to further study. Transmission electron microscopy showed the presence of the aggregates with the size range from 100 to 200 nm for the lipoplexes formed by **14c**, while lipid **14e** was found to form lipoplexes of irregular shapes and sizes.

The replacement of the hydrophobic spacer by hydrophilic one led to the new set of dimeric amphiphils **15a-d** possessing low toxicity. The amphiphiles **15a,b** were able to transfect the cells at the low N/P ratio, as well as in the presence of 30 and 50% serum (Bajaj et al., 2007b).

Due to the fact that lipids with ether bond are poorly degraded in the organism, new disulfide bond containing dimeric lipids **16a-c** were synthesized, able to degrade under the influence of intracellular reducing agents (Bajaj et al., 2008a). These lipids contain flexible hydrophobic and hydrophilic spacers, in addition to rigid hydrophobic spacers. The comparative analysis indicated that the TE of the lipids is decreases in the range **16c** > **16a** > **16b**. Thus, the hydrophilic flexible spacer in the lipid structure is essential for an effective transfection. The serum inhibited the activity of the lipids **16a-c**, as its negatively charged components compete with DNA for the binding to the cationic lipids, which results in the dissociation of the complexes and a decrease of the TE. In recent times, a new method for the synthesis of the dimeric lipids **17a-c** that contain cholesterol and spermine moieties and potentially posses the high TE was described (Petukhov et al., 2010).

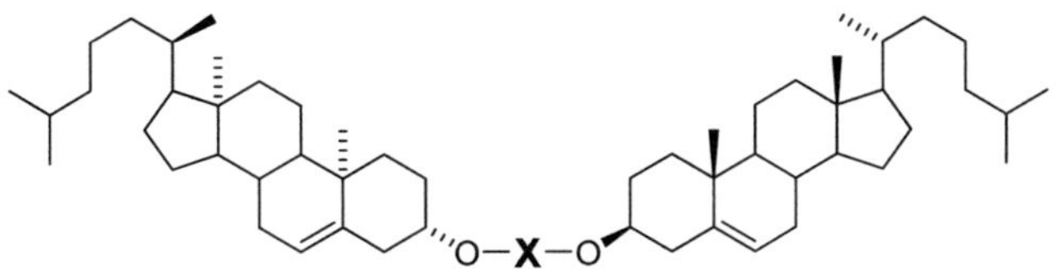

#	n	X
14a	3	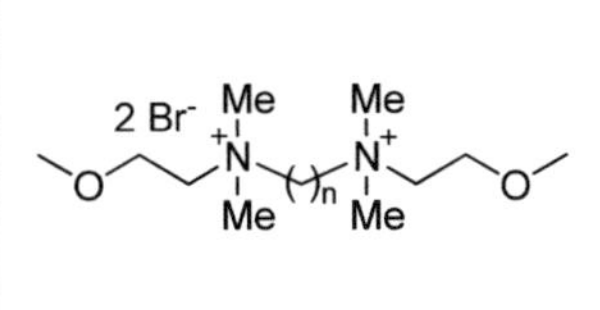
14b	4	
14c	5	
14d	6	
14e	12	
14f	3	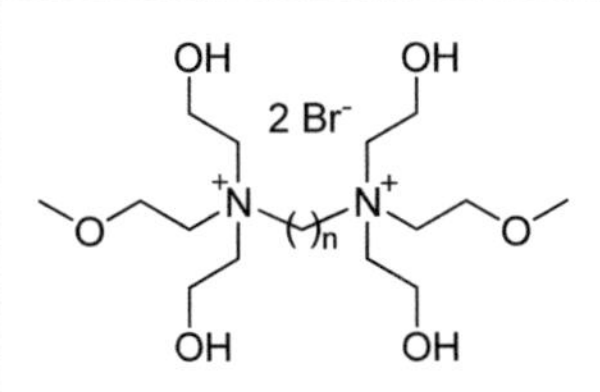
14g	4	
14h	5	
14i	6	
14k	12	

#	n	X
15a	1	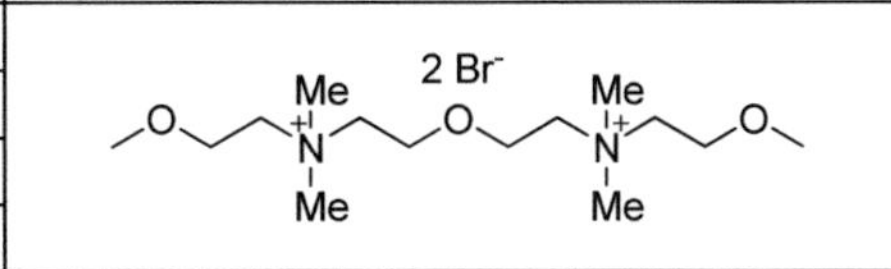
15b	2	
15c	3	
15d	5	
16a		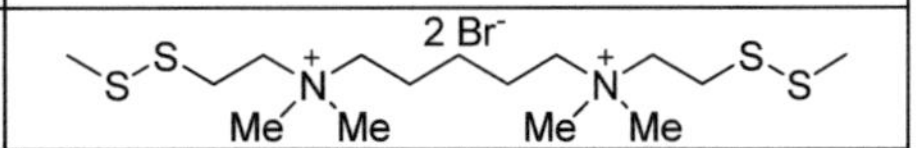
16b		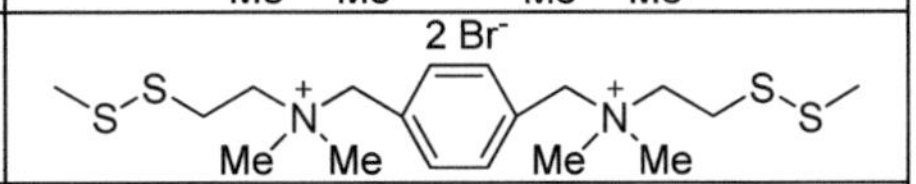
16c		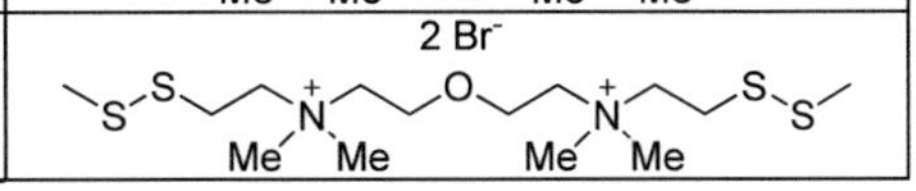

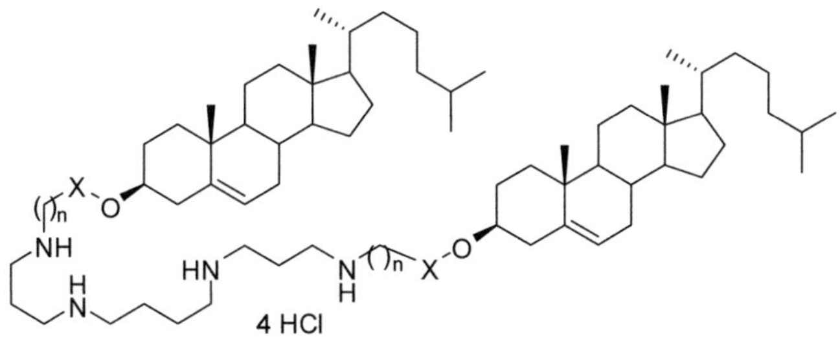

17a, X = C(O), n = 4
17b, X = C(O)NH, n = 4
17c, X = C(O)NH, n = 6

2.5 Polycationic lipids

Polycationic lipids contain a polar head that bears either several or multiple positive charges increasing their affinity to nucleic acids. Polyamines were successfully used as a component of polycationic lipids (Geall et al., 2000; Blagbrough et al., 2003; 2004; Oliver et al., 2004). Polyamines are a class of naturally occurring compounds that display excellent nucleic acid binding and condensing properties. It is well known that the overall positive charge of the lipoplexes is important for initiating cell entry and release of the complexed nucleic acid into the cell cytoplasm. Although the exact mechanism by which polycationic lipids mediate transfection requires more detailed investigation evidence in literature points towards the notion that the success of these reagents arises from a couple of factors: the abnormally low pKa's (pKa <7) of the polyamines, a direct result of the number of amino groups present and the methylene spacings between them (Stewart et al., 2001; Keller et al., 2003; Geall et al., 1999; 2000).

The effects of the regiochemical distribution of positive charges along the polyamine moiety in DNA condensing agents were studied (Geall et al., 2000). DNA condensation is dependent upon the number of positive charges, the regiochemical distribution of charges of polyamines (determined by the p*Ka* of each amino group), and the local salt concentration. A series of polyamine carbamates of cholesterol was prepared where both the charge and its regiochemical distribution have been varied along the polyamine moiety (**18a-f**) (Geall et al., 1999). Lipids **18a-f** were tested for transfection competence at three different N/P ratios (0.5:1, 1:1, 4:1), calculated taking into account the average charge per molecule at pH 7.4. It was found that the spermine based lipid **18a**, incorporating 3-4-3 methylene spacing along the polyamine moiety, has the highest TE, while lipid **18f** display the lowest TE. Geall and co-workers supposed that the four methylene spacing found in spermine, could have significant implications for DNA polyamine association and lipoplex formation.

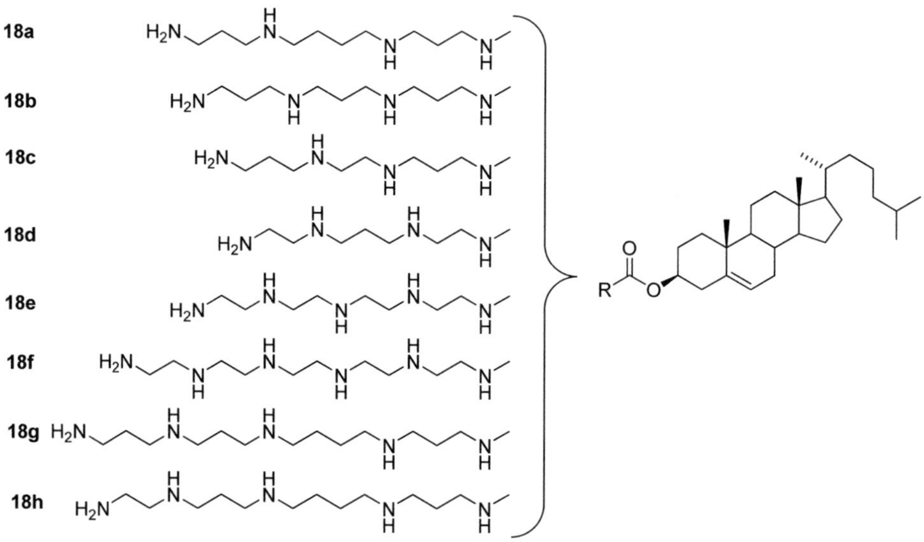

Recently second generation cationic liposomal systems that were formulated from polyamine analogues of DC-Chol and DOPE have been described (CDAN (**18d**), CDAD (**18a**), CTAP (**18g**), CTAH (**18h**)) (Cooper et al., 1998). Among the liposomal formulation tested the formulation from the novel pentaamine amphiphile CTAP (**18g**) and DOPE were shown to be approximately 400 times more efficient at mediating gene delivery to a mouse lung *in vivo* than DC-Chol/DOPE liposomes. CDAN (**18d**) is another cholesterol-based polyamine lipid with an unnaturally occurring 2–3–2 methylene spacing, which, in combination with DOPE forms an exceptionally effective transfection agent. Biophysical analyses show that CTAP/DOPE liposomes are effective *in vivo* because these liposomes are able to efficiently neutralise, condense and encapsulate nucleic acids into lipoplex particles and the unprotonated amine groups (p*K***a** < 8) presented in the polyamine at neutral pH that could have the capacity for endosome buffering, thereby facilitating nucleic acid escape from endosomes into the cytosol, like polyethylenimine (Stewart et al., 2001).
Recently a new solid-phase strategy to synthesize a library of cholesterol-based polyamine lipids in excellent yields (>87%) and purity was set forth (Oliver et al., 2004). The strategy employs 2-chlorotrityl chloride resin as a solid support and protecting group for one primary amine on the starting material, utilizing the high selectivity of 2-acetyldimedone as a protecting group for the second primary amine (Oliver et al., 2004).
Cationic liposomes CDAN (**18d**)/DOPE were tested as delivery systems for siRNAs (Spagnou et al., 2004). The results show that CDAN and DOPE with and without siRNA

confer low toxicity to mammalian cells. CDAN/DOPE-siRNA complexes exhibited a slower cellular uptake than Lipofectamine2000 based formulations. Intracellularly CDAN/DOPE-siRNA complexes appear to behave in a different fashion, accumulating in distinct but diffuse small non-lysosomal compartments for at least 5 h after transfection (Spagnou et al., 2004).

Recently, a new hepatotropic nontoxic lipid-based vector system for delivering chemically unmodified siRNA to the liver to inhibit Hepatitis B virus (HBV) propagation was described (Carmona et al., 2008). These anti-HBV formulations were created based on synthetic, self-assembly ABCD nanoparticle paradigm (Kostarelos & Miller, 2005). ABCD nanoparticles comprising nucleic acids, such as plasmid DNA (pDNA) or siRNA (A component) which are condensed with cationic liposomes (B component) to form AB core nanoparticles. An important feature of the assembly is the incorporation of an aminoxy cholesteryl lipid into these AB core nanoparticles in order to enable the quantitative chemoselective post-coupling of biocompatibility polymers (C component) and optional tissue-targeting ligands (D component) to the core nanoparticles. (Carmona et al., 2008). AB nanoparticles (70-80 nm in diameter) were initially formulated in an aqueous solution by mixing of siRNAs with cationic liposomes CDAN (**18d**)/DOPE/**19a** (40:50:10 molar ratio) or CDAN/DOPE/**19b** (40:50:10 molar ratio).

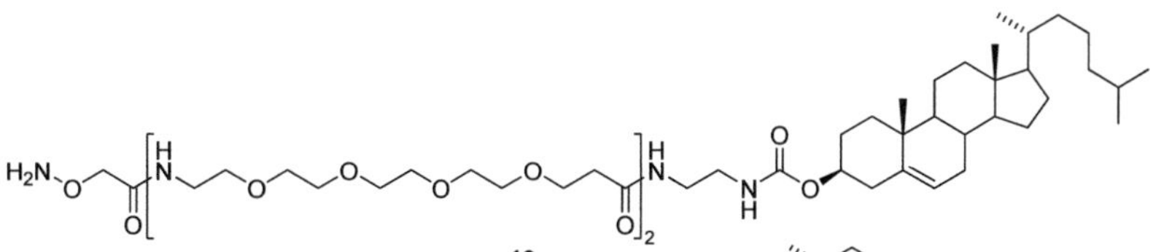

19a

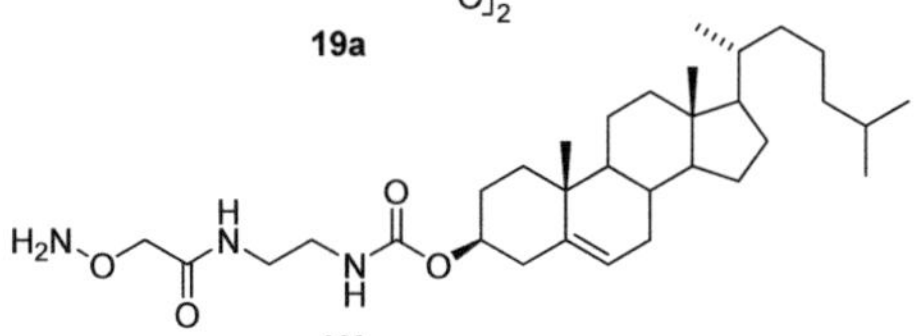

19b

Polyethylene glycol^{2000}-dialdehyde (C component), was coupled to AB particles under aqueous acidic conditions (pH 4). This surface post coupling was facilitated by a rapid, quantitative chemoselective aminoxy-aldehyde conjugation between the aminoxy functional group of aminoxy cholesteryl lipid and of the aldehyde functional groups of the C-component. The resulting oxime linkages are robust at pH 7; however at a level of pH 5.5 and below, they are prone to decomposition. The developed vectors administered intravenously, efficiently deliver unmodified siRNAs to murine livers leading to the strong suppression of HBV replication (Carmona et al., 2008).

The conjugates of guanidinium and cholesterol were synthesized with the yields of up to 61%, with the purpose of further improving the polar domain of cationic lipids (Vigneron et al., 1996). The guanidinium group can form with phosphate anions characteristic pairs stabilized by parallel zwitterionic hydrogen bonds. Moreover, the guanidinium group is also able to develop hydrogen bonding with nucleic bases, especially with guanine. The tertiary amine of compound **13b**, which is situated between two positive guanidinium groups and has probably a lower pKa, could also be able to buffer the acidic environment of late endosomes and of lysosomes, hence protecting the DNA against degradation. The lipid **13b** can be used *in vitro* without DOPE, and this permits the avoidance of the liposomes preparation step. Commonly used for the transfection **13b**-DNA complexes were found to form ordered aggregates characterized by a fingerprint-like structures, but not the concentric multilamellar vesicles demonstrated for the **13b**/DOPE–DNA complexes (Pitard et al., 1999).

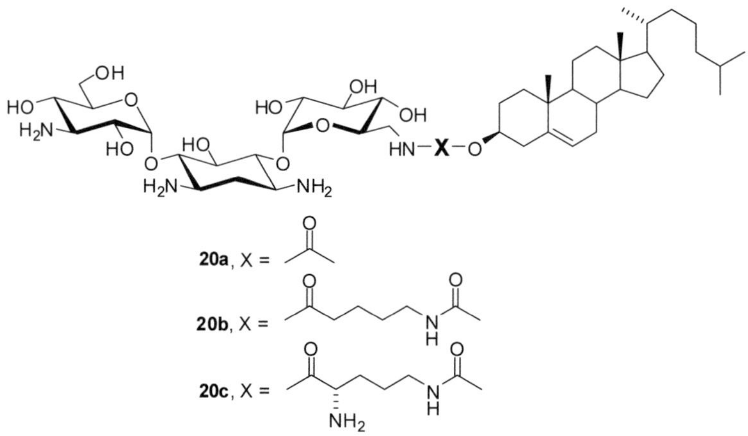

The analysis of transfection of a wide range of cell lines with **13b**/DOPE-DNA complexes revealed the high efficiency of this process, which is comparable with the commercially available transfectants and 10–20-fold exceeds the calcium phosphate precipitation protocol (Vigneron et al., 1996; Ouderhiri et al., 1997). Mediated by guanidinium-cholesterol lipids gene transfection is appropriate for the mammalian airway epithelium (Ouderhiri et al., 1997). The positive results of the transfection into primary human cells *in vitro* and into the mouse airways cells *in vivo* confirm the potential of the cationic lipids in relation to lung-directed gene therapy.

Aminoglycosides, natural polyamines that are known to bind to nucleic acids, represent a favorable scaffold for the synthesis of a variety of cationic lipids. The synthesis of a cationic cholesterol derivative of kanamycin A and its polyguanidinylated derivative was recently described (Belmont et al., 2002). The amino-sugar-based cationic lipid **20a** demonstrated a high level of TE in terms of gene transfection of a variety of mammalian cell lines when used either alone or as a part of a liposomal formulation with helper-lipid. In addition, colloidally stable kanamycin-cholesterol/DOPE lipoplexes were found to be efficient for gene transfection into the mouse airways *in vivo*.

Designed cholesterol-based kanamycin A analogues (**20b,c**) bearing various linkers between the aminoglycoside headgroup and the cholesterol moiety were prepared (Sainlos et al., 2005). It was successfully shown, that the length and nature of the spacer can affect the physicochemical and biological properties of the lipoplexes. The incorporation of a longer spacer into the structures of cholesterol derivatives of kanamycin A can yield the lipoplexes with improved in terms of TE physicochemical properties. The cholesterol derivatives **20b,c** were successfully used for the transfection of mouse airway epithelium *in vivo*. But the beneficial effects of the longer spacers observed *in vitro* with **20b,c** were not found *in vivo*, as only **20c** yielded levels of transgene expression higher than those obtained with **20a**.

2.6 Colesterol-PEI conjugates

Polyethyleneimine (PEI) is polycation widely used for DNA compaction and delivery. The high transfection efficiency of PEI was firstly demonstrated by Behr and co-workers (Boussif et al., 1995). PEI is well-known for its ability to compact DNA and to facilitate its early endosomal release, preventing the delivered DNA from degradation in the late endosomes (Kichler, 2004). The reason for the good transfection activity of PEI is the presence of the primary, secondary, and tertiary amino groups. These groups have different p*K*a values, which give the PEI a good buffer capacity, therefore not allowing a decrease in the pH value in the early endosomes (Kichler, 2004).

In literature several kinds of the PEI-cholesterol conjugates have been described. Kim and co-workers (Han et al., 2001) synthesized water-soluble lipopolymer (WLSP (**21a**)) in the reaction of the branched PEI (mw 1.8 kDa) and cholesteryl chloroformate. The average molecular weight of WSLP (**21a**) was approximately 2 kDa and the extent of modification with cholesterol was ~ 0.5. The WSLP (**21a**)-pDNA complexes were characterized by low toxicity *in vitro* and they induced the aggregation of erythrocytes to a lesser extent, as compared to PEI 25 kDa. WSLP (**21a**)-pDNA complexes demonstrated higher TE in both CT-26 and 293 T cells compared to PEI 25 kDa- or PEI 1.8 kDa-based formulations. As an experimental model for the estimation *in vivo* of the biological activity the authors used the antitumor activity of IL-12 coded by the pDNA transfected into the tumor cells. As a result of the injections of the WSLP (**21a**)-pDNA complexes into mice tumors a significant decrease in the tumor growth rate (~20% higher, as compared to the administration of the *naked DNA*) and of the level of metastasis formation were observed; resulting in higher survival rates of the animals after treatment (Mahato et al., 2001; Janat-Amsbury et al., 2005). Later data confirming the high efficacy of WSLP (**21a**) for the transfection of siRNA *in vitro* and *in vivo* were obtained (Kim et al., 2007).

The same authors endeavored to design a more effective transfection reagent based on branched PEI (bPEI) using chemically protected primary amine and conjugation of cholesterol at the secondary amino groups of PEI. However, contrary to expectations, the presence of the non-modified primary amino groups only resulted in a slight increase (1.5-fold) of the TE (Wang et al., 2002).

Kim and co-workers obtained partially contradictory data (Kim et al 2001). In this work a simple one-step synthetic procedure was used to yield myristyl and cholesterol derivatives of PEI having molecular mass 2 kDa. According to the obtained data these modified PEI efficiently transfected cell *in vitro* and displayed lower toxicity when compared to bPEI 2 kDa; however the compounds were less tolerated by cells than the parent bPEI 2 kDa.

Fewell and co-workers studied the properties of the PPC conjugates, containing the bPEI 1.8 kDa, cholesterol and PEG, where the PEGylation extent varied from 0.6 to 20 PEG molecules to one bPEI molecule (Fewell et al., 2005). The highest transfection efficiency *in vivo* was observed for the PPC conjugate, where the molar ratio bPEI:cholesterol:PEG was 1:1:2. When using the conjugates containing a large quantity of PEG molecules, a decrease of the reporter gene expression was observed. The variation of the number of the cholesterol residues in the conjugates was not performed: all the tested conjugates contained the bPEI and cholesterol at the ratio of 1:1. In order to study the TE of these molecules *in vivo* the authors used a biological model similar to the one described in (Mahato et al., 2001) and also demonstrated the efficient inhibition of the tumor growth.

Furgeson and co-workers also used linear PEI for the synthesis of new cholesterol-containing conjugates apart from bPEI. The polymer, obtained in the reaction of a low molecular weight lPEI (423 Da) with cholesterol chloroformate, was used for the preparation of the water insoluble liponanoparticles using DOPE as a lipid-helper (Furgeson et al., 2002). The *in vitro* TE of nanoparticle-pDNA complexes was ~4-fold higher, in comparison with bPEI 25 kDa.

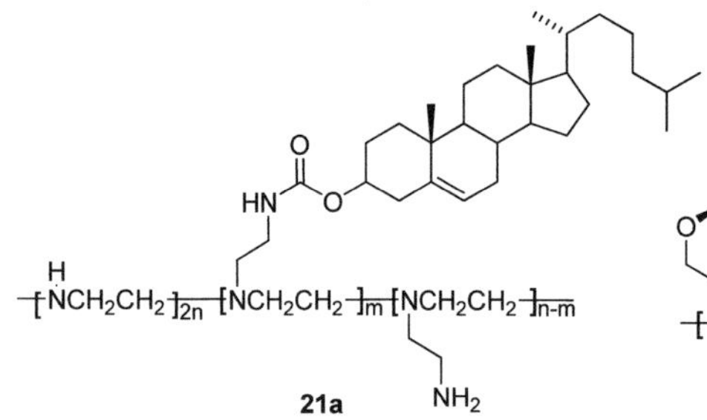

21a

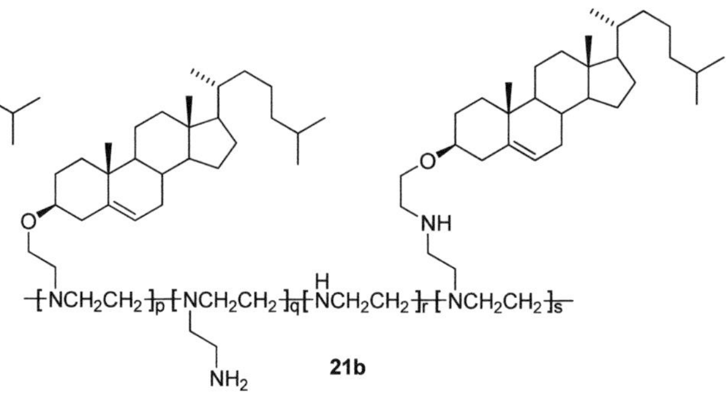

21b

T-shaped and L- (linear) shaped PEI 25 kDa conjugates with cholesterol (PEIC) were synthesized and thoroughly studied, revealing the improved transfection and reduced cytotoxic effect, partially a result of the sequestering of charged secondary amines of PEI, in the presence of cholesterol moiety (Furgeson et al., 2003). The modification extent of the PEI carrier in this study ranged from 1 to 2 cholesterol molecules per PEI. Polyplexes, formed by L- and T shapes PEICs with DNA possessed a higher TE *in vitro*, in comparison with the initial linear polymer; as well as the bPEI with the same molecular weight. The highest TE among the compounds tested was observed for L-PEIC: the expression of the reporter gene, delivered into the Renca cells using this conjugate was 32-fold higher in comparison with the expression observed in the presence of bPEI. The authors proposed that the differences in the TE depended on the conformational changes of the PEI molecule in the presence of the hydrophobic substitues. It was shown that the PEIC conjugates penetrated into the cells *via* the interaction with LDL receptors. The high TE of the LPC was confirmed *in vivo* in experiments with systemic and local administration of the polyplexes (Furgeson et al., 2004)
Multiple modifications of PEI's amines were commonly avoided, due to the importance of the cationic charge for DNA condensation and buffering capacity of the polymer. Therefore quantitative data characterizing the impact of cholesterol conjugation was not yet available. In connection with this, we attempted to find the optimal extent of modification of the 25 kDa PEI with cholesterol. Conjugates of PEI bearing a different number of cholesterol residues with 0.5 to 20% of amines modified were synthesized. We found that a small number of cholesterols attached to PEI (extent of modification was 0.5 or 1%) significantly increased the TE of the polymer, while extensively modified PEI-cholesterol conjugates demonstrated reduced TE, although possessing lower cytotoxicity (Gusachenko (Simonova) et al, 2009). TE studies were performed using different types of biologically active nucleic acids: single stranded oligonucleotide, plasmid DNA and siRNA duplex. The most promising conjugates in the series were found to be PEIC 0.5 and PEIC 1 demonstrating the best combination of TE with lower cytotoxicity.
The aforementioned PEI-cholesterol conjugates were prepared in the reaction of PEI, having various molecular weights and cholesteryl chloroformate. The PEI-lipid conjugates (**21b**) based on ether-linked cholesterol units were first described by Bhattacharya and co-workers (Bajaj et al., 2008b). Nine PEI-cholesterol-based conjugates having polymer amine backbone linked to the cholesterol unit via the ether link were synthesized. Three low molecular weight PEIs were used for the synthesis of these lipopolymers. The TE studies in HeLa cells showed a high potency and low cytotoxicity of these lipopolymers in comparison with the commercially available PEI. The TE of PEI 25 kDA decreased in the presence of a high percentage of serum, whereas PEI-cholesterol-based lipopolymers were discovered to be

effective, even in the presence of 50% of serum. The TE and cytotoxicity of the lipopolymers were found to depend on the percentage of cholesterol moieties and the molecular weight of PEI used for the synthesis of lipopolymers. Optimized lipopolymer-DOPE formulations exhibited a higher cell viability and high TE, which was unaffected by serum: the TE of the lipopolymers was obviously one of the highest among known non-viral delivery systems.

3. Physico-chemical properties of lipoplexes and their influence on the transfection efficiency

It is commonly known, that the efficiency of liposome-mediated gene delivery is determined not only by the structure of cationic and helper lipids or properties of the transfected plasmids, but also by the size of the lipoplex and its ζ-potential. The structure of the supramolecular DNA–lipid complexes is dependent upon both the external (pH, degree of hydration, temperature, and the presence of doubly charged cations, i.e., Ca^{2+}, Mg^{2+}) and internal factors. The physico-chemical properties can alter the lifetime, distribution, and the TE efficacy of lipoplexes. Thus, in order to shed more light on the mechanism of transfection and to elucidate the structure-activity relationships, it is necessary to investigate a number of physico-chemical parameters of the lipoplexes.

Using a set of physico-chemical methods, it was demonstrated that condensation and compactization of DNA by DC-Chol (**1a**)/DOPE cationic liposomes is a result of a strong entropically-driven surface electrostatic interactions. Fluorescence anisotropy results have revealed that low cationic lipid contents in the liposomes tend to favor more fluid bilayers; which in turn are potential advantages for transfecting cells. DC-Chol/DOPE-DNA lipoplexes are represented by supramolecular complexes with a different morphology: DNA-coated unilamellar lipoplexes, lipoplex nanostructures with thickened, flattened, and deformed walls, and also multilamellar lipoplexes with or without open bilayers (Rodriguez-Pulido et al., 2008). The effects of hydration and temperature on the structure of DC-Chol/DOPE–DNA lamellar lipoplexes were also investigated (Pozzi et al., 2006). The DNA complexation and condensation properties of two established cationic liposome formulations, CDAN (**18d**)/DOPE (50:50, *m*/*m*; Trojene™) and DC-Chol (**1a**)/DOPE (60:40, *m*/*m*), were studied by means of biophysical methods (Keller et al., 2003). The results provide a suitable framework for the understanding of why CDAN/DOPE cationic liposomes are exceptionally efficient, in comparison with other cationic lipid-based systems, at mediating cell transfection. The liposomes CDAN (**18d**)/DOPE formed the metastable lipoplexes, exhibiting greater transfection efficiency *in vitro* in the presence of 10% serum, in comparison to DC-Chol/DOPE liposomes. This metastability may be related to the unusually low p*K*a value of 5.7 of amino groups. In addition, it was supposed that CDAN (**18d**)/DOPE-pDNA particles may have a greater tendency to interact with negatively charged serum components and facilitate the DNA release from endosomes (Keller et al., 2003).

A critical factor in the lipid-mediated gene delivery is the structural and phase evolution of lipoplexes upon interaction and mixing with anionic cellular lipids (Tarahovsky et al., 2004; Koynova et al., 2005, 2006; Koynova & MacDonald, 2007). Such a structural rearrangement is supposed to play a central role in the DNA escape process; i.e. how DNA dissociates from lipoplexes and is released into the cytoplasm. The structural and phase evolution of lipoplexes upon interaction with lipid mixtures similar to real membranes and DNA release were investigated using liposomal formulations DC-Chol/DOPE, DC-Chol/DMPC, DOTAP/DOPC, DOTAP-DLPC, DOTAP/DOPE, prepared at different molar ratia. (Pozzi et al., 2009). It was shown that the most unstable lipoplexes (DOTAP/DOPC/DNA) rapidly release DNA, while the most stable ones (DC-Chol/DOPE/DNA) exhibit a lower degree of DNA release. Therefore, the results can be generalized as follows: the higher the structural stability, the lower the extent of DNA release. Using the SAXS technique it was demonstrated that the dilution of the DNA lattice takes place upon lipoplex interaction with anionic lipids, which is unequivocal proof of the charge neutralization of cationic lipids by anionic membranes (Banchelli et al., 2008; Lundqvist et al., 2008). Upon further interaction, disintegration of lipoplexes by anionic lipids as well as the formation of nonlamellar phases in lipoplex/anionic lipids mixtures are strongly affected by the shape coupling between lipoplexes and anionic lipids. Furthermore, coupling between the membrane charge densities of lipoplexes and anionic membranes contributes greatly to regulating the evolution of lipoplexes/anionic lipids mixtures and the release of plasmid DNA (Pozzi et al., 2009).

3.1 Influence of size

The data found in literature, describing the influence of the size of lipoplexes on the TE are contradictory. A number of researchers have argued that either size of the formed lipoplexes is not associated with TE, or that TE is not affected by initial lipoplex size (Han et al., 2008; Kearns et al., 2008; Malaekeh-Nikouei et al., 2009). Some researchers posit that large lipoplexes possess higher TE in comparison to the smaller ones. For instance, Ross et al. demonstrated that TE and cell uptake increased with the increase of the size of lipoplexes (Ross & Hui, 1999). The study of the CDAN(**18d**)/DOPE liposomes demonstrated the ability of the liposomes to form large complexes with plasmid DNA, which are characterized by the tendency for the sedimentation on the cell surface resulting in the increase of the TE (Keller et al., 2003). When siRNA was used as cargo for delivery into cells, the lipoplexes with a size between 60 and 400 nm were obtained and no influence of the lipoplex size on the efficacy of gene knockdown was observed (Spagnou et al., 2004). It was previously reported by Kawaura et al. that vesicles of a moderate size (0.4-1.4 micron) exhibit higher TE in terms of gene delivery (Kawaura et al., 1998). The data supporting the higher TE of the large lipoplexes were also reported by other researchers (Ding et al., 2008).

When the formation of complexes has been performed in physiological ionic strength conditions, compared with 40 mM Tris buffer, the size of lipoplexes can be significantly increased (Kearns et al., 2008). In contrast, the presence of serum could slightly decrease the size of the lipoplexes (Han et al., 2008).

Conversely, some researchers have demonstrated that smaller lipoplexes were more efficient (Salvati et al., 2006). We studied the correlation between the size of the cationic lipids **6a-f**/nucleic acid complexes and their TE (Medvedeva, et al., 2009). The ability of the cationic lipids to deliver plasmid DNA is dependent upon the size of the lipids/DNA complexes formed in solution, which is consistent with that the maximum endocytosis by non-specialized cells requires that the particle size is below 100 nm (Chen et al., 2007). The lipid **6a** formed the smallest complexes with the plasmid DNA, characterized by a narrow size distribution; this lipid exhibited the highest TE. The lipids **6b** and **6d** formed with plasmid DNA the complexes with a wide size distribution and a large fraction of small particles inferior to 50 nm; these lipids display moderate TE. A reduction in the size of liposomes, might facilitate their penetration through the physiological barriers, after the administration *in vivo*, in addition to the possibility of passively targeting the tumor sites, which is facilitated by the enhanced permeability of blood vessels and retention (EPR) effect (Gullotti & Yeo, 2009).

It was demonstrated that the size of latex particles has a significant effect upon the efficiency of cell uptake and the mode of the endocytic pathway (Rejman et al., 2004). Particles that have a size of 500 nm penetrated into the cell via the caveolae-mediated endocytosis. On the contrary, the microspheres having a diameter of 200 nm or less and preferred the clathrin-mediated endocytosis, were found to accumulate in the lysosomal compartment. The precise control of the size of lipoplexes is important for further intracellular fate of lipoplexes that determine by-turn their transfection efficiencies (Rejman et al., 2006).

3.2 Influence of surface charge

The colloidal stability of the lipoplexes is determined by the surface charged of the particles, which can be expressed as zeta potential (ξ-potential). The value of ξ-potential can be changed from negative to positive depending on the N/P ratio (ratio describing the number of the negatively-charged phosphate groups of the nucleic acid to the positively charged groups of the amphiphile). N/P ration contributes significantly to the delivery of nucleic acids into cells. The complexes having a neutral charge are usually characterized by a large size and a low TE, as a result of a tendency to form aggregates and to precipitate (Salvati et al., 2006). A small redundant positive charge of the lipoplexes facilitates the efficient interaction with the negatively charged components of the cell membrane, as well as the transport *via* the cell membrane.

A direct correlation was observed between the value of ξ-potential and TE, when studying the transfection in vitro. It was demonstrated that the cationic liposomes formed by lipid **2a** had the highest ζ-potential in comparison with liposomes formed by lipids **1a,b, 2b,c** and **3a,** and exhibited the highest TE with respect to HeLa, COS-7, and NIH 3T3 cells (Takeuchi et al., 1996). However the dependence of the structure of the lipid, ξ-potential and the TE was not always obvious (Kearns et al., 2008; Malaekeh-Nikouei et al., 2009).

3.3 Influence of physico-chemical parameters on the TE *in vivo*

The low transfection efficiency *in vivo* is one of factors that hinders the design of an efficient liposomal gene delivery systems. Negatively charged components of serum could interact with cationic liposome and compete with DNA for cationic liposome binding, leading to a decrease in TE. Other destructive effects of serum components attributed to its interaction with lipoplexes and early release of DNA from lipid shielding bilayer that reduces the TE. Moreover, the released nucleic acids could be recognized by Toll-like receptor expressed in B cells and dendritic cells; resulting in toxicity *via* induction of the cytokine production (Tousignant et al., 2000). Lipoplexes were reported to be generally more than 100 nm in diameter, as well as tend to self-aggregate in the blood stream, which resulting in limited passage through the vessel walls (Pouton & Seymour, 2001).

The difference between the optimal transfection parameters of *in vitro* and *in vivo* due to the profound difference of the biochemical characteristics between the cells and the organism, is the most severe problem associated with the use and practical implementation of cationic lipid or liposomes for the treatment of genetic and acquired diseases. In the case of monocationic lipids there is a single reference that the *in vivo* result corresponded to the *in vitro* one (Ding et al., 2008) and positively charged lipoplexes are significantly more effective than negatively charged ones. Other investigations revealed that the best TE *in vivo* corresponds to a low N/P ratio, small size of lipoplexes, and negative ξ-potential (Hattori et al., 2007; Gao & Hui, 2001). It is noteworthy when considering polycationic lipids, that lipoplexes that have a total negative charge and small size (200–300 nm) are optimal for both *in vitro* and *in vivo* transfection. (Stewart et al., 2001).

It was revealed that the efficient gene delivery by polycationic lipids (Cooper et al., 1998) *in vivo* requires the cationic liposome systems, which are able to bind DNA more tightly than for the *in vitro* delivery. In comparison to CDAN(**18d**)/DOPE and DC-Chol(**1a**)/DOPE liposomes, CTAP(**18g**)/DOPE was able to neutralize, condense and encapsulate nucleic acids into lipoplex particles with a high efficiency. SDS stimulated the DNA release from a lipoplex and revealed the structure-activity relationships between the TE and lipid shielding of DNA (Bajaj et al., 2008c). Low shielding could facilitate the release of DNA and its hydrolysis within the cells. Certainly, this characteristic could be expected to be useful *in vivo,* given the greater complexity of the extracellular environment *in vivo* as compared to *in vitro*. Caminiti and co-workers demonstrated that both unstable and lipoplexes that are too stable, result in a strong and poor DNA release respectively, and exhibit a low transfection efficiency (Caracciolo et al., 2007).

4. Acknowledgment

This research was supported by the Russian Academy of Science under the program "Molecular and Cell Biology"; The Russian Foundation for Basic Research (grants nos. 08-04-00753 and 09-03-00874), The Ministry of Science and Education (state contract P438 and P715).

5. References

Aissaoui, A., Martin, B., Kan, E., Oudrhiri, N., Hauchecorne, M., Vigneron, J.-P., Lehn, J.-M., Lehn, P. (2004) Novel cationic lipids incorporating an acid-sensitive acylhydrazone linker: synthesis and transfection properties. *J. Med. Chem.,* Vol. 47, No. 21, (October 2004), pp. 5210-5223, ISSN: 0022-2623

Ajmani, P.S., Hughes, J.A. (1999) [N-(N', N'-Dimethylaminoethane)-carbamoyl] cholesterol (DC-Chol)-mediated gene delivery to primary rat neurons: characterization and mechanism. *Neurochemical Research,* Vol. 24, No. 5, (November 1999), pp. 699-703, ISSN: 0364-3190

Bajaj, A., Kondaiah, P., Bhattacharya, S. (2007a) Design, synthesis, and in vitro gene delivery efficacies of novel cholesterol-based gemini cationic lipids and their serum compatibility: a structure-activity investigation. *J. Med. Chem.,* Vol. 50, No. 10, (May 2007), pp. 2432-2442, ISSN: 0022-2623

Bajaj, A., Kondaiah, P., Bhattacharya, S. (2007b) Synthesis and gene transfer activities of novel serum compatible cholesterol-based gemini lipids possessing oxyethylene-type spacers. *Bioconjugate Chem.,* Vol. 18, No. 5, (March 2007), pp. 1537-1546, ISSN: 1043-1802

Bajaj, A., Kondaiah, P., Bhattacharya, S. (2008a) Effect of the nature of the spacer on gene transfer efficacies of novel thiocholesterol derived gemini lipids in different cell lines: a structure–activity investigation. *J. Med. Chem.*, Vol. 51, No. 8, (April 2008), pp. 2533–2540, ISSN: 0022-2623

Bajaj, A., Kondaiah, P., Bhattacharya, S. (2008b) Synthesis and gene transfection efficacies of PEI-cholesterol-based lipopolymers. *Bioconjugate Chem.*, Vol. 19, No. 8, (July 2008), pp. 1640–1651, ISSN: 1043-1802

Bajaj, A., Mishra, S.K., Kondaiah, P., Bhattacharya, S. (2008c) Effect of the headgroup variation on the gene transfer properties of cholesterol based cationic lipids possessing ether linkage. *Biochimica et Biophysica Acta,* Vol. 1778, No. 5, (December 2008), pp. 1222–1236, ISSN: 0006-3002

Banchelli, M., Betti, F., Berti, D., Caminati, G., Bombelli, F.B., Brown, T., Wilhelmsson, L.M., Norden, B., Baglioni, P. (2008) Phospholipid membranes decorated by cholesterol-based oligonucleotides as soft hybrid nanostructures. *J. Phys. Chem., B.,* Vol. 112, No. 35, (August 2008), pp. 10942–10952, ISSN: 1520-6106

Belmont, P., Aissaoui, A., Hauchecorne, M., Oudrhiri, N., Petit, L., Vigneron, J.P., Lehn, J.M., Lehn, P. (2002) Aminoglycoside-derived cationic lipids as efficient vectors for gene transfection in vitro and in vivo. *J Gene Med.,* Vol. 4, No. 5, (September-October 2002), pp. 517–526, ISSN: 15212254

Belting, M., Sandgren, S., Wittrup, A. (2005) Nuclear delivery of macromolecules: barriers and carriers *Adv. Drug Deliv. Rev.,* Vol. 57, No. 4, (December 2005), pp. 505-527, ISSN: 0169-409X

Biswas, J., Bajaj, A., Bhattacharya, S. (2011) Membranes of cationic gemini lipids based on cholesterol with hydroxyl headgroups and their interactions with DNA and phospholipid. *J. Phys. Chem. B.,* Vol. 115, No. 3, (December 2011), pp. 478–486, ISSN: 1520-6106

Blagbrough, I.S., Geall, A.J., Neal, A.P. (2003) Polyamines and novel polyamine conjugates interact with DNA in ways that can be exploited in non-viral gene therapy. *Biochem. Society Transactions,* Vol. 31, No. 2, (April 2003), pp. 397-406, ISSN 0300-5127

Blagbrough, S., Adjimatera, N., Ahmed, O.A.A., Neal, A.P., Pourzand, C. (2004) *Spermine and lipopolyamines as gene delivery agents.* Society of chemical industry, neurotox'03: neurotoxicological targets from functional genomics and proteomics. D.J. Beadle, I.R. Mellor & P.N.R. Usherwood, editors, CHAPTER 16 ISBN: 0901001864

Blau, H.M., Springer, M.L. (1995) Gene therapy-a novel form of drug delivery. *N. Engl. J. Med.,* Vol. 333, No. 18, (November 1995), pp. 1204–1207, ISSN: 0028-4793

Boomer, J.A., Thompson, D.H., Sullivan, S.M. (2002) Formation of plasmid-based transfection complexes with an acid-labile cationic lipid: characterization of in vitro and in vivo gene transfer. *Pharmaceut. Res.,* Vol. 19, No. 9, (September 2002), pp. 1292-1301, ISSN: 0724-8741

Boussif, O., Lezoualc'h, F., Zanta, M.A., Mergny, M.D., Scherman, D., Demeneix, B., Behr, J.P. (1995) A versatile vector for gene and oligonucleotide transfer into cells in culture and in vivo: polyethylenimine. *Proc. Natl. Acad. Sci. U. S. A.,* Vol. 92, No. 16, (August 1995), pp. 7297-7301, ISSN: 0027-8424

Briane, D., Lesage, D., Cao, A., Coudert, R., Lievre, N., Salzmann, J.L., Taillandier, E. (2002) Cellular pathway of plasmids vectorized by cholesterol-based cationic liposomes. *J. Histochemistry and Cytochemistry,* Vol. 50, No. 7, (July 2002), pp. 983-991, ISSN: 0022-1554

Budker, V., Gurevich, V., Hagstrom, J.E., Bortzov, F., Wolff, J.A. (1996) pH-sensitive cationic liposomes: a new synthetic virus-like vector. *Nat. Biotechnol.,* Vol. 14, No. 6, (June 1996), pp. 760–764, ISSN: 1087-0156

Caplen, N.J., Kinrade, E., Sorgi, F., Gao, X., Gruenert, D., Geddes, D., Coutelle, C., Huang, L., Alton, E.W., Williamson, R. (1995) In vitro liposome-mediated DNA transfection of epithelial cell lines using the cationic liposome DC-chol/DOPE. *Gene Therapy,* Vol. 2, No 9, (November 1995), pp. 603-613, ISSN: 0969-7128

Caracciolo, G., Pozzi, D., Amenitsch, H., Caminiti, R. (2005) Multicomponent cationic lipid–DNA complex formation: role of lipid mixing. *Langmuir,* Vol. 21, No. 25, (December 2005), pp. 11582–11587, ISSN: 07437463

Caracciolo, G., Pozzi, D., Caminiti, R., Amenitsch, H. (2005), Lipid mixing upon deoxyribonucleic acid-induced liposomes fusion investigated by synchrotron small-angle x-ray scattering. *Appl. Phys. Lett.,* Vol. 87, pp. 133901–133903, ISSN: 0003-6951

Caracciolo, G., Pozzi, D., Caminiti, R., Marchini, C., Montani, M., Amici, A., Amenitsch, H. (2006) DNA release from cationic liposome/DNA complexes by anionic lipids. *Appl. Phys. Lett.,* Vol. 89, pp. 2339031–2339033, ISSN: 0003-6951

Caracciolo, G., Pozzi, D., Caminiti, R., Marchini, C., Montani, M., Amici, A., Amenitsch, H. (2007) Transfection efficiency boost by designer multicomponent lipoplexes. *Biochim. Biophys. Acta,* Vol. 1768, No. 9, (July 2007), pp. 2280–2292, ISSN: 0005-2736

Carmona, S., Jorgensen, M.R., Kolli, S., Crowther, C., Salazar, F.H., Marion, P.L., Fujino, M., Natori, Y., Thanou, M., Arbuthnot, P., Miller, A.D. (2009) Controlling HBV replication in vivo by intravenous administration of triggered PEGylated siRNA-nanoparticles. *Mol. Pharmaceutics,* Vol. 6, No. 3, (December 2008), pp. 706–717, ISSN 1543-8384

Chen, J., Tian, B., Yin, X., Zhang, Y., Hu, D., Hu, Z., Liu, M., Pan, Y., Zhao, J., Li, H., Hou, C., Wang, J., Zhang, Y. (2007) Preparation, characterization and transfection efficiency of cationic PEGylated PLA nanoparticles as gene delivery systems. *J. Biotechnology.* (February 2007), Vol. 130, No. 2, pp. 107–113, ISSN: 0168-1656

Choi, J.S., Lee, E.J., Jang, H.S., Park, J.S. (2001) New cationic liposomes for gene transfer into mammalian cells with high efficiency and low toxicity. *Bioconjugate Chem.,* Vol. 12, No. 1, (January-February 2001), pp. 108–113, ISSN: 1520-4812

Choi, S.H., Jin, S.-E., Lee, M.-K., Lim, S.-J., Park, J.-S. Kim, B.-G., Ahn, W.S., Kim, C.-K. (2008) Novel cationic solid lipid nanoparticles enhanced p53 gene transfer to lung cancer cells. *European Journal of Pharmaceutics and Biopharmaceutics,* Vol. 68, No. 3, (July 2007), pp. 545–554, ISSN: 0939-6411.

Cooper, R.G., Etheridge, C.J., Stewart, L., Marshall J., Rudginsky, S., Cheng, S.H., Miller, A.D. (1998) Polyamine analogues of 3β-[N-(N',N'-Dimethylaminoethane)carbamoyl]-cholesterol (DC-Chol) as agents for gene delivery *Chem. Eur. J.,* Vol. 4, No. 1, (January 1998), pp. 137-151, ISSN: 0947-6539

Crook, K., Stevenson B.J., Dubochet, M., Porteous, D.J. (1998) Inclusion of cholesterol in DOTAP transfection complexes increases the delivery of DNA to cells in vitro in the presence of serum. *Gene Ther.,* Vol. 5, No. 1, (January 1998), pp. 137–143, ISSN: 0969-7128

Dass, C.R. (2002) Biochemical and biophysical characteristics of lipoplexes pertinent to solid tumour gene therapy. *Int. J. Pharm.*, Vol. 241, No. 1, (July 2002), pp. 1–25, ISSN: 1811-7775

Ding, W.X., Hattori, Y., Higashiyama, K., Maitani, Y. (2008) Hydroxyethylated cationic cholesterol derivatives in liposome vectors promote gene expression in the lung. *Int. J. Pharm.*, Vol. 354, No. 1-2, (November 2008), pp. 196–203, ISSN: 0378-5173

El-Aneed, A. (2004) An overview of current delivery systems in cancer gene therapy. *J. Controlled Release,* Vol. 94, No. 1, (January 2004), pp. 1–14, ISSN: 0168-3659

Eliyahu, H., Barenholz, Y., Domb, A.J. (2005) Polymers for DNA delivery. *Molecules,* Vol. 10, No. 1, (January 2005), pp. 34-64, ISSN: 1420-3049

Escriou, V., Ciolina, C., Helbling-Leclerc, A., Wils, P., Scherman, D. (1998) Cationic lipid-mediated gene transfer: Analysis of cellular uptake and nuclear import of plasmid DNA. *Cell Biology and Toxicology,* Vol. 14, No. 2, (March 1998), pp. 95-104, ISSN: 0742-2091

Esposito, C., Masotti, A., Del Grosso, N., Malizia, D., Bianco, A., Bonadies, F., Napolitano, R., Ortaggi, G., Mossa, G. (2003) Function/structure correlation in novel pH-dependent cationic liposomes for glioma cells transfection in vitro. *C. R. Chimie,* Vol. 6, pp. 617–622, ISSN: 1631-0748

Farhood, H., Bottega, R., Epand, R.M., Huang, L. (1992) Effect of cationic cholesterol derivatives on gene transfer and protein kinase C activity. *Biochim. Biophys. Acta,* Vol. 1111, No. 2, pp. 239–246, ISSN: 1388-1981

Fewell, J.G., Matar, M., Slobodkin, G., Han, S.O., Rice, J., Hovanes, B., Lewis, D.H., Anwer, K. (2005) Synthesis and application of a non-viral gene delivery system for immunogene therapy of cancer. *J. Control Release.,* V. 109, No. 1-3, pp. 288-298, ISSN: 0168-3659

Furgeson, D.Y., Cohen, R.N., Mahato, R.I., Kim, S.W. (2002) Novel water insoluble lipoparticulates for gene delivery. *Pharm. Res.,* 2002. Vol. 19, No. 4, (April 2002), pp. 382-390, ISSN: 0724-8741

Furgeson, D.Y., Chan, W.S., Yockman, J.W., Kim, S.W. (2003) Modified linear polyethylenimine-cholesterol conjugates for DNA complexation. *Bioconjug. Chem.,* Vol. 14, No. 4, pp. 840-847, ISSN: 1043-1802

Furgeson, D.Y., Yockman, J.W., Janat, M.M., Kim, S.W. (2004) Tumor efficacy and biodistribution of linear polyethylenimine-cholesterol/DNA complexes. *Mol. Ther.,* Vol. 9, No.6, (Juny 2004), pp. 837-845, ISSN: 1525-0016

Ganta, S.H., Devalapally, A., Shahiwala, M., Amiji, J. (2008) A review of stimuli-responsive nanocarriers for drug and gene delivery. *Controlled Release,* Vol. 126, No. 3, (January 2008), pp. 187-204, ISSN: 0168-3659

Gao, X., Huang, L. (1991) A novel cationic liposome reagent for efficient transfection of mammalian cells. *Biochem. Biophys. Res. Commun.,* Vol. 179, No. 1, (August 1991), pp. 280–285, ISSN: 0006-291X

Gao, H., Hui, K.M. (2001) Synthesis of a novel series of cationic lipids that can act as efficient gene delivery vehicles through systematic heterocyclic substitution of cholesterol derivatives. *Gene Ther.,* Vol. 8, No. 11, (June 2001), pp. 855–863, ISSN: 0969-7128

Geall, A.J., Eaton, M.A.W., Baker, T., Catteral, C.l, Blagbrough, I.S. (1999) The regiochemical distribution of positive charges along cholesterol polyamine carbamates plays signi¢cant roles in modulating DNA binding affnity and lipofection. *FEBS Letters*, Vol. 459, No. 3, pp. 337-342. (October 1999), pp. 337-342, ISSN 0014-5793

Geall, A.J., Taylor, R.J., Earll, M.E., Eaton, M.A.W., Blagbrough, I.S. (2000) Synthesis of cholesterol-polyamine carbamates: pKa studies and condensation of calf thymus DNA. *Bioconjugate Chem.,* Vol. 11, No. 3, (June 2000), pp. 314–326, ISSN: 1520-4812

Ghosh, Y.K., Visweswariah, S.S., Bhattacharya, S. (2000) Nature of linkage between the cationic headgroup and cholesteryl skeleton controls gene transfection efficiency. *FEBS Letters,* Vol. 473, (April 2000), pp. 341-344, ISSN: 0014-5793

Ghosh, Y.K., Visweswariah, S.S., Bhattacharya, S. (2002) Advantage of the ether linkage between the positive charge and the cholesteryl skeleton in cholesterol-based amphiphiles as vectors for gene delivery. *Bioconjugate Chem.,* Vol. 13, No. 2, (June 2001), pp. 378-384, ISSN: 1043-1802

Gullotti, E., Yeo, Y. (2009) Extracellularly activated nanocarriers: a new paradigm of tumor targeted drug delivery. *Molecular Pharmaceutics,* Vol. 6, No. 4, (July-August 2009), pp. 1041–1051, ISSN: 1543-838

Guo, X., Szoka, F.C. (2003) Chemical approaches to triggerable lipid vesicles for drug and gene delivery. *Acc. Chem. Res.,* Vol. 36, No. 5, (May 2003), pp. 335-341, ISSN: 0001-4842

Gusachenko, (Simonova) O, Kravchuk, Y, Konevets, D, Silnikov, V, Vlassov, VV, Zenkova, MA. (2009) Transfection efficience 0f 25-kDa PEI-cholesterol conjugates with different levels of modification. *Journal of Biomaterials Science,* Vol. 20, No. 7-8, pp. 1091-1110, ISSN: 0920-5063

Han, So., Mahato, R.I., Kim, S.W. (2001) Water-soluble lipopolymer for gene delivery. *Bioconjug. Chem.,* Vol. 12, No. 3, (Juny 2001), pp. 337-345, ISSN: 1043-1802

Han, S.-E., Kang, H., Shima, G.Y., Suha, M.S., Kimc, S.J., Kimd, J.-S., Oh, Y.-K. (2008) Novel cationic cholesterol derivative-based liposomes for serum-enhanced delivery of siRNA. *International Journal of Pharmaceutics,* Vol. 353, No. 1-2, pp. 260–269, ISSN : 0378-5173

Hasegawa, S., Hirashima, N., Nakanishi, M. (2002) Comparative study of transfection efficiency of cationic cholesterols mediated by liposomes-based gene delivery. *Bioorganic & Medicinal Chemistry Letters,* Vol. 12, No. 9, (February 2022), pp. 1299–1302, ISSN: 0960-894x

Hattori, Y.W., Ding, Y., Maitani, J. (2007) Highly efficient cationic hydroxyethylated cholesterol-based nanoparticle-mediated gene transfer in vivo and in vitro in prostate carcinoma PC-3 cells. *Contr. Realease,* , Vol. 120, No. 1-2, (April 2007), pp. 122-130, ISSN: 0168-3659

Henriksen-Lacey, M., Christensen, D., Bramwell, V.W., Lindenstrøm, T., Agger, E. M., Andersen, P., Perrie, Y. (2011) Comparison of the depot effect and immunogenicity of liposomes based on dimethyldioctadecylammonium (DDA), 3-[N-(N',N'-dimethylaminoethane)carbomyl] cholesterol (DC-Chol), and 1,2-Dioleoyl-3-trimethylammonium propane (DOTAP): prolonged liposome retention mediates stronger Th1 responses. *Molecular Pharmaceutics,* Vol. 8, No. 1, (November 2010), pp. 153–161, ISSN: 1543-838

Hoekstra, D., Rejman, J., Wasungu, L., Shi, F., Zuhorn, I. (2007) Gene delivery by cationic lipids: in and out of an endosome. *Biochem. Soc. Trans.* Vol. 35, No. 1, (February 2007), pp. 68–71, ISSN: 0300-5127

Huang, Z., Li, W., MacKay, J.A., Szoka, F.C. (2005) Thiocholesterol-based lipids for ordered assembly of bioresponsive gene carriers. *Mol. Ther.*, Vol. 11, N. 3, (March 2005), pp. 409-417, ISSN: 1525-0016

Huang, L., Hung, M.-C., Wagner, E. (2005) *Non-viral vectors for gene therapy*. Part 1, Elsevier: Amsterdam. ISBN10: 012017653X / ISBN13: 9780120176533

Hui, S.W., Langner, M., Zhao, Y.L., Hurley, E., Chan, K. (1996) The role of helper lipids in cationic liposome-mediated gene transfer. *Biophys. J.*, Vol. 71, No. 2, (August 1996), pp. 590–599, ISSN: 0006-3495

Ilies, M., Seitz, W., Johnson, B., Ezell, E., Miller, A., Thompson, E., Balaban, A. (2006) Lipophilic pyrylium salts in the synthesis of efficient pyridinium-based cationic lipids, gemini surfactants, and lipophilic oligomers for gene delivery. *J. Med. Chem.*, V. 49, No. 13, (Juny 2006), pp. 3872–3887, ISSN: 1520-4804

Janát-Amsbury, M.M., Yockman, J.W., Lee, M., Kern, S., Furgeson, D.Y., Bikram, M., Kim, S.W. (2005) Local, non-viral IL-12 gene therapy using a water soluble lipopolymer as carrier system combined with systemic paclitaxel for cancer treatment. *J. Control Release.*, Vol. 101, No. 1-3, (January 2005), pp. 273-285, ISSN: 0168-3659

Karmali, P.P., Chaudhuri, A. (2007) Cationic liposomes as non-viral carriers of gene medicines: resolved issues, open questions, and future promises. *Medicinal Research Reviews*, Vol. 27, No. 5, pp. 696-722, ISSN: 0198-6325

Kawaura, C., Noguchi, A., Furuno, T., Nakanishi, M. (1998) Atomic force microscopy for studying gene transfection mediated by cationic liposomes with a cationic cholesterol derivative. *FEBS Letters*, Vol. 421, No. 1-2, (January 1998) pp. 69-72, ISSN: 0014-5793

Kearns M.D., Donkor, A.-M., Savva, M. (2008) Structure-transfection activity studies of novel cationic cholesterol-based amphiphiles. *Molecular pharmaceutics*, Vol. 5, No. 1, (December 2007), pp. 128–139, ISSN: 1543-8384

Keller, M., Jorgensen, M.R., Perouzel, E., Miller, A.D. (2003) Thermodynamic aspects and biological profile of CDAN/DOPE and DC-Chol/ DOPE lipoplexes. *Biochemistry*, Vol. 42, No. 20, (January 2003), pp. 6067-6077, ISSN: 0006-2960

Kerner, M., Meyuhas, O., Hirsch-Lerner, D., Rosen, L.J., Min, Z., Barenholz, Y. (2001) Interplay in lipoplexes between type of pDNA promoter and lipid composition determines transfection efficiency of human growth hormone in NIH3T3 cells in culture. *Biochim. Biophys. Acta*, Vol. 1532, No. 1-2, (April 2001), pp. 128-136, ISSN: 0006-3002

Kichler, A. (2004) Gene transfer with modified polyethylenimines. *J. Gene Med.*, Vol. 6, No. 1, (February 2004), pp. S3-10, ISSN: 15212254

Kim, S., Choi, J.S., Jang, H.S., Suh, H., ,Park, J. (2001) Hydrophobic modification of polyethyleneimine for gene trqansfectants. *Bull. Corean. Chem. Soc.*, Vol. 22, No. 10, pp. 1069-1075, ISSN 0253-2964

Kim, W.J., Chang, C.W., Lee, M., Kim, S.W. (2007) Efficient siRNA delivery using water soluble lipopolymer for anti-angiogenic gene therapy. *J. Control Release.*, Vol. 118, No. 3, (January 2007), pp. 357-363, ISSN: 0168-3659

Kirby, A.J., Camilleri, P., Engberts, J.B., Feiters, M.C., Nolte, R.J., Söderman, O., Bergsma, M., Bell, P.C., Fielden, M.L., García Rodríguez, C.L., Guédat, P., Kremer, A., McGregor, C., Perrin, C., Ronsin, G., van Eijk, M.C. (2003) Gemini surfactants: new synthetic vectors for gene transfection. *Angew. Chem.*, Vol. 42, No. 13, (April 2003), pp. 1448-1457, ISSN: 1433-7851

Kostarelos, K., Miller, A.D. (2005) Synthetic, self-assembly ABCD nanoparticles;a structural paradigm for viable synthetic non-viral vectors. *Chem. Soc. Rev.*, Vol. 34, No 11, pp. 970–994, ISSN 0306-0012

Koynova, R., Wang, L., Tarahovsky, Y., MacDonald, R.C. (2005) Lipid phase control of DNA delivery. *Bioconjugate Chem.*, V. 16, No. 6, (December 2005), pp. 1335–1339, ISSN: 1043-1802

Koynova, R., Wang, L., MacDonald, R.C. (2006) An intracellular lamellar- nonlamellar phase transition rationalizes the superior performance of some cationic lipid transfection agents *Proc. Natl. Acad. Sci. U. S. A.* Vol. 103, No. 39, (September 2006), pp. 14373–14378, ISSN: 0027-8424

Koynova, R., Macdonald, RC. (2007) Natural lipid extracts and biomembrane-mimicking lipid compositions are disposed to form nonlamellar phases, and they release DNA from lipoplexes most efficiently. *Biochim Biophys Acta,* (May 2007), Vol. 768, No. 10, pp. 2373-2382, ISSN: 0006-3002

Lesage, D, Cao, A, Briane, D, Lievre, N, Coudert, R, Raphael, M, Salzmann, J.L., Taillandier, E. (2002) Evaluation and optimization of DNA delivery into gliosarcoma 9L cells by a cholesterol-based cationic liposome. *Biochim Biophys Acta,* Vol. 1564, No. 2, pp. 393-402, ISSN: 0006-3002

Lin, A.J., Slack, N.L., Ahmad, A., George, C.X., Samuel, C.E., Safinya, C.R. (2003) Three-dimensional imaging of lipid gene-carriers: membrane charge density controls universal transfection behavior in lamellar cationic liposome-DNA complexes. *Biophys. J.*, Vol. 84, No. 5, (May 2003), pp. 3307–3316, ISSN: 0006-3495

Litzinger, D.C., Brown, J.M., Wala, I., Kaufman, S.A., Van, G.Y., Farrell, C. L., Collins, D. (1996) Fate of cationic liposomes and their complex with oligonucleotide in vivo. *Biochim. Biophys. Acta,* Vol. 1281, No. 2, pp. 139-149, ISSN: 0006-3002

Liu, Y., Mounkes, L.C., Liggitt, H.D., Brown, C.S., Solodin, I., Heath, T.D., Debs, R.J. (1997) Factors influencing the efficiency of cationic liposome-mediated intravenous gene delivery. *Nat. Biotech.*, Vol. 15, pp. 167–173, ISSN: 1087-0156

Lundqvist, M., Stigler, J., Elia, G., Lynch, I., Cedervall, T., Dawson, K.A. (2008) Nanoparticle size and surface properties determine the protein corona with possible implications for biological impacts. *Proc. Natl. Acad. Sci. U.S.A.,* Vol. 105, No. 38. (September 2008), pp. 14265-14270, ISSN: 0027-8424

Lv, H.T., Zhang, S.B., Wang, B., Cui, S.H., Yan, J. (2006) Toxicity of cationic lipids and cationic polymers in gene delivery. *J. Controlled Release,* Vol. 114, No. 1, pp. 100–109, ISSN: 0168-3659

Mahato, R.I., Lee, M., Han, S., Maheshwari, A., Kim, S.W. (2001) Intratumoral delivery of p2CMVmIL-12 using water-soluble lipopolymers. *Mol. Ther.,* Vol. 4, No. 2, (August 2001), pp. 130-138, ISSN: 1525-0016

Malaekeh-Nikouei, B., Malaekeh-Nikouei, M., Oskuee, R.K., Ramezani, M. (2009) Preparation, characterization, transfection efficiency, and cytotoxicity of liposomes containing oligoamine-modified cholesterols as nanocarriers to Neuro2A cells. *Nanomedicine*. Vol. 5, No. 4, (February 2009), pp. 457-462, ISSN: 1549-9634

Maslov, M.A., Morozova, N.G., Chizhik, E.I., Rapoport, D.A, Zenkova, M.A., Serebrennikova, G.A. (2010) Synthesis and delivery activity of new cationic cholesteryl glucosides. *Carbohydrate Research,* Vol. 345, No. 17, pp. 2438-2449, ISSN: 0008-6215

Medvedeva, D.A., Maslov, M.A., Serikov, R.N., Morosova, N.G., Serebrenikova, G.A., Sheglov, D.V., Latyshev, A.V., Vlassov, V.V., Zenkova, M.A. (2009) Novel cholesterol-based cationic lipids for gene delivery. *Journal of Medicinal Chemistry,* Vol. 52, No. 11, pp. 6558-6568, ISSN: 1520-4804

Mok, K.W.C., Cullis, P.R. (1997) Structural and fusogenic properties of cationic liposomes in the presence of plasmid DNA. *Biophys. J.*, Vol. *73*, No. 5, (March 1997), pp. 2534–2545, ISSN: 0006-3495

Mukherjee, S., Ghosh, R.N., Maxfield, F.R. (1997) Endocytosis. *Physiol. Rev.,* Vol. 77, No. 3, (July 1997), pp. 759-803, ISSN: 0031-9333

Muñoz-Ubeda, M., Rodríguez-Pulido, A., Nogales, A., Martín-Molina, A., Aicart, E., Junquera, E. (2010) Effect of lipid composition on the structure and theoretical phase diagrams of DC-Chol/DOPE-DNA lipoplexes. *Biomacromolecules,* Vol. 11, No. 12, (October 2010), pp. 3332–3340, ISSN 1525-7797

Moss, R.A., Li, J.-M. (1992) Bilayer-bridging bolaamphiphilic lipids *J. Am. Chem. Soc.,* Vol. 114, No. 23, pp. 9227-9229, ISSN: 0002-7863

Noguchi, A., Furuno, T., Kawaura, C., Nakanishi, M. (1998) Membrane fusion plays an important role in gene transfection mediated by cationic liposomes. *FEBS Lett.,* Vol. 433, No. 1-2, (August 1998), pp. 169-173, ISSN: 0014-5793

Okayama, R., Noji, M., Nakanishi, M. (1997) Cationic cholesterol with a hydroxyethylamino head group promotes significantly liposome-mediated gene transfection. *FEBS Letters,* Vol. 408, No. 2, (May 1997), pp. 232-234, ISSN: 0014-5793

Oliver, M., Jorgensen, M.R., Miller, A. (2004) The facile solid-phase synthesis of cholesterol-based polyamine lipids. *Tetrahedron Letter,* Vol. 45, No. 15, (February 2004), pp. 3105–3107, ISSN: 0040-4039

Ouderhiri, N, Vigneron, J.P., Peuchmaur, M., Leclerc, T, Lehn, J.M., Lehn, P. (1997) Gene transfer by guanidinium-cholesterol cationic lipids into airway epithelial cells in vitro and in vivo. *Proc Natl Acad Sci U S A,* Vol. 94, No. 5, (March 1997), pp. 1651-1656, ISSN: 0027-8424

Percot, A., Briane, D., Coudert, R., Reynier, P., Bouchema, N., Lie`vre, N., Hantz, E., Salzmann, J.L., Cao, A. (2004) A hydroxyethylated cholesterol-based cationic lipid for DNA delivery: effect of conditioning. *Int. J. Pharm.,* Vol. 278, No. 1, (June 2004), pp. 143–163, ISSN: 0378-5173

Petukhov, I.A., Maslov, M.A., Morozova, N.G., Serebrennikova, G.A. (2010) Synthesis of polycationic lipids based on cholesterol and spermine. *Russian Chemical Bulletin,* Vol. 59, No. 1, (January 2010), pp. 260-268, ISSN: 1066-5285

Pitard, B., Oudrhiri, N., Vigneron, J.P., Hauchecorne, M., Aguerre, O., Toury, R., Airiau, M., Ramasawmy, R, Scherman, D., Crouzet, J., Lehn, J.M., Lehn, P. (1999) Structural characteristics of supramolecular assemblies formed by guanidinium-cholesterol reagents for gene transfection. *Proc. Natl. Acad. Sci. USA,* Vol. 96, No. 6 (March 1999), pp. 2621-2626, ISSN: 0027-8424

Pouton, C.W., Seymou, L.W. (2001) Key issues in non-viral gene delivery, *Adv. Drug Deliv. Rev.,* Vol. 46, No. 1-3, (March 2001), pp. 187–203, ISSN: 0169-409X

Porter, C.D., Lukacs, K.V., Box, G., Takeuchi, Y., Collins, M.K. (1998) Cationic liposomes enhance the rate of transduction by a recombinant retroviral vector in vitro and in vivo. *J. Virol.*, Vol. 72, No. 6, (Juny 1998), pp. 832-4840, ISSN: 1743-422X

Pozzi, D., Amenitsch, H., Caminiti, R., Caracciolo, G. (2006) How lipid hydration and temperature affect the structure of DC-Chol–DOPE/DNA lipoplexes. *Chemical Physics Letters*, Vol. 422, pp. 439–445, ISSN: 0009-2614

Pozzi, D., Caracciolo, G., Caminiti, R., De Sanctis, S.C., Amenitsch, H., Marchini, C., Montani, M., Amici, A. (2009) Toward the rational design of lipid gene vectors: shape coupling between lipoplex and anionic cellular lipids controls the phase evolution of lipoplexes and the efficiency of DNA release. *Applied Materials&Interfaces*, Vol. 1, No. 10, (October 2009), pp. 2237–2249, ISSN 1944-8244

Rayburn, E.R., Zhang, R. (2008) Antisense, RNAi, and gene silencing strategies for therapy: mission possible or impossible? *Drug Discovery Today*, Vol. 13, No. 11-12, (June 2008), pp. 513-521, ISSN: 1359-6446

Rejman, J., Oberle, V., Zuhorn, I.S., Hoekstra, D. (2004) Size-dependent internalization of particles via the pathways of clathrin- and caveolae-mediated endocytosis. *Biochem J.*, Vol. 377, pp. 159–169, ISSN 0264-6021

Rejman, J., Conese, M., Hoekstra, D. (2006) Gene transfer by means of lipo- and polyplexes: role of clathrin and caveolae-mediated endocytosis. *Journal of liposome Research*, Vol. 16, No. 3, pp. 237-247, ISSN: 0898-2104

Reynier, P, Briane, D, Cao, A, Lievre, N, Naejus, R, Bissieres, P, Salzmann, J.L., Taillandier, E. (2002) In vitro and in vivo transfection of melanoma cells B16-F10 mediated by cholesterol-based cationic liposomes. *J Drug Target*, Vol. 10, No. 7, (November 2002), pp. 557-566, ISSN: 1029-2330

Rodríguez-Pulido, A, Ortega, F, Llorca, O, Aicart, E, Junquera, E. (2008) A physicochemical characterization of the interaction between DC-Chol/DOPE cationic liposomes and DNA. *J. Phys. Chem.. B*, Vol. 112, No. 39, (August 2008), pp. 12555–12565. ISSN: 1520-6106

Rolland, A.P. (1998) From genes to gene medicines: recent advances in nonviral gene delivery. *Crit. Rev. Ther. Drug Carrier Syst.*, Vol. 15, No. 2, pp. 143–198, ISSN: 0743-4863

Ross, P.C., Hui, S.W. (1999) Lipoplex size is a major determinant of in vitro lipofection efficiency. *Gene Therapy*, Vol. 6, No. 4, (April 2009), pp. 651–659, ISSN: 0969-7128

Sainlos, M., Hauchecorne, M., Oudrhiri, N., Zertal-Zidani, S., Aissaoui, A., Vigneron, J.-P., Lehn, J.-M., Lehn, P. (2005) Kanamycin A-Derived Cationic Lipids as Vectors for Gene Transfection. *ChemBioChem.*, 2005, Vol. 6, No. 6, (Juny 2005), pp. 1023 - 1033, ISSN: 1439-4227

Salvati, A., Ciani, L., Ristori, S., Martini, G., Masi, A., Arcangeli, A. (2006) Physico-chemical characterization and transfection efficacy of cationic liposomes containing the pEGFP plasmid. *Biophysical Chemistry*, Vol. 121, No. 1, (January 2006), pp. 21–29, ISSN: 0301-4622

Singh, R. S., Goncalves, C., Sandrin, P., Pichon, C., Midoux, P., Chaudhuri, A. (2004) On the gene delivery efficacies of pH-sensitive cationic lipids via endosomal protonation: a chemical biology investigation. *Chem. Biol.*, Vol. 11, No. 5, (May 2004), pp. 713-723, ISSN: 1074-5521

Sheng, R., Luo, T., Zhu, Y., Li, H., Sun, J, Chen, S, Sun, W., Cao, A. (2011) The intracellular plasmid DNA localization of cationic reducible cholesterol-disulfide lipids. *Biomatherials*, Vol. 32, No. 13, pp. 3507-3519, ISSN: 0142-9612

Simberg, D., Weisman, S., Talmon, Y., Faerman, A., Shoshani, T., Barenholz, Y. (2003) The role of organ vascularization and lipoplex-serum initial contact in intravenous murine lipofection. *J. Biol. Chem.*, Vol. 278, No. 41, (October 2003), pp. 39858-39865, ISSN: 0021-9258

Smith, J.G., Wedeking, T., Vernachio, J.H., Way, H., Niven, R.W. (1998) Characterization and in vivo testing of a heterogeneous cationic lipid–DNA formulation. *Pharm. Res.*, Vol. 15, No. 9, pp. 1356–1363, ISSN: 0724-874

Spagnou, S., Miller, A.D., Lipidic, M.K. (2004) Carriers of siRNA: Differences in the formulation, cellular uptake, and delivery with plasmid DNA. *Biochemistry*, Vol. 43, No. 42, (September 2004), 13348-13356, ISSN: 0006-2960

Solodin, I., Brown, C.S., Bruno, M.S., Chow, C.Y., Jang, E.H., Debs, R.J., Heath, T.D. (1995) A novel series of amphiphilic imidazolinium compounds for in vitro and in vivo gene delivery. *Biochemistry*, Vol. 34, No. 41, pp. 13537–13544, ISSN: 0006-2960

Song, Y.K., Liu, F., Chu, S., Liu D. (1997) Characterization of cationic liposome-mediated gene transfer in vivo by intravenous administration. *Hum. Gene. Ther.*, Vol. 8, No. 13, (September 1997), pp. 1585-1594, ISSN: 1043-0342

Sternberg, B, Hong, K., Zheng, W., Papahadjopoulos, D. (1998) Ultrastructural characterization of cationic liposome–DNA complexes showing enhanced stability in serum and high transfection activity in vivo. *Biochim. Biophys. Acta*, Vol. 1375, (October 1998), pp. 23–35, ISSN: 0006-3002

Stewart, L., Manvell, M., Hillery, E., Etheridge, C.J., Cooper, R.G., Stark, H., van-Heel, M, Preuss, M., Alton, EW.FW., Miller, A.D. (2001) Physico-chemical analysis of cationic liposome–DNA complexes (lipoplexes) with respect to in vitro and in vivo gene delivery efficiency. *J. Chem. Soc., Perkin Trans*, Vol. 2, (March 2001), pp. 624–632, ISSN: 1472-779x

Takeuchi, K, Ishihara, M, Kawaura, C, Noji, M, Furuno, T, Nakanishi, M. (1996) Effect of zeta potential of cationic liposomes containing cationic cholesterol derivatives on gene transfection. *FEBS Lett.*, Vol. 397, No. 2-3, (November 1996), pp. 207-209, ISSN: 0014-5793

Tang, F., Hughes, J.A. (1998). Introduction of a disulfide bond into a cationic lipid enhances transgene expression of plasmid DNA. *Biochem. Biophys. Res. Commun.* Vol. 242, No. 1, (January 1998), pp. 141-145, ISSN: 0006-291X

Tang, F., Hughes, J.A. (1999) Use of dithiodiglycolic acid as a tether for cationic lipids decreases the cytotoxicity and increases transgene expression of plasmid DNA in vitro. *Bioconjugate Chem.*, Vol. 10, No. 5, (September-October 1999), pp. 791-796, ISSN: 1043-1802

Tarahovsky, Y.S., Koynova, R., MacDonald, R.C. (2004) DNA release from lipoplexes by anionic lipids: correlation with lipid mesomorphism, interfacial curvature, and membrane fusion. *Biophys. J.*, V. 87, No.2, (August 2004), pp. 1054–1064, ISSN: 0006-3495

Templeton, N.S. (2010) Liposomes for gene transfer in cancer therapy. *Methods in Molecular Biology*, Vol. 651, pp. 271-278, ISSN: 1064-3745

Tousignant, J.D., Gates, A.L., Ingram, L.A., Johnson, C.L., Nietupski, J.B., Cheng, S.H., Eastman, S.J., Scheule, R.K. (2000) Comprehensive analysis of the acute toxicities induced by systemic administration of cationic lipid:plasmid DNA complexes in mice. *Hum Gene Ther.*, Vol. 11, No. 18, (December 2000), pp. 2493–513, ISSN: 1043-0342

Tseng, Y.-C., Mozumdar, S., Huang, L. (2009) Lipid-based systemic delivery of siRNA. *Advanced Drug Delivery Reviews,* Vol. 61, No. 9, (July 2009), pp. 721–731, ISSN: 0169-409X

Verma, I.M., Weitzman, M.D. (2005) Gene therapy: twenty-first century medicine. *Ann. Rev. Biochem.,* Vol. 74, pp. 711–738, ISSN: 0066-4154

Vigneron, J.P., Oudrhiri, N., Fauquet, M., Vergely, L., Bradley, J.C., Basseville, M., Lehn, P., Lehn, J.M. (1996) Guanidinium-cholesterol cationic lipids: Efficient vectors for the transfection of eukaryotic cells. *Proc. Natl. Acad. Sci. USA,* Vol. 93, No. 18, (September 1996), pp. 9682-9686, ISSN: 0027-8424

Wang, D.A., Narang, A.S., Kotb, M., Gaber, A.O., Miller, D.D., Kim, S.W., Mahato, R.I. (2002) Novel branched poly(ethylenimine)-cholesterol water-soluble lipopolymers for gene delivery. *Biomacromolecules,* V. 3, No. 6, (November-December 2002), pp. 1197-1207, ISSN: 1525-7797

Zabner, J., Fasbender, A.J., Moninger, T., Poellinger, K.A., Welsh, M.J. (1995) Cellular and molecular barriers to gene transfer by a cationic lipid. *J Biol Chem.,* Vol. 270, pp. 18997-9007, ISSN: 0021-9258

Zhdanov, R.I., Kutsenko, N.G., Podobed, O.V., Buneva, O.A., Tsvetkova, T.A., Konevets, D.N., Vlassov V.V. (1998) Cholesterol polyethylen/propylen/imines as mediators of transfection of eukaryotic cells for gene therapy. *Dokl. Akad. Nauk,* Vol. 361, pp. 695–699, ISSN: 0869-5652

Zhi, D., Zhang, S., Wang, B., Zhao, Y., Yang, B., Yu, S. (2010) Transfection efficiency of cationic lipids with different hydrophobic domains in gene delivery. *Bioconjugate Chem.,* Vol. 21, No 4, pp. 563–577, ISSN: 1043-1802

Zhu, M.-Z., Wu, Q.-H., Zhang, G., T. Ren, D. Liu, Guo, Q.-X. (2002) Synthesis and evaluation of cationic lipids bearing cholesteryl groups for gene delivery in vitro. *Bull. Chem. Soc. Jpn.,* Vol. 75, pp. 2207-2013, ISSN: 0009-2673

Zuidam, N.J., Barenholz, Y. (1998) Electrostatic and structural properties of complexes involving plasmid DNA and cationic lipids commonly used for gene delivery. *Biochim. Biophys., Acta.* Vol. 1368, No. 1, (January 1998), pp. 115–128, ISSN: 0006-3002

Zuidam, N.J., Hirsch-Lerner, D., Margulies, S., Barenholz, Y. (1999) Lamellarity of cationic liposomes and mode of preparation of lipoplexes affect transfection efficiency. *Biochim. Biophys. Acta,* Vol. 1419, No. 2, (July 1999), pp. 207-220, ISSN: 0006-3002

16

Polycation-Mediated Gene Delivery: The Physicochemical Aspects Governing the Process

Manuel Alatorre-Meda[1], Eustolia Rodríguez-Velázquez[2] and Julio R. Rodríguez[3]

[1]*Grupo de Física de Coloides y Polímeros, Departamento de Física de la Materia Condensada. Facultad de Física, Universidad de Santiago de Compostela*

[2]*Master student. Master en Ciencia y Tecnología de Materiales, Facultad de Física Universidad de Santiago de Compostela*

[3]*Grupo de Nanomateriales y Materia Blanda, Departamento de Física de la Materia Condensada. Facultad de Física, Universidad de Santiago de Compostela*

Spain

1. Introduction

1.1 Chapter objectives

Gene therapy is the process by which a foreign, corrective (or missing) gene is inserted toward biological tissues or cells aiming to alleviate symptoms or prevent disorders. Several clinical trials have demonstrated gene therapy as a promising option to treat diseases. However, therapeutic biological limitations (such as adverse immune responses of the body to incoming gene delivery systems) coupled with a poor understanding of the physicochemical motifs involved in the DNA compaction and delivery (transfection) processes have resulted in non-100% effective protocols. Aiming to contribute to a better understanding of the different physicochemical aspects of gene therapy, our group has committed for some years now to the physical chemistry characterization of the DNA compaction and transfection mediated by different kinds of compacting agents (vectors).

In this chapter, we present an overview of the results we have obtained during the last three years regarding the DNA compaction and transfection mediated by cationic-liposomes and -polymers (polycations). Two families of polycations, Chitosan and Poly (diallyldimethylammonium chloride) (pDADMAC), and one cationic lipid formulation extensively used worldwide in transfection assays, Metafectene® Pro (MEP), are studied as DNA vectors and compared with other systems already published. In particular, by varying the solution pH and polycation characteristics (chemical composition and molecular weight), we assess the influence of polycation-charge density (i.e., the mole fraction of the ionized groups along the polymer chain) and -valence (i.e., the total charge per polymer chain) on different parameters of the complexes formed that are important for gene therapy. The studied parameters include i) the hydrodynamic radius, R_H, ii) the stability with time, iii) the vector to DNA ratio at which complexation takes place iv) the ζ-potential, v) the binding energetics, vi) the morphology, and vii) the transfection efficiency. The physicochemical characterization was carried out by means of different experimental techniques including dynamic and static light scattering (DLS and SLS), electrophoretic mobility, isothermal titration calorimetry (ITC), transmission electron- and atomic force microscopy (TEM and AFM), and conductometry at 25 °C. Transfection experiments were conducted at standard culture conditions and evaluated by means of the β-galactosidase (β-gal) and luciferase assays at 25 °C. Outstanding results concerning the electrochemical and energetic features of the complexes with higher transfection efficiencies are fully discussed.

1.2 Gene therapy

The possibility to treat diseases by the insertion of genes into human cells and tissues has proposed gene therapy as the therapy of the 21st century (Verma & Somia, 1997). With the first clinical trial reported in the early 1990s (Anderson, 1990), protocols for several, diverse disorders have been conducted and promising results have been obtained (O'Connor & Crystal, 2006); however, a single protocol suitable to be applied as a routinely means to treat any particular disease is far to be achieved.

In practice, the entrance of naked, exogenous DNA to the cell nucleus results problematic due to different extra and intracellular barriers. On the one hand, systemic circulation of DNA is hindered by nuclease degradation (Nguyen et al., 2009). On the other hand, the electrolytic nature of DNA gives rise to electrostatic repulsions as DNA approaches to cells provided that both DNA and cell membranes are negatively charged (due to the phosphate groups distributed by the outside of the polymer helices and the several proteoglycans constituting the cell membranes) (Tros de Ilarduya et al., 2010). Also, once inside cells, steric restrictions are expected to hamper the DNA transportation to the cell nucleus given that mobility of free DNA based on diffusion in the cytoplasm is negligible (Dowty et al., 1995), possibly due to cytoskeletal elements within the cytoplasm that function as molecular sieves and prevent the diffusion of large molecules (Lubyphelps et al., 1987). Thus, for exogenous DNA to be properly transferred to living cells (and tissues), all these extra and intracellular barriers must be circumvented.

Current gene transfer protocols rely on the use of natural and synthetic DNA complexing agents, referred to as vectors or gene carriers, to compact, protect, and provoke a charge inversion of DNA, surpassing, by this way, the previously cited biological barriers. Vectors are either viral or non-viral. Viral delivery, also known as transduction, involves the packaging of DNA (or in some cases RNA) into a virus particle (Mancheño-Corvo & Martín-Duque, 2006). This procedure is, by far, the most effective one considering the high transfection efficiencies it renders; however, fundamental problems associated with viral vectors, including toxicity and immunogenicity, among others, have encouraged the investigation of safer gene delivery alternatives such as non-viral vectors (Verma & Somia, 1997).

Compared to viruses, non-viral transfection vectors possess many important advantages such as safety, versatility, ease of preparation, and, in some cases, the possibility to transfect DNA fragments of unlimited sizes (Orth et al., 2008). The first approaches using non-viral vectors as gene carriers come from the late 1980s when Felgner and coworkers started to try with cationic liposomes (Felgner et al., 1987). Cationic liposome-DNA complexes, also referred to as lipoplexes, form spontaneously after electrostatic interactions between the positively charged liposomes and the negatively charged DNA, producing physically stable formulations suitable to transfect relatively high amounts of plasmid DNA to cells in culture

(Felgner et al., 1987). Other non-viral vectors subsequently studied include surfactants, proteins (particularly histones), multivalent ions, nanoparticles, and polycations, all of which (also) form electrostatically driven DNA complexes (Gonzalez-Perez & Dias, 2009). In the following sections we explore representative gene delivery systems employing polycations and cationic liposomes as gene carriers.

1.3 Cationic-liposomes and -polymers for gene therapy

Polycations and cationic liposomes are the non-viral vectors most commonly studied for gene therapy due to the outstanding characteristics they present. In addition to the potential safety benefits, they offer, for instance, a great structural and chemical versatility for manipulating their physicochemical properties, vector stability upon storage and reconstitution, and a larger gene capacity to transfer DNA as compared to their viral and non-viral counterparts (Dias et al., 2002; Midoux et al., 2009; Tros de Ilarduya et al., 2010).
As mentioned before, cationic liposomes were the first class of non-viral vectors showing satisfactory transfection efficiencies. In the first work reporting on lipofection (the lipid-mediated DNA transfection process), Felgner and coworkers employed N-[1-(2,3-dioleyloxy)propyl]-N,N,N-trimethylammonium chloride (DOTMA), a synthetic cationic lipid, to transfect plasmid DNA to different cells lines in culture (Felgner et al., 1987). Major advantages of utilizing DOTMA containing liposomes were that DNA entrapment inside the lipoplexes was found to be of a 100%. Also, as suggested by fluorescence microscopy data, DOTMA demonstrated to facilitate fusion of the complexes with the plasma membrane of the studied culture cells, resulting in DNA transfer rates from 5- to >100-fold more effective (depending on the transfected cell line) than previous procedures such as the calcium phosphate or the DEAE-dextran transfection techniques (Kucherlapati & Skoultchi, 1984). However, a major drawback was that these liposomes were found to be cytotoxic (Felgner et al., 1987). Following the trail of this pioneering work, other cationic lipids and surfactants have also been tested over the years (Simberg et al., 2004). Unfortunately, the general perspective is that excessive positive charges, facilitating the electrostatic interactions with negatively charged DNA, also promote cytotoxicity. As a result, zwitterionic lipids such as dioleoylphosphatidylethanolamine (DOPE) and cholesterol are nowadays commonly implemented (Tros de Ilarduya et al., 2010).
Polycations (i.e., positively charged polyelectrolytes) are macromolecules attractive to gene therapy for various reasons. Firstly, provided the high charge density they bear, they are considered as the most efficient nucleic acid-condensing agents. Different to other kinds of non-viral vectors like trivalent ions and cationic surfactants, interacting with a few consecutive DNA monomers (bases) (Sarraguca & Pais, 2006), polycations interact with DNA bases that are significantly far apart, promoting bridging between different sites in the DNA chain or between different DNA chains (Dias et al., 2003).
Secondly, because of the strong DNA-polycation interactions, DNA-polycation complexes (polyplexes) are specially effective in what DNA charge masking and extracellular protection concerns (De Smedt et al., 2000). And thirdly, given that they can be functionalized, copolymerized or structurally modified, polycation constructs can be tailored to improve cell-specific therapeutic efficacy with reduced side effects (Ke & Young, 2010). Polycations most frequently studied as gene carriers include poly(L-lysine) (PLL) (G. Y. Wu & C. H. Wu, 1987), polyethylenimine (PEI) (Boussif et al., 1995), chitosan (Mumper et al., 1995), poly(β-amino ester)s (Lynn & Langer, 2000), and poly(amido amine) (PAMAM) dendrimers (Haensler & Szoka, 1993). Generally speaking, the basicity

and degree of protonation of polycationic vectors depend on their amount of primary, secondary, and tertiary amines, which greatly influences the cell toxicity, the escape of polyplexes from endosomes, and the transfection efficiency (Behr 1997).

1.4 Physicochemical aspects of relevance for gene therapy

Gene transfer to eukaryotic cells is a long process encompassing several successive steps. Plasmid DNA must be packaged into complexes/particles first. Next, the DNA-containing complexes/particles must associate with cells and become internalized into them by cellular uptake processes. Following uptake, DNA-containing complexes/particles must escape the endosomal compartment into the cytoplasm and release their DNA-cargo. Finally, DNA must translocate into the cell nucleus to be transcribed into mRNA and subsequently translated into protein antigen (Nguyen et al., 2009). For all these steps to successfully occur, the final characteristics of the lipo- and polyplexes to be employed must, undoubtedly, be studied and tailored. Of especial importance for complex formation and gene delivery, we can enumerate the following physicochemical aspects.

1.4.1 Size and surface charge

The ability of cationic vectors to condense DNA into nano-sized complexes is believed to be crucial for gene therapy (Sahay et al., 2010; Tros de Ilarduya et al., 2010). DNA compaction, also known as condensation, is a reversible coil to globule transition favored by the binding of cationic vectors to the negatively charged DNA phosphate groups (Bloomfield, 1997). When the number of neutralized charges reaches a critical value, DNA undergoes localized bending or distortion, which facilitates the formation of complexes with sizes much smaller (in the range of nanometers) than that of the DNA coil conformation (in the range of microns) (De Smedt et al., 2000; Wilson & Bloomfield, 1979). Analyzing the impact of experimental conditions on the resulting complex dimensions, several studies have demonstrated that parameters like type, size and modification of the cationic vector, the carrier/DNA charge ratio, and also the protocol of complex formation, can all exert a strong influence (Ogris et al., 1998). On the other hand, with respect to the role of complex size on the cellular internalization mechanism, it has been demonstrated that lipo- and polyplexes with sizes up to 200 nm are taken up by the clathrin-dependent pathway, whereas aggregates larger than 500 nm are internalized via clathrin-independent mechanisms (Rejman et al., 2004; Sahay et al., 2010).

Apart from a reduction in size, binding of cationic vectors to DNA also imparts a positive charge. Although this positive charge is important for both cellular-binding and -internalization, it might also be a cause for concern for in vivo applications since cationic complexes readily bind with serum proteins such as serum albumin, promoting aggregation and blood clearance (Tros de Ilarduya et al., 2010). Additionally, an excess of positive charge, commonly reflected by complexes formed at high vector to DNA ratios, might lead to cytotoxicity provided that negatively charged cell membranes are prone to be damaged in the presence of cationic, extracellular compounds (Thomas & Klibanov, 2003). Thus, a successful gene delivery procedure, pursuing a high transfection efficiency at the lowest possible cytotoxicity, should find a delicate balance in the complex surface charge, that is, the complex must possess a high enough positive charge so as to ensure a proper cell-complex association, but at the same time this necessary positive charge must not cause a lethal damage to the cell.

1.4.2 Structural organization

The DNA ordering inside lipoplexes has been reported in the form of four main conformations: one with a short-range lamellar structure composed of flat lipid bilayers and DNA packed between them (Battersby et al., 1998; Dias et al., 2002; Lasic et al., 1997; Radler et al., 1997; Salditt et al., 1997), another where the DNA molecules are encapsulated inside a lipid bilayer forming cylindrical complexes that are closely packed on a hexagonal network (Koltover et al., 1998), another where positively charged vesicles attach to the extended DNA molecule, the so-called "beads on a string" model (Felgner et al., 1987; Gershon et al., 1993; Ruozi et al., 2007; Sternberg et al., 1994), and a final one where DNA is expected to collapse and attach in the form of a globule into the outer surface of positively charged vesicles (Miguel et al., 2003). What can be drawn from all four cases, whatever the nature of the interactions, is that at dilute concentrations no structural change in the systems is present, namely vesicle or bilayer disruption, whereas at high concentrations the situation becomes different with vesicles tending to disrupt and flocculate (Dias et al., 2002; Radler et al., 1997; Salditt et al., 1997;). Concerning polyplexes, rod-like, globular, and toroidal DNA condensates are the morphologies most commonly observed (Carnerup et al., 2009; Danielsen et al., 2004).

1.4.3 Binding affinity

The capability of lipo- and polyplexes to avoid premature dissociation and promote the release of genetic material to the cytoplasm once inside the cell is strongly related to the binding affinity between the DNA and the vector in question (Prevette et al., 2007). Indeed, a strong binding affinity between DNA and its carrier entails a high DNA compaction and protection against degradation in the extracellular environment. However, following their escape from endosomes, the complexes need to approach the nucleus, as well as dissociate; as such, a high DNA-vector binding affinity might constitute a limiting step for transfection considering the difficulty in the separation of the DNA from its gene carrier (Tros de Ilarduya et al., 2010). For the case of polyplexes, presenting by far the highest degree of DNA binding affinity (and condensation), it is well accepted that the molecular weight (Mw) of the polycation (directly related to the cationic valence) is a key factor controlling the DNA-vector binding affinity and subsequent transfection. In general, lower Mw polycations yield higher DNA transfection efficiencies (Ziady et al., 1999) as the DNA dissociation from them is faster (Schaffer et al., 2000).

2. Polycation-mediated gene delivery: Our main results

As already mentioned, the present chapter concerns with the physicochemical characterization of the DNA compaction and transfection mediated by polycations and cationic liposomes. Two families of polycations, Chitosan and Poly (diallyldimethylammonium chloride) (pDADMAC), and one cationic lipid formulation extensively used worldwide in transfection assays, Metafectene® Pro (MEP), are characterized as DNA vectors. Important for the DNA complexation, the structural, electrochemical, and energetic aspects are assessed. Particular attention is paid to the effect of polycations charge density and valence on complex parameters such as i) the hydrodynamic radius, R_H, ii) the stability with time, iii) the vector to DNA ratio at which complexation takes place, iv) the ζ-potential, v) the energetics of binding, vi) the morphology, and vii) transfection efficiency.

It has to be noted that our characterizations were conducted as a function of two distinct cation-to-anion ratios reported in either molar (i.e., the N/P ratio, sections 2.1 and 2.2) or mass units (i.e., the L/D ratio, section 2.3). To get a complete description of the sample preparation, experimental procedures, and data analysis of the results here exposed, the reader is encouraged to consult our published papers (Alatorre-Meda et al., 2009; Alatorre-Meda et al., 2010a, 2010b; Alatorre-Meda et al., 2011). Outstanding results are presented below.

2.1 The DNA-chitosan system

Upon mixing, oppositely charged polyelectrolytes interact electrostatically and form complexes in a process that is promoted by an increase in entropy which is due to a release of counterions (Manning, 1978; Matulis et al., 2000). Accordingly, polycation molecular parameters such as charge density and valence have gained attention in recent reports (Danielsen et al., 2004; Maurstad et al., 2007).

The role of chitosan charge density is well established. It is accepted that the high charge density of chitosan at pHs below its pKa results beneficial for polyplex preparation, and also that its low charge density at pH 7.4 contributes to a low polyplex cytotoxicity and facilitates the intracellular release of DNA from the complex after its endocytotic cellular uptake (Strand et al., 2010). By contrast, the role of chitosan valence on transfection efficiency is contradictory. Namely, while several studies promote the use of high Mw chitosans (Huang et al., 2005; MacLaughlin et al., 1998), some other publications report that lower Mw chitosans are superior for gene transfer (Koping-Hoggard et al., 2003; Lavertu et al., 2006).

Aiming to draw general conclusions about the feasibility of using chitosan as a gene carrier, we characterized the DNA complexation and transfection mediated by three chitosans presenting different Mw (three different valences) at three different pHs of 5.0, 6.0, and 6.5 (three different charge densities). Table 1 summarizes the physical characteristics of the chitosans employed.

CHITOSAN	[η] (dl g^{-1})	Mw (kDa)	Label
Low viscous	4.42 $\pm$ 0.01	111 $\pm$ 2	C(689)
Middle viscous	7.85 $\pm$ 0.24	266 $\pm$ 14	C(1652)
Highly viscous	11.40 $\pm$ 0.24	467 $\pm$ 18	C(2901)

Table 1. Chitosans employed.

2.1.1 Chitosan to DNA complexation ratio, (N/P)c

Stable DNA-chitosan polyplexes, ensuring a complete DNA compaction, are usually formed when chitosan is added in molar excess relative to the negatively charged DNA; however, excessive positive charges might lead to cytotoxicity since negatively charged cell membranes are prone to be damaged in the presence of cationic, extracellular compounds (Thomas & Klibanov, 2003). Consequently, finding a molar ratio exhibiting stable complexes at the lowest possible chitosan concentration becomes important. Such a concentration, presenting this mandatory characteristic, is what we define as the chitosan to DNA complexation ratio (N/P)c.

a. Determination of the (N/P)c via static light scattering (SLS)

It is well accepted that linear, highly charged polyelectrolytes, at the dilute and semi-dilute regimes, can interact via a Coulombic repulsive potential which is strong enough to keep the polymer chains elongated and widely separated, although these interactions be partly screened by non-condensed counterions in solution (Manning, 1978). Polyelectrolytes in such concentration regimes produce in consequence very small scattering signals when irradiated with any source of light (Drifford & Dalbiez, 1984). The situation is rather distinct when polyelectrolytes interact one with each other or are complexed with external agents; in such a case they scatter higher amounts of light when irradiated (Drifford & Dalbiez, 1984). Based on these foundations we analyzed our polyplexes via SLS in order to follow the complexation process. SLS has proved to be a suitable tool to detect structural changes in linear biopolymers expected to be compacted provided that upon structural changes (such as the coil-globule transition observed during DNA compaction) they must scatter light to different extents.

To determine (N/P)c, we tested numerous chitosan/DNA formulations with varying N/P ratios (at a constant DNA concentration) in terms of the chitosan charge density and valence. What we found by SLS was that there exist, indeed, a molar ratio from which the structural conformation of the polyplexes remains apparently constant independently of further addition of chitosan (i.e., presenting non-accentuated changes in light scattering intensity). That molar ratio, defined as (N/P)c, proved to be strongly influenced by the chitosan charge density adopting values of around 1.5, 2.0, and 6.0 for the pHs of 5.0, 6.0, and 6.5, respectively. Our estimations, inferred from figure 1, can be discussed as follows.

Figure 1 presents the light scattering intensity of the DNA-C(1652) polyplexes as a function of the N/P ratio for the three studied pHs. This figure reflects various features worth analyzing. Interestingly, the system revealed plots similar in shape, but different in I values. The plots collected at pH 5.0 and 6.0 have I values one close to the other, whereas the plot at pH 6.5 has higher I values over the whole range of N/P studied. In all three plots three distinct regions can be identified, namely at $N/P = 0$, at $0 < N/P \lesssim 2$, and at $N/P > 2$. At $N/P = 0$, the system containing pure DNA shows the intensity at least five times lower than the samples at $N/P > 2$, indicating no aggregation. However, upon addition of chitosan to DNA, the intensity increases sharply with the maximum at N/P around 1-2 to finally level off at $N/P > 2$. This peculiar and interesting behavior observed when chitosan concentration in the system relative to DNA is around 1-2, is suggestive of the formation of some kind of complex structures between DNA and chitosan at this region, large in size, possibly aggregates that are responsible for the dispersion of higher amounts of light. Finally at $N/P > 2$, the intensity I reaches a constant value revealing the presence of well-formed, stable DNA-chitosan polyplexes with regular sizes. The N/P ratio marking the onset of the constant value in I is denoted as the (N/P)c. Very importantly, these results suggest that as the pH of the medium increases larger amounts of chitosans are required to completely compact the given amount of DNA. This phenomenon can be explained by the fact that at pHs close to its pKa (6.3–6.5), chitosan undergoes a decrease in its charge density due to the neutralization of its amino groups (Kumar et al., 2004), a feature that becomes even more pronounced for chitosans with higher molecular weights (higher valences) (MacLaughlin et al., 1998). Therefore, and having in mind that one of the driving forces of polyelectrolyte complexation is the release of counterions from the polyanion–polycation pair (Manning, 1978; Matulis et al., 2000), it is not strange that the binding affinity between DNA and chitosan lowered as the pH increased and got close to 6.5. Likewise, the highest intensities observed for the system at pH 6.5 over the whole range of N/P can be attributed to a lower chitosan solubility (also ascribed to pHs close to the pKa), a fact that leads to the formation of polyplexes of sizes larger than those at lower pHs, as described below (MacLaughlin et al., 1998; Mumper al., 1995). The DNA-C(689) and -C(2901) systems revealed the same behavior (data not included).

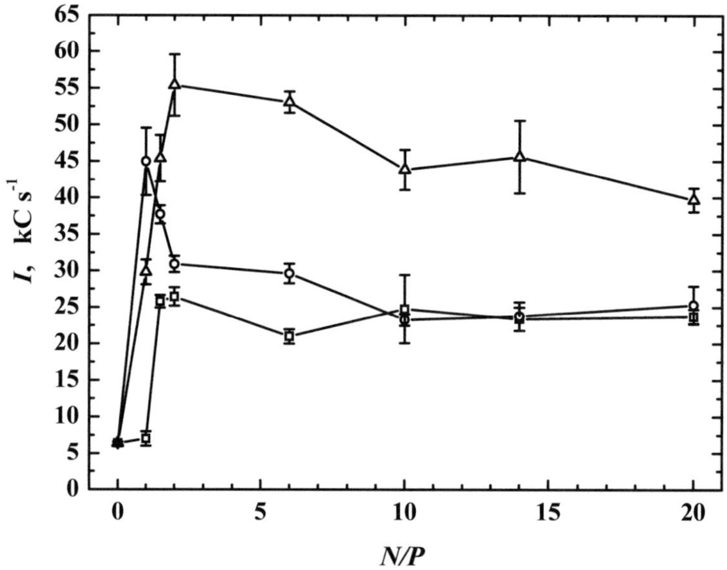

Adapted from (Alatorre-Meda et al., 2009).

Fig. 1. I vs. N/P of the DNA-C(1652) polyplexes at pH = 5.0 (squares), pH = 6.0 (circles), and pH = 6.5 (triangles).

b. Determination of the (N/P)c by conductometry

Electrostatic interactions between oppositely charged polyelectrolytes entail a release of counterions (Manning, 1978; Matulis et al., 2000). The tracking of this release by means of conductometry can be employed as a tool to characterize the DNA compaction process (Rodriguez-Pulido et al., 2008). To confirm the (N/P)c values obtained by SLS we measured the change in conductivity provoked by the addition of chitosan solutions to both, DNA and pure buffer solutions. Compared to those of SLS, the conductometry results, depicted in figure 2, reveal (N/P)c values slightly lower. Main findings as well as a possible explanation to the observed differences are exposed below.

Figure 2 presents a representative plot of the electrical conductivity, κ, as a function of the polycation concentration, recorded for C(2901) at pH 5.0. The filled and empty squares stand for the DNA and pure buffer reservoir solutions, respectively. As can be seen from this figure, in the buffer solution alone the conductivity increased linearly with the chitosan concentration (empty squares) indicating that no aggregation took place under the whole range of the polycation concentration. In the DNA solution (filled squares) by contrast, the conductivity grew linearly, however, with a clear change in slope at the chitosan concentration of 0.104 mM, corresponding to the N/P ratio of 0.82. A similar inflection in a conductivity plot during DNA compaction upon addition of a cationic vector has been observed elsewhere (Rodriguez-Pulido et al., 2008). The authors suggested that the increase in conductivity related to the counterion release from the polycation injected is accentuated by the release of counterions resulting from the complexation process (in our case Na^+ from DNA and $CH3COO^-$ from chitosan) thereby justifying a higher slope in the conductivity plot below the inflection point. On the other hand, once the inflection occurred, the lower slope can be attributed to the fact that only the counterions coming from the chitosan dissociation now contribute to the conductivity of the solution. This change in slope of the conductivity plot can in consequence be considered as the point from which DNA is compacted, namely (N/P)c (Rodriguez-Pulido et al., 2008).

Compared to the DNA compaction ratio we determined by SLS ((N/P)c ~ 1.5) , the lower ratio of N/P = 0.82 here depicted can be ascribed to the difference in ionic strength of the media used in both experiments and to the fact that contrary to SLS, in the conductometry experiment the complex formation was run at constant stirring.[1] The other two chitosans, C(689) and C(1652), although with slight differences in the conductivity values, revealed the inflection point at exactly the same N/P ratio as compared to C(2901) (plots not shown).

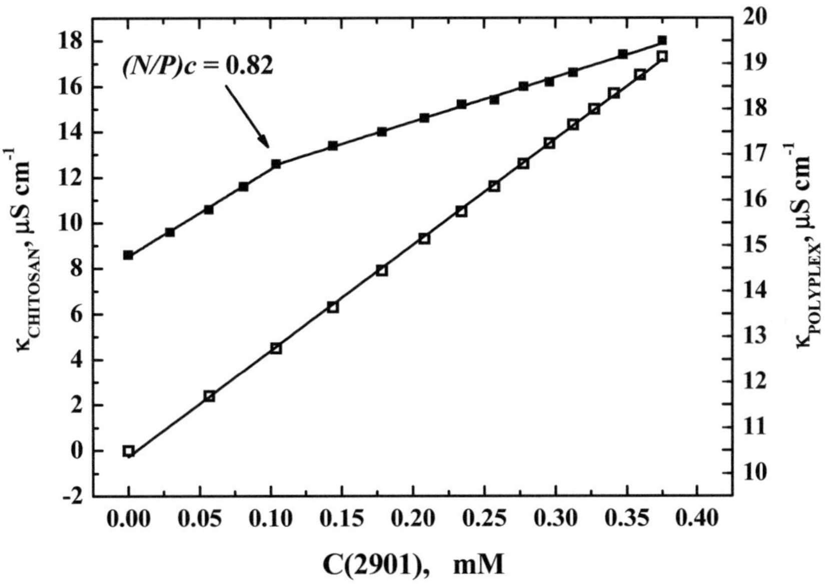

Fig. 2. Electrical conductivity, κ, vs. C(2901) concentration. Filled and empty squares stand for the addition of chitosan to a DNA and to a pure buffer solution, respectively. (Note the difference in scales).

[1] Sample preparation for conductometry experiments is described in (Alatorre-Meda et al., 2011). To consult the experimental conditions for SLS go to (Alatorre-Meda et al., 2009).

2.1.2 Time stability and size

To determine the time stability of the polyplexes, we measured by dynamic light scattering (DLS) the hydrodynamic radius, R_H, of a sample presenting an N/P > (N/P)c (more specifically, N/P = 6) during a period of 6 days at the three different pHs of interest. In general, the polyplexes, regardless of charge density and valence, presented constant sizes with fluctuations lower than a 10% (data not shown). Thus, and provided that small fluctuations as those observed in our measurements are most likely related to the nature of the DLS technique, the polyplexes can be considered as stable with time.

Considering their time stability, to calculate the characteristic size of the polyplexes we simply averaged the R_H values obtained along the testing time. The polyplex sizes thereby obtained were in the range of $187 \pm 21 < R_H < 246 \pm 13$ nm, in good agreement with results previously reported (Mumper et al., 1995). However, contrary to what we initially expected, the size of the polyplexes was found to be dependent on the chitosan valence, following a linear trend with the chitosan molecular weight.[2] Figure 3 depicts the average size of the polyplexes (regardless of chitosan charge density) as a function of the chitosan molecular weight.

Increasing trends in the complex size with polycation Mw, such as that observed in figure 3, are well documented in the literature. For the case of chitosan, it has been demonstrated that upon increasing in its chain length, the influence of the charge density with its correspondent entropy gain decrease. It is likely that the restriction of the polycation chain upon complexation becomes more important, giving rise to a different complexation behavior of high Mw chitosans compared to low Mw chitosans (Danielsen et al., 2004; Maurstad et al., 2007). Furthermore, the intuitive assumption that a higher Mw chitosan can interact better with DNA (due to its expected higher valence), and thus condense it more efficiently than a chitosan of a lower Mw is outweighed by the fact that a higher molecular weight chitosan is less soluble, and as a result, an increase in complex diameter or even complex aggregation may result (MacLaughlin et al., 1998; Mumper et al., 1995).

A general conclusion drawn throughout these sections is that an increased charge density of chitosan, resulting from a lowering of pH, leads to a greater binding affinity between chitosan and DNA as fewer chitosan is required to reach the complexation and the complexes thereby formed are more stable (Alatorre-Meda et al., 2009). Consequently, and in order to further understand the general aspects involved in the DNA-chitosan interactions, in subsequent studies we focused on working at acidic conditions exclusively (Alatorre-Meda et al., 2011). The influence of chitosan valence at those conditions on complex physicochemical properties other than size is described below.

2.1.3 Surface charge

For many polyplexes the cross-over from a negative to a positive ζ-potential occurs at or very close to the isoneutrality point (N/P)φ. (N/P)φ is defined as the point at which the N/P ratio of the polyplex equals 1, that is, the ratio where the negative charges of DNA are stoichiometrically neutralized by the positive charges of the polycation (De Smedt et al., 2000).

---

[2] In general, it is believed that polycations with higher charge densities and valences should produce smaller DNA complexes.

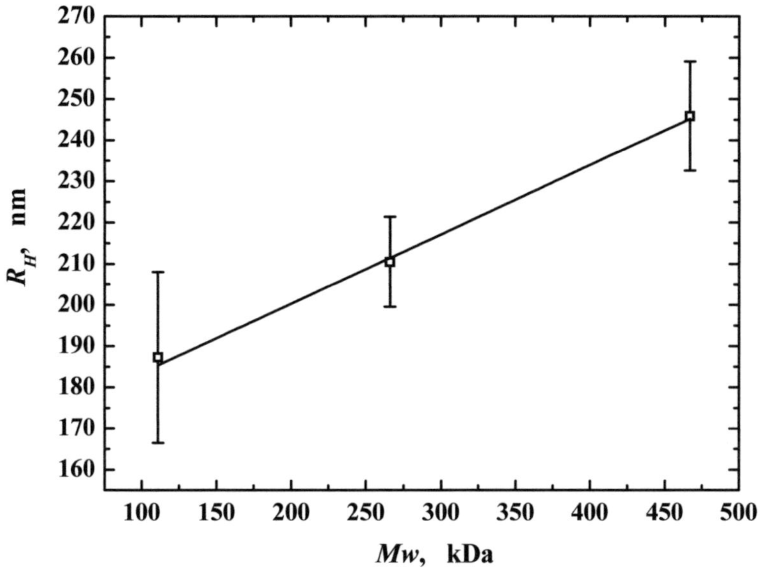

Reproduced from (Alatorre-Meda et al., 2009) with permission of Elsevier BV in the format Journal via Copyright Clearance Center.

Fig. 3. R_H of DNA-chitosan polyplexes, vs. Mw of chitosan.

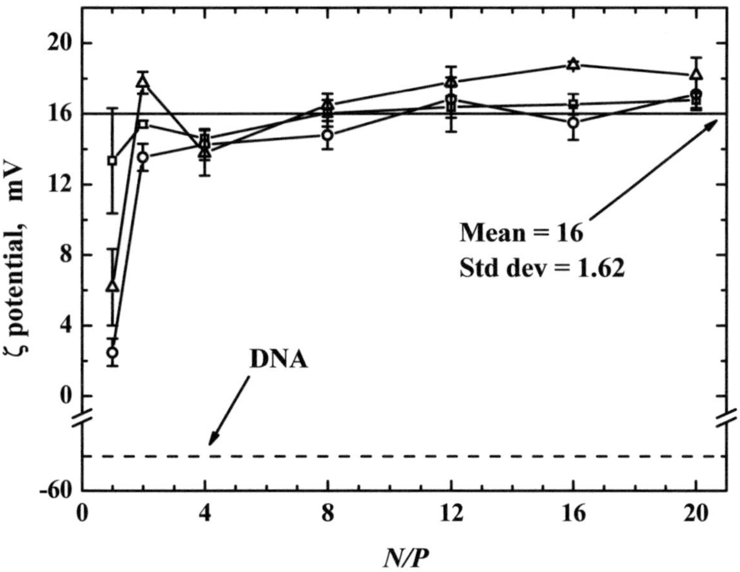

Reproduced from (Alatorre-Meda et al., 2011) with permission of Elsevier BV in the format Journal via Copyright Clearance Center.

Fig. 4. ζ-potential of DNA-chitosan polyplexes vs. N/P. DNA-C(689) (squares), DNA-C(1652) (circles), and DNA-C(2901) (triangles) are plotted. The dotted line stands for the DNA solution (ζ-potential = -55 mV).

In the present study, the characterization was done in the range $1 \leq N/P \leq 20$ for all polyplexes. The ζ-potential of the polyplexes is plotted as a function of N/P in figure 4. In general, all polyplexes presented a positive, stable ζ-potential from N/P ratios as low as (N/P)c confirming that DNA is completely compacted independently of further addition of chitosan. Main findings can be discussed as follows.

It can be seen from figure 4 that at N/P = 1 all polyplexes, in particular those formed with C(1652) and C(2901), reveal a lower ζ-potential as compared to the rest of compositions. The cationic vector-mediated DNA coil to globule transition demonstrated by other authors (Dias et al., 2005) in conjunction with the base line-absent DLS correlation functions we obtained for these systems at ratios $N/P \leq 1$ (Alatorre-Meda et al., 2009), may provide an explanation to this feature. Apparently, larger amounts of chitosan are needed to completely compact the DNA and in consequence populations entailing varying extents of DNA compaction are expected to be present in the bulk. On the other hand, at ratios higher than (N/P)ϕ, all polyplexes reach a plateau around 16mV regardless of chitosan Mw, which is in good agreement with other DNA-polycation systems (Tang & Szoka, 1997). This positive ζ-potential of the polyplexes suggests that the DNA compaction is completely achieved with chitosan chains probably pointing to the outer part of the polyplexes as inferred by other authors (Koping-Hoggard et al., 2003).

2.1.4 Structural organization

Imaging techniques can detect, localize, and analyze individual aggregates of a heterogeneous population, thereby revealing events that would otherwise be hidden. In this context transmission electron- and atomic force microscopy (TEM and AFM) are frequently used in parallel for the visual characterization of biological molecules (Arakawa et al., 1992; Lin & Goh, 2002). Figure 5 presents typical TEM (A) and AFM (B) images obtained for the DNA-C(689) polyplexes at N/P = 20. This figure reflects that the polyplexes adopt a peculiar brush-like conformation in which DNA is apparently confined to the interior of the complex although not fully compacted. The reason why of this polyplex conformation as well as the implications it might have on transfection are discussed below.

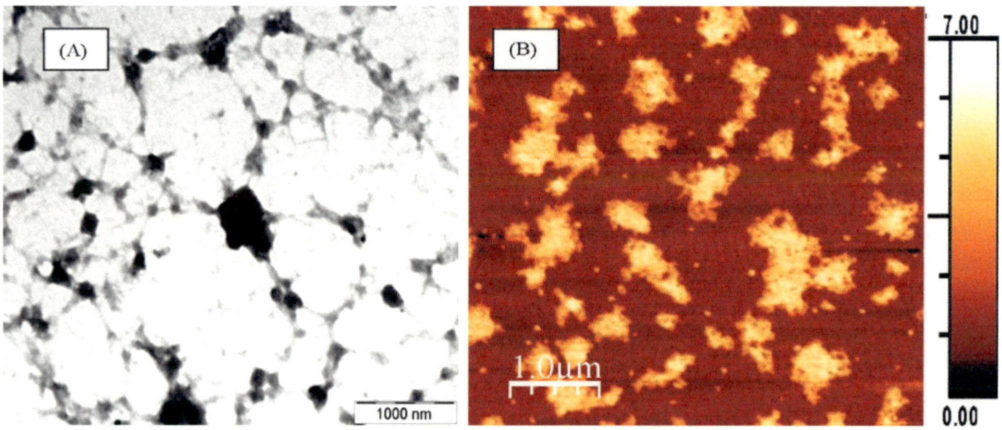

Reproduced from (Alatorre-Meda et al., 2011) with permission of Elsevier BV in the format Journal via Copyright Clearance Center.

Fig. 5. TEM (A) and height AFM (B) images of DNA-C(689) polyplexes, N/P = 20. The bar next to (B) represents the Z scale in nm.

It has been reported that the DNA complexation with chitosans might result in a blend of structures: toroids, rods, and globules, with the relative amounts of the different structures apparently depending on the actual chitosan, the charge ratio, and solution properties like pH and ionic strength (Danielsen et al., 2004; Maurstad et al. 2007). What we observe from figure 5A and B is a heterogeneous population of polyplexes with particle sizes ranging from 250 to 500 nm in good agreement with the DLS results (see section 2.1.2). Both images depict polyplexes with a brush-like conformation where globules/aggregates comprise a dense core that is surrounded by a "hairy" shell of polymer chains. This globular conformation has been reported as characteristic of the DNA complexation with high molecular weight chitosans (Mw> 100 kDa) (Danielsen et al., 2004; Maurstad et al., 2007); by contrast, complexes formed with lower molecular weight chitosans adopt toroid- and rod-like conformations (Maurstad et al., 2007). Similar brush-like structures were also obtained for the DNA complexation with transferrin-poly(l-lysine) conjugates. In this case, the complex morphology was found to depend on the conjugate to DNA ratio (Wagner et al., 1991). Carnerup and coworkers suggest that the significant morphological rearrangement undergone by DNA when it is condensed with low Mw polycations is because of the low charge density of the polycation in question (Carnerup et al., 2009). For toroidal aggregates to form, the electrostatic attraction has to be moderate; that is, a balance between mobility and high binding affinity of DNA to the polymer has to exist. In such a system, the condensed DNA chains will be able to arrange into a toroid. On the contrary, if the charge density of the polymer is too high (as expected for chitosan at pH 5), the DNA chains will entangle with the polymer ones, forming globular aggregates (Carnerup et al., 2009). Therefore, provided that our polyplexes proved to be stable (see section 2.1.2), the "not so tight" DNA complexation they present should be beneficial for DNA transfection (Tros de Ilarduya et al., 2010).

Very importantly, the morphological structure of our system depicted by TEM and AFM in conjunction with the markedly positive ζ-potentials obtained for the polyplexes at this high N/P ratio (see the previous section) appear to be in line with the core–shell structure proposed for polycation-excessive DNA complexes (A. V. Kabanov & V. A. Kabanov, 1998). This model states that DNA is condensed in the inner part of the polyplex by the binding of short segments of a large number of polycation chains, whereas the remaining segments of these same chains are expected to be free in the outer part of the polyplexes giving rise to markedly positive polyplex surface charges (A. V. Kabanov & V. A. Kabanov, 1998).

2.1.5 Binding affinity and complexation thermodynamics

Once the complex is released from the endosome, DNA must disassemble from its vector to be accessible to the cell machinery responsible for translating the enclosed information. For the case of polyplexes, the DNA decompaction (disassembly) is a process substantially dependent on i) the DNA-vector binding affinity, ii) the complexation thermodynamics, and iii) the solution conditions (Carlstedt et al., 2010; Prevette et al., 2007). Provided that acidic conditions demonstrated to be optimal for polyplex formation (see previous sections), we evaluated the DNA-chitosan binding affinity and complexation thermodynamics at a solution pH of 5.0. As depicted by isothermal titration calorimetry (ITC), lower valence chitosans demonstrated to have a higher binding affinity for DNA. Main results are described below.

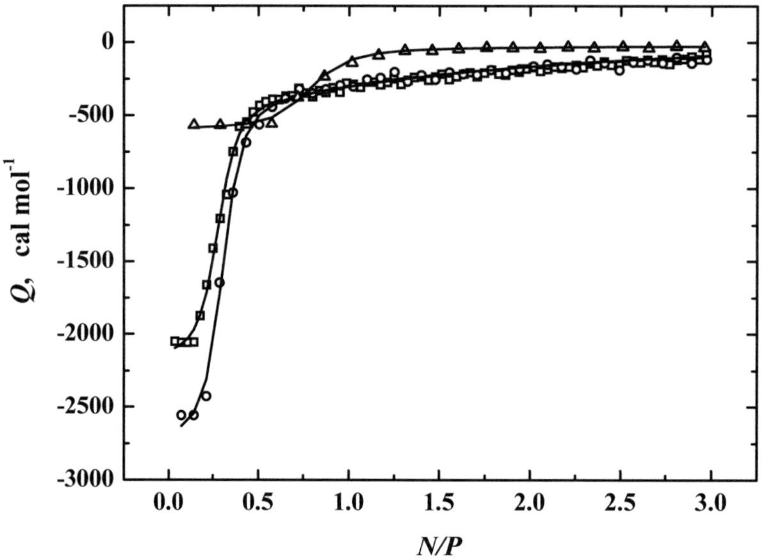

Fig. 6. Integrated heat of interaction of the titration of chitosan to DNA vs. N/P. Chitosans C(689) (squares), C(1652) (circles), and C(2901) (triangles) were titrated. Solid lines represent the two site model fitting to the experimental data.

Figure 6 shows the heat of interaction resulting from the titration of chitosan to DNA as a function of N/P. Supported on calorimetric measurements, it is well accepted that polyelectrolyte complex formation and coacervation are mainly entropically driven through the release of condensed counterions via the ion-exchange process in which an endothermic signal is recorded during the complex formation (de Kruif et al., 2004; Matulis et al., 2000). By contrast, in a result most commonly observed in the formation of protein–ligand complexes, it can be observed from figure 6 that for all experiments the injection of chitosan appears as a markedly negative signal at the beginning of the binding process followed by a gradual decrease in the released heat up until thermal equilibrium, that is, the complexation is exothermic. A similar decrease in the quantity of heat released on successive injections of titrant has been interpreted as an indicative of the progressive neutralization of charges in the reservoir molecule; meanwhile, the zone of the thermogram in which a plateau in the heat released is reached might be attributed to the complete DNA compaction (Bharadwaj et al., 2006). In this context, comparing the onset of the plateau yielded for the three chitosans during the DNA compaction it is clear that for C(2901) N/P~1, whereas for C(689) and C(1652) N/P~0.5. This result is consistent with those we observed by SLS (section 2.1.1) and ζ-potential (previous section) indicating that the use of higher valence chitosans, even at low pHs, apparently demands larger amounts of cationic polymer for DNA compaction. This is also supported by the 4–5-fold smaller enthalpic contribution rendered by C(2901) compared to its lower valence homologues (discussed below).

Table 2 summarizes the enthalpy, entropy, binding constant, and the stoichiometry of the DNA–chitosan interaction derived from the data fitting of figure 6.

chitosan	$K_1 \times 10^{-5}$ (M^{-1})	n_1	ΔH_1 (kcal mol^{-1})	ΔS_1 (kcal mol^{-1} K^{-1})
C(689)	29.9 ± 0.75	0.27 ± 0.03	-2.176 ± 0.23	0.022
C(1652)	29.0 ± 1.23	0.27 ± 0.05	-2.712 ± 0.12	0.020
C(2901)	4.82 ± 0.08	0.73 ± 0.01	-0.598 ± 0.07	0.024
chitosan	**$K_2 \times 10^{-5}$ (M^{-1})**	**n_2**	**ΔH_2 (kcal mol^{-1})**	**ΔS_2 (kcal mol^{-1} K^{-1})**
C(689)	0.095 ± 0.01	0.86 ± 0.02	-1.304 ± 0.16	0.014
C(1652)	0.011 ± 0.02	0.75 ± 0.04	-1.357 ± 0.12	0.014
C(2901)	0.009 ± 0.01	0.62 ± 0.07	-0.529 ± 0.02	0.012

Table 2. Thermodynamic parameters of the DNA-chitosan binding process. Sub-indices next to each parameter stand for the corresponding sites 1 and 2.

As can be observed from this table, the DNA binding constants obtained for all chitosans are on the order of 10^5 to 10^6 and 10^3 to 10^4 M^{-1} for the first and second class of binding sites, respectively. These results are in good agreement with previously reported values for other systems including cationic polymers (Nisha et al., 2004; Prevette, et al., 2007) and proteins (Engler et al., 1997; Milev et al., 2005). On the other hand, the decreasing values of the binding constants with the chitosan valence reveal that lower valence chitosans have a higher binding affinity for DNA. This is indicative that chitosan chains may undergo steric restrictions as Mw (valence) increases, restrictions that in turn apparently hamper the interpolyelectrolyte interactions (Danielsen et al., 2004; Maurstad et al., 2007). Concerning the enthalpy, it is well known that it results from a combination of electrostatics, conformational changes (especially for second binding sites), and hydrogen bonding interactions; therefore, ΔH cannot be strictly related to any one contribution. However, and despite the experimental evidence demonstrating that the binding enthalpy ΔH was negative, the DNA–chitosan complexation was proved to be entropically driven. This result is in good agreement with other electrostatic, polyelectrolyte associations promoted by the release of counterions and solvent upon attraction (Matulis et al., 2000; Prevette, et al., 2007; Srinivasachari et al., 2007).

2.1.6 Transfection efficiency

The potential of chitosans C(689) and C(2901) as DNA carriers towards HeLa cells was evaluated. Polyplexes and nanospheres with compositions in the range $1 \le N/P \le 18$ were tested. In addition, a MEP:DNA lipoplex (4:1 μL:μg) and naked DNA were measured as positive and negative controls, respectively. Although considerably lower compared to that of the DNA–MEP lipoplex, the transfection efficiency of the polyplexes was found to increase with chitosan valence as depicted by the β-galactosidase and luciferase expression assays. Main findings are described below.

Figure 7 shows the transfection efficiency of the polyplexes and controls as well as the protein content of the wells after lysation. Two features are observed from this figure. On the one hand, it is clear that polyplexes within the whole range of ratios rendered levels of β-galactosidase expression slightly higher than that of the negative control (DNA without polymer) with transfection efficiency being increased with chitosan valence. This result is somehow logical taking into account the lower binding affinity depicted by ITC assays for the DNA-C(2901) complex (see Table 2); that is, the DNA release from this complex in the interior of the cell is expected to be favored. On the other hand, compared to that of the DNA-MEP lipoplex, the transfection efficiency of the polyplexes is considerably lower.

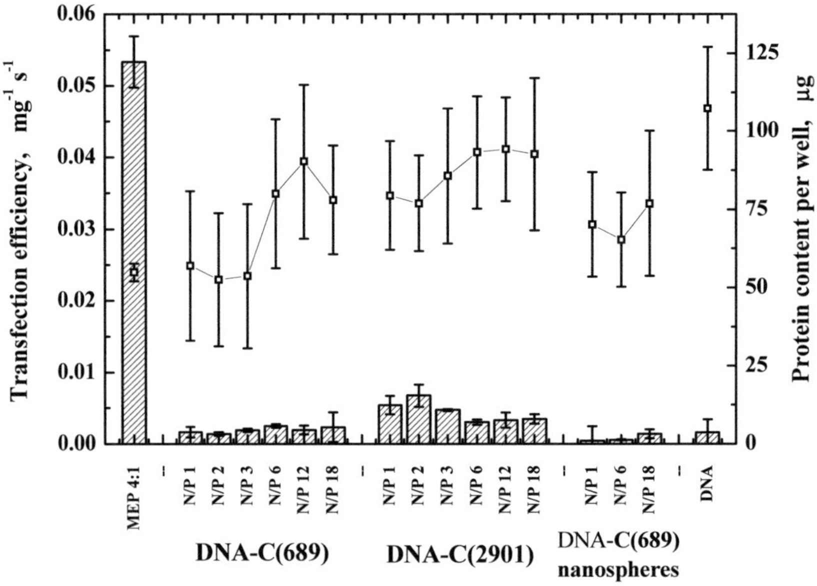

Fig. 7. Transfection efficiency of the DNA-chitosan complexes (columns) and protein content in wells after lysation (squares) vs. N/P.

Speculating that the low transfer rate of the polyplexes (compared to that of the lipoplex) might be related to cytotoxicity effects, the protein concentration was determined via the BCA assay. From figure 7 (right hand side axis) a comparable level of protein content for all formulations including the blanks was observed. Even if not totally conclusive regarding a measure of the cytotoxicity, this result shows that the cells proliferated approximately in the same way; consequently, the poor transfection efficiency shown by the DNA-chitosan polyplexes cannot be ascribed to cytotoxicity.

In the light of the transfection efficiency depicted by the polyplexes, a second kind of experiment was implemented. DNA-chitosan nanospheres were prepared following the protocol described by Mao and coworkers (Mao et al., 2001). The transfection efficiency results for C(689) are also plotted in figure 7. Compared to the polyplexes, no transfection improvement was observed, on the contrary, nanospheres in general showed a decreasing in gene expression yielding results only comparable to the naked DNA administration.

The luciferase assay was conducted in order to confirm the results obtained by the β-galactosidase assay. The transfection efficiency for all cases was similar to that observed in the β-galactosidase method. In general, naked DNA and complexes regardless of the N/P ratio and structure yielded a luminescence three orders of magnitude lower than that of the DNA–MEP lipoplex. Concerning the protein content determined by the BCA assay, the polyplexes and nanospheres rendered protein contents slightly higher than that of the DNA–MEP lipoplex (data not shown). In consequence, the transfection efficiency of polyplexes was confirmed to be low compared to that of the lipoplex.
In general, the low capacity of DNA to escape from complexes is regarded as one of the major limitations for the transfection efficiency of polyplexes (Midoux et al., 2009; Tros de Ilarduya et al., 2010). This feature has been ascribed to a number of factors. While some authors support that an excess of polycation, even in the presence of chloroquine, limits the protein expression due to in vitro cytotoxicity (Fischer et al., 2004), other authors affirm that the low tolerance of DNA to dissociate from polyplexes is presumably due to the bulky form they adopt in solution (Izumrudov et al., 1999). In our case the low transfection efficiency of the DNA–chitosan polyplexes compared to that of the lipoplex is most likely related to both the colloidal properties they exhibit and the DNA-chitosan binding affinity. On the one hand, the morphological structure depicted by TEM and AFM in conjunction with the markedly positive ζ-potentials obtained suggest a core–shell like polyplex structure with chitosan occupying the outer part of the complex (A. V. Kabanov & V. A. Kabanov, 1998). On the other hand, as mentioned before, chitosans presenting higher DNA binding affinities were found to yield lower transfection efficiencies.

2.1.7 Particular conclusions

In general, the DNA-chitosan polyplexes exhibited good colloidal properties such as sizes in the range of 180 to 250 nm, ζ-potentials of about 16 mV, and a stable core-shell like structural conformation. The influence of chitosan charge density and valence on all these physicochemical properties can be summarized as follows.

1. Role of chitosan charge density.

Chitosan charge density was found to play an important role on the complexation of DNA. Namely, as the solution pH got close to the chitosan pKa, the neutralization of the amino groups, entailing a decrease of chitosan charge density, resulted in a higher amount of chitosan needed for complexation. That is, the acidic conditions were found to be favorable for complex formation.

2. Role of chitosan valence.

Chitosan valence was found to be related to both the polyplex size and, more importantly, to the transfection efficiency. On the one hand, the hydrodynamic radii of complexes increased linearly with the chitosan Mw demonstrating that larger chitosan chains produce bulkier and less soluble polyplexes. On the other hand, in what we conceive as the main contribution of our investigations, we found that higher valence chitosans, exhibiting lower DNA binding affinities, yielded higher DNA transfection efficiencies.

2.2 The DNA-pDADMAC system

As stated before, cationic polymers most commonly studied as gene carriers include chitosan, PEI, PLL, poly(β-amino ester)s, and poly-(amidoamine) dendrimers. In addition,

because of its permanent cationic charge, poly(diallyldimethylammonium chloride) (pDADMAC) has recently been explored as well (Fischer et al., 2004; Krajcik et al., 2008).
pDADMAC is a water soluble cationic polymer. It is composed of mainly configurational isomers of pyrrolidinium rings and a small amount of pendant double bonds (Dautzenberg et al., 1998; Jaeger et al., 1996). With the pendent allylic double bonds being less reactive than those of the monomer, strictly linear macromolecules are formed at low conversions, but branching can proceed at high conversions as was demonstrated for commercial samples (Wandrey et al., 1999). Because of its physical structure pDADMAC is a highly flexible polymer compared to other polycations such as chitosan (Marcelo et al., 2005; Trzcinski et al., 2002). pDADMAC has been widely used in technical applications as a flocculant agent and as a composite for biosensors, which is because of its pH-independent cationic charge (Dautzenberg et al., 1998; Jaeger et al., 1996).

	Mw (kDa)	Label
Homopolymers	< 100	p(1, < 619)
	150	p(1, 929)
	275	p(1, 1703)
	450	p(1, 2786)
Copolymer	250	p(0.26, 668)

Table 3. pDADMACs employed. In p(x,y), x and y stand for charge density and valence, respectively.

In the present section we summarize outstanding results obtained in our laboratory describing relevant physicochemical characteristics of the DNA-pDADMAC complexes (Alatorre-Meda et al., 2010b). As done for chitosan in the previous section, we highlight the role of pDADMAC charge density and valence. Four homo-polymers (charge density = 1, with different valences) and one co-polymer, p(acrylamide-co-diallyldimethylammonium chloride) (coDADMAC) (charge density < 1, equivalent in valence to one of the homopolymers), were employed. Table 3 lists the cationic polymers characterized as gene carriers along with the nomenclature cited throughout this section.

2.2.1 DNA-pDADMAC characteristic ratios, (N/P)c and (N/P)*

Different to the chitosan system, the DNA-pDADMAC polyplexes exhibited two distinct characteristic ratios: the previously observed (N/P)c (i.e., the ratio from which DNA is compacted) and (N/P)*, an additional ratio from which the polyplexes adopt the most compact structure. Similarly to the DNA-chitosan polyplexes, (N/P)c was found to be dependent on the polycationic charge density, whereas (N/P)* proved to be a function of pDADMAC valence. Table 4 summarizes the characteristic ratios for each DNA-pDADMAC system together with the average size of the polyplexes formed (discussed in the next section). Our main findings can be described as follows.

(N/P)c was determined by means of conductometry. pDADMAC aliquots were injected to DNA and buffer solutions and the change in conductivity was recorded. Successive pDADMAC injections produced exactly the same outcome observed for the chitosan system; namely, a linear increment in conductivity for the buffer solution and an inflection in the conductivity plot for the DNA one (plots not shown). The ratio at which the conductivity inflection occurred is reported as (N/P)c (see section 2.1.1 for a complete explanation).

It is clear from table 4 that (N/P)c is governed by the charge density provided that polyplexes formed with pDADMAC homopolymers have complexation ratios lower than that of the polyplex formed with coDADMAC. This result confirms what we observed for chitosan not only with respect to the role of charge density but also regarding the (N/P)c values obtained which are very similar for both chitosan- and pDADMAC-based polyplexes (see section 2.1.1).

polymer	(N/P)c	(N/P)*	R_H (nm)
p(1, < 619)	0.7	4	79.4 + 2.1
p(1, 929)	0.6	2	87.0 + 6.9
p(1, 1703)	0.7	2	108.9 + 12.5
p(1, 2786)	0.6	1	112.6 + 9.7
p(0.26, 668)	1.5	2	199.8 + 23.5

Table 4. Characteristic N/P ratios and R_H of the DNA-pDADMAC polyplexes. (N/P)c and (N/P)* stand for the DNA compaction ratio (determined by conductometry) and for the ratio from which the size of the polyplexes remain constant (determined by DLS), respectively. R_H is the average of the recorded values in the range $(N/P)^* \leq N/P \leq 10$.

(N/P)* was found by DLS as a characteristic ratio from which the polyplexes adopt the most compact structure. As observed from table 4, the value of (N/P)* follows a decreasing trend with pDADMAC valence of the polyplexes, with p(1,619) and p(1,2786) showing the highest and the lowest (N/P)* values of 4 and 1, respectively. The interplay between (N/P)c and (N/P)* can be reasoned in terms of the different complexation states of DNA mediated by pDADMAC (Fischer et al., 2004).

2.2.2 Time stability and size

The characterization of the DNA-pDADMAC polyplexes in terms of size and time stability was carried out by means of DLS. The study was done in two steps. First, the hydrodynamic radii of the polyplexes, R_H, were determined at $0.2 \leq N/P \leq 10$. And second, the evolution of R_H with time was followed for the polyplexes at $N/P = 10$. R_H results are depicted in table 4. It is observed from table 4, that similarly to the chitosan systems, the size of the polyplexes was found to increase with pDADMAC valence, that is, the general assumption that the electrostatic interactions are outweighed to a certain extent by a decrease in the polycation solubility is confirmed (MacLaughlin et al., 1998; Mumper et al., 1995). Concerning the coDADMAC polyplex, it is clear that its size is ca. twice as big as those of the pDADMAC polyplexes. This outcome can be a consequence of an expected lower degree of DNA

compaction provided that the amount of positive charges in the polycation chain is lower, as also demonstrated for other systems encompassing non-ionic copolymers grafted to polycationic segments (Toncheva et al., 1998). Alternatively, the high hydrophilic capacity of acrylamide (AM) (Nuno-Donlucas et al., 2004) may allow larger amounts of water to be housed in the complex interior, resulting in bulkier polyplexes.
On the other hand, the time stability of the DNA-pDADMAC polyplexes was measured by following the time evolution of R_H for polyplexes at an N/P ratio of 10, as mentioned before. We observed that the sizes of the polyplexes formed with lower valence polymers remained practically constant during 7 days (ca. 85 nm). However, contrary to what we found with the chitosan systems, the DNA-p(1, 1703), -p(1, 2786), and -p(0.26, 668) polyplexes, whose initial sizes were above 100 nm, apparently underwent a structural change with time, resulting in a size reduction (data not shown). This structural rearrangement appeared to be valence-dependent since for the DNA-p(1,1703) system the size stabilization occurred from day 2 on, while for the DNA-p(1,2786) one it occurred from day 3 on. In general, it is theorized that both the branching of the pDADMAC polymer chain, expected to be present in a large extent (Wandrey et al., 1999), and the low stiffness of pDADMAC (Jaeger et al., 1989) are the main causes of such a behavior. Anyway, the final sizes of the homopolymer- and copolymer-based complexes were of ca. 85 and 120 nm, respectively.

2.2.3 Surface charge

In the present study, the ζ-potential characterization was done in the range $0.2 \leq N/P \leq 10$ for all polyplexes. Results are summarized in table 5. All polyplexes presented a positive, stable ζ-potential from N/P ratios as low as (N/P)c. As concluded for chitosan complexes, this result suggests a complete DNA compaction. Main findings are discussed below.

N/P	p(1, < 619)	p(1, 929)	p(1, 1703)	p(1, 2786)	p(0.26, 668)
0.2	-45.0 + 3.2	-44.3 + 1.9	-43.1 + 0.7	-39.9 + 3.0	-41.4 + 2.3
0.4	-44.6 + 1.4	-33.3 + 1.4	-35.4 + 2.2	-41.2 + 3.5	-35.5 + 1.3
0.6	-35.3 + 1.4	-34.3 + 3.5	-33.6 + 2.0	-40.6 + 1.3	-34.0 + 6.0
0.8	-29.0 + 5.5	-24.0 + 5.4	-16.4 + 12.0	-22.3 + 2.6	-24.0 + 1.6
1	7.7 + 0.8	10.5 + 0.8	10.1 + 0.5	11.8 + 1.1	-19.9 + 1.9
2	11.8 + 0.7	12.2 + 0.1	11.2 + 0.4	11.8 + 0.6	12.7 + 0.3
4	11.7 + 1.3	10.5 + 0.8	13.1 + 0.6	12.0 + 0.7	11.5 + 0.2
6	12.2 + 0.5	12.0 + 0.5	12.0 + 0.3	11.9 + 0.3	10.6 + 0.5
10	11.8 + 0.3	12.0 + 0.3	11.9 + 0.4	12.8 + 0.1	12.3 + 0.1

Table 5. ζ-potential of the DNA-pDADMAC polyplexes (in mV) measured at different N/P ratios.

The data in table 5 reveal that all polyplexes, regardless of pDADMAC valence, present a constant ζ-potential value of around 12 mV at N/P > (N/P)c, which is in good agreement with the chitosan systems. Of special interest for gene therapy is the fact that the presence of AM, expected to improve the polyplex biocompatibility, does not cause a decrease in the positive charge recommended for transfection. Very importantly, these constant ζ-potential values, irrespective of further addition of pDADMAC, are also suggestive of a polyplex core-shell conformation, as observed for the chitosan-mediated complexes (see section 2.1.3).

2.2.4 Structural organization

In order to illustrate the morphology of the polyplexes, tapping mode AFM in air was conducted. Figure 8 shows images of DNA polyplexes made with p(0.26, 668) (A), and with p(1, 2786) (B) at a constant ratio N/P = 10.

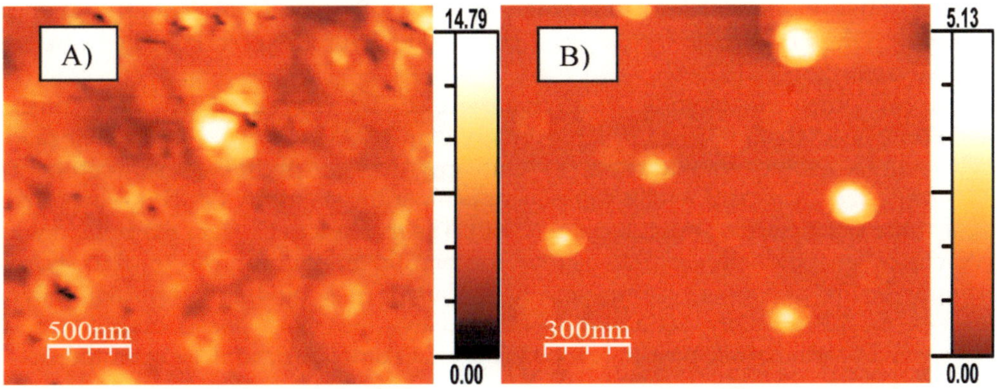

Reproduced from (Alatorre-Meda et al., 2010b) with permission of AMERICAN CHEMICAL SOCIETY in the format Journal via Copyright Clearance Center.

Fig. 8. Height AFM images of DNA polyplexes made with p(0.26, 668) (A), and with p(1, 2786) (B) at N/P = 10. Bars next to images represent the Z scale in nm.

Both figures depict high populations of well-defined toroids with sizes ranging from 125 to 250 nm and 80 to 200 nm for the DNA-p(0.26, 668) and the -p(1, 2786) polyplexes, respectively. As mentioned before, the toroidal conformation suggests a maximum DNA compaction. For the case of the pDADMAC polyplexes, this maximum DNA compaction seems logical given the permanent cationic charge of the polymer; however, for the case of the coDADMAC polyplex, such a high DNA compaction appears to be somehow counterintuitive in view of the fact that three molecules of non-ionic AM are present per each molecule of cationic charged DADMAC (Alatorre-Meda et al., 2010b). Concerning the smaller sizes depicted by AFM as compared to those displayed by DLS, it should be recalled that for the former technique the samples were dried before the measurement, that is, polyplexes apparently became dehydrated.

2.2.5 Binding affinity and complexation thermodynamics

As done for the DNA-chitosan polyplexes, ITC was performed to evaluate the DNA-pDADMAC binding affinity and complexation thermodynamics. Striking results were obtained as compared to the chitosan systems. Firstly, the DNA binding affinity of pDADMACs was found to be favored with valence; secondly, the complexation process was completed in three successive stages. Main results are discussed below.

Figure 9 shows the heat of interaction resulting from the titration of pDADMACs to DNA as a function of N/P. Three consecutive processes along the DNA-pDADMAC binding are observed. The first phase of binding occurred at N/P molar ratios lower than ~1, drawing a biphasic nature of the binding profiles for all polymers (except for p(1,<619)). As the polymer chains began to saturate the DNA, the slightly endothermic binding enthalpy decreased and reached an exothermic minimum at an N/P ratio of ~0.5. Similar slight endothermic heats have been ascribed to entropy-driven binding processes (Matulis et al., 2000; Srinivasachari et al., 2007) and ligand interactions with the DNA minor groove (Privalov et al., 2007) Concerning the reduction in the heat of interaction Q, it might result from the combination of both a decreased accessibility of binding sites to polymer molecules due to partial saturation of DNA molecules and from the dipole-dipole interactions between water molecules oriented favorably on adjacent DNA and polymer molecules (Strey et al., 1998). At this stage, bending of single DNA strand, bridging of neighboring DNA molecules by polymer chains and hydration can contribute to DNA collapse (Rau & Parsegian, 1992).

The second phase of binding was characterized by an additional post-transition endothermic heat which finished in a maximum for pDADMACs at an N/P molar ratio of ~0.75, with a subsequent decrease in enthalpy due to phosphate saturation. This endothermic heat increment with a subsequent peak or discontinuity has been suggested to represent the DNA collapse (Matulis et al., 2000). The increase in Q, from the zone in which DNA chains are partially saturated (the exothermic minimum) up to the observed maximum before phosphate saturation, is attributed to a binding of further polymer molecules to the partially saturated DNA. Finally, the third phase of binding was characterized by exothermic post-transition heats after complete phosphate saturation.

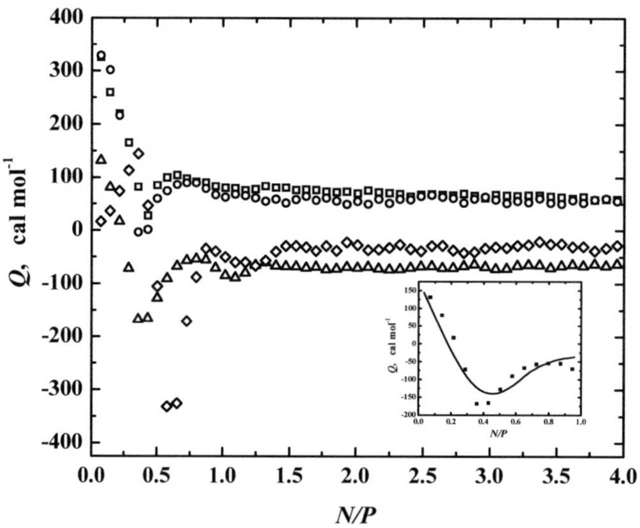

Reproduced from (Alatorre-Meda et al., 2010b) with permission of AMERICAN CHEMICAL SOCIETY in the format Journal via Copyright Clearance Center.

Fig. 9. Integrated heats of interaction of the titration of pDADMAC to DNA vs. N/P. Polymers p(1, <619) squares, p(1, 919) circles, p(1,1703) triangles, and p(1, 2786) diamonds were employed. The solid line in the inset represents the data fitting of the DNA-p(1, 1703) interaction.

Table 6 summarizes the enthalpy, entropy, binding constant, and the stoichiometry of the DNA–pDADMAC interaction derived from the data fitting of figure 9.

polymer	$K_1 \times 10^{-5}$ (M^{-1})	n_1	ΔH_1 (kcal mol^{-1})	ΔS_1 (kcal mol^{-1} K^{-1})
p(1, < 619)	1.02 ± 0.26	0.44 ± 0.12	0.26 ± 0.07	0.023
p(1, 929)	3.10 ± 0.48	0.39 ± 0.11	0.20 ± 0.07	0.026
p(1, 1703)	51.6 ± 0.31	0.28 ± 0.07	0.07 ± 0.01	0.030
p(1, 2786)	55.1 ± 0.26	0.28 ± 0.07	0.06 ± 0.01	0.031
p(0.26, 668)	1.72 ± 0.14	0.86 ± 0.13	0.17 ± 0.03	0.024
polymer	**$K_2 \times 10^{-5}$ (M^{-1})**	**n_2**	**ΔH_2 (kcal mol^{-1})**	**ΔS_2 (kcal mol^{-1} K^{-1})**
p(1, < 619)	0.06 ± 0.04	0.33 ± 0.10	2.34 ± 1.86	0.020
p(1, 929)	0.12 ± 0.07	0.26 ± 0.10	0.92 ± 0.74	0.022
p(1, 1703)	0.42 ± 0.08	0.15 ± 0.06	-0.40 ± 0.11	0.019
p(1, 2786)	0.43 ± 0.07	0.16 ± 0.06	-0.39 ± 0.11	0.020
p(0.26, 668)	0.17 ± 0.04	0.24 ± 0.04	-0.81 ± 0.07	0.020

Table 6. Thermodynamic parameters of the DNA-pDADMAC binding process. Sub-indices next to each parameter stand for the corresponding sites 1 and 2.

It can be observed from this table that the DNA binding constants obtained for all pDADMACs are on the order of 10^5-10^6 and 10^3-10^4 M^{-1} for the first and second class of binding sites, respectively. These global ranges are in good agreement with the DNA-chitosan binding data; however, it is clear that the present case exhibits an opposite behavior regarding the DNA binding affinity, namely, it increases with the polycationic valence. This opposite trend might be ascribed to the high water solubility of pDADMAC. That is, although higher valence pDADMACs produced bulkier polyplexes (see section 2.2.2), it appears that the ion-pair electrostatic interactions are not hindered at all by steric restrictions (see sections 2.1.1 and 2.1.5). On the other hand, concerning the energetic implications, the DNA binding with all polymers showed slight enthalpic contributions in both sites. This outcome depicts an entropically driven reaction typically observed in polyelectrolyte associations (Matulis et al., 2000; Prevette et al., 2007; Srinivasachari et al., 2007) where less favourable (more endothermic) ΔH values might be associated with breaking hydrogen bonds between polymer and water molecules (breaking a hydrogen bond in water corresponds to an enthalpy increase of 1.9 kcal/mol) (Silverstein et al., 2000).

2.2.6 Transfection efficiency

To determine the transfection efficiency of the DNA-pDADMAC polyplexes, we performed exactly the same protocols as those described for the chitosan systems (see section 2.1.6). Similarly to the chitosan complexes, the transfer rate of the pDADMAC polyplexes was very low compared to that of the DNA-MEP lipoplex. Even worse, polyplexes within the whole range of ratios rendered levels of β-galactosidase and luciferase expressions comparable to that of naked DNA (data not shown). Given that no cytotoxic effects can be argued

(Alatorre-Meda et al., 2010b), the low transfection efficiency demonstrated by pDADMAC (even lower than that of chitosan) might be ascribed to i) the polycation barrier occurring in the core-shell structure proposed (see section 2.1.4), ii) the high binding affinity depicted by ITC (high binding constants), and iii) the high degree of DNA compaction exhibited by the polyplexes (see sections 2.2.1 and 2.2.4).

2.2.7 Particular conclusions

In this section we described our most important findings regarding the characterization of pDADMAC as DNA carrier. In general, the DNA-pDADMAC polyplexes exhibited good colloidal properties such as sizes in the range of 80 to 200 nm, ζ-potentials of about 12 mV, and stable toroidal structural conformations. However, the transfection efficiency was found to be even lower than that of the DNA-chitosan complexes. The influence of pDADMAC charge density and valence on the physicochemical properties of the polyplexes can be summarized as follows.

1. Role of pDADMAC charge density.

pDADMAC charge density was found of play an important role on the DNA complexation ratio, (N/P)c. Our experiments demonstrated that the (N/P)c of pDADMACs polyplexes (pDADMAC charge density = 1) are lower than half the (N/P)c of the coDADMAC polyplex (coDADMAC charge density < 1).

2. Role of pDADMAC valence.

pDADMAC valence was found to increase i) the size of the polyplexes, ii) the ratio from which the sizes remain practically constant, (N/P)*, and iii) the DNA-pDADMAC binding affinity. In general, it is well accepted that higher valence polycations produce bulkier DNA polyplexes because of steric restrictions and solubility drops, giving support to our DLS results. However, our results demonstrate that the high water solubility and permanent cationic charge of pDADMAC apparently compensate such restrictions giving rise to higher binding affinities and lower (N/P)* ratios as the valence increases. Such high DNA-pDADMAC interactions proved to reduce the transfection efficiency (at least compared to the chitosan-mediated complexes). Finally, in what time stability concerns, higher valence pDADMACs were found to provoke a polyplex size reduction with time. This structural rearrangement may be related to both the branching of the pDADMAC polymer chain, expected to be present in a large extent, and the low stiffness of pDADMAC.

2.3 The DNA-MEP system

Metafectene® Pro (MEP) is a liposomal formulation that encompasses a mixture of a polyamine-lipid as the cationic group (average molecular weight of the repeat unit of 272.26 g mol^{-1}) and DOPE as the helper lipid. It belongs to a new class of transfection reagents based on the Repulsive Membrane Acidolysis technology (RMA) developed by Biontex laboratories GmbH (Bonetta 2005). Based on its high efficiency as transfection vector toward eukaryotic cells (Aluigi et al., 2007; Ibrahim & Kim, 2008; Kwon & Kim, 2008; Spinosa et al., 2008), MEP has been routinely used in our laboratories as a positive blank for DNA transfection assays. As observed in previous sections, compared to polyplexes formed with polycations chitosan and pDADMAC, the DNA-MEP lipoplexes yielded transfection rates markedly higher; therefore, it was of our interest to characterize the DNA-MEP complexation process from a physicochemical point of view attempting to elucidate the reason why of such a big difference in the transfection efficiencies.

The present section details the physical chemistry characterization of the interactions of MEP with DNA around the mass ratio recommended for transfection (L/D ~ 700). Aiming to establish a more general conclusion about the DNA-polyelectrolyte interactions, the experimental conditions implemented (salt concentration in buffer, pH, and temperature) were chosen to be similar to the other systems previously studied (Alatorre-Meda et al., 2010a). For simplicity and in order to use units consistent with the protocols established for transfection, all characterizations presented in this section are expressed in terms of the liposome to DNA mass ratio, L/D. Main results are exposed below.

2.3.1 MEP to DNA complexation ratio, (L/D)c

As done for chitosan polyplexes, the DNA-MEP complex formation was addressed via SLS. Depicted by a sharp increase in the scattering intensity, we determined the complexation ratio as (L/D)c ~ 600. Our main findings are described below.

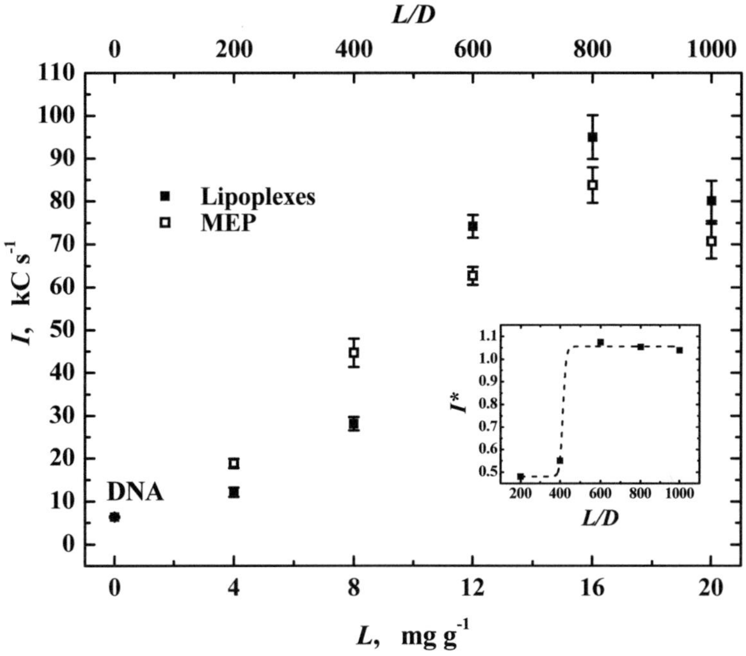

Reproduced from (Alatorre-Meda et al., 2010a) by permission of the PCCP Owner Societies.

Fig. 10. Average intensity of light scattered, I, by lipoplexes (filled squares) and by MEP (empty squares) as a function of the mass ratio L/D, and of the concentration L, respectively. The average intensity of light scattered by DNA is also included. The inset shows the average intensity scattered by lipoplexes normalized to the sum of the intensities scattered by MEP and by DNA in separate. The dotted line is a guide for the eye.

Figure 10 depicts the average intensity of the light scattered by lipoplexes as a function of the mass ratio L/D, and by MEP solutions in absence of DNA as a function of the concentration L. This figure shows that at L/D ~ 600 the intensity of light scattered by lipoplexes is roughly 50% lower than that scattered by their corresponding MEP solutions, whereas for (L/D) ≥ 600 this trend shifts, becoming higher the intensities scattered by the lipoplexes. An increment like this in the light scattered was observed along the DNA-

chitosan complexation process (see section 2.1.1). In that case, the increment in the scattering was attributed to the change in the particle structure, where the intensity of light scattered by the collapsed polymeric chains was confirmed to be higher than that scattered by the linear chains of DNA and chitosan before mixing. Nevertheless, in the present case the hydrodynamic radius of MEP scarcely changed after its mixing with DNA (see the following section), suggesting no change either in its vesicular conformation or in the coil conformation of DNA. Therefore, in our opinion the increase in intensity in the zone of $L/D \geq 600$ can only be explained in terms of a constructive interference that presumably arises when liposomes are connected one to each other by DNA coils (see section 2.3.4), where contrary to moving freely they start to move in ensemble. This assumption becomes clearer when the normalized intensity of the lipoplexes, ($I^* = I_{lipoplex}/(I_{DNA} + I_{MEP})$), is plotted as a function of the mass ratios (inset in Fig. 10).
The inset shows two well differentiated regions, one for $L/D < 600$ where DNA and MEP are expected not to interact, and other for $(L/D) \geq 600$ where, in good agreement with the zone suggested by Biontex Laboratories GmbH and demonstrated by transfection assays (Aluigi, et al., 2007; Ibrahim & Kim, 2008; Kwon & Kim, 2008; Spinosa et al., 2008), complexation occurs. On the other hand, the lowest intensity exhibited by pure DNA, as aforementioned, is a behavior characteristic of linear molecules in solution which are hardly detected by SLS (Drifford & Dalbiez, 1984).

2.3.2 Size and time stability

Particle sizes of both MEP and lipoplexes were measured via DLS in order to be compared. We found that the size of the MEP vesicles was equivalent to that of the lipoplexes, with the latter ones being slightly smaller (ca. 135 nm). It appears then, that as DNA comes in contact with MEP, the polyanion acts as a stabilizer of the liposomes, a result that has been observed for other polymer-vesicle interactions (Antunes et al., 2009; Rodriguez-Pulido et al., 2008). Very importantly, compared to the other DNA–cationic vector formulations here studied, in particular to the DNA–chitosan system (R_H up to 450 nm), the sizes depicted by the DNA–MEP complexes are considerably lower. This is believed to facilitate the cellular uptake (Tros de Ilarduya, et al., 2010).
To check the stability of the lipoplexes, we measured the time evolution of R_H of samples with $L/D \geq (L/D)c$. The magnitude of R_H during the testing time (7 days) changed less than a 10% in all cases, with the mean value and standard deviation lowering as the value of L/D increased (data not shown). Thus, the lipoplexes were validated as stable.

2.3.3 Surface charge

In order to elucidate the lipoplex charge at the transfection conditions, we studied the ζ-potential of the lipoplexes around the mass ratio recommended for transfection. To our surprise, the ζ-potential of the lipoplexes at the transfection conditions resulted to be negative (data not shown). This striking result finds support on the lipoplex structural conformation we detected by TEM and AFM (see next section) showing non-complexed DNA segments. Alternatively, as reported by others (Dias et al., 2002; Radler et al., 1997; Salditt et al., 1997), there must be a coexistence of DNA and lipoplexes in which, provided the negative ζ-potential, DNA is expected to be in excess.
Compared to cationic lipoplexes, negatively charged ones should offer advantages of decreased cytotoxicity and increased serum compatibility (Thakor et al., 2009); however, as

mentioned before, their cell internalization is problematic. Cell internalization of negatively charged particles often requires the presence of cell-specific ligands (attached to particle surface) for endocytosis to occur. Such ligands build the "bridge" between cellular membranes and particles otherwise absent in view of the electrostatic repulsions (Kono et al., 2001; Sahay et al., 2010; Simoes et al., 1998). By contrast, anionic particles not bearing cell-specific ligands are expected to enter cells during mitosis[3] (Khalil et al., 2006).

2.3.4 Structural organization

Figure 11 presents typical TEM (A and B) and AFM (C and D) images obtained for lipoplexes at L/D = 1000. This figure depicts non aggregated liposomes with DNA coils coming out from their surfaces seemingly connecting them; a feature that is more easily observed in the zooms shown in panels B and D. Such a morphology, referred to as the "beads on a string" conformation, has been observed not only for DNA-vesicle systems but also for DNA-micellar aggregates (Ruozi et al., 2007; Wang et al., 2007). In general, this structural conformation, occurring at low lipid to DNA ratios, is believed to appear because of packing and bending constraints on the long DNA molecules (Dan, 1998). Of importance for gene therapy, the exposed DNA sections are covered by a metastable, cylindrical lipid bilayer that protects DNA from inactivation or degradation (Sternberg et al., 1994).

2.3.5 Transfection efficiency

As observed in previous sections, compared to polyplexes formed with polycations chitosan and pDADMAC, the DNA-MEP lipoplex yielded transfection rates markedly higher. We speculate that the higher transfection efficiency of the MEP lipoplex must be related to a successful endosomal escape that is promoted simultaneously by a repulsive membrane acidolysis process and different conformational transitions adopted by DOPE upon pH changes (Bonetta 2005; Khalil et al., 2006; Tros de Ilarduya et al., 2010). Concerning the cell entrance mechanism our lipoplexes should display, we hypothesize mitosis as the most probable option given both the negative ζ-potential of the system and that, to our best knowledge, MEP does not contain any kind of cell-receptors. In this context, HeLa cells (the cells we worked with) are recognized as highly proliferating ones (Ota, et al.,2010). Importantly, as part of our protocols we seeded the cells at an 80-90% optical confluence so that transfection was practiced with the maximum possible number of healthy cells, assuring mitosis.[4]

2.3.6 Particular conclusions

Emphasizing the importance of studying the lipoplex formation under the same conditions at which transfection is practiced, our results point to a "beads on a string" complex conformation as depicted by i) the TEM and AFM micrographs revealing coils of DNA coming out from vesicle surface, ii) the ζ-potential results showing that the transfection mass ratios are well below isoneutrality, and iii) the practically constant vesicle sizes after complexation depicted by DLS. On the other hand, a sharp increase in the intensity of light

[3] Mitosis is also accepted as an important factor in the nuclear translocation of transgenes given that the integrity of the nuclear membrane is transiently lost, allowing their entrance (Khalil et al, 2006).

[4] It has to be noted that this very reasoning should be applied to the chitosan- and pDADMAC-mediated polyplexes.

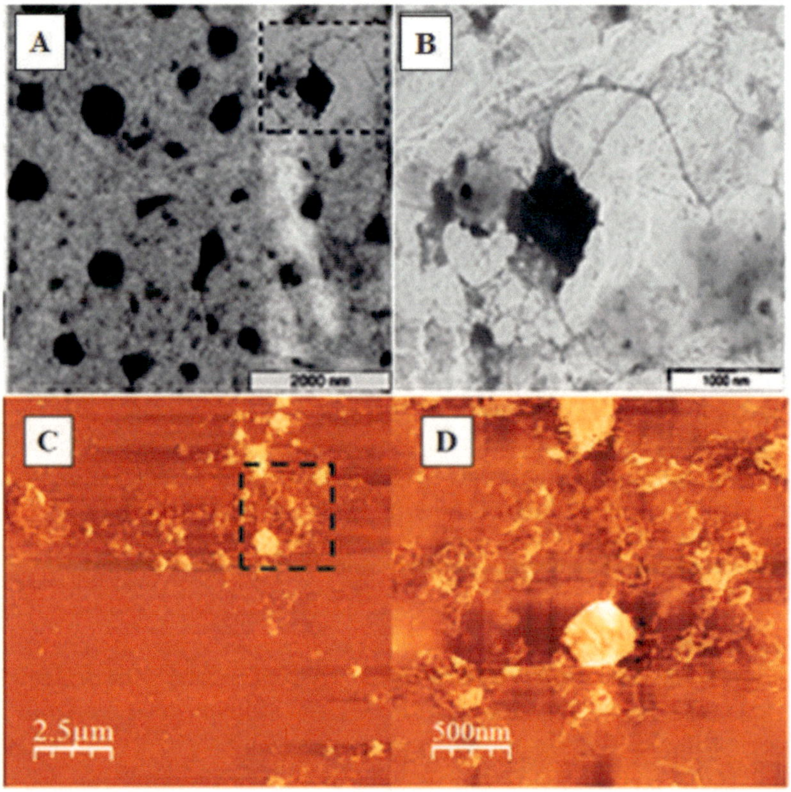

Reproduced from (Alatorre-Meda et al., 2010a) by permission of the PCCP Owner Societies.

Fig. 11. Typical TEM (A and B) and AFM (C and D) images obtained for DNA-MEP lipoplexes at L/D = 1000.

scattered by samples marks (L/D)c ~ 600 as the zone from which lipoplexes exist, validating the mass ratio recommended for transfection of (L/D) ~ 700. Finally, DLS results reveal lipoplexes with an average size of 135 nm that were stable within at least 7 days.

3. General conclusions and forthcoming work

In general, the DNA-chitosan and DNA-pDADMAC systems revealed good colloidal properties and similar physicochemical features as compared one to each other. They were able to condense DNA plasmids to form particles small and positive enough so as to be taken up to cells by endocytosis; however, the transfection efficiency they rendered was markedly lower than that of the DNA-MEP lipoplex. With the experimental results here presented it appears that this low transfection efficiency relies on the high DNA-polycation binding affinity coupled with the structural conformation the polyplexes adopt in solution. Additionally, repulsive membrane acidolysis processes and different conformational transitions adopted by DOPE upon pH changes confer the MEP lipoplex a successful endosomal escape not occurring during polyplex transfection.

In light of the obtained results a deeper understanding of both the complex internalization to cells and DNA release from complexes to the cytoplasm must, in our opinion, be achieved in order to improve the transfection process. In the context of the DNA release, special attention needs be paid to the development of strategies assuring a high degree of DNA-vector de-compaction. Interesting pioneering results stem from publications by González-Pérez and coworkers (Carlstedt et al., 2010; Gonzalez-Perez & Dias, 2009; Gonzalez-Perez et al., 2008).

4. Acknowledgment

M. A.-M. thanks the Ramón Areces foundation for his Post-Doctoral fellowship (Research project: 2010/CL509).

5. References

Alatorre-Meda, M.; González-Pérez, A. & Rodriguez, J. R. (2010). "DNA-Metafectene™ PRO complexation: A physical chemistry study. *Phys. Chem. Chem. Phys.*, Vol. 12, No. 27, (July 2010), pp. 7464-7472, ISSN 1463-9076.

Alatorre-Meda, M.; Taboada, P.; Hartl, F.; Wagner, T.; Freis, M. & Rodríguez, J. R. (2011). The influence of chitosan valence on the complexation and transfection of DNA: The weaker the DNA-chitosan binding the higher the transfection efficiency. *Colloids and Surfaces B: Biointerfaces,* Vol. 82, No. 1, (January 2011), pp. 54-62, ISSN 0927-7765.

Alatorre-Meda, M.; Taboada, P.; Krajewska, B.; Willemeit, M.; Deml, A.; Klösel, R. & Rodríguez, J. R. (2010). DNA-Poly(diallyldimethylammonium chloride) complexation and transfection efficiency. *J. Phys. Chem. B,* Vol. 114, No. 29, (July 2010), pp. 9356-9366, ISSN 1520-6106.

Alatorre-Meda, M.; Taboada, P.; Sabin, J.; Krajewska, B.; Varela, L. M. & Rodriguez, J. R. (2009). DNA-chitosan complexation: A dynamic light scattering study. *Colloids and Surfaces A: Physicochemical and Engineering Aspects,* Vol. 339, No. 1-3, (May 2009), pp. 145-152, ISSN 0927-7757.

Aluigi, M. G.; Hofreiter, S.; Falugi, C.; Pestarino, M. & Candiani, S. (2007). Efficiency of two different transfection reagents for use with human NTERA2 cells. *European Journal of Histochemistry,* Vol. 51, No. 4, (October 2007), pp. 301-304, ISSN 1121-760X.

Anderson, W. F. (1990). September 14, 1990: The beginning. *Human Gene Therapy,* Vol. 1, No. 4, (n.d. 1990), pp. 371-372, ISSN 1043-0342.

Antunes, F. E.; Marques, E. F.; Miguel, M. G. & Lindman, B. (2009). Polymer-vesicle association. *Advances in Colloid and Interface Science,* Vol. 147-48, No. Sp. Iss. SI, (March 2009), pp. 18-35, ISSN 0001-8686.

Arakawa, H.; Umemura, K. & Ikai, A. (1992). Protein images obtained by STM, AFM and TEM. *Nature,* Vol. 358, No. 6382, (July 1992) pp. 171-&, ISSN 0028-0836.

Battersby, B. J.; Grimm, R.; Huebner, S. & Cevc, G. (1998). Evidence for three-dimensional interlayer correlations in cationic lipid-DNA complexes as observed by cryo-electron microscopy. *Biochimica Et Biophysica Acta: Biomembranes,* Vol. 1372, No. 2, (July 1998), pp. 379-383, ISSN 0005-2736.

Behr, J. P. (1997). The proton sponge: A trick to enter cells the viruses did not exploit. *Chimia,* Vol. 51, No. 1-2, (January 1997), pp. 34-36, ISSN 0009-4293.

Bharadwaj, S.; Montazeri, R. & Haynie, D. T. (2006). Direct determination of the thermodynamics of polyelectrolyte complexation and implications thereof for electrostatic layer-by-layer assembly of multilayer films. *Langmuir,* Vol. 22, No. 14, (July 2006), pp. 6093-6101, ISSN 0743-7463.

Bloomfield, V. A. (1997). DNA condensation by multivalent cations. *Biopolymers,* Vol. 44, No. 3, (n.d. 1997), pp. 269-282, ISSN 0006-3525.

Bonetta, L. (2005). The inside scoop-evaluating gene delivery methods. *Nature Methods,* Vol. 2, No. 11, (November 2005), pp. 875-+, ISSN 1548-7091.

Boussif, O.; Lezoualch, F.; Zanta, M. A.; Mergny, M. D.; Scherman, D.; Demeneix, B. & Behr, J. P. (1995). A versatile vector for gene and oligonucleotide transfer into cells in culture and in-vivo: polyethylenimine. *PNAS,* Vol. 92, No. 16, (August 1995), pp. 7297-7301, ISSN 0027-8424.

Carlstedt, J.; Gonzalez-Perez, A.; Alatorre-Meda, M.; Dias, R. S. & Lindman, B. (2010). Release of DNA from surfactant complexes induced by 2-hydroxypropyl-beta-cyclodextrin. *International Journal of Biological Macromolecules,* Vol. 46, No. 2, (March 2010), pp. 153-158, ISSN 0141-8130.

Carnerup, A. M.; Ainalem, M. L.; Alfredsson, V. & Nylander, T. (2009). Watching DNA condensation induced by poly(amido amine) dendrimers with Time-Resolved Cryo-TEM. *Langmuir,* Vol. 25, No. 21, (November 2009), pp. 12466-12470, ISSN 0743-7463.

Dan, N. (1998). The structure of DNA complexes with cationic liposomes: cylindrical or flat bilayers? *Biochimica Et Biophysica Acta: Biomembranes,* Vol. 1369, No. 1, (February 1998), pp. 34-38, ISSN 0005-2736.

Danielsen, S.; Varum, K. M. & Stokke, B. T. (2004). Structural analysis of chitosan mediated DNA condensation by AFM: Influence of chitosan molecular parameters. *Biomacromolecules,* Vol. 5, No. 3, (May 2004), pp. 928-936, ISSN 1525-7797.

Dautzenberg, H.; Gornitz, E. & Jaeger, W. (1998). Synthesis and characterization of poly(diallyldimethylammonium chloride) in a broad range of molecular weight. *Macromolecular Chemistry and Physics,* Vol. 199, No. 8, (August 1998), pp. 1561-1571, ISSN 1022-1352.

de Kruif, C. G.; Weinbreck, F. & de Vries, R. (2004). Complex coacervation of proteins and anionic polysaccharides. *Current Opinion in Colloid & Interface Science,* Vol. 9, No. 5, (December 2004), pp. 340-349, ISSN 1359-0294.

De Smedt, S. C.; Demeester, J. & Hennink, W. E. (2000). Cationic polymer based gene delivery systems. *Pharmaceutical Research,* Vol. 17, No. 2, (February 2000), pp. 113-126, ISSN 0724-8741.

Dias, R. S.; Innerlohinger, J.; Glatter, O.; Miguel, M. G. & Lindman, B. (2005). Coil-globule transition of DNA molecules induced by cationic surfactants: A dynamic light scattering study. *J. Phys. Chem. B,* Vol. 109, No. 20, (May 2005), pp. 10458-10463, ISSN 1520-6106.

Dias, R. S.; Lindman, B. & Miguel, M. G. (2002). DNA interaction with catanionic vesicles. *J. Phys. Chem. B,* Vol. 106, No. 48, (December 2002), pp. 12600-12607, ISSN 1520-6106.

Dias, R. S.; Pais, A. A. C. C..; Miguel, M. G. & Lindman, B. (2003). Modeling of DNA compaction by polycations. *Journal of Chemical Physics,* Vol. 119, No. 15, (October 2003), pp. 8150-8157, ISSN 0021-9606.

Dowty, M. E.; Williams, P.; Zhang, G. F.; Hagstrom, J. E. & Wolff, J. A. (1995). Plasmid DNA entry into postmitotic nuclei of primary rat myotubes. *PNAS,* Vol. 92, No. 10, (May 1995), pp. 4572-4576, ISSN 0027-8424.

Drifford, M. & Dalbiez, J. P. (1984). Light-scattering by dilute-solutions of salt-free polyelectrolytes. *Journal of Physical Chemistry*, Vol. 88, No. 22, (n.d. 1984), pp. 5368-5375, ISSN 0022-3654.

Engler, L. E.; Welch, K. K. & JenJacobson, L. (1997). Specific binding by EcoRV endonuclease to its DNA recognition site GATATC. *Journal of Molecular Biology*, Vol. 269, No. 1, (May 1997), pp. 82-101, ISSN 0022-2836.

Felgner, P. L.; Gadek, T. R.; Holm, M.; Roman, R.; Chan, H. W.; Wenz, M.; Northrop, J. P.; Ringold, G. M. & Danielsen, M. (1987). Lipofection: A highly efficient, lipid-mediated DNA-transfection procedure. *PNAS*, Vol. 84, No. 21, (November 1987), pp. 7413-7417, ISSN 0027-8424.

Fischer, D.; Dautzenberg, H.; Kunath, K. & Kissel, T. (2004). Poly(diallyldimethylammonium chlorides) and their N-methyl-N-vinylacetamide copolymer-based DNA-polyplexes: Role of molecular weight and charge density in complex formation, stability, and in vitro activity. *International Journal of Pharmaceutics*, Vol. 280, No. 1-2, (August 2004), pp. 253-269, ISSN 0378-5173.

Gershon, H.; Ghirlando, R.; Guttman, S. B. & Minsky, A. (1993). Mode of formation and structural features of DNA cationic liposome complexes used for transfection. *Biochemistry*, Vol. 32, No. 28, (July 1993), pp. 7143-7151, ISSN 0006-2960.

Gonzalez-Perez, A. & Dias, R. S. (2009). Different strategies for controlling DNA conformation: Compaction and decompaction. *FBS*, Vol. E1, (June 2009), pp. 228-241, ISSN 1945-0494.

Gonzalez-Perez, A.; Dias, R. S.; Nylander, T. & Lindman, B. (2008). Cyclodextrin-surfactant complex: A new route in DNA decompaction. *Biomacromolecules*, Vol. 9, No. 3, (March 2008), pp. 772-775, ISSN 1525-7797.

Haensler, J. & Szoka, F. C. (1993). Polyamidoamine cascade polymers mediate efficient transfection of cells in culture. *Bioconjugate Chemistry*, Vol. 4, No. 5, (September 1993), pp. 372-379, ISSN 1043-1802.

Huang, M.; Fong, C. W.; Khor, E. & Lim, L. Y. (2005). Transfection efficiency of chitosan vectors: Effect of polymer molecular weight and degree of deacetylation. *Journal of Controlled Release*, Vol. 106, No. 3, (September 2005), pp. 391-406, ISSN 0168-3659.

Ibrahim, A. M. A. & Kim, Y. (2008). Transient expression of protein tyrosine phosphatases encoded in Cotesia plutellae bracovirus inhibits insect cellular immune responses. *Naturwissenschaften*, Vol. 95, No. 1, (January 2008), pp. 25-32, ISSN 0028-1042.

Izumrudov, V. A.; Zhiryakova, M. V. & Kudaibergenov, S. E. (1999). Controllable stability of DNA-containing polyelectrolyte complexes in water-salt solutions. *Biopolymers*, Vol. 52, No. 2, (n.d. 1999), pp. 94-108, ISSN 0006-3525.

Jaeger, W.; Gohlke, U.; Hahn, M.; Wandrey, C. & Dietrich, K. (1989). Synthesis and application of flocculating agents. *Acta Polymerica*, Vol. 40, No. 3, (March 1989), pp. 161-170, ISSN 0323-7648.

Jaeger, W.; Hahn, M.; Lieske, A.; Zimmermann, A. & Brand, F. (1996). Polymerization of water soluble cationic vinyl monomers. *Macromolecular Symposia*, Vol. 111, (December 1996), pp. 95-106, ISSN 1022-1360.

Kabanov, A. V. & Kabanov, V. A. (1998). Interpolyelectrolyte and block ionomer complexes for gene delivery: Physicochemical aspects. *Advanced Drug Delivery Reviews*, Vol. 30, No. 1-3, (March 1998), pp. 49-60, ISSN 0169-409X.

Ke, J. H. & Young T. H. (2010). Multilayered polyplexes with the endosomal buffering polycation in the core and the cell uptake-favorable polycation in the outer layer for enhanced gene delivery. *Biomaterials*, Vol. 31, No. 35, (December 2010), pp. 9366-9372, ISSN 0142-9612.

Khalil, I. A.; Kogure, K.; Akita, H. & Harashima, H. (2006). Uptake pathways and subsequent intracellular trafficking in nonviral gene delivery. *Pharmacological Reviews*, Vol. 58, No. 1, (March 2006), pp. 32-45, ISSN 0031-6997

Koltover, I.; Salditt, T.; Radler, J. O. & Safinya, C. R. (1998). An inverted hexagonal phase of cationic liposome-DNA complexes related to DNA release and delivery. *Science*, Vol. 281, No. 5373, (July 1998), pp. 78-81, ISSN 0036-8075.

Kono, K.; Torikoshi, Y.; Mitsutomi, M.; Itoh, T.; Emi, N.; Yanagie, H. & Takagishi, T. (2001). Novel gene delivery systems: complexes of fusigenic polymer-modified liposomes and lipoplexes. *Gene Therapy*, Vol. 8, No. 1, (January 2001), pp. 5-12, ISSN 0969-7128.

Koping-Hoggard, M.; Mel'nikova, Y. S.; Varum, K. M.; Lindman, B. & Artursson, P. (2003). Relationship between the physical shape and the efficiency of oligomeric chitosan as a gene delivery system in vitro and in vivo. *Journal of Gene Medicine*, Vol. 5, No. 2, (February 2003), pp. 130-141, ISSN 1099-498X.

Krajcik, R.; Jung, A.; Hirsch, A.; Neuhuber, W. & Zolk, O. (2008). Functionalization of carbon nanotubes enables non-covalent binding and intracellular delivery of small interfering RNA for efficient knock-down of genes. *Biochemical and Biophysical Research Communications*, Vol. 369, No. 2, (May 2008), pp. 595-602, ISSN 0006-291X.

Kucherlapati, R. & Skoultchi, A. I. (1984). Introduction of purified genes into mammalian-cells. *Crc Critical Reviews in Biochemistry*, Vol. 16, No. 4, (n.d. 1984), pp. 349-379, ISSN 0045-6411.

Kumar, M. N. V. R.; Muzzarelli, R. A. A.; Muzzarelli, C.; Sashiwa, H. & Domb, A. J. (2004). Chitosan chemistry and pharmaceutical perspectives. *Chemical Reviews*, Vol. 104, No.12, (December 2004), pp. 6017-6084, ISSN 0009-2665.

Kwon, B. & Kim, Y. (2008). Transient expression of an EP1-like gene encoded in Cotesia plutellae bracovirus suppresses the hemocyte population in the diamondback moth, Plutella xylostella. *Developmental and Comparative Immunology*, Vol. 32, No. 8, (n.d. 2008), pp. 932-942, ISSN 0145-305X.

Lasic, D. D.; Strey, H.; Stuart, M. C. A.; Podgornik, R. & Frederik, P. M. (1997). The structure of DNA-liposome complexes. *JACS*, Vol. 119, No. 4, (January 1997), pp. 832-833, ISSN 0002-7863.

Lavertu, M.; Methot, S.; Tran-Khanh, N. & Buschmann, M. D. (2006). High efficiency gene transfer using chitosan/DNA nanoparticles with specific combinations of molecular weight and degree of deacetylation. *Biomaterials*, Vol. 27, No. 27, (September 2006), pp. 4815-4824, ISSN 0142-9612.

Lin, A. C. & Goh, M. C. (2002). Investigating the ultrastructure of fibrous long spacing collagen by parallel atomic force and transmission electron microscopy. *Proteins-Structure Function and Genetics*, Vol. 49, No. 3, (November 2002), pp. 378-384, ISSN 0887-3585.

Lubyphelps, K.; Castle, P. E.; Taylor, D. L. & Lanni, F. (1987). Hindered diffusion of inert tracer particles in the cytoplasm of mouse 3T3 cells. *PNAS*, Vol. 84, No. 14, (July 1987), pp. 4910-4913, ISSN 0027-8424.

Lynn, D. M. & Langer, R. (2000). Degradable poly(β-amino esters): Synthesis, characterization, and self-assembly with plasmid DNA. *JACS,* Vol. 122, No. 44, (November 2000), pp. 10761-10768, ISSN 0002-7863.

MacLaughlin, F. C.; Mumper, R. J.; Wang, J. J.; Tagliaferri, J. M.; Gill, I.; Hinchcliffe, M. & Rolland, A. P. (1998). Chitosan and depolymerized chitosan oligomers as condensing carriers for in vivo plasmid delivery. *Journal of Controlled Release*, Vol. 56, No. 1-3, (December 1998), pp. 259-272, ISSN 0168-3659.

Mancheño-Corvo, P. & Martín-Duque, P. (2006). Viral gene therapy. *Clinical and Translational Oncology*, Vol. 8, No. 12, (n.d. 2006), pp. 858-867, ISSN 1699-048X.

Manning, G. S. (1978). Molecular theory of polyelectrolyte solutions with applications to electrostatic properties of polynucleotides. *Quarterly Reviews of Biophysics*, Vol. 11, No. 2, (n.d. 1978), pp. 179-246, ISSN 0033-5835.

Mao, H. Q.; Roy, K.; Troung-Le, V. L.; Janes, K. A.; Lin, K. Y.; Wang, Y.; August, J. T. & Leong, K. W. (2001). Chitosan-DNA nanoparticles as gene carriers: Synthesis, characterization and transfection efficiency. *Journal of Controlled Release,* Vol. 70, No. 3, (February 2001), pp. 399-421, ISSN 0168-3659.

Marcelo, G.; Tarazona, M. P. & Saiz, E. (2005). Solution properties of poly (diallyldimethylammonium chloride) (PDDA). *Polymer,* Vol. 46, No. 8, (March 2005), pp. 2584-2594, ISSN 0032-3861.

Matulis, D.; Rouzina, I. & Bloomfield, V. A. (2000). Thermodynamics of DNA binding and condensation: Isothermal titration calorimetry and electrostatic mechanism. *Journal of Molecular Biology*, Vol. 296, No. 4, (March 2000), pp. 1053-1063, ISSN 0022-2836.

Maurstad, G.; Danielsen, S. & Stokke, B. T. (2007). The influence of charge density of chitosan in the compaction of the polyanions DNA and xanthan. *Biomacromolecules*, Vol. 8, No. 4, (April 2007), pp. 1124-1130, ISSN 1525-7797.

Midoux, P.; Pichon, C.; Yaouanc, J. J. & Jaffres, P. A. (2009). Chemical vectors for gene delivery: A current review on polymers, peptides and lipids containing histidine or imidazole as nucleic acids carriers. *British Journal of Pharmacology,* Vol. 157, No. 2, (May 2009), pp. 166-178, ISSN 0007-1188.

Miguel, M. G.; Pais, A. A. C. C.; Dias, R. S.; Leal, C.; Rosa, M. & Lindman, B. (2003). DNA-cationic amphiphile interactions. *Colloids and Surfaces A: Physicochemical and Engineering Aspects*, Vol. 228, No. 1-3, (November 2003), pp. 43-55, ISSN 0927-7757.

Milev, S.; Bosshard, H. R. & Jelesarov, I. (2005). Enthalpic and entropic effects of salt and polyol osmolytes on site-specific protein-DNA association: The integrase Tn916-DNA complex. *Biochemistry,* Vol. 44, No. 1, (January 2005), pp. 285-293, ISSN 0006-2960.

Mumper, R. J.; Wang, J. J.; Claspell, J. M. & Rolland, A. P. (1995). Novel polymeric condensing carriers for gene delivery. *Proceedings of the International Symposium on Controlled Release Bioactive Materials*, Vol. 22, pp. 178-179.

Nguyen, D. N.; Green, J. J.; Chan, J. M.; Longer, R. & Anderson, D. G. (2009). Polymeric materials for gene delivery and DNA vaccination. *Advanced Materials,* Vol. 21, No. 8, (February 2009), pp. 847-867, ISSN 0935-9648.

Nisha, C. K.; Manorama, S. V.; Ganguli, M.; Maiti, S. & Kizhakkedathu, J. N. (2004). Complexes of poly(ethylene glycol)-based cationic random copolymer and calf thymus DNA: A complete biophysical characterization. *Langmuir*, Vol. 20, No. 6, (March 2004), pp. 2386-2396, ISSN 0743-7463.

Nuno-Donlucas, S. M.; Sanches-Diaz, J. C.; Rabelero, M.; Cortes-Ortega, J.; Luhrs-Olmos, C. C.; Fernandez-Escamilla, V. V.; Mendizabal, E. & Puig, J. E. (2004). Microstructured polyacrylamide hydrogels made with hydrophobic nanoparticles. *Journal of Colloid and Interface Science*, Vol. 270, No. 1, (February 2004), pp. 94-98, ISSN 0021-9797.

O'Connor, T. P. & Crystal, R. G. (2006). Genetic medicines: Treatment strategies for hereditary disorders. *Nature Reviews Genetics*, Vol. 7, No. 4, (April 2006), pp. 261-276, ISSN 1471-0056.

Ogris, M.; Steinlein, P.; Kursa, M.; Mechtler, K.; Kircheis, R. & Wagner, E. (1998). The size of DNA/transferrin-PEI complexes is an important factor for gene expression in cultured cells. *Gene Therapy*, Vol. 5, No. 10, (October 1998), pp. 1425-1433, ISSN 0969-7128.

Orth, P.; Weimer, A.; Kaul, G.; Kohn, D.; Cucchiarini, M. & Madry, H. (2008). Analysis of novel nonviral gene transfer systems for gene delivery to cells of the musculoskeletal system. *Molecular Biotechnology*, Vol. 38, No. 2, (February 2008), pp. 137-144, ISSN 1073-6085.

Ota, K.; Matsumiya, T.; Sakuraba, H.; Imaizumi, T.; Yoshida, H.; Kawaguchi, S.; Fukuda, S. & Satoh, K. (2010). Interferon-α2b induces $p21^{cip1/waf1}$ degradation and cell proliferation in HeLa cells. *Cell Cycle*, Vol. 9, No. 1, (January 2010), pp. 131-139, ISSN 1538-4101.

Prevette, L. E.; Kodger, T. E.; Reineke, T. M. & Lynch, M. L. (2007). Deciphering the role of hydrogen bonding in enhancing pDNA-Polycation interactions. *Langmuir*, Vol. 23, No. 19, (September 2007), pp. 9773-9784, ISSN 0743-7463.

Privalov, P. L.; Dragan, A. I.; Crane-Robinson, C.; Breslauer, K. J.; Remeta, D. P. & Minetti, C. (2007). What drives proteins into the major or minor grooves of DNA? *Journal of Molecular Biology*, Vol. 365, No. 1, (January 2007), pp. 1-9, ISSN 0022-2836.

Radler, J. O.; Koltover, I.; Salditt, T. & Safinya, C. R. (1997). Structure of DNA-cationic liposome complexes: DNA intercalation in multilamellar membranes in distinct interhelical packing regimes. *Science*, Vol. 275, No. 5301, (February 1997), pp. 810-814, ISSN 0036-8075.

Rau, D. C. & Parsegian, V. A. (1992). Direct measurement of the intermolecular forces between counterion-condensed DNA double helices: Evidence for long-range attractive hydration forces. *Biophysical Journal*, Vol. 61, No. 1, (January 1992), pp. 246-259, ISSN 0006-3495.

Rejman, J.; Oberle, V.; Zuhorn, I. S. & Hoekstra, D. (2004). Size-dependent internalization of particles via the pathways of clathrin-and caveolae-mediated endocytosis. *Biochemical Journal*, Vol. 377 (January 2004), pp. 159-169, ISSN 0264-6021.

Rodriguez-Pulido, A.; Aicart, E.; Llorca, O. & Junquera, E. (2008). Compaction process of calf thymus DNA by mixed cationic-zwitterionic liposomes: A physicochemical study. *J. Phys. Chem. B*, Vol. 112, No. 7, (February 2008), pp. 2187-2197, ISSN 1520-6106.

Ruozi, B.; Tosi, G.; Leo, E. & Vandelli, M. A. (2007). Application of atomic force microscopy to characterize liposomes as drug and gene carriers. *Talanta*, Vol. 73, No. 1, (August 2007), pp. 12-22, ISSN 0039-9140.

Sahay, G.; Alakhova, D. Y. & Kabanov, A. V. (2010). Endocytosis of nanomedicines. *Journal of Controlled Release*, Vol. 145, No. 3, (August 2010), pp. 182-195, ISSN 0168-3659.

Salditt, T.; Koltover, I.; Radler, J. O. & Safinya, C. R. (1997). Two-dimensional smectic ordering of linear DNA chains in self-assembled DNA-cationic liposome mixtures. *PRL*, Vol. 79, No. 13, (September 1997), pp. 2582-2585, ISSN 0031-9007.

Sarraguca, J. M. G. & Pais, A. A. C. C. (2006). Polyelectrolytes in solutions with multivalent salt. Effects of flexibility and contour length. *Phys. Chem. Chem. Phys.*, Vol. 8, No. 36, (n.d. 2006), pp. 4233-4241, ISSN 1463-9076.

Schaffer, D. V.; Fidelman, N. A.; Dan, N. & Lauffenburger, D. A. (2000). Vector unpacking as a potential barrier for receptor-mediated polyplex gene delivery. *Biotechnology and Bioengineering*, Vol. 67, No. 5, (March 2000), pp- 598-606, ISSN 0006-3592.

Silverstein, K. A. T.; Haymet, A. D. J. & Dill, K. A. (2000). The strength of hydrogen bonds in liquid water and around nonpolar solutes. *JACS*, Vol. 122, No. 33, (August 2000), pp. 8037-8041, ISSN 0002-7863.

Simberg, D.; Weisman, S.; Talmon, Y. & Barenholz, Y. (2004). DOTAP (and other cationic lipids): Chemistry, biophysics, and transfection. *Critical Reviews in Therapeutic Drug Carrier Systems*, Vol. 21, No. 4, (n.d. 2004), pp. 257-317, ISSN 0743-4863.

Simoes, S.; Slepushkin, V.; Gaspar, R.; de Lima, M. C. P. & Duzgunes, N. (1998). Gene delivery by negatively charged ternary complexes of DNA, cationic liposomes and transferrin or fusigenic peptides. *Gene Therapy*, Vol. 5, No. 7, (July 1998), pp. 955-964, ISSN 0969-7128.

Spinosa, M. R.; Progida, C.; De Luca, A.; Colucci, A. M. R.; Alifano, P. & Bucci, C. (2008). Functional characterization of Rab7 mutant proteins associated with Charcot-Marie-Tooth type 2B disease. *Journal of Neuroscience*, Vol. 28, No. 7, (February 2008), pp. 1640-1648, ISSN 0270-6474.

Srinivasachari, S.; Liu, Y. M.; Prevette, L. E. & Reineke, T. M. (2007). Effects of trehalose click polymer length on pDNA complex stability and delivery efficacy. *Biomaterials*, Vol. 28, No. 18, (June 2007), pp. 2885-2898, ISSN 0142-9612.

Sternberg, B.; Sorgi, F. L. & Huang, L. (1994). New structures in complex-formation between DNA and cationic liposomes visualized by freeze-fracture electron-microscopy. *Febs Letters*, Vol. 356, No. 2-3, (December 1994), pp. 361-366, ISSN 0014-5793.

Strand, S. P.; Lelu, S.; Reitan, N. K.; de Lange Davies, C.; Artursson, P. & Varum, K. M. (2010). Molecular design of chitosan gene delivery systems with an optimized balance between polyplex stability and polyplex unpacking. *Biomaterials*, Vol. 31, No. 5, (February 2010), pp. 975-87, ISSN 1878-5905.

Strey, H. H.; Podgornik, R.; Rau, D. C. & Parsegian, V. A. (1998). DNA-DNA interactions. *Current Opinion in Structural Biology*, Vol. 8, No. 3, (June 1998), pp. 309-313, ISSN 0959-440X.

Tang, M. X. & Szoka, F. C. (1997). The influence of polymer structure on the interactions of cationic polymers with DNA and morphology of the resulting complexes. *Gene Therapy*, Vol. 4, No. 8, (August 1997), pp. 823-832, ISSN 0969-7128.

Thakor, D. K.; Teng, Y. D. & Tabata, Y. (2009). Neuronal gene delivery by negatively charged pullulan-spermine/DNA anioplexes. *Biomaterials*, Vol. 30, No. 9, (March 2009), pp. 1815-1826, ISSN 0142-9612.

Thomas, M. & Klibanov, A. M. (2003). Non-viral gene therapy: polycation-mediated DNA delivery. *Applied Microbiology and Biotechnology*, Vol. 62, No. 1, (July 2003), pp. 27-34, ISSN 0175-7598.

Toncheva, V.; Wolfert, M. A.; Dash, P. R.; Oupicky, D.; Ulbrich, K.; Seymour, L. W. & Schacht, E. H. (1998). Novel vectors for gene delivery formed by self-assembly of DNA with poly(L-lysine) grafted with hydrophilic polymers. *Biochimica Et Biophysica Acta: General Subjects*, Vol. 1380, No. 3, (May 1998), pp. 354-368, ISSN 0304-4165.

Tros de Ilarduya, C.; Sun, Y. & Düzgünes, N. (2010). Gene delivery by lipoplexes and polyplexes. *European Journal of Pharmaceutical Sciences*, Vol. 40, No. 3, (June 2010), pp. 159-170, ISSN 0928-0987.

Trzcinski, S.; Varum, K. M.; Staszewska, D. U.; Smidsrod, O. & Bohdanecky, M. (2002). Comparative studies on molecular chain parameters of chitosans and poly(diallyldimethylammonium chloride): The stiffness B-parameter and the temperature coefficient of intrinsic viscosity. *Carbohydrate Polymers*, Vol. 48, No. 2, (May 2002), pp. 171-178, ISSN 0144-8617.

Verma, I. M. & Somia, N. (1997). Gene therapy: Promises, problems and prospects. *Nature*, Vol. 389, No. 6648, (September 1997), pp. 239-242, ISSN 0028-0836.

Wagner, E.; Cotten, M.; Foisner, R. & Birnstiel, M. L. (1991). Transferrin polycation DNA complexes: The effect of polycations on the structure of the complex and DNA delivery to cells. *PNAS*, Vol. 88, No. 10, (May 1991), pp. 4255-4259, ISSN 0027-8424.

Wandrey, C.; Hernandez-Barajas, J. & Hunkeler, D. (1999). Diallyldimethylammonium chloride and its polymers. *Radical Polymerisation Polyeletrolytes*, Vol. 145, (n.d. 1999), pp. 123-182, ISSN 0065-3195.

Wang, C. Z.; Li, X. F.; Wettig, S. D.; Badea, I.; Foldvari, M. & Verrall, R. E. (2007). Investigation of complexes formed by interaction of cationic gemini surfactants with deoxyribonucleic acid. *Phys. Chem. Chem. Phys.*, Vol. 9, No. 13, (n.d. 2007), pp. 1616-1628, ISSN 1463-9076.

Wilson, R. W. & Bloomfield, V. A. (1979). Counterion-induced condensation of deoxyribonucleic acid. A light-scattering study. *Biochemistry*, Vol. 18, No. 11, (May 1979), pp. 2192-2196, ISSN 0006-2960.

Wu, G. Y. & Wu, C. H. (1987). Receptor-mediated in vitro gene transformation by a soluble DNA carrier system. *JBC*, Vol. 262, No. 10, (April 1987), pp. 4429-4432.

Ziady, A. G.; Ferkol, T.; Dawson, D. V.; Perlmutter, D. H. & Davis, P. B. (1999). Chain length of the polylysine in receptor-targeted gene transfer complexes affects duration of reporter gene expression both in vitro and in vivo. *JBC*, Vol. 274, No. 8, (February 1999), pp. 4908-4916, ISSN 0021-9258.

17

Medical Polymer-Based Gene Therapy

Hu-Lin Jiang[1], You-Kyoung Kim[2], Chong-Su Cho[2]
and Myung-Haing Cho[1,3,4,5,6]
[1]*College of Veterinary Medicine, Seoul National University*
[2]*Department of Agricultural Biotechnology and Research Institute for Agriculture and Life Sciences, Seoul National University*
[3]*Department of Nanofusion Technology*
Graduate School of Convergence Science and Technology, Seoul National University
[4]*Advanced Institute of Convergence Technology, Seoul National University*
[5]*Graduate Group of Tumor Biology, Seoul National University*
[6]*Center for Food Safety and Toxicology, Seoul National University*
Korea

1. Introduction

Gene therapy provides great opportunities for treatment of diseases resulting from genetic disorders, infections, and cancer (Park, et al., 2006). Gene therapy has also been regarded as a suitable substitute for conventional protein therapy, since it can overcome inherent problems associated with administration of protein drugs in terms of bioavailability, systemic toxicity, *in vivo* clearance rate, and manufacturing cost (Ledley, 1996). Gene therapy refers to local or systemic administration of a nucleic acid construct capable of prevention, treatment, and even cure of disease through change of expression of genes responsible for the pathological condition (Bhavsar & Amiji, 2007). In theory, gene therapy is a simple concept that holds great promise as a cure for disease. However, in practice, considerable obstacles need to be overcome, including problems associated with safe and efficient gene delivery and stable gene expression. Many problems need to be solved in development of any gene therapy approach, including definition of cells that constitute the target, entry of DNA into those cells, expression of useful levels of gene product over an appropriate time period, and avoidance of the almost inevitable response of the host to the introduced materials, and so on (Grosshans, 2000, Smith, 1995).

Current gene therapy consists of two key factors: a gene that encodes a specific therapeutic protein, and a gene delivery system that controls delivery of gene expression plasmids to specific locations within the body (Mahato, et al., 1999, Park, et al., 2006). Due to several problems, including their instability in body fluids, non-specificity to target cells, degradation by enzymes, and low transfection efficiency, the lack of effective vectors is a major barrier to progress in gene therapy. Therefore, the ideal gene delivery method will be capable of high efficiency transfection of genes to a specific cell type; delivery to the nucleus, where it will become integrated into the host genome in a non-mutagenic fashion and be expressed or regulated; efficient transduction of cells, independent of the mitotic potential of the recipient; be non-infectious, non-toxic, and non-immunogenic; and be easy to manufacture and apply clinically (Chaum & Hatton, 2002).

Vehicles for gene delivery can be divided into two major groups: viral and non-viral vectors. Although such viral vectors have been commonly employed in clinical trials due to their high transfection efficiency, compared with non-viral vectors (Quong & Neufeld, 1998), their application to the human body is often frustrated by immunogenicity, potential infectivity, complicated production, and inflammation (Smith, 1995). Non-viral vectors involving use of cationic polymer and cationic lipid based carriers continue to enjoy a high profile due to the advantages offered by these systems, including safety, lower immunogenicity, and the ability to transfer larger DNA molecules, when compared with viruses (Anderson, 1998, Brown, et al., 2001). Previous efforts have focused primarily on cationic liposomes, such as *N*-[1-(2,3-dioleyloxy)propyl]-*N,N,N*-trimethyl ammonium chloride (DOTMA) (Felgner, et al., 1987), *N*-[1-(2,3-dioleoyloxy) propyl]-*N,N,N*-trimethyl ammonium ethyl sulphate (DOTAP) (Alexander & Akhurst, 1995), dimethylaminoethane-carbamoyl cholesterol (DC-Chol) and/or dioleoyl phosphatidylethanolamine (DOPE) (Farhood, et al., 1995) which incorporate with DNA and are transferred effectively into cell membranes. However, the major limitation of liposomes is their fast elimination from the bloodstream and localization in the reticuloendothelial system, primarily Kupfer cells of liver (Klibanov, et al., 1990). In addition, DNA/liposome complexes have been restricted due to cellular toxicity. Cellular changes, including cell shrinkage, reduced number of mitoses, and vacuolization of the cytoplasm (Friend, et al., 1996, Lappalainen, et al., 1994) and consequently leading to cell death via the apoptosis pathway, caused by lipoplexes, already been reported (Nguyen, et al., 2007). An alternative approach to development of non-viral vectors has been proposed for cationic polymers. In general, cationic polymers are widely accepted because of their ability for efficient condensation of DNA and interaction with cells due to the charge interaction between positively charged polymer/DNA complexes and negatively charged cellular membranes. Polymer/DNA complexes are more stable than those involving cationic lipids. In addition, they protect DNA against nuclease degradation (Jiang, et al., 2007, Jiang, et al., 2009).
Therefore, the objective of this chapter was to summarize the use of medical polymers, such as cyclodextrin, chitosan, polyethylenimine, poly(β-amino ester)s (PAEs), and their derivatives as non-viral vectors in the area of gene therapy.

2. Medical polymer-based gene therapy

2.1 Cyclodextrin

Cyclodextrins (CDs) are naturally occurring cyclic oligosaccharides composed of (1-4)-linked glucose units arising from enzymatic degradation of starch, which have been approved by the FDA for use as food additives (Mellet, et al., 2011). CDs comprised of 6, 7, and 8 glucose units are called α-, β-, and γ-CDs, respectively. Table. 1 shows the chemical structure and properties of α-, β-, and γ-CDs.
They feature a basket-shaped topology in which glucose hydroxyls orient to the outer space flanking the upper and lower rims, while methinic protons (H-5 and H-3), which point to the inner cavity cup-shaped cyclic oligomers of glucose, can form inclusion complexes with small, hydrophobic molecules (Forrest, et al., 2005). Due to their unique capability for formation of inclusion complexes in inner cavities, as well as many other favourable physicochemical and biological properties, natural CDs, and their derivatives have been applied in both drug delivery systems (Loftsson, et al., 2005, Uekama, et al., 1998) and gene delivery systems (Challa, et al., 2005, Dass, 2002, Redenti, et al., 2001).
The capability of CDs and their derivatives to interact with nucleotides is of great importance for exploitation of their properties of increasing resistance to nucleases as well

as delivery of genes. CDs can improve cellular uptake of genes and can also delay their degradation by increasing their stability against endonucleases. Zhao et al. reported that CDs can increase the cellular uptake of phosphorothioate ODNs (Zhao, et al., 1995). Cellular uptake of ^{35}S- and fluorescence-labeled antisense agents has been studied in human T cell leukemia cell lines (H9, CEM, or Molt-3) in the presence of CDs, including α-, β-, γCD, methyl-βCD, trimethyl sulfated βCD, HPγCD, HPβCD, hydroxyethyl βCD (HECD), trimethyl, sulfated βCD, and a mixture of various HPβCDs. Cellular uptake was found to be concentration and time dependent in the presence of CDs, and up to a two- and three-fold increase in cellular uptake was observed within 48 h. Interaction between βCD and cellular cholesterol in living cells was well reviewed by Zidovetzki et al. (Zidovetzki & Levitan, 2007). CDs can solve many of the problems associated with *in vivo* delivery of genetic materials, such as their limited ability to extravasate from the blood stream and traverse cellular membranes, high degree of susceptibility to endonucleases with potential toxicity of their breakdown products, polyanionic nature leading to nonspecific interactions with extracellular and intracellular cationic molecules, and potential immunogenicity (Challa, et al., 2005). For further efficient gene delivery, CDs were conjugated with cationic polymers. The most important feature of the CD-containing cationic polymer gene delivery system is that formation of polyplexes between polymers and DNA can be further modified by formation of inclusion complexes, since there are a large number of CD moieties (Davis & Brewster, 2004, Pack, et al., 2005). The first example of cationic polymers containing β-CD in the polymer backbone for gene delivery was reported by Davis and co-workers (Gonzalez, et al., 1999). β-CD containing cationic polymers efficiently condensed DNA to small particles and showed nontoxic and high gene transfection efficiency. The same group has developed a set of such CD-containing polymers and studied the structural effects of the polymers on gene delivery (Popielarski, et al., 2003, Reineke & Davis, 2003, 2003). In general, the CD-containing cationic polymers showed lower cytotoxicity and efficient gene transfection *in vitro*.

Chemical structure	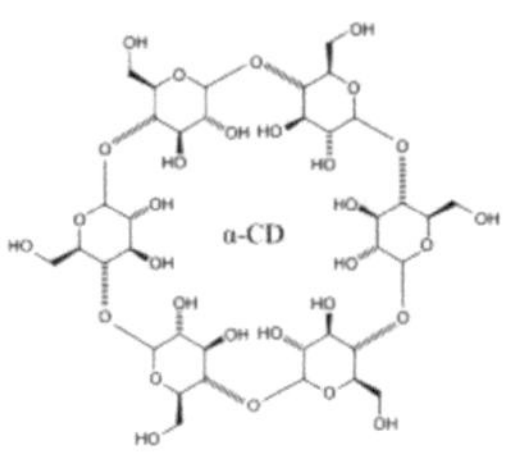	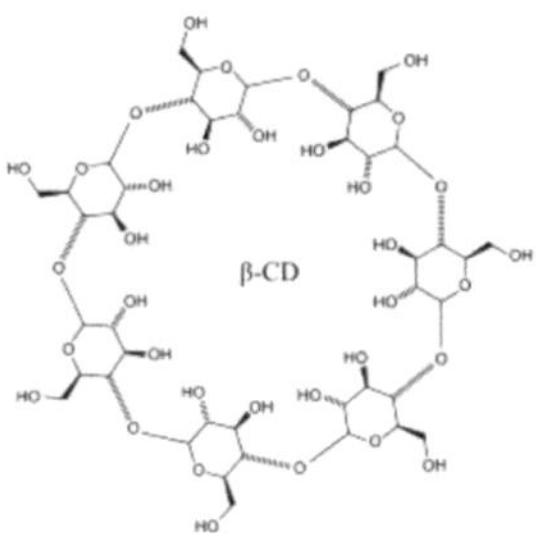	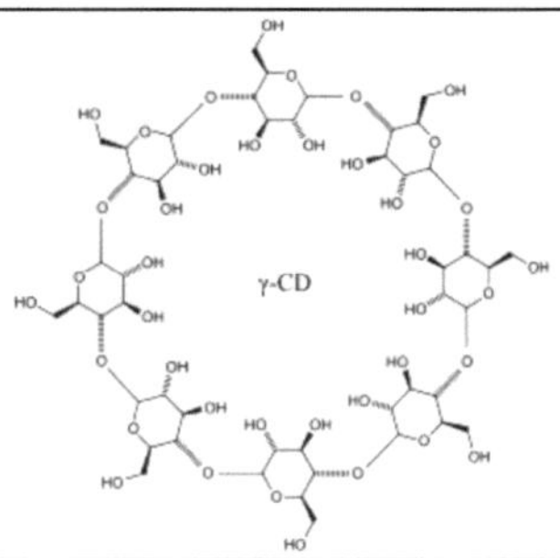
Cavity diameter (Å)	4.7 - 5.3	6.0 - 6.5	7.5 - 8.3
Molecular weight (Da)	972	1135	1297
Solubility (g/100 mL)	14.5	1.85	23.2

Table 1. Chemical structures and characterizations of CDs. CDs comprised of 6, 7, and 8 glucose units are called α-, β-, and γ-CDs, respectively.

The Uekama group synthesized dendrimer conjugates with α-, β-, and γ-CDs [Fig. 1], in anticipation of the following synergic effect; i.e., (1) dendrimer has the ability to complex with plasmid DNA (pDNA) and to enhance cellular uptake of pDNA and (2) CDs have a disruptive effect on biological membranes by complexation with membrane constituents, such as phospholipids and cholesterols (Arima, et al., 2001). Dendrimer-conjugated CD (CDE) provided the greatest transfection activity (approximately 100 times higher than those of dendrimer alone and the physical mixture of dendrimer and α-CD) in NIH3T3 fibroblasts and RAW264.7 macrophage cells (Arima, et al., 2001).

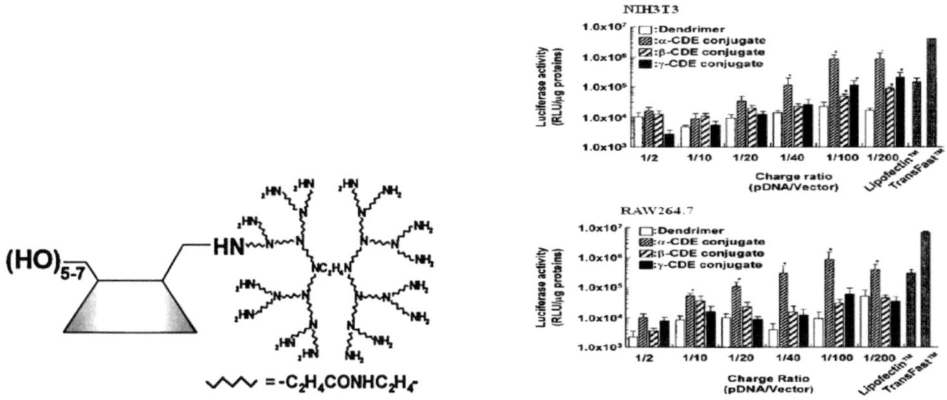

Fig. 1. Chemical structure of dendrimer-conjugated CD (left) and transfection efficiency of the complexes of pDNA/dendrimer or pDNA/CDE conjugates complexes at various charge ratios (right). [Source from Ref. (Arima, et al., 2001)].

They also studied the effect of dendrimer structure on gene transfection efficiency by preparation of CDEs with different dendrimer generations (Kihara, et al., 2002). The generation3 (G3) CDE showed the highest gene expression levels. More recently, the same group developed a lactose moiety-bearing CDE (Lac-α-CDE) for hepatocyte targeting (Arima, et al., 2010). Lac-α-CDE provided higher gene transfer activity than jetPEI™-Hepatocyte to hepatocytes with significantly fewer changes of blood chemistry values 12 h after intravenous administration in mice.

As shown in Fig. 2, Pun et al. synthesized linear and branched poly(ethylenimines) (PEIs) grafted with β-CD (CD-lPEI and CD-bPEI, respectively) by reaction of a mono-tosylated cyclodextrin with PEI amines and evaluated gene delivery ability as non-viral gene delivery agents *in vitro* and *in vivo* (Pun, et al., 2004).

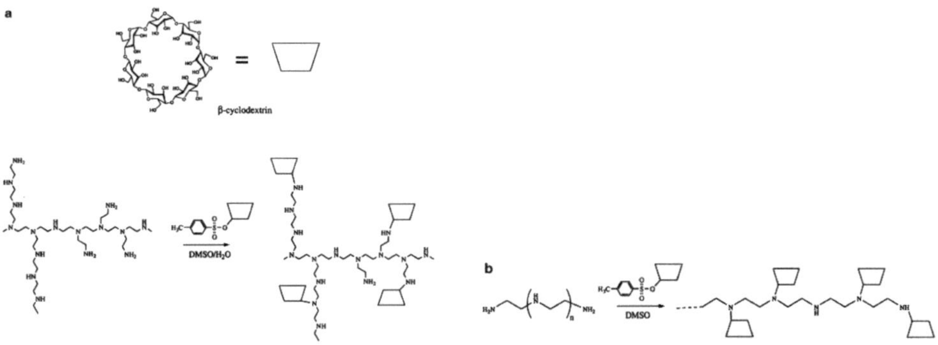

Fig. 2. (a) Synthesis of β-CD-bPEI. (b) Synthesis of β-CD-lPEI. [Source from Ref. (Pun, et al., 2004)].

Transfection efficiency of the polymers was impaired as cyclodextrin grafting increased, and toxicity was affected by cyclodextrin grafting due to the increasing polymer solubility, by capping primary amines, or by reducing polycation binding affinity [Fig. 3].

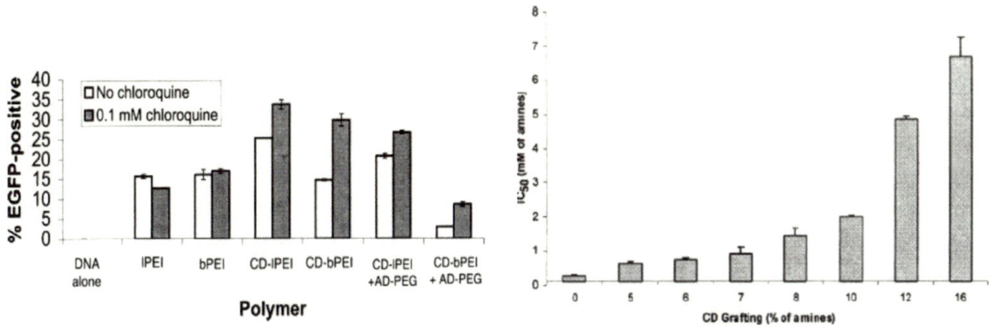

Fig. 3. Comparison of transgene expression from PEI and CD-PEI polymers in the presence or absence of 0.1 mM chloroquine (left) and effect of cyclodextrin grafting on CD-bPEI toxicity to PC3 cells (right). [Source from Ref. (Pun, et al., 2004)].

Recently, Huang et al. also used CDs for crosslinking of low MW branched PEI (MW 600) in order to form high MW cationic polymers (average MW 61K), which displayed lower cytotoxicity and high gene transfection in cultured cells (Huang, et al., 2006). As shown in Fig. 4, a series of new cationic star polymers were also synthesized by conjugation of multiple oligoethylenimine (OEI) arms onto an α-CD core as non-viral gene delivery vectors (Yang, et al., 2007).

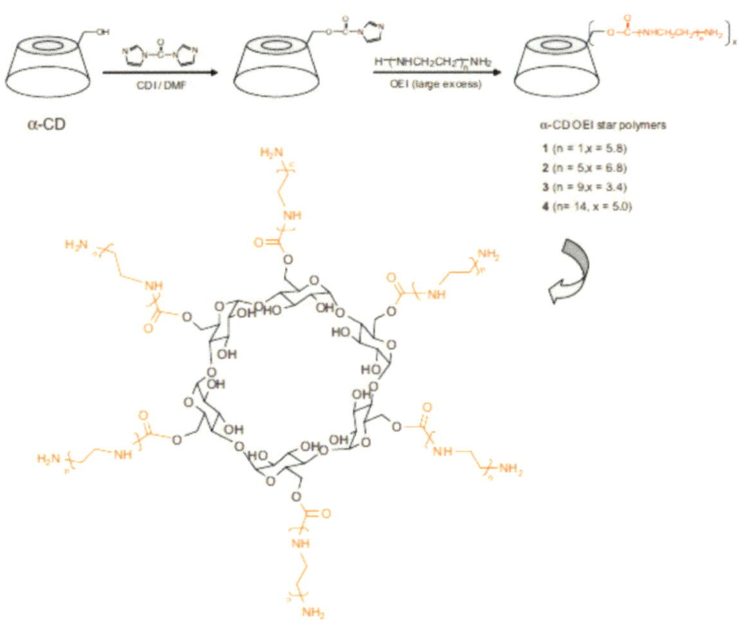

Fig. 4. Synthesis procedures and the structures of α-CD-OEI star polymers. [Source from Ref. (Yang, et al., 2007)].

All of the α-CD-OEI star polymers inhibited migration of pDNA on agarose gel through formation of complexes with pDNA, and the complexes formed nanoparticles with sizes ranging from 100-200 nm at N/P ratios of 8 or higher. Star polymers displayed much lower *in vitro* cytotoxicity than that of branched PEI 25 kD. α-CD-OEI star polymers showed excellent gene transfection efficiency in HEK293 and Cos7 cells. In general, transfection efficiency increased with an increase in OEI arm length. Star polymers with longer and branched OEI arms showed higher transfection efficiency. α-CD-OEI star polymers with different OEI arms have shown promise as new non-viral gene delivery vectors with low cytotoxicity and high gene transfection efficiency for use in future gene therapy applications.

In summary, CD-conjugated polymeric gene carriers showed enhanced transfection efficiency and reduced cytotoxicity, suggesting that CD is a material of potential interest for use in non-viral gene therapy, because these CD-conjugated polymeric gene delivery systems have been evaluated extensively in animal studies as well as clinical trials.

2.2 Chitosan

Chitosan [Fig. 5], a (1→4) 2-amino-2-deoxy-β-D-glucan, is a linear cationic polysaccharide derived by partial alkaline deacetylation of chitin, a polymer abundant in nature. The backbone of chitosan consists of two subunits, D-glucosamine and N-acetyl-D-glucosamine (Muzzarelli, 1997). It is a biocompatible, biodegradable polycationic polymer, which has minimum immunogenicity and low cytotoxicity (Mansouri, et al., 2004). Therefore, chitosan and chitosan derivatives may represent potentially safe cationic carriers for use in gene delivery.

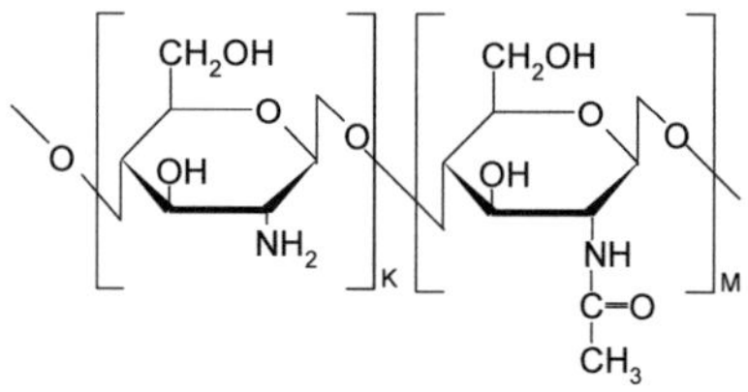

Fig. 5. Chemical structure of chitosan.

Factors including the degree of deacetylation, molecular weight, and charge of chitosan, and the media pH are important in determination of the transfection efficiency of polyplexes containing chitosan and DNA (Huang, et al., 2005, Ishii, et al., 2001, Lavertu, et al., 2006). The increased degree of deacetylation resulted in an increased level of DNA binding ability, and high transgene expression due to higher charge density along the chain (Kiang, et al., 2004, Lavertu, et al., 2006, Saranya, et al., 2011). The effect of the molecular weight of chitosan on complex formulation with DNA can be attributed to the chain entanglement effect (Kiang, et al., 2004). Chain entanglement contributes less to complex formulation as the molecular weight of chitosan decreases. The high molecular weight of chitosan resulted in easier entanglement of free DNA once the initial electrostatic interaction had occurred (Kiang, et al., 2004). Huang et al. reported that low molecular weight chitosan was less efficient at retaining DNA upon dilution, and, consequentially, less capable of protecting condensed DNA from degradation by DNase and serum components, and resulted in low transfection efficiency (Huang, et al., 2005). At acidic pH, below 5.5 or so, the primary amines in chitosan become positively charged due to the pKa value of chitosan around 6.3-6.4 (Li, et al., 1996). At this acidic pH, the primary amine groups are protonated, resulting in a cationic polymer of high charge density, which can form stable complexes with plasmid DNA, protecting DNA from nuclease degradation (Mao, et al., 2001).

N,N,N-trimethyl chitosan chloride (TMC) was synthesized in order to induce an increase of charge density and solubility of chitosan at physiological pH. TMC induced more effective condensation of DNA at physiological pH, compared with chitosan, and the transfection efficiency of TMC/DNA complex showed a 30-fold increase over that of chitosan/DNA (Thanou, et al., 2002). Of particular interest, the presence of fetal calf serum (FCS) did not affect the transfection efficiency of the chitoplexes, whereas the transfection efficiency of DOTAP-DNA complexes was decreased. Cells remained approximately 100% viable in the presence of chitosan oligomers, whereas viability of DOTAP treated cells decreased to about 50% in both cell lines (Thanou, et al., 2002). In addition, folate conjugated TMC (folate-TMC) was recently studied as a target gene delivery carrier (Zheng, et al., 2009). Transfection efficiency of folate-TMC/pDNA complexes in KB cells and SKOV3 cells (folate receptor over-expressing cell lines) increased with increasing N/P ratio and was enhanced up to 1.6-fold and 1.4-fold, compared with that of TMC/pDNA complexes; however, no significant difference was observed between transfection efficiencies of the two complexes in A549 cells and NIH/3T3 cells (folate receptor deficient cell lines), indicating that the increase in transfection efficiencies of folate-TMC/pDNA complexes were attributed to folate receptor mediated endocytosis (Zheng, et al., 2009).

PEGylation of proteins, drugs, and liposomes has been proven to be an effective approach in extending circulation in the blood stream (Patel, 1992). Therefore, in order to reduce the aggregation of complexes and increase circulation time, Jiang et al. synthesized and characterized chitosan-g-PEG [Fig. 6] as a gene carrier (Jiang, et al., 2006).

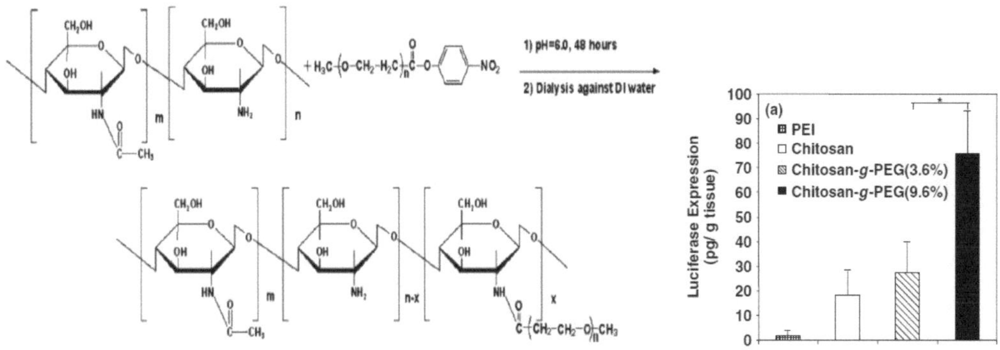

Fig. 6. Sythesis of chitosan-g-PEG polymers (left) and luciferase expression in rat liver after infusion of the complexes from common bile duct (right). [Source from Ref. (Jiang, et al., 2006)].

PEG grafting to chitosan efficiently shields the positive charge on the surface of chitosan/DNA complexes, improving particle stability in bile and serum; therefore, higher transfection efficiency was observed after infusion of the complexes through the bile duct [Fig. 6]. Chitosan-g-PEG mediated 3-fold higher luciferase expression in the liver than unmodified chitosan following intrabiliary infusion. Chitosan-g-PEG also exhibited slightly lower acute toxicity to the liver than chitosan.

Although chitosan showed good properties as a non-viral gene carrier, low transfection efficiency and low cell specificity of chitosan need to be overcome for clinical trials. Many research studies have been conducted for enhancement of transfection efficiency, such as pH-sensitive modification (Jiang, et al., 2007, Jones, et al., 2003, Kim, et al., 2003, Wong, et al., 2006), temperature-sensitive modification (Cho, et al., 2004, Dang, et al., 2006, Sun, et al., 2005), specific target ligand modification (Hashimoto, et al., 2006, Kim, et al., 2004, Kim, et al., 2006, Mansouri, et al., 2006, Wu & Wu, 1998, Zhang, et al., 2006) and so on. Among the chemical modifications of chitosan, PEI grafted chitosan showed some benefit due to high transfection efficiency. Wong et al. prepared PEI-graft-chitosan [Fig. 7] through cationic polymerization of aziridine in the presence of water-soluble oligo-chitosan (Wong, et al., 2006).

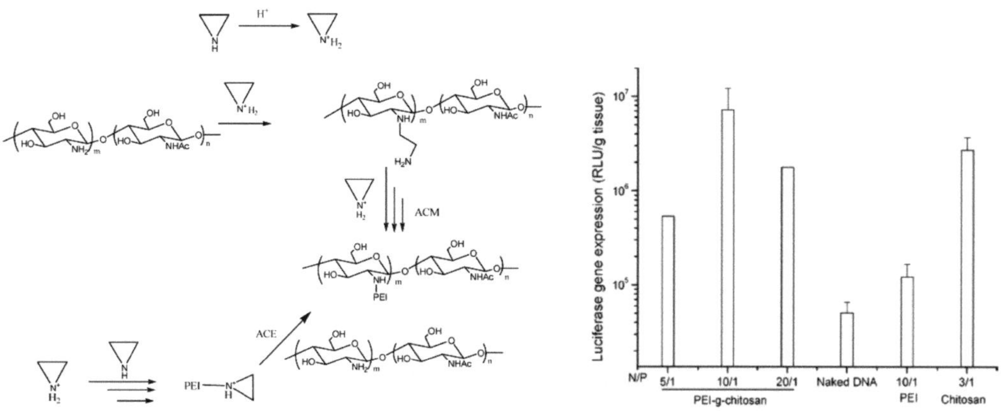

Fig. 7. Preparation of PEI-g-chitosan (left) and in vivo transfection efficiency of the complexes of PEI-g-chitosan/DNA in comparison with that of PEI (25 kDa) and chitosan after administration into common bile duct in rat liver (right). [Source from Ref. (Wong, et al., 2006)].

Results indicated that PEI-g-chitosan had a lower cytotoxicity than PEI 25K and PEI-g-chitosan showed higher transfection efficiency than PEI 25K both *in vitro* and *in vivo*. In addition, improved biocompatibility and long-term safety will be expected for PEI-g-chitosan due to the degradable chitosan main chain and short PEI side chains.

Wong et al. synthesized PEI-graft-chitosan using water-soluble chitosan; however, commercial chitosan is insoluble at neutral and alkaline pH values due to a weak base with a pKa value of the D-glucosamine residue of about 6.2-7.0. Using commercial chitosan, Cho's group synthesized a chitosan-g-PEI copolymer [Fig. 8] by an imine reaction between periodate-oxidized chitosan and an amine group of PEI (Jiang, et al., 2007).

In addition, the same group developed specific ligand-conjugated chitosan-g-PEI, such as galactosylated- (Jiang, et al., 2007), mannosylated- (Jiang, et al., 2009), and folate-conjugated (Jiang, et al., 2009). The specific ligand-conjugated chitosan-g-PEI showed low cytotoxicity and high transfection efficiency with specific cell targeting.

In summary, the transfection efficiency was dependent on the degree of deacetylation, molecular weight of the chitosan, and medium pH. Also, specific ligand-conjugation will increase the transfection efficiency depending on the targeting ability of the ligands. A number of *in vitro* and *in vivo* studies have shown that modified-chitosan is a suitable material for use in efficient non-viral gene therapy.

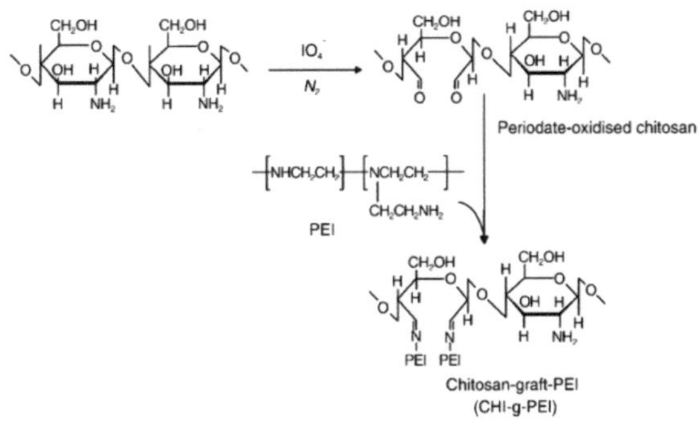

Fig. 8. Proposed reaction scheme for synthesis of CHI-g-PEI. [Source from Ref. (Jiang, et al., 2007)].

Similarly, according to Wong's results, the chitosan-g-PEI copolymer showed higher transfection efficiency and lower cytotoxicity than PEI 25K due to the buffering capacity of low moleculer weight PEI and biocompatible chitosan [Fig. 9].

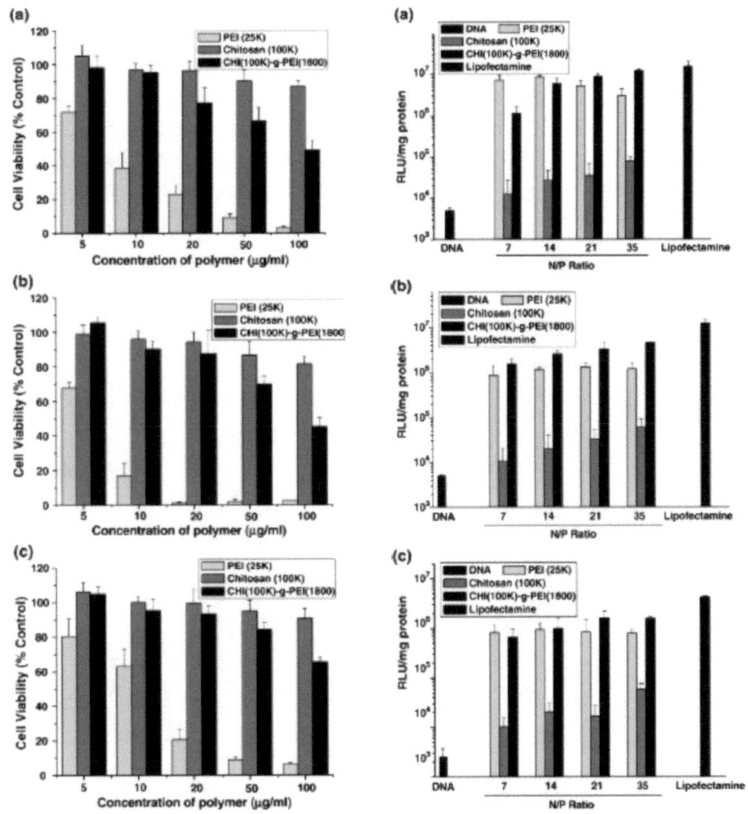

Fig. 9. Cytotoxicity of copolymer at various concentrations in different cell lines. (a) 293T, (b) HeLa and (c) HepG2 (left) and transfection efficiency of copolymer/DNA (pGL3-control) complex at various N/P ratios and in various cell lines. (a) 293T, (b) HeLa and (c) HepG2 (right). [Source from Ref. (Jiang, et al., 2007)].

2.3 Polyethylenimine (PEI)

PEI has received much attention due to its high transfection efficiency. In 1995, Behr's group made the first use of this polymer for delivery of DNA and oligonucleotides (Boussif, et al., 1995). As shown in Fig. 10, PEI exists in two principal forms, branched and linear, with a wide range of molecular weights (Lungwitz, et al., 2005).

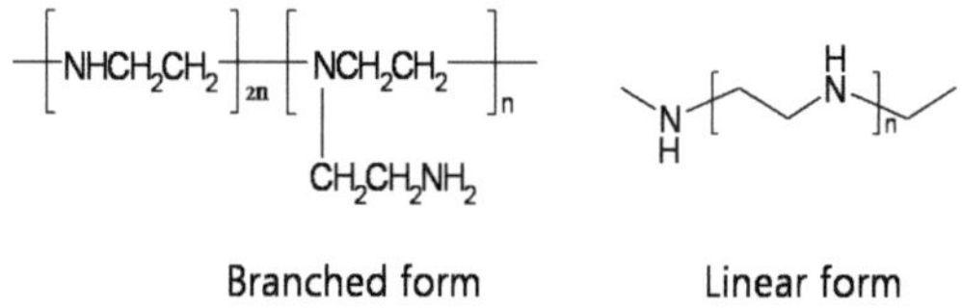

Fig. 10. Chemical structures of branched and linear PEI.

It is widely accepted that the high transfection ability of PEI is due to its high buffering capacity over a broad pH, which is called "the proton sponge effect" (Akinc, et al., 2005). In addition, the high content of primary amino groups enables chemical coupling of targeting moieties or intracellular active components; high density of positive charges in the molecule allows for a tight compaction of nucleic acids. However, high molecular weight of PEI shows high cytotoxicity, and when further decreasing the molecular weight, both cellular toxicity and transfection efficiency are decreased (Godbey, et al., 2001, Kunath, et al., 2003). One way to reduce toxicity of PEI is to reduce or mask the surface charge by attachment of vesicles with hydrophilic molecules, such as PEG. PEG chains of different length were used for modification of low-molecular weight PEIs (2 kDa), as well as high-molecular weight PEIs, such as the branched PEI (b-PEI) of 25 kDa [Fig. 11] (Petersen, et al., 2002) and the linear PEI (L-PEI) of 22 kDa (Kichler, et al., 2002). One beneficial effect of PEGylation is that PEG-PEI conjugates are less cytotoxic than non-modified polymers.

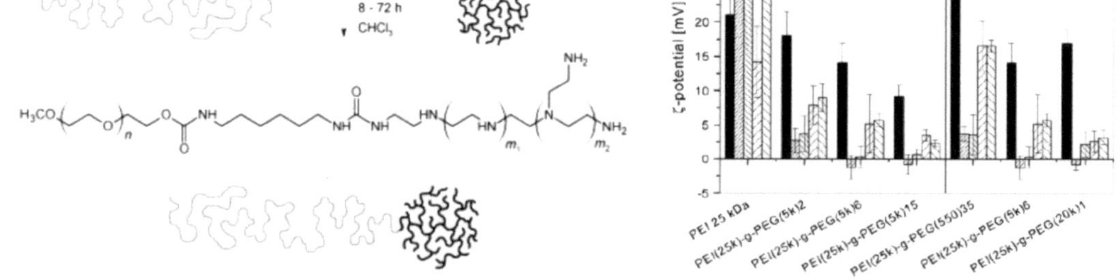

Fig. 11. Synthesis of bPEI-g-PEG copolymers (left) and zeta-potential of plasmid DNA complexes with PEI 25 kDa and bPEI-g-PEG block copolymers at different ionic strength and at different N/P ratios (right). [Source from Ref. (Petersen, et al., 2002)].

In all of the studies, covalent modification of PEI with PEG reduced the positive surface charge (zeta-potential) of the polyplexes, whereas it only marginally affected their size. However, PEGylation also reduces the DNA-binding capacity of the polymer and sterically hinders interactions of the polyplexes with the target cells. Therefore, in order to increase its usefulness, stealth technology must be combined with the use of ligands that allow specific cell targeting. Different types of ligands, such as sugar residues, peptides, proteins, and antibodies have been used for targeting of PEGylated PEI/DNA complexes [Table 2].

PEGylated PEI	
Ligand	**References**
Galactose	(Sagara & Kim, 2002)
Folate	(Benns, et al., 2002)
Transferrin	(Kursa, et al., 2003)
Epidermal growth factor	(Blessing, et al., 2001)

Table 2. Specific cell-targeting ligands conjugated with PEG-PEI.

Specific cell-targeting ligand-conjugated PEG-PEI showed low cytotoxicity and high transfection efficiency with specific cell targeting ability.

In summary, PEI is one of the successful and widely used gene delivery polymers, which has become the gold standard of non-viral gene delivery due to its high transfection efficiency. However, concerns over the cytotoxicity of PEI have to be solved for clinical trials. Cytotoxicity of PEI is dependent on its molecular weight; a lower molecular weight PEI has a lower cytotoxicity. Therefore, it is an attractive strategy by combination of lower molecular weight of PEI and biocompatible polymers as gene vectors for reduction of the toxicity of PEI. Also, similar to other cationic gene carriers, specific ligand-conjugation will be a way to increase transfection efficiency with specific cell-targeting.

2.4 Poly(β-amino ester)s (PAEs)

PAEs are one of the biodegradable cationic gene carriers. Biodegradable cationic PAEs are of interest both from the standpoint of mitigating the toxicity of conventional materials as well as a potential means through which to effect the timely release of DNA inside transfected cells (Lim, et al., 2000, Lim, et al., 2002, Luo & Saltzman, 2000). The Langer group has been particularly interested in PAEs as gene carriers, as they are easily synthesized via conjugate addition of either primary or bis(secondary) amine to diacrylate compounds, as shown in Fig. 12.

The Langer group reported a parallel approach suitable for synthesis of hundreds to thousands of structurally unique PAEs and application of these libraries to rapid and high throughput identification of new gene delivery agents and structure-function trends (Lynn, et al., 2001). The advantage of combinatorial chemistry and automated highthroughput synthesis is that it has revolutionized modern drug discovery by rapid synthesis and evaluation with greater precision. As shown in Fig. 13, 140 different PAEs (the set of 7 diacrylate monomers and 20 amine-based monomers) were synthesized as a screening library. Most of the PAEs showed low transfection efficiencies, compared with Lipofectamine 2000, a commercially available lipid-based vector system. However, B14 and G5 yielded higher gene transfection efficiencies. In particular, B14 showed higer transfection efficiency, compared with

Lipofectamine 2000, due to the high endosomal pH buffering capacity, similar to that of other imidazole-substituted polymers (Benns, et al., 2000, Pack, et al., 2000), suggesting that polymer B14 may be the more promising polymer as a gene delivery carrier.

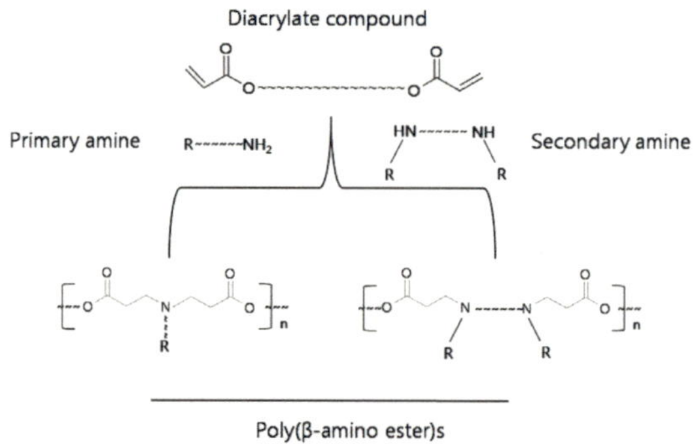

Fig. 12. Synthesis scheme of PAEs.

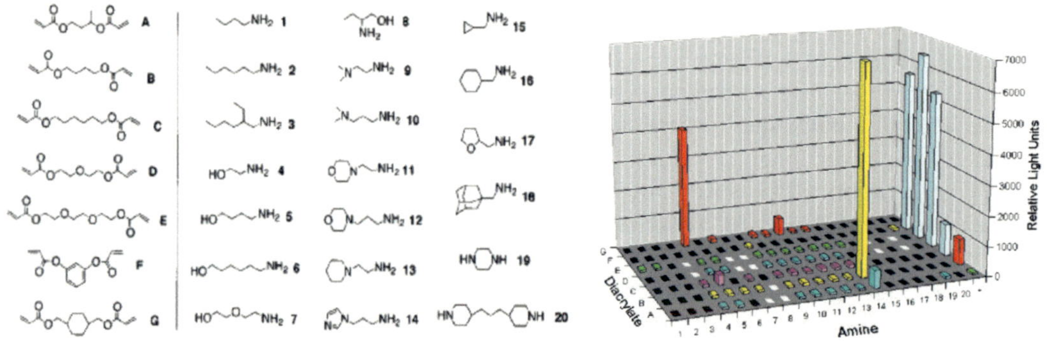

[Source from Ref. (Zugates, et al., 2006)].

Fig. 13. Diacrylate (A-G) and amine (1-20) monomers chosen for the synthesis of an initial screening library (left) and transfection data as a function of structure for an assay employing pCMV-Luc (600 ng/well, DNA/polymer = 1:20, right). [Source from Ref. (Lynn, et al., 2001)].

As shown in Fig. 14, using high throughput methods, over 2,350 PAEs were synthesized (Anderson, et al., 2003). Biodegradable PAEs demonstrated efficient transfection of cells and 26 of these polymers showed higher gene expression, compared with Lipofectamine 2000. Response to intracellular stimuli, such as pH, is a major advantage of a gene delivery system (Stayton, et al., 2005). Zugates et al synthesized new PAEs using a primary amine monomer, 2-(pyridyldithio)-ethylamine (PDA), speculating that pyridyldithio groups in these side chains display fast and selective reactivity with thiols without alteration of the charge density of the polymer backbone, as shown in Fig. 15 (Zugates, et al., 2006). This property of PDA-based PAEs further led to conjugation of cell-targeting peptides or ligands for targeted and site-specific delivery. As one potential application, they conjugated the mercaptoethylamine (MEA) and the RGDC peptide to PDA PAEs. MEA-based PAE has an advantage that it is sensitive to glutathione. The MEA-based polymer delivery system has demonstrated relative stability in the extracellular space; however, it is responsive to intracellular conditions in which partial unpacking is triggered.

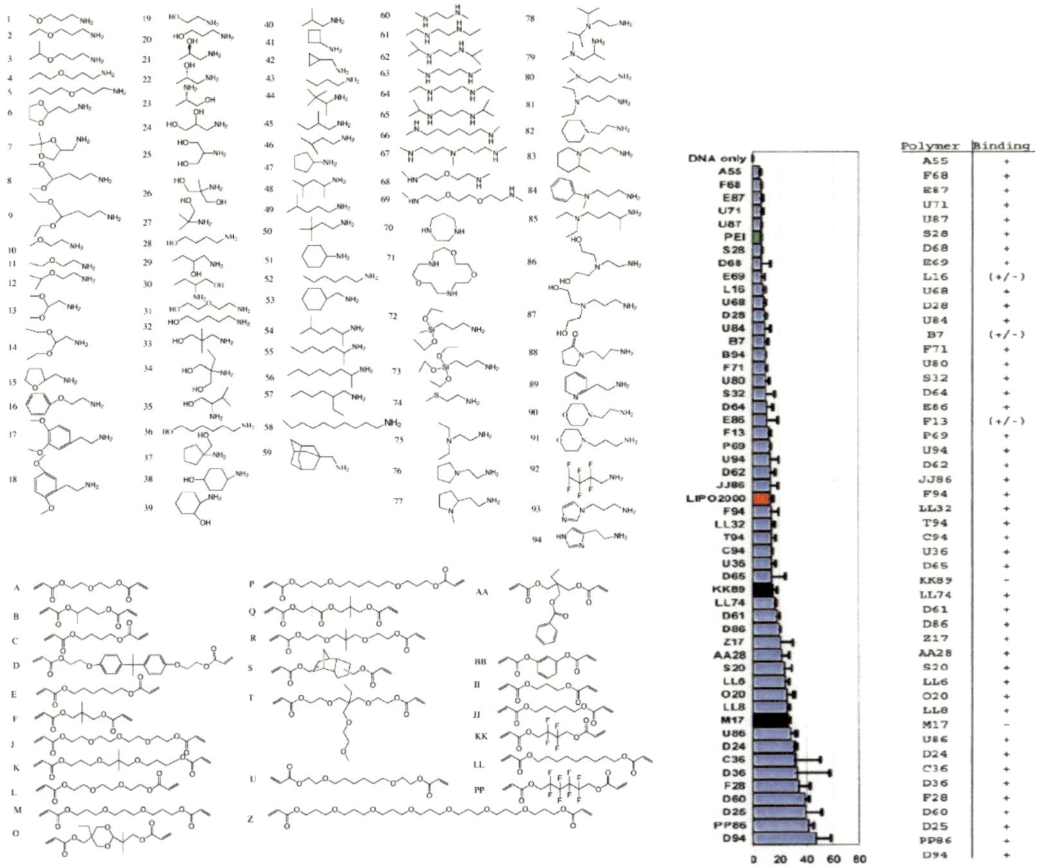

Fig. 14. Amino (numbers) and diacrylate (letters) monomers (left) and optimized transfection efficiency of the top 50 polymers relative to PEI and Lipofectamine 2000. [Source from Ref. (Anderson, et al., 2003)].

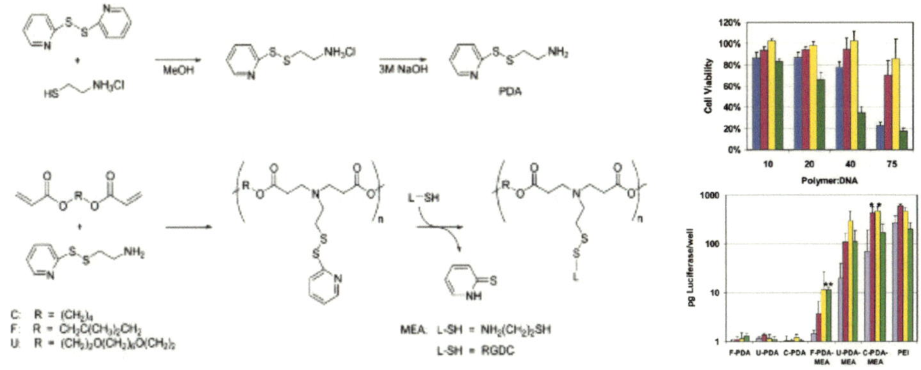

Fig. 15. Synthesis scheme of MEA (left) and cytotoxicity [C-PDA (blue), C-PDA-MEA (Redenti, et al.), 2-mercaptopyridine (2-MP, yellow), and PEI (green)] and transfection studies (right). [Source from Ref. (Zugates, et al., 2006)].

As shown in Fig. 16, Cho's group synthesized novel biodegradable PAEs composed of gamma-aminopropyl-triethoxysilane (APES) and poly (ethylene glycol) diacrylate (PEGDA) for gene delivery (Jere, et al., 2008).

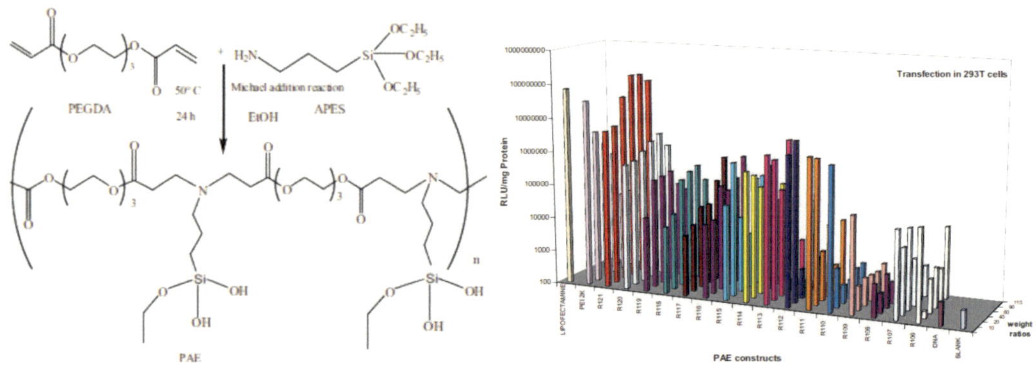

Fig. 16. Proposed reaction scheme for PAE copolymer (left) and transfection efficiency of PAE/DNA complexes in serum free-media at various mass ratios in a 293T cells (right). [Source from Ref. (Jere, et al., 2008)].

They reported that addition of PEGDA over APES resulted in a novel PAE, which shows high safety and transfection efficiency, especially in R121. PAE obtained from R121 showed good DNA binding and condensation with average particle sizes of 133 nm. In addition, PAE-mediated gene expression in the lung and liver was higher than that of the conventional PEI carrier. Of particular interest, non-invasive aerosol delivery induced higher gene expression in all organs, compared with an intravenous method, in an *in vivo* mice study (Park, et al., 2008). The same group developed a new PAE based on hydrophobic polycaprolactone (PCL) and low molecular weight branched PEI following the Michael addition reaction (Arote, et al., 2007). The synthesized PAE showed controlled degradation and was essentially non-toxic in all three cells (293T, HepG2 and HeLa) in contrast with PEI 25K. PAEs revealed much higher transfection efficiencies in three cell lines, compared with PEI 25K, and were also successfully transfected *in vivo*, compared with PEI 25K after aerosol administration. Targeting confers another important criterion in gene delivery. Recently, Arote et al. coupled folic acid moiety for a folate receptor targeting the PAE backbone using PEG (MW: 5000 Da) as a linker (Arote, et al., 2010). At the initial stage, folate-conjugated PAE revealed folate receptor-mediated endocytosis with elevated levels of luciferase expression in folate receptor positive cancer cell lines, suggesting application of specific ligand-modified PAE. They also developed folate-PEG-PAE (FP-PAE) as a gene carrier, which mediated high level folate receptor mediated endocytosis *in vitro* as well as *in vivo* [Fig. 17]. FP-PAE showed marked anti-tumor activity against folate receptor-positive human KB tumors in nude mice with no evidence of toxicity during and after therapy using the TAM67 gene. Anti-tumor activity with PAE without folic acid moiety (PEG-PAE, P-PAE) proved ineffective against a xenograft mice model with KB cells when administered at the same dose as that of FP-PAE, suggesting that FP-PAE is a highly effective gene carrier capable of producing a therapeutic benefit in a xenograft mice model without any signs of toxicity.

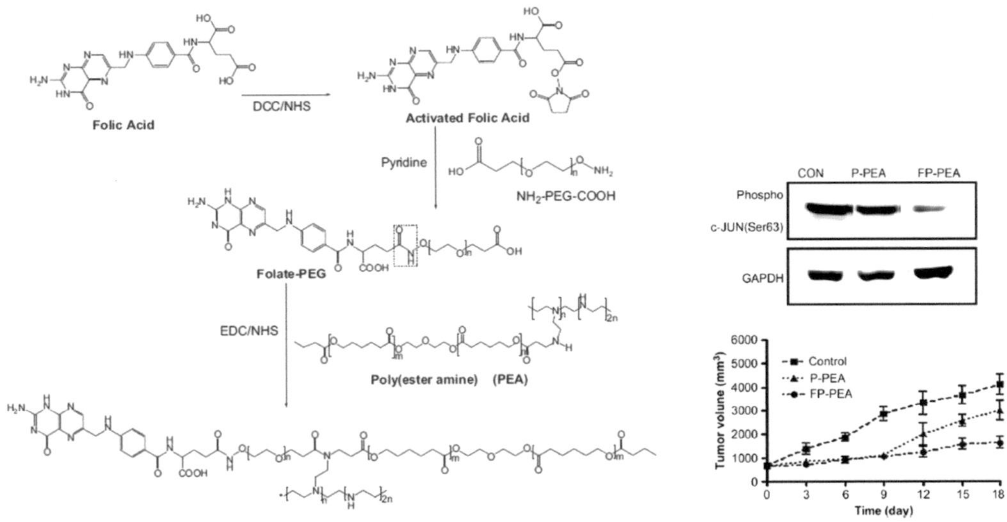

Fig. 17. Synthesis scheme of FP-PEA (left) and effect of FP-PEA/TAM67 complexes on tumor growth (right). Expression level of phospho-c-Jun and suppression of tumor growth by FP-PEA/TAM67 complexes. [Source from Ref. (Arote, et al., 2010)].

In summary, PAEs have excellent characteristics as gene carriers. PAEs comprise a class of degradable cationic polymers with many desirable properties in the context of gene delivery, including condensation of DNA into nanoscale-size particles, which facilitates cellular uptake of DNA and protects DNA from endogenous nucleases as well as efficient delivery of DNA with low toxicity. Tissue targeting, endosome disruption, and nuclear transport should be combined for development of an effective PAE for use in gene therapy. Also, extensive *in vitro* and *in vivo* evaluation and optimization of PAEs will provide valuable information for safe and efficient gene therapy applications.

3. Conclusion

Gene therapy shows tremendous promise for a broad spectrum of clinical applications. Development of a safe and efficient gene delivery system is one of the main challenges to be solved before this strategy can be adopted for routine use in clinical trails. In this chapter, medical polymers, including CD, chitosan, PEI, PAEs, and their derivatives as non-viral vectors in the area of gene therapy have been described. Although more development of structure-function relationships and fundamental research into cellular processes *in vitro* and *in vivo* should be performed for future direction of medical polymer based gene carriers, combination of these polymers will be a way to reduce toxicity and enhance tranfection efficiency. Also, selective tissue or cell targeting ligand conjugation will provide cell-specificity or improve transfection efficiency. Nowadays, multiple targeting gene therapy with multiple-functionalized genes and delivery system are possible. Suitable formulations of these polyplexes with low toxicity and high transfection efficiency must be chosen for *in vivo* use, which will allow for multiple applications of therapeutic genes; however, for this idea to be realized, much work lies ahead.

4. Acknowledgements

This work was partly supported by the R&D Program of MKE/KEIT (10035333, Development of anti-cancer therapeutic agent based on regulating cell cycle or cell death) as well as by the National Research Foundation (NRF-2011-0000380), Ministry of Education, Science and Technology (MEST) in Korea.

5. References

Akinc, A.; Thomas, M.; Klibanov, A. M. & Langer, R. (2005). Exploring polyethylenimine-mediated DNA transfection and the proton sponge hypothesis. *Journal of Gene Medicine,* Vol. 7, No. 5, (May 2005), pp. 657-663, ISSN 1099-498X

Alexander, M. Y. & Akhurst, R. J. (1995). Liposome-medicated gene transfer and expression via the skin. *Human Molecular Genetics,* Vol. 4, No. 12, (Dec 1995), pp. 2279-2285, ISSN 0964-6906

Anderson, D. G.; Lynn, D. M. & Langer, R. (2003). Semi-automated synthesis and screening of a large library of degradable cationic polymers for gene delivery. *Angewandte Chemie. International Ed. In English,* Vol. 42, No. 27, (Jul 14 2003), pp. 3153-3158, ISSN 1433-7851

Anderson, W. F. (1998). Human gene therapy. *Nature,* Vol. 392, No. 6679 Suppl, (Apr 30 1998), pp. 25-30, ISSN 0028-0836

Arima, H.; Kihara, F.; Hirayama, F. & Uekama, K. (2001). Enhancement of gene expression by polyamidoamine dendrimer conjugates with alpha-, beta-, and gamma-cyclodextrins. *Bioconjugate Chemistry,* Vol. 12, No. 4, (Jul-Aug 2001), pp. 476-484, ISSN 1043-1802

Arima, H.; Yamashita, S.; Mori, Y.; Hayashi, Y.; Motoyama, K.; Hattori, K.; Takeuchi, T.; Jono, H.; Ando, Y.; Hirayama, F. & Uekama, K. (2010). In vitro and in vivo gene delivery mediated by Lactosylated dendrimer/alpha-cyclodextrin conjugates (G2) into hepatocytes. *Journal of Controlled Release,* Vol. 146, No. 1, (Aug 17 2010), pp. 106-117, ISSN 1873-4995

Arote, R.; Kim, T. H.; Kim, Y. K.; Hwang, S. K.; Jiang, H. L.; Song, H. H.; Nah, J. W.; Cho, M. H. & Cho, C. S. (2007). A biodegradable poly(ester amine) based on polycaprolactone and polyethylenimine as a gene carrier. *Biomaterials,* Vol. 28, No. 4, (Feb 2007), pp. 735-744, ISSN 0142-9612

Arote, R. B.; Yoon, M. K.; Kim, T. H.; Jere, D.; Jiang, H. L.; Kim, Y. K.; Park, I. K. & Cho, C. S. (2010). Folate conjugated poly(ester amine) for lung cancer therapy. *Journal of Nanoscience and Nanotechnology,* Vol. 10, No. 5, (May 2010), pp. 3294-3298, ISSN 1533-4880

Benns, J. M.; Choi, J. S.; Mahato, R. I.; Park, J. S. & Kim, S. W. (2000). pH-sensitive cationic polymer gene delivery vehicle: N-Ac-poly(L-histidine)-graft-poly(L-lysine) comb shaped polymer. *Bioconjugate Chemistry,* Vol. 11, No. 5, (Sep-Oct 2000), pp. 637-645, ISSN 1043-1802

Benns, J. M.; Mahato, R. I. & Kim, S. W. (2002). Optimization of factors influencing the transfection efficiency of folate-PEG-folate-graft-polyethylenimine. *Journal of Controlled Release,* Vol. 79, No. 1-3, (Feb 19 2002), pp. 255-269, ISSN 0168-3659

Bhavsar, M. D. & Amiji, M. M. (2007). Polymeric nano- and microparticle technologies for oral gene delivery. *Expert Opin Drug Deliv,* Vol. 4, No. 3, (May 2007), pp. 197-213, ISSN 1742-5247

Blessing, T.; Kursa, M.; Holzhauser, R.; Kircheis, R. & Wagner, E. (2001). Different strategies for formation of pegylated EGF-conjugated PEI/DNA complexes for targeted gene delivery. *Bioconjugate Chemistry,* Vol. 12, No. 4, (Jul-Aug 2001), pp. 529-537, ISSN 1043-1802

Boussif, O.; Lezoualc'h, F.; Zanta, M. A.; Mergny, M. D.; Scherman, D.; Demeneix, B. & Behr, J. P. (1995). A versatile vector for gene and oligonucleotide transfer into cells in culture and in vivo: polyethylenimine. *Proceedings of the National Academy of Sciences of the United States of America,* Vol. 92, No. 16, (Aug 1 1995), pp. 7297-7301, ISSN 0027-8424

Brown, M. D.; Schatzlein, A. G. & Uchegbu, I. F. (2001). Gene delivery with synthetic (non viral) carriers. *International Journal of Pharmaceutics,* Vol. 229, No. 1-2, (Oct 23 2001), pp. 1-21, ISSN 0378-5173

Challa, R.; Ahuja, A.; Ali, J. & Khar, R. K. (2005). Cyclodextrins in drug delivery: an updated review. *AAPS PharmSciTech,* Vol. 6, No. 2, 2005), pp. E329-357, ISSN 1530-9932

Chaum, E. & Hatton, M. P. (2002). Gene therapy for genetic and acquired retinal diseases. *Survey of Ophthalmology,* Vol. 47, No. 5, (Sep-Oct 2002), pp. 449-469, ISSN 0039-6257

Cho, J. H.; Kim, S. H.; Park, K. D.; Jung, M. C.; Yang, W. I.; Han, S. W.; Noh, J. Y. & Lee, J. W. (2004). Chondrogenic differentiation of human mesenchymal stem cells using a thermosensitive poly(N-isopropylacrylamide) and water-soluble chitosan copolymer. *Biomaterials,* Vol. 25, No. 26, (Nov 2004), pp. 5743-5751, ISSN 0142-9612

Dang, J. M.; Sun, D. D.; Shin-Ya, Y.; Sieber, A. N.; Kostuik, J. P. & Leong, K. W. (2006). Temperature-responsive hydroxybutyl chitosan for the culture of mesenchymal stem cells and intervertebral disk cells. *Biomaterials,* Vol. 27, No. 3, (Jan 2006), pp. 406-418, ISSN 0142-9612

Dass, C. R. (2002). Vehicles for oligonucleotide delivery to tumours. *Journal of Pharmacy and Pharmacology,* Vol. 54, No. 1, (Jan 2002), pp. 3-27, ISSN 0022-3573

Davis, M. E. & Brewster, M. E. (2004). Cyclodextrin-based pharmaceutics: past, present and future. *Nature Reviews Drug Discovery,* Vol. 3, No. 12, (Dec 2004), pp. 1023-1035, ISSN 1474-1776

Farhood, H.; Serbina, N. & Huang, L. (1995). The role of dioleoyl phosphatidylethanolamine in cationic liposome mediated gene transfer. *Biochimica et Biophysica Acta,* Vol. 1235, No. 2, (May 4 1995), pp. 289-295, ISSN 0006-3002

Felgner, P. L.; Gadek, T. R.; Holm, M.; Roman, R.; Chan, H. W.; Wenz, M.; Northrop, J. P.; Ringold, G. M. & Danielsen, M. (1987). Lipofection: a highly efficient, lipid-mediated DNA-transfection procedure. *Proceedings of the National Academy of Sciences of the United States of America,* Vol. 84, No. 21, (Nov 1987), pp. 7413-7417, ISSN 0027-8424

Forrest, M. L.; Gabrielson, N. & Pack, D. W. (2005). Cyclodextrin-polyethylenimine conjugates for targeted in vitro gene delivery. *Biotechnology and Bioengineering,* Vol. 89, No. 4, (Feb 20 2005), pp. 416-423, ISSN 0006-3592

Friend, D. S.; Papahadjopoulos, D. & Debs, R. J. (1996). Endocytosis and intracellular processing accompanying transfection mediated by cationic liposomes. *Biochimica et Biophysica Acta,* Vol. 1278, No. 1, (Jan 12 1996), pp. 41-50, ISSN 0006-3002

Godbey, W. T.; Wu, K. K. & Mikos, A. G. (2001). Poly(ethylenimine)-mediated gene delivery affects endothelial cell function and viability. *Biomaterials,* Vol. 22, No. 5, (Mar 2001), pp. 471-480, ISSN 0142-9612

Gonzalez, H.; Hwang, S. J. & Davis, M. E. (1999). New class of polymers for the delivery of macromolecular therapeutics. *Bioconjugate Chemistry,* Vol. 10, No. 6, (Nov-Dec 1999), pp. 1068-1074, ISSN 1043-1802

Grosshans, H. (2000). Gene therapy--when a simple concept meets a complex reality. Review on gene therapy. *Funct Integr Genomics,* Vol. 1, No. 2, (Sep 2000), pp. 142-145, ISSN 1438-793X

Hashimoto, M.; Morimoto, M.; Saimoto, H.; Shigemasa, Y. & Sato, T. (2006). Lactosylated chitosan for DNA delivery into hepatocytes: the effect of lactosylation on the physicochemical properties and intracellular trafficking of pDNA/chitosan complexes. *Bioconjugate Chemistry,* Vol. 17, No. 2, (Mar-Apr 2006), pp. 309-316, ISSN 1043-1802

Huang, H.; Tang, G.; Wang, Q.; Li, D.; Shen, F.; Zhou, J. & Yu, H. (2006). Two novel non-viral gene delivery vectors: low molecular weight polyethylenimine cross-linked by (2-hydroxypropyl)-beta-cyclodextrin or (2-hydroxypropyl)-gamma-cyclodextrin. *Chemical Communications (Camb),* No. 22, (Jun 14 2006), pp. 2382-2384, ISSN 1359-7345

Huang, M.; Fong, C. W.; Khor, E. & Lim, L. Y. (2005). Transfection efficiency of chitosan vectors: effect of polymer molecular weight and degree of deacetylation. *Journal of Controlled Release,* Vol. 106, No. 3, (Sep 2 2005), pp. 391-406, ISSN 0168-3659

Ishii, T.; Okahata, Y. & Sato, T. (2001). Mechanism of cell transfection with plasmid/chitosan complexes. *Biochimica et Biophysica Acta,* Vol. 1514, No. 1, (Sep 3 2001), pp. 51-64, ISSN 0006-3002

Jere, D.; Yoo, M. K.; Arote, R.; Kim, T. H.; Cho, M. H.; Nah, J. W.; Choi, Y. J. & Cho, C. S. (2008). Poly (amino ester) composed of poly (ethylene glycol) and aminosilane prepared by combinatorial chemistry as a gene carrier. *Pharmaceutical Research,* Vol. 25, No. 4, (Apr 2008), pp. 875-885, ISSN 0724-8741

Jiang, H. L.; Kim, Y. K.; Arote, R.; Nah, J. W.; Cho, M. H.; Choi, Y. J.; Akaike, T. & Cho, C. S. (2007). Chitosan-graft-polyethylenimine as a gene carrier. *J Control Release,* Vol. 117, No. 2, (Feb 12 2007), pp. 273-280, ISSN 0168-3659

Jiang, H. L.; Kwon, J. T.; Kim, Y. K.; Kim, E. M.; Arote, R.; Jeong, H. J.; Nah, J. W.; Choi, Y. J.; Akaike, T.; Cho, M. H. & Cho, C. S. (2007). Galactosylated chitosan-graft-polyethylenimine as a gene carrier for hepatocyte targeting. *Gene Therapy,* Vol. 14, No. 19, (Oct 2007), pp. 1389-1398, ISSN 0969-7128

Jiang, H. L.; Kim, Y. K.; Arote, R.; Jere, D.; Quan, J. S.; Yu, J. H.; Choi, Y. J.; Nah, J. W.; Cho, M. H. & Cho, C. S. (2009). Mannosylated chitosan-graft-polyethylenimine as a gene carrier for Raw 264.7 cell targeting. *International Journal of Pharmaceutics,* Vol. 375, No. 1-2, (Jun 22 2009), pp. 133-139, ISSN 1873-3476

Jiang, H. L.; Xu, C. X.; Kim, Y. K.; Arote, R.; Jere, D.; Lim, H. T.; Cho, M. H.& Cho, C. S. (2009). The suppression of lung tumorigenesis by aerosol-delivered folate-chitosan-graft-polyethylenimine/Akt1 shRNA complexes through the Akt signaling pathway. *Biomaterials,* Vol. 30, No. 29, (Oct 2009), pp. 5844-5852, ISSN 1878-5905

Jiang, X.; Dai, H.; Leong, K. W.; Goh, S. H.; Mao, H. Q. & Yang, Y. Y. (2006). Chitosan-g-PEG/DNA complexes deliver gene to the rat liver via intrabiliary and intraportal infusions. *Journal of Gene Medicine,* Vol. 8, No. 4, (Apr 2006), pp. 477-487, ISSN 1099-498X

Jones, R. A.; Cheung, C. Y.; Black, F. E.; Zia, J. K.; Stayton, P. S.; Hoffman, A. S. & Wilson, M. R. (2003). Poly(2-alkylacrylic acid) polymers deliver molecules to the cytosol by pH-sensitive disruption of endosomal vesicles. *Biochemical Journal,* Vol. 372, No. Pt 1, (May 15 2003), pp. 65-75, ISSN 0264-6021

Kiang, T.; Wen, J.; Lim, H. W. & Leong, K. W. (2004). The effect of the degree of chitosan deacetylation on the efficiency of gene transfection. *Biomaterials,* Vol. 25, No. 22, (Oct 2004), pp. 5293-5301, ISSN 0142-9612

Kichler, A.; Chillon, M.; Leborgne, C.; Danos, O. & Frisch, B. (2002). Intranasal gene delivery with a polyethylenimine-PEG conjugate. *Journal of Controlled Release,* Vol. 81, No. 3, (Jun 17 2002), pp. 379-388, ISSN 0168-3659

Kihara, F.; Arima, H.; Tsutsumi, T.; Hirayama, F. & Uekama, K. (2002). Effects of structure of polyamidoamine dendrimer on gene transfer efficiency of the dendrimer conjugate with alpha-cyclodextrin. *Bioconjugate Chemistry,* Vol. 13, No. 6, (Nov-Dec 2002), pp. 1211-1219, ISSN 1043-1802

Kim, T. H.; Ihm, J. E.; Choi, Y. J.; Nah, J. W. & Cho, C. S. (2003). Efficient gene delivery by urocanic acid-modified chitosan. *Journal of Controlled Release,* Vol. 93, No. 3, (Dec 12 2003), pp. 389-402, ISSN 0168-3659

Kim, T. H.; Park, I. K.; Nah, J. W.; Choi, Y. J. & Cho, C. S. (2004). Galactosylated chitosan/DNA nanoparticles prepared using water-soluble chitosan as a gene carrier. *Biomaterials,* Vol. 25, No. 17, (Aug 2004), pp. 3783-3792, ISSN 0142-9612

Kim, T. H.; Nah, J. W.; Cho, M. H.; Park, T. G. & Cho, C. S. (2006). Receptor-mediated gene delivery into antigen presenting cells using mannosylated chitosan/DNA nanoparticles. *Journal of Nanoscience and Nanotechnology,* Vol. 6, No. 9-10, (Sep-Oct 2006), pp. 2796-2803, ISSN 1533-4880

Klibanov, A. L.; Maruyama, K.; Torchilin, V. P. & Huang, L. (1990). Amphipathic polyethyleneglycols effectively prolong the circulation time of liposomes. *FEBS Letters,* Vol. 268, No. 1, (Jul 30 1990), pp. 235-237, ISSN 0014-5793

Kunath, K.; von Harpe, A.; Fischer, D.; Petersen, H.; Bickel, U.; Voigt, K. & Kissel, T. (2003). Low-molecular-weight polyethylenimine as a non-viral vector for DNA delivery: comparison of physicochemical properties, transfection efficiency and in vivo distribution with high-molecular-weight polyethylenimine. *Journal of Controlled Release,* Vol. 89, No. 1, (Apr 14 2003), pp. 113-125, ISSN 0168-3659

Kursa, M.; Walker, G. F.; Roessler, V.; Ogris, M.; Roedl, W.; Kircheis, R. & Wagner, E. (2003). Novel shielded transferrin-polyethylene glycol-polyethylenimine/DNA complexes for systemic tumor-targeted gene transfer. *Bioconjugate Chemistry,* Vol. 14, No. 1, (Jan-Feb 2003), pp. 222-231, ISSN 1043-1802

Lappalainen, K.; Urtti, A.; Soderling, E.; Jaaskelainen, I.; Syrjanen, K. & Syrjanen, S. (1994). Cationic liposomes improve stability and intracellular delivery of antisense oligonucleotides into CaSki cells. *Biochimica et Biophysica Acta,* Vol. 1196, No. 2, (Dec 30 1994), pp. 201-208, ISSN 0006-3002

Lavertu, M.; Methot, S.; Tran-Khanh, N. & Buschmann, M. D. (2006). High efficiency gene transfer using chitosan/DNA nanoparticles with specific combinations of molecular weight and degree of deacetylation. *Biomaterials,* Vol. 27, No. 27, (Sep 2006), pp. 4815-4824, ISSN 0142-9612

Ledley, F. D. (1996). Pharmaceutical approach to somatic gene therapy. *Pharmaceutical Research,* Vol. 13, No. 11, (Nov 1996), pp. 1595-1614, ISSN 0724-8741

Li, J.; Revol, J. F. & Marchessault, R. H. (1996). Rheological Properties of Aqueous Suspensions of Chitin Crystallites. *Journal of Colloid and Interface Science,* Vol. 183, No. 2, (Nov 10 1996), pp. 365-373, ISSN 1095-7103

Lim, Y. B.; Han, S. O.; Kong, H. U.; Lee, Y.; Park, J. S.; Jeong, B. & Kim, S. W. (2000). Biodegradable polyester, poly[alpha-(4-aminobutyl)-L-glycolic acid], as a non-toxic gene carrier. *Pharmaceutical Research,* Vol. 17, No. 7, (Jul 2000), pp. 811-816, ISSN 0724-8741

Lim, Y. B.; Kim, S. M.; Suh, H. & Park, J. S. (2002). Biodegradable, endosome disruptive, and cationic network-type polymer as a highly efficient and nontoxic gene delivery carrier. *Bioconjugate Chemistry,* Vol. 13, No. 5, (Sep-Oct 2002), pp. 952-957, ISSN 1043-1802

Loftsson, T.; Jarho, P.; Masson, M. & Jarvinen, T. (2005). Cyclodextrins in drug delivery. *Expert Opininon on Drug Delivery,* Vol. 2, No. 2, (Mar 2005), pp. 335-351, ISSN 1742-5247

Lungwitz, U.; Breunig, M.; Blunk, T. & Gopferich, A. (2005). Polyethylenimine-based non-viral gene delivery systems. *European Journal of Pharmaceutics and Biopharmaceutics,* Vol. 60, No. 2, (Jul 2005), pp. 247-266, ISSN 0939-6411

Luo, D. & Saltzman, W. M. (2000). Synthetic DNA delivery systems. *Nature Biotechnology,* Vol. 18, No. 1, (Jan 2000), pp. 33-37, ISSN 1087-0156

Lynn, D. M.; Anderson, D. G.; Putnam, D. & Langer, R. (2001). Accelerated discovery of synthetic transfection vectors: parallel synthesis and screening of a degradable polymer library. *Journal of the American Chemical Society,* Vol. 123, No. 33, (Aug 22 2001), pp. 8155-8156, ISSN 0002-7863

Mahato, R. I.; Smith, L. C. & Rolland, A. (1999). Pharmaceutical perspectives of nonviral gene therapy. *Advances in Genetics,* Vol. 41, 1999), pp. 95-156, ISSN 0065-2660

Mansouri, S.; Lavigne, P.; Corsi, K.; Benderdour, M.; Beaumont, E. & Fernandes, J. C. (2004). Chitosan-DNA nanoparticles as non-viral vectors in gene therapy: strategies to improve transfection efficacy. *European Journal of Pharmaceutics and Biopharmaceutics,* Vol. 57, No. 1, (Jan 2004), pp. 1-8, ISSN 0939-6411

Mansouri, S.; Cuie, Y.; Winnik, F.; Shi, Q.; Lavigne, P.; Benderdour, M.; Beaumont, E. & Fernandes, J. C. (2006). Characterization of folate-chitosan-DNA nanoparticles for gene therapy. *Biomaterials,* Vol. 27, No. 9, (Mar 2006), pp. 2060-2065, ISSN 0142-9612

Mao, H. Q.; Roy, K.; Troung-Le, V. L.; Janes, K. A.; Lin, K. Y.; Wang, Y.; August, J. T. & Leong, K. W. (2001). Chitosan-DNA nanoparticles as gene carriers: synthesis, characterization and transfection efficiency. *Journal of Controlled Release,* Vol. 70, No. 3, (Feb 23 2001), pp. 399-421, ISSN 0168-3659

Mellet, C. O.; Fernandez, J. M. & Benito, J. M. (2011). Cyclodextrin-based gene delivery systems. *Chemical Society Reviews,* Vol. 40, No. 3, (Mar 22 2011), pp. 1586-1608, ISSN 1460-4744

Muzzarelli, R. A. (1997). Human enzymatic activities related to the therapeutic administration of chitin derivatives. *Cellular and Molecular Life Sciences,* Vol. 53, No. 2, (Feb 1997), pp. 131-140, ISSN 1420-682X

Nguyen, L. T.; Atobe, K.; Barichello, J. M.; Ishida, T. & Kiwada, H. (2007). Complex formation with plasmid DNA increases the cytotoxicity of cationic liposomes.

Biological and Pharmaceutical Bulletin, Vol. 30, No. 4, (Apr 2007), pp. 751-757, ISSN 0918-6158

Pack, D. W.; Putnam, D. & Langer, R. (2000). Design of imidazole-containing endosomolytic biopolymers for gene delivery. *Biotechnology and Bioengineering,* Vol. 67, No. 2, (Jan 20 2000), pp. 217-223, ISSN 0006-3592

Pack, D. W.; Hoffman, A. S.; Pun, S. & Stayton, P. S. (2005). Design and development of polymers for gene delivery. *Nature Reviews Drug Discovery,* Vol. 4, No. 7, (Jul 2005), pp. 581-593, ISSN 1474-1776

Park, M. R.; Kim, H. W.; Hwang, C. S.; Han, K. O.; Choi, Y. J.; Song, S. C.; Cho, M. H. & Cho, C. S. (2008). Highly efficient gene transfer with degradable poly(ester amine) based on poly(ethylene glycol) diacrylate and polyethylenimine in vitro and in vivo. *Journal of Gene Medicine,* Vol. 10, No. 2, (Feb 2008), pp. 198-207, ISSN 1099-498X

Park, T. G.; Jeong, J. H. & Kim, S. W. (2006). Current status of polymeric gene delivery systems. *Advanced Drug Delivery Reviews,* Vol. 58, No. 4, (Jul 7 2006), pp. 467-486, ISSN 0169-409X

Patel, H. M. (1992). Serum opsonins and liposomes: their interaction and opsonophagocytosis. *Critical Reviews in Therapeutic Drug Carrier Systems,* Vol. 9, No. 1, 1992), pp. 39-90, ISSN 0743-4863

Petersen, H.; Fechner, P. M.; Martin, A. L.; Kunath, K.; Stolnik, S.; Roberts, C. J.; Fischer, D.; Davies, M. C. & Kissel, T. (2002). Polyethylenimine-graft-poly(ethylene glycol) copolymers: influence of copolymer block structure on DNA complexation and biological activities as gene delivery system. *Bioconjugate Chemistry,* Vol. 13, No. 4, (Jul-Aug 2002), pp. 845-854, ISSN 1043-1802

Popielarski, S. R.; Mishra, S. & Davis, M. E. (2003). Structural effects of carbohydrate-containing polycations on gene delivery. 3. Cyclodextrin type and functionalization. *Bioconjugate Chemistry,* Vol. 14, No. 3, (May-Jun 2003), pp. 672-678, ISSN 1043-1802

Pun, S. H.; Bellocq, N. C.; Liu, A.; Jensen, G.; Machemer, T.; Quijano, E.; Schluep, T.; Wen, S.; Engler, H.; Heidel, J. & Davis, M. E. (2004). Cyclodextrin-modified polyethylenimine polymers for gene delivery. *Bioconjugate Chemistry,* Vol. 15, No. 4, (Jul-Aug 2004), pp. 831-840, ISSN 1043-1802

Quong, D. & Neufeld, R. J. (1998). DNA protection from extracapsular nucleases, within chitosan- or poly-L-lysine-coated alginate beads. *Biotechnology and Bioengineering,* Vol. 60, No. 1, (Oct 5 1998), pp. 124-134, ISSN 0006-3592

Redenti, E.; Pietra, C.; Gerloczy, A. & Szente, L. (2001). Cyclodextrins in oligonucleotide delivery. *Advanced Drug Delivery Reviews,* Vol. 53, No. 2, (Dec 17 2001), pp. 235-244, ISSN 0169-409X

Reineke, T. M. & Davis, M. E. (2003). Structural effects of carbohydrate-containing polycations on gene delivery. 2. Charge center type. *Bioconjugate Chemistry,* Vol. 14, No. 1, (Jan-Feb 2003), pp. 255-261, ISSN 1043-1802

Reineke, T. M. & Davis, M. E. (2003). Structural effects of carbohydrate-containing polycations on gene delivery. 1. Carbohydrate size and its distance from charge centers. *Bioconjugate Chemistry,* Vol. 14, No. 1, (Jan-Feb 2003), pp. 247-254, ISSN 1043-1802

Sagara, K. & Kim, S. W. (2002). A new synthesis of galactose-poly(ethylene glycol)-polyethylenimine for gene delivery to hepatocytes. *Journal of Controlled Release,* Vol. 79, No. 1-3, (Feb 19 2002), pp. 271-281, ISSN 0168-3659

Saranya, N.; Moorthi, A.; Saravanan, S.; Devi, M. P. & Selvamurugan, N. (2011). Chitosan and its derivatives for gene delivery. *International Journal of Biological Macromolecules,* Vol. 48, No. 2, (Mar 1 2011), pp. 234-238, ISSN 1879-0003

Smith, A. E. (1995). Viral vectors in gene therapy. *Annual Review of Microbiology,* Vol. 49, 1995), pp. 807-838, ISSN 0066-4227

Stayton, P. S.; El-Sayed, M. E.; Murthy, N.; Bulmus, V.; Lackey, C.; Cheung, C. & Hoffman, A. S. (2005). 'Smart' delivery systems for biomolecular therapeutics. *Orthodontics & Craniofacial Research,* Vol. 8, No. 3, (Aug 2005), pp. 219-225, ISSN 1601-6335

Sun, S.; Liu, W.; Cheng, N.; Zhang, B.; Cao, Z.; Yao, K.; Liang, D.; Zuo, A.; Guo, G. & Zhang, J. (2005). A thermoresponsive chitosan-NIPAAm/vinyl laurate copolymer vector for gene transfection. *Bioconjugate Chemistry,* Vol. 16, No. 4, (Jul-Aug 2005), pp. 972-980, ISSN 1043-1802

Thanou, M.; Florea, B. I.; Geldof, M.; Junginger, H. E. & Borchard, G. (2002). Quaternized chitosan oligomers as novel gene delivery vectors in epithelial cell lines. *Biomaterials,* Vol. 23, No. 1, (Jan 2002), pp. 153-159, ISSN 0142-9612

Uekama, K.; Hirayama, F. & Irie, T. (1998). Cyclodextrin Drug Carrier Systems. *Chemical Reviews,* Vol. 98, No. 5, (Jul 30 1998), pp. 2045-2076, ISSN 1520-6890

Wong, K.; Sun, G.; Zhang, X.; Dai, H.; Liu, Y.; He, C. & Leong, K. W. (2006). PEI-g-chitosan, a novel gene delivery system with transfection efficiency comparable to polyethylenimine in vitro and after liver administration in vivo. *Bioconjugate Chemistry,* Vol. 17, No. 1, (Jan-Feb 2006), pp. 152-158, ISSN 1043-1802

Wu, C. H. & Wu, G. Y. (1998). Receptor-mediated delivery of foreign genes to hepatocytes. *Advanced Drug Delivery Reviews,* Vol. 29, No. 3, (Feb 2 1998), pp. 243-248, ISSN 1872-8294

Yang, C.; Li, H.; Goh, S. H. & Li, J. (2007). Cationic star polymers consisting of alpha-cyclodextrin core and oligoethylenimine arms as nonviral gene delivery vectors. *Biomaterials,* Vol. 28, No. 21, (Jul 2007), pp. 3245-3254, ISSN 0142-9612

Zhang, H.; Mardyani, S.; Chan, W. C. & Kumacheva, E. (2006). Design of biocompatible chitosan microgels for targeted pH-mediated intracellular release of cancer therapeutics. *Biomacromolecules,* Vol. 7, No. 5, (May 2006), pp. 1568-1572, ISSN 1525-7797

Zhao, Q.; Temsamani, J. & Agrawal, S. (1995). Use of cyclodextrin and its derivatives as carriers for oligonucleotide delivery. *Antisense Research and Development,* Vol. 5, No. 3, (Fall 1995), pp. 185-192, ISSN 1050-5261

Zheng, Y.; Cai, Z.; Song, X.; Yu, B.; Bi, Y.; Chen, Q.; Zhao, D.; Xu, J. & Hou, S. (2009). Receptor mediated gene delivery by folate conjugated N-trimethyl chitosan in vitro. *International Journal of Pharmaceutics,* Vol. 382, No. 1-2, (Dec 1 2009), pp. 262-269, ISSN 1873-3476

Zidovetzki, R. & Levitan, I. (2007). Use of cyclodextrins to manipulate plasma membrane cholesterol content: evidence, misconceptions and control strategies. *Biochimica et Biophysica Acta,* Vol. 1768, No. 6, (Jun 2007), pp. 1311-1324, ISSN 0006-3002

Zugates, G. T.; Anderson, D. G.; Little, S. R.; Lawhorn, I. E. & Langer, R. (2006). Synthesis of poly(beta-amino ester)s with thiol-reactive side chains for DNA delivery. *Journal of the American Chemical Society,* Vol. 128, No. 39, (Oct 4 2006), pp. 12726-12734, ISSN 0002-7863

18

Chitosan and Its Modifications: Are They Possible Vehicles for Gene Therapy?

Ureporn Kedjarune-Leggat[1] and Peter A. Leggat[2]
[1]*Department of Oral Biology and Occlusion, Faculty of Dentistry*
Prince of Songkla University, Hat Yai, Songkhla
[2]*Anton Breinl Centre for Public Health and Tropical Medicine*
James Cook University, Townsville, Queensland
[1]*Thailand*
[2]*Australia*

1. Introduction

In gene therapy, the most important step is how to effectively deliver the therapeutic gene to the target cells or organ. At present, there are two methods, which are those using a viral and a non-viral vector system. The most common viral vectors that have been used include retroviruses, herpes simplex viruses, lentiviruses, adenoviruses and adeno-associated viruses (Oligino et al., 2000). The advantages of most viral vectors are high transfection efficiency and fast transcription of the foreign material inserted in the viral genome. However, a number of disadvantages have also been described, such as poor target-specificity, low capacity to incorporate foreign deoxyribonucleic acid (DNA) sequence to their genome (Mansouri et al., 2004), toxic and inflammatory effects, wild-type mutations, potential oncogenic effects (Lee et al., 1998), and, in particular, unwanted immune responses. In clinical trials of gene replacement therapy using viral vectors, significant adverse effects have been reported, including a fatal inflammatory response associated with adenoviral vector (Raper et al., 2003), and the development of acute leukaemia in recipients of ex-vivo, adenoviral vector-transduced hematopoietic cells (Woods et al., 2006). Intravenous adenoviral vector has also resulted in high liver toxicity due to uptake by hepatocytes or Kupffer cells of the liver reticular endothelial system, immediately following systemic administration.

2. Non-viral vectors for gene delivery

Due to the limitations and disadvantages of using viral vectors, there has been an ongoing search for an efficient safe vector for gene therapy, which has lead to the development of non-viral gene therapy. They have some advantages over viral methods, including simple large scale production and relatively low host immunogenicity. Previously, low levels of transfection and expression of the gene limited the usefulness of non-viral methods. However, recent advances in vector technology have been useful in yielding molecules and techniques with transfection efficiencies approaching or surpassing those of viral vectors. Table 1 provides examples of the main non-viral methods of gene delivery.

Non-viral method	Examples
Direct methods	Injection of naked DNA
Physical methods	Electoporation
	Gene gun
	Sonoporation
	Magnetofection
Chemical methods	Oligonucleotides
	Lipoplexes and polyplexes
	Dendrimers

Table 1. Examples of non-viral methods of gene delivery

Most non-viral vectors have no limitation in DNA size for packaging and they have the possibility of modification with ligands for tissue- or cell-specific targeting with low commercial cost and high reproducibility. Among these carriers, cationic lipids (lipoplexes) and cationic polymers (polycations) are primarily used, especially in *in vitro* gene transfection. Lipoplexes can form micelles or liposomes, which are multilayered structures, where the DNA is sandwiched between the cationic lipids. The lipoplexes present some problems due to their low physiological stability, reproducibility, and their toxicity of polar and hydrophobic moiety containing structure. *In vivo,* the intravenous administration of cationic lipid/DNA complexes presented significant problems, as these reagents can be quite toxic. On the other hand, polycations are more stable than lipoplexes and can protect DNA against nuclease degradation (Gao & Huang, 1996). Their structures also show more variability and versatility, including the possibility of incorporation of target-specific cellular receptors. Thus, modifications to these polymers, such as molecular weight (Mw), geometry (linear verses branched) and ligand attachment, can be easily undertaken successfully (Kim et al., 2007; Pack et al., 2005). Furthermore, they can compact DNA molecules to a relatively small particle size. However, the efficiency of gene delivery by both complexes is still relatively low, when compared to viral vectors. Polyethylenimine (PEI) is a cationic polymer that has been used for non-viral gene transfection for some time, but due to its toxicity and the variable results, it has not been widely accepted.

3. Chitosan as a non-viral carrier

At present, chitosan is the most prominent of the non-viral carriers being investigated. The biomaterial, chitosan, has interested many researchers around the world, particularly in relation to its ability to be a gene delivery vehicle or the ability to modify this biopolymer for the gene delivery vehicle. This is because of its properties of biodegradability, biocompatibility, and low toxicity, and because it can be modified for increasing transfection efficiency, as well as for targeting gene delivery development.

3.1 Molecular structure of chitosan

Chitosan (poly[β-(1-4)-2-amino-2-deoxy-D-glucopyranose]) is a deacetylation product of chitin (see Figure 1), a high Mw natural polymer found in the shells of marine crustaceans, such as shrimps (see Figure 2), as well as various insects, the internal structures of other invertebrates, and in the cell walls of fungi. It also provides an avenue for recycling of marine shellfish waste, which can now be "mined" for chitin and chitosan (Hayes et al., 2008).

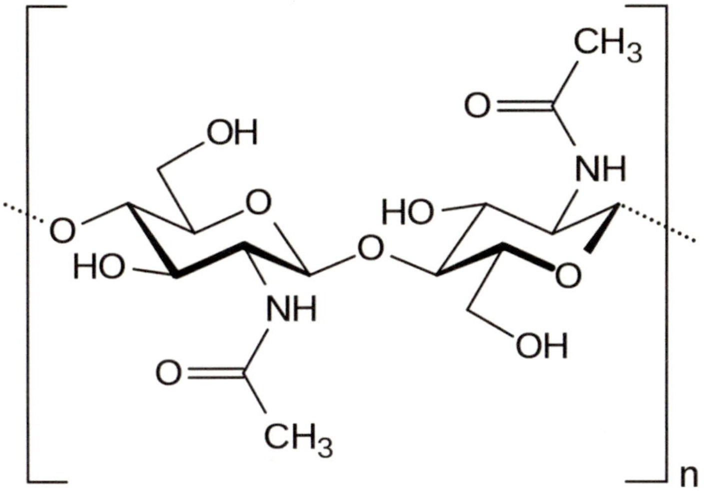

Fig. 1. Chemical structure of Chitin

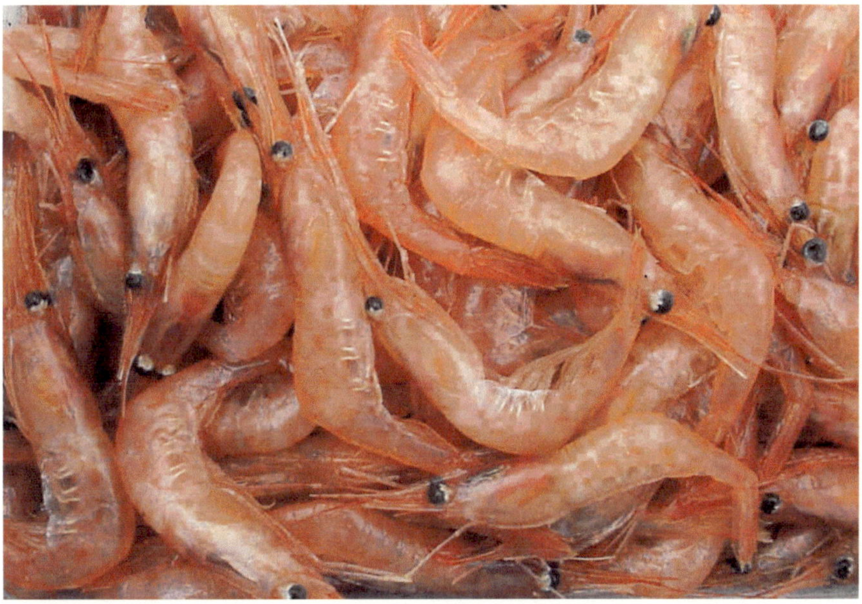

Fig. 2. Commercial chitosan is derived from the shells of shrimp and other sea crustaceans, including the Alaskan pink shrimp, pictured here (US National Oceanic and Atmosheric Administration, 2011)

Deacetylation of chitin can be performed by boiling chitin from crab or shrimp shells in sodium hydroxide after decolourisation with potassium permanganate (Van Der Lubben et al., 2001). Chitosan is a co-polymer of glucosamine and *N*-acetyl-D-glucosamine. When the number of N-acetylglucosamine units exceeds 50%, the biopolymer is called chitin; the term 'chitosan' is used to describe an N-acetyl-glucosamine unit content less than 50%. The chemical structure of chitosan is given in Figure 3.

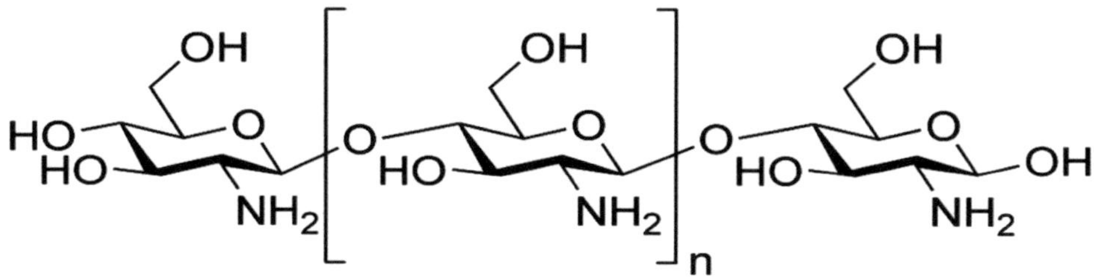

Fig. 3. Chemical structure of chitosan. It is a linear polysaccharide composed of randomly distributed β-(1-4)-linked D-glucosamine (deacetylated unit) and N-acetyl-D-glucosamine (acetylated unit)

3.2 Low toxicity of chitosan

Chitosan has low toxicity with an LD_{50} (lethal dose for 50% of test population) level in the same dose as sugar or salt (Arai, 1968). Toxicity tests reported the LD_{50} of chitosan in mice exceeded 16 g/kg. The molecular mass has minimal effect on cell viability, while the degree of deacetylation (DDA) of the polymer has greater effect on its toxicity (Richardson et al., 1999). DDA also affects the solubility, hydrophobicity and its ability to interact electrostatically with polyanions by affecting the number of protonatable amine groups of chitosan. Chitosan nanoparticles with lower DDA showed lower toxicity *in vitro* (Huang et al., 2004).

3.3 Applications of chitosan

Chitosan is a biodegradable polymer used in various industrial, biomedical and pharmaceutical applications due to its biocompatibility and the slow release of active molecules. Table 2 summarizes some of these broader applications. The novel properties of chitosan make it a versatile biomaterial for cell therapy, tissue engineering and gene therapy (Sui et al., 2006). Chitosan has a positive charge and hydrophilic character at an acidic pH. It is a continuum of primary aliphatic amine that can be protonated by acids; the pKa of the chitosan amine groups being around 6.3-6.5 (Kumar et al., 2004). The cationic amino groups on the C2 position of the repeating glucopyranose units of chitosan can interact electrostatically with the anionic groups (usually carboxylic acid groups) of other polyions to form polyelectrolyte complexes (Hamman, 2010). Many different polyanions from a natural origin (e.g. alginate, chondrotin sulfate or dextran sulphate) or from a synthetic orgin [e.g. poly(acrylic acid), polyphosphoric acid, or poly(L-lactide)] have been used to form polyelectrolyte complexes with chitosan, in order to provide the required physicochemical properties for design of specific drug delivery system, as well as specific target gene delivery (J. H. Park et al., 2010).

Usage	Examples of applications
Agricultural and horticultural	Natural biocontrol and elicitor
Water process engineering	Part of filtration process
Biomedical and pharmaceutical	Hemostatic agents
	Wound healing
	Tissue engineering
	Drug delivery
	Gene therapy

Table 2. Some applications of chitosan

4. Chitosan and gene delivery

Chitosan has been broadly studied as a promising non-viral vector for gene delivery (Bowman & Leong, 2006). This cationic polysaccharide can bind DNA between the positive charges of its amino groups and the negative charges of the phosphate groups of the DNA backbone in order to form nano- or microparticles. The interaction between chitosan and nucleic acids is electrostatic. The charge interaction is sufficiently strong that chitosan-DNA or small interfering ribonucleic acid (SiRNA) complex does not dissociate until it has entered the cell. Moreover, chitosan also protected nucleic acids from enzymatic degradation before entering the nucleus.

4.1 Transfection efficiency of chitosan

Tong et al. (2009) describes seven steps that should be overcome before the expression of exogenous DNA. They are complexation, *in vivo* administration, endocytosis, escape from endolysosome, release of DNA, trafficking through cytoplasm and finally importation of DNA into the nucleus. The transfection efficiency of chitosan itself is; however, relatively low, when compared to lipoplex or other methods. But this aminopolysaccharide can be modified for ease of DNA delivery, as well as for target gene delivery, which currently attracts many researchers to use chitosan and its modifications for gene delivery. Chitosan can be modified by ligand conjugation, such as transferrin-, folate- (folate and transferrin are over expressed in cancer cells), mannose- (target dendritic cells in tumor) and galactose (target Kupffer cells of the liver) conjugated chitosan, which can improve transfection efficiency of the targeted cells via receptor-mediated endocytosis (Duceppe & Tabrizian, 2010; Mao et al., 2010).

4.2 Factors affecting transfection efficiency

There are many factors that affect transfection efficiency. These include Mw, DDA, DNA complexes' charge ratio, pH and particle sizes, as well as the type of cell lines used.

4.2.1 Molecular weight (Mw)

High Mw chitosan can bind DNA tightly, which is due to the high number of positive charge of amino groups, but binding DNA tightly may give low transfection efficiency, due to not releasing the DNA to the nucleus after endocytosis to the cell. The Mw of chitosan also influences the size of the chitosan-DNA complexes, as the higher sizes of chitosan-DNA complexes can affect the cellular uptake. These factors lead to transfection efficiency (see review of Mao et al., 2010).

If the N/P ratio, which is the molar ratio between the amino groups of chitosan and the phosphate groups of DNA, was fixed, then the higher the Mw , the larger the chitosan-DNA complexes diameter (MacLaughlin et al., 1998). However, there have been differing conclusions proffered between the Mw of chitosan and transfection efficiency. Some studies have reported of high transfection efficiency with high Mw chitosan (Huang et al., 2005; Kiang et al., 2004; MacLaughlin et al., 1998). Other studies have reported that low Mw chitosan has better transfection efficiency (Koping-Hoggard et al., 2004; Lavertu et al., 2006; Supaprutsakul et al., 2010).

MacLaughlin et.al. (1998) synthesised depolymerised chitosan oligomers with a Mw from 7 - 92, but the transfection efficiency was much lower than at the higher Mw of 102 and 230 kDa, respectively, and being about 1000 times lower in transfection efficiency compared to lipofectamine™. Haung et al. (2005) also found a decreased A549 cellular uptake with the decreasing Mw or DDA of chitosan and a N/P ratio of 6 was used in that study. But the study of Supaprutsahul et al. (2010) revealed much higher transfection efficiency with the depolymerised chitosan at Mw ~16 kDa (or Mn ~ 6.5). This may be because of the different chitosan/DNA ratio, as the previous study used low N/P ratio, while Supaprutsakul et al. (2010) used chitosan/plasmid at an N/P ratio of about 56:1, which meant than a much higher amount of chitosan was used for the lower Mw. This was consistent with the study of Romøren et al. (2003), who found that low Mw chitosan was beneficial at the higher charge ratio of the complexes.

4.2.2 pH and degree of deacetylation (DDA)

The study of Lavertu et al. (2006) also found that the low Mw chitosan, which had a numeric average Mw (Mn) of about 10 and 80% DDA at N/P ratio 10:1, gave higher transfection efficiency at the same level as lipofectamine™ at pH 6.5. However, the very low Mw (1.9-7.7 kDa) chitosans with high DDA were found to form aggregates easily, even at very low charge ratios (Morris et al., 2008), and this might lower the transfection. However, the depolymerised LW chitosan in this study had only 54% DDA, which may reduce the problem of particles aggregation and, after cells uptake the chitosan-DNA nanoparticles, the DNA may be released from the nanoparticles more easily, as DNA binding efficacy was reduced as DDA was decreased (Kiang et al., 2004). Hence, many factors may have to be considered for improving transfection efficiency of chitosan, not only the ligand binding, but also the method of binding or conjugation, the size and morphology of the particles, the aggregation of the complexes, and especially the chitosan itself, as Mw, DDA and charge ratio, which may have to be adjusted.

4.2.3 Cell line dependency

Another factor, which may affect transfection efficiency of chitosan, is cell line dependency. Higher mitotic cell lines, such as cancer cells, usually have higher transfection efficiencies that lower proliferative rates of the cell line. This may be related to differences in cell physiology affecting the internalisation mechanism and subsequent internal trafficking of the vectors (Douglas et al., 2008). It has also been found that dividing cells have higher transfection ability compared to quiescent cells (Brunner et al., 2000) and higher levels of gene expression have been observed just before or during mitosis (Mortimer et al., 1999). This may explain why the immortalised cell line, with higher mitotic activity, has higher transfection ability than normal or primary cell lines. However, this factor requires further investigation.

4.3 Improving transfection efficiency

There have also some attempts to modify the chemical structure of chitosan to improve transfection efficiency, which have involved hydrophilic and hydrophobic modifications. The main purpose of hydrophilic modification of chitosan is to increase solubility and reduce sensitivity of chitosan-DNA complexes to pH, as well as reduce the chitosan-DNA complexes aggregation, which may improve transfection efficiency. The hydrophilic chitosan modification includes quaternised chitosan (Thanou et al., 2002), PEGylated (covalent attachment of polyethylene glycol polymer chains to another molecule) chitosan (Jiang et al., 2006) and low Mw soluble chitosan (Ercelen et al., 2006). Interestingly, Brannon-Peppas & Blanchette (2004) found that particles with more hydrophobic surfaces were also preferentially taken up by the liver, followed by the spleen and the lungs.

Hydrophobic modifications of chitosan have been performed in many studies. The main objectives of these modifications were increasing transfection efficiency by modulating complex interactions with cells, especially in the complexes' adsorption on the cell surfaces and cell uptake (Kurisawa et al., 2000). Some hydrophobic units also help in the dissociation between the chitosan DNA complexes to release DNA to enter the nucleus after cellular uptake, as well as protecting it from enzymatic degradation and facilitating intra cellular pDNA (plasmid DNA) association, which can enhance transfection efficiency. These hydrophobic modifications included deoxycholic chitosan, N-alkylated chitosan, thiolated chitosan and hybrid chitosan (Mao et al., 2010). The combination of hydrophilic and hydrophobic modification of chitosan structure has been another interesting area that looks highly promising for the development of high transfection efficiency in a non-viral vector, using chitosan as a core structure.

5. Chitosan and gene therapy

One of the significant applications of chitosan is in its application to gene therapy. It has a number of benefits. It has non-toxic, biodegradable and biocompatible with high cationic charge potential; protects DNA from degradation by nucleases; and has high yield transfection efficiency (Sui et al., 2006). Genetic material (DNA and RNA) has been explored for use as a treatment of genetic abnormalities or deficiencies, which is described as gene therapy. Gene therapy functions by transferring healthy genetic material or nucleic acid constructs, such as ribozymes, antisense molecules, decoy oligodeoxy nucleotides (ODNs), DNAzymes and siRNA, into diseased cells in an attempt to achieve a therapeutic effect that results in restoration of protein production, which was absent or deficient due to the pre-existing genetic disorder (Tan et al., 2009). But using small nucleic acid, such as DNAzymes and siRNA, has some limitations, since they are rapidly degraded in plasma and cellular cytoplasm and cannot passively diffuse through cellular membrane, which is due to the strong anionic charge of the phosphate backbone and the consequent electrostatic repulsion from the anionic cell membrane surface as well as limited size of cellular entrance. So, these small nucleic acids encapsulated with chitosan nanoparticles can reduce the limitations of these small nucleic acids.

5.1 Use of chitosan nanoparticles

The development of chitosan and its modification for non-viral gene delivery is also a target for gene therapy. This is because chitosan nanoparticles have a low toxicity and are taken up by endosomes allowing the DNA or nucleic acid to overcome the permeability barrier posed by epithelium and also to protect against enzymatic degradation. There are some studies that have attempted to use chitosan for cancer therapy. Chitosan itself was able to demonstrate growth inhibitory effects on cancer cells and has apoptosis effect on bladder tumour cells via caspase-3 activation (Tan et al., 2009). The various manufacturing processes for chitosan nano-/micro- particles/spheres (nanofabrication) has been described elsewhere (Masotti et al., 2009).

5.2 Use of siRNA loaded chitosan nanoparticles

In current developments in chitosan for gene therapy, there is an attempt to develop siRNA loaded chitosan nanoparticles to silence the target gene. This method can silence the gene by means of RNA interfering (RNAi). SiRNAs, usually containing 20-25 base pairs (see Figure

4), assemble into endoribonuclease containing complexes known as RNA-induced silencing complexes (RISCs).

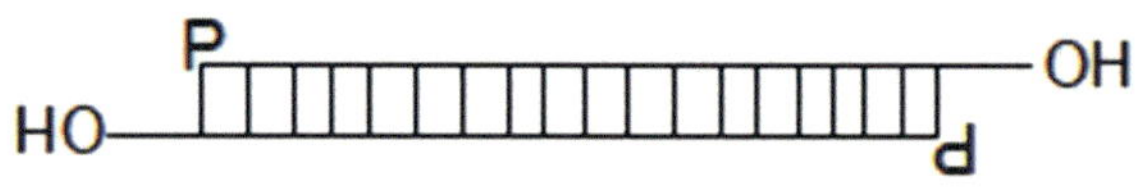

Fig. 4. Schematic representation of a siRNA molecule. SiRNA have a well-defined structure: a short (usually 21-nucleotide-long) double-strand of RNA with 2-nucleotide 3′ overhangs on either end (Alper, 2006).

The siRNA strands guide the RISCs to complementary RNA molecules leading to cleavage and destroy the target RNA (Manjunath & Dykxhoorn, 2010).
The mechanism of RNAi is described in Figure 5.

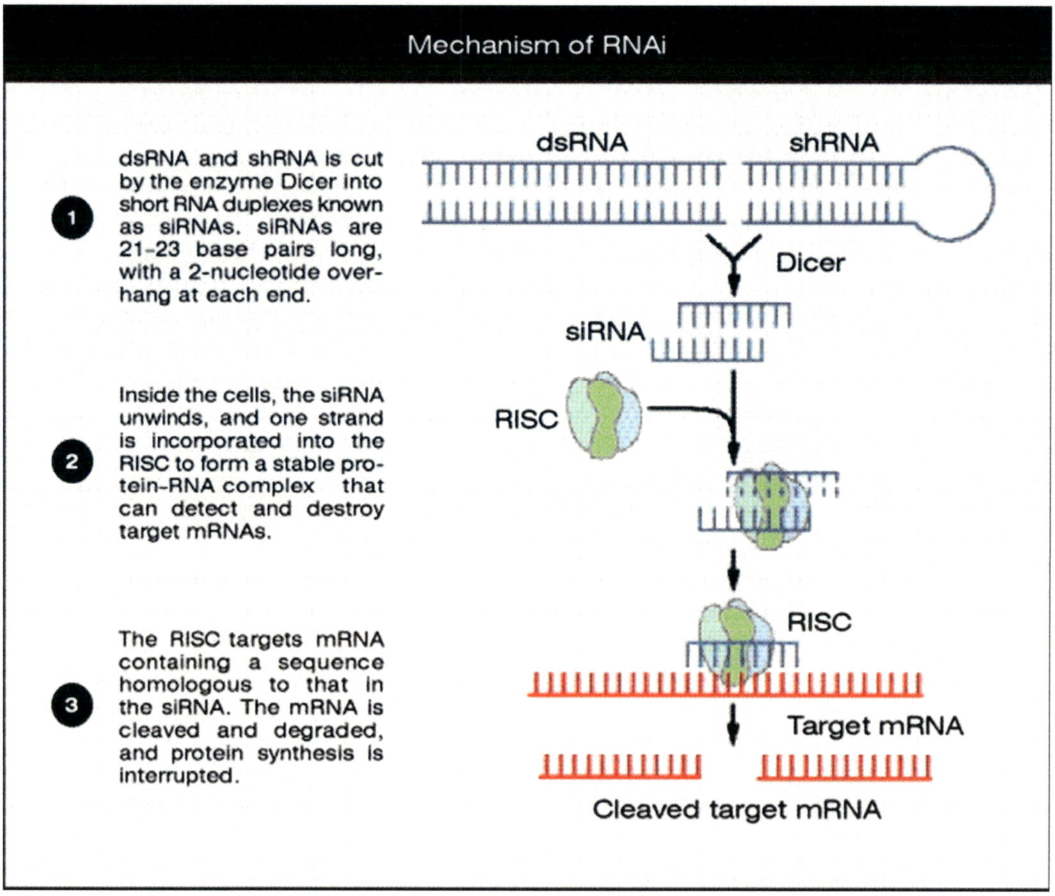

Fig. 5. Mechanism of RNAi (Hood, 2004). dsRNA=double stranded RNA; shRNA=small hairpin RNA (sequence of RNA that can be used to silence gene expression via RNA interference); mRNA=messenger RNA

This system is of interest to numerous researchers, as well as many pharmaceutical companies, since the efficient siRNA delivery system will have clinical therapeutic impact in gene therapy (Mao et al., 2010; Park et al., 2010; Rudzinski & Aminabhavi, 2010). However, further investigations are needed, especially *in vivo* experiments/clinical trials.

6. Limitations in the use of chitosan

There are some limitations in the use of chitosan for non-viral gene therapy. Firstly, there is a lack of knowledge of the pharmacokinetics of chitosan-nucleic acid complexes during uptake inside the body. When chitosan-DNA nanoparticles enter the body, they were quickly removed from the blood and deposited on different organs. Administration of larger nanoparticles results in a substantial increase of the particles in the lung with a subsequent decrease in the liver, indicating a strong dependence of the tissue distribution on particle size (Liu, 2007). However, more information on this topic is required. Secondly, there is a need for more studies in animals, including clinical trials.

Most of the studies in the past few years about chitosan and gene therapy continue to use an *in vitro* model; however, more studies have been performed using mouse model, as summarised in Table 3.

Route of transmission	Form of chitosan complexes	Target organ/ Disease	Study design	Reference
Utero gene transfer (injection in amniotic sacs)	Chitosan-DNA (reporter gene)	Expected route for fetal gene therapy	Mouse (murine)	Yang et al., 2008; Jang et al., in press
Local gene delivery via endovascular stent	Chitosan-DNA coated with dodecylated in endovascular stent	Expected route for diseased blood vessel wall	Mouse	Zhu et al., 2010
Local: inhalation	Chitosan-DNA (interferon-beta gene) complexes powder	Lung cancer	Mouse	Okamoto et al., 2010
Local: inhalation	Spray -freeze dry chitosan-DNA	Expected route for pulmonary gene therapy	Mouse	Mohri et al., 2010
Local: localized hydrogel by intra-tumoural injection	Chitosan-SiRNA	Expected route for multiple localized disease	Mouse models of melanoma and breast cancers	Han et al., 2010
Local: intra-tumoural injection	Chitosan-SiRNA design to down regulate RXFP1 expression	Prostate cancer	Mouse: xenograft model	Feng et al., 2010

Table 3. Summary of current animal experiments using chitosan as non-viral for gene therapy

Lastly, the route of transmission and target gene delivery are the major factors which contribute to the success in gene therapy, which still requires further investigation.
Table 4 summarises some attempts to modify the chitosan-nucleic acid complexes for target gene therapy.

Modification	Chitosan complexes	Conclusion	Study design	Reference
Folate mediated targeting induced by conjugating poly(ethylene glycol)-folate (PEG-FA) with arginine modified chitosan	PEG-FA-chitosan-DNA	The transfection efficiency was higher than PEI when transfected in KB cell line, which over expressed the folate receptor (FR) in presence of 10% foetal bovine serum (FBS).	*In vitro* (KB cell line)	Morris & Sharma, 2010
Arg-Gly-Asp (RGD) peptide-labelled chitosan nanoparticle (RGD-CH-NP) as a novel tumour targeted delivery system for short interfering RNA (siRNA).	RGD-CH–SiRNA nanoparticles	RGD-CH-NP is a novel and highly selective delivery system for siRNA with the potential for broad applications in human disease.	Orthotopic mouse models of ovarian carcinoma	Han et al., 2010
Antisense oligo-deoxynucleotides (asODN), using folic acid (FA) conjugated hydroxypropyl-chitosan	FA-Chtosan-asODN nanoparticles	Targeted antisense agent would be a potential approach to overcome tumour drug resistance.	*In vitro* (KB cell line)	Wang et al., 2010
Tumour- of adenoviral complexes targeting of Adenovirus (Ad)/chitosan-PEG-FA nanocomplexes formed by electrospining	Ad/chitosan-PEG-FA nano-complexes	Transduction efficiency of Ad/chitosan-PEG-FA was 57% higher than Ad/chitosan. This system aims for development of systemic administration of the vectors to target lesion.	*In vitro* (KB cell line)	Park et al., 2010

Table 4. Some modifications of chitosan for target gene therapy

7. Summary

An efficient gene delivery system is very important for gene therapy. Currently, the most efficient of these systems is a viral vector, which usually yields a transfection efficiency of more than 90%. However, by using a viral vector for gene therapy, there is a concern about the host versus vector immunological response, mutation and oncogenic effects; hence the need to develop a non-viral vector. There are many non-viral vectors; the high efficient one is cationic lipid, which gives high transfection efficiency, especially in tissue culture or *in vitro* conditions. *In vivo*, the intravenous administration of cationic lipid/DNA complexes presented significant problems, as these reagents can be quite toxic. PEI is another non-viral transfection material that has been used for some time, but due to its toxicity and the variable results, it has not been widely accepted.

Chitosan (poly[β-(1-4)-2-amino-2deoxy-D-glucopyranose]), a nontoxic biodegradable biopolymer, has been broadly studied as a promising non-viral vector for gene delivery. This cationic polysaccharide has been produced by partial deacetylation of chitin, a naturally polymer from crustacean shells. However, the transfection efficiency of chitosan itself is not efficient enough and depends on many factors such as Mw, DDA, DNA complexes charge ratio, pH and particle sizes, as well as the type of cells. There have been many attempts to modify chitosan in order to improve transfection efficiency. Some studies have revealed that low Mw chitosan, especially the product of oxidative depolymerisation from higher Mw chitosan with $NaNO_2$, had low cytotoxicity and improved solubility properties, as well as having potential for gene delivery both *in vitro* and *in vivo*. However, some studies have reported decreased transfection efficiency with lower Mw chitosan.

There have been other attempts modifying the chemical structure of chitosan. These have included introducing a hydrophilic group, such as coupling dextran, as well as incorporating poly (vinyl pyrolidone) into the galactosylated chitosan, which can reduce the aggregation of particles and increase transfection efficiency. Some studies have also using hydrophobic modification of chitosan, such as deoxycholic acid-modified chitosan, in order to increase transfection efficiency through enhancement of complex interaction with cells and cellular uptake of the particles. Chitosan can be modified by conjugation of chitosan-DNA complexes with ligands to target specific cell surface receptors, but these attempts have had variable results. Many factors may have to be considered for improving transfection efficiency of chitosan, not just ligand binding, but also the method of binding or conjugation, the size and morphology of the particles, the aggregation of the complexes, and especially the chitosan itself, as Mw, DDA and charge ratio may have to be adjusted.

The design criteria of the effective vector for non-viral gene therapy should also consider cost-effectiveness in synthesis and purification steps, serum stability and efficient packaging of large amount of the vector-nucleic acid complexes. Moreover, the route of administration of this vector to the target cells or tumour lesion, high transfection efficiency, specific target gene delivery should also be considered. Once the complexes enter the target cells, they have to escape from enzyme degradation. The complexes then release the therapeutic gene/ nucleic acid to the target organelle, such as DNA, which has to enter the nucleus, while siRNA functions in cytoplasm. This release has to occur without too many difficulties, which means that the bonding between the vectors and nucleic acid should not be too strong. Most importantly, these non-viral vectors have to be safe enough for the patient, including being non toxic to the host body, non-immunogenic and non pathogenic. Chitosan is now one of the candidate biomaterials for selection as an effective non-viral vector for gene therapy, especially as it is safe, cheap and easy to modify.

8. Acknowledgment

The authors wish to acknowledge the support of the World Safety Organization Collaborating Centre within the Anton Breinl Centre for Public Health and Tropical Medicine, James Cook University, Townsville, Queensland, Australia, for their kind support of this project.

9. References

Alper, J. (2006). Nanoparticles and siRNA-Partners on the pathway to new cancer therapies. *National Cancer Institute Alliance for Nanotechnology in Cancer Monthly Feature,* August: 1-3.

Arai, K., Kinumaki, T. & Fujitta, T. (1968) Toxicity of chitosan. *Bulletin of Tokai Regional Fisheries Research Laboratory,* 56: 89-94.

Brandon-Peppas, L & Brancehette, J. O. (2004). Nanoparticle and targeted systems for cancer therapy and diagnosis. *Advanced Drug Delivery Reviews,* 56: 1649-59.

Brunner, S., Sauer, T., Carotta, S., Cotton, M., Saltik, M. & Wagner, E. (2000). Cell cycle dependence of gene transfer by lipoplex, polyplex and recombinant adenovirus. *Gene Therapy,* 7(5): 401-7.

Bowman, K. & Leong, K.W. (2006). Chitosan nanoparticles for oral drug and gene delivery. *International Journal of Nanomedicine,* 1(2): 117-28.

Douglas, K.L., Piccirillo, C.A. & Tabrizian, M. (2008). Cell line-dependent internalization pathways and intracellular trafficking determine transfection efficiency of nanoparticle vectors. *European Journal of Pharmaceutics and Biopharmaceuticals,* 68(3): 676-87.

Duceppe, N. & Tabrizian, M. (2010). Advances in using chitosan-based nanoparticles for in vitro and in vivo drug and gene delivery. *Expert Opinion on Drug Delivery,* 7(10): 1191-207.

Ercelen, S., Zhang, X., Duportail, G., Grandfils, C., Desbrieres, J., Karaeva, S., Tikhonov, V., Mely, Y. & Babak, V. (2006). Physicochemical properties of low molecular weight alkylated chitosans: a new class of potential nonviral vectors for gene delivery. *Colloids and Surfaces B: Biointerfaces,* 51(2): 140-8.

Feng, S., Agoulnik, I.U., Truong, A., Li, Z., Creighton, C.J., Kaftanovskaya, E.M., Pereira, R., Han, H.D., Lopez-Berestein, G., Klonisch, T., Ittmann, M.M., Sood, A.K. & Agoulnik, A.I. (2010). Suppression of relaxin receptor RXFP1 decreases prostate cancer growth and metastasis. *Endocrine Related Cancer,* 17(4): 1021-33.

Gao, X. & Huang, L. (1996). Potentiation of cationic liposome-mediated gene delivery by polycations. *Biochemistry,* 35(3): 1027-36.

Hamman, J.H. (2010). Chitosan based polyelectrolyte complexes as potential carrier materials in drug delivery systems. *Marine Drugs,* 8(4): 1305-22.

Han, H.D., Mangala, L.S., Lee, J.W., Shahzad, M.M., Kim, H.S., Shen, D., Nam, E.J., Mora, E.M., Stone, R.L., Lu, C., Lee, S.J., Roh, J.W., Nick, A.M., Lopez-Berestein, G. & Sood, A.K. (2010). Targeted gene silencing using RGD-labeled chitosan nanoparticles. *Clinical Cancer Research,* 16(15): 3910-22.

Han, H.D., Mora, E.M., Roh, J.W., Nishimura, M., Lee, S.J., Stone, R.L., Bar-Eli, M., Lopez-Berestein, G. & Sood, A.K. (2011). Chitosan hydrogel for localized gene silencing. *Cancer Biology and Therapy,* 11(9): 839-45.

Hayes, M., Carney, B., Slater, J. & Brück, W. (2008). Mining marine shellfish wastes for bioactive molecules: chitin and chitosan. Part B: applications. *Biotechnology Journal,* 3(7): 878-89.

Hood, E. (2004). RNAi: What's all the noise about gene silencing? *Environmental Health Perspectives,* 114(4): A225-9. Assessed 23 April 2011. Available at: http://ehp.niehs.nih.gov/txg/members/2004/112-4/focus.html

Huang, M., Khor, E. & Lim, L.Y. (2004). Uptake and cytotoxicity of chitosan molecules and nanoparticles: effects of molecular weight and degree of deacetylation. *Pharmaceutical Research,* 21(2): 344-53.

Huang, M., Fong, C.W., Khor, E. & Lim, L.Y. (2005). Transfection efficiency of chitosan vectors: effect of polymer molecular weight and degree of deacetylation. *Journal of Controlled Release,* 106(3): 391-406.

Jiang, X., Dai, H., Leong, K.W., Goh, S.H., Mao, H.Q. & Yang, Y.Y. (2006). Chitosan-g-PEG/DNA complexes deliver gene to the rat liver via intrabiliary and intraportal infusions. *Journal of Gene Medicine,* 8(4): 477-87.

Kiang, T., Wen, J., Lim, H.W. & Leong, K.W. (2004). The effect of the degree of chitosan deacetylation on the efficiency of gene transfection. *Biomaterials* 25(22): 5293-301.

Kim, T.H., Jiang, H.L., Nah, J.W., Cho, M.H., Akaike, T. & Cho, C.S. (2007). Receptor-mediated gene delivery using chemically modified chitosan. *Biomedical Materials,* 2(3): S95-100.

Koping-Hoggard, M., Varum, K.M., Issa, M., Danielsen, S., Christensen, B.E., Stokke, B.T. & Artursson, P. (2004). Improved chitosan-mediated gene delivery based on easily dissociated chitosan polyplexes of highly defined chitosan oligomers. *Gene Therapy,* 11(19): 1441-52.

Kumar, M.N., Muzzarelli, R.A., Muzzarelli, C., Sashiwa, H. & Domb, A.J. (2004). Chitosan chemistry and pharmaceutical perspectives. *Chemical Reviews,* 104(12): 6017-84.

Kurisawa, M., Yokoyama, M. & Okano, T. (2000). Transfection efficiency increases by incorporating hydrophobic monomer units into polymeric gene carriers. *Journal of Controlled Release,* 68(1): 1-8.

Lavertu, M., Methot, S., Tran-Khanh, N. & Buschmann, M.D. (2006). High efficiency gene transfer using chitosan/DNA nanoparticles with specific combinations of molecular weight and degree of deacetylation. *Biomaterials,* 27(27): 4815-24.

Lee, K.Y., Kwon, I.C., Kim, Y.H., Jo, W.H. & Jeong, S.Y. (1998). Preparation of chitosan self-aggregates as a gene delivery system. *Journal of Controlled Release,* 51(2-3): 213-20.

MacLaughlin, F.C., Mumper, R.J., Wang, J., Tagliaferri, J.M., Gill, I., Hinchcliffe, M. & Rolland, A.P. (1998). Chitosan and depolymerized chitosan oligomers as condensing carriers for in vivo plasmid delivery. *Journal of Controlled Release,* 56(1-3): 259-72.

Manjunath, N. & Dykxhoorn, D.M. (2010). Advances in synthetic siRNA delivery. *Discovery Medicine,* 9(48): 418-30.

Mansouri, S., Lavigne, P., Corsi, K., Benderdour, M., Beaumont, E. & Fernandes, J.C. (2004). Chitosan-DNA nanoparticles as non-viral vectors in gene therapy: strategies to improve transfection efficacy. *European Journal of Pharmaceutics and Biopharmaceuticals,* 57(1): 1-8.

Mao, S., Sun, W. & Kissel, T. (2010). Chitosan-based formulations for delivery of DNA and siRNA. *Advanced Drug Delivery Reviews,* 62(1): 12-27.

Masotti, A. & Ortaggi, G. (2009). Chitosan micro- and nanospheres: fabrication and applications for drug and DNA delivery. *Mini-Reviews in Medicinal Chemistry,* 9(4): 463-9.

Mohri, K., Okuda, T., Mori, A., Danjo, K. & Okamoto, H. (2010). Optimized pulmonary gene transfection in mice by spray-freeze dried powder inhalation. *Journal of Controlled Release,* 144(2): 221-6.

Morris, V.B., Neethu, S., Abraham, T.E., Pillai, C.K. & Sharma, C.P. (2009). Studies on the condensation of depolymerized chitosans with DNA for preparing chitosan-DNA nanoparticles for gene delivery applications. *Journal of Biomedical Materials Research B: Applied Biomaterials,* 89B(2): 282-92.

Morris, V.B. & Sharma, C.P. (2010). Folate mediated in vitro targeting of depolymerised trimethylated chitosan having arginine functionality. *Journal of Colloid and Interface Science,* 348(2): 360-8.

Mortimer, I., Tam, P., MacLachlan, I., Graham, R.W., Saravolac, E.G. & Joshi, P.B. (1999). Cationic lipid-mediated transfection of cells in culture requires mitotic activity. *Gene Therapy,* 6(3): 403-11.

Okamoto, H., Shiraki, K., Yasuda, R., Danjo, K. & Watanabe ,Y. (2011). Chitosan-interferon-beta gene complex powder for inhalation treatment of lung metastasis in mice. *Journal of Controlled Release,* 150(2): 187-95.

Oligino, T.J., Yao, Q., Ghivizzani, S.C. & Robbins, P. (2000). Vector systems for gene transfer to joints. *Clinical Orthopaedics and Related Research,* 379(Suppl): S17-30.

Pack, D.W., Hoffman, A.S., Pun, S. & Stayton, P.S. (2005). Design and development of polymers for gene delivery. *Nature Reviews Drug Discovery,* 4(7): 581-93.

Park, J.H., Saravanakumar, G., Kim, K. & Kwon, I.C. (2010). Targeted delivery of low molecular drugs using chitosan and its derivatives. *Advanced Drug Delivery Reviews,* 62(1): 28-41.

Park, Y., Kang, E., Kwon, O.J., Hwang, T., Park, H., Lee, J.M., Kim, J.H. & Yun, C.O. (2010). Ionically crosslinked Ad/chitosan nanocomplexes processed by electrospinning for targeted cancer gene therapy. *Journal of Controlled Release,* 148(1): 75-82.

Raper, S.E., Chirmule, N., Lee, F.S., Wivel, N.A., Bagg, A., Gao, G.P., Wilson, J.M. & Batshaw, M.L. (2003). Fatal systemic inflammatory response syndrome in an ornithine transcarbamylase deficient patient following adenoviral gene transfer. *Molecular Genetics and Metabolism,* 80(1-2): 148-58.

Richardson, S.C., Kolbe, H.V. & Duncan, R. (1999). Potential of low molecular mass chitosan as a DNA delivery system: biocompatibility, body distribution and ability to complex and protect DNA. *International Journal of Pharmaceutics,* 178(2): 231-43.

Romøren, K., Pedersen, S., Smistad, G., Evensen, Ø., Thu, B.J. (2003). The influence of formulation variables on in vitro transfection efficiency and physicochemical properties of chitosan-based polyplexes. *International Journal of Pharmaceutics,* 261(1-2): 115-27.

Rudzinski, W.E. & Aminabhavi, T.M. (2010). Chitosan as a carrier for targeted delivery of small interfering RNA. *International Journal of Pharmaceutics,* 399(1-2): 1-11.

Shi, C., Zhu, Y., Ran, X., Wang, M., Yongping, S. & Cheng, T. (2006). Therapeutic potential of chitosan and its derivatives in regenerative medicine. *Journal of Surgical Research,* 133(2): 185-92.

Supaprutsakul, S., Chotigeat, W., Wanichpakorn, S. & Kedjarune-Leggat, U. (2010). Transfection efficiency of depolymerized chitosan and epidermal growth factor conjugated to chitosan-DNA polyplexes. *Journal of Materials Science: Materials in Medicine,* 21(5): 1553-61.

Tan, M.L., Choong, P.F. & Dass, C.R. (2009). Cancer, chitosan nanoparticles and catalytic nucleic acids. *Journal of Pharmacy and Pharmacology,* 61(1): 3-12.

Thanou, M., Florea, B.I., Geldof, M., Junginger, H.E. & Borchard, G. (2002). Quaternized chitosan oligomers as novel gene delivery vectors in epithelial cell lines. *Biomaterials,* 23(1): 153-9.

Tong, H., Shi, Q., Fernandes, J.C., Liu, L., Dai, K. & Zhang, X. (2009). Progress and prospects of chitosan and its derivatives as non-viral gene vectors in gene therapy. *Current Gene Therapy,* 9: 495-502.

US National Oceanic and Atmosheric Administration. (2011) Alaskan pink shrimp (*Pandalus eous*). Accessed 22 April 2011. Available from: http://www.afsc.noaa.gov/race/media/photo_gallery/invert_files/Alaskan_pink_shrimp.htm

Van Der Lubben, I.M., Konings, F.A., Borchard, G., Verhoef, J.C. & Junginger, H.E. (2001). In vivo uptake of chitosan microparticles by murine Peyer's patches: visualization studies using confocal laser scanning microscopy and immunohistochemistry. *Journal of Drug Targeting,* 9(1): 39-47.

Wang, J., Tao, X., Zhang, Y., Wei, D. & Ren, Y. (2010). Reversion of multidrug resistance by tumor targeted delivery of antisense oligodeoxynucleotides in hydroxyproply-chitosan nanoparticles. *Biomaterials,* 31(15: 4426-33.

Woods, N.B., Bottero, V., Schmidt, M., von Kalle, C. & Verma, I.M. (2006). Gene therapy: therapeutic gene causing lymphoma. *Nature,* 440(7088): 1123.

Yang, P.T., Jia, W. & Skarsgard, E.D. (2008). In utero gene delivery using chitosan-DNA nanoparticles in mice. *Clinical and Investigative Medicine,* 31(4 Suppl.): S25.

Yang, P.T., Hoang L., Jia, W.W. & Sharsgard, E.D. (2011). In utero gene delivery using chitosan-DNA nanoparticles in mice. *Journal of Surgical Research,* (in press)

Zhu, D., Jin, X., Leng, X., Wang, H., Bao, J., Liu, W., Yao, K. & Song, C. (2010). Local gene delivery via endovascular stents coated with dodecylated chitosan-plasmid DNA nanoparticles. *International Journal of Nanomedicine,* 5(1): 95-102.

19

Chitosan-DNA/siRNA Nanoparticles for Gene Therapy

Qin Shi[1], Marcio J. Tiera[2], Xiaoling Zhang[3], Kerong Dai[3], Mohamed Benderdour[1] and Julio C. Fernandes[1]

[1]*Orthopedic Research Laboratory, Hôpital du Sacré-Cœur de Montréal Université de Montréal*

[2]*Departamento de Quimica e Ciencias Ambientais, UNESP-Universidade Estadual Paulista- Brazil*

[3]*The key laboratory of Stem Cell Biology, Institute of Health Sciences Shanghai Jiao Tong University School of Medicine (SJTUSM) & Shanghai Institutes for Biological Sciences (SIBS), Chinese Academy of Sciences (CAS)*

[1]*Canada*

[2]*Brazil*

[3]*China*

1. Introduction

Human diseases can be treated by the transfer of therapeutic genes (transgene) into specific cells or tissues of patients to correct or supplement defective, causative genes. Gene therapy offers a solution to controlled and specific delivery of genetic materials (DNA and RNA) to targeted cells. The success of gene therapy depends on the ability to deliver these therapeutic materials to targeted site. Viral vectors (e.g. adenovirus) are very effective in term of transfection efficiency, but they have limitations *in vivo*, particularly by their safety concern and non tissue-specific transfection. Non-viral gene transfer systems are limited by their lower gene transfer efficiency, low tissue specificity and transient gene expression.

Chitosan is a polysaccharide usually obtained from deacetylation of chitin, which may be extracted from various sources, particularly from exoskeletons of arthropods such as crustaceans. The goal of this chapter is to introduce the readers to chitosan as a DNA/small interfering RNA (siRNA) delivery vector, as well as different variable strategies to improve cellular transfection and its potential clinical application. the first section is to present of chapter (section 1). The second section presents the discussion about barriers to DNA/siRNA delivery *in vitro* and *in vivo*. It is important to have a clear overview of obstacles to the *in vivo* treatment with DNA/siRNAs. Different *in vivo* administration routes will encounter different physiological barriers, and complications may be furthered by different cells in organs and tissues (section 2). The third section provides the readers with an understanding of the key steps of cellular internalization of DNA/siRNA non-viral vectors. Internalization of non-viral vector-based DNA/siRNA delivery system into cells typically occurs through endocytosis (section 3). the fourth section describes chitosan as a vector for gene therapy (section 4) followed by chitosan structure and physicochemical behaviour (section 5), general strategies for chitosan modification (section 6), chitosan-DNA delivery system (section 7), chitosan-siRNA delivery system (section 8), and potential applications of chitosan–DNA/siRNA nanoparticles (section 9). Our current research will be summarized in the section of conclusion.

2. Barriers to gene delivery using non-viral vectors

2.1 Viral gene vectors

Gene transfer can occur through 2 delivery systems: viral or non-viral vectors. Viral gene therapy consists of using viral vectors which, given their structure and mechanisms of action, are good candidates or models to carry therapeutic genes efficiently, leading to long-term expression. Viruses are obvious first choices as gene transport. They have the natural ability to enter cells and express their own proteins. Nowadays, most viral vectors used are retroviruses, herpes virus, adenoviruses and lentiviruses. Unfortunately, certain viral vectors (for example, adenoviruses) can elicit a robust cellular immune response against viral and some transgenic proteins, so their use has been limited to studies in immune-compromised animals (Seiler et al., 2007). Adeno-associated viruses (AAV), which have been considered safe, appear to be immunogenic in several experimental settings (Vandenberghe & Wilson, 2007) and in a clinical trial (Mingozzi & High, 2007). Some serious adverse events have occurred with viral gene therapy. One patient died of fatal systemic inflammatory response syndrome after adenoviral gene transfer in 1999 (Raper et al., 2003). Two children developed leukemia-like clonal lymphocyte proliferation after recombinant retroviral gene transfer in 2000 (Hacein-Bey-Abina et al., 2003), and 1 of them died after unsuccessful chemotherapy late in 2004. Attention focused recently on the tragic death of a young female patient in a gene therapy study (intra-articular injection of AAV vectors) of severe RA in 2007 (Kaiser, 2007).

2.2 Non-viral gene vectors

Non-viral gene transfer systems offer several potential advantages over virus vectors. They are non-infectious, relatively non-immunogenic, have low acute toxicity, can accommodate large DNA plasmids or RNA, and may be produced on a large scale (Castanotto & Rossi, 2009; Gary et al., 2007). Non-viral gene therapy has been explored by physical approaches (transfer by gene gun, electroporation, ultrasound-facilitated and hydrodynamic delivery) as well as chemical approaches (cationic lipid-mediated gene delivery and cationic polymer-mediated gene transfer). Numerous chemical non-viral gene transfer systems have been proposed, including naked DNA, cationic liposomes, histones, and polymers (Gao et al., 2007; Ulrich-Vinther, 2007). The main drawback of non-viral vectors as gene carriers is their typically low transfection efficiency (Gao et al., 2007; Giannoudis et al., 2006). Furthermore, the *in vivo* delivery of non-viral liposome/plasmid DNA complex triggers an immune response (Sakurai et al., 2008). Non-viral gene therapy with cationic liposomes has already been tested in clinical trials that dealt with the treatment of inherited genetic disorders (for example, cystic fibrosis) (Hyde et al., 2000) and cancer (Ramesh et al., 2001). Synthetic and natural cationic polymers (positively-charged) have been widely used to carry DNA or siRNA (both negatively-charged) and condense it into small particles, facilitating cellular internalization via endocytosis through charge-charge interactions with anionic sites on cell surfaces. Although existing non-viral vectors have been found to enable DNA expression after *in vivo* delivery, the efficiency and duration of ensuing gene expression have proven to be unsatisfactory. Research efforts to improve the *in vivo* DNA-delivery efficacy of non-viral vectors are ongoing.

2.3 Barriers to DNA delivery

Systemic gene delivery involves a systemic approach in which exogenous genes are delivered to cells in a certain tissues, and secreted gene products are released into the circulatory system where they could modulate disease processes throughout the body. Systemic non-viral gene delivery has become an attractive alternative to viral vectors because of their safety, versatility and ease of preparation (Li & Huang, 2006). Genes can be delivered systemically (intramuscularly, intravenously, subcutaneously or, in animals, intraperitoneally). Otherwise, hydrodynamic-based gene delivery through systemic DNA injection offers a convenient, efficient and powerful means for high-level gene expression in animals (Liu & Knapp, 2001; Suda & Liu, 2007). This method is expected to be evaluated in patients soon (Romero et al., 2004). The limitations of the systemic approach to gene therapy are essentially the advantages of local delivery: exposure of non-target tissues to the therapeutic agent may have toxic effects or may compromise the immune system of the patient. Certain proteins will likely require very high levels of synthesis to achieve therapeutic function.

Ideally, gene therapy must protect DNA against degradation by nucleases in intercellular matrices so that the availability of macromolecules is not affected. Transgenes should be brought across the plasma membrane and into the nucleus of targeted cells but should have no detrimental effects. Hence, interaction with blood components, vascular endothelial cells and uptake by the reticuloendothelial system must be avoided. For DNA-based gene therapy to succeed, small-sized systems must internalize into cells and pass to the nucleus. Also, flexible tropisms allow applicability to a range of disease targets. Last but not least, such systems should be able to escape endosome-lysosome processing for endocytosis.

2.4 Barriers to siRNA delivery

The discovery of small interfering RNAs (siRNAs) has given renewed vision to the treatment of incurable diseases and genetically-associated disorders. Short double stranded (ds) RNA of 21-23 bp was cleaved by the RNAse III-like protein Dicer and incorporated into RNA-induced silencing complexes (RISC) (Hammond et al., 2000). Chemically-synthesized siRNAs and short hairpin RNA (shRNA) expression plasmids, which are sequence-specific for mRNA targeting, are methods commonly employed to mimic Dicer cleavage (Chen et al., 2007). However, siRNAs are susceptible to nuclease destruction and cannot penetrate the cell membrane because of their highly-charged backbone. An effective delivery system would enclose siRNA in carriers for protection and transport to the cytoplasm of targeted cells but should have no detrimental effects such as specific and non-specific off-targeted effects. Off-target effects can be divided into two categories: specific and non-specific off-targeted effects. Off-targeted effects may cause inflammation including interferon response, cell toxicity, and unintended gene knockdown.

Turning siRNA into drugs is a 3-step process. The design and *in vitro* screening of target siRNAs are followed by incorporating stabilizing chemical modifications in lead siRNAs, as required, and end in the selection as well as *in vivo* evaluation of delivery technologies that are appropriate for the target cell type/organ and disease setting (Vaishnaw et al., 2010). After nearly 10 years of study and development, many problems have been resolved, such as improving the stability of siRNAs, and avoiding 2 types of off-target effects. A recent anti-influenza study showed that the anti-viral activity of siRNA as found to be due to active siRNA. However, a different non-targeting control siRNA also had significant anti-viral activity (Mook et al., 2007). siRNA targeting vascular endothelial growth factor for patients with age-related macular degeneration (AMD) are currently in clinical trial. But further study showed that the inhibition is a siRNA classic effect, which is sequence- and target-independent (Jackson & Linsley, 2010). The off-target effect can be minimized by optimizing the rules and algorithms for siRNA design (Vaishnaw et al., 2010). However, several other factors limit the utility of siRNAs as therapeutic agents, such as competition with endogenous RNA, induction of immune responses, degradation in lysosomes after endocytosis (Dominska & Dykxhoorn, 2010; Wang et al., 2010). Unprotected, naked siRNAs are relatively unstable in blood and serum and have short half-lives *in vivo* (Gao et al., 2009). Naked siRNAs do not freely cross cellular membranes because of their large molecular weight (~13 kDa) and strong anionic charge. They are rapidly degraded by nuclease. Physiological barriers hinder siRNAs from reaching their targets, thereby reducing their therapeutic efficacy. Moreover, siRNA molecules have unfavorable physicochemical properties (negative charge, large molecular weight and instability). Therefore, they need delivery systems to overcome physiological obstacles and prolong vascular circulation by reducing renal clearance, protecting them from serum nucleases, improving their effective bio-distribution as well as targeted cellular uptake with endosomal escape and, finally, promoting trafficking to the cytoplasm and loading onto RISC. Therefore, delivery systems are required to facilitate siRNA access to intracellular sites of action.Barriers to siRNA delivery depend on the targeted organ and routes of administration. For example, intravenous (IV) administration is the most commonly used technique. The endothelial wall in the vasculature presents the primary delivery barrier to siRNAs. The endothelial barrier is often altered by inflammatory processes (e.g., RA, infection) (Moghimi et al., 2005). siRNAs leave a blood vessel to enter tissue. After reaching target cells, they undergo internalization via endocytosis, escape from endosomes, and release into the cytosol and, finally, load onto RISC. At the same time, siRNAs undergo elimination. The mononuclear phagocyte system is responsible for removing circulating foreign particles from the bloodstream by the phagocytosis of resident macrophages (Moghimi et al., 2005).

3. Cellular internalization of non-viral vector delivery system

There are seven steps should be overcome before the expression of exogenous DNA. They are (1) complexation, (2) *in vivo* administration, (3) endocytosis, (4) escape from endolysosome, (5) release of DNA, (6) trafficking through cytoplasm and (7) finally import of DNA into nucleus. (If siRNA is used as exogenous nucleotide, the last two steps can be ignored; but if vector-expressed siRNA is used, the process remains the same.) During each step, many factors may come into play, inducing toxicity, immunogenicity or affecting transfection efficiency. (1) During complexation, the non-viral vectors-DNA interaction is driven mainly by the electrostatic interaction between the polycation and the charged phosphate groups leading to reversible linear to globule transition of DNA. The ability of the non-viral vectors to condense DNA into nanoparticles is often critical for transfection efficiency since DNA must be protected from DNase degradation. (2) Different *in vivo* administration routes will meet different physiological barriers. Therefore, it is suggested that the corresponding primary cells and similar physiological barriers should be tested *in vitro* as far as possible, before *in vivo* administration is attempted. (3) The following step is to reach its target, the cell by endocytosis. In this respect it is well accepted that the polyelectrolyte complex polycation-DNA exhibiting a net positive charge binds to negatively charged cell membrane. (4) After the internalization the following crucial step in gene delivery with cationic polymers is the escape of the polymer/DNA complexes from the endosome. (5) The inefficient release of the DNA/polymer complex from endocytic vesicles into the cytoplasm is indicated as one of the primary causes of poor gene delivery. (6) and (7) the following step, the nuclear envelope is the ultimate obstacle to the nuclear entry of plasmid DNA. This obstacle is also considered crucial and two main mechanisms were proposed to explain how plasmid DNA enters into the nucleus: (i) a passive DNA entry into the nucleus during cell division when the nuclear membrane is temporarily disintegrated or (ii) an active transport of the DNA through the nuclear pores.

4. Chitosan as a vector for gene therapy

Cationic polymers, such as chitosan, are promising candidates for DNA transport in non-viral delivery systems (Kean & Thanou, 2010; Tong et al., 2009). Chitosan, a linear polysaccharide composed of randomly distributed β-(1-4)-linked D-glucosamine (deacetylated unit) and N-acetyl-D-glucosamine (acetylated unit), and has once been considered as an attractive gene transfer candidate for its superior biocompatibility, superior biodegradability and low cell toxicity. In recent years, with more researching methods involved, a more accurate and subtle view on the process of the entry of chitosan/DNA complexes into the cell nucleus has been developed. The enabling characteristics of Chitosan-DNA nanoparticles include biocompatibility, multiple ligand affinity, and a capacity of taking up large DNA fragments, while remaining small in size (Techaarpornkul et al., 2010). Chitosan and its derivatives, as favorable non-viral vectors involved in plasmid DNA delivery, have attracted attention in the field of siRNA delivery *in vitro* and *in* vivo (Andersen et al., 2009; Howard et al., 2009). Chitosan was once believed to be less effective than most other non-viral vectors because of its low stability and buffering capacity. However, recent technological advances in the chemical modification of chitosan have instituted improvements of its transfection efficiency without disturbing its biocompatibility and biodegradability. It has been demonstrated that transfection level is closely related to the molecular weight of polymers (Godbey et al., 1999). Chitosan (10-150 kDa), with a specific degree of deacetylation, allows maximum transgenic expression *in vitro* (Lavertu et al., 2006). Another strategy for improving transfection is to take advantage of the mechanism of ligand-mediated uptake by cells to promote targeting and internalization, enhancing transfection efficiency. Ligand-mediated transfection has been shown to facilitate DNA internalization into cells via membrane receptors both *in vitro* and *in vivo.* Cell-specific ligand modification such as galactose, transferrin, folate and mannose can also effectively enhance the specificity of transfection through receptor-mediated endocytosis. Galactose ligand modification has been used to target HepG2 cells through the interaction with asialoglycoprotein receptors (ASGP-R) (Gao et al., 2003). A transferrin receptor is found on many mammalian cells, therefore it can be used as a universal ligand (Dautry-Varsat, 1986). Folate is not only over-expressed on macrophage surfaces, but is also over-expressed on many human cancer cell surfaces (Lee et al., 2006). Antigen presenting cells (APCs), the ideal targets of DNA vaccine, such as macrophages and immature dendritic cells are the target cells of mannose ligand (Kim et al., 2006). The specificity of these modifications can be demonstrated through ligand competitive inhibition experiments.

The low stability, low buffering capacity and low cell-specificity have also hindered its clinical applications. However, as a nature resource-based polysaccharide, chitosan has more functional groups that can be chemically modified than other cationic polymers, thus has many more potential chemical derivatives to overcome the deficiencies. Chitosan has been experimentally modified using hydrophilic, hydrophobic, pH-sensitive, thermosensitive and cell-specific ligand groups for enhancement of transfection efficiency (Ishii et al., 2001). The degree of deacetylation (DDA) and the molecular weight (MW) of chitosan or its derivatives, can affect the ultimate transfection efficiency. Most chitosan/DNA complexes are highly deacetylated (above 80%), because chitosan with a high degree of deacetylation exhibits an increased DNA binding efficacy (Kiang et al., 2004). Through chain entanglement, chitosan with a higher MW (longer chain length) can become more readily enmeshed with free DNA, once the initial electrostatic interaction has occurred. But it will also delay the disassociation of chitosan and DNA (Huang et al., 2005). Consequently, low MW chitosan requires a higher charge ratio to stably condense DNA for the same DDA, and a lower DDA requires a higher charge ratio to stably condense DNA at equal MW (Lavertu et al., 2006). The charge ratio for minimum complexation can be determined by agarose gel electrophoresis.

5. Chitosan structure and physicochemical behaviour

The structure of chitin and chitosan correspond to those of poly [β(1→4)-2-acetamido-2-deoxy-d-glucopyranose] and poly[β(1→4)-2-amino-2-deoxy-d-glucopyranose], respectively (Figure 1). Chitosan is mainly manufactured from crustaceans (crab, krill and crayfish) primarily because a large amount of the crustacean exoskeleton is available as a byproduct of food processing. However, depending on the organism considered chitin can adopt polymorphic structures denominated alpha (α), beta (β) and gamma (γ) chitin (Jang et al., 2004).The polymorphism of chitin is due to different arrangements of chitin chains in the lamellas that constitute the crystalline portions. Alpha (α) chitin found in arthropods corresponds to an antiparallel chain packing at which intramolecular and intermolecular hydrogen bonding is favored. β-Chitin, typically extracted from squid pens, is less widely used although it can have higher reactivity than that of α-chitin. The parallel arrangement of the lamellas is responsible for a loose-packing fashion with weak intermolecular interactions. In the gamma (γ) chitin structure arrangements, beta and alpha occur, i.e., two lamellas in a parallel arrangement is intercalated by a lamella arranged in antiparallel packing (Roberts, 1992). The source from which chitosan is prepared is considered very important since chitosan derived from β-chitin exhibits higher reactivity than that derived from α-chitin (Kuritia et al., 1994; Shimojohay 1998).

In general the isolation of chitin from crustacean shell waste consists of three basic steps: demineralization (DM-calcium carbonate and calcium phosphate separation), deproteinization (DP-protein separation), and decolorization (DC-removal of pigments). These three steps are the standard procedure for chitin production (No et al., 1989). Chitosan is obtained after hydrolysis of the acetamide groups of chitin. However in the commercialized samples both units are commonly found, since chitosans having high deacetylation degrees (DA> 99%) are obtained only through of successive hydrolysis with strong bases as KOH and NaOH, and the degree of deacetylation is strongly dependent of the alkali concentration and temperature (Figure.1). The source of chitin and the deacetylation process can change dramatically the properties of the final product and the deacetylation in alkaline medium leads to the depolimerization (Domard & Rinaudo, 1983; Tolaimate et al., 2000). However it has been reported that chitin extracted from squid pens can be hydrolyzed under conditions that it allows obtaining chitosans of high molecular weight (Tolaimate et al., 2003).

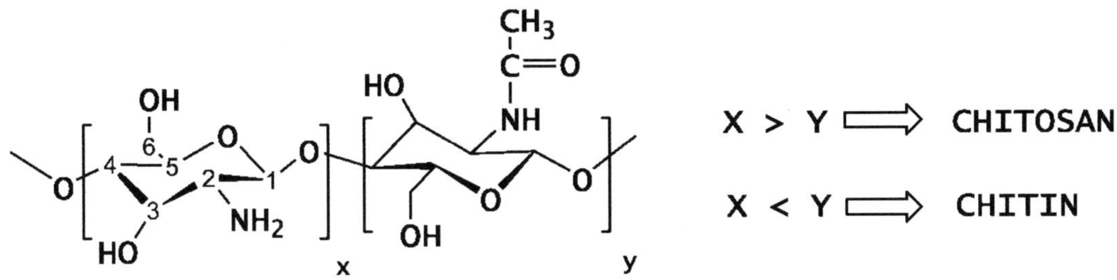

Fig. 1. Chemical structure of chitin and chitosan. In the 2-amino-2-deoxy-d-glucopyranose ring is shown the commonly used numbering for the carbon atoms.

The homopolymer is a weak base with a pKa value of the D-glucosamine residue of about 6.3 and is therefore insoluble at neutral and alkaline pH values. In acidic mediums, the amine groups will be positively charged, conferring to the polysaccharide a high charge density. As in all polyelectrolytes, the dissociation constant of chitosan is not constant, but depends on the degree of dissociation at which it is determined. The pka value can be calculated using the Katchalsky's equation (Roberts, 1992).

$$Pk_a = pH + \log [(1-\alpha)/\alpha] = pK_0 - \varepsilon\Delta\psi(\alpha)/kT$$

Where $\Delta\psi$ is the difference in electrostatic potential between the surface of the polyion and the reference, α is the degree of dissociation, k is Boltzman's constant, T is the temperature and ε is the electron charge. Extrapolation of the pK_a values to $\alpha = 1$, where the polymer is uncharged and hence the electrostatic potential becomes zero, makes possible the value of the intrinsic dissociation constant of the ionizable groups, pK_0, to be determined. The value obtained does not depend of the degree of *N*-acetylation, whereas the pKa value is dependent on this parameter, since the electrostatic potential will be varied depending of amount of the free amino groups. The pK_0 value is called the intrinsic pK_a of the chitosan. However chitosans of low molecular weight having degrees of deacetylation higher than 0.4 are also easily soluble in weakly acidic solvents such as acetic acid and formic acid (Lee et al., 1995).

The physicochemical behavior in aqueous solution is highly dependent of pH and degree of acetylation and has received more attention only recently. Bertha et al. working on chitosans from 95 to 175kDa have recently determined the radius of gyration of chitosan (R_G) (Bertha et al., 1998a; 2002b). The R_G is an alternative measure of the size of the polymer chain and it can be measured by light scattering measurements. R_G express the square mean radius of each one of the elements of the chain measured from its center of gravity. The study established the relationship between the molecular weight and radius of gyration (R_G) of chitosan in aqueous solution, and the author indicated that chitosan behaved more like a Gaussian coil instead of the worm-like chain model found in common polyelectrolytes. At the same time the presence of *N*- acetyl groups on the chitosan backbone imparts hydrophobic properties. Schatz et al. (Schatz et al., 2003) have studied homogeneous series of chitosans with different degrees of acetylation and almost the same degree of

polymerization in ammonium acetate buffer. Their results indicate that the aqueous solution behavior depends only on the degree of acetylation (DA). Three distinct domains of DA were defined and correlated to the different behaviors of chitosans: (i) a polyeletrolyte domain for DA below 20%; (ii) a transition domain between DA = 20% and 50% where chitosan loses its hydrophilicity; (iii) a hydrophobic domain for DAs over 50% where polymer associations can arise. Conformations of chitosan chains varying from 160 to 270kDa were studied by the calculations of the persistence lengths (L(p)). The average value was found to be close to 5 nm, in agreement with the wormlike chain model, but no significant variation of L(p) with the degree of acetylation was noticed. Pa et al. (Pa & Yu, 2001) have also reported that that the particle sizes of chitosan molecules in dilute acetic acid/water solutions increased with decreasing pH value. SLS data also demonstrated that the second virial coefficient (A_2) increased with decreasing pH value, suggesting that solubility of chitosan in water increased with increasing acetic acid concentration. Signini et al. (Signini et al., 2000) have also shown that acid-free aqueous solutions of chitosan hydrochloride of variable ionic strengths (0:06 M $\leq \mu \leq$ 0.3 M) are free of aggregation as evaluated by the values of the Huggins constants ($0.31 \leq k \leq 0.63$).
As other polysaccharides the biodegradation and biocompatibility are important properties of chitosan making it an attractive polymer for a variety of biomedical and pharmaceutical applications. Besides the degradation by chitinases (Hung et al., 2002), chitosanases (Kuroiwa et al., 2003), papain (Kumar et al., 2004; Lin et al., 2002; Muzzarelli et al., 2002; Terbojevich et al., 1996) and other proteases (Kumar et al., 2004), partially acetylated chitosan may be also degraded by lyzosymes of the human serum (Varurn et al., 1997), by oxidative-reductive depolymerization (Mao et al., 2004) and by acid hydrolysis reactions (Lee et al., 1999). In the acid hydrolysis the protonation of the glycosidic oxygen is recognized as the first step of the mechanism, which leads to formation of a cyclic carbonium -oxonium ion, yielding after the addition of water the reducing sugar end group (Sinnott et al., 1990; Yip & Withers, 2004). Besides enzymatic and acid hydrolysis the alkaline treatment with ultrasonication can be used to obtain either chitosan of decreasing molecular weight (Tang et al., 2003) or oligomers having a few glucosamine units (Tsaih et al., 2003).

6. General strategies for chitosan modification

In the chitosan structure two groups are particularly susceptible to react through nucleophilics attacks, i.e., the free amine and/or acetamide groups, and the hydroxyl groups linked to the glucopyranose ring. The hydroxyl groups can be modified by substitution of the hydrogen atoms but their reactivities are smaller than that of the amino group. Various procedures targeting the hydroxyl groups employ a sequence of protection/deprotection reactions aiming to obtain derivatives with a well defined structure (Kuitra, 2001). On the other hand under appropriated conditions a variety of other reactions can be easily conducted to selectively modify the free amine groups. The literature presents a wide range of procedures to target the amine group aiming to improve the properties of chitosan for a particular purpose. The modifications include those aiming the separation technologies of chiral molecules (Franco et al., 2001), recovery of metals (Guibal, 2004; Varma et al., 2004), antimicrobial activity (Rabea et al., 2003), anti tumoral carriers (Kato et al., 2004), biomedical applications (Berge et al., 2004a; 2004b) and vectors for gene therapy (Janes et al., 2001; Sinha et al., 2004; Liu et al., 2002; Borchard et al., 2001). Kumar et al (Kumar et al., 2004) and Kurita (Kurta, 2001) reviewed the procedures for the modification of chitosan.

Many strategies have been deployed to improve transfection efficiency, taking into account the biological steps involved in gene delivery. Modifications of chitosan structure to impart properties to NPs, such as to increase endosomal escape (Jiang et al., 2010; Yu et al., 2010), attaching of ligands to mediate cell internalization or to promote the nuclear entry of DNA, are among the most common ways. Figure 2 shows representative structures from these chitosan derivatives tested as carriers for gene therapy. A variety of nucleophilic reactions targeting the groups linked to the glucopyranose ring have been employed to improve the properties of chitosan.

Poly (ethylene glycol) (PEG) has been widely used for attaching to chitosan due to its hydrophilicity and biocompatibility. In general, the terminal hydroxyl group of methoxy poly(ethylene glycol) is modified to generate PEG derivatives able to promote nucleophilic displacements targeting the amino groups of chitosan (Harris et al., 1984; Aiba et al, 1993; Saito et al., 1997; Ouchi et al., 1998). Chitosan nanospheres modified by introducing PEG_{5000} chains to amine groups were more stable during lyophilization (Leong et al., 1998). These chitosan-DNA nanospheres were effective in tranfecting 293 cells but not HeLa cells, and tranfection efficiency was not affected by PEG derivatization.

Polymers can also be attached to the chitosan main chain using different routes. Poly(vinyl pyrrolidone) (PVP) was also grafted on galactosylated chitosan (GCPVP) and displayed improved physicochemical properties over unmodified chitosan (Park et al., 2003). PVP with a single terminus carboxylic group was coupled to galactosylated chitosan via formation of an amide bond between the amino *complex* group of GC and the terminal carboxyl group of the PVP. The terminal carboxyl group of PVP was activated by the *N*-hydroxysuccinimide (NHS)/EDC. The binding strength of GCPVP 10k/DNA was superior to that of GCPVP 50k/DNA, which was attributed to its higher flexibility because of its smaller size. However, DNase I protection of GCPVP 10k/DNA complex was inferior to that of GCPVP 50k/DNA. The DNA-binding property was shown to be dependent on the MW of chitosan and the composition of PVP (Park et al., 2003). The reaction of chitosan with methoxy poly(ethylene glycol) iodide (mPEG, Mn 2 kDa) in an alkalinized suspension was recently used by Yu *et al.* to attach PEG (Yu et al., 2010). This derivative was subsequently modified by attaching poly(ethylenimine) to the amino groups (Figure 2). Other approaches successfully employed to attach PEI to chitosan were an imine reaction between periodate-oxidized chitosan and amine groups of low MW PEI (Jiang et al., 2007) and the cationic polymerization of aziridine in the presence of water-soluble oligo-chitosan (Wong et al., 2006).

A series of new degradable cationic polymers composed of biocompatible chitosan backbones and poly((2-dimethyl amino) ethylmethacrylate) (P(DMAEMA)) side chains were recently synthesized via atom transfer radical polymerization (ATR) (Ping et al., 2010). This synthesis was carried out by introducing alkyl halide initiators onto chitosan, followed by the reaction with DMAEMA. Bromoisobutyryl-terminated chitosan (CS-Br initiators) was prepared via the reaction of primary amines of chitosan with carboxyl group of 2-bromo-2-methylpropionic acid (BMPA), which was previously converted into reactive esters (succinimidyl intermediates) in the presence of EDAC and NHS. The reactive esters underwent nucleophilic substitution reactions with the amine groups of chitosan to form a stable amide linkage and produce the resultant CS-Br initiators for DMAE polymerization (Ping et al., 2010).

The activation of carboxylic groups is one of the most commonly used procedures to attach different ligands and peptides to chitosan chain. Arginine-modified trimethylated chitosans labeled with folic acid have been prepared by activation of the acid group of arginine using EDC/NHS (Morris et al., 2010). The same procedure was utilized by Gao et al and it has proven to increase the transfection efficiency (Gao et al., 2008) and chitosan properties (Liu et al., 2004). A similar procedure was utilized to attach a short peptide (SP) (Sun et al., 2010) to chitosan. The peptide was further combined with GFP/luciferase reporter gene pDNA to form SP-CS/DNA complex. The NPs were able to transfect multiple cell lines, and the results revealed that, compared with CS, SP-CS could intensively augment transfection efficiency nearly to the level of Lipofectamine 2000 (Sun et al., 2010). Reactions targeting the hydroxyl groups are uncommon, however Sato et al. have prepared 6-Amino-6-deoxychitosan from 6-deoxy-6-halo-N-phthaloylchitosan via 6-azidation. The product had high stereoregularity because of the effective and regioselective reactions (Saito et al., 2004; Satoh et al., 2007).

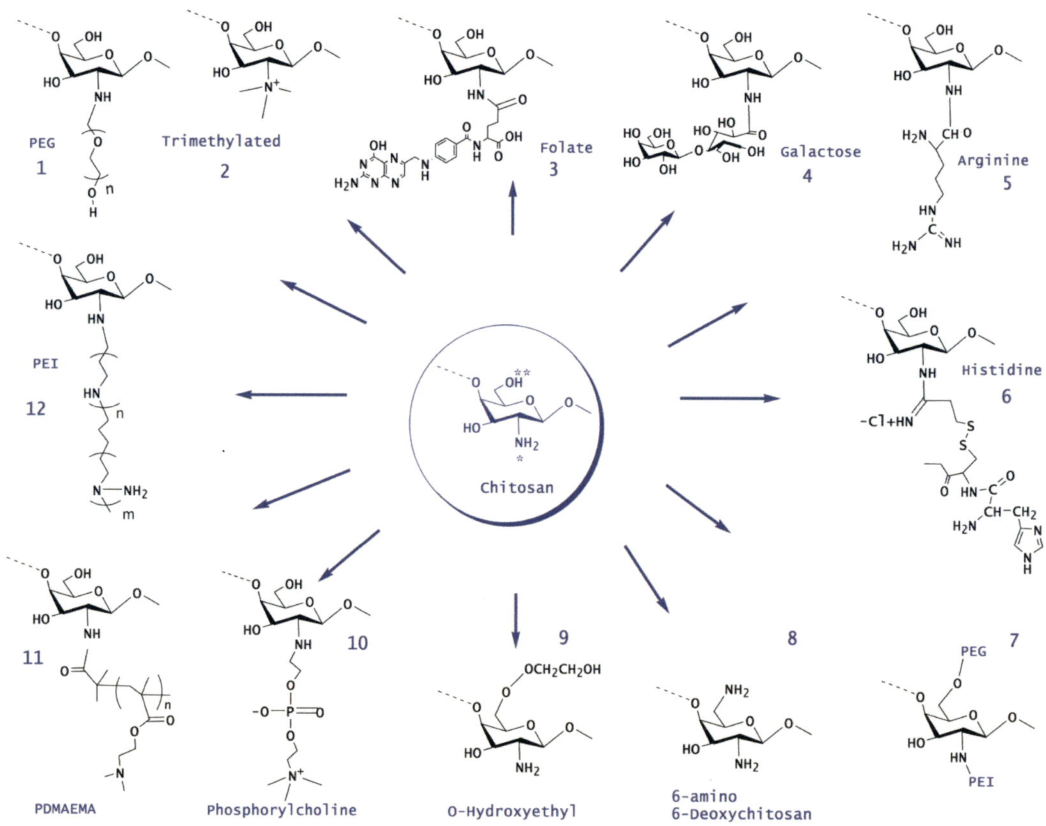

Fig. 2. Chemical structures of chitosan and its derivatives; **1.** PEG (Harris et al., 1984); **2.** trimethylated (Zeng et al., 2007); **3.** folic acid (Mansouri et al., 2006; Fernandes et al., 2008); **4.**galactosylated (Park et al., 2001); **5.** Arginine (Morris et al., 2010); **6.** histidine; **7.** PEI and PEG grafts (Yu et al., 2010); **8.** 6-amino 6-deoxychitosan (Saito et al., 2004; Satoh et al., 2007); **9.** O-hydroethyl (Kwon et al., 2003); **10.** Phosphorylcholine (Case et al., 2009; Tiera et al., 2006); **11.** grafted PDMAEMA (Ping et al., 2010); **12.** PEI (Jiang et al., 2007; Wong et al., 2006).

7. Chitosan-DNA delivery system

Chitosan-DNA gene delivery methods must achieve sufficient efficiency in the transportation of therapeutic genes across various extracellular and intracellular barriers. These barriers include interactions with blood components, vascular endothelial cells and uptake by the reticuloendothelial system. Furthermore, the degradation of therapeutic DNA by serum nucleases is a potential obstacle for functional delivery to target cells. DNA should escape from endosomes and traffic to enter the nucleus. Many factors, including the degree of deacetylation (DDA) and the molecular weight (MW) of the chitosan, the pH of the serum, the charge ratio (in some conditions, it equals the ratio of N/P, 'N': the content of Nitrogen atom in cationic polymer; 'P': the content of Phosohorus atom in DNA or RNA) of chitosan to DNA or RNA and the cell type can all affect the transfection efficiency of chitosan during each step of the process. The pKa value of chitosan is around 6.3-6.4, below which the protonated amines in the chitosan structure facilitate their binding to negatively charged DNA. Sato et al. showed the highest transfection efficiency can be obtained at pH 6.8 to 7.0. When pH of the transfection medium increases to 7.4, the transfection efficiency dramatically decreases due to the dissociation of the free plasmid from the complex (Sato et al., 2001).

Even if chitosan/DNA complexes display high transfection efficiency *in vitro*, their transfection efficiency *in vivo* may be low. Chitosan and its derivatives have become of great interest in the field of controlled release due to their favorable biocompatibility and biodegradability. Thiolated chitosan, which can be oxidized to form inter- and intra-molecular disulfide bonds, allowing the crosslinking of chitosan, shows a significant enhancement of transfection over that of lipofectin (Lee et al., 2007). Chitosan microspheres for micro-encapsulation of adenoviral vectors has been achieved by ionotropic coacervation of chitosan, using bile salts as counter-anions (Lameiro et al., 2006). A 3-D scaffold composed of chitosan-gelatin complexes with entrapped DNA has been proposed as a promoter of cartilage regeneration (Xia et al., 2004).

Although hydrophobic modification is not cell-specific, it can also enhance the attachment of complexes on cell surfaces and the subsequent cell uptake. Amphiphobic deoxycholic acid-modified chitosan oligosaccharide (DACO) nanoparticles showed superior gene condensation and high gene transfection efficiency, even in the presence of serum (Chae et al., 2005). After endocytosis, the endosome containing the complexes has to fuse with a lysosome to form an endolysosome. At this point, the complexes will meet a harsh acidic and multienzymatic environment. Nanocomplexes that are successfully protected against dissociation and degradation will finally escape from the endolysosome and enter the cytoplasm. PEI, a classic synthetic polymer with many amino groups to absorb protons (called a proton sponge mechanism), was found to have a better endolysosome buffering ability and caused a quicker release from the endolysosome in its intact form than did chitosan (Kim et al., 2005). The chemical modifications, such as urocanic acid (UA) (Kim et al., 2003), PEI-graft-chitosan (Wong et al., 2006), chitosan-graft-PEI (Jiang et al., 2007), poly(propyl acrylic acid) (PPAA) (Jones et al., 2003), trimethyl chitosan (Germershaus et al., 2008), have similar effects to PEI. Such modifications can be called pH-sensitive modifications that will not only enhance the escape of chitosan/DNA complexes from endolysosome but also enhance the stability of complexes in different pH situations.

The dissociation of chitosan/DNA complexes and subsequent release of DNA is also a very important step for its rate-limiting effect (Schaffer et al., 2000). Hydrophobic modification, such as deoxycholic acid modification (Lee et al., 1998), or 5β-cholanic acid modification (Yoo et al., 2005), can attenuate the electrostatic attractions between cationic polymers and anionic DNA. It is actually a contradiction between the stability and dissociation ability of complexes. A temperature-sensitive modification of poly(N-isopropylacrylamide) (PNIPAAm) can control the dissociation of PNVLCS (N-isopropylacrylamide/vinyl laurate copolymer with chitosan) complexes with DNA by a temporary reduction in the culture temperature to 20℃ (Sun et al., 2005)

The cytoplasm, a mesh-like network of microfilaments and microtubules, will limit the diffusion of complexes or DNA about 500-1000-fold. Adenovirus particles naturally bind to dynein and are actively transported towards the nuclear pore complexes once they are inside the cytoplasm. Prior to entry into the nucleus, the viruses dissociate into smaller structures and use their attached transport factors such as importins or karyopherins which have nuclear localization signals (NLS) to recognize the nuclear pore complex (NPC) (Whittaker & Helenius, 1998). Justin Hanes et al. used a new method called multiple particles tracking (MPT) to quantify the intracellular transport of non-viral DNA nanocarriers. They found that PEI/DNA complexes can accumulate in the perinuclear area through a subdiffusive transport, which is a combination of diffusive transport and active transport. This discovery is a dispute to the common belief that non-viral vectors go through the cell cytoplasm in a slow random way. Further investigation showed that actively transported complexes of PEI/DNA are in endosomes undergoing motor protein-driven movement guided by microtubules or physically associated with the motor proteins themselves (Suh et al., 2003). As to chitosan and its derivatives, however, few studies have examined how they pass through the highly structured cytoplasm and eventually enter into the nucleus.

8. Chitosan-siRNA delivery system

siRNA silencing technology is exploited in a wide range of biological studies, but has also become one of the most challenging therapeutic strategies. However, because of its poor delivery and susceptibility to nuclease degradation, siRNA-based approaches need a protective delivery system. A variety of polymer formulations have been proposed in the literature as potential carriers (De Fougerolles 2008; Gary et al., 2007; Zhang et al., 2007). Polymer molecular weight, change density, N/P ratio (ratio of protonatable polymer amine groups to nucleic acid phosphate groups) and ionic strength of the medium can affect electrostatic binding between siRNA and cationic polymers. Research over the years has revealed that chitosan is one of the desirable polymeric carriers of siRNA because of its natural biocompatibility, biodegradability, nontoxicity, and high nuclease resistance. The effects of different chitosan (114-kDa or more)-siRNA complexes on transfection activity have been observed previously (Katas et al., 2008; Katas & Alpar, 2006; Liu et al., 2007; Rojanarata et al., 2008). Higher MW and DDA are desirable characteristics for the formation of chitosan nanoparticles, as higher MW chitosan molecules are long and flexible while higher DDA enhances its electrostatic interaction with siRNAs, thus synergically reducing the size of complexes and increasing their stability (Liu et al., 2007). A high charge ratio also enhances the stability of complexes because the loosely bound excess chitosan on the outer surface of nanoparticles can promote binding and uptake across anionic cell surfaces and also provide subsequent protection against siRNA degradation within endosome compartments (Liu et al., 2007). The method of complexation also affects the gene-silencing activity of chitosan/siRNA complexes. Haliza Katas et al. studied the difference between simple complexation, ionic gelation (siRNA entrapment) and adsorption of siRNA onto the surface of preformed chitosan nanoparticles. Ionic gelation gave the strongest stability and the most efficient gene-silencing activity among the three methods tested. For the involvement of tripolyphosphate (TPP) ions during the complexation of ionic gelation, pH became one of the factors that mostly affected the gene-silencing activity. The decrease of pH resulted in a reduction in the charge number of TPP, which subsequently led to the need for more TPP ions for cross-linking of the chitosan by electrostatic forces (Katas & Alpar, 2006). Rojanarata et al. reported that chitosan-thiamine pyrophosphate (TPP)-mediated siRNA enhanced green fluorescent protein (EGFP) gene silencing efficiency depended on the molecular weight and weight ratio of chitosan and siRNA. The chitosan-TPP-siRNA complex with the lowest molecular weight of chitosan (20 kDa) at a weight ratio of 80 showed the strongest inhibition of gene expression (Rojanarata et al., 2008). A novel study of chitosan/siRNA nanoparticles with fluorescent quantum dots was taken to silence HER2/neu and achieved desirable silencing effects (Tahara et al., 2008; Tan et al., 2007). In the field of controlled release, chitosan coating PLGA nanospheres with a high loading efficiency of siRNAs were found to reduce the initial burst of nucleic acid release and to prolong release at later stages, without changing the release pattern (Tahara et al., 2008). Kenneth A. Howard found that the chitosan-based system had the ability for endosome escape through the proton sponge mechanism, because the endosomolytic agent chloroquine did not increase the effect of RNA interference (Howard et al., 2006). In terms of *in vivo* administration of chitosan/siRNAs complexes, only a few studies are available. Nasal administration to silence EGFP expression of the endothelial cells distributed in the bronchioles of transgenic EGFP mouse model has been successfully achieved without showing any adverse effects (Howard et al., 2006). Cross-linking of hyaluronan and chitosan has proven to have a higher efficiency of transfection in ocular tissue over unmodified chitosan (de la Fuente et al., 2008).

9. Potential application of chitosan-DNA/siRNA nanoparticles

Gene therapy offers new possibilities for the clinical management of different disease conditions that are difficult to treat by traditional surgical or medical means. In the last decade, extensive improvements have been made to optimize gene therapy and have been tested on several disease conditions. The success of chitosan-DNA nanoparticles for delivery plasmid DNA to mucosal surfaces such as the oral and nasal mucosa has already shown (Bivas-Benita et al., 2003; Chen et al., 2004; Khatri et al., 2008). Oral delivery is most attractive due to easy administration. The oral delivery of peptide, protein, vaccine and nucleic acid-based biotechnology products is the greatest challenge facing the drug delivery industry. Mice were fed with plasmid pCMVβ (containing LacZ gene), whether it was wrapped by chitosan or no. The study demonstrated that oral chitosan-DNA nanoparticles can efficiently deliver genes to enterocytes, and may be used as a useful tool for gene transfer (Chen et al., 2004). Hepatitis B virus infection is a major global health concern and is the most common cause of chronic liver disease, new generation of HBV vaccines are urgently needed in order to overcome problems encountered with the immunization of immunocompromised people and more importantly with the potential of using active immunotherapy in treating chronic patients. DNA vaccines have the potential to eliminate many of the limitations of current vaccine technologies. Chitosan nanoparticles loaded with plasmid DNA encoding surface protein of Hepatitis B virus. Nasal administration of such nanoparticles resulted in serum anti-HBsAg titre that was less compared to that elicited by naked DNA and alum adsorbed HBsAg, but the mice were seroprotective within 2 weeks and the immunoglobulin level was above the clinically protective level (Khatri et al., 2008). Particulate mucosal delivery systems that encapsulate protein or plasmid DNA encoding antigens have been widely explored for their ability to induce an immune response. Oral delivery of vaccines using chitosan as a carrier material appears to be beneficial for inducing an immune response against *Toxoplasma gondii*. Chitosan microparticles as carriers for GRA-1 protein vaccine were prepared. It was shown that priming with secreted dense granule protein 1 (GRA1) protein vaccine loaded chitosan particles and boosting with GRA1 pDNA vaccine resulted in high anti-GRA1 antibodies, characterized by a mixed IgG2a/IgG1 ratio (Bivas-Benita et al., 2003). The application of chitosan-based delivery system as ocular gene carriers, there is evidence of their ability to transfect the ocular cells in vitro. This capacity of chitosan nanoparticles to transfect the cells, was found to be highly dependent on the molecular weight of chitosan. Only chitosan of low molecular weight (10-12 kDa) was able to transfect plasmid DNA in both cell lines derived from the human cornea and the conjunctives (De la Fuente et al., 2008). In Utero delivery of chitosan-DNA results in postnatal gene expression, and shows promise for non-viral gene transfer in animal models of fetal gene therapy (Yang et al., 2010). The intravenous and intratracheal solutions and the intratracheal powder of pCMV-Muβ encoding murine interferon-β were administered the day after the inoculation of mice with CT26 cells. Lung weight and the number of pulmonary nodules at day 21 were significantly suppressed by the three formulations at a dose of 10 μg (N/P = 5). Reducing the dose to 1 μg resulted in a loss of effect by the intravenous solution (Okamoto et al., 2010). These findings showed that therapeutic gene powders are promising for gene therapy to treat lung cancer or metastasis.

siRNA gene therapy research has focused on several types of viral vectors: adeno-associated viruses (AAV), adenoviruses, retroviruses, lentiviruses, and herpes simplex viruses. siRNA therapeutics have been assessed in numerous diseases, including genetic and viral diseases, cancer, as well as non-lethal disorders, such as arthritis and osteoporosis. Among these viral vectors, lentiviruses have progressed to clinical trials on metastatic melanoma and HIV infection (Baker, 2010a; 2010b). siRNA-based gene therapy has already been tested in clinical trials dealing with the treatment of age-related macular degeneration, viral infection, skin disorders and cancer. Cancer treatment is by the most important proposed application of gene therapy and many clinical trials using gene therapy are under investigation. Non-viral vectors including chitosan derivatives have been used in animal model, but clinical trials are lagging due to low transfection efficiency. Anderson et al. (Andersen et al., 2008) demonstrated that silencing of pro-inflammatory TNFα in the RAW 246.7 murine macrophage cell line was achieved by using lyophilized chitosan/siRNA. Compared to research in vitro with chitosan-based systems, in vivo research is still in the developmental stage. Only a few studies are avaible which *in vivo* demonstration of chitosan/siRNA nanocomplexes in silencing gene expression in animals. Howard et al. (Howard et al., 2009) demonstrated that chitosan nanopaticles contains an anti-TNFα siRNA knock downed efficiently of TNFα expression in primary peritoneal macrophages in vitro. Downregulation of TNFα-induced inflammatory responses arrested systemic and local inflammation in collagen-induced arthritic mice after intraperitoneal injection of chitosan/anti-TNFα siRNA nanoparticles, thereby presenting a novel strategy for arthritis treatment.

10. Conclusion

Clinical trials on gene therapy are limited to naked DNA or plasmid DNAs/siRNA delivered by viral vectors. Among non-viral vectors for DNA and siRNA delivery, chitosan and its derivatives are promising alternatives to viral vectors for targeting DNA and siRNA to specific cells. Chitosan has once been considered as an attractive gene transfer candidate for its superior biocompatibility, superior biodegradability and low cell toxicity, but the low stability, low buffering capacity and low cell-specificity have also hindered its clinical applications. To date, however, no clinical trials of chitosan-DNA or siRNA therapy have been performed. Chitosan-based gene therapy remains in the experimental stage due to low transfection efficacy. Many key challenges were involved in DNA and siRNA delivery to targeted cells using chitosan-based carriers. As a nature resource-based polysaccharide, chitosan has more functional groups that can be chemically modified than do the other cationic polymers, thus has many more potential chemical derivatives to make up these deficiencies. Parameters are critical to achieve favourable transfection efficiency and include degree of deacetylation, molecular weight, pH and N/P ratio. For example, a low molecular weight, high degree of deacetylation, small particle size and a moderate, positive, surface zeta potential along with a high N/P ration are advantageous to achieve high siRNA transfection efficiency. Recent technological advances in the chemical modification of chitosan have instituted improvements of its transfection efficiency without disturbing its biocompatibility and biodegradability.

Our work on gene coding for IL-lRa in dogs (Pelletier et al., 1997) and rabbits (Fernandes et al., 1999) was our previous study with the protein itself. We have improved a non-viral intraarticular transfection technique using lipofection and have tested it in osteoarhtritis animal models. These were the very first published articles in the literature that demonstrated the efficacy of gene therapy in osteoarthritis models *in vivo*. Our recent work on polymeric nanoparticles has led us to develop a much safer and effective system for in vitro transfection of embryonic kidney cells, as well as adult mesenchymal stem cells (Corsi et al., 2003). This new system has been successfully tested in muscle and skin tissues *in vivo* in mice and holds great promise for future application on the field of gene therapy and tissue engineering. We developed a second-generation nanovector by successfully coupling folic acid to the polymer (Mansouri et al., 2006). One strategy for improving transfection is to take advantage of the mechanism of folate-mediated uptake by cells to promote targeting and internalization, hence improving transfection efficiency. Folate-mediated transfection has been shown to facilitate DNA internalization into cells via membrane receptors both *in vitro* and *in vivo* (Sudimack & Lee, 2000). Expression of folate receptor (FR)-β in synovial mononuclear cells and CD14+ cells from patients with RA was described by 1999 (Nakashima-Matsushita et al., 1999). Articular macrophages isolated from rats with adjuvant-induced arthritis overexpress FRs and exhibit significantly higher binding capacity for folate conjugates than macrophages obtained from healthy rats (Turk et al., 2002). The wide distribution of FRs at the surface of activated macrophages in rheumatoid arthritis allows the use of folate as potential ligand for folate-targeted chitosan gene therapy. Our laboratory demonstrated that folate-chitosan DNA nanoparticle containing IL-1Ra has been shown to play a role to prevent abnormal osteoblast metabolism and bone damage in this adjuvant-induced arthritis model (Fernandes et al., 2008). It also allows a significant decrease of the inflammation in the rats' paw compared to untreated rats, proving indirectly the efficacy of the IL-1Ra protein treatment. Various inflammation markers (IL-1β and PGE_2)

showed a significant decrease in muscle and serum after the injection of the IL-1Ra protein demonstrating by direct evidence the efficacy of the administration technique to deliver efficient nanoparticles. Therefore, we have already shown it is possible to do gene therapy with IL-1Ra to decrease arthritis and have a positive effect on inflammation.

11. Acknowledgments

This work was supported by the grants from National Natural Science Foundation of China (No. 30811120440 and 30911120261), The Ministry of Science and Technology of China (No. S2011GR0323), Shanghai International Collaboration Foundation (No. 08410701800) and Canadian Institutes of Health Research (CCI-92212, CCL-99636 and CCM 104888). Dr Fernandes and Dr Benderdour are research scholars of *Fonds de la Recherche en santé du Québec* (FRSQ). Dr Tiera holds a post-PH D scholarship from UNESP - Brazil.

12. References

Alexander, B.L.; Ali, R.R.; Alton, E.W.; Bainbridge, J.W.; Braun, S.; Cheng, S.H.; Flotte, T.R.; Gaspar, H.B.; Grez, M.; Griesenbach, U.; Kaplit,t M.G.; Ott, M.G.; Seger, R.; Simons, M.; Thrasher, A.J.; Thrasher, A.Z. & Ylä-Herttuala, S. (2007). Progress and prospects: gene therapy clinical trials (part 1). *Gene Ther.*, 14, 1439-1447, ISSN 0969-7128

Aiba, S. (1993). Reactivity of partially N-acetylated chitosan in aqueous media, *Makromolekulare Chemie.*, 194(1), 65–75, ISSN 0025-116X

Andersen, M.O.; Howard, K.A. & Kjems, J. (2009). RNAi using a chitosan/siRNA nanoparticle system: in vitro and in vivo applications. *Methods Mol. Biol.*, 555, 77-86, ISSN 1064-3745

Andersen, M.O.; Howard, K.A.; Paludan, S.R.; Besenbacher, F. & Kjems,J. (2008). Delivery of siRNA from lyophilized polymeric surfaces. *Biomaterials*, 29, 506-512, ISSN 1043-1802

Baker, M. (2010a). RNA interference: From tools to therapies. *Nature*, 464, 1225, ISSN 0028-0836

Baker, M. (2010b). RNA interference: Homing in on delivery. *Nature*, 464, 1225-1228. ISSN 0028-0836

Berger, J.; Reist, M.; Mayer, J.M.; Felt, O. & Gurny, R. (2004). Structure and interactions in chitosan hydrogels formed by complexation or aggregation for biomedical applications. *Eur. J. Pharm. Biopharm.*, 57, 35-52, ISSN 0928-0987

Berger, J.; Reist, M.; Mayer, J.M.; Felt, O.; Peppas, N.A. & Gurny, R. (2004). Structure and interactions in covalently and ionically crosslinked chitosan hydrogels for biomedical applications. *Eur. J. Pharm. Biopharm.*, 57, 19-34, ISSN 0928-0987

Bertha, G.; Dautzenberg, H. & Peter, M.G. (1998). Physico-chemical characterization of chitosans varying in degree of acetylation. *Carbohydr. Polym.*, 36, 205-216, ISSN 0144-8617

Bertha, G. & Dautzenberg, H. (2002). The degree of acetylation of chitosans and its effect on the chain conformation in aqueous solution. *Carbohydr. Polym.*, 47, 39-51, ISSN 1043-1802

Bivas-Benita, M.; Laloup, M.; Versteyhe, S.; Dewit, J.; De, B.J.; Jongert, E. & Borchard, G. (2003). Generation of Toxoplasma gondii GRA1 protein and DNA vaccine loaded chitosan particles: preparation, characterization, and preliminary in vivo studies. *Int. J. Pharm.*, 266, 17-27, ISSN 0378-5173.

Borchard, G. (2001). Chitosans for gene delivery. *Adv. Drug Deliv. Rev.*, 52, 145-150, ISSN 0169-409X

Casé, A.H.; Picola, I.P.D.; Zaniquelli, M.E.D.Z.; Fernandes, J.C.; Sebastião Taboga, R.; Winnik, F.M. & Tiera, M.J. (2009). Physicochemical characterization of nanoparticles formed between DNA and phosphorylcholine substituted chitosans, *J. Colloid. Interface. Sci.*, 336, 125–133, ISSN 0021-9797

Castanotto, D. & Rossi, J.J. (2009). The promises and pitfalls of RNA-interference-based therapeutics. *Nature*, 457, 426-433, ISSN 0028-0836

Chae, S.Y.; Son, S.; Lee, M.; Jang, M.K. & Nah, J.W. (2005). Deoxycholic acid-conjugated chitosan oligosaccharide nanoparticles for efficient gene carrier. *J. Control Release*, 109, 330-344. ISSN 0168-3659

Chen, J.; Yang, W.L.; Li, G.; Qian, J.; Xue, J.L.; Fu, S.K. & Lu, D.R. (2004). Transfection of mEpo gene to intestinal epithelium in vivo mediated by oral delivery of chitosan-DNA nanoparticles. *World J. Gastroenterol.*, 10, 112-116, ISSN 1007-9327

Chen, M.; Granger, A.J.; Vanbrocklin, M.W.; Payne, W.S.; Hunt, H.; Zhang, H.; Dodgson, J.B. & Holmen, S.L. (2007). Inhibition of avian leukosis virus replication by vector-based RNA interference. *Virology*, 365, 464-472, ISSN 0042-6822

Corsi. K.; Chellat, F.; Yahia, L. & Fernandes, J.C. (2003). Mesenchymal stem cells, MG63 and HEK293 transfection using chitosan-DNA nanoparticles. *Biomaterials,* 24:1255-64, ISSN 0142-09612

Dautry-Varsat, A. (1986). Receptor-mediated endocytosis: the intracellular journey of transferrin and its receptor. *Biochimie*, 68, 375-381, ISSN 0300-9084

De Fougerolles, A.R. (2008). Delivery vehicles for small interfering RNA in vivo. *Hum. Gene Ther.*, 19, 125-132, ISSN 1043-0342

De la Fuente, M.; Seijo, B. & Alonso, M.J. (2008). Bioadhesive hyaluronan-chitosan nanoparticles can transport genes across the ocular mucosa and transfect ocular tissue. *Gene Ther.*, 15, 668-676, ISSN 0969-7128

Domard, A. & Rinaudo, M. (1983). Preparation and characterization of fully deacetylated chitosan. *Int. J. Biol. Macromol.*, 5, 49–53, ISSN 0141-8130

Dominska, M. & Dykxhoorn, D.M. (2010). Breaking down the barriers: siRNA delivery and endosome escape. *J. Cell Sci.*, 123, 1183-1189, ISSN 1477-9137

Fernandes, J.; Tardif, G.; Martel-Pelletier, J., Lascau-Coman, V., Dupuis, M., Moldovan, F., Sheppard, M., Krishnan, B.R. & J.P. (1999). In vivo transfer of interleukin-1 receptor antagonist gene in osteoarthritic rabbit knee joints: prevention of osteoarthritis progression. *Am. J. Pathol.*, 154, 1159-69, ISSN 1525-2191

Fernandes, J.C.; Wang, H.; Jreyssaty, C.; Benderdour, M.; Lavigne, P.; Qiu, X.; Winnik, F.M.; Zhang, X.; Dai, K. & Shi, Q. (2008). Bone-protective effects of nonviral gene therapy with folate-chitosan DNA nanoparticle containing interleukin-1 receptor antagonist gene in rats with adjuvant-induced arthritis. *Mol. Ther.*, 16, 1243-1251, ISSN 1525-0016

Franco, P.; Senso, A.; Oliveros, L. & Minguillon, C. (2001). Covalently bonded polysaccharide derivatives as chiral stationary phases in high-performance liquid chromatography. *J. Chromatogr. A*, 906, 155-170, ISSN 0021-9673

Gao, S.; Chen, J.; Xu, X.; Ding, Z.; Yang, Y.H.; Hua, Z. & Zhang, J. (2003). Galactosylated low molecular weight chitosan as DNA carrier for hepatocyte-targeting. *Int. J. Pharm.*, 255, 57-68, ISSN 0378-5173

Gao, S.; Dagnaes-Hansen, F.; Nielsen, E.J.; Wengel, J.; Besenbacher, F.; Howard, K.A. & Kjems, J. (2009). The effect of chemical modification and nanoparticle formulation on stability and biodistribution of siRNA in mice. *Mol. Ther.*, 17, 1225-1233, ISSN 1525-0016

Gao, X.; Kim, K.S. & Liu, D. (2007). Nonviral gene delivery: what we know and what is next. *AAPS. J.*, 9, E92-104, ISSN 1550-7416

Gao, Y.; Xu, Z.H.; Chen, S.W.; Gu, W.W.; Chen, L.L. & Li, Y.P. (2008). Arginine-chitosan/DNA self-assemble nanoparticles for gene delivery: In vitro characteristics and transfection efficiency. *Int. J. Pharm.*, 359, 241-246, ISSN 0378-5173

Gary, D.J.; Puri, N. & Won, Y.Y. (2007). Polymer-based siRNA delivery: perspectives on the fundamental and phenomenological distinctions from polymer-based DNA delivery. *J. Control Release*, 121, 64-73, ISSN 0168-3659

Germershaus, O.; Mao, S.; Sitterberg, J.; Bakowsky, U. & Kissel, T. (2008). Gene delivery using chitosan, trimethyl chitosan or polyethylenglycol-graft-trimethyl chitosan block copolymers: establishment of structure-activity relationships in vitro. *J. Control Release*, 125, 145-154, ISSN 0168-3659

Giannoudis, P.V.; Tzioupis, C.C. & Tsiridis, E. (2006). Gene therapy in orthopaedics. *Injury*, 37 Suppl 1, S30-S40, ISSN 0020-1383

Godbey, W.T.; Wu, K.K. & Mikos, A.G. (1999). Size matters: molecular weight affects the efficiency of poly(ethylenimine) as a gene delivery vehicle. *J. Biomed. Mater. Res.*, 45, 268-275, ISSN 1549-3296

Guibal, E. (2004). Interactions of metal ions with chitosan-based sorbents: a review. *Separ. Purific. Techn.*, 38, 43-74, ISSN 1383-5866

Guo, T.; Zhao, J.; Chang, J.; Ding, Z.; Hong, H.; Chen, J. & Zhang, J. (2006). Porous chitosan-gelatin scaffold containing plasmid DNA encoding transforming growth factor-beta1 for chondrocytes proliferation. *Biomaterials*, 27, 1095-1103, ISSN 0142-9612

Hacein-Bey-Abina, S.; von, K.C.; Schmidt, M.; Le, D.F.; Wulffraat, N.; McIntyre, E.; Radford, I.; Villeval, J.L.; Fraser, C.C.; Cavazzana-Calvo, M. & Fischer, A. (2003). A serious adverse event after successful gene therapy for X-linked severe combined immunodeficiency. *N. Engl. J Med*, 348, 255-256, ISSN 0028-4793

Hammond, S.M.; Bernstein, E.; Beach, D. & Hannon, G.J. (2000). An RNA-directed nuclease mediates post-transcriptional gene silencing in Drosophila cells. *Nature*, 404, 293-296, ISSN 0028-0836

Harris, J.M., Struk, E.C., Case, M.G., Paley, M.S., Yalpani, M., Van Alstin, J.M. & Brooks, D.E. (1984). Synthesis and Characterization of Poly(ethylene Glycol) Derivatives. J. Polym. Sci. Polym. Chem. Ed. 22, 341–352, ISSN 0360-6376

Hillaireau, H. & Couvreur, P. (2009). Nanocarriers' entry into the cell: relevance to drug delivery. *Cell Mol. Life Sci.*, 66, 2873-2896, ISSN 1420-682X

Howard, K.A., Paludan, S.R., Behlke, M.A., Besenbacher, F., Deleuran, B. & Kjems, J. (2009). Chitosan/siRNA nanoparticle-mediated TNF-alpha knockdown in peritoneal macrophages for anti-inflammatory treatment in a murine arthritis model. *Mol. Ther.*, 17, 162-168, ISSN 1525-0016

Howard, K.A., Rahbek, U.L., Liu, X., Damgaard, C.K., Glud, S.Z., Andersen, M.O., Hovgaard, M.B., Schmitz, A., Nyengaard, J.R., Besenbacher, F. & Kjems, J. (2006). RNA interference in vitro and in vivo using a novel chitosan/siRNA nanoparticle system. *Mol. Ther.*, 14, 476-484, ISSN 1525-0016

Huang, M., Fong, C.W., Khor, E. & Lim, L.Y. (2005). Transfection efficiency of chitosan vectors: effect of polymer molecular weight and degree of deacetylation. *J. Control Release*, 106, 391-406, ISSN 0168-3659

Hung, T.H.; Chang, Y.M.; Sung, H.Y. & Chang, C.T. (2002). Purification and characterization of hydrolase with chitinase and chitosanase activity from commercial stem bromelain, *J. Agric. Food Chem.*, 50, 4666-4673, ISSN 0021-8561

Hyde, S.C., Southern, K.W., Gileadi, U., Fitzjohn, E.M., Mofford, K.A., Waddell, B.E., Gooi, H.C., Goddard, C.A., Hannavy, K., Smyth, S.E., Egan, J.J., Sorgi, F.L., Huang, L., Cuthbert, A.W., Evans, M.J., Colledge, W.H., Higgins, C.F., Webb, A.K. & Gill, D.R. (2000). Repeat administration of DNA/liposomes to the nasal epithelium of patients with cystic fibrosis. *Gene Ther.*, 7, 1156-1165, ISSN 0969-7128

Ishii, T., Okahata, Y. & Sato, T. (2001). Mechanism of cell transfection with plasmid/chitosan complexes. *Biochim. Biophys. Acta*, 1514, 51-64, ISSN 0006-3002

Jackson, A.L. & Linsley, P.S. (2010). Recognizing and avoiding siRNA off-target effects for target identification and therapeutic application. *Nat. Rev. Drug. Discov.*, 9, 57-67, ISSN 1474-1776

Janes, K.A.; Calvo, P. & Alonso, M.J. (2001). Polysaccharide colloidal particles as delivery systems for macromolecules. *Adv. Drug Deliv. Rev.*, 47, 83–97, ISSN 0169-409X

Jang, M.K.; Kong, B.G; Jeong, Y.I.; Lee, C.H. & Nah, J.W. (2004). Physicochemical Characterization of α-Chitin, β-Chitin, and γ-Chitin Separated from Natural Resources. *J. Polym. Sci. Pol. Chem.*, 42, 3423–3432, ISSN 1099-0518.

Jiang, H.L., Kim, Y.K., Arote, R., Nah, J.W., Cho, M.H., Choi, Y.J., Akaike, T. & Cho, C.S. (2007). Chitosan-graft-polyethylenimine as a gene carrier. *J. Control Release*, 117, 273-280, ISSN 0168-3659

Jiang, H.L.; Kim, Y.K.; Lee, S.M.; Park, M.R.; Kim, E.M.; Jin, Y.M.; Arote, R.; Jeong, H.J.; Song, S.C.; Cho, M.H. & Cho, C.S. (2010). Galactosylated chitosan-g-PEI/DNA complexes-loaded poly(organophosphazene) hydrogel as a hepatocyte targeting gene delivery system. *Arch. Pharm. Res.*, 33, 551, ISSN 0253-6269

Jones, R.A., Cheung, C.Y., Black, F.E., Zia, J.K., Stayton, P.S., Hoffman, A.S. & Wilson, M.R. (2003). Poly(2-alkylacrylic acid) polymers deliver molecules to the cytosol by pH-sensitive disruption of endosomal vesicles. *Biochem. J.*, 372, 65-75, ISSN 0264-6021

Kaiser, J. (2007). Clinical research. Death prompts a review of gene therapy vector. *Science*, 317, 580. ISSN 0036-8075

Katas, H. & Alpar, H.O. (2006). Development and characterisation of chitosan nanoparticles for siRNA delivery. *J. Control Release*, 115, 216-225, ISSN 0168-3659

Katas, H., Chen, S., Osamuyimen, A.A., Cevher, E. & Oya, A.H. (2008). Effect of preparative variables on small interfering RNA loaded Poly(D,L-lactide-co-glycolide)-chitosan submicron particles prepared by emulsification diffusion method. *J. Microencapsul.*, 25, 541-548, ISSN 0265-2048

Kato, Y.; Onishi, H. & Machida, Y. (2004). *N*-succinyl-chitosan as a drug carrier: water-insoluble and water-soluble conjugates. *Biomaterials*, 25, 907-915, ISSN 0142-9612

Kean, T. & Thanou, M. (2010). Biodegradation, biodistribution and toxicity of chitosan. *Adv. Drug Deliv. Rev.*, 62, 3-11. ISSN 0169-409X

Khatri, K., Goyal, A.K., Gupta, P.N., Mishra, N. & Vyas, S.P. (2008). Plasmid DNA loaded chitosan nanoparticles for nasal mucosal immunization against hepatitis B. *Int. J. Pharm.*, 354, 235-241, ISSN 0378-5173

Kiang, T., Wen, J., Lim, H.W. & Leong, K.W. (2004). The effect of the degree of chitosan deacetylation on the efficiency of gene transfection. *Biomaterials*, 25, 5293-5301, ISSN 1043-1802

Kim, T.H., Ihm, J.E., Choi, Y.J., Nah, J.W. & Cho, C.S. (2003). Efficient gene delivery by urocanic acid-modified chitosan. *J. Control Release*, 93, 389-402, ISSN 0168-3659

Kim, T.H., Kim, S.I., Akaike, T. & Cho, C.S. (2005). Synergistic effect of poly(ethylenimine) on the transfection efficiency of galactosylated chitosan/DNA complexes. *J. Control Release*, 105, 354-366, ISSN 0168-3659

Kim, T.H., Nah, J.W., Cho, M.H., Park, T.G. & Cho, C.S. (2006). Receptor-mediated gene delivery into antigen presenting cells using mannosylated chitosan/DNA nanoparticles. *J. Nanosci. Nanotechnol.*, 6, 2796-2803, ISSN 1533-4880

Kumar, M.N.V.R.; Muzzarelli, R.A.A.; Muzzarelli, C.; Sashiwa, H. & Domb, A.J. (2004). Chitosan chemistry and pharmaceutical perspectives. *Chem. Rev.*, 104, 6017-6084, ISSN 0009-2665

Kumar, A.B.V. & Tharanathan, R.N. (2004). A comparative study on depolymerization of chitosan by proteolytic enzymes, *Carbohydr. Polym.* 58, 275-283, ISSN 0144-8617

Kumar, A.B.V.; Varadaraj, M. C.; Lalitha, R.G. & Tharanathan, R.N. (2004). Low molecular weight chitosans: preparation with the aid of papain and characterization, *Biochim. Biophys. Acta-Gen. Sub.* 1670, 137-146, ISSN 0304-4165

Kurita. K. (2001). Controlled functionalization of polysaccharide chitin. *Prog. Polym. Sci.*, 26, 1921-1971, ISSN 0340-255X

Kurita, K.; Ishii, S.; Tomita, K.; Nishimura, S.I. & Shlmoda, K. (1994) Reactivity characteristics of squid beta-chitin as compared with those of shrimp chitin: High potentials of squid chitin as a starting material for facile chemical modifications. *J. Polym. Sci. Pol. Chem.*, 32, 1027-1032, ISSN 1099-0518

Kuroiwa, T.; Ichikawa, S.; Sato, S. & Mukataka, S. (2003). Improvement of the yield of physiologically active oligosaccharides in continuous hydrolysis of chitosan using immobilized chitosanases. *Biotechn. Bioeng.*, 84 , 121-127, ISSN 0006-3592.

Kwon, S.; Park, J.H.; Chung, H.; Kwon, I.C. & Jeong, S.Y. (2003). Physicochemical Characteristics of Self-Assembled Nanoparticles Based on Glycol Chitosan Bearing 5β-Cholanic Acid. *Langmuir*, 19, 10188-10193, ISSN 0743-7463

Lameiro, M.H., Malpique, R., Silva, A.C., Alves, P.M. & Melo, E. (2006). Encapsulation of adenoviral vectors into chitosan-bile salt microparticles for mucosal vaccination. *J. Biotechnol.*, 126, 152-162, ISSN 0168-1656

Lavertu, M., Methot, S., Tran-Khanh, N. & Buschmann, M.D. (2006). High efficiency gene transfer using chitosan/DNA nanoparticles with specific combinations of molecular weight and degree of deacetylation. *Biomaterials,* 27, 4815-4824, ISSN 1043-1802

Lee, K.Y.; Ha, W.S. & Park, W.H. (1995) Blood compatibility and biodegradability of partially *N*-acylated chitosan derivatives. *Biomaterials,* 16, 1211-1216, ISSN 1043-1802

Lee, K.Y., Kwon, I.C., Kim, Y.H., Jo, W.H. & Jeong, S.Y. (1998). Preparation of chitosan self-aggregates as a gene delivery system. *J. Control Release,* 51, 213-220, ISSN 0168-3659

Lee, D., Lockey, R. & Mohapatra, S. (2006). Folate receptor-mediated cancer cell specific gene delivery using folic acid-conjugated oligochitosans. *J. Nanosci. Nanotechnol.,* 6, 2860-2866, ISSN 1533-4880

Lee, D., Zhang, W., Shirley, S.A., Kong, X., Hellermann, G.R., Lockey, R.F. & Mohapatra, S.S. (2007). Thiolated chitosan/DNA nanocomplexes exhibit enhanced and sustained gene delivery. *Pharm. Res.,* 24, 157-167, ISSN 0724-8741

Lee, M.Y.; Var, F.; Shin-ya, Y.; Kajiuchi, T. & Yang, J.W. (1999). Optimum conditions for the precipitation of chitosan oligomers with DP 5–7 in concentrated hydrochloric acid at low temperature. *Proc. Biochem,* 34, 493–500, ISSN 1359-5113

Leong, K.W.; Mao, H.Q.; Truong-Le, V.L.; Roy, K.; Walsh, S.M. & August, J.T. (1998). DNA-polycation nanospheres as non-viral gene delivery vehicles. *J. Control Release.,* 53, 183–193, ISSN 0168-3659

Li, S.D. & Huang, L. (2006). Gene therapy progress and prospects: non-viral gene therapy by systemic delivery. *Gene Ther.,* 13, 1313-1319, ISSN 0969-7128

Lin, H.; Wang, H. Y.; Xue, C.H. M. Y, (2002). Preparation of chitosan oligomers by immobilized papain. *Enzyme Microbial Technology,* 31,588-592, ISSN 0141- 0229

Liu, D. & Knapp, J.E. (2001). Hydrodynamics-based gene delivery. *Curr. Opin. Mol. Ther.,* 3, 192-197, ISSN 1093-4715

Liu, X., Howard, K.A., Dong, M., Andersen, M.O., Rahbek, U.L., Johnsen, M.G., Hansen, O.C., Besenbacher, F. & Kjems, J. (2007). The influence of polymeric properties on chitosan/siRNA nanoparticle formulation and gene silencing. *Biomaterials,* 28, 1280-1288, ISSN 1043-1802

Liu, W.G.; Zhang, J.R.; Cao, Z.Q.; Xu, F.Y. & Yao, K.D. (2004). A chitosan-arginine conjugate as a novel anticoagulation biomaterial. *J. Mater. Sci. Mater. Med.,* 15, 1199–1203, ISSN 0957-4530.

Liu, W.G. & Yao, K.D. (2002). Chitosan and its derivatives—a promising non-viral vector for gene transfection. *J. Control Release,* 83, 1-11, ISSN 0168-3659

Mansouri, S.; Cui, Y.; Winnik, F.; Shi, Q.; Benderdour, M.; Lavigne, P.; Beaumont, E. & Fernandes, J.C. (2006). Characterization of Folate-Chitosan-DNA nanoparticles for gene therapy. *Biomaterials,* 27, 2060-2065, ISSN 0142-9612

Mao, S.; Shuai, X.; Unger, F. Simona, M., Kissel, D., & Bi, T. (2004). The depolymerization of chitosan: effects on physicochemical and biological properties. *Int. J. Pharm.,* 281, 45–54, ISSN 0378-5173

Mingozzi, F. & High, K.A. (2007). Immune Responses to AAV in Clinical Trials. *Curr. Gene Ther.,* 7, 316-324, ISSN 1566-5232

Moghimi, S.M., Hunter, A.C. & Murray, J.C. (2005). Nanomedicine: current status and future prospects. *FASEB J.,* 19, 311-330, ISSN 0892-6638

Mook, O.R., Baas, F., de Wissel, M.B. & Fluiter, K. (2007). Evaluation of locked nucleic acid-modified small interfering RNA in vitro and in vivo. *Mol. Cancer Ther.*, 6, 833-843, ISSN 1535-7163

Morris, V.B. & Sharma C.P. (2010). Folate mediated in vitro targeting of depolymerised trimethylated chitosan having arginine functionality. *J. Coll. Interf. Sci.*, 348, 360-368, ISSN 0021-9797

Muzzarelli, R.A.A.; Terbojevich, M.; Muzzarelli, C. & Francescangeli, O. (2002). Chitosans depolymerized with the aid of papain and stabilized as glycosylamines. *Carbohydr. Polym.*, 50, 69-78, ISSN 0144-8617

Nakashima-Matsushita, N., Homma, T., Yu, S., Matsuda, T., Sunahara, N., Nakamura, T., Tsukano, M., Ratnam, M. & Matsuyama, T. (1999). Selective expression of folate receptor beta and its possible role in methotrexate transport in synovial macrophages from patients with rheumatoid arthritis. *Arthritis Rheum.*, 42, 1609-1616, ISSN 1529-0131

No, H.K. & Meyers, S.P. (1989). Crawfish chitosan as a coagulant in recovery of organic compounds from seafood processing streams. *J. Agric. Food Chem.* 37, 580-583, ISSN 0021-8561

Okamoto, H., Shiraki, K., Yasuda, R., Danjo, K. & Watanabe, Y. (2010). Chitosan-interferon-beta gene complex powder for inhalation treatment of lung metastasis in mice. *J. Control Release.* 2010 Dec 23. [Epub ahead of print, ISSN 0168-3659

Ouchi, T.; Nishizawa, H. & Ohya, Y. (1998). Aggregation phenomenon of PEG-grafted chitosan in aqueous solution. *Polymer,* 39, 5171-5175, ISSN 0032-3861

Pa, J.H. & Yu T.L. (2001). Light scattering study of chitosan in acetic acid aqueous solutions. *Macromol. Chem. Phys.*, 202, 985-991, ISSN 1022-1352

Park, I.K.; Ihm, J.E.; Park, Y.H.; Choi Y.J.; Kim, S.I.; Kim W.J.; Akaike, T. & Cho, C.S. (2003). Galactosylated chitosan (GC)-graft-poly(vinyl pyrrolidone) (PVP) as hepatocyte-targeting DNA carrier Preparation and physicochemical characterization of GC-graft-PVP/DNA complex. *J. Control Release*, 86: 349-359, ISSN 0168-3659.

Park, I.K., Park, Y.H., Shin, B.A., Choi, E.S., Kim, Y.R., Akaike, T. & Cho, C.S. (2000). Galactosylated chitosan-graft-dextran as hepatocyte-targeting DNA carrier. *J. Control Release,* 69, 97-108, ISSN 0168-3659

Pelletier, J.P., Caron, J.P., Evans, C., Robbins, P.D., Georgescu, H.I., Jovanovic, D., Fernandes, J.C. & Martel-Pelletier, J. (1997). In vivo suppression of early experimental osteoarthritis by interleukin-1 receptor antagonist using gene therapy. Arthritis Rheum., 40, 1012-9, ISSN 1529-0131

Ping, Y.A.; Liu, C.D.; Tang, G.P.; Li, J.S.; Li, J.; Yang, W.T. & Xu, F.J. (2010). Functionalization of chitosan via atom transfer radical polymerization for gene delivery. *Adv. Funct. Mater.*, 20, 3106–3116, ISSN 1616-3028

Rabea, E.I.; Badawy, M.E.T.; Stevens, C.V.; Smagghe, G. & Steurbaut, W. (2003). Chitosan as Antimicrobial Agent: applications and mode of action. *Biomacromolecules,* 4, 1457-1465, ISSN 1525-7797

Ramesh, R., Saeki, T., Templeton, N.S., Ji, L., Stephens, L.C., Ito, I., Wilson, D.R., Wu, Z., Branch, C.D., Minna, J.D. & Roth, J.A. (2001). Successful treatment of primary and disseminated human lung cancers by systemic delivery of tumor suppressor genes using an improved liposome vector. *Mol. Ther.*, 3, 337-350, ISSN 1525-0016

Raper, S.E., Chirmule, N., Lee, F.S., Wivel, N.A., Bagg, A., Gao, G.P., Wilson, J.M. & Batshaw, M.L. (2003). Fatal systemic inflammatory response syndrome in a ornithine transcarbamylase deficient patient following adenoviral gene transfer. *Mol. Genet. Metab,* 80, 148-158, ISSN 1096-7192

Richardson, S.C., Kolbe, H.V. & Duncan, R. (1999). Potential of low molecular mass chitosan as a DNA delivery system: biocompatibility, body distribution and ability to complex and protect DNA. *Int. J. Pharm.,* 178, 231-243, ISSN 0378-5173

Roberts, G.A.F. (1992). *Chitin Chemistry,* Mc Millan Press Ltd, London, ISBN 0333524179

Rojanarata, T., Opanasopit, P., Techaarpornkul, S., Ngawhirunpat, T. & Ruktanonchai, U. (2008). Chitosan-thiamine pyrophosphate as a novel carrier for siRNA delivery. *Pharm. Res.,* 25, 2807-2814. ISSN 0724-8741

Romero, N.B., Braun, S., Benveniste, O., Leturcq, F., Hogrel, J.Y., Morris, G.E., Barois, A., Eymard, B., Payan, C., Ortega, V., Boch, A.L., Lejean, L., Thioudellet, C., Mourot, B., Escot, C., Choquel, A., Recan, D., Kaplan, J.C., Dickson, G., Klatzmann, D., Molinier-Frenckel, V., Guillet, J.G., Squiban, P., Herson, S. & Fardeau, M. (2004). Phase I study of dystrophin plasmid-based gene therapy in Duchenne/Becker muscular dystrophy. *Hum. Gene Ther.,* 15, 1065-1076. ISSN 1043-0342

Sakurai, H., Kawabata, K., Sakurai, F., Nakagawa, S. & Mizuguchi, H. (2008). Innate immune response induced by gene delivery vectors. *Int. J Pharm.,* 354, 9-15, ISSN 0378-5173

Saito, H.; Wu, Sato, T.; Nagasaki, T.; Sakairi, N. & Shinkai, S. (2004). 6-Amino-6-deoxychitosan (2004) Preparation and application as plasmid vector in COS-1 cells. *Chem. Lett.,* 33: 340-341, ISSN 0366-7022

Saito, H.; Wu, X.; Harris, J.M. & Hoffman, A.S. (1997). Graft copolymers of poly(ethylene glycol) (PEG) and chitosan. *Macromol. Rapid Commun.,* 18, 547-550, ISSN 1022-1336

Sato, T., Ishii, T. & Okahata,Y. (2001). In vitro gene delivery mediated by chitosan. effect of pH, serum, and molecular mass of chitosan on the transfection efficiency. *Biomaterials,* 22, 2075-2080, ISSN 0142-9612

Satoh, T.; Kakimoto, S.; Kano, H.; Nakatani, M.; Shinkai, S. & Nagasaki, T. (2007). In vitro gene delivery to HepG2 cells using galactosylated 6-amino-6-deoxychitosan as a DNA carrier. *Carbohydr. Res.,* 342, 1427–1433, ISSN 0008-6215

Schaffer, D.V., Fidelman, N.A., Dan, N. & Lauffenburger, D.A. (2000). Vector unpacking as a potential barrier for receptor-mediated polyplex gene delivery. *Biotechnol. Bioeng.,* 67, 598-606, ISSN 0006 3592

Schatz, C.; Viton, C.; Delair, T.; Pichot, C. & Domard, A. (2003). Typical physicochemical behaviors of chitosan in aqueous solution. *Biomacromolecules,* 4, 641-648, ISSN 1525-7797

Seiler, M.P., Cerullo, V. & Lee, B. (2007). Immune response to helper dependent adenoviral mediated liver gene therapy: challenges and prospects. *Curr. Gene Ther.,* 7, 297-305, ISSN 1566-5232

Shimojohay, M.; Fukushimab, K. & Kurita. K. (1998). Low-molecular-weight chitosans derived from P-chitin: preparation, molecular characteristics and aggregation activity. *Carbohydr. Polym.,* 35, 223-231, ISSN 0144-8617

Signini, R.; Desbrieres, J. & Campana Filho, S.P. (2000). On the stiffness of chitosan hydrochloride in acid-free aqueous solutions. *Carbohydr. Polym.* 43, 351–357. ISSN 1043-1802

Sinha, V.R.; Singla, A.K.; Wadhawan, S.; Kaushik, R.; Kumria, R.; Bansal, K. & Dhawan, S. (2004). Chitosan microspheres as a potential carrier for drugs. *Int. J. Pharm. 274,* 1-33, ISSN 0378-5173

Sinnott, M.L. (1990). Catalytic mechanism of enzymic glycosyl transfer. *Chem. Rev.*, 90, 1171–1202, ISSN 0009-2665

Suda, T. & Liu, D. (2007). Hydrodynamic gene delivery: its principles and applications. *Mol. Ther.*, 15, 2063-2069, ISSN 1525-0016

Sudimack, J. & Lee, R.J. (2000). Targeted drug delivery via the folate receptor. *Adv. Drug Deliv. Rev.*, 41, 147-162, ISSN 0169-409X

Suh, J., Wirtz, D. & Hanes, J. (2003). Efficient active transport of gene nanocarriers to the cell nucleus. *Proc. Natl. Acad. Sci. U. S. A*, 100, 3878-3882. ISSN 2227 8424

Sun, S., Liu, W., Cheng, N., Zhang, B., Cao, Z., Yao, K., Liang, D., Zuo, A., Guo, G. & Zhang, J. (2005). A thermoresponsive chitosan-NIPAAm/vinyl laurate copolymer vector for gene transfection. *Bioconjug. Chem.*, 16, 972-980, ISSN 1043-1802

Sun, B.; Zhao, R.L.; Kong, F.Q.; Ren, Y.P.; Zuo, A.J.; Liang, D.C.; Zhang, J.Y. (2010). Phosphorylatable short peptide conjugation for facilitating transfection efficacy of CS/DNA complex. *Int. J. Pharm.*, 397: 206-210, ISSN 0378-5173

Tahara, K., Sakai, T., Yamamoto, H., Takeuchi, H. & Kawashima, Y. (2008). Establishing chitosan coated PLGA nanosphere platform loaded with wide variety of nucleic acid by complexation with cationic compound for gene delivery. *Int. J. Pharm.*, 354, 210-216, ISSN 0378-5173

Tan, W.B., Jiang, S. & Zhang,Y. (2007). Quantum-dot based nanoparticles for targeted silencing of HER2/neu gene via RNA interference. *Biomaterials,* 28, 1565-1571, ISSN 1043-1802

Tang, E.S.K.; Huang, M. & Lim, L.Y. (2003). Ultrasonication of chitosan and chitosan nanoparticles. *Int. J. Pharm.*, 265,103–114, ISSN 0378-5173

Techaarpornkul, S., Wongkupasert, S., Opanasopit, P., Apirakaramwong, A., Nunthanid, J. & Ruktanonchai, U. (2010). Chitosan-mediated siRNA delivery in vitro: effect of polymer molecular weight, concentration and salt forms. *AAPS. PharmSciTech.,* 11, 64-72, ISSN 1530-9932

Terbojevich, M.; Cosani, A. & Muzzarelli, R.A.A. (1996). Molecular parameters of chitosans depolymerized with the aid of papain, *Carbohydr. Polym.*, *29,* 63-68, ISSN 0144-8617

Tiera, M.J.; Qiu, X.P.; Bechaouch, S.; Shi, Q.; Fernandes, J.C. & Winnik, F.M. (2006). Synthesis and Characterization of Phosphorylcholine-Substituted Chitosans Soluble in Physiological pH Conditions. *Biomacromolecules*, 7, 3151-3156, ISSN 1525-7797

Tolaimate, A.; Desbrieres, J.; Rhazi, M.; Alagui, A.; Vincendon, M. & Vottero, P. (2000). On the influence of deacetylation process on the physicochemical characteristics of chitosan from squid chitin. *Polymer,* 41, 2463–2469, ISSN 0032-3861

Tolaimate, A.; Desbrieres, J.; Rhazia, M. & Alagui, A. (2003). Contribution to the preparation of chitins and chitosans with controlled physico-chemical properties, *Polymer,* 44, 7939–7952. ISSN 0032-3861

Tong, H., Qin, S., Fernandes, J.C., Li, L., Dai, K. & Zhang, X. (2009). Progress and prospects of chitosan and its derivatives as non-viral gene vectors in gene therapy. *Curr. Gene Ther.*, 9, 495-502, ISSN 1566-5232

Tsaih, M.L. & Chen, R.H. (2003). Effect of degree of deacetylation of chitosan on the kinetics of ultrasonic degradation of chitosan. *J. Appl. Polym. Sci.* 90, 3526-3531, ISSN 0021-8995

Turk, M.J., Breur, G.J., Widmer, W.R., Paulos, C.M., Xu, L.C., Grote, L.A. & Low, P.S. (2002). Folate-targeted imaging of activated macrophages in rats with adjuvant-induced arthritis. *Arthritis Rheum.,* 46, 1947-1955, ISSN 1529-0131

Ulrich-Vinther, M. (2007). Gene therapy methods in bone and joint disorders. Evaluation of the adeno-associated virus vector in experimental models of articular cartilage disorders, periprosthetic osteolysis and bone healing. *Acta Orthop Suppl,* 78, 1-64, ISSN 1745-3674

Vaishnaw, A.K., Gollob, J., Gamba-Vitalo, C., Hutabarat, R., Sah, D., Meyers, R., de, F.T. & Maraganore, J. (2010). A status report on RNAi therapeutics. *Silence.,* 1, 14, ISSN 1758-907X

Vandenberghe, L.H. & Wilson, J.M. (2007). AAV as An Immunogen. *Curr. Gene Ther.,* 7, 325-333, ISSN 1566-5232

Wang, J., Lu, Z., Wientjes, M.G. & Au, J.L. (2010). Delivery of siRNA Therapeutics: Barriers and Carriers. *AAPS. J.,* 12(4):492-503, ISSN 1550-7416

Whittaker, G.R. & Helenius, A. (1998). Nuclear import and export of viruses and virus genomes. *Virology,* 246, 1-23, ISSN 0042-6822

Wong, K., Sun, G., Zhang, X., Dai, H., Liu, Y., He, C. & Leong, K.W. (2006). PEI-g-chitosan, a novel gene delivery system with transfection efficiency comparable to polyethylenimine in vitro and after liver administration in vivo. *Bioconjug. Chem.,* 17, 152-158, ISSN 1043-1802

Varma, A.J.; Deshpande, S.V. & Kennedy, J.F. (2004). Metal complexation by chitosan and its derivatives: a review. *Carbohydr. Polym.*, 55, 77-93, ISSN 0144-8617

Varurn, K.M.; Myhr, M.M.; Hjerde, R.J.N. & Smidsrod, O. (1997). In vitro degradation rates of partially *N*-acetylated chitosans in human serum, *Carbohydr. Res.*, 299, 99- 101, ISSN 0144-8617

Xia, W., Liu, W., Cui, L., Liu, Y., Zhong, W., Liu, D., Wu, J., Chua, K. & Cao, Y. (2004). Tissue engineering of cartilage with the use of chitosan-gelatin complex scaffolds. *J Biomed Mater Res B Appl Biomater.*, 15:71(2), 373-80, ISSN 1552-4973

Yang, P.T., Hoang, L., Jia, W.W. & Skarsgard, E.D. (2010). In Utero Gene Delivery Using Chitosan-DNA Nanoparticles in Mice. *J. Surg. Res.,* 2010 Jun 12. [Epub ahead of print], ISSN 0022-4804

Yip, V.L.Y. & Withers, S.G. (2004). Nature's many mechanisms for the degradation of oligosaccharides. *Org. Biol. Chem.*, 2, 2707–2713.

Yoo, H.S., Lee, J.E., Chung, H., Kwon, I.C.& Jeong, S.Y. (2005). Self-assembled nanoparticles containing hydrophobically modified glycol chitosan for gene delivery. *J. Control Release,* 103, 235-243, ISSN 0168-3659

Yu, B., Zhao, X., Lee, L.J. & Lee, R.J. (2009). Targeted delivery systems for oligonucleotide therapeutics. *AAPS. J.,* 11, 195-203, ISSN 1550-7416

Yu, Y.Y.; Wang, Z.; Cai, L.; Wang, G.; Yang, X.; Wan, X.P.; Xu, X.H.; Li, Y. & Gao R. (2010). Synthesis and characterization of methoxy poly(ethylene glycol)-O-chitosan-polyethylenimine for gene delivery. *Carbohydr. Polym.* 81: 269-274, ISSN 0144-8617

Zeng, J.M.; Wang, X. & Wang, S. (2007). Self-assembled ternary complexes of plasmid DNA, low molecular weight polyethylenimine and targeting peptide for nonviral gene delivery into neurons. *Biomaterials,* 28: 1443-1451, ISSN 0142-9612

Zelphati, O., Uyechi, L.S., Barron, L.G. & Szoka, F.C., Jr. (1998). Effect of serum components on the physico-chemical properties of cationic lipid/oligonucleotide complexes and on their interactions with cells. *Biochim. Biophys. Acta,* 1390, 119-133.

Zhang, S., Zhao, B., Jiang, H., Wang, B. & Ma, B. (2007). Cationic lipids and polymers mediated vectors for delivery of siRNA. *J. Control Release,* 123, 1-10, , ISSN 0168-3659

Zhang, Y., Chen, J., Zhang, Y., Pan, Y., Zhao, J., Ren, L., Liao, M., Hu, Z., Kong, L. & Wang, J. (2007). A novel PEGylation of chitosan nanoparticles for gene delivery. *Biotechnol. Appl. Biochem.,* 46, 197-204, ISSN 0885-4513

20

Toxicity of Polymeric-Based Non-Viral Vector Systems for Pulmonary siRNA Application

Andrea Beyerle[1,2], Thomas Kissel[2] and Tobias Stoeger[1,2]
[1]*Comprehensive Pneumology Center, Institute of Lung Biology and Disease Helmholtz Zentrum, München*
[2]*Department of Pharmaceutics and Biopharmacy, Philipps-University Marburg Germany*

1. Introduction

Nanomedicine has the potential of clinical benefit by combination of engineering technologies and materials (Schatzlein, 2006). Development of nanometre scaled therapeutics which provides new and improved properties by specifically targeting the site of action and causing low level of side effects would be a big challenge to treat patients with severe and live-threatening diseases like cancer. Gene therapy provides a new way to treat patients and a lot of effort is made to improve the clinical benefit. But current gene therapy is still experimental and has not proven success in the clinics. Nevertheless there is a need for new approaches to treat „undruggable" disease sites and there are some clinical trials ongoing which using RNA inference (RNAi) as therapeutic mechanism (Table 1).

2. Gene silencing by siRNAs

2.1 RNA interference

RNA interference (RNAi), the Nobel Prize winning mechanism for gene silencing (Fire *et al.*, 1998), raises nowadays increasing attention of many researchers as a new way to treat life-threatening diseases like cancer (Akhtar, 2006) or other genetic disorders like cystic fibrosis (Griesenbach and Alton, 2009) or viral infection as respiratory syncytial virus (RSV) (Ge *et al.*, 2004) and as an in vitro research tool to investigate mechanisms which are involved in those diseases. Small interfering RNA (siRNA) duplexes of 19-23 base pairs could trigger sequence specific gene silencing in mammalian cells (Caplen *et al.*, 2001; Elbashir *et al.*, 2001; Hannon and Rossi, 2004; Meister *et al.*, 2004; Mello and Conte, 2004). The siRNAs are double stranded molecules, consisting of a guide strand that is perfectly complementary to a target mRNA and a passenger strand. Core components of this siRNA-mediated post-transcriptional silencing include the RNAse III enzyme Dicer and its co-factor transactivating response RNA-binding protein (TRBP) along with the Argonaute family of proteins, in particular Argonaute 2 (Ago 2) (Meister *et al.*, 2004), which is the catalytic engine of the RNA induced silencing complex (RISC). Dicer converts dsRNA into 21-25 nucleotide duplexes with 3′ 2nt overhangs. The siRNA is incorporated into one or more of the Argonaute proteins in RISC for sequence specific target degradation or translational inhibition (Tuschl *et al.*, 1999). In general, perfect or near perfect base pairing between the siRNA guide strand and the target mRNA is required for Ago2 cleavage to occur. In

Company	siRNA	Target	Disease/ Disorder	Status	Administration / Formulation	Remarks
Acuity Pharmaceuticals (Opko Health)	Bevasiranib (Cand5)	VEGF	AMD, DME	Phase II	intravitreal injection, free siRNA	-
Alnylam Pharmaceuticals	ALN-RSV-01 ALN-RSV-02	RSV Pediatric RSV	RSV Pediatric RSV	Phase IIb	aerosolized siRNA, free siRNA	-
	ALN-VSP02	KSP and VEGF	Liver cancer	Phase I	i.v., free siRNA	-
Silence Therapeutics	Atu027	PKN3	Advanced solid cancer	Phase I	i.v., free siRNA	-
Sirna Therapeutics (Calando Pharmaceuticals)	CALAA-01	RRM2	Solid tumor cancer	Phase I	i.v., Cyclodextrin-adamantan-PEG-transferrin nanocomplex.	-
Sirna Therapeutics (TransDerm Inc.)	TD101	PC keratin K6a	Pachyonychia congenita	Phase Ib	Injection into a callus on the bottom of one foot, free siRNA	-
Sirna Therapeutics	AGN211745 (Sirna-027)	VEGFR1	AMD, CNV & AMD	Phase II	intravitreal injection, free siRNA	-
Quarks Pharmaceuticals	I5NP (QPI-1002)	p53	Delayed graft function, Kidney transplantation	Phase I Phase II	i.v., free siRNA	-
	QPI-1007	Caspase 2	Chronic optic nerve atrophy Non-Arteritic Anterior Ischemic Optic Neuropathy	Phase I	intravitreal injection, free siRNA	-
Tekmira Pharmaceuticals Corporation	PRO-040201	APOB	Hypercholesterolemia	Phase I	i.v., liposomal formulation	study has been terminated due to potential for immune stimulation to interfere with further dose escalation

Silenseed Ltd	siG12D LODER (Local Drug EluteR)	KRAS G12D	Pancreatic cancer	Phase I	miniature biodegradable polymeric matrix, placed in the tumor using an endoscopic ultrasound biopsy needle	-

source: http://clinicaltrials.ifpma.org/no_cache/en/search-trials-ongoing/all/index.htm,

Table 1. Summary of ongoing clinical trials for siRNA delivery,
abbreviations used: AMD: age related macular degeneration; APOB: apolipoprotein B; CNV: choroidale neovascularization; DME: diabetic macular edema; i.v.: intravenous; KSP: kinesin spindle protein; PC: pachyonychia congenital; PKN3: protein kinase N3; RRM2: ribonucleotide reductase M2 polypeptide; RSV: respiratory syntical virus; VEGF: vascular endothelial growth factor

laboratory work and in clinical trials siRNAs are most often chemically synthesized, bypassing the Dicer cleavage step for entry into RISC and avoiding any immune responses and toxicity which is described for long double stranded RNAs (dsRNAs) (Behlke, 2008).
RNAi has widely been used in drug development and several phase I and II clinical trials (Table 1) are ongoing. However, for therapeutic applications still some concerns and challenges need to be overcome, e.g. off-target effects, innate immune response and most importantly specific delivery into the cytoplasm of target cells.

3. Small interfering RNAs (siRNA)

siRNAs are very attractive for therapy because they are easily designed and synthesized, and their versatility allows simultaneous use of multiple siRNAs or change of sequences to accommodate virus mutations. The negative charge of siRNA and their size of around 14 kDa make it difficult to cross the cell membrane without any carrier. There are various delivery strategies under investigation, which includes nanoparticular systems consisting of polymers and/or lipids of different compositions and with or without any conjugation like antibodies or ligands for achieving the most specific way to the target side of action. Davis et al. showed 2008 first evidence for RNAi mechanism of action in human with their self-assembling, cyclodextrin polymer-based nanoparticle system (CALAA-01) targeting the riboucleotide reductase subunit 2 (RRM2) which could be used for therapy of different types of cancers (Heidel *et al.*, 2007; Davis, 2009; Davis *et al.*, 2010). At the same time Zimmermann, MacLachlan and colleagues reported successful siRNA delivery using a different approach for delivery (Zimmermann *et al.*, 2006). They introduced so-called stable nucleic acid lipid particles (SNALP) generated by ethanol dilution technique and showed for the first time in non-human primate a successful targeting of ApoB in the liver (Soutschek *et al.*, 2004; Morrissey *et al.*, 2005; Zimmermann *et al.*, 2006). Ge and co-workers (Ge *et al.*, 2004) used PEI 25 kDa to complex and protect siRNA specific to influenza virus genes and they showed successful reduction of influenza virus infection in mice. Alton et al. gave first evidence for successful gene therapy by using a lipid-based system to delivery CFTR DNA in cystic fibrosis patients (Alton *et al.*, 1999). Thus, gene therapy approaches still need improvements regarding specific targeting and successful delivery of the nucleic acid but clinical trials are ongoing and preclinical testing are conducted for different kind of diseases (Table 1).

4. Non-viral vector systems for siRNA delivery

RNA interference (RNAi) based therapeutics represent a fundamentally new way to treat human disease by addressing targets that are otherwise "undruggable" with existing medicines (Novina and Sharp, 2004; de Fougerolles *et al.*, 2007). The goal of RNAi-based therapy represents the activation of selective mRNA cleavage for efficient gene silencing. There are two possibilities to harness the endogenous pathway: either i) by using viral vector to express short hairpin RNA (shRNA) that resembles miRNA precursors, or (ii) by introducing siRNAs that mimic Dicer cleavage product into the cytoplasm. Synthetic siRNAs utilize the naturally occurring RNAi pathway in a manner that is consistent and predictable, thus making them particularly attractive as therapeutics. Since they enter RNAi pathway later, siRNAs are less likely to interfere with gene regulation by endogenous miRNAs (Jackson *et al.*, 2003; Grimm *et al.*, 2006). The most important characteristics for effective design and selection of siRNAs are potency, specificity, and nuclease stability. Two types of off-target effects need to be avoided or minimized: i) silencing of genes sharing partial homology to the siRNA and ii) immune stimulation induced by recognition of certain siRNAs by the innate immune system. The activation of the innate immune systems by siRNA could be induced by recognition of dsRNAs by the serine/threonine protein kinase receptor (PKR) (Schlee *et al.*, 2006). This pathway is normally triggered by dsRNAs that are more than 30 nucleotides long, but at higher concentrations also siRNAs may be able to activate this pathway resulting in global translational blockade and cell death. The potential to activate toll-like receptors (TLRs) in the endosomal compartment is more likely to occur after siRNA delivery due to recognition of specific nucleotide sequence motifs (e.g. GU) by TLRs. TLR activation could trigger the production of type I interferons and pro-inflammatory cytokines, and induce nuclear factor kappa B (NF-kB) activation (Hornung *et al.*, 2005; Judge *et al.*, 2005). For example, the presence of 2'-O-methyl modifications within the siRNA duplex could abrogate the binding to TLR7 in endosomes and abolish immunostimulatory response. In addition, these modifications also reduce sequence-dependent off-target silencing and may be particularly beneficial in enhancing siRNA target specificity (Judge *et al.*, 2006; Robbins *et al.*, 2008; Robbins *et al.*, 2009).

Due to increasing mortality and morbidity caused by several lung diseases, RNAi strategies have attracted particular attention and the lung as target organ provides an attractive tool because of the accessibility via non-invasive routes, e.g. nasal or pulmonary applications. The clinical success of siRNA-mediated interventions critically depends upon the safety and efficacy of the delivery methods and agents. Naked siRNAs are degraded in human plasma with a half-life of minutes (Layzer *et al.*, 2004; Choung *et al.*, 2006). Thus, the search for optimized nanocarriers to deliver siRNA is still under intensive investigation. The negative charge and chemical degradability of siRNA under physiologically relevant conditions make its delivery a major challenge (Gary *et al.*, 2007). Depending on their origin, two types of positively charged carriers could be distinguished: i) lipid-based and ii) polymeric-based carrier systems. Both systems provided several advantages to deliver siRNA. Liposome formation agents like Lipofectamine 2000 (Dalby *et al.*, 2004; Santel *et al.*, 2006) and cardiolipin analogues (Chien *et al.*, 2005; Pal *et al.*, 2005) have been successfully used for the delivery of siRNA. Negatively charged nucleic acids and positively charged lipids spontaneously form

nanoparticles, known as lipoplexes, of 50-200 nm in diameter (Sitterberg *et al.,* 2010). Interaction with serum components represents one of the major hurdles that influence the performance when used systemically (Zuhorn *et al.*, 2007). Recently, lipid-mediated delivery of siRNA against apolipoprotein B (ApoB) has been used to target ApoB mRNA to the (Soutschek *et al.*, 2004; Zimmermann *et al.*, 2006). The in vivo use of cationic lipids especially by i.v. administration presents significant problems as these reagents can be quite toxic. Despite problems with i.v. use, cationic lipids are employed for i.p. injection (Verma *et al.*, 2003; Flynn *et al.*, 2004; Miyawaki-Shimizu *et al.*, 2006), for CNS injection (Hassani *et al.*, 2005; Luo *et al.*, 2005) or in topical epithelial surface application (Maeda *et al.*, 2005; Palliser *et al.*, 2006) and intratracheal (Griesenbach *et al.*, 2006). Toxicity varies with the precise chemical composition of the lipids employed dose, and the delivering route. Variations in chemical composition can have a large impact on the functional properties of cationic lipid mixtures (Spagnou et al., 2004), and lipoplex/liposomal preparations have been devised with decreased toxicity that are more compatible with i.v. administration. Liposomes can be modified with ligands such as folate or small peptides, which assist with delivery and help target specific cell types or tissues (Meyerhoff, 1999; Dubey *et al.*, 2004). Through the use of neutral polyethylene glycol-substituted surfaces and other approaches, liposomes can be stabilized and made more "stealthy" showing reduced clearance and improved pharmacokinetics (Oupicky *et al.*, 2002; Moghimi and Szebeni, 2003). These kinds of lipid nanoparticles have been successfully used to deliver antisense oligonucleotides and siRNAs in vivo (Braasch *et al.*, 2003; Chien *et al.*, 2005).
Similar to the lipid-based non viral vector systems, the positive charges of polycations allow an efficient interaction with siRNAs to form so-called polyplexes, which can bind onto cell plasma membrane and be endocytosed. In contrast to the lipid-based systems that rely on the fusogenic property of the liposomes to mediate endosomal escape, polymeric carriers such as poly(ethylene imine) (PEI) use the so-called "proton-sponge" effect to enhance endosomal release of endocytosed polyplexes (Boussif *et al.*, 1995; Behr, 1997; Akinc *et al.*, 2005; Demeneix and Behr, 2005; Nel *et al.*, 2009). According to this mechanism, the deprotonated amines with different pK_a values confer a buffer effect over a wide range of pH. This buffering may protect the siRNA from degradation in the endosomal compartment during maturation of the early endosomes to late endosomes and their subsequent fusion with the lysosomes. The buffering property also allows the polycation to escape from the endosome. At lower pH the buffering capacity causes an influx of chloride ions and water into the endosomes, which burst due to osmotic pressure and facilitating intracellular release of PEI - siRNA polyplexes. PEI has been used for many years to facilitate nucleic acid delivery (Boussif *et al.*, 1995; Demeneix and Behr, 2005). However, due to toxicity and variable performance it has not found generalized acceptance as a delivery tool for either antisense oligonucleotides or siRNAs. Nevertheless, PEI can be used as a prototype for formulation of more complex particles with improved properties (Kim and Kim, 2009).

5. PEI-based non-viral vector systems

Polyethylene imine (PEI) is a simple repetition of the 43 Da CH_2-CH_2-NH ethylene imine motifs. It can be synthesized from ethylene imine (aziridine) via ring opening polymerization or by hydrolysis of poly(2-ethyl-2-oxazolium), leading to branched or linear polymeric backbones, respectively (Godbey *et al.*, 1999). PEI represents one of the most comprehensive investigated cationic polymer for gene delivery in vitro and in vivo (Godbey *et al.*, 1999; Fischer *et al.*, 2002; Brus *et al.*, 2004; Neu *et al.*, 2005; Gary *et al.*, 2007). PEI 25 kDa serves as gold standard for in vitro transfection experiments (Godbey *et al.*, 2000). The mechanism of cell entry and action for gene delivery is intensively analyzed. To enhance the endosomal release of endocytosed polyplexes PEI uses the so-called "proton-sponge" effect (Boussif *et al.*, 1995; Behr, 1997) Due to the high buffer capacity of PEI amino groups in PEI molecules will be protonated at lower pHs like in the endosomal-lysosomal environment, additional chloride influx into the vesicles increases the osmolarity and the vesicles begin to swell and under the increased osmotic pressure the vesicle will be disrupted and the nucleic acid protected from PEI will be released into the cytoplasm (Godbey *et al.*, 1999; Akinc *et al.*, 2005; Nel *et al.*, 2009). PEI has been used for many years to facilitate nucleic acid delivery (Demeneix and Behr, 2005). However, due to toxicity and variable performance a lot of research is undertaken to reduce the toxicity of PEI and maintain or improve the efficacy and specificity by modification PEI backbone and/or conjugation of hydrophilic molecules like polyethylene glycol (PEG) (Petersen *et al.*, 2002a; Petersen *et al.*, 2002b), disulfide linkages (Breunig *et al.*, 2008), or for specific targeting molecules like transferrin, galactose, TAT-peptide, RGD-motifs (Ogris *et al.*, 1999; Kunath *et al.*, 2003a; Kunath *et al.*, 2003b; Kleemann *et al.*, 2005). Other approaches are reduction of the molecular weight of PEI 25 kDa or purification of PEI 25 kDa via gel filtration (Boeckle *et al.*, 2004; Urban-Klein *et al.*, 2005; Werth, 2006; Fahrmeir *et al.*, 2007) or using instead of the branched PEI 25 kDa the linear form PEI22kDa (Breunig *et al.*, 2005). Thomas and colleagues showed that full deacylation of linear PEI dramatically improves the efficacy but on cost of increased cytotoxicity due to increased numbers of protonatable nitrogens in the PEI molecule (Thomas *et al.*, 2005).

6. Modifications of PEI

Modifications of PEI with the hydrophilic poly(ethylene glycol) (PEG) reduces dramatically the cytotoxicity of PEI 25 kDa but in part on cost of efficacy and increased immunomodulatory and proinflammatory effects (Kichler *et al.*, 2002; Petersen *et al.*, 2002b; Mao *et al.*, 2005; Glodde *et al.*, 2006; Beyerle *et al.*, 2010a; Beyerle *et al.*, 2010b). PEG provides polyplexes with improved solubility, lower surface charge, diminished aggregation, lower cytotoxicity, and possibly improved "stealth effect" in the bloodstream.

Glodde et al. synthesized a series of PEG-PEI copolymers and found that the molecular weight of PEG was found to be the major determinant of polyplex size, via its influence on particle aggregation and polyplex stability (Glodde *et al.*, 2006). Transfection efficiency was correlated to polyplex stability and low molecular weight PEI 2 kDa grafted with PEG showed higher activity than their counterparts with high molecular weight PEI 25 kDa (Williams *et al.*, 2006). In contrast, Petersen and Mao showed good transfection efficiencies for PEI 25 kDa - PEG copolymers with high molecular weight PEG and low numbers of grafting on PEI backbone compare to low molecular weight PEG with high grafting numbers on PEI 25 kDa (Mao *et al.*, 2005; Merkel *et al.*, 2009; Beyerle *et al.*, 2011a).

Grayson and colleagues investigated the siRNA transfection efficacy of different PEI polymers (branched 800 Da, branched 25 kDa and linear 22 kDa) in HeLa derivative cell line (Grayson *et al.*, 2006). They showed that the siRNA delivery and activity was mainly dependent on the biophysical and structural characteristics of the polyplexes and only

25 kDa PEI was able to effective deliver siRNA. The authors explained the high activity of PEI25kDa/siRNA with good stability of polyplexes, small size, and positively surface charge, but nevertheless the cytotoxicity was highest for PEI 25 kDa.
Succinylated PEI polymers for complexation of siRNA were introduced by Wagner and colleagues which showed 10-fold lower toxicity and higher knockdown efficacy compare to pure PEI polyplexes (Zintchenko *et al.*, 2008).

7. Toxicity of PEI-based non-viral vector systems

Synthetic polymers and nanomaterials display selective phenotypic effects in cells and in the body that affect signal transduction mechanisms involved in inflammation, differentiation, proliferation, and apoptosis. When physically mixed or covalently conjugated with cytotoxic agents, bacterial DNA or antigens, polymers can drastically alter specific genetically controlled responses to these agents (Kabanov, 2006). These effects, in part, result from cooperative interactions of polymers and nanomaterials with plasma cell membranes and trafficking of polymers and nanomaterials to intracellular organelles. Cells and whole organism responses to these materials can be phenotype or genotype dependent. In selected cases, polymer agents can bypass limitations to biological responses imposed by the genotype, for example, phenotypic correction of immune response by polyelectrolytes. Overall, these effects are relatively benign as they do not result in cytotoxicity or major toxicities in the body. Collectively, however, these studies support the need for thoroughly assessing pharmacogenomic effects of polymer materials to maximize clinical outcomes and understand the pharmacological and toxicological effects of polymer formulations of biological agents, i.e. polymer genomics. In addition, it is well described in the literature that cationic nanoparticles disrupt lipid bilayers (Hong *et al.*, 2006; Leroueil *et al.*, 2008), induce oxidative stress inside the cell as a result of cell-type interplay and cause in some cases acute lung inflammation when administered intratracheally (Tan and Huang, 2002; Beyerle *et al.*, 2010b; Beyerle *et al.*, 2011a and Beyerle *et al.*, 2011c). Intensive efforts will have to focus on the issue of cytotoxicity to obtain more insight in the exact mechanisms behind, which are multidimensional and largely depend on the application route as well as the formulation that is delivered. Therefore, tissue specific toxicity profiles are still needed and represent a great implement in improving non-viral delivery systems.

8. General toxicity

Hornung et al. described that any rupture or leakage of the endosomal or lysosomal membrane will release cathepsin B, which leads to an inflammasome activation associated with IL-1 production and apoptosis (Hornung *et al.*, 2008). Beyerle et al. found that application PEI/siRNA complexes caused release of proinflammatory cytokines like IL-6, G-CSF, TNF-a, IP-10 in murine lung cell lines (Beyerle *et al.*, 2010a; Beyerle *et al.*, 2010b; Beyerle *et al.*, 2011a and Beyerle *et al.*, 2011c). Cytokine release upon PEI/nucleic acid polyplex treatment has been also described by Gautam and Kawakami et al. (Gautam *et al.*, 2001; Kawakami *et al.*, 2006). Cubillos-Ruis and co-workers investigated linear PEI/siRNA complexes for antitumor immunity and identified linear PEI as TLR 5 agonist of mouse and human. They found that linear PEI/siRNA complexes induced a pattern of inflammatory cytokines which are triggered in vivo by flagellin in a TLR5 dependent manner (Cubillos-

Ruiz *et al.*, 2009). Thus, for in vivo use a lot of effort should be made to avoid the high proinflammatory effects caused by the rupture or leakage of the endosome caused by PEI. Godbey classified PEI-mediated toxicity in an immediate toxicity, associated with free PEI and a delayed form, connected with cellular processing of PEI/DNA polyplexes (Godbey *et al.*, 2001). To form stable and protective PEI nucleic acid polyplexes an excess of PEI polymer is needed, 60-80% PEI remains in a free form after nucleic acid escape and is mainly attributed to PEI toxicity. The high positively charged PEI molecule is able to disrupt cell membranes, disruption of the endosome is on one hand favourable with respect to the intended cytoplasmatic delivery, but on the other hand disruption of other cell membranes (e.g., lysosomal membranes, mitochondrial membrane, plasma membrane) is not favourable as it will cause stress responses or even apoptotic or necrotic cell death. In this context it has been shown that PEI causes apoptosis in an unspecific manner in all kinds of cells (Beyerle *et al.*, 2010a; Merkel *et al.*, 2011) which should be avoided with regard to human use. Therefore, a purification approach of the PEI polymer before and after complexation with nucleic acid is one possibility to reduce PEI-related toxicity (Boeckle *et al.*, 2004; Werth, 2006; Fahrmeir *et al.*, 2007).

9. Lung toxicity

Espescially, when regarding the lung as target organ the activation of the inflammosome should be avoided. Lung targeting could in general be achieved by systemic delivery or pulmonary delivery. Pulmonary delivery enhances siRNA retention in the lungs, lowers the dose of siRNA required for efficient delivery, and therefore implicates reduced systemic toxic effects, and due to lower nuclease activity in the lung siRNA stability is increased. RNAi can be used to treat or prevent diseases affecting the lungs, such as lung cancer (Li and Huang, 2006; Tong, 2006; Jere *et al.*, 2008; Ren *et al.*, 2009; Zamora-Avila *et al.*, 2009), various types of respiratory infectious diseases (Ge *et al.*, 2004; Fulton *et al.*, 2009; DeVincenzo *et al.*, 2010), airway inflammatory diseases (Lee and Chiang, 2008; Seguin and Ferrari, 2009), and cystic fibrosis (Pison *et al.*, 2006).

Beyerle and co-workers investigated the effects of PEGylation on cytotoxicity and cell-compatibility of different PEG-PEI copolymers in murine lung cell lines and found a clear structure-function relationship (Fig. 1).

The higher the degree of PEGylation on PEI25kDa with low molecular weight PEG, the stronger was the reduction of cytotoxicity and oxidative stress, but the proinflammatory potential of PEI remained high (Beyerle *et al.*, 2010b). The same group evaluated the pulmonary toxicity of PEI/siRNA complexes and found at day three after intratracheal delivery still high numbers of neutrophils and high levels of proinflammatory cytokines in the airspace of polyplex treated mice (Beyerle *et al.*, 2011a and Beyerle *et al.*, 2011c). The higher inflammatory potential but lower toxicity of PEI modifications is still an issue to be overcome when targeting pulmonary diseases. There is an urgent need to balance the efficacy and toxicity of such nucleic acid carriers.

10. Toxicogenomics of PEI-based non-viral vector systems

Toxicogenomic and genotoxic information of non-viral vector systems is rare, but of great concern when nowadays focusing personalized medicine. Gene delivery systems should be

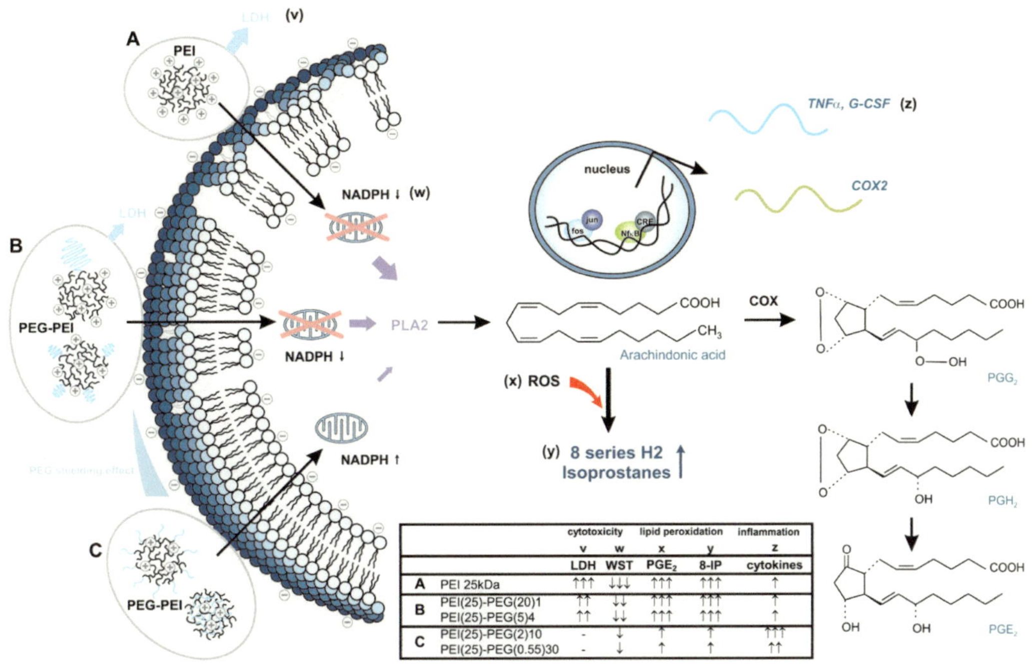

		cytotoxicity		lipid peroxidation		inflammation
		v	w	x	y	z
		LDH	WST	PGE_2	8-IP	cytokines
A	PEI 25kDa	↑↑↑	↓↓↓	↑↑↑	↑↑↑	↑
B	PEI(25)-PEG(20)1	↑↑	↓↓	↑↑↑	↑↑↑	↑
	PEI(25)-PEG(5)4	↑↑	↓↓	↑↑↑	↑↑↑	↑
C	PEI(25)-PEG(2)10	-	↓	↑	↑	↑↑↑
	PEI(25)-PEG(0.55)30	-	↓	↑	↑	↑↑

Fig. 1. Structure-function-relationships of PEG-PEI copolymers
Overview of the structure-function relationships of PEG modified PEI copolymers (B-C) in comparisonto PEI 25kDa (A) with regard to cytotoxic (v,w), oxidative stress (x,y) and proinflammatory responses (z). Arrows represent the up- or downregulation of the investigated molecules.

able to pass through biological membranes/barriers and transfer the desired information to target sites with minimal impact on the integrity of the target cell or tissue (Forrest and Pack, 2002; Omidi *et al.*, 2008). Viral vectors possess high efficacy accompanied by stimulation of the immune systems which is a limitation of these systems to deliver nucleic acids and human use. Therefore, non-viral vector systems should overcome these adverse side effects and represent safer and more efficient alternatives with improved bioavailability and reduced cellular toxicity in the clinics (Akhtar *et al.*, 2000; Somia and Verma, 2000; Panyam and Labhasetwar, 2003). It has been shown that cationic polymers and lipid-based transfection reagents could elicit cellular gene expression changes and complexation with siRNA increased these changes (Omidi *et al.*, 2003; Omidi *et al.*, 2005; Fedorov *et al.*, 2006; Hollins *et al.*, 2007; Tagami *et al.*, 2007; Tagami *et al.*, 2008). Beyerle et al. analyzed the expression changes of genes related to cytotoxicity, inflammation and oxidative stress in a pathway focused qRT-PCR array system upon treatment with different PEI-PEG copolymers in murine lung epithelial cells (LA-4 cell line) and could show that PEGylated PEI copolymers altered the gene expression profile on cost of upregulation of genes involved in inflammatory and oxidative stress processes while PEI 25 kDa mainly induced genes related to cytotoxicity and apoptosis (Beyerle *et al.*, 2010a). In addition, the potential of PEI and PEI-PEG copolymers to induce DNA damage and therefore their genotoxic potential was investigated in a lung epithelial cell line derived from the MutaMouse, but no indication for genotoxicity of PEI 25 kDa and PEI-PEG copolymers was observed (Beyerle *et al.*, 2011b). These investigations showed that PEI uptake causes cellular oxidative stress which affects the cytoplasmatic compartment with subsequent gene expression responses, but PEI not necessarily penetrate the nuclear membrane and cause DNA damage.

11. Conclusion

In conclusion, for development of safe and efficient non-viral vector systems a lot of investigations are needed before enter clinical trials. In our book chapter we mainly focused on PEI-related polymers for siRNA delivery to the lungs and gave an overview of the ongoing research in this field with a great focus on toxicity. To improve the toxicity profile of such carriers for pulmonary application one of the biggest challenge is to overcome the inflammatory response besides reduction of the overall cytotoxicity. Future studies should implement basic toxicity testing like evaluation of cytotoxicity (cell viability, LDH release, erythrocytes aggregation, apoptosis), inflammation (cytokine release, gene regulation, in vivo analysis of relevant tissues and cells or liquids), oxidative stress (lipid mediators, GSH levels) before extensively improving the efficacy of such carriers.

12. References

Akhtar, S. (2006). Non-viral cancer gene therapy: beyond delivery. *Gene Ther* 13, 739-740.

Akhtar, S., Hughes, M. D., Khan, A., Bibby, M., Hussain, M., Nawaz, Q., Double, J., and Sayyed, P. (2000). The delivery of antisense therapeutics. *Adv Drug Deliv Rev* 44, 3-21.

Akinc, A., Thomas, M., Klibanov, A. M., and Langer, R. (2005). Exploring polyethylenimine-mediated DNA transfection and the proton sponge hypothesis. *J Gene Med* 7, 657-663.

Alton, E. W., Stern, M., Farley, R., Jaffe, A., Chadwick, S. L., Phillips, J., Davies, J., Smith, S. N., Browning, J., Davies, M. G., Hodson, M. E., Durham, S. R., Li, D., Jeffery, P. K., Scallan, M., Balfour, R., Eastman, S. J., Cheng, S. H., Smith, A. E., Meeker, D., and Geddes, D. M. (1999). Cationic lipid-mediated CFTR gene transfer to the lungs and nose of patients with cystic fibrosis: a double-blind placebo-controlled trial. *Lancet* 353, 947-954.

Behlke, M. A. (2008). Chemical modification of siRNAs for in vivo use. *Oligonucleotides* 18, 305-319.

Behr, J. (1997). The proton sponge: A trick to enter cells the viruses did not exploit. *Chimica* 51, 34-36.

Beyerle, A., Braun, A., Banerjee, A., Ercal, N., Eickelberg, O., Kissel, T., and Stoeger, T. (Biomaterials 2011c, in press). Inflammtory response to pulmonary application of PEI-based siRNA nanocarriers in mice.

Beyerle, A., Braun, A., Merkel, O., Koch, F., Kissel, T., and Stoeger, T. (2011a). Comparative in vivo study of poly(ethylene imine)/siRNA complexes for pulmonary delivery in mice. *J Control Release*. 151(1):51-6.

Beyerle, A., Irmler, M., Beckers, J., Kissel, T., and Stoeger, T. (2010a). Toxicity pathway focused gene expression profiling of PEI-based polymers for pulmonary applications. *Mol Pharm* 7, 727-737.

Beyerle, A., Long, A. S., White, P., Kissel, T. H., and Stoeger, T. (2011b). Poly(ethylene imine) nanocarriers do not induce mutations nor oxidative DNA damage in vitro in MutaMouse FE1 cells. *Mol Pharm*. 8(3):976-81

Beyerle, A., Merkel, O., Stoeger, T., and Kissel, T. (2010b). PEGylation affects cytotoxicity and cell-compatibility of poly(ethylene imine) for lung application: structure-function relationships. *Toxicol Appl Pharmacol* 242, 146-154.

Boeckle, S., von Gersdorff, K., van der Piepen, S., Culmsee, C., Wagner, E., and Ogris, M. (2004). Purification of polyethylenimine polyplexes highlights the role of free polycations in gene transfer. *J Gene Med* 6, 1102-1111.

Boussif, O., Lezoualc'h, F., Zanta, M. A., Mergny, M. D., Scherman, D., Demeneix, B., and Behr, J. P. (1995). A versatile vector for gene and oligonucleotide transfer into cells in culture and in vivo: polyethylenimine. *Proc Natl Acad Sci U S A* 92, 7297-7301.

Braasch, D. A., Jensen, S., Liu, Y., Kaur, K., Arar, K., White, M. A., and Corey, D. R. (2003). RNA interference in mammalian cells by chemically-modified RNA. *Biochemistry* 42, 7967-7975.

Breunig, M., Hozsa, C., Lungwitz, U., Watanabe, K., Umeda, I., Kato, H., and Goepferich, A. (2008). Mechanistic investigation of poly(ethylene imine)-based siRNA delivery: disulfide bonds boost intracellular release of the cargo. *J Control Release* 130, 57-63.

Breunig, M., Lungwitz, U., Liebl, R., Fontanari, C., Klar, J., Kurtz, A., Blunk, T., and Goepferich, A. (2005). Gene delivery with low molecular weight linear polyethylenimines. *J Gene Med* 7, 1287-1298.

Brus, C., Petersen, H., Aigner, A., Czubayko, F., and Kissel, T. (2004). Physicochemical and biological characterization of polyethylenimine-graft-poly(ethylene glycol) block copolymers as a delivery system for oligonucleotides and ribozymes. *Bioconjug Chem* 15, 677-684.

Caplen, N. J., Parrish, S., Imani, F., Fire, A., and Morgan, R. A. (2001). Specific inhibition of gene expression by small double-stranded RNAs in invertebrate and vertebrate systems. *Proc Natl Acad Sci U S A* 98, 9742-9747.

Chien, P. Y., Wang, J., Carbonaro, D., Lei, S., Miller, B., Sheikh, S., Ali, S. M., Ahmad, M. U., and Ahmad, I. (2005). Novel cationic cardiolipin analogue-based liposome for efficient DNA and small interfering RNA delivery in vitro and in vivo. *Cancer Gene Ther* 12, 321-328.

Choung, S., Kim, Y. J., Kim, S., Park, H. O., and Choi, Y. C. (2006). Chemical modification of siRNAs to improve serum stability without loss of efficacy. *Biochem Biophys Res Commun* 342, 919-927.

Cubillos-Ruiz, J. R., Engle, X., Scarlett, U. K., Martinez, D., Barber, A., Elgueta, R., Wang, L., Nesbeth, Y., Durant, Y., Gewirtz, A. T., Sentman, C. L., Kedl, R., and Conejo-Garcia, J. R. (2009). Polyethylenimine-based siRNA nanocomplexes reprogram tumor-associated dendritic cells via TLR5 to elicit therapeutic antitumor immunity. *J Clin Invest* 119, 2231-2244.

Dalby, B., Cates, S., Harris, A., Ohki, E. C., Tilkins, M. L., Price, P. J., and Ciccarone, V. C. (2004). Advanced transfection with Lipofectamine 2000 reagent: primary neurons, siRNA, and high-throughput applications. *Methods* 33, 95-103.

Davis, M. E. (2009). The first targeted delivery of siRNA in humans via a self-assembling, cyclodextrin polymer-based nanoparticle: from concept to clinic. *Mol Pharm* 6, 659-668.

Davis, M. E., Zuckerman, J. E., Choi, C. H., Seligson, D., Tolcher, A., Alabi, C. A., Yen, Y., Heidel, J. D., and Ribas, A. (2010). Evidence of RNAi in humans from systemically administered siRNA via targeted nanoparticles. *Nature* 464, 1067-1070.

de Fougerolles, A., Vornlocher, H. P., Maraganore, J., and Lieberman, J. (2007). Interfering with disease: a progress report on siRNA-based therapeutics. *Nat Rev Drug Discov* 6, 443-453.

Demeneix, B., and Behr, J. P. (2005). Polyethylenimine (PEI). *Adv Genet* 53, 217-230.

DeVincenzo, J., Lambkin-Williams, R., Wilkinson, T., Cehelsky, J., Nochur, S., Walsh, E., Meyers, R., Gollob, J., and Vaishnaw, A. (2010). A randomized, double-blind, placebo-controlled study of an RNAi-based therapy directed against respiratory syncytial virus. *Proc Natl Acad Sci U S A* 107, 8800-8805.

Dubey, P. K., Mishra, V., Jain, S., Mahor, S., and Vyas, S. P. (2004). Liposomes modified with cyclic RGD peptide for tumor targeting. *J Drug Target* 12, 257-264.

Elbashir, S. M., Harborth, J., Lendeckel, W., Yalcin, A., Weber, K., and Tuschl, T. (2001). Duplexes of 21-nucleotide RNAs mediate RNA interference in cultured mammalian cells. *Nature* 411, 494-498.

Fahrmeir, J., Gunther, M., Tietze, N., Wagner, E., and Ogris, M. (2007). Electrophoretic purification of tumor-targeted polyethylenimine-based polyplexes reduces toxic side effects in vivo. *J Control Release* 122, 236-245.

Fedorov, Y., Anderson, E. M., Birmingham, A., Reynolds, A., Karpilow, J., Robinson, K., Leake, D., Marshall, W. S., and Khvorova, A. (2006). Off-target effects by siRNA can induce toxic phenotype. *Rna* 12, 1188-1196.

Fire, A., Xu, S., Montgomery, M. K., Kostas, S. A., Driver, S. E., and Mello, C. C. (1998). Potent and specific genetic interference by double-stranded RNA in Caenorhabditis elegans. *Nature* 391, 806-811.

Fischer, D., von Harpe, A., Kunath, K., Petersen, H., Li, Y., and Kissel, T. (2002). Copolymers of ethylene imine and N-(2-hydroxyethyl)-ethylene imine as tools to study effects of polymer structure on physicochemical and biological properties of DNA complexes. *Bioconjug Chem* 13, 1124-1133.

Flynn, M. A., Casey, D. G., Todryk, S. M., and Mahon, B. P. (2004). Efficient delivery of small interfering RNA for inhibition of IL-12p40 expression in vivo. *J Inflamm (Lond)* 1, 4.

Forrest, M. L., and Pack, D. W. (2002). On the kinetics of polyplex endocytic trafficking: implications for gene delivery vector design. *Mol Ther* 6, 57-66.

Fulton, A., Peters, S. T., Perkins, G. A., Jarosinski, K. W., Damiani, A., Brosnahan, M., Buckles, E. L., Osterrieder, N., and Van de Walle, G. R. (2009). Effective treatment of respiratory alphaherpesvirus infection using RNA interference. *PLoS One* 4, e4118.

Gary, D. J., Puri, N., and Won, Y. Y. (2007). Polymer-based siRNA delivery: perspectives on the fundamental and phenomenological distinctions from polymer-based DNA delivery. *J Control Release* 121, 64-73.

Gautam, A., Densmore, C. L., and Waldrep, J. C. (2001). Pulmonary cytokine responses associated with PEI-DNA aerosol gene therapy. *Gene Ther* 8, 254-257.

Ge, Q., Filip, L., Bai, A., Nguyen, T., Eisen, H. N., and Chen, J. (2004). Inhibition of influenza virus production in virus-infected mice by RNA interference. *Proc Natl Acad Sci U S A* 101, 8676-8681.

Glodde, M., Sirsi, S. R., and Lutz, G. J. (2006). Physiochemical properties of low and high molecular weight poly(ethylene glycol)-grafted poly(ethylene imine) copolymers and their complexes with oligonucleotides. *Biomacromolecules* 7, 347-356.

Godbey, W. T., Barry, M. A., Saggau, P., Wu, K. K., and Mikos, A. G. (2000). Poly(ethylenimine)-mediated transfection: a new paradigm for gene delivery. *J Biomed Mater Res* 51, 321-328.

Godbey, W. T., Wu, K. K., and Mikos, A. G. (1999). Poly(ethylenimine) and its role in gene delivery. *J Control Release* 60, 149-160.

Godbey, W. T., Wu, K. K., and Mikos, A. G. (2001). Poly(ethylenimine)-mediated gene delivery affects endothelial cell function and viability. *Biomaterials* 22, 471-480.

Grayson, A. C., Doody, A. M., and Putnam, D. (2006). Biophysical and structural characterization of polyethylenimine-mediated siRNA delivery in vitro. *Pharm Res* 23, 1868-1876.

Griesenbach, U., and Alton, E. W. (2009). Gene transfer to the lung: lessons learned from more than 2 decades of CF gene therapy. *Adv Drug Deliv Rev* 61, 128-139.

Griesenbach, U., Kitson, C., Escudero Garcia, S., Farley, R., Singh, C., Somerton, L., Painter, H., Smith, R. L., Gill, D. R., Hyde, S. C., Chow, Y. H., Hu, J., Gray, M., Edbrooke, M., Ogilvie, V., MacGregor, G., Scheule, R. K., Cheng, S. H., Caplen, N. J., and Alton, E. W. (2006). Inefficient cationic lipid-mediated siRNA and antisense oligonucleotide transfer to airway epithelial cells in vivo. *Respir Res* 7, 26.

Grimm, D., Streetz, K. L., Jopling, C. L., Storm, T. A., Pandey, K., Davis, C. R., Marion, P., Salazar, F., and Kay, M. A. (2006). Fatality in mice due to oversaturation of cellular microRNA/short hairpin RNA pathways. *Nature* 441, 537-541.

Hannon, G. J., and Rossi, J. J. (2004). Unlocking the potential of the human genome with RNA interference. *Nature* 431, 371-378.

Hassani, Z., Lemkine, G. F., Erbacher, P., Palmier, K., Alfama, G., Giovannangeli, C., Behr, J. P., and Demeneix, B. A. (2005). Lipid-mediated siRNA delivery down-regulates exogenous gene expression in the mouse brain at picomolar levels. *J Gene Med* 7, 198-207.

Heidel, J. D., Yu, Z., Liu, J. Y., Rele, S. M., Liang, Y., Zeidan, R. K., Kornbrust, D. J., and Davis, M. E. (2007). Administration in non-human primates of escalating intravenous doses of targeted nanoparticles containing ribonucleotide reductase subunit M2 siRNA. *Proc Natl Acad Sci U S A* 104, 5715-5721.

Hollins, A. J., Omidi, Y., Benter, I. F., and Akhtar, S. (2007). Toxicogenomics of drug delivery systems: Exploiting delivery system-induced changes in target gene expression to enhance siRNA activity. *J Drug Target* 15, 83-88.

Hong, S., Leroueil, P. R., Janus, E. K., Peters, J. L., Kober, M. M., Islam, M. T., Orr, B. G., Baker, J. R., Jr., and Banaszak Holl, M. M. (2006). Interaction of polycationic polymers with supported lipid bilayers and cells: nanoscale hole formation and enhanced membrane permeability. *Bioconjug Chem* 17, 728-734.

Hornung, V., Bauernfeind, F., Halle, A., Samstad, E. O., Kono, H., Rock, K. L., Fitzgerald, K. A., and Latz, E. (2008). Silica crystals and aluminum salts activate the NALP3 inflammasome through phagosomal destabilization. *Nat Immunol* 9, 847-856.

Hornung, V., Guenthner-Biller, M., Bourquin, C., Ablasser, A., Schlee, M., Uematsu, S., Noronha, A., Manoharan, M., Akira, S., de Fougerolles, A., Endres, S., and Hartmann, G. (2005). Sequence-specific potent induction of IFN-alpha by short interfering RNA in plasmacytoid dendritic cells through TLR7. *Nat Med* 11, 263-270.

Jackson, A. L., Bartz, S. R., Schelter, J., Kobayashi, S. V., Burchard, J., Mao, M., Li, B., Cavet, G., and Linsley, P. S. (2003). Expression profiling reveals off-target gene regulation by RNAi. *Nat Biotechnol* 21, 635-637.

Jere, D., Xu, C. X., Arote, R., Yun, C. H., Cho, M. H., and Cho, C. S. (2008). Poly(beta-amino ester) as a carrier for si/shRNA delivery in lung cancer cells. *Biomaterials* 29, 2535-2547.

Judge, A. D., Bola, G., Lee, A. C., and MacLachlan, I. (2006). Design of noninflammatory synthetic siRNA mediating potent gene silencing in vivo. *Mol Ther* 13, 494-505.

Judge, A. D., Sood, V., Shaw, J. R., Fang, D., McClintock, K., and MacLachlan, I. (2005). Sequence-dependent stimulation of the mammalian innate immune response by synthetic siRNA. *Nat Biotechnol* 23, 457-462.

Kabanov, A. V. (2006). Polymer genomics: an insight into pharmacology and toxicology of nanomedicines. *Adv Drug Deliv Rev* 58, 1597-1621.

Kawakami, S., Ito, Y., Charoensit, P., Yamashita, F., and Hashida, M. (2006). Evaluation of proinflammatory cytokine production induced by linear and branched polyethylenimine/plasmid DNA complexes in mice. *J Pharmacol Exp Ther* 317, 1382-1390.

Kichler, A., Chillon, M., Leborgne, C., Danos, O., and Frisch, B. (2002). Intranasal gene delivery with a polyethylenimine-PEG conjugate. *J Control Release* 81, 379-388.

Kim, W. J., and Kim, S. W. (2009). Efficient siRNA delivery with non-viral polymeric vehicles. *Pharm Res* 26, 657-666.

Kleemann, E., Neu, M., Jekel, N., Fink, L., Schmehl, T., Gessler, T., Seeger, W., and Kissel, T. (2005). Nano-carriers for DNA delivery to the lung based upon a TAT-derived peptide covalently coupled to PEG-PEI. *J Control Release* 109, 299-316.

Kunath, K., Merdan, T., Hegener, O., Haberlein, H., and Kissel, T. (2003a). Integrin targeting using RGD-PEI conjugates for in vitro gene transfer. *J Gene Med* 5, 588-599.

Kunath, K., von Harpe, A., Fischer, D., and Kissel, T. (2003b). Galactose-PEI-DNA complexes for targeted gene delivery: degree of substitution affects complex size and transfection efficiency. *J Control Release* 88, 159-172.

Layzer, J. M., McCaffrey, A. P., Tanner, A. K., Huang, Z., Kay, M. A., and Sullenger, B. A. (2004). In vivo activity of nuclease-resistant siRNAs. *Rna* 10, 766-771.

Lee, C. C., and Chiang, B. L. (2008). RNA interference: new therapeutics in allergic diseases. *Curr Gene Ther* 8, 236-246.

Leroueil, P. R., Berry, S. A., Duthie, K., Han, G., Rotello, V. M., McNerny, D. Q., Baker, J. R., Jr., Orr, B. G., and Holl, M. M. (2008). Wide varieties of cationic nanoparticles induce defects in supported lipid bilayers. *Nano Lett* 8, 420-424.

Li, S. D., and Huang, L. (2006). Targeted delivery of antisense oligodeoxynucleotide and small interference RNA into lung cancer cells. *Mol Pharm* 3, 579-588.

Luo, M. C., Zhang, D. Q., Ma, S. W., Huang, Y. Y., Shuster, S. J., Porreca, F., and Lai, J. (2005). An efficient intrathecal delivery of small interfering RNA to the spinal cord and peripheral neurons. *Mol Pain* 1, 29.

Maeda, Y., Fukushima, K., Nishizaki, K., and Smith, R. J. (2005). In vitro and in vivo suppression of GJB2 expression by RNA interference. *Hum Mol Genet* 14, 1641-1650.

Mao, S., Shuai, X., Unger, F., Wittmar, M., Xie, X., and Kissel, T. (2005). Synthesis, characterization and cytotoxicity of poly(ethylene glycol)-graft-trimethyl chitosan block copolymers. *Biomaterials* 26, 6343-6356.

Meister, G., Landthaler, M., Patkaniowska, A., Dorsett, Y., Teng, G., and Tuschl, T. (2004). Human Argonaute2 mediates RNA cleavage targeted by miRNAs and siRNAs. *Mol Cell* 15, 185-197.

Mello, C. C., and Conte, D., Jr. (2004). Revealing the world of RNA interference. *Nature* 431, 338-342.

Merkel, O. M., Beyerle, A., Beckmann, B. M., Zheng, M., Hartmann, R. K., Stoger, T., and Kissel, T. H. (2011). Polymer-related off-target effects in non-viral siRNA delivery. *Biomaterials* 32, 2388-2398.

Merkel, O. M., Beyerle, A., Librizzi, D., Pfestroff, A., Behr, T. M., Sproat, B., Barth, P. J., and Kissel, T. (2009). Nonviral siRNA delivery to the lung: investigation of PEG-PEI polyplexes and their in vivo performance. *Mol Pharm* 6, 1246-1260.

Meyerhoff, A. (1999). U.S. Food and Drug Administration approval of AmBisome (liposomal amphotericin B) for treatment of visceral leishmaniasis. *Clin Infect Dis* 28, 42-48; discussion 49-51.

Miyawaki-Shimizu, K., Predescu, D., Shimizu, J., Broman, M., Predescu, S., and Malik, A. B. (2006). siRNA-induced caveolin-1 knockdown in mice increases lung vascular permeability via the junctional pathway. *Am J Physiol Lung Cell Mol Physiol* 290, L405-413.

Moghimi, S. M., and Szebeni, J. (2003). Stealth liposomes and long circulating nanoparticles: critical issues in pharmacokinetics, opsonization and protein-binding properties. *Prog Lipid Res* 42, 463-478.

Morrissey, D. V., Lockridge, J. A., Shaw, L., Blanchard, K., Jensen, K., Breen, W., Hartsough, K., Machemer, L., Radka, S., Jadhav, V., Vaish, N., Zinnen, S., Vargeese, C., Bowman, K., Shaffer, C. S., Jeffs, L. B., Judge, A., MacLachlan, I., and Polisky, B. (2005). Potent and persistent in vivo anti-HBV activity of chemically modified siRNAs. *Nat Biotechnol* 23, 1002-1007.

Nel, A. E., Madler, L., Velegol, D., Xia, T., Hoek, E. M., Somasundaran, P., Klaessig, F., Castranova, V., and Thompson, M. (2009). Understanding biophysicochemical interactions at the nano-bio interface. *Nat Mater* 8, 543-557.

Neu, M., Fischer, D., and Kissel, T. (2005). Recent advances in rational gene transfer vector design based on poly(ethylene imine) and its derivatives. *J Gene Med* 7, 992-1009.

Novina, C. D., and Sharp, P. A. (2004). The RNAi revolution. *Nature* 430, 161-164.

Ogris, M., Brunner, S., Schuller, S., Kircheis, R., and Wagner, E. (1999). PEGylated DNA/transferrin-PEI complexes: reduced interaction with blood components, extended circulation in blood and potential for systemic gene delivery. *Gene Ther* 6, 595-605.

Omidi, Y., Barar, J., and Akhtar, S. (2005). Toxicogenomics of cationic lipid-based vectors for gene therapy: impact of microarray technology. *Curr Drug Deliv* 2, 429-441.

Omidi, Y., Barar, J., Heidari, H. R., Ahmadian, S., Yazdi, H. A., and Akhtar, S. (2008). Microarray analysis of the toxicogenomics and the genotoxic potential of a cationic lipid-based gene delivery nanosystem in human alveolar epithelial a549 cells. *Toxicol Mech Methods* 18, 369-378.

Omidi, Y., Hollins, A. J., Benboubetra, M., Drayton, R., Benter, I. F., and Akhtar, S. (2003). Toxicogenomics of non-viral vectors for gene therapy: a microarray study of lipofectin- and oligofectamine-induced gene expression changes in human epithelial cells. *J Drug Target* 11, 311-323.

Oupicky, D., Ogris, M., Howard, K. A., Dash, P. R., Ulbrich, K., and Seymour, L. W. (2002). Importance of lateral and steric stabilization of polyelectrolyte gene delivery vectors for extended systemic circulation. *Mol Ther* 5, 463-472.

Pal, A., Ahmad, A., Khan, S., Sakabe, I., Zhang, C., Kasid, U. N., and Ahmad, I. (2005). Systemic delivery of RafsiRNA using cationic cardiolipin liposomes silences Raf-1 expression and inhibits tumor growth in xenograft model of human prostate cancer. *Int J Oncol* 26, 1087-1091.

Palliser, D., Chowdhury, D., Wang, Q. Y., Lee, S. J., Bronson, R. T., Knipe, D. M., and Lieberman, J. (2006). An siRNA-based microbicide protects mice from lethal herpes simplex virus 2 infection. *Nature* 439, 89-94.

Panyam, J., and Labhasetwar, V. (2003). Biodegradable nanoparticles for drug and gene delivery to cells and tissue. *Adv Drug Deliv Rev* 55, 329-347.

Petersen, H., Fechner, P. M., Fischer, D., and Kissel*, T. (2002a). Synthesis, Characterization, and Biocompatibility of
Polyethylenimine-graft-poly(ethylene glycol) Block Copolymers. *Macromolecules* 35, 6867-6874.

Petersen, H., Fechner, P. M., Martin, A. L., Kunath, K., Stolnik, S., Roberts, C. J., Fischer, D., Davies, M. C., and Kissel, T. (2002b). Polyethylenimine-graft-poly(ethylene glycol) copolymers: influence of copolymer block structure on DNA complexation and biological activities as gene delivery system. *Bioconjug Chem* 13, 845-854.

Pison, U., Welte, T., Giersig, M., and Groneberg, D. A. (2006). Nanomedicine for respiratory diseases. *Eur J Pharmacol* 533, 341-350.

Ren, X. L., Xu, Y. M., Bao, W., Fu, H. J., Wu, C. G., Zhao, Y., Li, Z. K., Zhang, J., Li, S. Q., Chen, W. Q., Wang, T., Zhang, R., Zhang, L. H., Qian, G. S., Chen, S. Y., Jia, L. T., and Yang, A. G. (2009). Inhibition of non-small cell lung cancer cell proliferation and tumor growth by vector-based small interfering RNAs targeting HER2/neu. *Cancer Lett* 281, 134-143.

Robbins, M., Judge, A., Ambegia, E., Choi, C., Yaworski, E., Palmer, L., McClintock, K., and MacLachlan, I. (2008). Misinterpreting the therapeutic effects of small interfering RNA caused by immune stimulation. *Hum Gene Ther* 19, 991-999.

Robbins, M., Judge, A., and MacLachlan, I. (2009). siRNA and innate immunity. *Oligonucleotides* 19, 89-102.

Santel, A., Aleku, M., Keil, O., Endruschat, J., Esche, V., Fisch, G., Dames, S., Loffler, K., Fechtner, M., Arnold, W., Giese, K., Klippel, A., and Kaufmann, J. (2006). A novel siRNA-lipoplex technology for RNA interference in the mouse vascular endothelium. *Gene Ther* 13, 1222-1234.

Schatzlein, A. G. (2006). Delivering cancer stem cell therapies - a role for nanomedicines? *Eur J Cancer* 42, 1309-1315.

Schlee, M., Hornung, V., and Hartmann, G. (2006). siRNA and isRNA: two edges of one sword. *Mol Ther* 14, 463-470.

Seguin, R. M., and Ferrari, N. (2009). Emerging oligonucleotide therapies for asthma and chronic obstructive pulmonary disease. *Expert Opin Investig Drugs* 18, 1505-1517.

Sitterberg, J., Ozcetin, A., Ehrhardt, C., and Bakowsky, U. (2010). Utilising atomic force microscopy for the characterisation of nanoscale drug delivery systems. *Eur J Pharm Biopharm* 74, 2-13.

Somia, N., and Verma, I. M. (2000). Gene therapy: trials and tribulations. *Nat Rev Genet* 1, 91-99.

Soutschek, J., Akinc, A., Bramlage, B., Charisse, K., Constien, R., Donoghue, M., Elbashir, S., Geick, A., Hadwiger, P., Harborth, J., John, M., Kesavan, V., Lavine, G., Pandey, R. K., Racie, T., Rajeev, K. G., Rohl, I., Toudjarska, I., Wang, G., Wuschko, S., Bumcrot, D., Koteliansky, V., Limmer, S., Manoharan, M., and Vornlocher, H. P. (2004). Therapeutic silencing of an endogenous gene by systemic administration of modified siRNAs. *Nature* 432, 173-178.

Spagnou, S., Miller, A. D., and Keller, M. (2004). Lipidic carriers of siRNA: differences in the formulation, cellular uptake, and delivery with plasmid DNA. *Biochemistry* 43, 13348-13356.

Tagami, T., Barichello, J. M., Kikuchi, H., Ishida, T., and Kiwada, H. (2007). The gene-silencing effect of siRNA in cationic lipoplexes is enhanced by incorporating pDNA in the complex. *Int J Pharm* 333, 62-69.

Tagami, T., Hirose, K., Barichello, J. M., Ishida, T., and Kiwada, H. (2008). Global gene expression profiling in cultured cells is strongly influenced by treatment with siRNA-cationic liposome complexes. *Pharm Res* 25, 2497-2504.

Tan, Y., and Huang, L. (2002). Overcoming the inflammatory toxicity of cationic gene vectors. *J Drug Target* 10, 153-160.

Thomas, M., Lu, J. J., Ge, Q., Zhang, C., Chen, J., and Klibanov, A. M. (2005). Full deacylation of polyethylenimine dramatically boosts its gene delivery efficiency and specificity to mouse lung. *Proc Natl Acad Sci U S A* 102, 5679-5684.

Tong, A. W. (2006). Small RNAs and non-small cell lung cancer. *Curr Mol Med* 6, 339-349.

Tuschl, T., Zamore, P. D., Lehmann, R., Bartel, D. P., and Sharp, P. A. (1999). Targeted mRNA degradation by double-stranded RNA in vitro. *Genes Dev* 13, 3191-3197.

Urban-Klein, B., Werth, S., Abuharbeid, S., Czubayko, F., and Aigner, A. (2005). RNAi-mediated gene-targeting through systemic application of polyethylenimine (PEI)-complexed siRNA in vivo. *Gene Ther* 12, 461-466.

Verma, U. N., Surabhi, R. M., Schmaltieg, A., Becerra, C., and Gaynor, R. B. (2003). Small interfering RNAs directed against beta-catenin inhibit the in vitro and in vivo growth of colon cancer cells. *Clin Cancer Res* 9, 1291-1300.

Werth, S., Urban-Klein, B., Dai L., Höbel S., Grzelinski M., Bakowsky U., Czubayko F., Aigner A. (2006). A low molecular weight fraction of polyethylenimine (PEI) displays increased trasnfection efficiency of DNA and siRNA in fresh or lyophilized complexes. *J Control Rel* 112, 257-270.

Williams, J. H., Sirsi, S. R., Latta, D. R., and Lutz, G. J. (2006). Induction of dystrophin expression by exon skipping in mdx mice following intramuscular injection of antisense oligonucleotides complexed with PEG-PEI copolymers. *Mol Ther* 14, 88-96.

Zamora-Avila, D. E., Zapata-Benavides, P., Franco-Molina, M. A., Saavedra-Alonso, S., Trejo-Avila, L. M., Resendez-Perez, D., Mendez-Vazquez, J. L., Isaias-Badillo, J., and Rodriguez-Padilla, C. (2009). WT1 gene silencing by aerosol delivery of PEI-RNAi complexes inhibits B16-F10 lung metastases growth. *Cancer Gene Ther* 16, 892-899.

Zimmermann, T. S., Lee, A. C., Akinc, A., Bramlage, B., Bumcrot, D., Fedoruk, M. N., Harborth, J., Heyes, J. A., Jeffs, L. B., John, M., Judge, A. D., Lam, K., McClintock, K., Nechev, L. V., Palmer, L. R., Racie, T., Rohl, I., Seiffert, S., Shanmugam, S., Sood, V., Soutschek, J., Toudjarska, I., Wheat, A. J., Yaworski, E., Zedalis, W., Koteliansky, V., Manoharan, M., Vornlocher, H. P., and MacLachlan, I. (2006). RNAi-mediated gene silencing in non-human primates. *Nature* 441, 111-114.

Zintchenko, A., Philipp, A., Dehshahri, A., and Wagner, E. (2008). Simple modifications of branched PEI lead to highly efficient siRNA carriers with low toxicity. *Bioconjug Chem* 19, 1448-1455.

Zuhorn, I. S., Engberts, J. B., and Hoekstra, D. (2007). Gene delivery by cationic lipid vectors: overcoming cellular barriers. *Eur Biophys J* 36, 349-362.

21

PAMAM Dendrimer as Potential Delivery System for Combined Chemotherapeutic and MicroRNA-21 Gene Therapy

Xuan Zhou, Yu Ren, Xubo Yuan, Peiyu Pu and Chunsheng Kang
Department of Neurosurgery, Laboratory of Neuro-Oncology, Tianjin Medical University
Tianjin research center of basic medical science, Tianjin medical university
First Department of Head and Neck Cancer
Tianjin Medical University Cancer Institute & Hospital
School of Materials Science & Engineering, Tianjin University
China

1. Introduction

Chemotherapeutic drugs are fundamental in cancer management and are responsible for most cases of adjuvant treatment in patients after surgical procedures. However, the median overall survival does not increase in patients treated by concurrent chemo-radiotherapy. Consequently, further studies that could enhance the therapeutic effect should be encouraged [1].

Although the biological functions of microRNAs (miRNA) are not completely revealed, there is growing evidence that miRNA pathways are a new mechanism of gene regulation in both normal and diseased conditions [2]. Recent evidence has shown that miRNA mutations or aberrant expression patterns correlate with various diseases, such as cancer, viral infections, cardiovascular and indicates that miRNAs can function as tumor suppressors and oncogenes and oretically become a target to enhance the chemotherapeutic effect in cancer therapy.

However, although much work has been accomplished, the development of an efficient delivery system still remain a major challenge for the wide application of miRNA. In the following sections -- after a brief introduction of the miRNA strategies -- the potential and contributions of dendrimers in the development of effective non-viral delivery systems for combined the microRNA therapy with drug delivery will be discussed.

2. MicroRNA strategy

MicroRNAs (miRNAs) are a class of naturally occurring small non-coding RNAs, approximately 22 nucleotides in length, that target protein-coding mRNAs at the post-transcriptional level [4]. Generally, mature miRNAs are integrated into a protein–RNA complex called a microRNA RNPs (similar to the RISCs (RNA-induced silencing complexes) for siRNA). miRNAs bind through partial sequence homology to the 3_-untranslated regions (3'-UTRs) of target genes. Because of this unique feature, a single miRNA has multiple targets. It is thought that more than 30% of human genes are posttranscriptionally regulated by miRNAs [5]. miRNAs have diverse functions in biological processes, including the regulation of cellular proliferation, differentiation, and cell death. As dysregulation of these biological processes frequently occur in human cancer, miRNAs may, therefore, play a critical role in the process of tumorigenesis.

This regulatory mechanism was first shown in the developmental processes in worms, flies, and plants [6]. Subsequently, miRNAs have been shown to have important roles in many physiological processes of mammalian systems by influencing cell apoptosis, development, and metabolism through regulation of critical signaling molecules including cytokines, growth factors, transcription factors, and pro-apoptotic and anti-apoptotic proteins. Increasing number of miRNAs have been identified in the human genome and they are collectively called the miRNome [7]. Accumulating evidence shows the potential involvement of altered regulation of miRNAs in initiation and progression in a wide range of human cancers. Altered expression profiles of miRNAs are associated with genetic and epigenetic alterations including deletion, amplification, point mutation, and aberrant DNA methylation.

2.1 miR-21 general aspects

MiR-21 has been identified as the best hit in a number of miRNA profiling studies designed for the detection of miRNAs dysregulated in human cancer [8]. MiR-21 could suppress several tumor suppressor proteins translation, including PTEN, PDCD4, TMP1 and p53, to mediated cancer cell malignant phenotype alternation [9-10]. MiR-21 was emerging as key regulators of multiple pathways involved in tumorgenesis and may become the next targeted therapies in human cancers [11]. Previously we identified miR-21's aberrant expression in glioblastoma(GBM), and we focused on in what way miR-21 regulated GBM development and progression. Thus, in the current chapter, we manage to elucidate the view point that miR-21 was an effective molecule with great potential of human cancer gene therapy; of course, we will take miR-21's biological role to GBM as an example.

Recent reports suggested that miR-21 functions as an oncogene in human cancers. Ciafre` et alprofiled the expression of 245 miRNAs in 10 glioblastoma (GBM) cell lines and nine freshly resected GBM samples and observed that miR-21 was overexpressed in human brain tumors [12]. It was shown that when miR-21 was suppressed, cell growth inhibition and caspase-dependent apoptosis were observed in A172, U87, LN229, and LN308 cells. It has been shown that miR-21 modulates breast cancer cell anchorage-independent growth through suppressing TMP1 expression. In human colorectal, breast cancer, and renal cell carcinoma, miR-21 contributes to invasion and metastasis cell by inhibiting Pdcd4 mRNA at the post-transcription level. A recent study showed that miR-21 targets PTEN gene through a binding site on the 3'-UTR in hepatocellular carcinoma [13]. PTEN has been shown to be a critical tumor suppressor gene that is commonly inactivated in GBM by deletion, mutation, or attenuated expression. Thus, increased expression of miR-21 may contribute to the attenuated expression of PTEN in GBM.

2.2 miR-21 was up regulated in GBM cell lines and tissue samples

Microarray assay was used to screen the miRNA expression status in GBM cell lines. Data showed miR-21 exhibited a 7.0-fold increase relative to normal brain tissue [14]. In addition,

in-situ hybridization (ISH) of surgery resected glioma samples proved that miR-21 displayed varying degrees of intensity in glioma with different grades and the positive rate increased with the ascending order of the glioma WHO grade. In hence, it was important to note that miR-21 ISH was conducted at both the tissue level and the cellular level to indicate that miR-21 disregulation could be a marker to predict the outcome of glioma patients.
To identify miR-21 that was abnormal upregulated in high-grade gliomas, we used ISH to test miR-21 insitu expression in human non-neoplastic brain tissues, I~II grade gliomas, grade III gliomas (anaplastic gliomas, AAs) and GBMs.
Our group showed that miR-21 was over expressed in 57 of 60 glioma samples and miR-21 was detected in the cytoplasm of the neoplastic cells of all the positive cases. MiR-21 displayed varying degrees of intensity in glioma with different grades and the positive rate increased with the ascending order of the WHO grade. There were 27 of 30 (90%) in WHO I and II gliomas, 15 of 15 (100%) in AAs and GBMs, whereas miR-21 was rarely detected in control brain tissues. The first indication of miR-21's aberrant expression came from the miRNA profiling of human glioblastoma. Compared to normal brain tissue, miR-21 relative expression was seven to eleven folds in low-grade astrocytomas, AAs and GBMs. Besides providing the consistent data to the previous study, it is important to note that miR-21 ISH was conducted at both the tissue level and the cellular level to indicate that miR-21 disregulation could be a marker to predict the outcome of glioma patients.

2.3 miR-21 regulated GBM cell growth in vitro and in vivo

To evaluate the significance of miR-21 overexpression in glioma cells, we used a loss-of-function antisense approach. An As-miR-21 oligonucleotide (ODN) was used to knock down miR-21 expression in U251 and LN229 cells. RT-realtime PCR results determined that the relative expression level of miR-21 in As-miR-21 ODN-treated U251 cell was 6.25% ($P<0.01$) and 12.5% for LN229 cells ($P<0.01$) compared with their control cells, respectively. In addition, LNA-based in situ hybridization showed that transfection of a scrambled ODN had no effect on miR-21 expression. In contrast, the cy3 red fluorescence signal in As-miR-21-transfected U251 cells was lower (Figure 1B). These data suggested that As-miR-21 can specifically inhibit the endogenous miR-21 expression in U251 and LN229 cells.
The GBM cell growth inihibitory effect (MTT assay) of decreased miR-21 reached maximum three days post transfection. G1 phase blockage was observed to indicate cell cycle distribution changed significantly after miR-21 inhibitory. Additionally, the Annexin V positive early phase apoptotic cells were significantly increased in cells transfected with AS-miR-21 as compared to that in parental cells and cells treated with scrambled ODN.
The in vitro experiments suggest that miR-21 is a potential target for therapy in GBM. To further confirm this, we performed a proof-of-principle experiment using a U251 glioma xenograft model and a lipofectamine-mediated gene therapy approach. The xenograft tumors volume suppression indicated that miR-21 contributed a lot to U251 GBM cell proliferation in vivo. Pathological examination found micro-vessel density indicated that was and evaluated miR-21 expression by in situ hybridization and cellular apoptosis by TUNEL assay.
Despite the apparently predominance of microRNA in cancer therapy, several problems have to be overcome for successful clinical application. They show a poor stability towards nuclease activity, low intracellular penetration and low bioavailability. Although chemical modifications were brought to the basic microRNA, their sensitivity to degradation and poor intracellular penetration is still hampering their widespread clinical applications. In fact, the major bottleneck in the development of miRNA strategy is the delivery of these

macromolecules to the target cells, tissues or organs. Therefore the development of more efficient delivery systems is regarded as one of the most promising strategies to solve these pharmaceutical hurdles. Specifically, delivery vectors must be designed to effectively complex with nucleic acid molecules and aid in overcoming intracellular barriers such as endosomal escape and cytoplasmic vector dissociation. For that reason, improvements on effective delivery have progressed rapidly. Among the different approaches under study, dendrimers are attracting a great interest for their well defined structure and great versatility in their chemistry that offer a unique platform for the rational design of efficient antisense delivery systems.

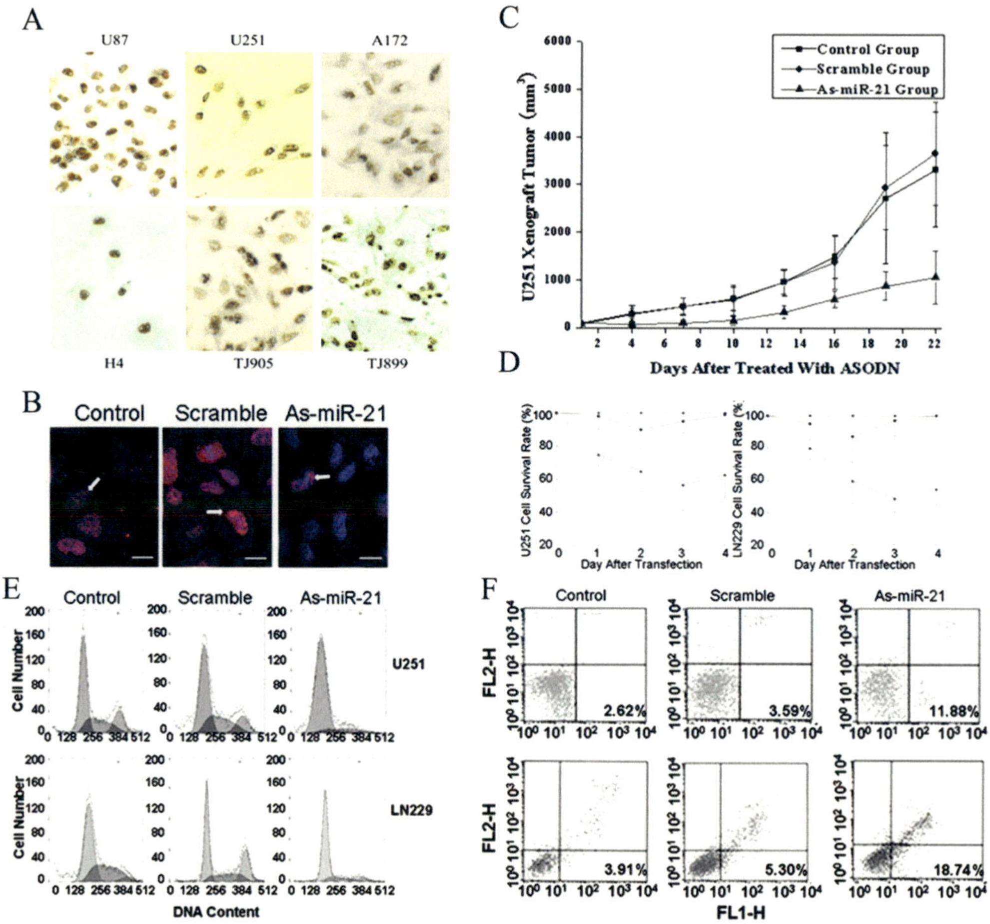

Fig. 1. The effect of miR-21 knockdown on U251 and LN229 GBM cell proliferation. (A) miR-21 was overexpressed in six glioma cells. (B) In situ examination of miR-21 expression in U251 cells. Arrows highlight miR-21 in situ expression in U251 cells. Bar¼20 mm. (C、 D) MTT cell proliferation assay. miR-21 knockdown in U251 and LN229 GBM inhibits cell proliferation in vitro and in vivo. (E) Cell-cycle profiles after PI staining. miR-21 knockdown induced G1 arrest in both U251 and LN229 GBM cells. (F). As-miR-21 and scramble ODN-transfected U251 and LN229 GBM cells were analyzed using FCM to determine cell-cycle status.

3. Polyamidoamine (PAMAM) dendrimers

Recently, a great deal of attention has been given to polyamidoamine (PAMAM) dendrimers; these are one of the most appropriate candidates for suitable carrier systems. PAMAM dendrimers represent an exciting new class of macromolecular architecture called dense star polymers. Unlike classical polymers, dendrimers have a high degree of molecular uniformity, a narrow molecular weight distribution, specific size and shape character [15]. The terminal amine groups of PAMAM dendrimers can be modified with different functionalities and can be linked with various biomolecules. These unique structural features of PAMAM dendrimers make them ideal nanoplatforms to conjugate biologically important substances.

3.1 PAMAM dendrimer in gene transfection

Gene therapy is a promising approach for the treatment of cancer because it enables the production of bioactive agents or the cessation of abnormal functions in the tumor cell. However, the success of gene therapy requires efficient and safe transfer systems because of the degradation of the delivered gene in the systemic circulation.

A variety of molecules including polymers, lipids, and peptides have been studied for their effectiveness as delivery vectors for DNA and RNA molecules. Successful delivery vectors must exhibit a combination of functional attributes. Polymeric carrier molecules should be cationic to complex with nucleic acids, possess a high buffering capacity, exhibit low cytotoxicity, and also contain chemically reactive groups that can be modified for the addition of targeting moieties or other groups.

As a non-viral gene delivery carrier, highly branched, dendritic polymers including poly(amidoamine) (PAMAM) have recently attracted interest as nucleic acid delivery vectors. Previous work has demonstrated that dendrimers can bind to DNA and RNA molecules and mediate modest cellular delivery of these nucleic acids. (PAMAM) dendrimers have attracted great interest due to their high efficacy in vitro gene delivery because of their branched structure. These dendritic polymers bear primary amine groups on their branched surface, which can bind DNA, compact it into polyplexes, and promote the cellular uptake of genes. Therefore, PAMAM dendrimers show high levels of transfection in a wide variety of cultured cells, especially in fractured form of G5 (commercially named SuperFect). Enhanced transfection efficiency has been reported by surface modification of PAMAM with L-arginine. Moreover, the primary amines located on the surface of PAMAM make it possible to conjugate suitable ligands, such as Transferrin, for efficient brain-targeting gene delivery.

Studies that focus on the cell entry mechanisms for several nonviral vectors, including PAMAM dendrimers [16]. The cationic surface charge imparted to the complex through high dendrimer–DNA charge ratios is required for subsequent interaction with the anionic glycoproteins and phospholipids that reside on the cell membrane surface. This interaction initiates the interior movement of the dendrimer–DNA complex into the cell cytosol, either by passive transport caused by membrane perturbations or by endocytosis. Complexes formed without an excess cationic surface charge do not mediate high gene transfection efficiency, which furnishes support for the importance of the initial electrostatic interaction between the complex and cell membrane. Studies following the incorporation of radiolabeled DNA and/or dendrimer components into cells established that the uptake in most cells was primarily via an active endocytosis mechanism. Cells preincubated with inhibitors of endocytosis (i.e. cytochalasin B and deoxyglucose) or cellular metabolism (i.e. sodium azide) reduced the uptake that corresponded to lower transgene expression, regardless of cell type.

These dendrimers as nanocarriers possess the following advantages: (1) neutral surface of the dendrimer for low cytotoxicity; (2) existence of cationic charges inside the dendrimer (not on the outer surface) resulting in highly organized compact nanoparticles, which can potentially protect nucleic acids from degradation. Noteworthly, surface modified QPAMAM-NHAc dendrimer demonstrated enhanced cellular uptake of siRNA when compared with the internally cationic QPAMAM-OH dendrimer (degree of quaternization 97%).

George's study shows PEG-G5 and PEG-G6 dendrimers, with PEG conjugation molar ratio at 8% (PEG to surface amine per PAMAM), can facilitate dramatic intramuscular gene delivery in neonatal mice [17]. Park's group concluded that di-arginine conjugation to PAMAM dendrimers can improve polyplex stability, ntra-nuclear localization, and transfection efficiency but also induce charge density- and generation-dependent cytotoxicity. Therefore, a novel strategy for highly densed arginine conjugation maintaining low cytotoxicity will be needed for the development of efficient gene delivery carriers [18].

3.2 PAMAM dendrimer as drug delivery system

Polymeric drug delivery can improve bioavailability and efficacy of therapeutics with intrinsically poor water solubility and high toxicity. Dendrimers, a class of highly branched polymers, are effective drug delivery vehicles due to their monodispersity and nanoscopic size. With each increase in dendrimer generation, the diameter increases linearly while the number of surface groups increases exponentially. These high density surface groups can be conjugated to drug molecules, targeting moieties and imaging agents, rendering dendrimers a versatile drug delivery platform. In addition, surface groups on dendrimers can be modified to modulate cytotoxicity and permeation across biological barriers.

During their synthesis, PAMAM dendrimers can be produced that are either anionic or cationic in nature, with "full generations" (ie. G1, G2) having amine terminal groups and "half generations" (ie, G0.5, G1.5) possessing carboxylic acid terminal groups. The size and charge of PAMAM dendrimers impact their cytotoxicity and transepithelial transport, with cationic dendrimers showing higher toxicity in vitro. Due to their intrinsically low cytotoxicity and appreciable transepithelial permeation characteristics across Caco-2 monolayers and everted rat intestinal sac models, anionic dendrimers show distinct advantages as vehicles for oral drug delivery, with higher generation dendrimers showing the greatest potential because of their large number of modifiable surface groups.

PAMAM has well-defined internal cavities and an open architecture, guest molecules can become directly encapsulated into the macromolecule interior through hydrophobic interactions. Drug-polymer conjugates are potential candidates for the selective delivery of anticancer agents to tumor tissue. The main advantages of conjugating drugs to polymeric carriers include an increase in water solubility of low soluble or insoluble drugs, and therefore, enhancement of drug bioavailability, protection of drug from deactivation and preservation of its activity during circulation, a reduction in antigenic activity of the drug leading to a less pronounced immunological body response, and the ability to provide passive or active targeting of the drug specifically to the site of its action.

Surface-modified dendrimers were predicted to enhance pilocarpine bioavailability [19]. The anticancer drugs adriamycin and methotrexate were encapsulated into PAMAM dendrimers (i.e. G=3 and 4) which had been modified with PEG monomethyl ether chains (i.e. 550 and 2000 Da respectively) attached to their surfaces. A similar construct involving PEG chains and PAMAM dendrimers was used to deliver the anticancer drug 5-fluorouracil. Encapsulation of 5-fluorouracil into G=4 increase in the cytotoxicity and permeation of dendrimers.

Dendrimers have ideal properties which are useful in targeted drug-delivery system. One of the most effective cell-specific targeting agents delivered by dendrimers is folic acid PAMAM dendrimers modified with carboxymethyl PEG5000 surface chains revealed reasonable drug loading, a reduced release rate and reduced haemolytic toxicity compared with the non-PEGylated dendrimer. A third-generation dendritic unimolecular micelle with indomethacin entrapped as model drug gives slow and sustained in vitro release, as compared to cellulose membrane control [20]. Controlled release of the Flurbiprofen could be achieved by formation of complex with amine terminated generation 4 (G4) PAMAM Dendrimers [21]. The results found that PEG-dendrimers conjugated with encapsulated drug and sustained release of methotrexate as compare to unencapsulated drug.

4. Multifunctional dendrimer nanodevices: In vitro and in vivo testing

4.1 Target gene therapy to rat C6 glioma cells rhrough folate receptor-PAMAM

Despite the progress in the PAMAM mediated gene delivery, few studies have investigated the suitability of PAMAM dendrimers for ASODN delivery in vivo, especially for brain gliomas. The purpose of the present study is to evaluate whether in vivo gene delivery by folate-PAMAM (G5) conjugates can inhibit the development of gliomas. We selected the EGFR gene as an antisense target and the rat C6 intracranial glioma model for the in vivo study. Synthetic foliated (FA-)PAMAM was complexed with EGFR ASODN, and then the gene transfection efficacy, dynamic uptake, and biological effects of the FA-PAMAM delivery system on C6 rat glioma cells were investigated both in vitro and in vivo. Our results showed that the FA-PAMAM dendrimer conjugates transported EGFR-ASODNs into glioma cells in vitro, and yielded a favorable therapeutic effect in vivo on administration by local perfusion. Therefore, FA-PAMAM may represent a potential delivery system for short oligonucleotides in glioma-targeted therapy [22].

We chose G5 PAMAM as the gene vector in the present study because its many surface amine groups enable efficient complex formation with ASODNs through charge-based interactions. Western blot analysis demonstrated the binding of G5 PAMAM to ASODNs, with an optimum ASODN/PAMAM ratio of 16:1. TEM analysis revealed that the complexes were >70 nm in size, and this small size likely enabled the efficient transfer of ASODNs to cells that we observed by flow cytometry. We used ASODNs directly labeled with fluorescent probes, such that flow cytometry directly reflected the uptake of the ASODN by the tumor. ASODN uptake mediated by PAMAM increased twofold in comparison with oligofectamine. The high uptake of ASODNs resulted in significant down-regulation of EGFR, suggesting that PAMAM mediated high efficiency transfection of C6 tumor cells with ASODNs. This high transfection efficiency can be attributed to not only the small size of the complexes, but also to the 'proton sponge' effect of PAMAM,31 in which the acidification of tertiary amino groups on PAMAM in the endosome increases the osmotic pressure within the endosome, leading to the release of ASODNs into cytoplasm.

However, while nonderivatized PAMAM achieves high efficiency transfection, its low targeting efficiency needs to be improved. One strategy to achieve this is the derivatization of PAMAM with ligands. Various ligands such as folic acid, transferring, and lactoferrin have been conjugated to PAMAM, thus enabling efficient gene targeting to tumors or brain. We chose folic acid as the functional ligand with which to modify PAMAM because of its low immunogenicity, unlimited availability, functional stability, defined conjugation chemistry, and a favorable nondestructive cellular internalization pathway.23 More importantly, the receptor for folic acid is a cell-proliferation protein that is overexpressed in many types of cancer cells.32 - 34 The expression levels of folate receptor in tumors have been reported to be 100 - 300 times higher than those observed in normal tissue.35 Although some ambiguity surrounds the expression level of the folate receptor in brain tumors,36 our results demonstrate that conjugation with folic acid enhanced the uptake of ASOND/PAMAM complexes by tumor cells and resulted in greater inhibition of EGFR expression in comparison with the native dendrimer. The in vivo study also demonstrates the superiority of FAPAMAM over either PAMAM or oligofectamine as a vector for mediating ASODN gene therapy. Dynamic contrast MRI scanning indicated significant suppression of tumor growth 2 weeks after C6 cell implantation (Fig. 2), which prolonged the survival time of rats in the FA-PAMAM-mediated therapeutic groups.

In the first place, we evaluated the efficiency of folate-PAMAM dendrimers conjugates (FA-PAMAM) for the in situ delivery of therapeutic antisense oligonucleotides (ASODN) that could inhibit the growth of C6 glioma cells. Folic acid was coupled to the surface amino groups of G5-PAMAM dendrimer (G5D) through a 1-[3-(dimethylamino)propyl]-3-ethylcarbodiimide bond, and ASODNs corresponding to rat epidermal growth factor receptor (EGFR) were then complexed with FA-PAMAM. At an ASODN to PAMAM ratio of 16:1, agarose electrophoresis indicated that antisense oligonucleotides were completely complexed with PAMAM or FA-PAMAM. The ASODN transfection rates mediated by FA-PAMAM and PAMAM were superior to oligofectamine, resulting in greater suppression of EGFR expression and glioma cell growth. Stereotactic injection of EGFR ASODN:FA-PAMAM complexes into established rat C6 intracranial gliomas resulted in greater suppression of tumor growth and longer survival time of tumor-bearing rats compared with PAMAM and oligofectamine-mediated EGFR-ASODN therapy. The current study demonstrates the suitability of folate-PAMAM dendrimer conjugates for efficient EGFR ASODN delivery into glioma cells, wherein they release the ASODN from the FA-PAMAM to knock down EGFR expression in C6 glioma cells, both in vitro and in vivo. FA-PAMAM may thus represent a novel delivery system for short oligonucleotides in glioma-targeted therapy.

4.2 Co-delivery of as-mir-21 and 5-fu by poly(amidoamine) dendrimer attenuates human glioma cell growth in vitro

The efficacy of conventional chemotherapy is limited owing to the low therapeutic index of many anticancer drugs, as well as intrinsic or acquired drug resistance. To circumvent these difficulties, novel therapeutic strategies have been developed, and one attractive strategy is the combination of gene therapy with chemotherapy.

MicroRNAs have been demonstrated to be deregulated in different types of cancer. miR-21 is a key player in the majority of cancers. Down-regulation of miR-21 in glioblastoma cells leads to repression of cell growth, increased cellular apoptosis and cell-cycle arrest, which can theoretically enhance the chemotherapeutic effect in cancer therapy.

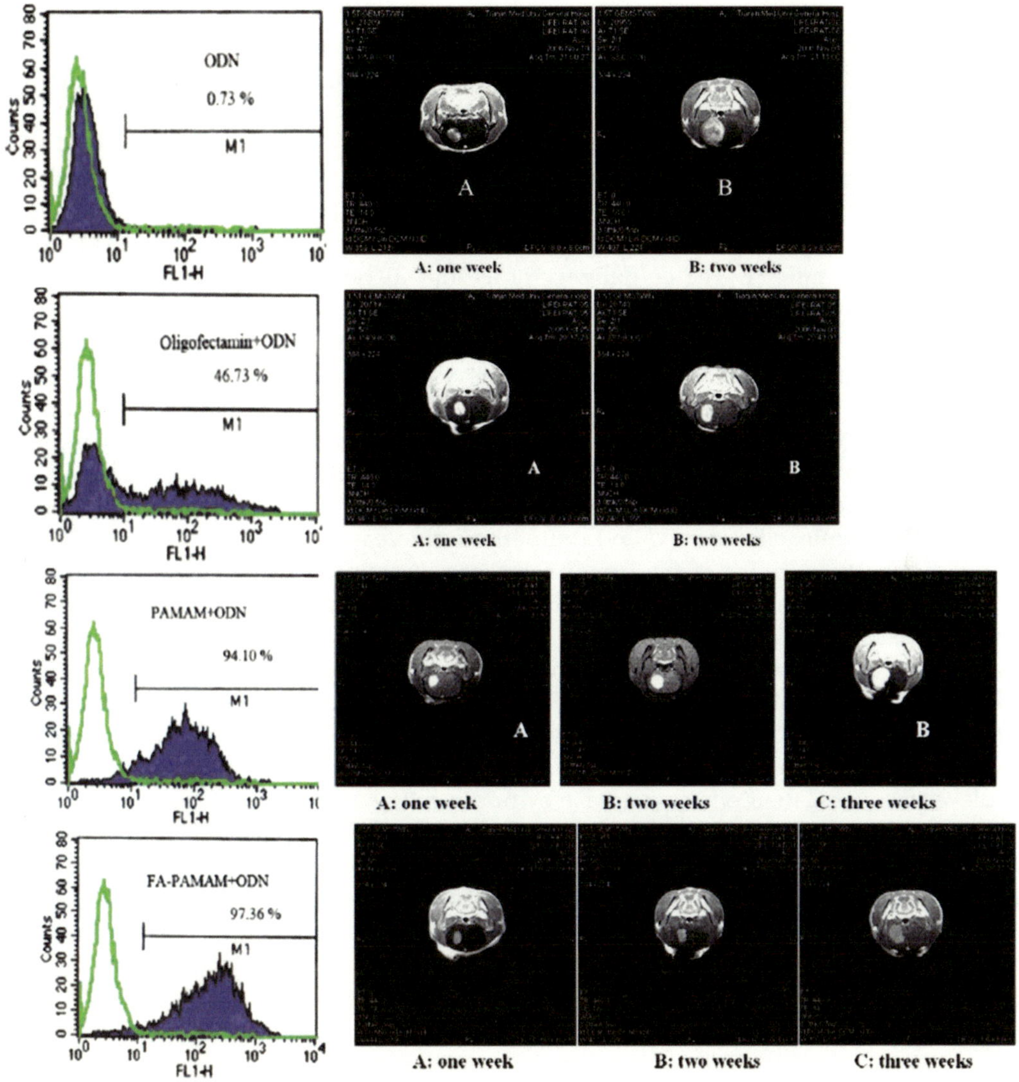

Fig. 2. Contrast-enhanced coronal MR images of representative animals in the ASODN, Oligofectamine/ASODN, PAMAM/ASODN, FA-PAMAM/ASODN group at 1, 2, and 3weeks after tumor xenograft. Four animals in PAMAM/ASODN and FA-PAMAM/ASODN reached the 3-week time point, preventing a valid statistical comparison at that interval. The tumor in this animal is smaller in diameter and less contrast-enhanced than the one in the animal without gene therapy.

With positively charged primary amino groups on the surface, the PAMAM dendrimer can feasibly interact with biomolecules to form complexes through charge-based interactions, and protect them from rapid degradation by cellular endo- and exonucleases. Thus, the PAMAM dendrimer may be suitable for gene transfer or oligonucleotide delivery. Besides, because PAMAM has well-defined internal cavities and an open architecture, guest molecules can become directly encapsulated into the macromolecule interior through hydrophobic interactions. In this study, the poly(amidoamine) (PAMAM) dendrimer was employed as a carrier to co-deliver antisense-miR-21 oligonucleotide (as-miR-21) and 5-fluorouracil (5-FU) to achieve delivery of as-miR-21 to human glioblastoma cells and enhance the cytotoxicity of 5-FU antisense therapy.

Taking advantage of hydrogen-bond interaction, we encapsulated 5-FU in the PAMAM nanoparticles simply by a membrane dialysis method. the encapsulation efficiency and loading efficiency of the drug were determined by UV spectroscopy to be 66.21 and 31.77%, respectively. Through their charge-based interactions, 5-FU-PAMAM could conjugate with as-miR-21. The co-delivery of as-miR-21 not only significantly improved the cytotoxicity and chemosensitivity of 5-FU and dramatically increased the apoptotic percentage of the U251 cells but also brought down the migration ability of the tumor cells. The inhibitory effect toward brain tumors was evaluated by MTT assay, and measurements of cell apoptosis and invasion using the human brain glioma cell line U251. PAMAM could be simultaneously loaded with 5-FU and as-miR-21, forming a complex smaller than 100 nm in diameter. Both the chemotherapeutant and as-miR-21 could be efficiently introduced into tumor cells. The co-delivery of as-miR-21 significantly improved the cytotoxicity of 5-FU and dramatically increased the apoptosis of U251 cells, while the migration ability of the tumor cells was decreased. These results suggest that our co-delivery system may have important clinical applications in the treatment of miR-21-overexpressing glioblastoma.

We report the anticancer potential of a combination of 5-FU treatment and antisense miR-21 technology using PAMAM dendrimers. PAMAM dendrimers, an available co-carrier of chemotherapeutant and as-miR-21, could effectively deliver 5-FU and as-miR-21 simultaneously, forming complexes smaller than 100 nm in diameter. The small size of the complexes facilitated their effective uptake by tumor cells, so the chemotherapeutant and as-miR-21 could be synchronously introduced to glioma cell for combined actions. The co-delivery of as-miR-21 significantly improved the cytotoxicity of 5-FU and dramatically increased the level of apoptosis of U251 cells; it also decreased the migration abilities of the tumor cells. Our results provide invaluable information regarding the future application of drug - polymer complexes combined with gene therapy for cancer treatments. Taken together, our findings suggest that the combination of 5-FU treatment and as-miR-21 might be a potential clinical strategy for cancer chemotherapy [23].

4.3 MicroRNA-21 inhibitor sensitizes human glioblastoma cells to taxol using PAMAM dendrimer

Chemotherapeutic drugs are fundamental in cancer management and are responsible for most cases of adjuvant treatment in patients with GBMs after surgical procedures. Recently, much attention has been focused on the use taxol on glioma, both in experimental studies and in clinical trails [24]. However, the median overall survival did not increase in patients treated by concurrent chemoradiotherapy.

The successful of anti-cancer treatment are often limited by the development of drug resistance. Consequently, further studies that could enhance the therapeutic effect of taxol should be encouraged.Recent work has highlighted the involvement of non-coding RNAs, microRNAs(miRNAs) in cancer development, and their possible involvement in the evolution of drug resistance has been proposed.

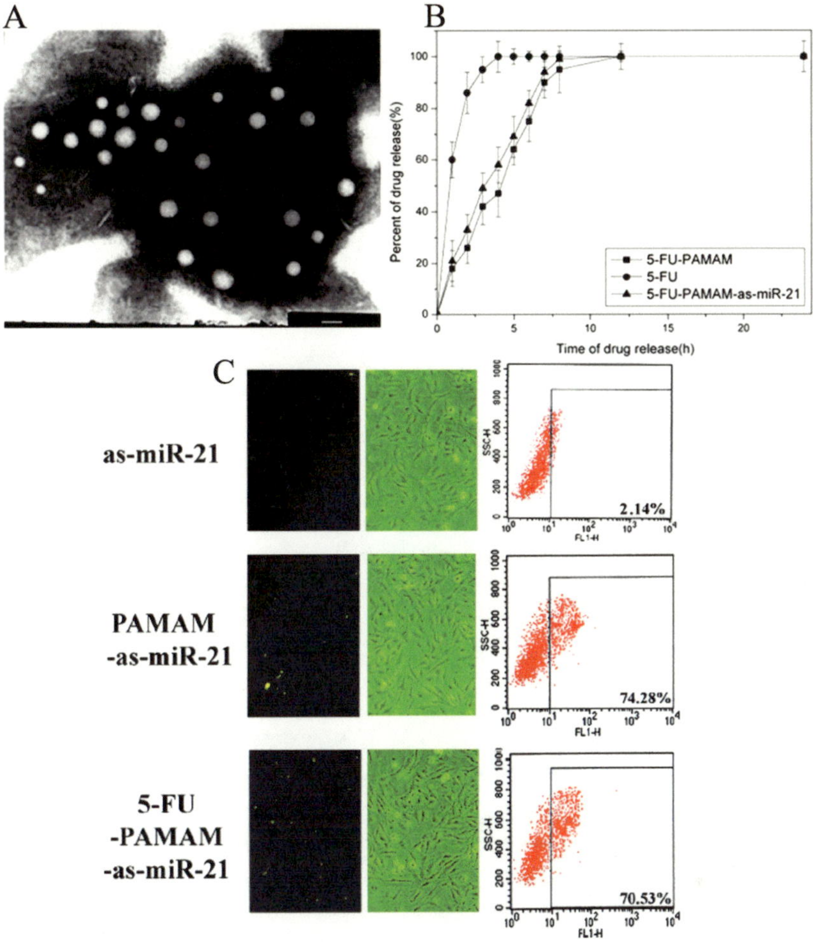

Fig. 3. Characterization of 5-FU/PAMAM/As-miR-21 complex. TEM image of 5-FU-PAMAM-as-miR-21 complex, N/P = 16. Magnification 58 000×, scale bar = 100 nm (A). Release profiles of 5-FU from PAMAMand PAMAM-as-miR-21 complexes compared with free 5-FU (B). Cell uptake detected by flow cyctometry and fluorescent microscopy image of U251 cells after transfection with different complexes (C).

Substantial data indicate that the oncogene microRNA 21 (miR-21) is significantly elevated in glioblastoma multiforme (GBM) and regulates multiple genes associated with cancer cell proliferation, apoptosis, and invasiveness. Thus, miR-21 can theoretically become a target to enhance the chemotherapeutic effect in cancer therapy. So far, the effect of downregulating miR-21 to enhance the chemotherapeutic effect to taxol has not been studied in human GBM.
In this study, we combine taxol chemotherapy and miR-21 inhibitor treatment via polyamidoamine (PAMAM) dendrimers vector to evaluate the effects of combination therapy on suppression of glioma cells. The result indicated that the miR-21 inhibitor can decrease the proliferation of both U251 and LN229 cells and increase the cells' sensitivity to taxol treatment. The taxol concentration causing 50% growth inhibition (IC50) of U251 cells is 400 nmol/mL; whereas, in combination with the miR-21 inhibitor (20 μmol/L) the IC50

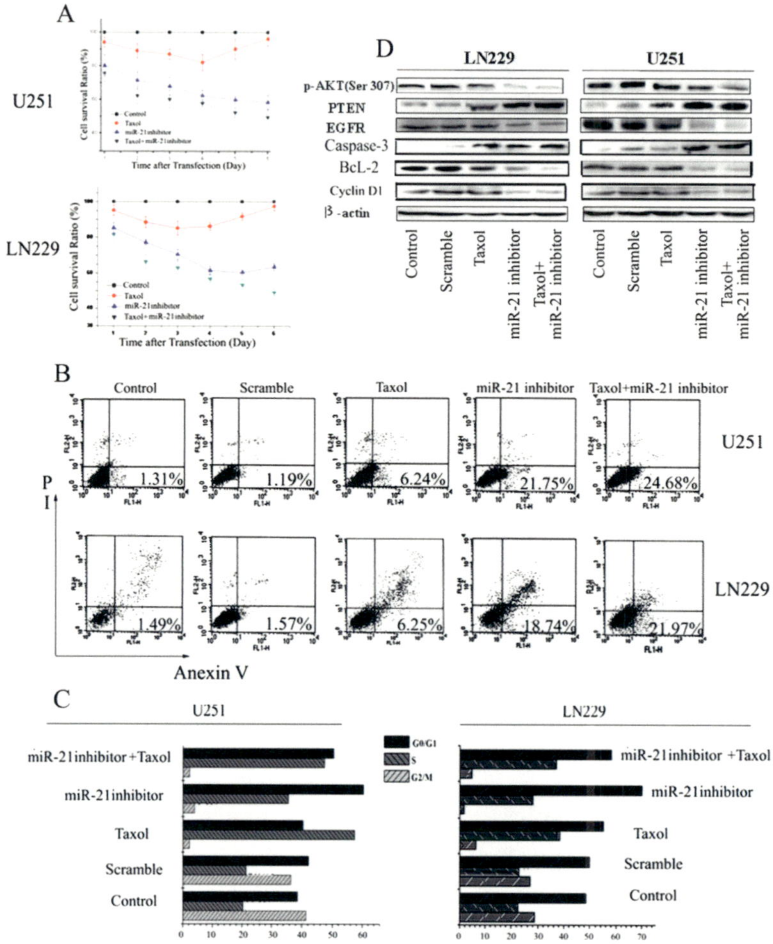

Fig. 4. Effect of the miR-21 inhibitor on the chemo-sensitivity of U251 and LN229 cells to taxol treatment. The growth of U251 and LN229 cells were inhibited by the miR-21 inhibitor, taxol only, and the indicated combinations. The cells were treated with the miR-21 inhibitor complexed to PAMAM for 6 h at 37°C. The medium was then replaced with media containing various concentrations of taxol. After 72 h of incubation, an MTT assay was performed. Absorbance at 570 nm was normalized to the control (untreated cells) to determine cell viability. Each value represents the mean ±SD from triplicate determinations. An aqueous solution of taxol (circles) and miR-21 inhibitor-loaded PAMAM (triangle) was incubated with human glioblastoma U251 and LN229 cells for six days. Druginduced decrease in cell numbers was measured using the MTT assay. The miR-21 inhibitor enhanced taxol induced apoptosis. Flow cytometry analyses of propidium iodide-stained cells were performed in triplicate (B). miR-21 inhibitor and taxol induce G1 and S phase arrest on cell cycle distribution. U251 and LN229 cells were treated with the miR-21 inhibitor and taxol alone or in combination, and cell cycle distributions were detected by Flow cytometry 48 h later (C). Evaluation of the expression of PTEN, EGFR, STAT3, and p-STAT3 in human glioblastoma LN229 and U251 cell lines. Western blot of protein extracts from cells treated with the miR-21 inhibitor or taxol, alone or combination (D). The expression of b-actin was examined to ensure uniform protein loading in all lanes.

was 60 nmol/mL. Taxol can also increase the efficacy of the miR-21 inhibitor. For example, combination treatment reduced cell viability to 20% compared with 86% viability for miR-21 inhibitor gene therapy alone. In LN229 cells, combination treatment with 20 μ mol/L of the miR-21 inhibitor reduced the IC50 of taxol from 820 to 160 nmol/L . It is worth noting that the miR-21 inhibitor additively interacted with taxol on U251cells and synergistically on LN229 cells.

Taxol treatment also increased the percentage of apoptotic cancer cells in miR-21 inhibitor transfected cells compared with control cells. Furthermore, treatment of the miR-21 inhibitor-transfected cells with the anti-cancer drugs taxol resulted in significantly reduced cell viability and invasiveness compared with control cells. These results indicated that the miR-21 plays an important role in the resistance of brain cancer cells to chemotherapeutic drugs. Therefore, miR-21 inhibitor gene therapy combined with taxol chemotherapy might represent a promising novel therapeutic approach for the treatment of glioblastoma.

Thus, the miR-21 inhibitor might interrupt the activity of EGFR pathways, independently of PTEN status. Meanwhile, the expression of STAT3 and p-STAT3 decreased to relatively low levels after miR-21 inhibitor and taxol treatment. The data strongly suggested that a regulatory loop between miR-21 and STAT3 might provide an insight into the mechanism of modulating EGFR/STAT3 signaling [25].

5. Conclusion

MiR-21 was one of the most frequently overexpressed miRNA in human glioblastoma (GBM) cell lines which can serve as a therapeutic target for glioblastoma. We validated that downregulation of miR-21 inhibited the growth of GBM cell lines and induced apoptosis. These effects were only partially dependent on PTEN, highlighting the existence of multiple, and possibly yet unknown, targets of miR-21. Inhibition of miR-21 also suppressed EGFR and Akt activity. These observations were confirmed in in vivo xenograft experiments that showed the potential clinical relevance of miR-21-targeting agents. Targeting miR-21 by antisense or small-molecule compounds may represent new targeted therapeutic strategies for human cancers, including gliomas.

PAMAM dendrimer has been reported to be good gene delivery candidate. Although the biological effects obtained from in vitro analysis of PAMAM and FA-PAMAM are approximate, our in vivo study implies that FAPAMAM is functionally effective for gene delivery into three-dimensional tissues. This may be due to folate-mediated targeting of ASODNs to folate receptor-expressing cells in solid tumors. Stereotactic administration, which enables FA-PAMAM-ASODNs to be injected directly into a tumor, may also produce better results than intravenous injection. Site-specific delivery remains the best choice to overcome gene delivery side effects and to increase its efficacy.

Next, we exhibit the anticancer potential of a combination of 5-FU treatment and antisense miR-21 technology using PAMAM dendrimers. PAMAM dendrimers, an available co-carrier of chemotherapeutant and as-miR-21, could effectively deliver 5-FU and as-miR-21 simultaneously, forming complexes smaller than 100 nm in diameter. The small size of the complexes facilitated their effective uptake by tumor cells, so the chemotherapeutant and as-miR-21 could be synchronously introduced to glioma cell for combined actions. The co-delivery of as-miR-21 significantly improved the cytotoxicity of 5-FU and dramatically increased the level of apoptosis of U251 cells; it also decreased the migration abilities of the tumor cells. Our results provide invaluable information regarding the future application of

drug–polymer complexes combined with gene therapy for cancer treatments. Taken together, our findings suggest that the combination of 5-FU treatment and as-miR-21 might be a potential clinical strategy for cancer chemotherapy.
Furthermore, the miR-21 inhibitor could enhance the chemo-sensitivity of human glioblastoma cells to taxol via PAMAM dendrimer. A combination of miR-21 inhibitor and taxol could be an effective therapeutic strategy for controlling. The above data suggested that in both the PTEN mutant U251 cell line and the PTEN wild-type LN229 cells, miR-21 blockage could increase the chemosensitivity to taxol. It is worth noting that the miR-21 inhibitor additively interacted with taxol on U251cells and synergistically on LN229 cells. Thus, the miR-21 inhibitor might interrupt the activity of EGFR pathways, independently of PTEN status. The miR-21 inhibitor enhanced the chemo-sensitivity of human glioblastoma cells to taxol and combination of the miR-21 inhibitor and taxol could be an effective therapeutic strategy for suppressing the growth of GBM.
the growth of GBM by inhibiting STAT3 expression and phosphorylation.

6. Acknowledgements

This work was financially supported by the China National Natural Scientific Fund (51073118 and 30971136), the Tianjin Science and Technology Committee (09JCZDJC17600, 10JCYBJC12500), and a Program for New Century Excellent Talents in University (NCET-07-0615).

7. References

Minniti G, et al. (2009). Chemotherapy for glioblastoma: current treatment and future perspectives for cytotoxic and targeted agents. *Anticancer Res*, Vol.29, No.12, (2009 Dec) pp: 5171-84, ISSN: 0250-7005

Santos-Rebouças CB,et al (2010). MicroRNAs: macro challenges on understanding human biological functions and neurological diseases. *Curr Mol Med*. Vol.10, No.8, (2010 Nov) pp: 692-704, ISSN: 1566-5240

Kaneda Y. (2010). Update on non-viral delivery methods for cancer therapy: possibilities of a drug delivery system with anticancer activities beyond delivery as a new therapeutic tool. *Expert Opin Drug Deliv*. Vol.7, No.9, (2010 Sep), pp: 1079-93, ISSN: 1742-5247.

He L, Hannon GJ. (2004) MicroRNAs: small RNAs with a big role in gene regulation. *Nat Rev Genet*. Vol. 5, No. 7, (2004 Jul), pp: 522-31 , ISSN: 1471-0056

Bartel DP. (2004). MicroRNAs: genomics, biogenesis, mechanism, and function. *Cell*. Vol. 116, No. 2, (2004 Jan), pp: 281-97, ISSN: 2155-1790

Akbergenov R, et al (2006). Molecular characterization of geminivirus-derived small RNAs in different plant species. *Nucleic Acids Res*, Vol.34, (2006 Jan) pp: 462–471, ISSN: 0305-1048

Valeri N, et al (2009). Epigenetics, miRNAs, and human cancer: a new chapter in human gene regulation. *Mamm Genome*, Vol. 20, No. 9-10, (2009 Sep-Oct), pp: 573-80 , ISSN: 0938-8990

Selcuklu SD, Donoghue MT, Spillane C (2009). miR-21 as a key regulator of oncogenic processes. *Biochem Soc Trans*. Vol. 37, No. 4, (2009 Aug), pp: 918-25, ISSN: 0300-5127

Zhu S, et al (2007). MicroRNA-21 targets the tumor suppressor gene tropomyosin 1 (TPM1). *J Biol Chem*, Vol. 282, No.19, (2007 May), pp: 14328–14336, ISSN: 0021-9258

Asangani IA, et al (2008). MicroRNA-21 (miR-21) post-transcriptionally downregulates tumor suppressor Pdcd4 and stimulates invasion, intravasation and metastasis in colorectal cancer. *Oncogene*, Vol. 27, No. 15, (2008 Apr), pp: 2128–2136, ISSN: 0950-9232

Moore LM, Zhang W. Targeting miR-21 in glioma: a small RNA with big potential. Expert Opin Ther Targets. Vol. 14, No.11, (2010 Nov r), pp: 1247-57, ISSN: 1472-8222

Ciafre` SA, et al. Extensive modulation of a set of microRNAs in primary glioblastoma. *Biochem Biophys Res Commun* Vol. 334 , No.4 , (2005 Sep), pp: 1351–1358 , ISSN: 0006-291X

Meng F, et al (2007). MicroRNA-21 regulates expression of the PTEN tumor suppressor gene in human hepatocellular cancer. *Gastroenterology*, Vol. 133, No. 2, (2007 Aug), pp: 647–658, ISSN: 0016-5085

Malzkorn B, et al (2010). Identification and functional characterization of microRNAs involved in the malignant progression of gliomas. *Brain Pathol.* Vol.20, No.3, (2010 May), pp: 539-50, ISSN: 1015-6305

Baker JR Jr (2009). Dendrimer-based nanoparticles for cancer therapy. *Hematology Am Soc Hematol Educ Program*. pp: 708-19 , ISSN: 1520-4391

Eichman JD, et al (2000). The use of PAMAM dendrimers in the efficient transfer of genetic material into cells. *Pharm Sci Technolo Today*, Vol. 3, No. 7, (2000 Jul), pp: 232-245, ISSN: 1461-5347

Qi R, et al (2009). PEG-conjugated PAMAM dendrimers mediate efficient intramuscular gene expression. *AAPS J*. Vol. 11 , No. 3, (2009 Sep) pp: 395-405, ISSN: 1550-7416

Kim TI, et al (2009). Comparison between arginine conjugated PAMAM dendrimers with structural diversity for gene delivery systems. *J Control Release*. Vol. 136, No. 2, (2009 Jun) pp: 132-9, ISSN: 0168-3659

Tolia,G.T et al (2008). The role of dendrimers in drug delivery, Pharmaceut. Tech., Vol. 32, No.11, (2008 Nov) pp:88-98, ISSN:

Patri, A.K., Majoros and. Baker, J.R., (2002). Dendritic polymer macromolecular carriers for drug delivery, *Curr. Opin. Chem. Biol.* Vol. 6, No. 4, (2002 Aug) pp: 466-71, ISSN: 1367-5931

Asthana ,A.,et al, 2005 . Poly (amidoamine) (pamam) dendritic nanostructures for controlled site specific delivery of acidic anti-inflammatory active ingredient, *AAPS PharmSciTech*. Vol. 6 , No. 3, (2005 Oct) pp: E536-42, ISSN: 1530-9932

Kang C, et al (2010). Evaluation of folate-PAMAM for the delivery of antisense oligonucleotides to rat C6 glioma cells in vitro and in vivo. *J Biomed Mater Res A*. (2010 May), Vol. 93 , No. 2, pp: 585-94, ISSN: 1549-3296

Ren Y, et al (2010). Co-delivery of as-miR-21 and 5-FU by poly(amidoamine) dendrimer attenuates human glioma cell growth in vitro. *J Biomater Sci Polym Ed*. Vol. 21 , No. 3, (2010 Mar) pp: 303-14., ISSN: 0920-5063

Karmakar S, et al (2007). Combination of all- trans retinoic acid and taxol regressed glioblastoma T98G xenografts in nude mice. *Apoptosis*, Vol.12, No.11, (2007 Nov) pp: 2077-87, ISSN: 1360-8185.

Ren Y, et al (2010). MicroRNA-21 inhibitor sensitizes human glioblastoma cells U251 (PTEN-mutant) and LN229 (PTEN-wild type) to taxol. *BMC Cancer*. Vol. 10 , (2010 Jan) pp: 27, ISSN: 1471-2407

22

Nanomedicine Based Approaches to Cancer Diagonsis and Therapy

Roderick A. Slavcev, Shawn Wettig and Tranum Kaur
School of Pharmacy, University of Waterloo, Ontario
Canada

1. Introduction

Pharmaceutical nanoparticles were first described in 1970s, and the term "nanotechnology" is now commonly used to refer to the fabrication of new materials with nanoscale dimensions between 1 and 100 nm (Thrall 2004). Several types of nanometer scale systems such as nanoparticles, nanospheres, nanotubes, nanogels and molecular conjugates are being investigated (Lemieux et al. 2000;Liu et al. 2007;Ravi et al. 2004). The field of nanomedicine aims to use the properties and physical characteristics of nanomaterials which have been extensively investigated as novel intravascular or cellular probes for both diagnostic (imaging) and therapeutic purposes (drug/gene delivery). The sub-micron size of nanoparticle delivery systems confers distinct advantages as compared to large sized systems including targeted delivery, higher and deeper tissue penetrability, greater cellular uptake and greater ability to cross the blood-brain barrier (Kreuter et al. 1995;Vinogradov et al. 2002;Vogt et al. 2006). Therapeutic transgene(s) encoded by plasmid or chemically modified DNA can be dissolved, entrapped, chemically conjugated, encapsulated or adsorbed to the surface of nanoparticles. There are, broadly, two main types of nanosized particles with different inner structures: A. Nanoparticle/Nanosphere: Matrix composed of entangled oligomer or polymer units; and B. Nanocapsule: Reservoir consisting of a hydrophobic core surrounded by a polymer wall. Lipids can also be used to generate liposomes or micelles (discussed in detail later). These nanodevices can confer protection to the DNA against a variety of degradative and destabilizing factors, and enhance delivery efficiency to the cells while minimizing the toxic effects.

Nanoparticles are expected to play a critical role in the innovation and development of future cancer treatment modalities. Recent research has developed functional nanoparticles that are covalently linked to biological molecules such as peptides, proteins, nucleic acids, or small-molecule ligands (Alivisatos 2004;Chan et al. 2002;Michalet et al. 2005). Medical applications have also appeared, such as the use of superparamagnetic iron oxide nanoparticles as a contrast agent in the detection of lymph node prostate cancer (Harisinghani et al. 2003) and the use of polymeric nanoparticles for targeted gene delivery to tumor vasculatures (Hood et al. 2002). Target-specific drug/gene delivery and early diagnosis is currently a high priority R&D area, and one in which nanomedicine will inevitably make critical contributions. Current modalities of diagnosis and treatment of various diseases, especially cancer, have major limitations such as poor sensitivity or specificity and high drug toxicities respectively. The success of nanoparticle delivery systems will ultimately depend on the ability to efficiently deliver the gene of interest and express a therapeutic gene(s) in tumor cells in a targeted manner in order to mitigate toxicity. This chapter examines current existing nanoparticle-based gene therapy approaches to cancer treatment, and assesses their therapeutic utility.

2. Nanobased cancer treatment strategies

Most neoplasm's are derived from multiple mutations and rarely can be controlled through the targeting of a single mutation. The efficacy of gene therapy in tumor treatment will undoubtedly rely upon the simultaneous targeting of multiple cellular processes or the ability to invoke various antitumor responses. Current clinical trials in cancer exploit a variety of different treatment approaches. Tumor suppressor modalities compensate for a genetic mutation via gene transfer or replacement of an altered tumor suppressor gene (e.g. *p53, BRCA1*). Molecular chemotherapy, involves the transfer of a suicide gene (e.g. Herpes Simplex Virus-thymidine kinase [*HSV-tk*], CD::upp) targeted to specific tissues by extracellular tumor/tissue targeting strategies, and/or via tissue-specific expression. The delivered gene then makes the cell susceptible to a prodrug (e.g. gancyclovir, 5-FC) making tumor-specific expression critical. Tumor immunotherapy involves the gene transfer of cytokines (e.g. IL-2, IL-12) that impart antitumor immunomodulatory properties. Oncofactor inhibition strategies such as growth factor inhibition and oncogene inhibition (e.g. erb-B2 silencing) aim to prevent tumor progression by inhibiting key growth factors. Anti-angiogenesis therapy seeks to destroy the vasculature supplying the tumor in the hopes of starving it of essential nutrients to diminish or prevent its progression. Multi Drug Resistance associated genes strategies, involve knocking down gene associated with or conferring MDR, such as *PRP-4* and *survivin* to improve chemosensitivity. We will examine in detail each of these strategies.

2.1 Tumor suppressor gene therapy

As a critical player in cancer onset, *p53* has come to the forefront of oncological research and is now recognized to be the single most frequently inactivated gene in human cancers (Ning et al. 2011;Olivier et al. 2002;Olivier et al. 2010). The *p53* gene enforces a variety of anticancer functions by encouraging cells to arrest or die in the face of DNA damage, hypoxia, oxidative stress, excessive mitogenic stimuli or denuded telomers. In addition, the protein influences several biological functions such as involvement in cell cycle regulation, programmed cell death, senescence, differentiation and development, transcription, DNA replication, DNA repair and maintenance of genomic stability. Thus, it's not surprising that *p53* is regarded as the "*Guardian of the Genome*" in preventing human neoplasia (Lane 1992). *P53* protein has emerged as a key tumor suppressor protein in cellular stress response pathways. The *p53* gene, mapped to chromosome 17p13.1, consists of 11 exons spanning over 20 kb of DNA encoding a 393 amino acid and 53 kDa nuclear protein. Its structure consists of an acidic N-terminus with a transactivation domain, a hydrophobic central DNA-binding core and a basic C-terminus with regulatory and oligomerization domains (Hainaut and Vahakangas 1997). Although greater than 90% of the isolated mutations in this gene have been localized to the DNA binding site of *p53*, coded by exons 5 to 8; some mutations have also been reported outside the evolutionary conserved regions (Hainaut and Hollstein

2000). The *p53* gene product is a sequence-specific nuclear transcription factor that binds to defined consensus sites within DNA as a tetramer and affects the transcription of its target genes. These target genes are involved in critical cell processes such as:

1. Growth arrest: P21, Gadd45 and 14-3-3σ.
2. DNA repair: *P53R2*.
3. Apoptosis: Bax, Bcl-xL, Fas, FasL, DR5/Killer, Apaf-1, Puma and Noxa.

The loss of *p53* function is of relevance to a broad array of cancer types, including 15–50% of breast cancer cases, 25–70% of metastatic prostate cancers, 25–75% of lung cancers, 33–100% of head and neck cancers and 60-80% advanced ovarian cancers (Ruley, 1996). Furthermore, the null mutation of the gene imparts strongly unfavorable prognosis when associated within human ovarian, lung, colon and breast cancer cases. *P53* also represses genes involved in tumor angiogenesis, and recent evidence suggests that tumor cells possessing a wild-type *p53* allele are more sensitive to chemotherapeutic agents and radiation than *p53* null mutants (Lowe et al. 1994). The pleiotropic abnormalities imparted by deficient *p53* in a significant fraction of human cancers make it one of the primary candidates for cancer gene therapy, whereby the effective expression or replacement of *p53* may re-establish cell growth control, restore appropriate responses to DNA-damaging agents (e.g. chemotherapy and radiotherapy) and preclude tumor angiogenesis. In human neoplasia's that express the wild-type protein, aberrations of p53 regulators, such as MDM2, account for p53 inhibition. For this reason, improved understanding of the p53 pathway should lead to better diagnosis and treatment of cancer in the future.

The *p53* gene therapeutic, Gendicine, is currently approved in China and its US counterpart, Advexin, has shown activity in number of clinical trials. In more conventional approaches a range of small drug like molecules targeting the *p53* mediated system have been developed and several are now in clinical trials. Of critical importance has been the development of small-molecule inhibitors of the p53–Mdm2 protein interaction such as the Nutlins (Vassilev 2004), which have shown activity against human xenografts in preclinical models. Therefore, designing small-molecule inhibitors of the *p53*-MDM2 protein-protein interaction is a promising strategy for the treatment of cancers retaining wild-type *p53* (Lauria et al. 2010). Advanced structural approaches have provided compelling support for the idea that some *p53* mutants can be targets for small molecules that would cause them to regain wild-type function (Joerger et al. 2006). Many adenoviral vectors with cancer specific conditional replication properties have been preclinically evaluated to date. Most promising among these are: i) the Ad dl1520 that possesses a deletion of the 55-kd E1B gene limiting growth to only *p53*-deficient tumor cells. This strategy has shown preclinical efficacy against *p53*-deficient nude mouse-human ovarian carcinomatosis xenografts (Vasey et al. 2002); and ii) the integrin-targeted Ad5-D24RGD and serotype 3 receptor-targeted Ad5/3-D24 that possesses a 24 bp deletion in the retinoblastoma binding site of E1A, conferring selective replication in cancer cells that are deficient in the Rb/p16 pathway.

2.2 Molecular chemotherapy

Suicide gene therapy/molecular chemotherapy is a new experimental form of cancer chemotherapy that is currently being evaluated in human trials (Bhaumik 2011; Onion et al. 2009;Xu et al. 2009). This approach involves intra-tumoral delivery of genes encoding enzymes that convert nontoxic prodrugs into toxic anti-metabolites. Two suicide genes that are being evaluated in the clinic are the *Escherichia coli* CD (*codA* cytosine deaminase) and

HSV-1 *tk* (thymidine kinase) genes, which confer sensitivity to 5-FC (5-flourocytosine) and GCV , respectively. The rationale behind the suicide gene therapy approach is that after "targeted" transfer of these genes to the tumor, only tumor and neighboring cells will be rendered sensitive to their cytotoxic action. A variety of tumor models have demonstrated that both the CD/5-FC (by inhibiting thymidylate synthase) and HSV-1 *tk*/GCV prodrug systems (by inhibiting DNA chain elongation) can enhance the efficacy of radiation therapy, resulting in significantly better tumor control and/or cure (Rogulski et al., 1997). Suicide gene therapy is a particularly attractive approach to the treatment of cancer as it is essentially a tumor-targeted chemotherapy. As such, the systemic toxicity commonly associated with, and a major limitation of, conventional chemotherapy is avoided. Using a pair of adenoviral vectors that express a *CD*/HSV-1 *tk* fusion gene without or with the wt human *p53* gene, it has been found that co-expression of *p53* did not enhance the cytotoxicity of *CD*/5-FC or HSV-1 *tk*/GCV suicide gene therapies using the SK-OV-3 and Hep3B tumor models *in vitro* or *in vivo* (Xie et al., 1999). This notion is consistent with the fact that *CD*/5-FC and HSV-1 *tk*/GCV suicide gene therapies have demonstrated effectiveness against a variety of tumors that lack functional *p53* (e.g., SK-OV-3, Hep3B, 9L, WiDr, U251, DU145, PC-3, C33A, and many others). Azatian et al. (Azatian et al. 2009) investigated the effectiveness of HSV-*tk* activation as gene therapy for gastroesophageal junction and gastric adenocarcinomas using a stress-inducible Grp78 promoter. The gastric adenocarcinoma cell line MKN-74/*tk* cells were completely killed when cultured with 1 µg/ml GCV for 10 days. Cell viability was also significantly lower under glucose starvation conditions when HSV-*tk* expression was regulated by the Grp78 promoter . Furthermore, non-viral approaches are being investigated for use in combination with suicide gene therapy for treatment of various carcinomas. Using transferrin lipoplexes, prepared from cationic liposomes and cholesterol, significant tumor reduction was achieved upon intratumoral delivery of HSV-*tk* or *CD* genes, followed by intraperitoneal injection of GCV or 5-FC, respectively (Neves et al. 2009). Enhanced apoptosis, the recruitment of NK cells, CD4 and CD8 T-lymphocytes and an increase in the levels of several cytokines/chemokines were observed within the tumors. These observations suggest that suicide gene therapy with lipoplexes modifies the tumor microenvironment, and leads to the recruitment of immune effector cells that can act as adjuvants in reducing the tumor size.

2.3 Immunomodulatory strategies

Tumor cells alter antigen presentation on their surface compromising recognition by the immune system and immunosurveillance evasion. Tumor immunotherapy strategies aim to boost the anti-tumor immune response by stimulating the cell-mediated arm of the immune system (Wojtowicz-Praga 1997). Gene therapy approaches to enhance immune responses include delivery of cytokines to the tumor, administration of tumor vaccines based on tumor-associated antigens (TAAs), upregulation of Major Histocompatibitlity Complexes (MHC)(Nabel et al. 1993) or co-stimulatory molecules, and inhibition of immunosuppressive molecules. Many cytokines activate the immune system, including interleukins (IL) 2, 4, 7, 12 and 18, interferon γ (IFN-γ), tumor necrosis factor α (TNF-α), and granulocyte–macrophage colony-stimulating factor (GM-CSF), which are among the most potent inducers of anti-tumor activity in a variety of preclinical studies. More recently, some exciting new cytokines have been characterized, such as IL-21, IL-23, IL-27, and their immunomodulatory and antitumor effects *in vitro* and *in vivo* suggest that they may have considerable promise for future immunotherapy protocols (Weiss et al. 2007). Recent studies using animal models have shown that genetically modified tumor cells expressing cytokines such as IL-2, IL-4, IL-6, IFN-γ or GM-CSF were capable of inducing an immune response against preexisting tumors (Connor et al. 1993). In preclinical models and clinical trials, cytokines have been delivered to melanoma lesions by intratumoral injection of naked DNA, recombinant viral vectors and transduced tumor cells and fibroblasts (Sun et al. 1998). Initial clinical trials evaluating the systemic delivery of IL-2 and TNF-α were complicated by significant systemic toxicity (Rosenberg 1999), thereby generating interest in gene transfer strategies that limit cytokine production to the tumor milieu. Preclinical studies employing TAAs to generate tumor vaccines have been promising, and seem to suggest that immunization with recombinant, virus-encoding TAAs can confer suppression of growth in pre-established tumors and the production of specific cytotoxic T lymphocyte responses. However, conversion to clinical trials has failed to show significant efficacy.

The cytokine IFN-γ has been shown to up-regulate MHC expression, antigen processing, antigen processing and presentation expression in many cell populations, including dendritic cells, B cells, macrophages, and endothelial cells, producing more potent antigen presenting cells (APCs), as IFN-γ can induce multiple gene expressions that are related to MHC processing and presentation. Dendritic cells (DCs) play a vital role in the initiation of immune response as professional antigen presenting cells to T cells promoting $CD8^+$ T-cell-mediated cytotoxic responses. Reported research in animal studies indicates that vaccine immunity may represent a promising alternative therapy for cancer patients. However, broad clinical utility has yet to be achieved, owing to the low transfection efficiency of DCs (Chen et al. 2010b). Different formulations of liposomes have been designed to improve the uptake by DCs through different receptor-mediated routes. These formulations include liposomes prepared with mannosylated phosphatidylethanolamine (Man-PE), trimethyl ammonium propane, and phosphatidylserine targeted to mannose receptor (MR), negatively charged surface proteins and phosphatidylserine receptor (PSR) of DCs, respectively. Several other immunomodulatory clinical trials are under way with cytokines currently comprising 18.3% of immunotherapy clinical trials (http://www.wiley.com/legacy/wileychi/genmed/clinical/). Table 1 provides a list of various types of genes currently involved in various gene therapy clinical trials. A number of other monoclonal antibodies; namely EC90, Removab, and CNTO-95 which target FOLR1, EpCAM and α-integrin (CD51), respectively are in Phase I/II studies, and indicate that further clinical investigation in this area is warranted (Bell-McGuinn et al. 2011;Kowalski et al. 2010).

2.4 Oncofactor inhibition strategies

2.4.1 Growth factor inhibition

The epidermal growth factor receptor (EGFR) belongs to the proto-oncogene family, which consists of four structurally-related transmembrane receptors (i.e., EGFR, ErbB2, ErbB3, and ErbB4) and is a key therapeutic target in the treatment of many types of cancer. The most extensively studied growth factors are ErbB1 (Javle et al. 2010) and ErbB2 (Nihira 2003). These ErbB/EGF receptors are tyrosine kinases and play important physiologic roles in cell proliferation, survival, adhesion, motility, invasion, and angiogenesis. High expression of EGF receptor protein is observed in several types of cancer including breast, bladder, colon, lung and gastric cancers, making them potential targets for targeted therapies, which represent some of the most successful therapeutic approaches to date (Iqbal et al. 2011;Lai et al. 2009;Yarom and Jonker 2011).

Gene type	Gene Therapy Clinical Trials	
	Number	%
Adhesion molecule	10	0.6
Antigen	334	20.7
Antisense	13	0.8
Cell cycle	8	0.5
Cell protection/Drug resistance	19	1.1
Cytokine	317	18.5
Deficiency	136	7.9
Growth factor	128	7.5
Hormone	8	0.5
Marker	54	3.2
Oncogene regulator	11	0.6
Oncolytic virus	37	2.2
Porins, ion channels, transporters	12	0.7
Receptor	113	6.6
Replication inhibitor	74	4.3
Ribozyme	6	0.4
siRNA	11	0.6
Suicide	144	8.4
Transcription factor	28	1.6
Tumor suppressor	150	8.8
Viral vaccine	6	0.4
Others	26	1.5
Unknown	49	2.9
Total	1714	

Table 1. List of various types of genes presently involved in various gene therapy clinical trials (Source: http://www.wiley.com/legacy/wileychi/genmed/clinical/).

Gefitinib and Erlotinib are small molecules that exert their function by inhibiting the intracellular tyrosine kinase domain of EGFR. Recently, the southwest oncology group

study S0413, a phase II trial of lapatinib was conducted as first-line therapy in patients with advanced or metastatic gastric cancer. Median (95% CI) time to treatment failure was 1.9 (1.6-3.1) months and overall survival (OS) was 4.8 (3.2-7.4) months. Lapatinib is well tolerated, with modest single-agent activity in advanced/metastatic gastric cancer patients. Potential molecular correlatives such as HER2, interleukin (IL)-8 and genomic polymorphisms IL-8, and vascular endothelial growth factor correlated with OS (Iqbal et al. 2011). Similarly, in other Phase II studies with single agent Gefitinib or Erlotinib only modest activity was observed. Gefitinib cytotoxic combinations are also currently under examination (Wagner et al. 2007). Further, very recently it was observed that direct covalent coupling of antibodies to glutaraldehyde activated nanoparticles is an appropriate method to achieve cell-type specific drug carrier systems based on polymeric nanoparticles that have potential to be applied for targeted chemotherapy in EGFR positive cancer (Aggarwal et al. 2011).
Trastuzumab (trade name Herceptin) is the first anticancer drug generated by Genentech, Inc. whose use as a treatment for breast cancer patients is decided based on the status of the HER2 gene amplification/HER2 protein over-expression. The development and standardization of an HER2 test was a key strategy in clinical development of this drug, since appropriate selection of patients with HER2 over-expression was critical for success. This also highlights the important and evolving era of personalized and targeted therapies. In the clinic, the success of imatinib (Gleevec®, STI571) and trastuzumab, both firsts of their kind, spurred further development of new, second-generation drugs that target kinases in cancer. Further, these targeted drugs combined with chemotherapeutic drugs are found effective and well tolerated in nanoparticle based drug delivery (e.g. albumin-bound paclitaxel combined with carboplatin and trastuzumab or as trastuzumab-dextran iron oxide nanoparticles) for the treatment of cancer (Conlin et al. 2010).

2.4.2 Signal transduction (P13K/AKT/mTOR pathway) inhibition

Phosphoinositide 3-kinase (PI3K) is a major signaling component downstream of growth factor receptor tyrosine kinases (RTKs). PI3K catalyzes the production of the lipid second messenger phosphatidylinositol-3,4,5-triphosphate (PIP3) at the cell membrane. PIP3 in turn contributes to the recruitment and activation of a wide range of downstream targets, including the serine-threonine protein kinase Akt (also known as protein kinase B). The PI3K-Akt-mTOR signaling pathway regulates many normal cellular processes including cell proliferation, survival, growth, and motility—processes that are critical for tumorigenesis. Components of this pathway are frequently abnormal in a variety of tumors, making them an attractive target for anti-cancer therapy. In contrast to *p53* and other tumor-suppressor pathways, the PI3K pathway is activated in cancer, making this an optimal target for therapy as it is easier to inhibit activation events than to replace lost tumor-suppressor function. Studies have demonstrated that phosphorylative activation via the mTOR pathway results in increased G1 cell cycle progression, cell survival, and tumor cell proliferation (Campbell et al. 2004;Vega et al. 2006). The mTOR pathway has been shown in preclinical studies to play a role in the carcinogenesis of breast, ovary and prostate as well as gastrointestinal malignancies. Novel analogs of rapamycin (temsirolimus, everolimus, and deforolimus), which have improved pharmaceutical properties, have been designed for oncology indications. Clinical trials of these analogs have already validated the importance of mTOR inhibition as a novel treatment strategy for several malignancies (Gibbons et al. 2009).

2.4.3 Oncogene inhibition

Gene therapy has also been employed in a reversed approach, namely by inhibition of oncogenes. The use of vectors to express anti-sense (ODN), ribozymes or small interfering RNAs (siRNA) to silence a variety of oncogenes has enabled genetic loss-of-function studies in tissue culture systems. Gene expression can be disrupted at the transcriptional (triplex DNA) or translational (antisense DNA or short inference RNA) level (Braasch et al. 2002). In the triplex DNA-based antigene approach, transcription is disrupted by the binding of a triplex-forming oligonucleotide at the promoter region of a target gene. In the antisense strategy, the oligonucleotide (ON) molecule corresponding to a target gene is delivered inside a cell where it binds to its complementary, targeted messenger RNA (mRNA), to produce a partially double-stranded ON/mRNA complex. Extensive work in this area has already led to one antisense ON product approved for local therapy of cytomegalovirus retinitis (Vitravene) and nearly twenty others in late-stage clinical trials (Cheung et al. 2010).

Silencing of specific mRNA using double stranded RNA oligonucleotides represents one of the newest technologies for suppressing a specific gene product. Small interfering RNA (siRNA) are 21 nucleotides long, double stranded RNA fragments that are identical in sequence to the target mRNA. Silencing of specific gene targets, such as cancer-associated mutations in oncogenes and their amplification in tumors therefore represents promising therapeutic approach in treating cancer, and strategies focusing on classic oncogenes (such as *bcl-2*, *ras* and *HER-2/neu*) have been extensively explored in esophageal, breast, ovarian and other carcinomas. Other candidate targets may include genes associated with cell proliferation, metastasis, angiogenesis, and drug resistance. Very recently, Liang et al., (2011) showed that DNA vector-based Stat3-specific RNA interference (si-Stat3) blocks Stat3 signalling which was delivered by hydroxyapatite nanoparticles and suppresses mouse prostate tumor growth *in vivo*. In this study, the Stat3 downstream genes Bcl-2, VEGF and cyclin D1 were also strongly downregulated in the tumor tissues that also displayed significant increases in Bax expression and Caspase3 activity (Liang et al. 2011). While the application of antisense technology to the treatment of human cancer is conceptually straightforward, selection of appropriate gene targets is an important parameter in the potential success of siRNA cancer therapies (Ashihara 2010), and in practice there are many complicated, mechanistically based questions that must be considered. Importantly, folding of target RNAs or their association with specific proteins in the cell often prevents the ON molecules from binding to their targets. In addition, silencing of such genes must not affect the functions of normal cells.

2.5 Anti-angiogenic therapy

The ability of solid tumors to grow locally, and subsequently disseminate to distant organs, is dependent upon the formation of new blood vessels (Azad et al. 2008) and involves angiogenic factors such as vascular endothelial growth factor (VEGF). VEGF plays an important role in the proliferation of cancer cells, angiogenesis and vascular permeability in peritoneal dissemination. BevacizumAb, the only United States Food and Drug Administration (FDA)-approved anti-VEGF agent, is a monoclonal antibody that inhibits the binding of VEGF to VEGF receptors. CBO-P11, a cyclo-peptide, has proven to specifically bind to receptors of VEGF and may be used as targeting ligand for tumor angiogenesis. Deshayes et al., (2011) investigated the conjugation of CBO-P11 on the surface of poly(vinylidene fluoride) nanoparticles using the copper(I)-catalyzed Huisgen 1,3-dipolar cycloaddition known as a "click" reaction. Nanoparticles were found to be spherical, dense, monodisperse and stable. No cytotoxicity was observed after four days of incubation demonstrating the biocompatibility of nanoparticles. Fluorescence highlighted the specific interaction of these functionalized nanoparticles for VEGF receptors, suggesting that the targeting peptide bioactivity was retained (Deshayes et al. 2011). Therapies based on mAb targeting and blocking of vascular endothelial growth factor, such as that conferred by the monoclonal bevacizumAb, have clearly demonstrated remarkable antitumor efficacy, although the mechanism of action here is not well understood. Combined treatment of bevacizumAb with Sorafenib (a small molecular inhibitor of several tyrosine protein kinases such as VEGFR and PDGFR) resulted in partial response or disease stabilization for ≥ 4 months (median, 6 months; range, 4 to 22+ months) in 22 (59%) of 37 assessable patients with advanced solid tumors .

Matrix metalloproteases (MMPs) are a family of more than 20 zinc and calcium dependent enzymes that degrade all major basement membrane and extracellular matrix components. These enzymes also promote tumor invasion and metastasis, regulating host defense mechanisms and normal cell function. They are well adapted to serve as signaling conduits in the tumor-stromal microenvironment given their crucial roles in the complex processes of tissue invasion, blood vessel homeostasis, and metastasis. Specifically, MMP-1, MMP-2 and MMP-9 mRNA expression in multivariate analyses has been correlated with a well-characterized clinical significance in solid tumors but have no such role in effusions, suggesting the clinical role of MMP is limited to solid lesions. MMP inhibitors (MMPIs) are expected to be useful for the treatment of diseases such as cancer, osteoarthritis, and rheumatoid arthritis. A vast number of MMPIs have been developed in recent years. With the failure of these inhibitors in clinical trials, more efforts have been directed to the design of specific inhibitors with different Zn-binding groups (Tu et al. 2008).

2.6 Multidrug resistance inhibition/gene transfer strategies

Cancer cells counter the influx of a chemotherapeutic by draining the drug from cells, deactivating the protein that transports the drug across cell walls, restoring DNA breaks, or developing some other mechanism to deactivate the drug. Multidrug resistance continues to be a major problem in the management of cancer and knockdown of drug resistance associated genes such as MDR1 (ABCB1), survivin, and pre-mRNA processing factor-4 (PRP-4) has been attempted in cancer cell lines. PRP-4 belongs to the serine/threonine protein kinase family, plays a role in pre-mRNA splicing and cell mitosis whereas survivin, a member of the inhibitor of apoptosis family of proteins, is implicated in both apoptosis inhibition and cell cycle control. Recently, Chen et al., (2010) developed two nanoparticle formulations, cationic liposome-polycation-DNA (Whitmore et al. 1999) and anionic liposome-polycation-DNA (LPD-II), for systemic co-delivery of doxorubicin (Dox) and a therapeutic small interfering RNA (siRNA) to multiple drug resistance (Hesdorffer et al. 1998) tumors. In this study, they have provided four strategies to overcome drug resistance. First, the investigators formed the LPD nanoparticles with a guanidinium-containing cationic lipid, i.e. N,N-distearyl-N-methyl-N-2-(N'-arginyl) aminoethyl ammonium chloride, which can induce reactive oxygen species, down-regulate MDR transporter expression, and increase Dox uptake. Second, to block angiogenesis and increase drug penetration, the authors have further formulated LPD nanoparticles to co-deliver vascular endothelial growth factor siRNA and Dox. An enhanced Dox uptake and a therapeutic effect were observed when combined with vascular endothelial growth factor siRNA in the nanoparticles. Third, to avoid P-glycoprotein-mediated drug efflux, they further designed another delivery vehicle, LPD-II, which showed much higher entrapment efficiency of Dox than LPD. Finally, the authors delivered a therapeutic siRNA to inhibit MDR transporter. Three daily intravenous injections of therapeutic siRNA and Dox (1.2 mg/kg) co-formulated in either LPD or LPD-II nanoparticles showed a significant improvement in tumor growth inhibition (Chen et al. 2010a). Numerous other similar studies highlights a potential clinical use for these multifunctional nanoparticles with an effective delivery property and a function to overcome drug resistance in cancer.

3. Delivery systems

Over the past 20 years, a variety of techniques have been developed for encapsulating both conventional drugs (such as anticancer drugs and antibiotics) and new genetic drugs (plasmid DNA containing therapeutic genes, antisense oligonucleotides and small interfering RNA) within nanoparticles. Nanoparticle delivery systems for gene delivery possess useful inherent attributes, including a diameter of approximately 100 nm or less, a high drug-to-lipid ratio (in the case of lipid based systems), excellent retention of the encapsulated drug, and a long (> 6 h) circulation lifetime. These properties permit nanoparticles to protect their contents during circulation, prevent contact with healthy normal tissues, and accumulate at sites of disease.

3.1 Viral and non-viral delivery systems

A major impediment to the successful application of gene therapy for the treatment of a range of diseases is not a paucity of therapeutic genes, but the lack of an efficient non-toxic gene delivery system. Gene delivery is generally accomplished using one of two categories of delivery vector: 1) Viral delivery vectors derived from engineered retrovirus, adenovirus, herpesvirus, lentivirus or hybrid retro/adeno virus), and 2) Non-viral (synthetic) vectors comprised of polymers and lipids, naked DNA, plasmid-protein conjugates. Other (physical as opposed to chemical) methods include microneedle coating, gene gun, and ultrasound/microbubble-mediated gene delivery.

Viral vectors account for nearly 75% of all clinical trials conducted thus far (http://www.wiley.co.uk/genetherapy/ clinical). These vectors are essentially viruses that have been genetically modified to remove any replication/pathogenic genes, and instead encode a gene of interest (Hesdorffer et al. 1998). This strategy preserves the viruses highly efficient ability to infect cells, while eliminating/attenuating toxicity. The most commonly used viral vectors are retroviral, adenoviral, adeno-associated viral and herpes simplex viral-based (Young et al. 2006). Although Vitravene, an antisense oligonucleotide-based product, is the only gene delivery product approved so far by US-FDA, there are several other products in late stages of clinical trials. Gendicine, an adenovirus encoding the *p53* gene, developed by SiBiono GeneTech Co., Ltd., was recently approved by China's state Food and Drug Administration, for the treatment of head and neck squamous cell carcinoma. Virus-based treatments tend to maximize efficiency of gene transfer, often at the cost of safety, while non-viral options generally capitalize on a higher safety profile, but usually at the expense of Gene of Interest (GOI) expression efficiency. Many viruses including retroviruses, adenoviruses, herpes simplex viruses, adeno-associated viruses (AAV) and pox viruses have been modified to eliminate their toxicity, maintain their high gene transfer capability and long term gene expression.

However, despite these advantages, there are currently major limitations to the use of viruses as gene delivery vectors. These include the limited carrying capacity of transgenic materials (i.e. size of plasmid) since the packaging capacity of viral vectors (usually up to 5 kb) is constrained; the potential for oncogenesis due to chromosomal integration or activation of oncogenes/inactivation of oncogene regulators; the generation of infectious viruses due to recombination; and concerns regarding instability that challenge production and storage.

The potentially hazardous nature of viral vectors has been observed in a number of gene therapy-related patient mortalities in various clinical trials. Patient complications to date have included the rejection of DNA carriers, resulting in immune response that have led to already one death, Jesse Gelsinger, who died in 1999 from a rare metabolic disorder during a gene-therapy clinical trial at the University of Pennsylvania (Branca 2005;Ledford 2007;Stolberg 1999;Wilson 2010). DNA constructs need to be optimized to carry minimal immunogenic components without compromising both efficient and long-term transgene expression. In this context, technology employing minimal immunological defined gene expression technology (MIDGE) represents a promising future alternative to conventional plasmids in terms of biosafety, improved gene transfer, potential bioavailability, minimal size and low immunogenicity associated with these chemically engineered miniDNA vectors. MIDGEs are non-viral, lcc (linear covalently closed) miniplasmids synthesized *in vitro* via a patented chemical modification of linear open (lo). These plasmids confer the advantage of a minimal coding sequence that relieves complications from expression of additional unwanted genes and CpG motifs that have a 20-fold higher occurrence in bacterial cells. MIDGE lcc plasmid transfection expression was reported to increase luciferase transgene expression from 2.5 to 17 fold *ex vivo* compared to circular covalently closed (ccc), isogenic forms in a tissue-dependent manner (Schakowski et al. 2007) . In addition, the mean numbers of MIDGE vector molecules per cell was also found to be significantly higher, suggesting that linear lcc plasmids transfect cells more efficiently. MIDGE technology has already been applied, with promising results, to the development of a Leishmania DNA vaccine and a colon carcinoma treatment. Here, therapy was based on IL-2 delivery to specific tumor cell lines *ex vivo*, and revealed 2 to 4 fold higher relative transgene expression compared to the ccc control (Schakowski et al. 2001). In combination, the existing studies employing lcc DNA systems suggest that lcc DNA is superior to lo DNA in transfection efficiency, and to ccc DNA in transgene expression. Purified TelN (closely related to Tel) was previously reported to generate lcc plasmids *in vitro* in (*pal*-related) *telRL*-dependent manner and was shown to successfully deliver EGFP to human embryonal kidney cells *in vitro,* as well as IL-12 in an untargeted manner to inhibit metastasis formation in B16F10C57BL/6 melanoma model mice *in vivo* (Heinrich et al. 2002).

At present, our laboratory is involved in design, and construction of bacteriophage-encoded recombination systems to generate linear covalently closed (lcc) DNA mini-vectors. Conditional expression recombinase systems *in vivo* in *E. coli* provide a one step production system for step minivectors from specialized parental plasmids. The exploitation of this recombination system allows us to generate lcc miniplasmids that should have a preferential safety profile, preventing viable vector-chromosome, single recombination products in mammalian cells. In theory, the integration of covalently closed linear exogenous DNA into double-stranded (ds) DNA breaks is unlikely due to the unavailability of terminal ends, and a vector single recombination event into a target chromosome should theoretically result in the disruption of the chromosome, killing the cell (see Figure 1).

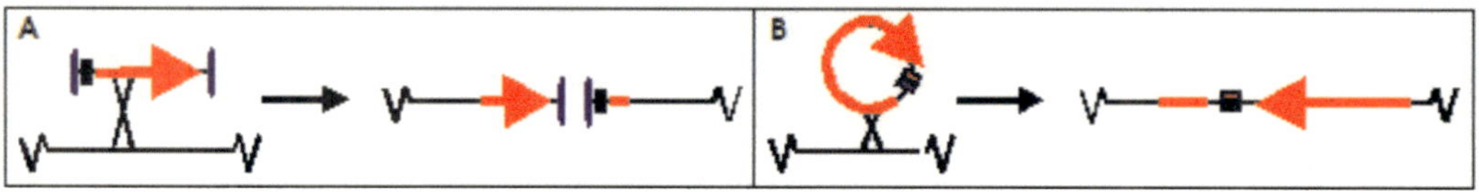

Fig. 1. Plasmid Integration Events: A miniplasmid that undergoes a single recombination event with the host chromosome should be rare due to the removal of all elements except the gene of interest. Any integration events by: A. A lcc miniplasmid should result in chromosomal disruption that is likely lethal and cannot be replicated or segregated; B. A ccc miniplasmid can integrate without disrupting the host chromosome.

Non-viral gene delivery is emerging as a realistic alternative to the use of viral vectors with the potential to have a significant impact on clinical therapies. Synthetic vectors provide flexibility in formulation design and can be tailored to the size and topology of the DNA cargo and the specific route of vector administration, and can be delivered selectively to a specific tissue type through the incorporation of a targeting ligand. Compared to viral vectors, synthetic vectors are potentially less immunogenic, relatively easy to produce in clinically relevant quantities, and are associated with fewer safety concerns (Liu and Huang 2002). As a result of these advantages, their use has rapidly moved from transfection of cell cultures to clinical cancer gene therapy applications.

Synthetic vectors designed for parenteral administration encompass a wide range of formulations. These include unmodified (naked) DNA, which is designed for direct intra-tissue injection, cationic polymer-DNA complexes, cationic lipid-DNA complexes, and cationic polymer-lipid-DNA ternary complexes (lipopolyplexes), which are mostly aimed at systemic administration.

3.1.1 Naked DNA

The simplest employed method of transgene delivery is the injection of naked DNA. It shows very little dissemination and transfection at distant sites following delivery and can be re-administered multiple times into mammals (including primates) without inducing an antibody response against itself (i.e., no anti-DNA antibodies generated) (Wolff and Budker, 2005). The simplicity of this approach is offset by serious limitations such as inefficient uptake of the therapeutic gene into the target cells and rapid clearance of the DNA from the circulation. Direct *in vivo* gene transfer with naked DNA was first demonstrated by efficient transfection of myofibers following injection of mRNA or pDNA into skeletal muscle (Wolff JA, 1990). This novel approach was heralded as a superior method of *in vivo* transfection and its application was later advanced to confer high level expression in hepatocytes in mice by the rapid injection of naked DNA in large volumes into the tail vein (Zhang et al., 1999). This hydrodynamic tail vein (HTV) procedure has proven very useful not only to gene expression studies, but also more recently for the delivery of siRNA (Lewis et al., 2002; McCaffrey et al., 2002). Ultrasound-mediated eruption of polyethyleneglycol (PEG)-modified liposomes loaded with naked plasmid-DNA is also a feasible and efficient technique for gene delivery (Negishi et al. 2010).

3.1.2 Cationic liposomes

Cationic liposomes are one of the most efficient, and among the most widely used non-viral vector systems. They are composed of positively charged lipid bilayers that can be complexed to DNA through electrostatic interactions resulting in complexes, termed lipoplexes. The application of cationic liposomes to gene therapy was first described in 1987 by Felgner (Felgner et al. 1987). The lipoplexes are generally composed of a positively charged lipidic component (see Figure 2), such as dioleylpropyltrimethylammonium chloride, dioleoyl triethylammonium propane (DOTAP), or dimethylaminoethane carbamoyl cholesterol (DC-Chol), that is capable of complexing and condensing the DNA (Giatrellis et al. 2009). Most lipoplex formulations include a "helper" lipid, such as dioleoylphosphatidyl-ethanolamine (DOPE, as seen in Figure 2), or cholesterol that provides added stability to the lipoplexes and enhances DNA release from endosomal compartments. While transfection activity of lipoplexes is shown to vary depending on their DNA/cationic lipid ratio, it is necessary for them to be positively charged to interact with the negatively charge cell membranes and exhibit transfection activity. Lipoplex uptake occurs through endosome formation (via a number of mechnisms including caveosomes, clathrin dependent, etc.), followed by disruption of the endosomal membrane by fusion with, or incorporation of the lipoplex lipids resulting in DNA release.

The advantages of liposomes in delivery system designs include their simplicity in preparation, ability to complex relatively large amounts of DNA, versatility for use with any size or type of DNA/RNA, ability to transfect non-dividing cells and overall stability (Dutta et al. 2010). In addition, lipids are non-immunogenic allowing for repeated administration without adverse immunologic reaction(Barron et al. 1999). The primary disadvantages of lipoplex delivery vectors include low tumor transfection efficiency and lack of tumor specificity.

In order to enhance gene transfection, based upon structure-activity relationship, various gemini surfactants (Gemini surfactants consist of two hydrophobic chains and two polar headgroups linked chemically by a spacer group) have been designed. In order to enhance gene transfection based upon structure-activity relationship, various gemini surfactants have been designed, synthesized and tested for gene delivery in our laboratory (Donkuru et al. 2010;Wang and Wettig 2011;Wettig et al. 2007a;Wettig et al. 2007b;Wettig and Verrall 2001). Recent reports have shown that obstacles can be overcome by exploiting receptor-mediated endocytosis for highly efficient internalization of ligands naturally employed by eukaryotic cells. Advances along this line include the conjugation of mAbs ("immunoliposomes"), ligands such as growth factors, or hormones to liposomes to confer targeting capability. Nanoparticle based anti-cancer gene/drug delivery first reached clinical trial in mid 1980s and the first nanomedicine Doxil® (liposomal encapsulated doxorubicin) was marketed in 1995. Other example of liposome-mediated drug delivery include daunorubicin (Daunoxome), which is also currently being marketed as liposome delivery systems. Numerous new nanoparticle based cancer gene therapy systems are under development.

3.1.3 Polyplexes

Polyplexes differ from lipoplexes in that they are comprised of charged complexes of plasmid DNA and a cationic polymer, such as poly-L-lysine (PLL), polyethylenimine, polyamidoamine (starburst) dendrimers, and chitosan with a net positive charge (See Figure 2). Cationic polymers differ from cationic lipids primarily in that they do not contain a hydrophobic moiety and are completely soluble in water. A wide variety of cationic polymers that transfect cells *in vitro* have been characterized (Midoux et al., 2008). A key determinant of polyplex gene transfer efficiency is the positive (on amine nitrogen atoms in the polymer) to negative charge ratio or the related negative to positive (N/P) ratio. Given their polymeric nature, cationic polymers can be synthesized in different lengths, with different geometry (linear versus branched), and with substitutions or additions of functional groups with relative ease and flexibility, which opens the way to extensive structure/function relationship studies.

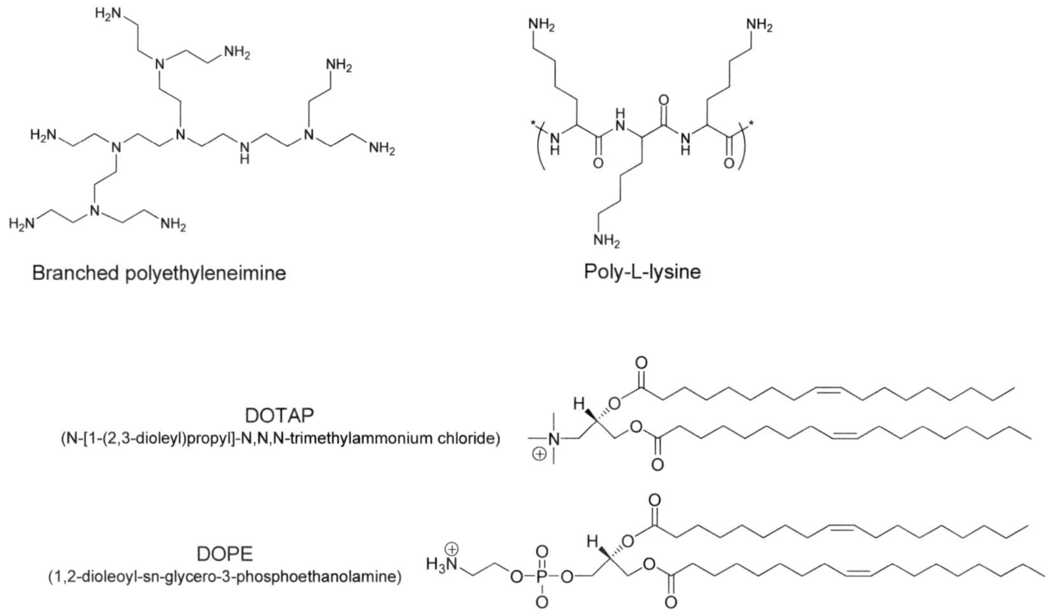

Fig. 2. Examples of commonly used lipids (DOPE and DOTAP) and polymers (PEI and poly-L-lysine) in gene therapy.

Polymer-based nanoparticles are now widely used for gene and drug delivery and targeted therapy. One of the most widely applied cationic polymers used for DNA transfections is polyethyleneimine (Choosakoonkriang et al. 2003). DNA complexation with PEI, has not been found to result in an alteration of DNA conformation, remaining essentially in the B form, and the utility of PEI as a gene delivery vector has been demonstrated in numerous studies (Jere et al. 2009;Moore et al. 2009). High molecular weight PEI has been shown to be one of the most successful polymeric vectors due to the large number of protonatable amine groups that result in an enhanced ability to escape from the endosome following uptake by the cell via the so-called "proton sponge" effect. This benefit is contrasted by the high level of cellular toxicity also imparted by the number of amine groups within the polymer. Attempts to overcome this increased level of toxicity have involved using low molecular weight PEI; however, transfection efficiencies are directly correlated with decreases in molecular weight while the tendency to aggregate can increase with decreasing polymer molecular weight. Another successful strategy has involved the shielding of the polyethylenimine/DNA core with a shell of polyethylene glycol (PEG). This approach results in the formation of a dense hydrophilic outer surface of the complexes, reducing hydrophobic interactions with serum proteins and components of the reticulo-endothelial system (RES). In addition to decreasing toxicity of the polyplexes, this strategy also confers increased biocirculation times and therefore, further increases transfection efficiencies. [Please see van Vlerken et al. 2007 for a recent review of PEG modification of nanocarriers]. The presence of the terminal alcohol groups in this PEG outer shell also provides sites for further modification that have been conjugated to various types of targeting ligands, including glycoprotein, transferring, carbohydrates, folate and epidermal growth factors, facilitating tissue-specific gene delivery (Guo and Lee 1999;Han et al. 1999;Lai et al. 2009). Such complexes have been found to mediate efficient gene transfer into tumor cell lines in a receptor-dependent and cell-cycle-dependent manner. While the modifications described here have resulted in significant improvements in both the transfection efficiencies and toxicity profiles of polycation-based transfection vectors, a number of questions relating to mechanisms of endosome escape (Tros, I et al. 2010), structure-activitiy relationships, pharmacokinetics, and *in-vitro* vs *in-vivo* application remain (Jere et al. 2009). Overall, while proving to be a very promising strategy toward gene therapy design, polyplex systems still require much further testing and improvement prior to entering clinical trials (Midoux et al., 2008).

3.1.4 Lipopolyplexes

Lipopolyplexes (lipid-polymer-DNA complexes or LPDs) combine plasmid DNA with both a cationic polymer and liposomes via electrostatic interactions. In general, these vectors are compact particles that exhibit superior colloidal stability, reduced cytotoxicity, and provide elevated transfection efficiency compared to either polyplexes or lipoplexes alone. The cationic polymer may be covalently linked to the liposomes (e.g. lipopolylysine) or be non-covalently incorporated into a ternary lipid–polymer–DNA complex by a charge-mediated self-assembly process. The polycation component facilitates the optimal condensation of plasmid DNA, whereas lipidic components, to which targeting ligands can be attached, further stabilize the vector formulation and mediate the efficient endosomal escape of the vector following cellular internalization. LPD particles prepared using protamine as the cationic polymer and DOTAP/Chol cationic liposomes have been reported to inhibit tumor growth following i.v. administration in mice (Whitmore et al. 1999). Both *in vitro* and *in vivo* studies have demonstrated improved outcomes of (liposomes/protamine/DNA) LPD-mediated gene transfer over conventional liposomes (El-Aneed 2004) . It is believed that the small size of LPD (100 to 250 nm, which is almost three to five times less than conventional lipoplexes) will facilitate endocytosis and increase the *in vivo* circulating half life.

4. Challenges in nanoparticle based gene therapy

To facilitate efficient gene expression, delivered plasmid DNA must initially circumnavigate various barriers to cellular and nuclear entry as seen in Figure 3. The lipoplex/polyplex must first be internalized by the cell membrane,for which there are many different possible routes including receptor mediated endocytosis, pinocytosis and phagocytosis (Godbey and Mikos 2001). Receptor-mediated endocytosis or clathrin-dependent internalization is the most common of these and can be exploited to engineer polyplexes to express attached ligands to facilitate this process (Morille et al. 2008).

Pinocytosis is the process by which cells internalize liquids which contain suspended or soluble particles. Untargeted polyplexes that interact with the cell membrane electrostatically may be internalized via this pathway . Phagocytosis is another possible method of internalization involving the ingestion of larger particles greater than 0.5 μm in diameter.

Targeting and internalization of microspheres to phagocytic cells *in vivo* can be achieved through size exclusion. It is important to note that internalization mechanisms may also be largely dependent on the cell type, the vector used, and the process parameters of that a particular vector system (Duncan et al. 2006). On the cellular level, many complexes become buried in the endolysosomal compartment or are degraded in the cytoplasm. After internalization occurs, the lipoplex/polyplex is believed to be most commonly contained within an endocytic vesicle after which it is transferred to late endosomes and lysosomes. In these compartments the pH rapidly changes to the range of 4.5–6, and in order for successful transfection to occur the DNA must find a way to escape from these structures and reach the nucleus as DNA that remains in these cellular compartments is readily degraded (Pack et al. 2005). The final obstacle in the DNA vector's journey is the double bilayer membrane surrounding the nucleus, or nuclear membrane. While small molecules may gain access to the nucleus directly through its network of pores, larger molecules must be internalized by specific nuclear import proteins. This process is largely dependent on the size of the DNA and its conformation. As such, in the absence of specialized enhancer sequences, nuclear import of plasmids is limited to actively dividing cells undergoing mitosis.

In gene therapy studies, nuclear localization signal (NLS) peptides have been investigated as facilitators of nuclear transport with the aim of enhancing transgene expression. In order to improve overall transfection specificity and efficiency it is necessary to optimize intracellular trafficking of the DNA complex as well as the performance after systemic administration (Schatzlein 2001). Properties of vector such as size, shape, and surface characteristics can also have a major impact on its pharmacokinetic properties and delivery efficiency. For most nanoparticles, it is unknown what size and/or charge of nanoparticles could lead to defects in DNA transcription and chromosomal damage and aberration. However, there are indications that certain types of nanoparticles are capable of causing DNA damage, where the composition and the coating of nanoparticles are likely the key factors imparting genotoxic effects.

With respect to systematic *in vivo* applications, nanocarrier approaches face additional hurdles. First, despite advances in using PEG or other hydrophilic polymers for extracellular stability to prolong their circulation in the blood stream, a large fraction of the injected dose of nanoparticles accumulates in the liver and is taken up by hepatic phagocytes. Second, due to the vascular endothelial barrier, nanoparticles can only reach certain tissues such as the liver, spleen, and some types of tumors as a result of enhanced permeability and retention (an effect due to the presence of fenestrated endothelium in tumor blood vessels i.e passive targeting) effect, where the nanoparticles tend to accumulate in tumor tissues much more than in normal tissues. However, nanoparticles cannot, or rarely access, parenchymal cells in most normal tissues as they are simply excluded by the endothelial barrier. Thus, many potential disease targets cannot at present be addressed by existing nanocarrier approaches.

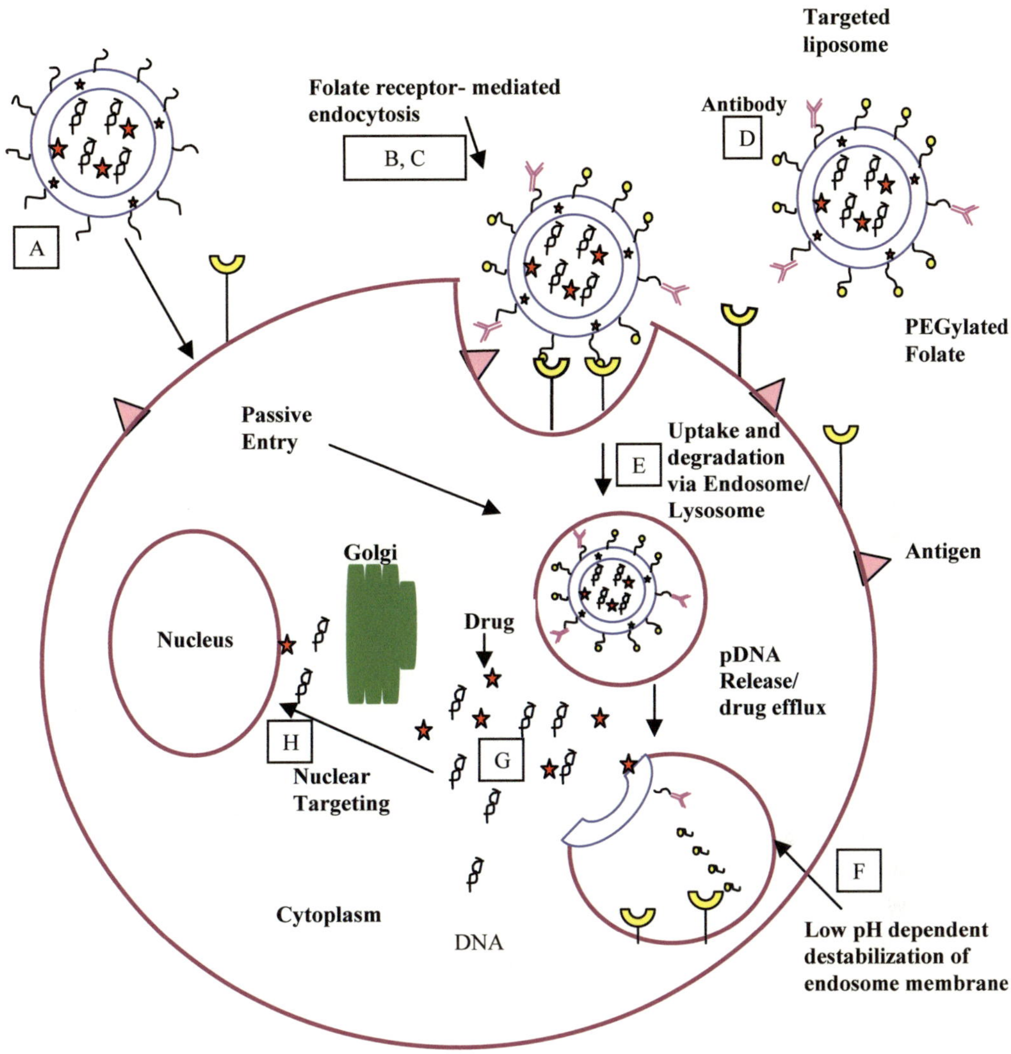

Fig. 3. A schematic generalized diagram of folate receptor/ non-receptor mediated non-viral delivery system: The tethers connecting the folate to the lipid headgroups consist of 250 Å long polyethyleneglycol spacers. Condensation/ complexation of DNA-based therapeutics with DNA delivery vector; (B, C) Non-specific adsorption to cell membrane and cellular internalization via non-receptor mediated (passive entry) or folate-receptor (folate tittered PEGylated liposome's shown in yellow balls and encapsulated drugs as red stars) mediated endocytosis pathway; (D) Monoclonal antibody-antigen complex mediated endocytosis pathway; (E) Uptake and degradation via endosome. lysosome; (F) Low pH dependent destabilization of endosome membrane; (G) Cytoplasmic release of plasmid DNA and drug efflux; (H) Nuclear targeting via nuclear localization signals, transcription and transgene expression.

4.1 Targeted nanomedicine

Construction of organ-targeted gene delivery vectors is a promising route to improve the safety and efficacy of nanomedicine based cancer gene therapy. There are a variety of 'vector targeting' strategies, that can be accomplished using transcriptional targeting, transductional targeting, or ideally, a combination of these. While transcriptional targeting refers to the use of gene regulatory elements (promoters and enhancers) to restrict gene expression to specific cells, transductional targeting refers to the delivery of DNA to specific cells. Targeted gene expression has been analyzed using tissue-specific promoters (breast-, prostate-, and melanoma-specific promoters) and disease-specific promoters (carcinoembryonic antigen, HER-2/neu, Myc-Max response elements, DF3/MUC). The addition of a ligand (i.e., folate, transferrin, RGD peptide, among others) to the nanoparticle surface, thus targeting the DNA to cells *in vivo* has been demonstrated quite successfully. Folate-receptor-targeted liposomes have proven effective in delivering doxorubicin *in vivo* and have been found to bypass multidrug resistance in cultured tumor cells (Immordino et al. 2006). Hong et al., (2010) exploited the possibility of combination of the functions of passive and active targeting by transferring-PEGlyated nanoparticles (Tf-PEG-NP), as well as sustained drug release in tumor by PEGylated drug for most efficient tumor targeting and anti-tumor effects enhancement. Such Tf-PEG-NP loaded with PEGylated drug conjugates could be one of the promising strategies in nanomedicine to deliver anti-tumor drugs to tumor (Hong et al. 2010). Further enhancement of the therapeutic index may also be achieved by overcoming barriers both at cellular and nuclear levels. In gene therapy studies, nuclear localization signal peptides have been investigated as facilitators of nuclear transport with the aim of enhancing transgene expression. Selective tumor targeting with minimal toxicity using folate modified, incorporating nuclear localization signal represents a popular approach. In recent years, Poly(ε-caprolactone)/poly(ethylene glycol) (PCL/PEG) copolymers which are biodegradable and amphiphilic, are also emerging as a potential nanoplatform for anticancer agent delivery (Gou et al. 2011).

5. Nanobased cancer diagnosis approaches

Current problems and unmet needs in translational oncology include (i) advanced technologies for tumor imaging and early detection, (ii) new methods for accurate diagnosis and prognosis, (iii) strategies to overcome the toxicity and adverse side effects of chemotherapy drugs, and (iv) basic discovery in cancer biology leading to new knowledge for treating aggressive and lethal cancer phenotypes such as bone metastasis. Advances in these areas will undoubtedly form the major cornerstones for a future medical practice of personalized oncology. Cancer detection, diagnosis, and therapy will be tailored to each individual's tumor molecular profile and used in predictive oncology, whereby genetic/molecular markers will play an essential role in the prediction of disease development, progression, and clinical outcomes.

The probability of a successful treatment modality increases dramatically if tumor cells can be selectively removed before they evolve to their mature stages and metastases production. As such, novel and more sensitive diagnostic tools like metallic and semiconducting nanoparticles are being developed with the aim of improving the early and noninvasive detection of rising malignancies and the accuracy of tumor tissue localization. Paramagnetic nanoparticles, quantum dots, nanoshells and nanosomes represent some of these new technologies, used for diagnostic purposes (See Figure 4). Compared to conventional materials, inorganic nanomaterials provide several advantages such as simple preparative processes and precise control over their shape, composition and size. These systems provide promising potential not only in diagnostics, but also as delivery systems for therapeutic agents and are discussed in detail below.

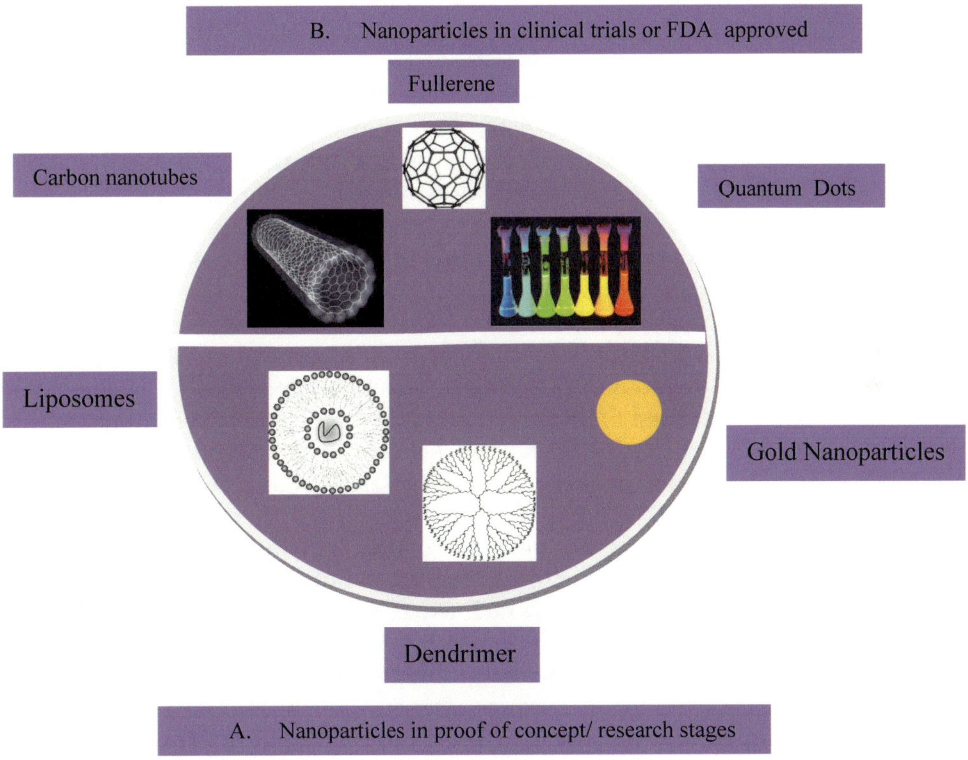

Fig. 4. Nanoparticles used in cancer diagnosis and treatment. Liposomes contain amphiphilic molecules, which have hydrophobic and hydrophilic groups that self-assemble in water. Gold nanoparticles are solid metal particles that are conventionally coated with drug molecules, proteins, or oligonucleotides. Quantum dots consist of a core-and-shell structure (e.g., CdSe coated with zinc and sulfide with a stabilizing molecule and a polymer layer coated with a protein). Fullerenes (typically called "buckyballs" because they resemble Buckminster Fuller's geodesic dome) and carbon nanotubes have only carbon-to-carbon bonds.

5.1 Quantum dots

Quantum Dots (QDs) are a unique class of light emitting semiconductor nanoparticles ranging from 2-10 nanometers in diameter and are becoming highly popular for biological imaging due to their high intensity and stable fluorescence profile (most QDs are approximately 10–20× brighter than organic dyes). QDs usually consist of a CdSe core surrounded by a inorganic shell composed of ZnS (Pinaud et al. 2010). For biological imaging applications, they are given hydrophilic coatings of PEG or multiple carboxylate groups.

Compared to the commercially available organic dyes and fluorescent proteins used in medical imaging, QDs provide many advantages (Park et al. 2009;Pic et al. 2010;Rogach and Ogris 2010;Yong et al. 2009). The first and foremost important feature is the long-term photostability of QD imaging probes, which opens the possibility of investigating the dynamics of cellular processes over time, such as continuously tracking cell migration, differentiation, and metastasis. In addition, QD emission wavelengths are size-tunable and extend from visible to near infrared (NIR) (650 nm to 950 nm), to take advantage of the improved tissue penetration depth and reduced background fluorescence at these wavelengths. For example, CdSe/ZnS QDs of approximately 2 nm in diameter produce a blue emission, while QDs approximately 7 nm in diameter emit red light. While fluorescence imaging is often limited by the poor transmission of visible light through biological tissue, there is a NIR optical window in most biological tissue that is suitable for deep tissue optical imaging, where only a few organic dyes emit brightly in this region and generally suffer from photobleaching. In contrast, the novel optical properties of QDs allow the synthesis of bright and stable fluorescent labels that emit in the near infra red spectrum by adjusting their size and composition.

Surface functionalization using peptides, proteins and antibodies, confers the ability of QDs to provide high biological compatibility and capacity to target and image tumors in living subjects through the rapid readout of fluorescence imaging. Moreover, QDs allow imaging of deeper tissues and is also used to image lymph nodes and blood vessels in tissues. A key property for *in vivo* imaging is the unusual QD Stokes shift (measured by the distance between excitation and emission peaks), which can be as large as 300-400nm depending on the wavelength of the excitation light, which can be used to further improve the detection sensitivity. Organic dye signals with a small stoke shift are often buried by strong tissue autofluorescene, whereas QD signal with large Stokes shift are clearly detectable above the background. Unlike traditional dyes which usually show a broad emission band, QDs exhibit narrow sharp emission peaks and broadband absorption, which are ideal for multiplexed multicolor imaging. QDs are thus able to increase the number of labels that can be used simultaneously in a single system. The effective brightness per probe particle is also superior with quantum dots as evidenced by their large molar absorption cross-sections which are a consequence of their nanometer size and composition. Different from "soft" organic nanoparticles (e.g., polymers, micelles, liposomes), inorganic nanomaterials with rigid cores usually show inefficient extravasation inside tumors. A number of reports suggest that QDs tend to stay within the tumor vasculatures without getting into the interstitial space or tumor cells, reducing the nonspecific tumor cell labeling in angiogenesis imaging (Liu and Peng 2010). The long term photostability and superior brightness of QDs make them appealing for live animal targeting and imaging. These properties have made QDs a topic of intensive interest in cancer biology, molecular imaging, and molecular profiling.

The ability to functionalize as well as control the surface of quantum dots with specific linkers and multi-functional molecules is critical for nanoparticle-based gene therapy. Currently, QDs are used both as a transfection vector as well as a fluorescence label in RNA interference research. Quantum dot conjugates have been successfully used for targeted silencing of bcr/abl gene by RNA interference in human myelogenous leukemia K562 cells (Zhao et al. 2010). In addition, Derfus et al., (2007) using PEGlyated quantum dot core as a scaffold, and conjugating siRNA and tumor-homing peptides (F3) to functional groups on the particle's surface found that the homing peptide was required for targeting internalization by tumor cells, and that siRNA cargo could be co-attached without affecting the function of the peptide (Derfus et al. 2007). Using an EGFP model system, the role of conjugation chemistry was also investigated, with siRNA attached to the particle by disulfide cross-linkers showing greater silencing efficiency than when attached by a non-reducible thioether linkage. Delivery of these F3/siRNA-QDs to EGFP-transfected HeLa cells and release from their endosomal entrapment led to significant knockdown of EGFP signal. By designing the siRNA sequence against a therapeutic target (e.g., oncogene) instead of EGFP, this technology may be ultimately adapted to simultaneously treat and image metastatic cancer. These nanoprobes could be used for both active and passive targeting. Therefore, in future research, QDs can be seen as multi-functional platforms focusing on targeted delivery, high transfection efficiency, and multi-modal imaging/tracking and treatment of cancer as shown in Figure 5.

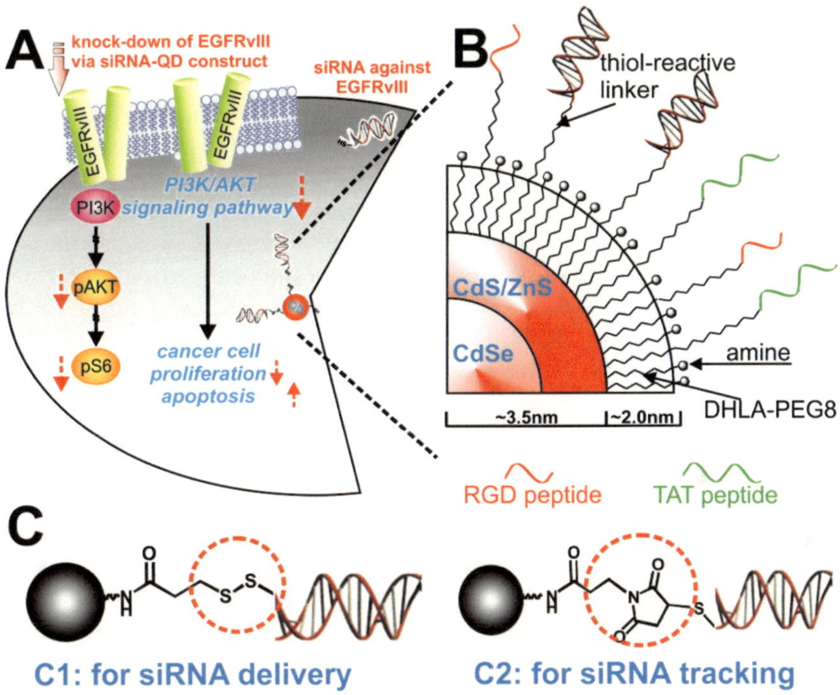

Fig. 5. (A): Quantum dots as a multi-functional nanoplatform to deliver siRNA and to elucidate of EGFR knockdown effect of PI3K signaling pathway in brain tumor cells. (B): Detailed structural information of multifunctional siRNA-QDs: CdSe as core with ZnS capping along with thiol reactive linker for siRNA conjugation as well as RGD peptides as shown in red and TAT peptides as shown in green. In order to make QD constructs water-soluble and suitable for conjugating with siRNA, hydrophobic ligands are displaced with a dihydrolipoic acid (DHLA) derivatized with an amine terminated polyethylene glycol (PEG) spacer. (C): Two different strategies for the siRNA-QD conjugate. (C1) Linker for attaching siRNA to QDs through a disulfide linkage which are easily reduced within the cells to release the siRNA. (C2) Linker for covalently conjugating siRNA to QDs which enable tracking of siRNA-QDs within the cells. (Taken from: Jung et al. 2010).

However, there have been some QD concentration dependent toxicity and distribution concerns. QDs have been shown to remain in liver, lymph nodes and bone marrow of mice for 1 month after tail injection, despite of its low affinity to cells and tissues (Ballou et al. 2004;Ballou et al. 2009). Recently, the hydrophilic QDs (diameter <10 nm) have attracted more attention for *in vivo* applications, due to the rapid renal clearance of QDs, minimizing the potential toxicity to the system (Park et al. 2009). Recently, Peng and co-workers developed InAs/InP/ZnSe core/shell/shell QDs with high quantum yield (76%) of NIR fluorescence, ultrasmall hydrodynamic sizes (< 10 nm), and the biocompatibility desired for *in vivo* applications (Liu and Peng 2010). These novel QDs have obviously lower intrinsic toxicity compared to commercial Cd-containing NIR emitting QDs and showed significantly improved circulation half-life with reduced RES uptake. NIR-emitting QDs demonstrate exceptional brightness and fluorescent quantum yields. Also, once capped with a chemically stable shell, QDs can exhibit remarkable photostability, providing continuous fluorescent singles for long-term imaging applications. Other types of novel QDs with entirely different compositions and photoluminescence mechanism such as silicon QDs and carbon dots have also emerged as potential probes in bioimaging applications. Further, typical fluorescence images of a single QD shows changes in emission intensity. The intensity time trace illustrates the random alternation between "on" and "off" states, which is known as blinking and it is a signature feature of an individual QD. Also, reducing size of QDs has proven difficult because of decreased colloidal stability and increased nonspecific interactions. Other major limitations include reproducibility in production, proper control of surface functionality, bulky surface coatings (PEG, multiple antibodies, ampiphilic molecules) which leads to restrictions on studying spatially confined, crowded regions of the cell and may also perturb the behavior of the labeled molecules. Quantum dots are not yet approved for use in humans and much more research is needed in future for this growing field.

5.2 Carbon nanotubes

Molecular imaging exploits the specific recognition of labeled probes to their biological targets in conventional imaging techniques to monitor biological processes at the molecular level with improved specificity and sensitivity. Conventional clinical cancer imaging techniques, such as X-ray, CT and MRI, do not possess sufficient spatial resolution for early detection of the disease. Positron emission tomography (PET) is a highly sensitive and accurate imaging technology that relies on changes in tissue biochemistry and metabolism. It is the most valuable means we have so far to identify early-stage alterations in molecular biology, often before there is any morphologic change. Nevertheless, fluoro-desoxy-glucose (FDG), the most commonly used PET tracer in clinical oncology (more than 95% of the molecular imaging procedures make use of FDG at present), is not a specific tracer for malignant diseases but for increased metabolism. Therefore, it is imperative to develop new tools for early cancer diagnosis.

CNTs have been explored in almost every single cancer treatment modality, including drug delivery, lymphatic targeted chemotherapy, thermal therapy, photodynamic therapy, and gene therapy. Based on their structure, CNTs can be classified into two general categories: single-walled (SWNTs), which consist of one layer of cylinder graphene (diameter 0.4-2 nm) and multi-walled (MWNTs), which contain several concentric graphene sheets (diameter 2-100 nm). CNTs have unique physical and chemical properties such as high aspect ratio, ultralight weight, high mechanical strength, high electrical conductivity, and high thermal conductivity (Ji et al. 2010). Carbon nanotubes are the strongest and stiffest materials yet discovered in terms of tensile strength and elastic modulus respectively. As CNTs are intrinsically not water soluble, modification through chemical functionalization can increases the solubility of carbon nanotubes in aqueous solutions.

Imaging functionalities and therapeutics can be incorporated on the same nanoparticle for multifunctional cancer imaging and treatment. SWNT-paclitaxel (PTX) conjugates also showed higher efficacy in suppressing tumor growth than clinical Taxol alone in a murine 4T1 breast cancer model, owing to prolonged blood circulation time and enhanced permeability and retention (EPR) in the tumor (Feazell et al. 2007). Besides, with very high surface area per unit weight, SWNTs provide higher capacity of drug loading, compared to that reported for conventional liposomes and dendrimer drug carriers. Doxorubicin, a commonly used cancer chemotherapy drug, can be loaded on the surface of PEGylated SWNTs with remarkably high loading, up to 4 g of drug per 1 g of nanotube, owing to the ultrahigh surface area of SWNTs. Further, the intrinsic stability and structural flexibility of CNTs may prolong the circulation time as well as improve the bioavailability of drug molecules conjugated to them. Surface-enhanced Raman spectroscopy of carbon nanotubes opens up a method of protein microarray with detection sensitivity down to 1 fmol/L. *In vitro* and *in vivo* toxicity studies reveal that highly water soluble and serum stable nanotubes are biocompatible, nontoxic, and potentially useful for biomedical applications. However, nonfunctionalized nanotubes are toxic to cells and animals and therefore one has to be cautious about the safety aspects of CNTs. If well functionalized, nanotubes may be excreted mainly through the biliary pathway in feces.

Carbon nanotube-based drug delivery has shown promise in various *in vitro* and *in vivo* experiments including delivery of small interfering RNA (siRNA), paclitaxel and doxorubicin (Liu et al. 2009). Multiwalled PEGylated carbon nanotubes are found to be successful, effective and do not alter particle sizes and zeta potentials of carbon nanotubes after PEGylation (Ilbasmis-Tamer et al. 2010). In addition, the propensity to absorb the body transparent NIR radiation also envisages photothermal and photoacoustic therapy using nanotubes.

5.3 Gold and other nanoparticles for cancer diagnosis

Thermal ablation therapy is one the most promising of methods in cancer treatment but is limited by incomplete tumor destruction and damage to adjacent normal tissues. Current radiofrequency ablation techniques require invasive needle placement and are limited by accuracy of targeting. Use of nanoparticles has refined noninvasive thermal ablation of tumors, and several nanomaterials have been used for this purpose. These include gold nanomaterials, iron nanoparticles, magnetic nanoparticles, carbon nanotubes and affisomes (thermosensitive liposomes). Heating of the particles can be induced by magnets, lasers, ultrasound, photodynamic therapy and low-power X-rays. The clinical trials include studies of designed nanoparticles such as the thermosensitive liposomal doxorubicin (Thermodox®) as a novel activated therapy using radiofrequency ablation (Wang and Thanou 2010). As gold nanoparticles have evolved other gold structures have also been suggested. Nanorods, with the appropriate PEG stealth layer, are being developed as an improved means of hyperthermia. By attaching monoclonal antibodies (mAbs), which can recognize a specific cancer cell, to gold nanoparticles or nanorods are also used in cancer detection. Gold nanoparticles conjugated to anti-epidermal growth factor receptor (El-Sayed et al. 2006) mAbs specifically and homogeneously bind to the surface of the cancer cells with 600% greater affinity than to the noncancerous cells. This specific and homogeneous binding is found to give a relatively sharper surface plasma resonance (Hinz et al. 2006) absorption band with a red shifted maximum compared to that observed when added to the noncancerous cells . Surface plasma resonance scattering imaging or SPR absorption spectroscopy generated from antibody conjugated gold nanoparticles may be useful in molecular biosensor techniques for the diagnosis and investigation of cancer cells *in vivo* and *in vitro*.

These inorganic nanoparticles represent a different class of nanoparticles that are usually much smaller, 5–40 nm and they do not have the flexibility observed in liposomes and polymeric nanoparticles. Inorganic nanoparticles have made their appearance in cancer therapy during the last decades in a number of applications. The main type of inorganic nanoparticles—the iron oxide nanoparticles, has been used for imaging tumor (Wang and Thanou 2010). The main advantage of magnetic nanoparticles is their ability to be visualised by Magnetic Resonance (MR) imaging. Additionally, iron oxide nanoparticles can be guided to target sites (i.e. tumor) using external magnetic field and they can be also heated to provide hypethermia for cancer therapy. Yu et al. reported thermally cross-linked superparamagnetic iron oxide nanoparticles that could carry a Cy5.5 near infra-red probe (dual imaging) and doxorubicin for the imaging and treatment of cancer. The nanoparticles substantially diminished tumor size and provided the proof of concept that they can combine several modalities for maximum antitumor effect (Yu et al. 2010). Magnetic nanoparticles have been used in the development of dual purpose probes for the *in vivo* transfection of siRNA. The iron nanoparticles deliver siRNA at the same time as imaging their own accumulation in tumor sites. Hence, multifunctional nanoparticles have emerged that are capable of cancer targeting and simultaneous cancer imaging and therapy.

Metal nanoshells are another class of nanoparticles with tunable optical resonances. Metal nanoshells consist of a spherical dielectric core nanoparticle, in this case silica, which is surrounded by a thin metal shell, such as gold. These particles possess a highly tunable plasmon resonance, a resonant phenomenon whereby light induces collective oscillations of conductive metal electrons at the nanoshell surface. Nanoshells derived from gold provide an attractive system for imaging applications owing to the established ease of preparation, chemical inertness, good biocompatibility, and surface functionalization. Further, nanoparticle based near infrared imaging (NIR) is steadily presenting itself as a powerful diagnostic technique with the real potential to serve as a minimally invasive, nonionizing method for sensitive, deep tissue diagnostic imaging that are not prone to the rapid photobleaching and instability of their organic counterparts. NIR laser treatment of the bulk tissue selectively heats and destroys the nanoshell-laden tumor regions within the tissue, while leaving surrounding tissue intact. Nanoshells are currently evaluated in a number of clinical settings after a 5-year period of intensive preclinical development. Such development of nanoshells included the combination of nanoshells with cancer antibodies. Anti-HER2 antibody conjugated onto nanoshells provides the potential of combining antibody therapy with imaging and hyperthermia. NIR dye-encapsulating nanoparticles also demonstrate improved optical performances compared to unencapsulated organic fluorophores. Specifically, the encapsulation shields the dye molecules from unfavorable environmental influences that normally hinder fluorescence signals, thereby enhancing quantum yields, emission brightness, and fluorescent lifetime. While, at present, these NIR nanoparticulates appear to be superior in terms of optical performances, they are marred by their heavy metal composition and high propensity for toxicity. It is therefore reasonable to be concerned about the ineffectual clearance and long-term accumulation in untargeted organs and tissues of these particulates for *in vivo* use.

6. Conclusion

With the understanding of the genetic origins of certain cancers, an entirely new approach to the treatment of this disease has evolved, employing nanoparticle-based gene therapy. Numerous nanoparticle based cancer gene therapy strategies are already in clinical trials. The key to the success of any new therapeutic is to maximize safety without compromising efficacy, which has led to growing interest in non-viral gene delivery systems (such as liposomes) over the viral gene delivery systems. Grafting biorecognition molecules (ligands, antibodies) onto the nanoparticles (i.e active targeting) aims to improve targeting by specific cell uptake and using hydrophilic polymer coating, PEG, which aims to further enhance biocompatibility. To overcome other challenges of gene therapy, such as escape from endosome and other nuclear and cytosolic barriers, next generation vectors are being designed with use of gene regulatory elements (promoters and enhancers) to restrict gene expression to specific cells, along with nuclear localization signal peptides for nuclear targeting.

There has been substantial interest in dual purpose nanoparticle based gene therapy for both diagnostic (imaging) and therapeutic purposes (drug/gene delivery). Newer technologies for cancer detection/diagnosis using metallic and semiconducting nanoparticles are also under intense investigation. These nanoparticles for *in vivo* application targeting cancer are amenable to different size structures and possess tunable properties. Quantum dots possess unique size- and composition- dependent optical and electrical properties. In addition to quantum dots, carbon nanotubes, paramagnetic nanoparticles, nanoshells and nanosomes represent just a few of these novel technologies, used for both diagnostic and delivery purposes.

The imminent research challenge facing investigators moving forward is the expansion of the knowledge and understanding of the chemical and physical properties associated with these nanoparticle systems toward the design of superior cancer therapy modalities that maximize efficiency of treatment, while maintaining a superior safety profile.

7. References

Aggarwal,S., Yadav,S. and Gupta,S. (2011) EGFR targeted PLGA nanoparticles using gemcitabine for treatment of pancreatic cancer. *J. Biomed. Nanotechnol.* 7, 137-138.

Alivisatos,P. (2004) The use of nanocrystals in biological detection. *Nat. Biotechnol.* 22, 47-52.

Ashihara,E. (2010) [RNA interference for cancer therapies]. *Gan To Kagaku Ryoho.* 37, 2033-2041.

Azad,N.S., Posadas,E.M., Kwitkowski,V.E., Steinberg,S.M., Jain,L., Annunziata,C.M., Minasian,L., Sarosy,G., Kotz,H.L., Premkumar,A., Cao,L., McNally,D., Chow,C., Chen,H.X., Wright,J.J., Figg,W.D. and Kohn,E.C. (2008) Combination targeted therapy with sorafenib and bevacizumab results in enhanced toxicity and antitumor activity. *J. Clin. Oncol.* 26, 3709-3714.

Azatian,A., Yu,H., Dai,W., Schneiders,F.I., Botelho,N.K. and Lord,R.V. (2009) Effectiveness of HSV-tk suicide gene therapy driven by the Grp78 stress-inducible promoter in esophagogastric junction and gastric adenocarcinomas. *J. Gastrointest. Surg.* 13, 1044-1051.

Ballou,B., Ernst,L.A., Andreko,S., Fitzpatrick,J.A., Lagerholm,B.C., Waggoner,A.S. and Bruchez,M.P. (2009) Imaging vasculature and lymphatic flow in mice using quantum dots. *Methods Mol. Biol.* 574, 63-74.

Ballou,B., Lagerholm,B.C., Ernst,L.A., Bruchez,M.P. and Waggoner,A.S. (2004) Noninvasive imaging of quantum dots in mice. *Bioconjug. Chem.* 15, 79-86.

Barron,L.G., Uyechi,L.S. and Szoka,F.C., Jr. (1999) Cationic lipids are essential for gene delivery mediated by intravenous administration of lipoplexes. *Gene Ther.* 6, 1179-1183.

Bell-McGuinn,K.M., Matthews,C.M., Ho,S.N., Barve,M., Gilbert,L., Penson,R.T., Lengyel,E., Palaparthy,R., Gilder,K., Vassos,A., McAuliffe,W., Weymer,S., Barton,J. and Schilder,R.J. (2011) A phase II, single-arm study of the anti-alpha5beta1 integrin antibody volociximab as monotherapy in patients with platinum-resistant advanced epithelial ovarian or primary peritoneal cancer. *Gynecol. Oncol.* [Epub ahead of print]-doi:10.1016/j.ygyno.2010.12.362.

Bhaumik,S. (2011) Advances in Imaging Gene-Directed Enzyme Prodrug Therapy. *Curr. Pharm. Biotechnol.* 12 (4):497-507.

Braasch,D.A. and Corey,D.R. (2002) Novel antisense and peptide nucleic acid strategies for controlling gene expression. *Biochemistry.* 41, 4503-4510.

Branca,M.A. (2005) Gene therapy: cursed or inching towards credibility? *Nat. Biotechnol.* 23, 519-521.

Campbell,I.G., Russell,S.E., Choong,D.Y., Montgomery,K.G., Ciavarella,M.L., Hooi,C.S., Cristiano,B.E., Pearson,R.B. and Phillips,W.A. (2004) Mutation of the PIK3CA gene in ovarian and breast cancer. *Cancer Res.* 64, 7678-7681.

Chan,W.C., Maxwell,D.J., Gao,X., Bailey,R.E., Han,M. and Nie,S. (2002) Luminescent quantum dots for multiplexed biological detection and imaging. *Curr. Opin. Biotechnol.* 13, 40-46.

Chen,Y., Bathula,S.R., Li,J. and Huang,L. (2010a) Multifunctional nanoparticles delivering small interfering RNA and doxorubicin overcome drug resistance in cancer. *J. Biol. Chem.* 285, 22639-22650.

Chen,Y.Z., Yao,X.L., Tabata,Y., Nakagawa,S. and Gao,J.Q. (2010b) Gene carriers and transfection systems used in the recombination of dendritic cells for effective cancer immunotherapy. *Clin. Dev. Immunol.* 2010, 565-643.

Choosakoonkriang,S., Lobo,B.A., Koe,G.S., Koe,J.G. and Middaugh,C.R. (2003) Biophysical characterization of PEI/DNA complexes. *J. Pharm. Sci.* 92, 1710-1722.

Conlin,A.K., Seidman,A.D., Bach,A., Lake,D., Dickler,M., D'Andrea,G., Traina,T., Danso,M., Brufsky,A.M., Saleh,M., Clawson,A. and Hudis,C.A. (2010) Phase II trial of weekly nanoparticle albumin-bound paclitaxel with carboplatin and trastuzumab as first-line therapy for women with HER2-overexpressing metastatic breast cancer. *Clin. Breast Cancer.* 10, 281-287.

Connor,J., Bannerji,R., Saito,S., Heston,W., Fair,W. and Gilboa,E. (1993) Regression of bladder tumors in mice treated with interleukin 2 gene-modified tumor cells. *J. Exp. Med.* 177, 1127-1134.

Derfus,A.M., Chen,A.A., Min,D.H., Ruoslahti,E. and Bhatia,S.N. (2007) Targeted quantum dot conjugates for siRNA delivery. *Bioconjug. Chem.* 18, 1391-1396.

Deshayes,S., Maurizot,V., Clochard,M.C., Baudin,C., Berthelot,T., Esnouf,S., Lairez,D., Moenner,M. and Deleris,G. (2011) "Click" Conjugation of Peptide on the Surface of Polymeric Nanoparticles for Targeting Tumor Angiogenesis. *Pharm. Res.*

Donkuru,M., Badea,I., Wettig,S., Verrall,R., Elsabahy,M. and Foldvari,M. (2010) Advancing nonviral gene delivery: lipid- and surfactant-based nanoparticle design strategies. *Nanomedicine. (Lond).* 5, 1103-1127.

Duncan,R., Ringsdorf,H. and Satchi-Fainaro,R. (2006) Polymer therapeutics--polymers as drugs, drug and protein conjugates and gene delivery systems: past, present and future opportunities. *J. Drug Target.* 14, 337-341.

Dutta,T., Jain,N.K., McMillan,N.A. and Parekh,H.S. (2010) Dendrimer nanocarriers as versatile vectors in gene delivery. *Nanomedicine.* 6, 25-34.

El-Aneed,A. (2004) An overview of current delivery systems in cancer gene therapy. *J. Control Release.* 94, 1-14.

El-Sayed,I.H., Huang,X. and El-Sayed,M.A. (2006) Selective laser photo-thermal therapy of epithelial carcinoma using anti-EGFR antibody conjugated gold nanoparticles. *Cancer Lett.* 239, 129-135.

Feazell,R.P., Nakayama-Ratchford,N., Dai,H. and Lippard,S.J. (2007) Soluble single-walled carbon nanotubes as longboat delivery systems for platinum(IV) anticancer drug design. *J. Am. Chem. Soc.* 129, 8438-8439.

Felgner,P.L., Gadek,T.R., Holm,M., Roman,R., Chan,H.W., Wenz,M., Northrop,J.P., Ringold,G.M. and Danielsen,M. (1987) Lipofection: a highly efficient, lipid-mediated DNA-transfection procedure. *Proc. Natl. Acad. Sci. U. S. A.* 84, 7413-7417.

Giatrellis,S., Nikolopoulos,G., Sideratou,Z. and Nounesis,G. (2009) Calorimetric study of the interaction of binary DMTAP/DOTAP cationic liposomes with plasmid DNA. *J. Liposome Res.* 19, 220-230.

Gibbons,J.J., Abraham,R.T. and Yu,K. (2009) Mammalian target of rapamycin: discovery of rapamycin reveals a signaling pathway important for normal and cancer cell growth. *Semin. Oncol.* 36 Suppl 3:S3-S17., S3-S17.

Godbey,W.T. and Mikos,A.G. (2001) Recent progress in gene delivery using non-viral transfer complexes. *J. Control Release.* 72, 115-125.

Gou,M., Wei,X., Men,K., Wang,B., Luo,F., Zhao,X., Wei,Y. and Qian,Z. (2011) PCL/PEG Copolymeric Nanoparticles: Potential Nanoplatforms for Anticancer Agent Delivery. *Curr. Drug Targets.* [Epub ahead of print].

Guo,W. and Lee,R.L. (1999) Receptor-targeted gene delivery via folate-conjugated polyethylenimine. *AAPS. PharmSci.* 1, E19.

Hainaut,P. and Hollstein,M. (2000) p53 and human cancer: the first ten thousand mutations. *Adv. Cancer Res.* 77, 81-137.

Hainaut,P. and Vahakangas,K. (1997) p53 as a sensor of carcinogenic exposures: mechanisms of p53 protein induction and lessons from p53 gene mutations. *Pathol. Biol. (Paris).* 45, 833-844.

Han,J., Lim,M. and Yeom,Y.I. (1999) Receptor-mediated gene transfer to cells of hepatic origin by galactosylated albumin-polylysine complexes. *Biol. Pharm. Bull.* 22, 836-840.

Harisinghani,M.G., Barentsz,J., Hahn,P.F., Deserno,W.M., Tabatabaei,S., van de Kaa,C.H., de la,R.J. and Weissleder,R. (2003) Noninvasive detection of clinically occult lymph-node metastases in prostate cancer. *N. Engl. J. Med.* 19;348, 2491-2499.

Heinrich,J., Schultz,J., Bosse,M., Ziegelin,G., Lanka,E. and Moelling,K. (2002) Linear closed mini DNA generated by the prokaryotic cleaving-joining enzyme TelN is functional in mammalian cells. *J. Mol. Med.* 80, 648-654.

Hesdorffer,C., Ayello,J., Ward,M., Kaubisch,A., Vahdat,L., Balmaceda,C., Garrett,T., Fetell,M., Reiss,R., Bank,A. and Antman,K. (1998) Phase I trial of retroviral-mediated transfer of the human MDR1 gene as marrow chemoprotection in patients undergoing high-dose chemotherapy and autologous stem-cell transplantation. *J. Clin. Oncol.* 16, 165-172.

Hinz,T., Buchholz,C.J., van der,S.T., Cichutek,K. and Kalinke,U. (2006) Manufacturing and quality control of cell-based tumor vaccines: a scientific and a regulatory perspective. *J. Immunother.* 29, 472-476.

Hong,M., Zhu,S., Jiang,Y., Tang,G., Sun,C., Fang,C., Shi,B. and Pei,Y. (2010) Novel anti-tumor strategy: PEG-hydroxycamptothecin conjugate loaded transferrin-PEG-nanoparticles. *J. Control Release.* 141, 22-29.

Hood,J.D., Bednarski,M., Frausto,R., Guccione,S., Reisfeld,R.A., Xiang,R. and Cheresh,D.A. (2002) Tumor regression by targeted gene delivery to the neovasculature. *Science.* 296, 2404-2407.

Ilbasmis-Tamer,S., Yilmaz,S., Banoglu,E. and Degim,I.T. (2010) Carbon nanotubes to deliver drug molecules. *J. Biomed. Nanotechnol.* 6, 20-27.

Immordino,M.L., Dosio,F. and Cattel,L. (2006) Stealth liposomes: review of the basic science, rationale, and clinical applications, existing and potential. *Int. J. Nanomedicine.* 1, 297-315.

Iqbal,S., Goldman,B., Fenoglio-Preiser,C.M., Lenz,H.J., Zhang,W., Danenberg,K.D., Shibata,S.I. and Blanke,C.D. (2011) Southwest Oncology Group study S0413: a phase II trial of lapatinib (GW572016) as first-line therapy in patients with advanced or metastatic gastric cancer. *Ann. Oncol.* [Epub ahead of print] doi:-10.1093/annonc/mdr021.

Javle,M.M., Shroff,R.T., Xiong,H., Varadhachary,G.A., Fogelman,D., Reddy,S.A., Davis,D., Zhang,Y., Wolff,R.A. and Abbruzzese,J.L. (2010) Inhibition of the mammalian target of rapamycin (mTOR) in advanced pancreatic cancer: results of two phase II studies. *BMC. Cancer.* 10:368., 368.

Jere,D., Jiang,H.L., Arote,R., Kim,Y.K., Choi,Y.J., Cho,M.H., Akaike,T. and Cho,C.S. (2009) Degradable polyethylenimines as DNA and small interfering RNA carriers. *Expert. Opin. Drug Deliv.* 6, 827-834.

Ji,S.R., Liu,C., Zhang,B., Yang,F., Xu,J., Long,J., Jin,C., Fu,D.L., Ni,Q.X. and Yu,X.J. (2010) Carbon nanotubes in cancer diagnosis and therapy. *Biochim. Biophys. Acta.* 1806, 29-35.

Jiang,N., Wang,J., Wang,Y., Yan,H. and Thomas,R.K. (2005) Microcalorimetric study on the interaction of dissymmetric gemini surfactants with DNA. *J. Colloid Interface Sci.* 284, 759-764.

Joerger,A.C., Ang,H.C. and Fersht,A.R. (2006) Structural basis for understanding oncogenic p53 mutations and designing rescue drugs. *Proc. Natl. Acad. Sci. U. S. A.* 103, 15056-15061.

Kaur,T., Slavcev,R.A. and Wettig,S.D. (2009) Addressing the challenge: current and future directions in ovarian cancer therapy. *Curr. Gene Ther.* 9, 434-458.

Kowalski,M., Entwistle,J., Cizeau,J., Niforos,D., Loewen,S., Chapman,W. and MacDonald,G.C. (2010) A Phase I study of an intravesically administered immunotoxin targeting EpCAM for the treatment of nonmuscle-invasive bladder cancer in BCGrefractory and BCG-intolerant patients. *Drug Des Devel. Ther.* 4:313-20., 313-320.

Kreuter,J., Alyautdin,R.N., Kharkevich,D.A. and Ivanov,A.A. (1995) Passage of peptides through the blood-brain barrier with colloidal polymer particles (nanoparticles). *Brain Res.* 674, 171-174.

Lai,M.D., Yen,M.C., Lin,C.M., Tu,C.F., Wang,C.C., Lin,P.S., Yang,H.J. and Lin,C.C. (2009) The effects of DNA formulation and administration route on cancer therapeutic efficacy with xenogenic EGFR DNA vaccine in a lung cancer animal model. *Genet. Vaccines. Ther.* 7, 2.

Lane,D.P. (1992) Cancer. p53, guardian of the genome. *Nature.* 358, 15-16.

Lauria,A., Tutone,M., Ippolito,M., Pantano,L. and Almerico,A.M. (2010) Molecular modeling approaches in the discovery of new drugs for anti-cancer therapy: the investigation of p53-MDM2 interaction and its inhibition by small molecules. *Curr. Med. Chem.* 17, 3142-3154.

Ledford,H. (2007) Death in gene therapy trial raises questions about private IRBs. *Nat. Biotechnol.* 25, 1067.

Lemieux,P., Vinogradov,S.V., Gebhart,C.L., Guerin,N., Paradis,G., Nguyen,H.K., Ochietti,B., Suzdaltseva,Y.G., Bartakova,E.V., Bronich,T.K., St-Pierre,Y., Alakhov,V.Y. and Kabanov,A.V. (2000) Block and graft copolymers and NanoGel copolymer networks for DNA delivery into cell. *J. Drug Target.* 8, 91-105.

Liang,Z.W., Guo,B.F., Li,Y., Li,X.J., Li,X., Zhao,L.J., Gao,L.F., Yu,H., Zhao,X.J., Zhang,L. and Yang,B.X. (2011) Plasmid-based Stat3 siRNA delivered by hydroxyapatite nanoparticles suppresses mouse prostate tumor growth in vivo. *Asian J. Androl.* [Epub ahead of print], doi:10.1038/aja.2010.167.

Liu,F. and Huang,L. (2002) Development of non-viral vectors for systemic gene delivery. *J. Control Release.* 78, 259-266.

Liu,Y., Miyoshi,H. and Nakamura,M. (2007) Nanomedicine for drug delivery and imaging: a promising avenue for cancer therapy and diagnosis using targeted functional nanoparticles. *Int. J. Cancer.* 120, 2527-2537.

Liu,Z. and Peng,R. (2010) Inorganic nanomaterials for tumor angiogenesis imaging. *Eur. J. Nucl. Med. Mol. Imaging.* 37 Suppl 1, S147-S163.

Liu,Z., Tabakman,S., Welsher,K. and Dai,H. (2009) Carbon Nanotubes in Biology and Medicine: In vitro and in vivo Detection, Imaging and Drug Delivery. *Nano. Res.* 2, 85-120.

Lowe,S.W., Bodis,S., McClatchey,A., Remington,L., Ruley,H.E., Fisher,D.E., Housman,D.E. and Jacks,T. (1994) p53 status and the efficacy of cancer therapy in vivo. *Science.* 266, 807-810.

Michalet,X., Pinaud,F.F., Bentolila,L.A., Tsay,J.M., Doose,S., Li,J.J., Sundaresan,G., Wu,A.M., Gambhir,S.S. and Weiss,S. (2005) Quantum dots for live cells, in vivo imaging, and diagnostics. *Science.* 307, 538-544.

Moore,N.M., Sheppard,C.L. and Sakiyama-Elbert,S.E. (2009) Characterization of a multifunctional PEG-based gene delivery system containing nuclear localization signals and endosomal escape peptides. *Acta Biomater.* 5, 854-864.

Morille,M., Passirani,C., Vonarbourg,A., Clavreul,A. and Benoit,J.P. (2008) Progress in developing cationic vectors for non-viral systemic gene therapy against cancer. *Biomaterials.* 29, 3477-3496.

Nabel,G.J., Nabel,E.G., Yang,Z.Y., Fox,B.A., Plautz,G.E., Gao,X., Huang,L., Shu,S., Gordon,D. and Chang,A.E. (1993) Direct gene transfer with DNA-liposome complexes in melanoma: expression, biologic activity, and lack of toxicity in humans. *Proc. Natl. Acad. Sci. U. S. A.* 90, 11307-11311.

Negishi,Y., Endo-Takahashi,Y., Suzuki,R., Maruyama,K. and Aramaki,Y. (2010) [Development of gene delivery system into skeletal muscles by bubble liposomes and ultrasound]. *Yakugaku Zasshi.* 130, 1489-1496.

Neves,S., Faneca,H., Bertin,S., Konopka,K., Duzgunes,N., Pierrefite-Carle,V., Simoes,S. and Pedroso de Lima,M.C. (2009) Transferrin lipoplex-mediated suicide gene therapy of oral squamous cell carcinoma in an immunocompetent murine model and mechanisms involved in the antitumoral response. *Cancer Gene Ther.* 16, 91-101.

Nihira,S. (2003) Development of HER2-specific humanized antibody Herceptin (trastuzumab). *Nippon Yakurigaku Zasshi.* 122, 504-514.

Ning,X., Sun,Z., Wang,Y., Zhou,J., Chen,S., Chen,D. and Zhang,H. (2011) Docetaxel plus trans-tracheal injection of adenoviral-mediated p53 versus docetaxel alone in patients with previously treated non-small-cell lung cancer. *Cancer Gene Ther.* [Epub ahead of print], doi:10.1038/cgt.2011.15.

Olivier,M., Eeles,R., Hollstein,M., Khan,M.A., Harris,C.C. and Hainaut,P. (2002) The IARC TP53 database: new online mutation analysis and recommendations to users. *Hum. Mutat.* 19, 607-614.

Olivier,M., Hollstein,M. and Hainaut,P. (2010) TP53 mutations in human cancers: origins, consequences, and clinical use. *Cold Spring Harb. Perspect. Biol.* 2, a001008.

Onion,D., Patel,P., Pineda,R.G., James,N. and Mautner,V. (2009) Antivector and tumor immune responses following adenovirus-directed enzyme prodrug therapy for the treatment of prostate cancer. *Hum. Gene Ther.* 20, 1249-1258.

Pack,D.W., Hoffman,A.S., Pun,S. and Stayton,P.S. (2005) Design and development of polymers for gene delivery. *Nat. Rev. Drug Discov.* 4, 581-593.

Park,J.H., Gu,L., von,M.G., Ruoslahti,E., Bhatia,S.N. and Sailor,M.J. (2009) Biodegradable luminescent porous silicon nanoparticles for in vivo applications. *Nat. Mater.* 8, 331-336.

Patil,S.D., Rhodes,D.G. and Burgess,D.J. (2005) DNA-based therapeutics and DNA delivery systems: a comprehensive review. *AAPS. J.* 7, E61-E77.

Pic,E., Pons,T., Bezdetnaya,L., Leroux,A., Guillemin,F., Dubertret,B. and Marchal,F. (2010) Fluorescence imaging and whole-body biodistribution of near-infrared-emitting quantum dots after subcutaneous injection for regional lymph node mapping in mice. *Mol. Imaging Biol.* 12, 394-405.

Pinaud,F., Clarke,S., Sittner,A. and Dahan,M. (2010) Probing cellular events, one quantum dot at a time. *Nat. Methods.* 7, 275-285.

Ravi,K.M., Hellermann,G., Lockey,R.F. and Mohapatra,S.S. (2004) Nanoparticle-mediated gene delivery: state of the art. *Expert. Opin. Biol. Ther.* 4, 1213-1224.

Rogach,A.L. and Ogris,M. (2010) Near-infrared-emitting semiconductor quantum dots for tumor imaging and targeting. *Curr. Opin. Mol. Ther.* 12, 331-339.

Rosenberg,S.A. (1999) A new era of cancer immunotherapy: converting theory to performance. *CA Cancer J. Clin.* 49, 70-3, 65.

Schakowski,F., Gorschluter,M., Buttgereit,P., Marten,A., Lilienfeld-Toal,M.V., Junghans,C., Schroff,M., Konig-Merediz,S.A., Ziske,C., Strehl,J., Sauerbruch,T., Wittig,B. and Schmidt-Wolf,I.G. (2007) Minimal size MIDGE vectors improve transgene expression in vivo. *In Vivo.* 21, 17-23.

Schakowski,F., Gorschluter,M., Junghans,C., Schroff,M., Buttgereit,P., Ziske,C., Schottker,B., Konig-Merediz,S.A., Sauerbruch,T., Wittig,B. and Schmidt-Wolf,I.G. (2001) A novel minimal-size vector (MIDGE) improves transgene expression in colon carcinoma cells and avoids transfection of undesired DNA. *Mol. Ther.* 3, 793-800.

Schatzlein,A.G. (2001) Non-viral vectors in cancer gene therapy: principles and progress. *Anticancer Drugs.* 12, 275-304.

Sinha,N. and Yeow,J.T. (2005) Carbon nanotubes for biomedical applications. *IEEE Trans. Nanobioscience.* 4, 180-195.

Stolberg,S.G. (1999) The biotech death of Jesse Gelsinger. *N. Y. Times Mag.* 136-150.

Sun,Y., Jurgovsky,K., Moller,P., Alijagic,S., Dorbic,T., Georgieva,J., Wittig,B. and Schadendorf,D. (1998) Vaccination with IL-12 gene-modified autologous melanoma cells: preclinical results and a first clinical phase I study. *Gene Ther.* 5, 481-490.

Thrall,J.H. (2004) Nanotechnology and medicine. *Radiology.* 230, 315-318.

Tros,d., I, Sun,Y. and Duzgunes,N. (2010) Gene delivery by lipoplexes and polyplexes. *Eur. J. Pharm. Sci.* 40, 159-170.

Tu,G., Xu,W., Huang,H. and Li,S. (2008) Progress in the development of matrix metalloproteinase inhibitors. *Curr. Med. Chem.* 15, 1388-1395.

van Vlerken,L.E., Vyas,T.K. and Amiji,M.M. (2007) Poly(ethylene glycol)-modified nanocarriers for tumor-targeted and intracellular delivery. *Pharm. Res.* 24, 1405-1414.

Vasey,P.A., Shulman,L.N., Campos,S., Davis,J., Gore,M., Johnston,S., Kirn,D.H., O'Neill,V., Siddiqui,N., Seiden,M.V. and Kaye,S.B. (2002) Phase I trial of intraperitoneal injection of the E1B-55-kd-gene-deleted adenovirus ONYX-015 (dl1520) given on days 1 through 5 every 3 weeks in patients with recurrent/refractory epithelial ovarian cancer. *J. Clin. Oncol.* 20, 1562-1569.

Vassilev,L.T. (2004) Small-molecule antagonists of p53-MDM2 binding: research tools and potential therapeutics. *Cell Cycle.* 3, 419-421.

Vega,F., Medeiros,L.J., Leventaki,V., Atwell,C., Cho-Vega,J.H., Tian,L., Claret,F.X. and Rassidakis,G.Z. (2006) Activation of mammalian target of rapamycin signaling pathway contributes to tumor cell survival in anaplastic lymphoma kinase-positive anaplastic large cell lymphoma. *Cancer Res.* 66, 6589-6597.

Vinogradov,S.V., Bronich,T.K. and Kabanov,A.V. (2002) Nanosized cationic hydrogels for drug delivery: preparation, properties and interactions with cells. *Adv. Drug Deliv. Rev.* 54, 135-147.

Vogt,A., Combadiere,B., Hadam,S., Stieler,K.M., Lademann,J., Schaefer,H., Autran,B., Sterry,W. and Blume-Peytavi,U. (2006) 40 nm, but not 750 or 1,500 nm, nanoparticles enter epidermal CD1a+ cells after transcutaneous application on human skin. *J. Invest Dermatol.* 126, 1316-1322.

Wagner,U., du,B.A., Pfisterer,J., Huober,J., Loibl,S., Luck,H.J., Sehouli,J., Gropp,M., Stahle,A., Schmalfeldt,B., Meier,W. and Jackisch,C. (2007) Gefitinib in combination with tamoxifen in patients with ovarian cancer refractory or resistant to platinum-taxane based therapy--a phase II trial of the AGO Ovarian Cancer Study Group (AGO-OVAR 2.6). *Gynecol. Oncol.* 105, 132-137.

Wang,H. and Wettig,S.D. (2011) Synthesis and aggregation properties of dissymmetric phytanyl-gemini surfactants for use as improved DNA transfection vectors. *Phys. Chem. Chem. Phys.* 13, 637-642.

Wang,M. and Thanou,M. (2010) Targeting nanoparticles to cancer. *Pharmacol. Res.* 62, 90-99.

Weiss,J.M., Subleski,J.J., Wigginton,J.M. and Wiltrout,R.H. (2007) Immunotherapy of cancer by IL-12-based cytokine combinations. *Expert. Opin. Biol. Ther.* 7, 1705-1721.

Wettig,S.D., Badea,I., Donkuru,M., Verrall,R.E. and Foldvari,M. (2007a) Structural and transfection properties of amine-substituted gemini surfactant-based nanoparticles. *J. Gene Med.* 9, 649-658.

Wettig,S.D. and Verrall,R.E. (2001) Thermodynamic Studies of Aqueous m-s-m Gemini Surfactant Systems. *J. Colloid Interface Sci.* 235, 310-316.

Wettig,S.D., Wang,C., Verrall,R.E. and Foldvari,M. (2007b) Thermodynamic and aggregation properties of aza- and imino-substituted gemini surfactants designed for gene delivery. *Phys. Chem. Chem. Phys.* 9, 871-877.

Whitmore,M., Li,S. and Huang,L. (1999) LPD lipopolyplex initiates a potent cytokine response and inhibits tumor growth. *Gene Ther.* 6, 1867-1875.

Wilson,R.F. (2010) The death of Jesse Gelsinger: new evidence of the influence of money and prestige in human research. *Am. J. Law Med.* 36, 295-325.

Wojtowicz-Praga,S. (1997) Reversal of tumor-induced immunosuppression: a new approach to cancer therapy. *J. Immunother.* 20, 165-177.

Xu,F., Li,S., Li,X.L., Guo,Y., Zou,B.Y., Xu,R., Liao,H., Zhao,H.Y., Zhang,Y., Guan,Z.Z. and Zhang,L. (2009) Phase I and biodistribution study of recombinant adenovirus vector-mediated herpes simplex virus thymidine kinase gene and ganciclovir administration in patients with head and neck cancer and other malignant tumors. *Cancer Gene Ther.* 16, 723-730.

Yarom,N. and Jonker,D.J. (2011) The role of the epidermal growth factor receptor in the mechanism and treatment of colorectal cancer. *Discov. Med.* 11, 95-105.

Yong,K.T., Hu,R., Roy,I., Ding,H., Vathy,L.A., Bergey,E.J., Mizuma,M., Maitra,A. and Prasad,P.N. (2009) Tumor targeting and imaging in live animals with functionalized semiconductor quantum rods. *ACS Appl. Mater. Interfaces.* 1, 710-719.

Young,L.S., Searle,P.F., Onion,D. and Mautner,V. (2006) Viral gene therapy strategies: from basic science to clinical application. *J. Pathol.* 208, 299-318.

Yu,M.K., Park,J., Jeong,Y.Y., Moon,W.K. and Jon,S. (2010) Integrin-targeting thermally cross-linked superparamagnetic iron oxide nanoparticles for combined cancer imaging and drug delivery. *Nanotechnology.* 21, 415102.

Zhao,Y., Zhao,L., Zhou,L., Zhi,Y., Xu,J., Wei,Z., Zhang,K.X., Ouellette,B.F. and Shen,H. (2010) Quantum dot conjugates for targeted silencing of bcr/abl gene by RNA interference in human myelogenous leukemia K562 cells. *J. Nanosci. Nanotechnol.* 10, 5137-5143.

23

Toxicogenomics of Nonviral Cationic Gene Delivery Nanosystems

Yadollah Omidi, Vala Kafil and Jaleh Barar
Research Center for Pharmaceutical Nanotechnology
Faculty of Pharmacy, Tabriz University of Medical Sciences, Tabriz
Iran

1. Introduction

To date, both viral and nonviral vectors have been exploited for delivery of gene-based therapies to target cells/tissues. Despite high efficiency of the viral vectors (e.g., retroviruses and adenoviruses), these vectors appear to be immunogenic and potentially harmful when used in clinical gene therapy protocols (Ferber, 2001b). Besides, the preparation and purification of the viral vectors appear to be laborious, cost-prohibitive and not amenable to industrial-scale manufacture. Nonviral vectors such as cationic lipids (CLs) and cationic polymers (CPs) have been categorized as advanced materials and their low immunogenicity, lack of pathogenicity, and ease of pharmacologic production continue to make them attractive alternatives to viral vectors (Medina-Kauwe et al., 2005). However, these vectors may also suffer from relatively low levels of gene transfer compared to viruses. Thus, the drive to advance these vectors continues resulting in considerable progresses in improved transfection efficiency. Nonviral vectors (in particular cationic gene delivery systems) are able to bind and enter the target cells, however they yield low gene expression. No substantial information is available on interactions of these vectors with cellular biomolecules. Since these medicaments tend to act at genomic levels, thus understanding the genomic impacts of the nonviral vectors may help develop more efficient gene delivery systems. Nonetheless, this needs recruitment of high throughput screening methodologies.

To date, exploitation of the "omics" concepts (e.g., genomics, proteomics and metabolomics) is going to change the face of pharmacotherapy towards significantly more advanced and efficient pharmaceuticals (e.g., gene based nanomedicines) with minimal adverse consequences (Aardema & MacGregor, 2002). Enormous efforts have also been devoted for application of the global gene expression profiling in pharmacologic and toxicological investigations. The gene expression profiling technology has been primarily exploited for identification of underlying mechanisms for toxicity of pharmaceuticals and their genomic signatures, by which the safety liabilities can be determined and manifestations of undesired genotoxicity can be prohibited (Suter et al., 2004; Yang et al., 2004).

This methodology can be successfully used for the discovery and development of any chemicals and pharmaceuticals including gene delivery nanosystems. The main focus of the current book chapter is to provide some useful information about "genocompatibility" and "toxicogenomics" of the nonviral vectors using global gene expression profiling techniques i.e. DNA microarray.

2. Gene therapy challenges and dilemmas

The principle of gene therapy possesses undeniable therapeutic advantages over the conventional therapeutic modalities that are basically dependent upon exploitation of small molecules or biological pharmaceuticals. These advantages are: 1) specific or selective treatment of diseased cells/tissue, 2) minimal adverse consequences, 3) correction of the genetic cause of a disease, and 4) long-term treatment after single application (Rubanyi, 2001). Basically, to silence/suppress a target gene or to correct a genetic defect, the gene-based therapeutics such as oligodeoxynuleutides (ODNs), plasmid DNA, ribozymes, DNAzymes or short interfering RNA (siRNA) need to be shuttled to the target site. Delivery of gene-based therapeutics has been also advanced by development and implementation of various strategies, including: biological (e.g., viral vectors), physical (e.g., microinjection and electroporation, gene gun, ultrasound, and hydrodynamic delivery), and chemical (e.g., non-viral vectors) approaches. However, gene transfer into various target cells still faces major obstacles including poor delivery efficiency, cellular toxicity, immunogenicity and oncogenicity, as well as short-term transgenic expression and poor expression levels.

The first clinical test of gene therapy was accomplished a decade ago with the transfer of the missing "adenosine deaminase" gene into lymphocytes isolated from patients with severe combined immune-deficiency syndrome (i.e., as ex-vivo gene therapy approach). However, despite the early promising prophecy on the high effectiveness of gene therapy, the existing clinical experience indicate insufficient therapeutic efficacy coupled with increasing safety concerns and ethical issues (Verma & Somia, 1997). In some cases, aptamer-based genomedicines (e.g., Pegaptanib sodium, Macugen™) have been successfully utilized for treatment of the age related macular degeneration (Barar et al., 2008). Gendicine™ is an adenoviral p53-based gene medicine that was approved by the Chinese FDA in 2003 for treatment of head and neck cancer, while Advexin™ (a similar gene therapy approach from Introgen) was turned down by the US FDA in 2008. In fact, the death of Jesse Gelsinger in a gene therapy experiment in 1999 imposed a significant setback to gene therapy research in the United States, however many scientists aimed to resolve problems associated with the gene therapy strategies. In 2006, an international group of scientists announced the successful use of gene therapy to treat two adult patients for a disease affecting myeloid cells (Ott et al., 2006). Also in 2007, the world's first gene therapy trial for inherited retinal disease was announced for treatment of Leber's congenital amaurosis which is a inherited blinding disease caused by mutations in the RPE65 gene (Maguire et al., 2008). It should be evoked that the performance and pathogenicity of viral vectors (e.g., retroviruses, lentiviruses, adenoviruses, and adeno-associated viruses) and nonviral vectors have been evaluated in animal models. Promising results form the basis for clinical trials to treat genetic disorders and acquired diseases, however vector development/advancement remains a seminal concern for improved gene therapy technologies (Verma & Weitzman, 2005). Fundamentally, an ideal gene delivery method should protect the transgene against degradation, transport the transgene into the cytoplasm and then nucleus of target cells with little undesired detrimental effects (Gao et al., 2007).

Results obtained from *in vitro* studies have revealed that treatment of cells with antisense oligonucleotides (As-ODNs) for a period of only a few hours can bestow the desired effects of As-ODNs, while animal experiments demand repeated administration through multiple injections for prolonged exposure to As-ODNs. Despite promising results of some in vivo studies with free As-ODNs, improved delivery systems are essential to increase the efficacy of As-ODNs and to reduce its amount and frequency of administration (Hughes et al., 2001). Successful delivery of desired genes are important for both *ex vivo*, where cells undergo gene therapy in culture prior to implantation into the patient, or *in vivo* gene therapy where nucleic acids are administered directly to the patient to attain the desired gene change. Preferably, in either approach, only the therapy-intended gene expression changes should occur. However, this is not always the case, for example viral vectors are known to be efficient delivery systems for nucleic acids but can also induce immunogenic responses (Audouy et al., 2002; Ferber, 2001a; Ferber, 2001b). Hence, several nonviral gene delivery nanosystems such as cationic polymer- or lipid-based formulations have been developed for nucleic acid delivery. These cationic nanostructures can readily condense DNA into complexes and form polyplexes/lipoplexes to be used for *ex vivo* and *in vivo* gene therapy.

Although the CPs/CLs can principally enhance the delivery and improve the biological end-point of genomic-therapeutics, they often exert cytotoxicity depending on delivery system and target cell/tissue (Pedroso de Lima et al., 2001). Thus, both transfection efficiency evaluation and safety assessment are essential for gene transfer with these gene therapy vectors. A number of factors may affect the efficacy and safety of nonviral vector-mediated gene transfer; in particular their structural properties and type of target cells and tissue. It should be noticed that as various target cells may display different responses, the transfection efficacy and safety of vectors should be carefully optimized upon types of target cells and target organs. Once transfection accomplished, specific attention should be given to the genotoxicity potentials of gene-based medicines. Surprisingly, no substantial information is available about the genomic signature of the cationic delivery systems. We have previously investigated the potential of the commercially available nonviral vectors (e.g., Polyamidoamine (PAMAM) dendrimers such as Polyfect™ (PF) and Superfect™ (SF)) and lipids (e.g., Lipofectin™ (LF) and Oligofectamine™ (OF)) on global gene expression within human epithelial A431 and A549 cells by exploiting the cDNA microarray technology (Barar et al., 2009; Omidi et al., 2003; Omidi et al., 2005a; Omidi et al., 2005b; Omidi et al., 2008). These investigations revealed occurrence of inadvertent nonspecific gene expression changes within target cells upon treatments with these cationic gene delivery nanosystems. These findings led us to screen series of lipid- or polymer-based non-viral vectors for their toxicogenomic and genomic toxicity potentials in target cells.

Fig. 1 represents schematic illustrations of polymer/lipid based micro/nano systems used for delivery of genes/drugs.

3. Cellular trafficking and toxicity of polycationic nanostructures

For achievement of an efficient systemic delivery of gene-based nanomedicines, various factors appear to play crucial role, including: 1) the physicochemical characteristics of the gene-based therapies, 2) the effects of biological environment, 3) the functionality of membranes and barriers, and 4) the biological impacts of cellular microenvironment.

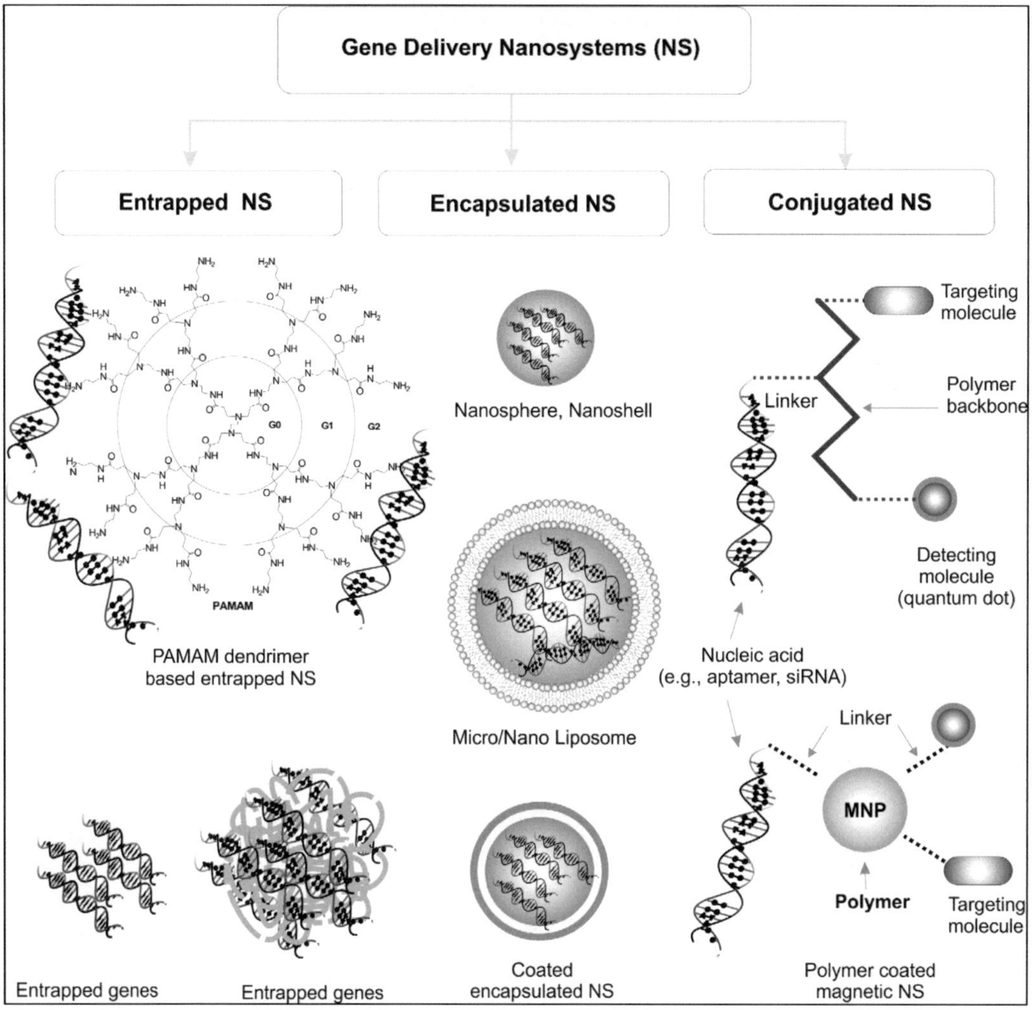

Fig. 1. Schematic representation of various polymer based gene delivery nanosystems. To prepare gene medicine nanosystems (NS) nucleic acids (e.g., antisense, siRNA, and aptamer) are generally entrapped, encapsulated or conjugated with polymers. Genes can be conjugated to magnetic nanoparticles (MNP) and quantum dots for concurrent detection and therapy.

Within the circulation system, blood cells, proteins, enzymes and serum components may bind to the genomedicines and cause instability and lowered transfection efficiency (Konopka et al., 2005). In addition, the circulating gene therapies must circumvent the immune system clearance and cross the capillary endothelial cells to reach the target cells/tissue. Once inside the target cells (normally via receptor-mediated endocytosis pathway), the genomedicine must overcome the subcellular and/or biomolecular impacts. In fact, the amphipathic sheet like lipid bilayer architecture of the biological membranes along with the integrated proteins separate cells from their environment and form the boundaries of different organelles inside the cells, at which exchange of materials among the different parts of a cell is controlled (Omidi & Gumbleton, 2005). Nonviral vectors may bind to cells by means of one or both of two types of cell binding interaction machineries, i.e. receptor and non-receptor mediated bindings (Medina-Kauwe et al., 2005). At cellular level, trafficking of the gene-based nanomedicines is basically performed through vesicular transportation pathways, in which they may engineer their own escape from demise in the lysosome. Endocytosis of macromolecular nanomedicines occurs through various cellular pathways, including clathrin coated pits, caveolae membranes and lipid rafts (Conner & Schmid, 2003; Spang, 2008). More likely, these complexes enter cells through nonspecific exploitation of these endocytic machineries, presumably mainly involving clathrin-mediated endocytic pathway. This route initiates and stabilizes membrane curvature formation, in which the adaptor proteins bind to clathrin pits and augment the inward pull of the membrane towards the cytoplasm leading to vesicle formation (Young, 2007).

It has been evidenced that the N-1(-(2,3-dioleoyloxy)propyl)-N,N,N-trimethylammoniummethylsulphate (DOTAP) lipoplexes are internalized by cells solely via clathrin-mediated endocytosis, however PEI polyplexes were shown to be internalized both by clathrin-mediated and caveolae-mediated endocytosis (Rejman et al., 2005). Once inside the cytoplasm, DNA is released from vesicular compartment upon physicochemical properties of the genomedicine. The endosomal escape of DNA at an early stage of endocytosis is deemed to be critical for cytosolic DNA delivery and determination of overall transfection efficiency. Among CPs and CLs, fusogenic lipid dioleoylphosphatidylethanolamine (DOPE) as a helper lipid for liposome-based DNA delivery were reported to induce membrane fusion between the endosome and the liposome and result in membrane destabilization and release of DNA into the cytoplasm (Farhood et al., 1995). Such destabilization of the vesicular membrane further highlights the interaction of cationic lipids with cellular compartments. This inadvertent nonspecific interaction may be exacerbated for *in vivo* systemic gene, which requires high and potentially toxic doses of nonviral vectors. Utilization of the cell-specific ligands or antibodies were reported to lower the cytotoxicity, while facilitating tissue targeting (Rawat et al., 2007), in which the ligand choice is largely dictated by whether or not the target receptor undergoes vesicular trafficking and the endocytic pathway used by the vector is dependent upon the targeting ligand as well as cell type. The structural architecture of the gene delivery nanosystems was shown to be important from gene expression changes viewpoints (Omidi et al., 2005b), which is also largely dependent upon cell type, in particular the membrane lipid composition and membrane phase state (Kabanov, 2006). Adsorption of polycations such as poly(N -ethyl-4-vinylpyridinium) salts (PEVP) in liposomic biomembranes was shown to induce flip-flop of negatively charged lipids (e.g., cardiolipin, phosphatidylserine, and phosphatidic acid) from the inner to the outer leaflet of the liquid liposomal membrane, but not in solid membranes (Yaroslavov et al., 1994; Yaroslavov et al., 2006). Among polycations, starburst PAMAM dendrimers and PEI appeared to elicit the most dramatic increase in membrane permeability by interacting the membranous biomolecules and forming holes in lipid membranes (Hong et al., 2006; Leroueil et al., 2007). Such structures could function as gates, through which the lipid molecules can be transported across the biomembranes (Kabanov, 2006). Fig. 2 represents cytotoxicity of linear and branched PEI in A431 cells (Kafil & Omidi, 2011).

Upon differences in cell types, the polyions can bind to the cellular compartments and accordingly induce compartmentalization within certain areas of the membranes and inadvertently trigger various signaling paths. Furthermore, nanoscaled defects were shown to be induced by PAMAM dendrimers through removing lipid from the fluid domains at a significantly greater rate than for the gel domains (Erickson et al., 2008). This reinforces a possibility of compartmentalization of synthetic polymers within different membrane domains as well as a differential effect of polymers on functional systems in the membranes that consecutively provoke inadvertent cytoplasmic/nucleic consequences directly and indirectly via secondary messengers such as G proteins.

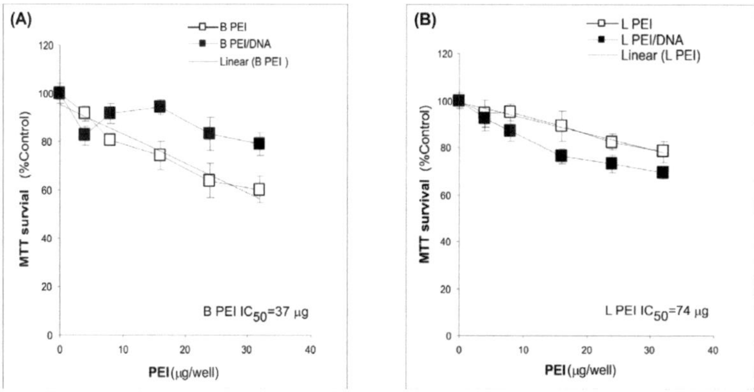

Fig. 2. Cytotoxicity of polyethylenimine (25 kDa) polymers in A431 cells evaluated by MTT assay. A) Cytotoxicity of B PEI with IC_{50}=37 µg. B) Cytotoxicity of LPEI with IC_{50}=74 µg. BPEI: Branched polyethylenimine; LPEI: linear polyethylenimine; adapted with permission from (Kafil & Omidi, 2011).

Fischer et al. (2003) monitored cytotoxicity of various polycationic gene delivery systems in L929 mouse fibroblasts using MTT assay and the release of the cytosolic enzyme lactate dehydrogenase (LDH). They showed a pattern for cellular toxicity as follow, poly(ethylenimine)=poly(L-lysine)>poly(diallyl-dimethyl-ammonium chloride)>diethylaminoethyl-dextran>poly(vinyl pyridinium bromide)>Starburst dendrimer>cationized albumin>native albumin. These researchers, interestingly, confirmed the molecular weight and the cationic charge density of the polycations as key parameters for the interaction with the cell membranes and accordingly the cell damage (Fischer et al., 2003). Besides, interaction of dendrimers with erythrocyte membrane proteins was shown to trigger echinocytosis (Domanski et al., 2004), while the cationic liposomes are less cytotoxic than dendrimers. The toxicity by CLs appeared to be dependent upon the type of cationic lipid macromolecule, concentration, molecular weight and the presence of DNA, where complexation of the polycations with DNA resulted in reduced tissue damage. However, Gebhart et al. (2001) showed increased cytotoxicity in the cos-7 cells upon complexation of various polymers with DNA (Gebhart & Kabanov, 2001).

Filion et al. (1997) have performed an important body of work by evaluating the toxicity of liposomes, formulated with various cationic lipids, towards murine macrophages and T lymphocytes and the human monocyte-like U937 cell line. They reported occurrence of pronounced toxicity by cationic liposomes formulated from DOPE and cationic lipids based on diacyltrimethylammonium propane (dioleoyl-, dimyristoyl-, dipalmitoyl-, disteroyl-: DOTAP, DMTAP, DPTAP, DSTAP) or dimethyldioctadecylammonium bromide (DDAB) in the phagocytic cells (macrophages and U937 cells), but not within non-phagocytic T lymphocytes. They also showed the rank order of toxicity as follows: DOPE/DDAB > DOPE/DOTAP > DOPE/DMTAP > DOPE/DPTAP > DOPE/DSTAP.

Once complexed with nucleic acid (e.g., antisense oligonucleotide or plasmid vector), lipoplexes revealed marginally reduced toxicity towards macrophages (Filion & Phillips, 1997b). Furthermore, since cationic lipids display intrinsic anti-inflammatory activity, they should be cautiously utilized as a gene delivery system to transfer nucleic acids for gene therapy *in vivo*.

DNA microarray technology has advanced and accelerated the identification process for mechanistic toxicology to illuminate genomic aspects of toxicology that could consequently postulate early effect within targets cells/tissues upon exposure to the toxicants (de et al., 2004). Recently, an interesting study was performed to compare different commercially available cationic liposome–DNA lipoplexes (Masotti et al., 2009), and it was reported that the lipoplex size and cationic lipid to DNA ratio are the two main parameters affecting the transfection efficiency of lipoplexes. The lipofection efficiency was determined mainly by lipoplex size, but not by the extent of lipoplex–cell interactions including binding, uptake or fusion. In the presence or absence of serum, lipoplex size was found to be a major factor determining lipofection efficiency. These researchers concluded that, by controlling lipoplex size, an efficient lipid delivery system may be achieved for *in vitro* and *in vivo* gene therapy.

Florea et al. (2002) evaluated PEIs with different molecular weights for their efficiency in transfecting undifferentiated COS-1 and well-differentiated human submucosal airway epithelial Calu-3 cells and showed that transfection efficiency was dependent upon the cell types, but not molecular weights. These researchers reported that gene transfer by PEI was 3 orders of magnitude more effective in COS-1 than in Calu-3 cells, perhaps because of secretion of mucins by Calu-3 cells (Florea et al., 2002). However, the larger molecular weights of PEI were also shown to yield the highest transfection efficiency in EA.hy 926 cell line derived from a fusion of the human A549 cell line with human umbilical vein endothelial cells, HUVEC (Godbey et al., 2001). Two types of cytotoxicities in process of PEI -mediated cell transfection have been reported: 1) an immediate toxicity associated with free PEI, 2) a delayed toxicity associated with cellular processing of PEI/DNA complexes (Godbey et al., 1999; Godbey et al., 2001). The immediate toxicity seems to occur upon interaction of the free PEIs with negatively charged serum proteins (e.g., albumin) and red blood cells (cytotoxic effects), while the delayed toxicity by PEI/DNA complex appeared to be closely related to the release of DNA (genomic effects). In cell culture, free PEI interacts with cellular components and inhibits normal cellular process. It causes several changes to cells, which include cell shrinking, reduced number of mitoses and vacuolization of the cytoplasm. We have observed significant genotoxicity impacts induced by PEI in A431 cells (Kafil & Omidi, 2011) and xenografted mice (our unpublished data).

Toxicity impacts of nanostructured materials have been recently reviewed (Nel et al., 2006), while many aspects of this issue (in particular at genomics/protemics levels) still remains unresolved. As a result, necessity of analysis of toxicogenomics of the nanoscaled advanced biomaterials is very clear. It will direct us towards development of safe pharmaceutical formulations with maximal efficiency and wide therapeutic index yet displaying minimal toxicity profiles since the conventional assessment of toxicity solely provide preliminary information with little devotion to the global genomic/proteomic impacts (Hollins et al., 2007; Kabanov et al., 2005; Kabanov, 2006; Omidi et al., 2005a). If this is the case, then the gene and drug delivery paradigms are going to stumble upon new era to deal with "functionalized excipients".

4. Genocompatibility and toxicogenomics of polycationic nanostructures

To pursue the genomic impacts of any gene based medicine, it is necessary to exploit high throughput screening methodologies (e.g., DNA microarray) for evaluation of global gene changes induced by the gene medicine or any other chemicals/compounds. Such genome based impact could be termed as "genotoxicity" or "toxicogenomics".

The DNA microarray technology combines standard molecular techniques with high-throughput screening to monitor the expression of up to ~40000 genes, which may provide a means for toxicity prediction prior to classical toxicological endpoints such as histopathology or clinical chemistry (Goldsmith & Dhanasekaran, 2004). In gene silencing experiments, such approach may allow a genomic characterization of delivery systems leading to identification of possible incompatibilities with intended target genes or biological effects of the gene based medicine. This may allow screening of compatible or useful delivery systems early in drug development that could subsequently save time and money in pre-clinical and clinical studies (Fielden & Kolaja, 2006; Lettieri, 2006).

Cytotoxicity and genotoxicity potentials of CPs and CLs are going to be well acknowledged, and accordingly these cationic nanosystems should undergo a rigorous genocompatibility evaluation prior to *in vitro* and *in vivo* exploitation (Kabanov, 2006; Omidi et al., 2005a). These systems alone or in combination with biologically active molecules (e.g., siRNA, antisense, aptamer) are able to alter cell signaling and biological responses in cells and organisms, emerging a cluster of genomic and post genomic consequences. In general, toxic responses to these kinds of nanomaterials are deemed to be very profound, in which various signaling pathways such as oxidative stress, immune responses and apoptosis pathways may be involved in response to generation of reactive oxygen species in the membranes (Kabanov, 2006). Cationic liposomes, irrespective of complexation with DNA, can downregulate the synthesis of pro-inflammatory mediators such as nitric oxide (NO) and tumor necrosis factor-alpha (TNF-alpha) in lipopolysaccharide (LPS)/interferon-gamma (IFN-gamma)-activated macrophages (Filion & Phillips, 1997a; Filion & Phillips, 1997b). Under the oxidative stress, cells may undergo the Nrf-2 signaling or the pro-inflammatory signaling cascades such as mitogen-activated protein kinase (MAPK) and nuclear factor kB (NFkB) cascades and eventually a programmed cell death may occur (Kabanov, 2006). Certain proteins such as protein kinase C (PKC) may also be affected detrimentally by cationic amphiphiles (Aberle et al., 1998), which function as PKC inhibitors and may inevitably result in inadvertent toxicity. It seems that the cationic amphiphiles with steroid backbones can exert more potent inhibitors of PKC than their straight-chain analogues, resulting in greater toxic impacts (Bottega & Epand, 1992). Polycations such as PEI formulated with plasmid DNA and administered to mouse lungs was reported to activate the p38 pathway involved in endocytosis, phagocytosis and hydrogen peroxide production. The observed *in vitro* and *in vivo* toxicity of such PEI polyplex formulations appeared to link to a general stress reaction, inflammatory responses, cell cycle regulation and DNA damage repair (Regnstrom et al., 2006). To obtain a complete image, it is essential to recruit high throughput screening methods such as DNA microarray.

5. DNA microarray technology

Practically, in the exploring stage, the expression of ~40,000 gene spots and replicates can be simultaneously analyzed on a couple of glass array in a single experiment by means of microarray technology. However, for accomplishment of a significant correlation between the gene expression profiles and their functionality expression, it is important to implement substantial complementary investigations to verify the results at the molecular level and as a result extend our understanding of gene expression patterns and molecular pathways.

Microarray technology can be exploited to attain a wealth of data that can be used to develop a more complete understanding of gene expression, which can be used for transcriptional regulation and interactions as well as functional genomics. Despite its successful *in vitro* cell-based implementation, application of this technology for *in vivo* investigations is deemed to be more sophisticated because of complexity of cytotoxicity and genotoxicity studies, which can be confounded by a number of variables such as type of target organ, effect of pharmacokinetics and/or pharmacodynamics parameters (Lobenhofer et al., 2001). Since its advent and application in life sciences, microarray has been widely applied for molecular/biological studies. In fact, a large number of indexed articles in various data banks (e.g., MEDLINE/PubMed) highlight the importance of microarray technology in post-genomics era.

Fig. 3 shows a schematic illustration of step-wise processes of the DNA microarray technology.

Technically, DNA microarray can be generated in two different types including printing pre-synthesized cDNAs (500–2000 bp) or synthesizing short oligonucleotides (20–50 bases) onto glass microscope slides, in which gene spots include either fully sequenced genes of known function or collections of partially sequenced cDNA derived from expressed sequence tags (ESTs) corresponding to the messenger RNAs of unknown genes. For example in practice, one may compare two different cells/tissues from untreated (UT) versus treated (T). For gene expression profiling, normally total RNA is extracted from the untreated and treated samples. Using an indirect labeling methodology, they are converted to labeled cDNA (e.g., with aminoallyle-dUTP). The aminoallyle-dUTP-cDNA is then labeled with cyanine dye (e.g., Cy3 or Cy5). The Cy3 and Cy5 labeled aminoallyle-dUTP-cDNA from UT and T samples are hybridized on a single glass array, which is subjected to several washing steps, scanning with an appropriate scanner (e.g., using RS Reloaded™, TECAN, Switzerland) and data mining (e.g., using GeneMath™ software; Applied Maths, Sint-Martens-Lathem, Belgium); for detailed information reader is directed to see (Hegde et al., 2000; Omidi et al., 2005b; Omidi et al., 2008).

For microarray analysis, significantly upregulated and/or downregulated genes can be identified using traditional method (gene expression changes with a fixed cutoff threshold usually in 2 fold) to infer significance differences (i.e., the so called "fold change method"). The resultant data are normally presented as scatter plots of treated (T) versus untreated (UT) control. To reach this stage, data need to undergo a number of processes called as "transformation" and "normalization" to minimize the experimental erroneousness (i.e., the so called "data mining"). Since a scatter plot of T versus UT genes would cluster along a straight line, normalization of this type of data is equivalent to calculating the best-fit slope using regression techniques and adjusting the intensities so that the calculated slope is one. In many experiments, the intensities are nonlinear, and local regression techniques are more suitable, such as Locally WEighted Scatterplot Smoothing (LOWESS) regression (Berger et al., 2004; Chen et al., 2003).

In our studies, we have successfully exploited both approaches to study the impacts of the nonviral vectors (CPs and CLs based formulation) on global gene expression experiments. To get the significant alterations in gene expression, we rejected the arrays showing non-

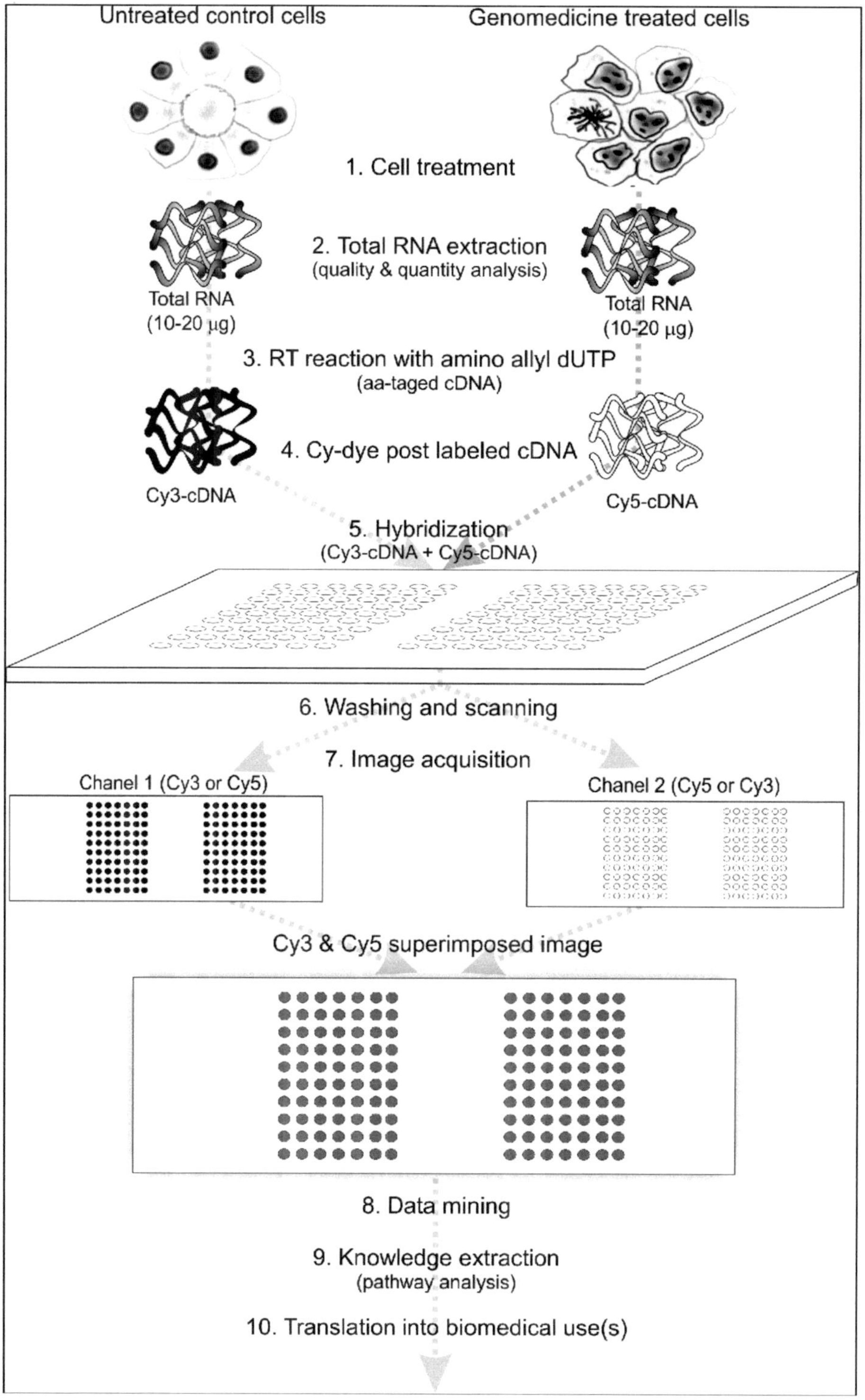

Fig. 3. Schematic illustration of step-wise process of DNA microarray methodology.

equal intensity or variable intensity of control gene spots in replicates on the same slide or between slides in dye-flipping experiments (Hollins et al., 2007; Omidi et al., 2003; Omidi et al., 2005b; Omidi et al., 2008). Data for each gene were typically reported as an "expression ratio" or as the base 2 logarithm (log_2) of the expression ratio of T to UT control. Genes were assumed to be up regulated or downregulated if they revealed an expression ratio of >2 and <0.5 (or >1 and <-1 for log_2 transformed data), respectively.

Based on our findings, the starburst PAMAM dendrimer alone or as complexed with DNA can elicit inadvertent gene expression changes. We also found that the linear and branched PEI (25 kDa) are able to induce gene expression changes in A431 cells, as shown in Fig. 4 (our unpublished data).

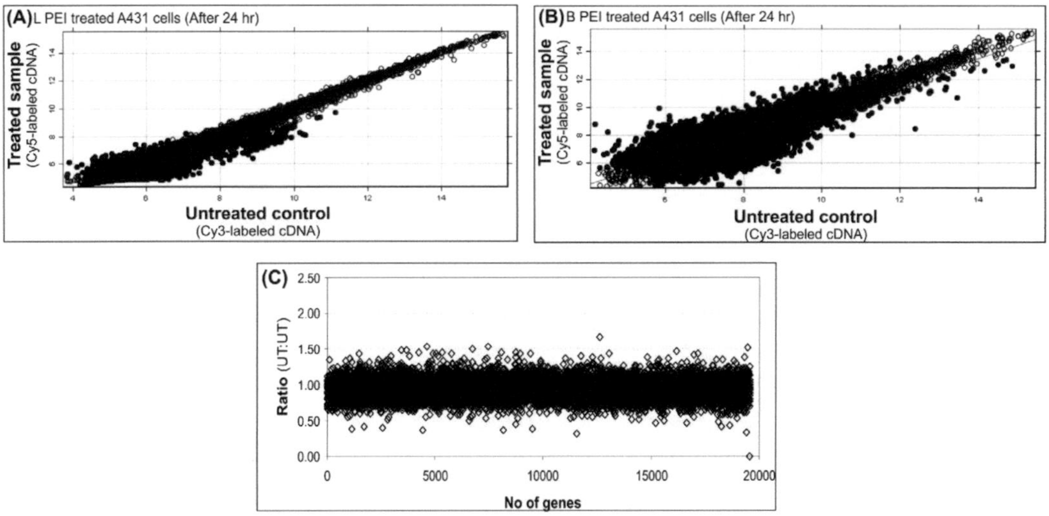

Fig. 4. Scatter plots of gene expression changes induced by cationic linear (A) and branched (B) PEI (25 kDa) in A431 cells. Data represent Log2 transformed gene expression values for large arrays housing 20000 genes. Above 2-fold change in expression of treated to untreated is indicated by bold circles and unchanged genes by unfilled circles. Panel C represents gene expression changes ratio between untreated A431 cells from different experiment. BPEI: branched polyethylenimine; LPEI: linear polyethylenimine (our unpublished data produced by Omidi et al.).

In the case of arrays with thousands of spots, one needs to employ the "feature reduction" or "dimension reduction" to find the minimum number of the features (i.e., genes or maybe even the conditions) that can best describe the data and the classification using statistical methods such as principal component analysis (PCA), correspondence analysis (CA), multi-dimensional scaling (MDS), and cluster analysis, reader is directed to see the following citation (Hegde et al., 2000; Quackenbush, 2001; Quackenbush, 2002). Of the dimension reduction methods, PCA is the most widely used method as a tool in exploratory data analysis, which involves a mathematical procedure that transforms a number of possibly correlated variables into a smaller number of uncorrelated variables called principal components. PCA ignores the dimensions in which data do not vary significantly and it is closely related to factor analysis.

6. Pathway analysis for functional genomics and gene ontology

To understand the functions of the genomic changes, one needs to implement appropriate methods on knowledge extraction from DNA microarray data. Such aim can be performed by means of "pathway analysis" (PA), which should be towards functional enrichment for establishing networks between genes. In fact, understanding the expression dynamics of gene networks helps us infer innate complexities and phenomenological networks among genes. Likewise, studying the regulation patterns of genes in groups, using clustering and classification methods may help us understand different pathways in the cell, their functions, regulations and the way one component in the system affects the other one. For pathway analysis, one of the most widely used methods is comparing the gene list to a pathway which gives a p value as a result. Basically, such scoring enrichment methods compare a list of the genes to that of a pathway and count the hits, so that the greater the number of the hits, the greater the score and the enrichment (Curtis et al., 2005). GenMAPP is an open source package that allows users to visualize microarray and proteomics data in the context of biological pathways (freely available at http://www.genmapp.org/). It represents biological pathways in a special file format called 'MAPPs' which are independent of the gene expression data. It is used to group genes by any organizing principle (e.g., apoptosis pathways). In addition, the gene set enrichment analysis (GSEA) is a novel method that uses all the data on the microarray in the order of expression, determining whether a priori defined set of genes shows statistically significant, concordant differences between two biological states such as phenotypes (Subramanian et al., 2005). In 2003, Hosack et al. developed a powerful software named, "the Expression Analysis Systematic Explorer" (EASE), which is customizable software for rapid biological interpretation of gene lists resulted by "omics" technology such as toxicogenomics, proteomics, or other high-throughput genomic data, in particular DNA microarray gene expression profiles. In fact, the biological themes returned by EASE recapitulate manually determined themes in previously published gene lists and are robust to varying methods of normalization, intensity calculation and statistical selection of genes (Hosack et al., 2003). We have largely exploited EASE to rapidly searching the Genbank in order to find the functional 'themes' in our microarray experiments. We have found various functional themes for the upregulated or downregulated genes induced by CLs in human epithelial cells, mainly: signal transducer activity, catalytic activity, response to external stimulus, cell growth and/or maintenance, cell cycle, response to biotic stimulus, regulation of programmed cell death, humoral immune response, cellular defense response, positive regulation of biosynthesis, negative regulation of cell proliferation, regulation of interferon-gamma biosynthesis, transcription factor binding, DNA repair, regulation of nucleocytoplasmic transport, apoptosis, apoptosis inhibitor activity, positive regulation of apoptosis, nuclease activity, transcriptional elongation regulator activity, regulation of caspase activation, response to oxidative stress, DNA damage response, and cell-mediated immune response (Omidi et al., 2005a).

As a secondary goal of array experiments it necessitates to look for groups of genes that behave similarly across a series of treatments (i.e. clustering analysis). There are a number of methodologies for clustering that can be employed upon experimental and statistical objectives; for clustering methods see citations (Azuaje, 2003; Sturn et al., 2002; Yang et al., 2001). In our studies on toxicogenomics of gene delivery systems, we have used softwares such as GeneSight™ or GeneMath™gene expression to present data as a single linkage

Hierarchical clustering plot. The algorithm used subjects the expression intensity ratio of treated versus untreated samples to single-linkage Hierarchical clustering (by means of Euclidean distance metric) analyses in order to arrange each gene with its related group members exhibiting a similar ratio of change in expression. We have shown that some overexpressed - or underexpressed genes display not only a similar pattern of expression but also a related cellular functionality and themes (e.g. apoptotic related genes) (Omidi et al., 2003; Omidi et al., 2005a). Such Hierarchical clustering maybe considered as a "genomic signature" of any chemical.

Taken all these facts together, surprisingly, still little information is available upon specific genomic effects elicited by chemicals within various cells/tissues despite implementing the "omics" technology for discovery of intrinsic genomic signature of chemicals/compounds in various targets. As a result, extensive investigations are yet to be performed to get sufficient information on genetic-signature of chemical and pharmaceuticals in target cells/tissues. Accordingly, many individuals and some organizations have attempted to accomplish such aim. For example, the Comparative Toxicogenomics Database (CTD) is a useful platform providing insights into complex chemical-gene and protein interaction networks (http://ctd.mdibl.org/about) that can be used for successfully advancement of novel pharmaceuticals.

7. Genomic impacts of cationic lipids

To date, cationic lipids have been the most widely used delivery system for delivery of nucleic acids both *in vitro* and *in vivo*. For example, Lipofectin™ is the 1:1 mixture of DOTMA and DOPE. It is the first cationic lipid formulation that was received widespread attention. We found that cationic liposomes such as LF and OF, at concentrations routinely used to obtain efficient delivery of gene based medicines, were able to induce gene expression changes in human epithelial A431 cells (Table 1). Such alterations in gene expressions appeared to be largely dependent upon the physicochemical characteristics of the lipid, wherein OF elicited greater gene expression than LF, i.e., up to 16% of the genes studied (Omidi et al., 2003). We speculate that the surface charge may play a key role in terms of such genotoxicity. In these cells, we witnessed that the affected genes were functionally involved in various cellular processes such as cell proliferation, differentiation and apoptosis. The upregulated or downregulated genes include some important genes such as bcl-2-related protein a1 (BCL2A1), caspase 8 isoform c (CASP8), heat shock protein 70 (HSP70) and 60 (HSP60), annexin a2 (ANXA2), and tubulin beta 5 (TUBB5) (Omidi et al., 2003). Up regulation of caspase-8 clearly impart activation of procaspases and caspases that may provoke activity of a series of apoptotic signaling cascades such as electron carrier protein cytochrome C, adaptor protein Apaf-1, Bcl-2 family, p53 and various transcription factors (Kanduc et al., 2002). Given that the heat shock protein 70 acts as an inhibitor of apoptosis (Li et al., 2000), it's upregulation by OF in A431 cells is deemed to be a cellular compensatory or defense response. We assume that cells recognize the xenobiotics upon their biological properties. To examine such concept, we compared OF genotoxicities within two epithelial cell lines (i.e., A431 and A549 cells).

In A549 cells, the genomic impacts were intriguingly dissimilar compared to that of A431 cells (Table 1). Further, we observed some commonalities in gene expression modulation between two different cell lines (Omidi et al., 2008). Upon EASE analyses, the changes in gene expression fell into a number of various functional genomic ontologies. For example, the upregulated genes by OF nanoliposomes included the genes involved in apoptosis, oxidative stress and external/biotic stimulus (e.g., IL9R, DUSP1, CSK, CSE1L); while the downregulated genes were related to the cell growth and/or cell maintenance, cell proliferation and apoptosis (e.g., SEP6, PSMA4).

Gene ID (Accession No.)	Gene description	LF-A431	OF-A431	OF-A549
NM_004417	Dual specificity phosphatase 1; DUSP1	–	+	+
NM_033356	Caspase 8, isoform c; CASP8	NC	+	NC
NM_002467	V-mycmyelocytomatosis viral oncogene homolog (avian); MYC	NC	+	NC
NM_004049	Bcl2-related protein a1; BCL2A1	NC	+	NC
NM_003195	Transcription elongation factor a (sii), 2; TCEA2	NC	+	NC
NM_001983	Excision repair cross-complementing rodent repair deficiency, complementation group 1 (includes overlapping antisense sequence); ERCC1	NC	+	NC
NM_004094	Eukaryotic translation initiation factor 2, subunit 1 (alpha, 35kd); EIF2S1	NC	+	NC
NM_000994	Rbosomal protein l32; RPL32	NC	+	NC
NM_001274	Chk1 checkpoint homolog (s. pombe); CHEK1	NC	+	NC
NM_002849	Protein tyrosine phosphatase, receptor type, r; PTPRR	NC	+	NC
NM_002156	Heat shock 60kd protein 1 (chaperonin); HSPD1	NC	+	+
NM_002957	Retinoid x receptor, alpha; RXRA	NC	+	NC
NM_001242	Cd27 antigen; TNFRSF7	NC	+	NC
NM_006083	Red protein; IK	NC	+	NC
L12723	Heat shock protein 70; HSP70	NC	+	+
NM_004383	C-src tyrosine kinase; CSK	NC	+	+
NM_004635	Mitogen-activated protein kinase-activated protein kinase 3; MAPKAPK3	NC	+	NC
NM_005546	Il2-inducible t-cell kinase; ITK	NC	+	NC
NM_006235	Pou domain, class 2, associating factor 1; POU2AF1	NC	+	NC
NM_002623	Prefoldin 4; PFDN4	NC	NC	NC
NM_001316	Cse1 chromosome segregation 1-like (yeast); CSE1L	NC	NC	+
NM_002953	Ribosomal protein s6 kinase, 90kd, polypeptide 1; RPS6KA1	NC	NC	NC
NM_000660	Transforming growth factor, beta 1; TGFB1	NC	NC	NC
NM_000043	Apoptosis (apo-1) antigen 1; TNFRSF6	NC	NC	NC
NM_001961	Eukaryotic translation elongation factor 2; EEF2	NC	NC	NC
NM_001786	Cell division cycle 2 protein, isoform 1; CDC2	NC	NC	NC
NM_021103	Thymosin beta, TMSB10	NC	NC	NC
NM_004315	N-acylsphingosineamidohydrolase (acidceramidase);	–	NC	NC

Gene ID (Accession No.)	Gene description	LF-A431	OF-A431	OF-A549
	ASAH			
NM_002026	Fibronectin 1, isoform 1 preproprotein; FN1	–	NC	NC
NM_001238	Cyclin e1, isoform 1; CCNE1	NC	NC	NC
NM_002186	Interleukin 9 receptor; IL9R	NC	NC	+
NM_002945	Replicationprotein a1 (70kd); RPA1	NC	NC	NC
NM_003875	Guanine monophosphate synthetase; GMPS	–	NC	NC
NM_000887	Integrinalpha x precursor; ITGAX	NC	NC	+
NM_000075	Cyclin-dependent kinase 4, isoform 1; CDK4	NC	NC	–
NM_032959	Dna directed rna polymerase ii polypeptide j, isoform b; POLR2J	NC	NC	+
NM_000970	Ribosomal protein l6; RPL6	–	NC	NC
NM_005319	H1 histone family, member 2; H1F2	NC	NC	NC
NM_002592	Proliferating cell nuclear antigen; PCNA	–	NC	NC
NM_020300	Microsomal glutathione s-transferase 1; MGST1	NC	NC	NC
NM_021065	H2a histone family, member g; H2AFG	NC	–	NC
NM_004832	Glutathione-s-transferase like; GSTTLP28	NC	–	NC
NM_006087	Tubulin, beta, 5; TUBB5	NC	–	NC
NM_002789	Proteasome (prosome, macropain) subunit, alpha type, 4; PSMA4	NC	–	–
NM_005566	Ldha	NC	–	NC
NM_015129	Septin 6; SEP6	NC	–	–
NM_004039	Annexin a2; ANXA2	NC	–	NC

Table 1. Gene expression changes induced by cationic liposomes in A431 and A549 cells. LF: Lipofectin™ ; OF: Oligofectamine™; NC: no changes; +: upregulation; –: downregulation; adapted with permission (Barar et al., 2009).

For example, among the genes upregulated by OF in A549 cells (but not A431 cells), the IL9R gene encodes IL9 receptor protein which is a cytokine receptor that specifically mediates the biological effects of IL9. The ligand binding of this receptor leads to the activation of various JAK kinases and STAT proteins, which connect to different biologic responses, in particular some genetic studies, suggested an association of this gene with the development of asthma (Gaga et al., 2007).

The heat shock proteins 60 and 70 as well as c-src tyrosine kinase (CSK) were observed to be upregulated in both cell lines (Table 1). Of these, the heat shock proteins family of molecular chaperones appears to act in protein folding, translocation, and assembly into complexes; while CSK is mainly involved in protein-tyrosine kinase activity as well as protein metabolism and modifications. Once looked at the overlapped activities of these genes, we found that they are cooperating mostly to activate the binding activity - we speculate that these genes somehow are collaborating perhaps in terms of protein folding and binding.

Since liposomal formulations are being explored for pulmonary drug/gene delivery, and thus their ability to activate IL9R should be assessed when used clinically for lung gene therapy. The CSK along with some other genes were upregulated in A549 cells treated with cationic lipids similar to what we observed previously in A431 cells (Omidi et al., 2003) and is mainly involved in cell growth and/or cell maintenance. The SEP6 and PSMA4 were downregulated genes by OF in both cell lines. The SEP6 gene is a member of the septin family of GTPases. Members of this family are required for cytokinesis. One version of pediatric acute myeloid leukemia is the result of a reciprocal translocation between chromosomes 11 and X, with the breakpoint associated with the genes encoding the mixed-lineage leukemia and septin 2 proteins. This gene encodes four transcript variants encoding three distinct isoforms. An additional transcript variant has been identified, but its biological validity has not been determined. The PSMA4 is a multicatalytic proteinase complex with a highly ordered ring-shaped 20S core structure. They are distributed throughout eukaryotic cells at a high concentration and cleave peptides in an ATP/ubiquitin-dependent process in a non-lysosomal pathway.

Because of the gene expression commonalities and distinctions between the two cell lines, we conceptualized that these cells may respond to the cationic lipid "OF" differently upon their cellular characteristics. These cells appeared to undergo somewhat adaptation upon exposure to xenobiotics, as a result of which they could dynamically respond as expressing/activating related cellular elements for recognition and internalization of the cationic lipid. Of interest, we found that the genotoxicity elicited by the cationic lipid nanosystems were largely dependent upon the structural architecture and/or physicochemical properties of the cationic lipid since no extensive overlap was observed in the gene expression profile induced by either LF or OF in A431 cells. Besides, the responsiveness of the target cells to the lipids could be different since the transfection efficiency is significantly depended upon the target cells and lipids used. Likewise, Filion and Phillips (1997) reported high toxicity rate elicited by some cationic lipids in phagocytic cells such as macrophages and U937 cells, but not in non-phagocytic T lymphocytes.

Taken all these findings together, it seems that for attaining detailed characterization of the toxicogenomics of these lipid delivery systems (based on their molecular structure), the gene expression patterns/profiles need to be determined in different cell types perhaps with known cell surface architecture.

8. Genomic impacts of cationic polymers

Despite plethora of investigations on application of polymers in drug/gene delivery, surprisingly, little attention has been devoted about possible biofunction of polymer *per se* in particular genomic effects. Many researchers have now consensus upon functionalities of polymers, and accordingly new domains of polymer science such as "polymer genomics", "polymer genocompatibly" and "polymer genotoxicity" have been arisen. To examine the polymer genocompatibly concept, we have previously reported that starburst PAMAM dendrimers (i.e., PF and SF) as well as polypropylene imine (PPI) dendrimers (e.g., DAB8 and DAB16) can inadvertently induce alterations in gene expression (Hollins et al., 2007; Omidi et al., 2005b). These dendrimers have been successfully exploited for delivery of gene based medicines. Of these dendrimers, we have previously shown dramatic alteration in gene expression induced by DAB16 dendrimer in A431 and A549 cells (Omidi et al., 2005b).

Table 2 represents the gene expression changes by DAB polymers in A431 and A549 cells. Of the altered genes in A431 cells, some are related to cell defense and response to stress (e.g., ALOX5, TNFRSF7) and apoptosis (e.g., TNFRSF7). In A549 cells, some of the altered genes

Gene ID (Accession No.)	Description	A431 cells		A549 cells	
		DAB8	DAB16	DAB16	DAB16:DNA
NM_006716	Activator of s phase kinase; ASK	NC	–	NC	NC
NM_000034	Aldolase a; ALDOα	NC	NC	NC	NC
NM_004039	Annexin a2; ANXα2	NC	+	NC	NC
NM_000698	Arachidonate 5-lipoxygenase; ALOX5	NC	–	NC	NC
NM_004049	Bcl2-related protein a1; BCL2α1	NC	NC	NC	+
NM_000591	Cd14 antigen precursor; CD14	NC	NC	+	NC
NM_001242	Cd27 antigen; TNFRSF7	NC	–	NC	NC
NM_001786	Cell division cycle 2 protein, isoform 1; CDC2	NC	NC	–	NC
NM_003467	Chemokine (c-x-c motif), receptor 4 (fusin); CXCR4	NC	NC	NC	–
NM_001274	Chk1 checkpoint homolog (s. pombe); CHEK1	NC	NC	NC	–
NM_004383	C-src tyrosine kinase; CSK	NC	NC	NC	–
NM_003914	Cyclin a1; CCNα1	NC	NC	+	NC
NM_001239	Cyclin h; CCNH	NC	NC	–	NC
NM_000075	Cyclin-dependent kinase 4, isoform 1; CDK4	NC	+	NC	NC
NM_001801	Cysteine dioxygenase, type i; CDO1	NC	NC	NC	–
NM_004417	Dual specificity phosphatase 1; DUSP1	NC	–	NC	+
NM_003875	Guanine monophosphate synthetase; GMPS	NC	–	NC	+
NM_021065	H2a histone family, member g; H2AFG	NC	+	NC	NC
NM_002156	Heat shock 60kd protein 1 (chaperonin); HSPD1	NC	–	NC	NC
NM_000879	Interleukin 5 (colony-stimulating factor, eosinophil); IL5	NC	NC	NC	–
NM_002186	Interleukin 9 receptor; IL9R	NC	NC	+	NC
NM_002358	Mad2-like 1; MAD2L1	NC	NC	NC	+
NM_002424	Matrix metalloproteinase 8 preproprotein; MMP8	NC	NC	NC	–
NM_000245	Met proto-oncogene precursor; Met	+	NC	–	NC
NM_004315	N-acylsphingosine amidohydrolase (acid ceramidase); ASAH	NC	NC	NC	+
NM_006235	Pou domain, class 2, associating factor 1; POU2AF1	NC	NC	NC	–
NM_000946	Primase, polypeptide 1 (49kd); PRIM1	NC	NC	NC	+
NM_002592	Proliferating cell nuclear antigen; PCNA	NC	NC	–	NC
NM_000532	Propionyl coenzyme a carboxylase, beta polypeptide; PCCβ	NC	–	NC	NC
NM_002789	Proteasome (prosome, macropain)	NC	+	NC	NC

Gene ID (Accession No.)	Description	A431 cells		A549 cells	
		DAB8	DAB16	DAB16	DAB16:DNA
	subunit, alpha type, 4; PSMα4				
NM_002796	Proteasome (prosome, macropain) subunit, beta type, 4; PSMβ4	NC	NC	–	NC
NM_002737	Protein kinase c, alpha; PRKCα	NC	NC	NC	–
NM_006083	Red protein; IK	NC	–	NC	NC
NM_002914	Replication factor c (activator 1) 2 (40kd); RFC2	NC	NC	NC	–
NM_002947	Replicationprotein a3 (14kd); RPα3	NC	–	NC	NC
NM_002957	Retinoid x receptor, alpha; RXRα	NC	NC	+	NC
NM_007209	Ribosomal protein l35; RPL35	NC	NC	NC	+
NM_033301	Ribosomal protein l8; RPL8	NC	–	NC	NC
NM_003139	Signal recognition particle receptor ('docking protein'); SRPR	NC	NC	NC	+
NM_003072	Swi/snf related, matrix associated regulator of chromatin, SMARCA4	NC	–	NC	–
NM_003236	Transforming growth factor, alpha; TGFα	NC	NC	+	NC
NM_000660	Transforming growth factor, beta 1; TGFβ1	NC	NC	NC	+
NM_003292	Translocated promoter region (to activated met oncogene); TPR	NC	NC	+	NC
NM_006087	Tubulin, beta, 5; TUBβ5	NC	+	NC	NC
NM_003299	Tumor rejection antigen (gp96) 1; TRA1	NC	NC	+	NC
NM_006826	Tyrosine 3-monooxygenase/tryptophan 5-monooxygenase activation protein, theta polypeptide; YWHAQ	NC	–	NC	NC

Table 2. Gene expression changes by DAB polymers in A431 and A549 cells. NC: no changes; +/-: up/down regulation; adapted with permission from (Omidi et al., 2005b).

were in association with cell defense, DNA repair/damage and apoptosis (e.g., CCNH; ERCC1; PCNAM, CD14).

With a particular interest on toxicogenomic of the DBA16:DNA nanoparticles in A549 cells, expression changes (upregulation/downregulation) were found for some important genes (i.e., TGFβ1,BCL2α1, IL5, CXCR4 and PCKα). Of these, TGFβ1 is a member of a super-family of multifunctional cytokines that regulate cell proliferation, differentiation, and apoptosis (Chiarugi et al., 1997; Haufel et al., 1999), while the BCL2 protein family is involved in a wide variety of cellular activities that also act as anti- and pro-apoptotic regulators. The protein encoded by BCL2 is able to reduce the release of pro-apoptotic cytochrome c from mitochondria and block caspase activation which is the main apoptosis pathway. Further, this gene is a direct transcription target of NF-KAPPAβ in response to inflammatory mediators, and has been shown to be upregulated by different extracellular signals, such as granulocyte-macrophage colony-stimulating factor (GM-CSF), CD40, phorbol ester and inflammatory cytokine TNF and IL1, which suggests a cyto-protective function that is essential for lymphocyte activation as well as cell survival; reader is directed to see following citations (May et al., 1994; Ruvolo et al., 2001). The upregulation of TGFβ1 and BCL2α conceivably imply incitement of apoptosis in A549 cells upon treatments with DAB16:DNA polyplexes.

It was also found that the altered genes induced by PF, DAB16 and OF in A431 cells shows some commonalities and differences in pattern, presumably due to their positive charge and structural architecture. In A431 cells, treated with either DAB8 or DAB16 resulted in ~13% and ~7% similar and opposite patterns of gene expression changes, respectively. For example, BCL2α1 which acts as anti- and pro-apoptotic regulator was largely affected by DAB16 compared to DAB8. This could be due to higher surface charge and/or interaction capacity of DAB16. Similar pattern was seen for proteasomeα4, but Met proto-oncogene revealed opposite pattern. Once DAB16 was tested in different cell line (i.e., A549 cells), similar and opposite patterns of gene expression changes were ~11% and ~9%, respectively. Intriguingly, upregulation of some important genes (e.g., IL9R, TGFα) was seen solely in A549 cells, but not in A431 cells. It can be speculated that A549 cells can show greater response than A431 cells. Hence, these dendrimers could potentially affect cell growth and immune response of cells by altering the expression of some related genes at doses which did not distinctly modify cell viability (Table 2). It should be also evoked that the identity of the genes whose expression was significantly altered (i.e. the "gene signature" of the delivery system) was markedly different in the two cell lines, despite the similar expression of the majority of the genes (80%) that remained unaffected (Akhtar & Benter, 2007).

Table 3 shows the gene expression of some selected genes induced by branched and linear polyethylenimine (BPEI and LPEI, respectively) in A431 cells. These data solely present the upregulated and downregulated genes, similarly induced by these cationic polymers, while there are a large number of genes showed opposite pattern (data not shown). Based on these results, it was found that the alterations in gene expression by BPEI were significantly greater than LPEI. We contemplate that this could be because of the greater interaction of BPEI with subcellular biomolecules.

To examine the late effect of BPEI in target cells, we evaluated gene expression pattern of caspases genes in A431 cells as a time series approache (i.e., immediately after transfection, 24 h and 48 h after transfection). Fig. 5 represents the gene expression profile of selected caspase pathway genes in A431 cells treated with BPEI, showing significant impacts of BPEI even 48 h after treatment. Of these genes, as previously mentioned, caspase 8 play a key role in apoptosis.

These findings directed us to examine some other cationic polymers such as PAMAM and PEI. Upon our examination on SF and PF, we found that PF induced gene expression changes much greater than SF. This could be due to differences in dendrimers architecture. Significant decrease in gene expression changes were observed upon PF complexation with a DNA at the supplier recommended ratio of 10:1 (w/w) of PF:DNA. Reduced in number, but not in nature and magnitude, of expressed genes were observed upon PF:DNA complexation. In treated A431 cells with cationic dendrimer PF or cationic lipid OF, opposite and similar patterns of gene expression changes were 20% and 16%, respectively (Barar et al., 2009).

Function	Gene ID	T/UT ratio		
		BPEI	LPEI	
gi:407955 - membrane-associated protein hem-1	M58285	4.10	1.95	+
gi:7106883 - HSPC247	AF151081	2.74	1.98	+
gi:13569894 - diaphanous homolog 3; DIAPH3	NM_030932	2.23	2.44	+
gi:14010613 - methylmalonyl-coa epimerase	AF364547	2.13	2.21	+
gi:14248538 - STONIN2	AF255309	2.10	2.13	+
gi:188560 - prepro-mullerian inhibiting substance	K03474	2.10	2.69	+
gi:285915 - epimorphin	D14582	2.07	3.17	+
gi:7109206 - four alpha helix cytokine; ZCYTO10	AF224266	1.99	2.00	+
gi:558098 - protein kinase c-theta; PRKCT	L01087	1.97	1.93	+
gi:9843747 - putative pyroglutamyl-peptidase i; PGPEP1	AJ278828	1.93	2.82	+
gi:22041589 - similar to data source:sptr, source key:q9h4b3, evidence:iss~homolog to mucolipidin~putative; loc255231	XM70908	0.58	0.25	-
gi:14588660 - histidase; hal	AB042217	0.57	0.27	-
gi:10439114 - homo sapiens cdna: flj22644 fis, clone hsi07088; unnamed protein product.	AK026297	0.53	0.26	-
gi:10944321 - myozenin; MYOZ	AF240633	0.53	0.26	-
gi:2613124 - small cell vasopressin subtype 1b receptor	AF030512	0.52	0.26	-
gi:20278870 - delta 4 progesterone receptor; pr	AB084248	0.46	0.26	-
gi:7020101 - cdna clone unnamed protein product	AK000183	0.45	0.27	-
gi:7209599 - melatonin 1b receptor	AB033598	0.44	0.26	-
gi:307425 - nerve terminal protein; SNAP	L19760	0.43	0.25	-
gi:18182679 - nkg2d	AF461811	0.41	0.25	-
gi:347133 - succinate dehydrogenase flavoprotein subunit; SDH	L21936	0.39	0.23	-
gi:2738815 - p2y1 receptor; p2yr1	AF018284	0.28	0.26	-
gi:21928730 - seven transmembrane helix receptor	AB065731	0.26	0.27	-
gi:3088552 - cystatin-related epididymal spermatogenic protein; cres	AF059244	0.24	0.24	-
gi:22048232 - similar to riken cdna 2610027o18; KIAA1393	XM_050793	0.21	0.22	-

Table 3. Gene expression changes of selected genes induced by branched and linear polyethylenimine (BPEI and LPEI, respectively) in A431 cells (our unpublished data produced by Omidi et al.). +/-: up/down regulation

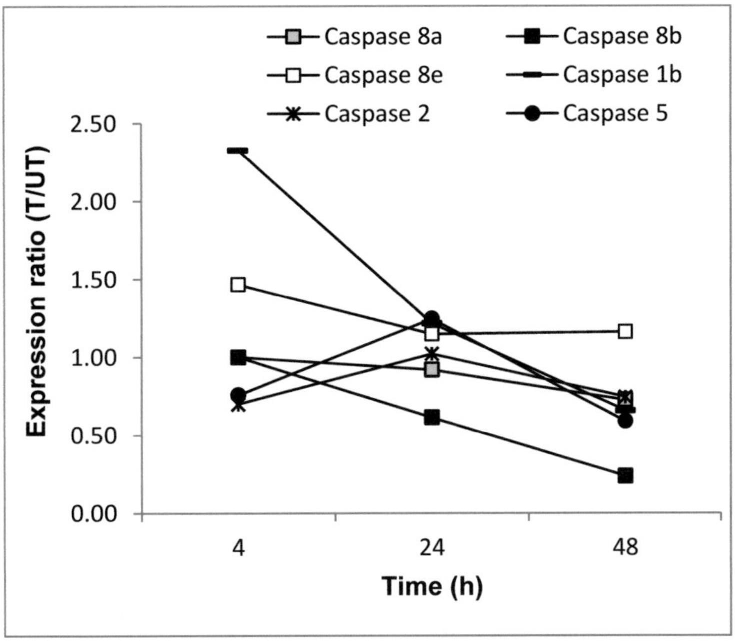

Fig. 5. Gene expression ratio of selected caspase pathway genes in A431 cells treated with BPEI after 4, 24 and 48 h (our unpublished data produced by Omidi et al.).

Likewise, Pluronic® block copolymers were shown to cause various functional alterations in cells through interacting with cellular biomolecules and thus affecting various cellular functions such as mitochondrial respiration, ATP synthesis, activity of drug efflux transporters, apoptotic signal transduction, and transcriptional activation of gene expression both *in vitro* and *in vivo* (Batrakova & Kabanov, 2008). This polymer is able to enhance expression of reporter genes under the control of cytomegalovirus promoter and NF-KB response element in stably and transiently transfected mouse fibroblasts and myoblasts *in vitro*. It has been shown that these block copolymers are able to act as biological response modifying agents through upregulating the transcription of genes via activation of selected signaling pathways such as NF-KB (Sriadibhatla et al., 2006).

Furthermore, Pluronic® P85 (P85) was reported to promote transport of the pDNA to the nucleus in cells transiently transfected with DNA/PEI polyplex (Kabanov, 2006). It has also been successfully exploited for DNA vaccine delivery, however some investigations revealed that P85 simultaneously increase transgene expression and activate immunity, in which P85 alone and P85:DNA complexes were shown to increase the systemic expansion of CD11c+ (DC), and local expansion of CD11c+, CD14+ (macrophages) and CD49b+ (natural killer) cell populations. DNA/P85 polyplex can also increase maturation of local DC (CD11c+ CD86+, CD11c+ CD80 +, and CD11c+ CD40+ (Gaymalov et al., 2009). Thus, the activation of immunogenes in the antigen-presenting cells by P85:DNA complexes can highlight new insights for these kinds of polymers.

In addition, Pluronic® can cause some alterations in HSP68 expression, suggesting that this polymer may affect stress-related pathways or there is a cross-talk between the stress and other pathways activated by the copolymer (Sriadibhatla et al., 2006). These results are in accord with what we have observed for some other cationic polymers or lipids. Pluronic®

(a mixture of Pluronic L61 and F127; also called as SP1017) has been reported to deliver plasmid DNA in skeletal and cardiac muscle, as well as in solid tumors. Unlike other polycations, Pluronic® does not bind and condense the nucleic acids, it does not protect DNA from degradation or facilitate transport of the DNA into the cell and its effects involve transcriptional activation of gene expression (Kabanov, 2006). The effect of Pluronic® was reported to be related to the activation of gene expression by activating the NF-κB and p53 signaling pathways, in which pro-apoptotic AP-l gene that is frequently regulated by the NF-κB system, was not responsive. This, perhaps, indicates that Pluronic-mediated influence on transcription is selective and it is not a result of a general nonspecific activation of immune defense system such as NO-mediated burst (Kabanov, 2006). Nonetheless, to ensure about this supposition, it is essential to recruit global gene expression screening methods such as microarray technology as we have witnessed dramatic alterations in gene expression *in vitro* and *in vivo* upon treatment with different polymers using microarray technology. Kabanov's group has reported that Pluronic block copolymers interact with biomembranes and induce gene expressions through mechanisms that differ from the delivery of the DNA into the cell. They also questioned whether upregulation of expression of genes delivered into cells can also take place by other nonviral polymer-based gene delivery systems? We have observed that various polymers, in particular polycations, are able to alter gene expressions related to immune response and cell defense (Barar et al., 2009; Hollins et al., 2007; Omidi et al., 2008).

It appears that the cytotoxicity of nonviral vectors is largely dependent upon the cationic nature of the vector, which attains different level to different structural architecture. For cationic lipid, the cytotoxic effects are mainly determined by the structure of its hydrophilic group (Prokop & Davidson, 2008), e.g. the quaternary ammonium amphiphiles are more toxic than their tertiary amine counterparts. Such toxicity (due to positive charge of the head group) can be reduced by importing a heterocyclic ring such as imidazolium or pyridinium.

The biodegradability potential of the advanced nanobiomaterials are also determined their toxicity. For example, poly(lactic-co-glycolic acid) nanoparticles elicit very low level of cytotoxicity and toxicogenomic compared to cationic polymers, but not the modified PLGA-grafted poly(L-lysine) nanosystems (Omidi & Davaran, 2011).

Surprisingly, the effect of hydrophobic chain on toxicity has not been adequately addressed to date even though it is deemed that the hydrophobic moieties may disrupt the integrity of lipid bilayer. Like cationic lipid, cationic polymers with acid-labile linkage can be rapidly degraded and less toxic. It has been reported that the toxicity of polymers (e.g., PEI, PLL or dendrimers) increases with high molecular weight (Bieber & Elsasser, 2001). Polymers synthesized by linking low molecular weight with acid-labile show low toxicity (Li et al., 2004). The creation of amphiphilic cationic polymer based on PEI or PLL, by linking PEG or other groups, reduces toxicity without compromising the gene delivery efficiency (Zhang et al., 2008).

Upon our observations the biodegradable cationic polymers (e.g., polysaccharides) which display high degree of biodegradability possess low toxicity, thus we speculate that they may be extensively used for *in vivo* transfection in the future. Further, high transfection efficiency and low toxicity can be obtained by the addition of co-lipids or co-polymers (PEGylation). Water soluble lipopolymer, to combine the advantages of both cationic polymer and liposome, seems to be our next approach for optimized gene transfer. Besides, adding cell-specific biomolecules (e.g. aptamer, peptide ligands, antibodies or nanobodies) to gene transfer vectors potentially improve the specific problem by permitting lower and safer vector doses while facilitating tissue targeting.

9. Concluding remarks

Synthetic lipids or polymers used for gene delivery may impose selective "phenotypic effects" in cells by affecting cell signaling involved in various biological functions such as cell defense, inflammation, differentiation, proliferation and apoptosis. It is believed that these effects result basically from their interactions with cell membranes, intracellular organelles and subcellular biomolecules, as a result the target cells can respond to these effects phenotypically or genotypically. In some cases, these effects can be relatively benign as they do not induce sever cytotoxic effects, while in the case of nonviral cationic vectors it is not the case since the interaction of the polycationic gene delivery nanosystems with target cells is significantly greater than non-cationic polymers. It is now deemed that one unifying property of polycationic gene delivery nanosystems is their potential to interact with cellular/subcellular biomolecules, upon which profound changes in various cell processes may occur. From this standpoint, it becomes clear that these polycations are able to penetrate into cells and reach different critical subcellular targets and induce inventible biological functions, for which the nanoscaled range of sizes is an important factor. Different cell types as biological targets may response differently, and even modify the activities of such nanomaterials. While the genome-based therapeutics (e.g., oligonucleotides and gene silencing siRNAs) have already been lined up for clinical trials (up to 1700 trials), our knowledge is lacking upon genomic signature of such gene based medicines. As concluding statement, it is suggested that the inadvertent intrinsic genomic signature of nonviral delivery systems should be assessed and taken into consideration for a gene therapy trial since gene silencing/stimulation experiments are to target a specific gene while the gene delivery system may potentially mask or interfere with the desired genotype and/or phenotype end-point of gene therapy. The upregulation or downregulation of genes induced by gene delivery systems or any other drug carriers and excipients appears to instigate a new directionality such as "functional excipients". But, this approach simply represents the gene expression changes which are solely based on intensities of expressed genes for various signaling pathways, while we should look for ways to correlate such gene expression intensities with functional genomics.

10. References

Aardema, M.J. & MacGregor, J.T. (2002). Toxicology and genetic toxicology in the new era of "toxicogenomics": impact of "-omics" technologies. *Mutat.Res.*, Vol.499, No.1, (January 2002), pp. 13-25, ISSN 0027-5107

Aberle, A.M.; Tablin, F.; Zhu, J.; Walker, N.J.; Gruenert, D.C. & Nantz, M.H. (1998). A novel tetraester construct that reduces cationic lipid-associated cytotoxicity. Implications for the onset of cytotoxicity. *Biochemistry*, Vol.37, No.18, (1998), pp. 6533-6540, ISSN 0006-2960

Akhtar, S. & Benter, I. (2007). Toxicogenomics of non-viral drug delivery systems for RNAi: potential impact on siRNA-mediated gene silencing activity and specificity. *Adv.Drug Deliv.Rev.*, Vol.59, No.2-3, (March 2007), pp. 164-182, ISSN 0169-409X

Audouy, S.A.; de Leij, L.F.; Hoekstra, D. & Molema, G. (2002). In vivo characteristics of cationic liposomes as delivery vectors for gene therapy. *Pharm Res*, Vol.19, No.11, (2002), pp. 1599-1605, ISSN 1043-6618

Azuaje, F. (2003). Clustering-based approaches to discovering and visualising microarray data patterns. *Brief.Bioinform.*, Vol.4, No.1, (March 2003), pp. 31-42, ISSN 1467-5463

Barar, J.; Hamzeiy, H.; Mortazavi-Tabatabaei, S.A.; Hashemi-Aghdam, S.E. & Omidi, Y. (2009). Genomic signature and toxicogenomics comparison of polycationic gene delivery nanosystems in human alveolar epithelial A549 cells. *Daru*, Vol.17, No.3, (2009), pp. 139-147, ISSN 1560-8115

Barar, J.; Javadzadeh, A.R. & Omidi, Y. (2008). Ocular novel drug delivery: impacts of membranes and barriers. *Expert.Opin.Drug Deliv.*, Vol.5, No.5, (May 2008), pp. 567-581, ISSN 1742-5247

Batrakova, E.V. & Kabanov, A.V. (2008). Pluronic block copolymers: evolution of drug delivery concept from inert nanocarriers to biological response modifiers. *J.Control Release*, Vol.130, No.2, (September 2008), pp. 98-106, ISSN 0168-3659

Berger, J.A.; Hautaniemi, S.; Jarvinen, A.K.; Edgren, H.; Mitra, S.K. & Astola, J. (December 2004). Optimized LOWESS normalization parameter selection for DNA microarray data. *BMC.Bioinformatics.*, Vol.5, No.1, (December 2004), pp. 194, ISSN 1471-2105

Bieber, T. & Elsasser, H.P. (2001). Preparation of a low molecular weight polyethylenimine for efficient cell transfection. *Biotechniques*, Vol.30, No.1, (2001), pp. 74-77, ISSN 0736-6205

Bottega, R. & Epand, R.M. (1992). Inhibition of protein kinase C by cationic amphiphiles. *Biochemistry*, Vol.31, No.37, (September 1992), pp. 9025-9030, ISSN 0006-2960

Chen, Y.J.; Kodell, R.; Sistare, F.; Thompson, K.L.; Morris, S. & Chen, J.J. (2003). Normalization methods for analysis of microarray gene-expression data. *J.Biopharm.Stat.*, Vol.13, No.1, (February 2003), pp. 57-74, ISSN 1054-3406

Chiarugi, V.; Magnelli, L. & Cinelli, M. (1997). Complex interplay among apoptosis factors: RB, p53, E2F, TGF-beta, cell cycle inhibitors and the bcl2 gene family. *Pharmacol Res*, Vol.35, No.4, (1997), pp. 257-261, ISSN 1043-6618

Conner, S.D. & Schmid, S.L. (2003). Regulated portals of entry into the cell. *Nature*, Vol.422, No.6927, (March 2003), pp. 37-44, ISSN 0028-0836

Curtis, R.K.; Oresic, M. & Vidal-Puig, A. (2005). Pathways to the analysis of microarray data. *Trends Biotechnol.*, Vol.23, No.8, (August 2005), pp. 429-435, ISSN 0167-7799

de, L.F.; Bertholet, V. & Remacle, J. (2004). DNA microarrays as a tool in toxicogenomics. *Comb.Chem.High Throughput.Screen.*, Vol.7, No.3, (May 2004), pp. 207-211, ISSN 1386-2073

Domanski, D.M.; Bryszewska, M. & Salamonczyk, G. (2004). Preliminary evaluation of the behavior of fifth-generation thiophosphate dendrimer in biological systems.

Biomacromolecules., Vol.5, No.5, (September 2004), pp. 2007-2012, ISSN 1525-7797

Erickson, B.; Dimaggio, S.C.; Mullen, D.G.; Kelly, C.V.; Leroueil, P.R.; Berry, S.A.; Baker, J.R., Jr.; Orr, B.G. & Banaszak Holl, M.M. (2008). Interactions of Poly(amidoamine) Dendrimers with Survanta Lung Surfactant: The Importance of Lipid Domains. *Langmuir, Vol.24, No.19, (September 2008), pp. 11003-11008, ISSN 0743-7463*

Farhood, H.; Serbina, N. & Huang, L. (1995). The role of dioleoyl phosphatidylethanolamine in cationic liposome mediated gene transfer. *Biochim.Biophys.Acta*, Vol.1235, No.2, (May 1995), pp. 289-295, ISSN 0006-3002

Ferber, D. (2001). Gene therapy. Repair kits for faulty genes. *Science*, Vol.294, No.5547, (2001), pp. 1639, ISSN 0036-8075

Ferber, D. (2001). Gene therapy. Safer and virus-free? *Science*, Vol.294, No.5547, (2001), pp. 1638-1642, ISSN 0036-8075

Fielden, M.R. & Kolaja, K.L. (2006). The state-of-the-art in predictive toxicogenomics. *Curr.Opin.Drug Discov.Devel.*, Vol.9, No.1, (January 2006), pp. 84-91, ISSN 1367-6733

Filion, M.C. & Phillips, N.C. (1997a). Anti-inflammatory activity of cationic lipids. *Br.J.Pharmacol.*, Vol.122, No.3, (October 1997), pp. 551-557, ISSN 0007-1188

Filion, M.C. & Phillips, N.C. (1997b). Toxicity and immunomodulatory activity of liposomal vectors formulated with cationic lipids toward immune effector cells. *Biochim Biophys Acta*, Vol.1329, No.2, (1997), pp. 345-356, ISSN 0006-3002

Fischer, D.; Li, Y.; Ahlemeyer, B.; Krieglstein, J. & Kissel, T. (2003). In vitro cytotoxicity testing of polycations: influence of polymer structure on cell viability and hemolysis. *Biomaterials*, Vol.24, No.7, (2003), pp. 1121-1131, ISSN 0142-9612

Florea, B.I.; Meaney, C.; Junginger, H.E. & Borchard, G. (2002). Transfection efficiency and toxicity of polyethylenimine in differentiated Calu-3 and nondifferentiated COS-1 cell cultures. *AAPS PharmSci*, Vol.4, No.3, (2002), pp. E12, ISSN 1530-9932

Gaga, M.; Zervas, E.; Grivas, S.; Castro, M. & Chanez, P. (2007). Evaluation and management of severe asthma. *Curr.Med Chem.*, Vol.14, No.9, (2007), pp. 1049-1059, ISSN 0929-8673

Gao, X.; Kim, K.S. & Liu, D. (2007). Nonviral gene delivery: what we know and what is next. *AAPS.J.*, Vol.9, No.1, (2007), pp. E92-104, ISSN 1550-7416

Gaymalov, Z.Z.; Yang, Z.; Pisarev, V.M.; Alakhov, V.Y. & Kabanov, A.V. (2009). The effect of the nonionic block copolymer pluronic P85 on gene expression in mouse muscle and antigen-presenting cells. *Biomaterials*, Vol.30, No.6, (February 2009), pp. 1232-1245,

Gebhart, C.L. & Kabanov, A.V. (2001). Evaluation of polyplexes as gene transfer agents. *J Control Release*, Vol.73, No.2-3, (2001), pp. 401-416, ISSN 0168-3659

Godbey, W.T.; Wu, K.K. & Mikos, A.G. (1999). Poly(ethylenimine) and its role in gene delivery. *J Control Release*, Vol.60, No.2-3, (1999), pp. 149-160, ISSN 0168-3659

Godbey, W.T.; Wu, K.K. & Mikos, A.G. (2001). Poly(ethylenimine)-mediated gene delivery affects endothelial cell function and viability. *Biomaterials*, Vol.22, No.5, (2001), pp. 471-480, ISSN 0142-9612

Goldsmith, Z.G. & Dhanasekaran, N. (2004). The microrevolution: applications and impacts of microarray technology on molecular biology and medicine (review). *Int.J.Mol.Med.*, Vol.13, No.4, (April 2004), pp. 483-495, ISSN 1107-3756

Haufel, T.; Dormann, S.; Hanusch, J.; Schwieger, A. & Bauer, G. (1999). Three distinct roles for TGF-beta during intercellular induction of apoptosis: a review. *Anticancer Res*, Vol.19, No.1A, (1999), pp. 105-111, ISSN 0250-7005

Hegde, P.; Qi, R.; Abernathy, K.; Gay, C.; Dharap, S.; Gaspard, R.; Hughes, J.E.; Snesrud, E.; Lee, N. & Quackenbush, J. (2000). A concise guide to cDNA microarray analysis. *Biotechniques*, Vol.29, No.3, (September 2000), pp. 548-562, ISSN 0736-6205

Hollins, A.J.; Omidi, Y.; Benter, I.F. & Akhtar, S. (2007). Toxicogenomics of drug delivery systems: Exploiting delivery system-induced changes in target gene expression to enhance siRNA activity. *J.Drug Target*, Vol.15, No.1, (January 2007), pp. 83-88, ISSN 1061-186X

Hong, S.; Leroueil, P.R.; Janus, E.K.; Peters, J.L.; Kober, M.M.; Islam, M.T.; Orr, B.G.; Baker, J.R., Jr. & Banaszak Holl, M.M. (2006). Interaction of polycationic polymers with supported lipid bilayers and cells: nanoscale hole formation and enhanced membrane permeability. *Bioconjug.Chem.*, Vol.17, No.3, (May 2006), pp. 728-734, ISSN 1043-1802

Hosack, D.A.; Dennis, G., Jr.; Sherman, B.T.; Lane, H.C. & Lempicki, R.A. (2003). Identifying biological themes within lists of genes with EASE. *Genome Biol*, Vol.4, No.10, (2003), pp. R70, ISSN 1474-760X

Hughes, M.D.; Hussain, M.; Nawaz, Q.; Sayyed, P. & Akhtar, S. (2001). The cellular delivery of antisense oligonucleotides and ribozymes. *Drug Discov Today*, Vol.6, No.6, (2001), pp. 303-315, ISSN 1359-6446

Kabanov, A.V.; Batrakova, E.V.; Sriadibhatla, S.; Yang, Z.; Kelly, D.L. & Alakov, V.Y. (2005). Polymer genomics: shifting the gene and drug delivery paradigms. *J.Control Release*, Vol.101, No.1-3, (January 2005), pp. 259-271, ISSN 0168-3659

Kabanov, V.A. (2006). Polymer Genomics: An Insight into Pharmacology and Toxicology of Nanomedicines. *Adv Drug Deliv Rev*, Vol.58, No.15, (2006), pp. 1597-1621, ISSN 0169-409X

Kafil, V. & Omidi, Y. (2011). Cytotoxic impacts of linear and branched polyethylenimine nanostructures in A431 cells. *BioImpacts*, Vol.1, No.1, (2011), pp. pp. 23-30, ISSN 2228-5652

Kanduc, D.; Mittelman, A.; Serpico, R.; Sinigaglia, E.; Sinha, A.A.; Natale, C.; Santacroce, R.; Di Corcia, M.G.; Lucchese, A.; Dini, L.; Pani, P.; Santacroce, S.; Simone, S.; Bucci, R. & Farber, E. (2002). Cell death: apoptosis versus necrosis (review). *Int J Oncol*, Vol.21, No.1, (2002), pp. 165-170, ISSN 1019-6439

Konopka, K.; Fallah, B.; Monzon-Duller, J.; Overlid, N. & Duzgunes, N. (2005). Serum-resistant gene transfer to oral cancer cells by Metafectene and GeneJammer:

application to HSV-tk/ganciclovir-mediated cytotoxicity. *Cell Mol.Biol.Lett.*, Vol.10, No.3, (2005), pp. 455-470, ISSN 1425-8153

Leroueil, P.R.; Hong, S.; Mecke, A.; Baker, J.R., Jr.; Orr, B.G. & Banaszak Holl, M.M. (2007). Nanoparticle interaction with biological membranes: does nanotechnology present a Janus face? *Acc.Chem.Res.*, Vol.40, No.5, (May 2007), pp. 335-342, ISSN 0001-4842

Lettieri, T. (2006). Recent applications of DNA microarray technology to toxicology and ecotoxicology. *Environ.Health Perspect.*, Vol.114, No.1, (January 2006), pp. 4-9, ISSN 0091-6765

Li, C.Y.; Lee, J.S.; Ko, Y.G.; Kim, J.I. & Seo, J.S. (2000). Heat shock protein 70 inhibits apoptosis downstream of cytochrome c release and upstream of caspase-3 activation. *J Biol Chem*, Vol.275, No.33, (2000), pp. 25665-25671, ISSN 0021-9258

Li, W.; Huang, Z.; Mackay, J.A.; Grube, S. & Szoka, F.C., Jr. (2004). Low-pH-sensitive poly(ethylene glycol) (PEG)-stabilized plasmid nanolipoparticles: effects of PEG chain length, lipid composition and assembly conditions on gene delivery. *J.Gene Med*, Vol.7, No.1, (October 2004), pp. 67-79, ISSN 1099-498X

Lobenhofer, E.K.; Bushel, P.R.; Afshari, C.A. & Hamadeh, H.K. (2001). Progress in the application of DNA microarrays. *Environ.Health Perspect.*, Vol.109, No.9, (September 2001), pp. 881-891, ISSN 0091-6765

Maguire, A.M.; Simonelli, F.; Pierce, E.A.; Pugh, E.N., Jr.; Mingozzi, F.; Bennicelli, J.; Banfi, S.; Marshall, K.A.; Testa, F.; Surace, E.M.; Rossi, S.; Lyubarsky, A.; Arruda, V.R.; Konkle, B.; Stone, E.; Sun, J.; Jacobs, J.; Dell'Osso, L.; Hertle, R.; Ma, J.X.; Redmond, T.M.; Zhu, X.; Hauck, B.; Zelenaia, O.; Shindler, K.S.; Maguire, M.G.; Wright, J.F.; Volpe, N.J.; McDonnell, J.W.; Auricchio, A.; High, K.A. & Bennett, J. (2008). Safety and efficacy of gene transfer for Leber's congenital amaurosis. *N.Engl.J.Med.*, Vol.358, No.21, (May 2008), pp. 2240-2248, ISSN 0028-4793

Masotti, A.; Mossa, G.; Cametti, C.; Ortaggi, G.; Bianco, A.; Grosso, N.D.; Malizia, D. & Esposito, C. (2009). Comparison of different commercially available cationic liposome-DNA lipoplexes: Parameters influencing toxicity and transfection efficiency. *Colloids Surf.B Biointerfaces.*, Vol.68, No.2, (February 2009), pp. 136-144,

May, W.S.; Tyler, P.G.; Ito, T.; Armstrong, D.K.; Qatsha, K.A. & Davidson, N.E. (1994). Interleukin-3 and bryostatin-1 mediate hyperphosphorylation of BCL2 alpha in association with suppression of apoptosis. *J Biol Chem*, Vol.269, No.43, (1994), pp. 26865-26870, ISSN 0021-9258

Medina-Kauwe, L.K.; Xie, J. & Hamm-Alvarez, S. (2005). Intracellular trafficking of nonviral vectors. *Gene Ther.*, Vol.12, No.24, (December 2005), pp. 1734-1751, ISSN 0969-7128

Nel, A.; Xia, T.; Madler, L. & Li, N. (2006). Toxic potential of materials at the nanolevel. *Science*, Vol.311, No.5761, (February 2006), pp. 622-627, ISSN 0036-8075

Omidi, Y.; Barar, J. & Akhtar, S. (2005a). Toxicogenomics of cationic lipid-based vectors for gene therapy: impact of microarray technology. *Curr.Drug Deliv.*, Vol.2, No.4, (October 2005), pp. 429-441, ISSN 1567-2018

Omidi, Y.; Barar, J.; heidari, H.R.; Ahmadian, S.; Ahmadpour Yazdi, H. & Akhtar, S. (2008). Microarray Analysis of the Toxicogenomics and the Genotoxic Potential of a Cationic Lipid-Based Gene Delivery Nanosystem in Human Alveolar Epithelial A549 Cells. *Toxicology Mechanisms and Methods*, Vol.18, No.4, (2008), pp. 369-378, ISSN 1537-6524

Omidi, Y. and Davaran, S. (2011). Impacts of biodegradable polymers: towards biomedical applications, In: *Handbook of Applied Biopolymer Technology: Synthesis, Degradation and Applications*, Sharma, S. and Mudhoo, A., pp. 388-418, Royal Society of Chemistry (RSC), ISBN 978-1-84973-151-5, London

Omidi, Y. and Gumbleton, M. (2005). Biological Membranes and Barriers, In: *Biomaterials for Delivery and Targeting of Proteins Nucleic Acids*, Mahato, R. I., pp. 232-274, CRC Press, ISBN 0849323347, New York

Omidi, Y.; Hollins, A.J.; Benboubetra, M.; Drayton, R.; Benter, I.F. & Akhtar, S. (2003). Toxicogenomics of non-viral vectors for gene therapy: a microarray study of lipofectin- and oligofectamine-induced gene expression changes in human epithelial cells. *J Drug Target*, Vol.11, No.6, (2003), pp. 311-323, ISSN 1061-186X

Omidi, Y.; Hollins, A.J.; Drayton, R.M. & Akhtar, S. (2005b). Polypropylenimine dendrimer-induced gene expression changes: the effect of complexation with DNA, dendrimer generation and cell type. *J.Drug Target*, Vol.13, No.7, (August 2005), pp. 431-443, ISSN 1061-186X

Ott, M.G.; Schmidt, M.; Schwarzwaelder, K.; Stein, S.; Siler, U.; Koehl, U.; Glimm, H.; Kuhlcke, K.; Schilz, A.; Kunkel, H.; Naundorf, S.; Brinkmann, A.; Deichmann, A.; Fischer, M.; Ball, C.; Pilz, I.; Dunbar, C.; Du, Y.; Jenkins, N.A.; Copeland, N.G.; Luthi, U.; Hassan, M.; Thrasher, A.J.; Hoelzer, D.; von, K.C.; Seger, R. & Grez, M. (2006). Correction of X-linked chronic granulomatous disease by gene therapy, augmented by insertional activation of MDS1-EVI1, PRDM16 or SETBP1. *Nat.Med.*, Vol.12, No.4, (April 2006), pp. 401-409, ISSN 1078-8956

Pedroso de Lima, M.C.; Simoes, S.; Pires, P.; Faneca, H. & Duzgunes, N. (2001). Cationic lipid-DNA complexes in gene delivery: from biophysics to biological applications. *Adv Drug Deliv Rev*, Vol.47, No.2-3, (2001), pp. 277-294, ISSN 0169-409X

Prokop, A. & Davidson, J.M. (2008). Nanovehicular intracellular delivery systems. *J.Pharm.Sci.*, Vol.97, No.9, (September 2008), pp. 3518-3590,

Quackenbush, J. (2001). Computational analysis of microarray data. *Nat.Rev.Genet.*, Vol.2, No.6, (June 2001), pp. 418-427, ISSN 1471-0056

Quackenbush, J. (2002). Microarray data normalization and transformation. *Nat Genet*, Vol.32 Suppl (2002), pp. 496-501, ISSN 1061-4036

Rawat, A.; Vaidya, B.; Khatri, K.; Goyal, A.K.; Gupta, P.N.; Mahor, S.; Paliwal, R.; Rai, S. & Vyas, S.P. (2007). Targeted intracellular delivery of therapeutics: an overview. *Pharmazie*, Vol.62, No.9, (September 2007), pp. 643-658, ISSN 0031-7144

Regnstrom, K.; Ragnarsson, E.G.; Fryknas, M.; Koping-Hoggard, M. & Artursson, P. (2006). Gene expression profiles in mouse lung tissue after administration of two cationic polymers used for nonviral gene delivery. *Pharm.Res.*, Vol.23, No.3, (March 2006), pp. 475-482, ISSN 1043-6618

Rejman, J.; Bragonzi, A. & Conese, M. (2005). Role of clathrin- and caveolae-mediated endocytosis in gene transfer mediated by lipo- and polyplexes. *Mol.Ther.*, Vol.12, No.3, (September 2005), pp. 468-474, ISSN 1525-0016

Rubanyi, G.M. (2001). The future of human gene therapy. *Mol Aspects Med*, Vol.22, No.3, (2001), pp. 113-142, ISSN 0098-2997

Ruvolo, P.P.; Deng, X. & May, W.S. (2001). Phosphorylation of Bcl2 and regulation of apoptosis. *Leukemia*, Vol.15, No.4, (2001), pp. 515-522, ISSN 0887-6924

Spang, A. (2008). The life cycle of a transport vesicle. *Cell Mol.Life Sci.* (August 2008), ISSN 1420-682X

Sriadibhatla, S.; Yang, Z.; Gebhart, C.; Alakhov, V.Y. & Kabanov, A. (2006). Transcriptional activation of gene expression by pluronic block copolymers in stably and transiently transfected cells. *Mol.Ther.*, Vol.13, No.4, (April 2006), pp. 804-813, ISSN 1525-0016

Sturn, A.; Quackenbush, J. & Trajanoski, Z. (2002). Genesis: cluster analysis of microarray data. *Bioinformatics.*, Vol.18, No.1, (January 2002), pp. 207-208, ISSN 1367-4803

Subramanian, A.; Tamayo, P.; Mootha, V.K.; Mukherjee, S.; Ebert, B.L.; Gillette, M.A.; Paulovich, A.; Pomeroy, S.L.; Golub, T.R.; Lander, E.S. & Mesirov, J.P. (2005). Gene set enrichment analysis: a knowledge-based approach for interpreting genome-wide expression profiles. *Proc.Natl.Acad.Sci.U.S.A*, Vol.102, No.43, (October 2005), pp. 15545-15550, ISSN 0027-8424

Suter, L.; Babiss, L.E. & Wheeldon, E.B. (2004). Toxicogenomics in predictive toxicology in drug development. *Chem.Biol.*, Vol.11, No.2, (February 2004), pp. 161-171, ISSN 1074-5521

Verma, I.M. & Somia, N. (1997). Gene therapy -- promises, problems and prospects. *Nature*, Vol.389, No.6648, (September 1997), pp. 239-242, ISSN 0028-0836

Verma, I.M. & Weitzman, M.D. (2005). Gene therapy: twenty-first century medicine. *Annu.Rev.Biochem.*, Vol.74 (2005), pp. 711-738, ISSN 0066-4154

Yang, Y.; Blomme, E.A. & Waring, J.F. (2004). Toxicogenomics in drug discovery: from preclinical studies to clinical trials. *Chem.Biol.Interact.*, Vol.150, No.1, (November 2004), pp. 71-85, ISSN 0009-2797

Yang, Y.H.; Buckley, M.J. & Speed, T.P. (2001). Analysis of cDNA microarray images. *Brief.Bioinform.*, Vol.2, No.4, (December 2001), pp. 341-349, ISSN 1467-5463

Yaroslavov, A.A.; Kul'kov, V.E.; Polinsky, A.S.; Baibakov, B.A. & Kabanov, V.A. (1994). A polycation causes migration of negatively charged phospholipids from the inner to outer leaflet of the liposomal membrane. *FEBS Lett.*, Vol.340, No.1-2, (1994), pp. 121-123, ISSN 0014-5793

Yaroslavov, A.A.; Melik-Nubarov, N.S. & Menger, F.M. (2006). Polymer-induced flip-flop in biomembranes. *Acc.Chem.Res.*, Vol.39, No.10, (October 2006), pp. 702-710, ISSN 0001-4842

Young, A. (2007). Structural insights into the clathrin coat. *Semin.Cell Dev.Biol.*, Vol.18, No.4, (August 2007), pp. 448-458, ISSN 1084-9521

Zhang, X.; Pan, S.R.; Hu, H.M.; Wu, G.F.; Feng, M.; Zhang, W. & Luo, X. (2008). Poly(ethylene glycol)-block-polyethylenimine copolymers as carriers for gene delivery: effects of PEG molecular weight and PEGylation degree. *J.Biomed.Mater.Res.A*, Vol.84, No.3, (March 2008), pp. 795-804, ISSN 1549-3296

24

Nano-Particulate Calcium Phosphate as a Gene Delivery System

Babak Mostaghaci[1,2], Arash Hanifi[3], Brigitta Loretz[1] and Claus-Michael Lehr[1,4]

[1]Dept. of Drug Delivery (DDEL), Helmholtz-Institute for Pharmaceutical Research Saarland (HIPS), Helmholtz Centre for Infectious Research (HZI) Saarland University, Saarbruecken

[2]Biomaterials Group, Materials Engineering Department Isfahan University of Technology, Isfahan

[3]Tissue Imaging and Spectroscopy Lab, Bioengineering Department Temple University, Philadelphia, PA

[4]Department of Biopharmaceutics and Pharmaceutical Technology Saarland University, Saarbruecken

[1,4]Germany

[2]Iran

[3]USA

1. Introduction

Four decades ago, calcium phosphate systems were introduced for in-vitro gene delivery applications. Recently, many studies have been conducted regarding the different applications of these systems in delivering genes to different cell types for therapeutic purposes. Although there are important limitations of using calcium phosphates in gene delivery, there is a high interest in using this type of gene delivery system. This is because of the significant biocompatibility of calcium phosphates, easy synthesis methods of this system, and intrinsic characteristics of calcium phosphates that increase the transfection efficiency. The combination of these properties are rarely seen in other gene delivery systems.

This chapter aims to localise calcium phosphate nanoparticles among the most common non-viral gene delivery systems. It also reviews the history of using calcium phosphates in gene delivery applications and the efforts made to make this system suitable for further clinical applications.

1.1 Non-viral gene delivery

The application of non-viral systems increased considerably after it was shown that using viral systems can result in several problems including difficulty in production, limited opportunity for repeated administrations due to acute inflammatory response, and delayed humoral or cellular immune responses. Insertional mutagenesis is also a potential issue for some viral systems that integrate foreign DNA into the genome (Al-Dosari & Gao, 2009). Although viral systems such as retrovirus, adenovirus, and adeno-associated virus are potentially efficient, non-viral systems have some advantages in that they are less toxic, less immunogenic, and easier to prepare (Nishikawa & Huang, 2001).

A lot of research has been conducted to find suitable non-viral systems. An ideal gene delivery method needs to meet 3 major criteria:

i. It should protect the transgene against degradation by nucleases in intercellular matrices.
ii. It should be able to carry the transgene across the cell membrane and into the nucleus of targeted cells.
iii. It should have no detrimental effects (Gao et al., 2007).

Recently, various materials have been introduced as potential gene delivery systems. Three groups of substances are more advantageous in this application. These three groups are:

i. Cationic polymers (like polyethyleneimine (Kichler et al., 2001; Kircheis et al., 2001; Wightman et al., 2001), dendrimers (Tang et al., 1996; Zinselmeyer et al., 2002; Dufes et al., 2005), chitosan (Lee et al., 1998; Koping-Hoggard et al., 2001; Loretz & Bernkop-Schnurch, 2006) and poly-L-lysine (Trubetskoy et al., 1992; Benns et al., 2000));
ii. Lipids (like liposomes (Alton et al., 1993; Templeton et al., 1997; Templeton & Lasic, 1999));
iii. Inorganic materials (like calcium phosphates (Liu et al., 2005) and silica nanoparticles (Kneuer et al., 2000; Csogor et al., 2003; Sameti et al., 2003)).

However, some limitations accompany the use of most of these systems including cell toxicity, immune response and low tranfection efficiency.

1.2 Inorganic vectors

Inorganic systems have been used in in-vitro gene delivery for many years, but their clinical application has been developed mostly in the last decade when amino-functionalized silica was introduced. Researchers at Saarland University showed that amino-functionalized silica exhibits good gene tranfection efficiency in addition to its suitable biocompatibility (Kneuer et al., 2000; Csogor et al., 2003; Sameti et al., 2003). Because of this, several studies have been conducted on using amino-funtionalized silica as a gene delivery system (Bharali et al., 2005; Roy et al., 2005; Klejbor et al., 2007; Choi et al., 2008). Research was also conducted on using silica in combination with other polymers for gene delivery. Results demonstrated that making composites of certain polymers with silica nanoparticles could enhance transfection efficiency due to the dense nature of silica nanoparticles (Luo et al., 2004).

There is an increasing interest in mesoporous silica for drug/gene delivery applications because of their higher capacity and of the potential for tailored release of the active molecule. Some studies have been conducted on functionalized or non-functionalized mesoporous silica but the research on using this type of inorganic systems is still ongoing (Park et al., 2008; Slowing et al., 2008).

Some studies have been done on using functionalized gold nanoparticles as a gene delivery system. The results demonstrated the feasibility of using this approach, but further research is needed in this new area (Liang et al., 2010; Niidome et al., 2011).

In addition to calcium phosphate, (their gene delivery application is reviewed in this chapter), other inorganic systems have also been studied regarding in-vitro gene delivery to

targeted cells. Silica nanotubes (Namgung et al., 2011), zirconia (Tan et al., 2007), carbon nanotubes (Pantarotto et al., 2004) and layered double hydroxides (Choy et al., 2008) are some examples of these inorganic systems. However, their low transfection efficacy limits their use. Table 1 summarizes inorganic nanoparticles properties.
The following sections discuss calcium phosphates; one of the most important groups of inorganic non-viral gene delivery systems.

2. Calcium phosphate

The work of Graham and Van Der Eb completed in 1973 shows the first application of calcium phosphate in condensation of genetic materials. The brilliant results of their research were that calcium phosphate could condense DNA and increase the transfection efficiency with a relatively simple procedure (Graham & Van Der EB, 1973a). This first research led to vast application of this technology in in-vitro gene delivery because of the demonstrated easy preparation method and proper results.
In order to have a better understanding of calcium phosphate gene delivery properties, first we shall have a look at the structure and characteristics of the calcium phosphate family.

2.1 Calcium phosphates family

Calcium phosphate-based bioceramics have been used in medicine and dentistry for decades. Applications include dental implants, percutaneous devices, periodontal treatment, alveolar ridge augmentation, orthopedics, maxillofacial surgery, otolaryngology and spinal surgery (Hench, 1991).
Bone is a natural nano-composite composed of organic (40%) and inorganic (60%) components. The inorganic constituent of bone is made up of biological apatites, which provide strength to the skeleton and act as a storehouse for calcium, phosphorus, sodium, and magnesium. These biological apatites are structurally similar, though not identical, to the mineral apatite hydroxyapatite (HAp, $Ca_{10}(PO_4)_6(OH)_2$). Hydroxyapatite is the most ubiquitous and well-known phase of calcium phosphate. It has the Ca/P ratio of 1.67 (Narayan et al., 2004). Different phases of calcium phosphate ceramics are used depending upon whether a resorbable or bioactive material is desired. The stable phases of calcium phosphate ceramics depend considerably upon temperature and the presence of water, either during processing or use in the environment (See Fig. 1) (Hench, 1991).
Going through aforementioned properties, it can be realized that the calcium phosphates family includes several members with different characteristics. Calcium phosphate ratio, Ca/P, has been found as the best way to distinguish among these members. In table 2 these members are shown based on their Ca/P ratio.

2.2 Properties

Calcium phosphates being light in weight, chemically stable and compositionally similar to the mineral phase of the bone are preferred as bone graft materials in hard tissue engineering. They are composed of ions commonly found in physiological environment, which make them highly biocompatible. Many research works demonstrated the biocompatibility of calcium phosphates in-vitro and in-vivo. In addition, these bioceramics are also resistant to microbial attack, pH changes, and solvent conditions (Thamaraiselvi & Rajeswari, 2004; Kalita et al., 2007). Degradation properties are very important, especially in the application of calcium phosphates related to drug delivery. It has been shown that

Kind of nanoparticle	Chemical Composition	Typical Size Range	Solubility in μgL^{-1}	Comments
Cadmium Sulfide	CdS	2–5 nm	0.69 ngL^{-1}	toxic, fluorescent, semiconducting
Calcium Phosphate	$Ca_{10}(PO_4)_6OH_2$ (hydroxyapatite)	10–100 nm	6.1 mg L^{-1}	biodegradable, biocompatible; may be made fluorescent by incorporation of lanthanides; cations and anions may be substituted
Carbon Nanotubes	C_n	diameter of a few nm and length of a few mm	0	Not biodegradable, hollow; may be covalently functionalized to improve solubility and may be loaded with molecules
Cobalt-Platinum	$CoPt_3$	3–10 nm	≈ 0	ferromagnetic or superparamagnetic; toxic in uncoated form
Gold	Au	1–50 nm	≈ 0	easily covalently functionalized, for example, with thiols
Iron Oxide (Magnetite)	Fe_3O_4	5–20 nm	≈ 0	ferromagnetic or superparamagnetic; harmful for cells in uncoated form; solubility increases with falling pH
Layered Double Hydroxide	$Mg_6Al_2(CO_3)(OH)_{16} \cdot 4 H_2O$ (hydrotalcite)	50–200 nm	moderate, increases below pH 5–6	high selective anion exchange capacity; biodegradable in slightly acidic environment; cations can be substituted
Nickel	Ni	5–100 nm	≈ 0	immunogenic, toxic
Silica	$SiO_2 \cdot nH_2O$	3–100 nm	ca. 120 mg SiO_2 L^{-1} (for silica particles)	Biodegradable; available also in micro- or mesoporous form (e.g., zeolites); easily functionalizable, for example, by chlorosilanes
Silver	Ag	5–100 nm	≈ 0	Bactericidal; dissolution product (Ag^+) potentially harmful for cells
Zinc Oxide	ZnO	3–60 nm	1.6 to 5 mg L^{-1}	fluorescent, semiconducting
Zinc Sulfide	ZnS	3–50 nm	67 ngL^{-1}	fluorescent, semiconducting

Table 1. Some key properties of inorganic nanoparticles which are used for transfection in cell biology (Reprinted from (Sokolova & Epple, 2008)).

different crystalline phases of calcium phosphate present different degradation properties. Table 3 summarizes the solubility properties and stability pH range of calcium phosphate.

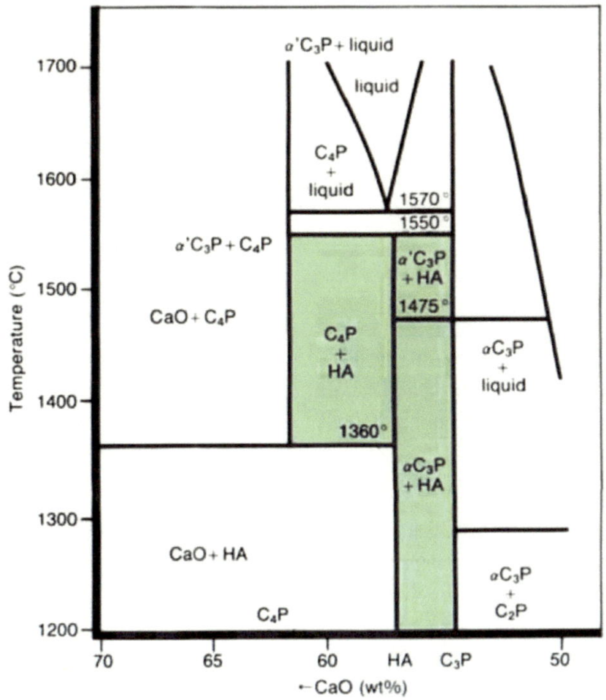

Fig. 1. Calcium phosphate phase equilibrium diagram with 500 mmHg partial pressure of water. Shaded area is the processing range to yield HAp (Hench, 1991).

Ca/P	Name	Formula
2	Tetracalcium phosphate	$Ca_4O(PO4)_2$
1.67	Hydroxyapatite	$Ca_{10}O(PO4)_6(OH)_2$
N/A*	Amorphous calcium phosphate	$Ca_{10-x}H_{2x}(PO4)_6(OH)_2$
1.50	Tricalcium phosphate (α, β, γ)	$Ca_3(PO_4)_2$
1.33	Octacalcium phosphate	$Ca_8H_2(PO_4)_6.5H_2O$
1	Dicalcium phosphate dihydrate	$CaHPO_4.2H_2O$
1	Dicalcium phosphate	$CaHPO_4$
1	Calcium pyrophosphate (α, β, γ)	$Ca_2P_2O_7$
1	Calcium pyrophosphate dihydrate	$Ca_2P_2O_7.2H_2O$
0.7	Heptacalcium phosphate	$Ca_7(P_5O_{16})_2$
0.67	Tetracalcium dihydrogen phosphate	$Ca_4H_2P_6O_{20}$
0.5	Monocalcium phosphate monohydrate	$Ca(H_2PO_4)_2.H_2O$
0.5	Calcium metaphosphate (α, β, γ)	$Ca(PO_3)_2$

*N/A = not applicable

Table 2. Various calcium phosphates with their respective Ca/P atomic ratios (Reprinted from (Vallet-Regi & Gonzalez-Calbet, 2004)).

Phases	Solubility at 25 °C, -log (K_{sp})	pH Stability Range in aqueous solution at 25 °C
Hydroxyapatite (HAp)	116.8	9.5-12
β-Tricalcium Phosphate (β-TCP)	28.9	Cannot be precipitated from aqueous solutions.
α-Tricalcium Phosphate (α-TCP)	25.5	Cannot be precipitated from aqueous solutions.
Tetracalcium Phosphate (TTCP)	38-44	Cannot be precipitated from aqueous solutions.
Dicalcium Phosphate Dehydrate (DCPD)	6.59	2.0 – 6.0
Dicalcium Phosphate Anhydrate (DCPA)	6.90	Stable at temperatures above 100 °C
Amorphous Calcium Phosphate (ACP)	Cannot be measured precisely. However, the following values were reported: 25.7 ± 0.1 (pH 7.40), 29.9 ± 0.1 (pH 6.00), 32.7 ± 0.1 (pH 5.28)	Always metastable. The composition of a precipitate depends on the solution pH value and composition.
Calcium-deficient Hydroxyapatie (CDHA)	≈ 85.1	6.5-9.5

Table 3. Solubility and pH stability of different phases of calcium phosphates (Reprinted from (Kalita et al., 2007)).

2.3 Calcium phosphate nanoparticles

With the introduction of smaller calcium phosphate particles, it has become possible to use them in advanced fields of biomedicine. Calcium phosphate nanoparticles, with a size about 100 nm, are highly biocompatible. These particles are able to penetrate the outer membrane of cells and bacteria. Calcium phosphate nanoparticles could be utilized in different fields of biomedicine such as drug delivery, gene delivery, and imaging (Epple et al., 2010). Also, to produce high quality HAp bioceramics for artificial bone substitution, ultrafine HAp powder is usually employed. Nano-HAp powder results in easy handling, casting, and sintering leading to an excellent sintered body in the bioceramics preparation process (Cao et al., 2005).

3. Calcium phosphate nanoparticles as gene delivery vector

3.1 Historical view

Previously, it is mentioned that the first use of calcium phosphate in gene delivery application was conducted by Graham and Van Der EB in 1973. In this study, calcium phosphate was used for transfecting cells with Adenovirus 5 DNA to assay infectivity. (Graham & Van Der EB, 1973a). They diluted Adenovirus 5 DNA in a buffer containing Na_2HPO_4. Then, calcium chloride was added and the mixture was incubated with KB Cells. Using labeled DNA they concluded that by adding the calcium precursor in the experiment, the uptake of DNA increased and DNA showed a better stability against enzymatic degradation (Fig. 2). It was reported that this technique gave a 100 fold increase in efficiency over the DEAE-dextran method for human adenovirus DNA.

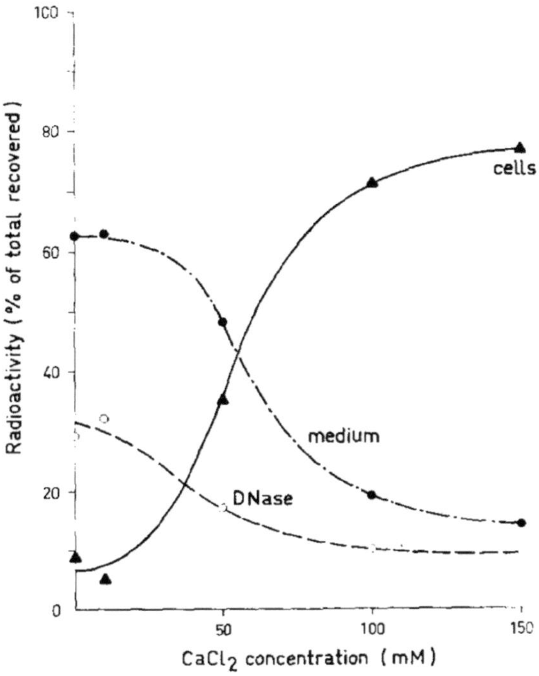

Fig. 2. Effect of $CaCl_2$ on adsorption of ^{14}C-Ad5 DNA to KB cells. KB cells were exposed to MEM-Tris containing DNA plus $CaCl_2$ at various concentrations. The curves represent the fraction of radioactivity recovered in the medium (●), in the DNase digest (O), or in the SDS lysate of the cells (▲) (Graham & Van Der EB, 1973a).

With the same methodology, this group conducted another study to transform rat kidney cells with the DNA of human adenovirus 5. In Fig. 3 the transfected area is clearly visible as contained small, round, densely packed cells characteristic of adenovirus transformation. This work claimed that the "calcium technique" was a suitable system to study transformation by adenovirus DNA and the efficiency of transformation, though not high, appeared to be reasonably reproducible (Graham & Van Der EB, 1973b).

In another study, Graham, Veldhuisen and Wilkie used the aforementioned technique to investigate the infectivity of herpes simplex virus type I (HSV-I) (Graham et al., 1973). In 1975, Abrahams and Van Der EB made a transformation of rat kidney cells and mouse 3T3 cells by DNA from Simian Virus 40 using "calcium technique". They stated that this technique for in-vitro transformation was reproducible (Abrahams & Van Der Eb, 1975). Later, Van Der EB and Graham successfully used "calcium technique" to determine the ability to transform primary baby rat kidney (BRK) cells with specific fragments of human adenoviruses 2 and 5 DNAs (Van Der EB et al., 1977).

In 1976, Stow and Wilkie reported that treatment of cells with dimethyl sulphoxide (DMSO) after injection with "Herpes Simplex Virus DNA"/calcium phosphate complex could lead to a significant increase in the number of plaques obtained. These researchers proposed that DMSO could initiate the plaque formation. It was interesting that in other method (DEAE-dextran) using DMSO did not exhibit that significant enhancement (Fig. 4) (Stow & Wilkie, 1976).

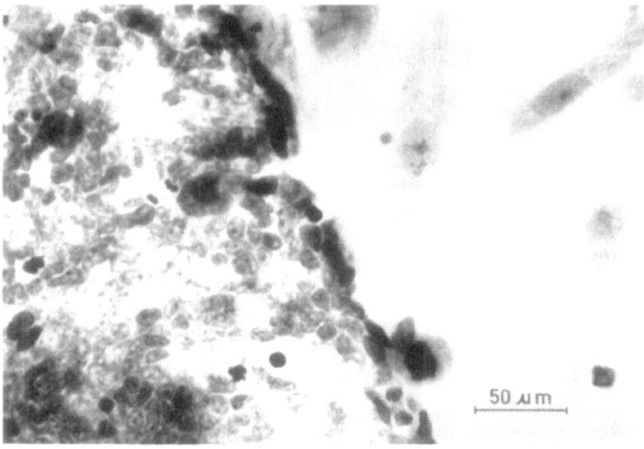

Fig. 3. Part of transformed colony resulting from exposure of primary rat kidney cells to Adenovirus 5 DNA+ $CaCl_2$ 22 days previously. Three normal cells can be seen to the right of the photograph. Giemsa stain (Graham & Van Der EB, 1973b).

During the 1980's, the calcium phosphate method for in-vitro gene delivery had become a common method. In 1981, some of the parameters that affect the transformation procedure by calcium phosphate system had been investigated by Corsaro and Pearson (Corsaro & Pearson, 1981). First, to confirm the work of Stow and Wilkie in 1976, they performed a study on the effect of rinsing the complex of DNA/calcium phosphate with DMSO. They also added an additional variable to this experiment which was the exposure time of DNA/calcium phosphate complex to cells. They claimed that when suboptimal DNA exposure time is applied (e.g. 4-12 hours), the DMSO rinse increases the transformation frequency. However, rinsing with DMSO had no effect when the optimal condition was utilized. They concluded that exposure to DMSO offers no significant advantage.

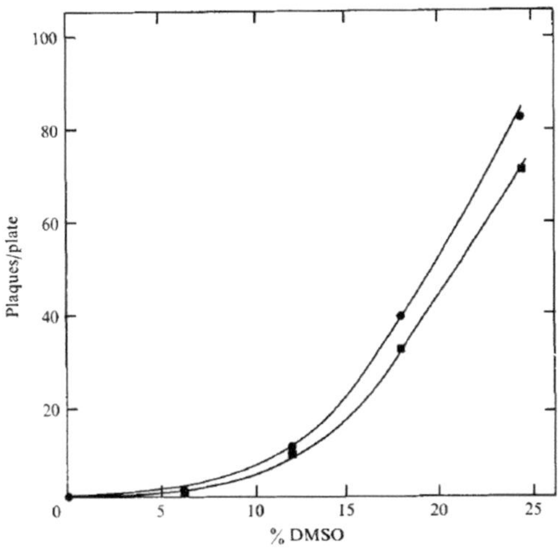

Fig. 4. The effect of DMSO concentration on the enhancement of HSV-I DNA infectivity. Varying concentration of DMSO dissolved in HeBS (●) or eagle's medium (■) (Stow & Wilkie, 1976).

Regarding the formation of DNA/calcium phosphate precipitates, they found that it is critical to add the solution of DNA/$CaCl_2$ to the HEPES-phosphate buffer rather than in the reverse order. Also, they claimed that it is important to add the solution drop-wise, rather than directly (Corsaro & Pearson, 1981).
In 1982, a research group at Yale University conducted research on the mechanism for entry of DNA/calcium phosphate complex in to mammalian cells by electron microscopy and fluorescent dyes (Loyter et al., 1982a; Loyter et al., 1982b).
Electron microscopy and filter hybridization studies revealed that most of the DNA strands enter by phagocytosis. The effect of different drugs and respiratory inhibitors on the entry of DNA was also investigated (Table 4, Fig. 5). Results showed phagocytosis of DNA is inhibited both by respiratory inhibitors and drugs, such as Colcemid, which disassemble microtubules. They concluded that the uptake of DNA/calcium phosphate resembles "receptor mediated" phagocytosis. Also it was seen that ATP-depleted and cold treated cells were not able to adsorb the complex. Thus the authors claimed that the phagocytosis of DNA/calcium phosphate complex is an energy- and temperature-dependent process (Loyter et al., 1982a).

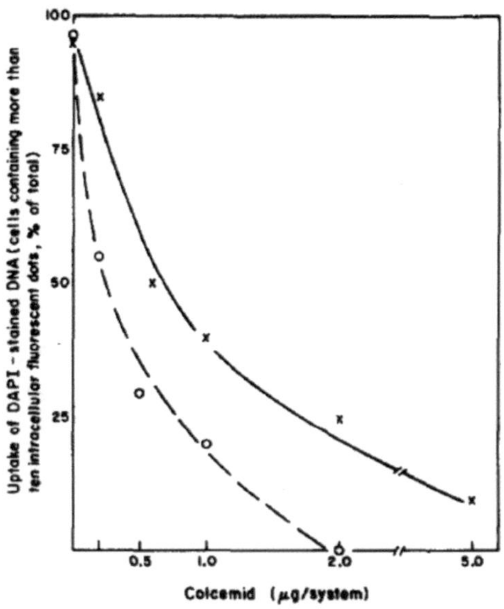

Fig. 5. Effect of increasing concentration of Colcemid on the entry of DAPI-stained DNA/calcium phosphate complexes into *Ltk-* cells (Loyter et al., 1982a).

These researchers also claimed that the pH of the formation of the DNA/calcium phosphate complexes is crucial for successful gene transfer. Studies on the effect of pH and DNA concentration on the entry of fluorescent dye-labeled DNA into cells showed that only during the calcium phosphate complexes formation in the pH rang of 7.1 to 7.5 could fluorescent spots be visualized in the cytoplasm of recipient cells. For the complexes formed above pH = 7.5 no entry to cells could be detected (Fig. 6A).
On the other hand, the DNA/calcium phosphate ratio is important on the adsorption of the complexes. When higher concentrations of DNA was utilized with the constant concentration of calcium phosphate, adsorption was not affected, whereas the appearance of cytoplasmic florescence was drastically reduced (Fig. 6B) (Loyter et al., 1982b).

System	Effect of DNA Entry
Drugs	
Cytochalasin B (1-4 µg/ml)	No effect
Colcemid (5 µg/ml)	Complete inhibition
DMSO (10%, 10-30 min)	No effect
Respiratory inhibitors	
2 deoxyglucose	Partial inhibition
NaN_3	Partial inhibition
NaF	Partial inhibition
NaF + 2 deoxyglucose	Complete inhibition
NaN_3 + 2 deoxyglucose	Complete inhibition

Table 4. The effect of various drugs and respiratory inhibitors on introduction of DNA into *Ltk- Aprt-* cells (Reproduced from (Loyter et al., 1982a)).

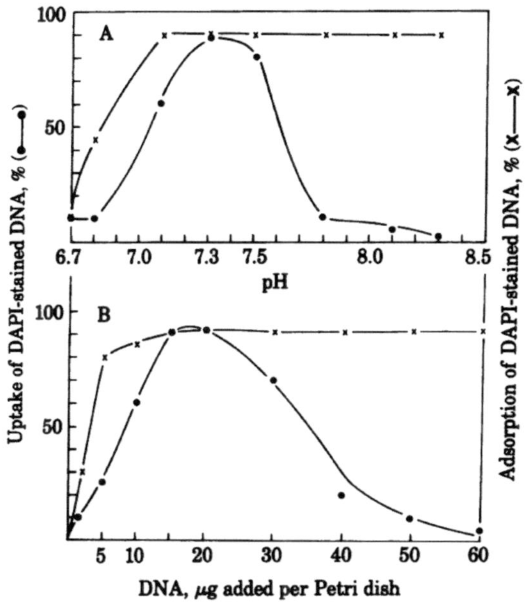

Fig. 6. Adsorption (cells containing adsorbed fluorescent dots) and uptake (cells containing more than 10 intracellular fluorescent dots) of DAPI-stained DNA as a function of the pH of the DNA/calcium phosphate complex (A) and DNA concentration in DNA/calcium phosphate complex (B) (Loyter et al., 1982b).

One of the limitations of calcium phosphate systems in gene delivery applications is that most of the input DNA is degraded before it reaches the nucleus of the cell, where gene expression and DNA replication take place. In 1983, Luthman and Magnusson conducted research on increasing the efficiency of transfection by inhibiting the lysosomal degradation using Chloroquine as a lysosomotropic compound. For this purpose they used a conventional procedure for transfection with calcium phosphate, but they added Chloroquine to the growth medium of the cells. In Fig. 7 the effect of Chloroquine concentration on transfection efficiency using DNA/calcium phosphate complexes can be seen. The authors concluded that when Chloroquine treatment was effective, it increased the fraction of cells that could be successfully transfected. They claimed that this conclusion was supported by the results of experiments in which cells were transfected with linear forms of viral DNA. In that case, in Chloroquine treated cells, the number of DNA molecules which had re-circularized and were able to replicate was much larger than untreated cells (Luthman & Magnusson, 1983).

With the same approach, in 1984 a research group in Norway used different inhibitors of intracellular degradation (such as 3-methyl adenine, NH_4Cl, FCPP and etc.) and claimed that the frequency of transformation was increased due to increasing the cytoplasmic level of exogenous DNA (Table 5) (Ege et al., 1984).

In 1987, Chen and Okayama introduced a new method for gene delivery with calcium phosphate systems. The aim of their work was the formation of DNA/calcium phosphate complexes gradually in medium during incubation with cells. They found that in this method the crucial factors that affect the transfection efficiency are the pH of the buffer used for calcium phosphate precipitation (optimized pH was 6.95) and the CO_2 level during the incubation of DNA with cells. They also found that the amount and the form of DNA are important factors. It was observed that circular DNA has better efficiency than linear DNA but, the reason for this phenomenon was not clear at that time. The authors claimed that the efficiency of their method is comparable to the efficiency of other common transfection systems of that time (Chen & Okayama, 1987).

In 1990 Orrantia and Chang investigated the intracellular distribution of DNA after the DNA/calcium phosphate complexes move into the cells. Results showed that only a small fraction of internalized DNA could be found in the nucleus, the target place for gene delivery. In the enriched nuclear fraction, the mouse cells retained 6.4% of internalized DNA while the human cells retained only 2.2% (Fig. 8).

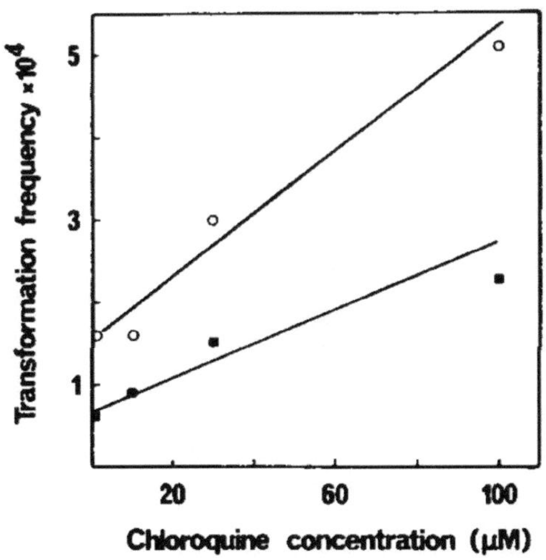

Fig. 7. Effect of Chloroquine concentration on transfection efficiency. Rat-1 cultures were transfected by co-precipitating calcium phosphate and polyoma DNA, 20 ng (■) and 100 ng (o) (Luthman & Magnusson, 1983).

Addition	Concentration	Transformation Frequency after 6 hours
None, no DNA		0
None, DNA alone		4
DNA + glycerol	17 %	10
DNA + DMSO	20 %	22
DNA + NH_4Cl	20 mM	64
DNA + FCPP	1 μM	50
DNA + Procaine	10 mM	3
DNA + chloroquine	100 μM	5
DNA + monensin	5 mM	1
DNA + 3-methyl adenine	5 mM	46

Table 5. Effect of different compounds on the transformation frequency of rat 2 *tk*- cells transfected with pAGO DNA 6 hours after incubation of the indicated compounds with the cells (reproduced from (Ege et al., 1984)).

The authors concluded that transfection with DNA/calcium phosphate is a procedure with low efficiency partly because most of the endocytosed DNA is quickly degraded and excreted to the cytosol (Orrantia & Chang, 1990).
In 1994, O'Mahoney and Adams modified the calcium phosphate transfection procedure described by Chen and Okayama in 1987 and claimed that they reached a reliable and reproducible method with high transfection efficiency. They claimed that the critical factor in this method is the standing time of the DNA/$CaCl_2$/BES-buffered saline prior to addition to cultured cells. They concluded that in the optimal condition it is possible to reach 100% efficiency (Omahoney & Adams, 1994).

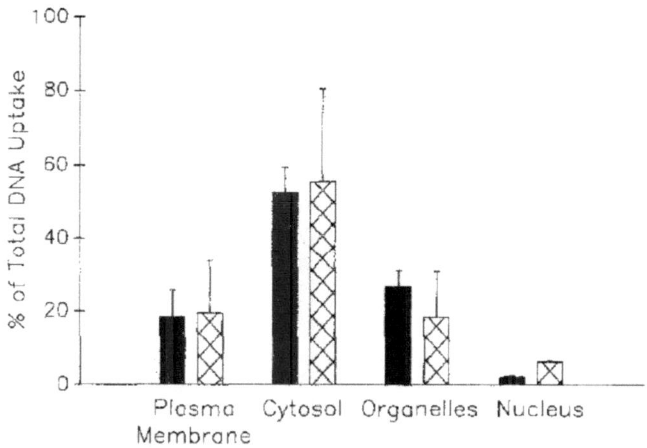

Fig. 8. Distribution of internalized DNA in subcellular fractions from human and mouse cells. Cultured Cells were transfected with ^{32}P-labeled high-molecular-weight DNA/calcium phosphate for 4 h. ■: Human primary fibroblast cells, ☒: Transformed mouse Ltk- cells (Orrantia & Chang, 1990).

In 1996, a research group in Taiwan conducted some research works on electrochemical properties of DNA/calcium phosphate complexes. The study focused on the variation of zeta potential with changes in pH for calcium phosphate and DNA/calcium phosphate complexes. The point of zero charge (pzc) and isoelectric point (iep) were found to be at pH 7.09 and 7.0, respectively. With addition of plasmid DNA, both pzc and iep points shifted to higher values of 7.18 and 7.15, respectively (Yang & Yang, 1996a).

In their other research on this topic, they revealed that the pH of the formation of DNA/calcium phosphate complexes and the concentration of DNA within the complexes were the crucial factor for the entry of these complexes to cells. The results of their study showed that optimum transfection efficiency occurred in the region close to the iep of DNA-calcium phosphate co-precipitates of pH 7.15 and close to the maximum flocculation of this colloidal system. The enhanced cell transformation efficiency occurred at pH 7.01. The zeta potentials of the DNA co-precipitates prepared in the absence of DMEM and calf serum were determined to lie between 11 and 21 mV. Preparation within these limits resulted in an efficient internalization of the DNA/calcium phosphate complexes, and for endocytosis to occur (Yang & Yang, 1996b).

In 2004, Jordan and Wurm investigated the methods that were applied previously for gene delivery with calcium phosphate particles by different authors. They stated that all of the numerous variations of the protocol found in the literature are based on the same principle—a spontaneous precipitation that occurs in supersaturated solutions. Although a wide range of conditions will lead to precipitates, high transfection efficiencies are only obtained within a narrow range of optimized parameters that assure certain properties of the precipitate. Finally, they concluded that despite a rapidly growing choice of efficient transfection reagents, this method remains highly attractive due to its highly biocompatible nature (Jordan & Wurm, 2004).

3.2 Current studies

Research on using calcium phosphate nanoparticles for gene delivery application is still continuing. Researchers perform a lot of new experiments to optimize the parameters involved in gene delivery with calcium phosphate nanoparticles. We have tried to review some of these studies in this chapter.

A research group in the University of Duisburg-Essen, proposed a method to prepare multi-shell calcium phosphate/DNA particles. They utilized a simple method to prepare multi-shell calcium phosphate as illustrated in Fig. 9.

They prepared different nanoparticles and showed that with multi-shell calcium phosphate/DNA nanoparticles the transfection efficiency is increased due to the protection of DNA against nuclease enzymes (Fig. 10). Moreover, the authors claimed that in contrast with conventional calcium phosphate, these particles could be stored for weeks without loss of their transfection efficiency (Sokolova et al., 2006).

They also showed that the standard calcium phosphate method selectively unbalanced intracellular calcium homeostasis while it remained at low control levels after transfection using nanoparticles. They concluded that with using DNA-functionalized calcium phosphate nanoparticles, cells are able to cope with the associated calcium uptake and therefore proved their method to be a superior transfection method (Neumann et al., 2009).

Hanifi et al. conducted some research on the feasibility of using strontium and magnesium substituted calcium phosphate in gene delivery applications. They prepared the particles via a simple sol-gel route. They obtained some particles with nano-size structure, high specific surface area, and a high dissolution rate (Fig. 11). The zeta potential (Table 6) was increased in comparison with simple calcium phosphate. They concluded that due to increased surface charge and solubility, these novel systems could increase the gene transfection efficiency (Hanifi et al., 2010a; Hanifi et al., 2010b).

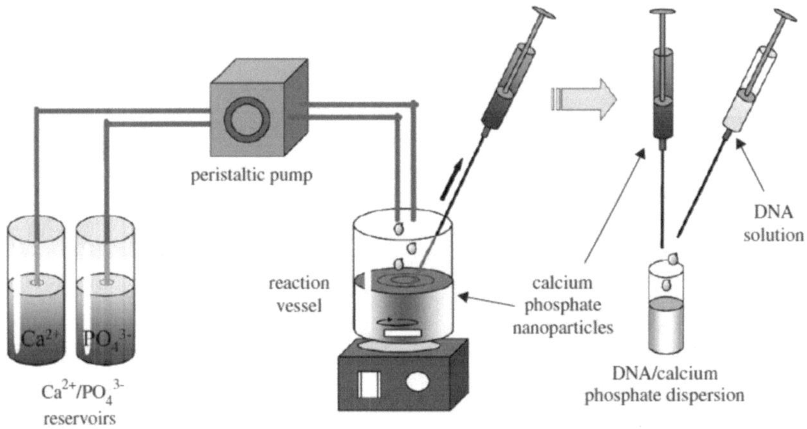

Fig. 9. Schematic set-up of the apparatus used for preparation of DNA-functionalized calcium phosphate nanoparticles. Calcium nitrate and diammonium hydrogen phosphate solutions are mixed in a vessel to form a precipitate. A part of the dispersion is taken with a syringe and mixed with DNA solution in an Eppendorf tube (Sokolova et al., 2006).

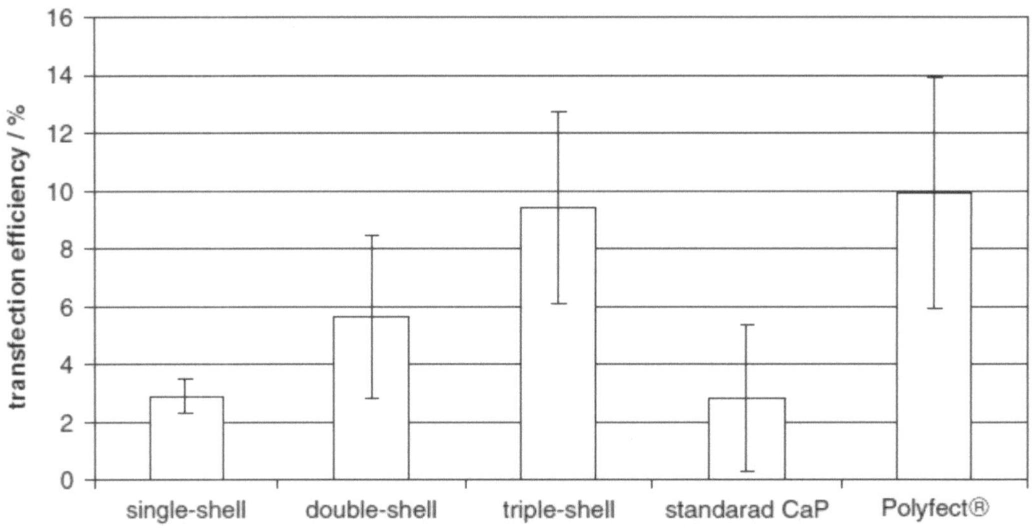

Fig. 10. Comparison of the transfection efficiency of multi-shell calcium phosphate/DNA by different methods. There are significant differences between single-shell and triple-shell ($P<0.01$) and triple-shell and the standard calcium phosphate methods ($P<0.05$) (Sokolova et al., 2006).

Recently there has been an approach to incorporate other agents or materials with calcium phosphate to improve its function as a gene delivery system. Stabilizing with bis-phosphonate (Giger et al., 2011), coating with lipids (Zhou et al., 2010), incorporating in alginate hydrogel (Krebs et al., 2010) and association with Adenovirus (Toyoda et al., 2000) are some examples for this approach.

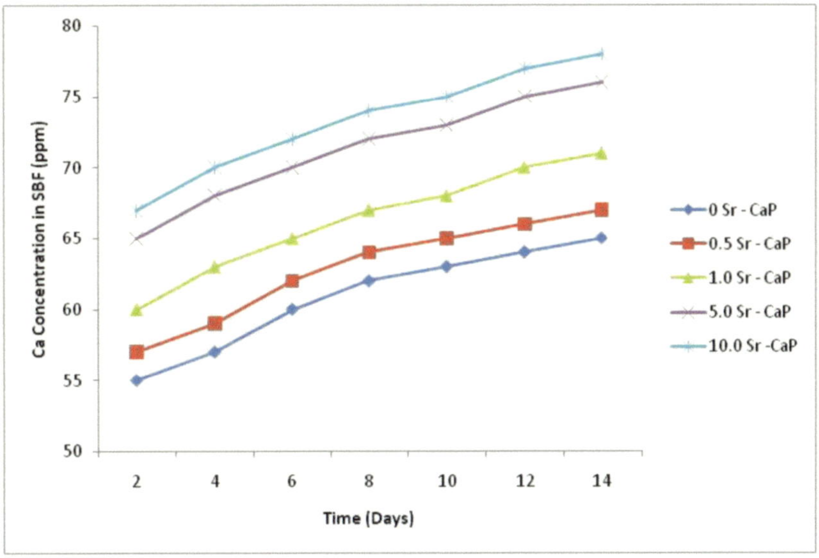

(a)

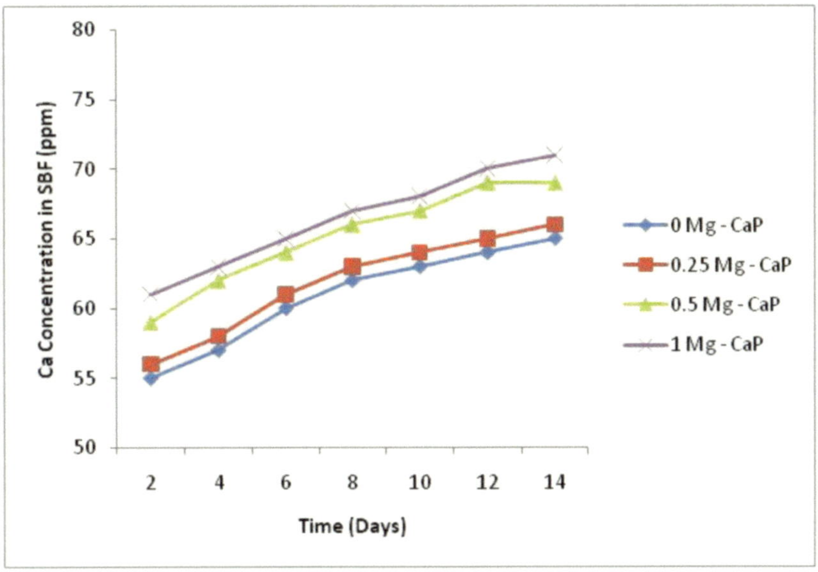

(b)

Fig. 11. Concentration of Ca^{++} ions in SBF solution after predicted period of time. A: Sr-CaP, B: Mg-CaP (Not Published).

Sample composition	Zeta potential (mV)
Sr-Substituted CaP	
0.0Sr-CaP	4.5±0.1
0.5Sr-CaP	5.0±0.2
1.0Sr-CaP	6.1±0.1
5.0Sr-CaP	7.3±0.3
10.0Sr-CaP	7.8±0.2
Mg-Substituted CaP	
0.0Mg-CaP	3.2±0.5
0.25Mg-CaP	6.7±0.4
0.50Mg-CaP	7.5±1
1.0Mg-CaP	8±0.8

Table 6. Surface charge of Sr and Mg substituted calcium phosphate nanoparticles (Reproduce from (Hanifi et al., 2010a; Hanifi et al., 2010b)).

4. Conclusion

Nano-particulate calcium phosphate has shown several interesting advantages in biomedical applications because of its biocompatibility and easy preparation process. The DNA condensation characteristic of nano-particulate calcium phosphate makes it a potential choice for gene therapy system applications. Nano-particulate calcium phosphates are able to condense DNA strands, carry them in the blood, deliver the genetic material to target cells, and move them into cells resulting in reasonable transcription.

Therefore, there is a common agreement among most of the works regarding gene delivery application on utilizing the calcium phosphate to deliver the gene into the nucleus; the final target of gene therapy methods. Because of the advantages of the DNA/calcium phosphate complex, it is one of the highly appealing systems currently studied, although it has been used in in-vitro gene delivery for many years already. The translation of its application into clinical therapy methods requires more work.

Researchers need to solve the instability of calcium phosphate in physiological conditions. If calcium phosphate/DNA complexes degrade in the blood circuit, it cannot be used in most of the clinical gene delivery applications. The other problem is the low transfection efficiency, which currently limits the application of the system. There are controversial reports about the transfection efficiency of calcium phosphate/DNA system, mostly because of instability and the complicated nature of calcium phosphate in solution. Once these problems are overcome by adequate novel technologies, the excellent biocompatibility and biodegradability of calcium phosphate remains as a major advantage.

5. References

Abrahams, P. J. & Van Der Eb, A. J. (1975). In vitro transformation of rat and mouse cells by DNA from simian virus 40. *J Virol*, 16, 1, pp. 206-209

Al-Dosari, M. S. & Gao, X. (2009). Nonviral Gene Delivery: Principle, Limitations, and Recent Progress. *Aaps Journal*, 11, 4, pp. 671-681

Alton, E. W. F. W., Middleton, P. G., Caplen, N. J., Smith, S. N., Steel, D. M., Munkonge, F. M., Jeffery, P. K., Geddes, D. M., Hart, S. L., Williamson, R., Fasold, K. I., Miller, A. D., Dickinson, P., Stevenson, B. J., Mclachlan, G., Dorin, J. R. & Porteous, D. J. (1993). Noninvasive Liposome-Mediated Gene Delivery Can Correct the Ion-Transport Defect in Cystic-Fibrosis Mutant Mice. *Nature Genetics*, 5, 2, pp. 135-142

Benns, J. M., Choi, J. S., Mahato, R. I., Park, J. S. & Kim, S. W. (2000). pH-sensitive cationic polymer gene delivery vehicle: N-Ac-poly(L-histidine)-graft-poly(L-lysine) comb shaped polymer. *Bioconjugate Chemistry*, 11, 5, pp. 637-645

Bharali, D. J., Klejbor, I., Stachowiak, E. K., Dutta, P., Roy, I., Kaur, N., Bergey, E. J., Prasad, P. N. & Stachowiak, M. K. (2005). Organically modified silica nanoparticles: A nonviral vector for in vivo gene delivery and expression in the brain. *Proceedings of the National Academy of Sciences of the United States of America*, 102, 32, pp. 11539-11544

Cao, L. Y., Zhang, C. B. & Huang, H. F. (2005). Synthesis of hydroxyapatite nanoparticles in ultrasonic precipitation. *Ceramics International*, 31, 8, pp. 1041-1044

Chen, C. & Okayama, H. (1987). High-Efficiency Transformation of Mammalian-Cells by Plasmid DNA. *Molecular and Cellular Biology*, 7, 8, pp. 2745-2752

Choi, E. W., Shin, I. S., Lee, C. W. & Youn, H. Y. (2008). The effect of gene therapy using CTLA4Ig/silica-nanoparticles on canine experimental autoimmune thyroiditis. *Journal of Gene Medicine*, 10, 7, pp. 795-804

Choy, J.-H., Park, M. & Oh, J.-M. (2008). Gene and Drug Delivery System with Soluble Inorganic Carriers, In: *NanoBioTechnology : bioinspired devices and materials of the future*, O. Shoseyov and I. Levy, pp. 349-367, Humana Press, Totowa, N.J.

Corsaro, C. M. & Pearson, M. L. (1981). Enhancing the Efficiency of DNA-Mediated Gene-Transfer in Mammalian-Cells. *Somatic Cell Genetics*, 7, 5, pp. 603-616

Csogor, Z., Nacken, M., Sameti, M., Lehr, C. M. & Schmidt, H. (2003). Modified silica particles for gene delivery. *Materials Science & Engineering C-Biomimetic and Supramolecular Systems*, 23, 1-2, pp. 93-97

Dufes, C., Uchegbu, I. F. & Schatzlein, A. G. (2005). Dendrimers in gene delivery. *Advanced Drug Delivery Reviews*, 57, 15, pp. 2177-2202

Ege, T., Reisbig, R. R. & Rogne, S. (1984). Enhancement of DNA-Mediated Gene-Transfer by Inhibitors of Autophagic-Lysosomal Function. *Experimental Cell Research*, 155, 1, pp. 9-16

Epple, M., Ganesan, K., Heumann, R., Klesing, J., Kovtun, A., Neumann, S. & Sokolova, V. (2010). Application of calcium phosphate nanoparticles in biomedicine. *Journal of Materials Chemistry*, 20, 1, pp. 18-23

Gao, X., Kim, K. S. & Liu, D. X. (2007). Nonviral gene delivery: What we know and what is next. *Aaps Journal*, 9, 1, pp. E92-E104

Giger, E. V., Puigmarti-Luis, J., Schlatter, R., Castagner, B., Dittrich, P. S. & Leroux, J. C. (2011). Gene delivery with bisphosphonate-stabilized calcium phosphate nanoparticles. *J Control Release*, 150, 1, pp. 87-93

Graham, F. L. & Van Der EB, A. J. (1973a). New Technique for Assay of Infectivity of Human Adenovirus 5 DNA. *Virology*, 52, 2, pp. 456-467

Graham, F. L. & Van Der EB, A. J. (1973b). Transformation of Rat Cells by DNA of Human Adenovirus-5. *Virology*, 54, 2, pp. 536-539

Graham, F. L., Veldhuis.G & Wilkie, N. M. (1973). Infectious Herpesvirus DNA. *Nature-New Biology*, 245, 148, pp. 265-266

Hanifi, A., Fathi, M. H. & Sadeghi, H. M. M. (2010a). Effect of strontium ions substitution on gene delivery related properties of calcium phosphate nanoparticles. *Journal of Materials Science-Materials in Medicine*, 21, 9, pp. 2601-2609

Hanifi, A., Fathi, M. H., Sadeghi, H. M. M. & Varshosaz, J. (2010b). Mg2+ substituted calcium phosphate nano particles synthesis for non viral gene delivery application. *Journal of Materials Science-Materials in Medicine*, 21, 8, pp. 2393-2401

Hench, L. L. (1991). Bioceramics - from Concept to Clinic. *Journal of the American Ceramic Society*, 74, 7, pp. 1487-1510

Jordan, M. & Wurm, F. (2004). Transfection of adherent and suspended cells by calcium phosphate. *Methods*, 33, 2, pp. 136-143

Kalita, S. J., Bhardwaj, A. & Bhatt, H. A. (2007). Nanocrystalline calcium phosphate ceramics in biomedical engineering. *Materials Science & Engineering C-Biomimetic and Supramolecular Systems*, 27, 3, pp. 441-449

Kichler, A., Leborgne, C., Coeytaux, E. & Danos, O. (2001). Polyethylenimine-mediated gene delivery: a mechanistic study. *Journal of Gene Medicine*, 3, 2, pp. 135-144

Kircheis, R., Wightman, L. & Wagner, E. (2001). Design and gene delivery activity of modified polyethylenimines. *Advanced Drug Delivery Reviews*, 53, 3, pp. 341-358

Klejbor, I., Stachowiak, E. K., Bharali, D. J., Roy, I., Spodnik, I., Morys, J., Bergey, E. J., Prasad, P. N. & Stachowiak, M. K. (2007). ORMOSIL nanoparticles as a non-viral gene delivery vector for modeling polyglutamine induced brain pathology. *Journal of Neuroscience Methods*, 165, 2, pp. 230-243

Kneuer, C., Sameti, M., Haltner, E. G., Schiestel, T., Schirra, H., Schmidt, H. & Lehr, C. M. (2000). Silica nanoparticles modified with aminosilanes as carriers for plasmid DNA. *International Journal of Pharmaceutics*, 196, 2, pp. 257-261

Koping-Hoggard, M., Tubulekas, I., Guan, H., Edwards, K., Nilsson, M., Varum, K. M. & Artursson, P. (2001). Chitosan as a nonviral gene delivery system. Structure-property relationships and characteristics compared with polyethylenimine in vitro and after lung administration in vivo. *Gene Therapy*, 8, 14, pp. 1108-1121

Krebs, M. D., Salter, E., Chen, E., Sutter, K. A. & Alsberg, E. (2010). Calcium phosphate-DNA nanoparticle gene delivery from alginate hydrogels induces in vivo osteogenesis. *J Biomed Mater Res A*, 92, 3, pp. 1131-1138

Lee, K. Y., Kwon, I. C., Kim, Y. H., Jo, W. H. & Jeong, S. Y. (1998). Preparation of chitosan self-aggregates as a gene delivery system. *Journal of Controlled Release*, 51, 2-3, pp. 213-220

Liang, X. J., Guo, S. T., Huang, Y. Y., Jiang, Q. A., Sun, Y., Deng, L. D., Liang, Z. C., Du, Q. A., Xing, J. F., Zhao, Y. L., Wang, P. C. & Dong, A. J. (2010). Enhanced Gene Delivery and siRNA Silencing by Gold Nanoparticles Coated with Charge-Reversal Polyelectrolyte. *Acs Nano*, 4, 9, pp. 5505-5511

Liu, T., Tang, A., Zhang, G. Y., Chen, Y. X., Zhang, J. Y., Peng, S. S. & Cai, Z. M. (2005). Calcium phosphate nanoparticles as a novel nonviral vector for efficient trasfection of DNA in cancer gene therapy. *Cancer Biotherapy and Radiopharmaceuticals*, 20, 2, pp. 141-149

Loretz, B. & Bernkop-Schnurch, A. (2006). In vitro evaluation of chitosan-EDTA conjugate polyplexes as a nanoparticulate gene delivery system. *Aaps Journal*, 8, 4, pp. E756-E764

Loyter, A., Scangos, G., Juricek, D., Keene, D. & Ruddle, F. H. (1982a). Mechanisms of DNA Entry into Mammalian-Cells .2. Phagocytosis of Calcium-Phosphate DNA Coprecipitate Visualized by Electron-Microscopy. *Experimental Cell Research*, 139, 1, pp. 223-234

Loyter, A., Scangos, G. A. & Ruddle, F. H. (1982b). Mechanisms of DNA Uptake by Mammalian-Cells - Fate of Exogenously Added DNA Monitored by the Use of Fluorescent Dyes. *Proceedings of the National Academy of Sciences of the United States of America-Biological Sciences*, 79, 2, pp. 422-426

Luo, D., Han, E., Belcheva, N. & Saltzman, W. M. (2004). A self-assembled, modular DNA delivery system mediated by silica nanoparticles. *Journal of Controlled Release*, 95, 2, pp. 333-341

Luthman, H. & Magnusson, G. (1983). High-Efficiency Polyoma DNA Transfection of Chloroquine Treated-Cells. *Nucleic Acids Research*, 11, 5, pp. 1295-1308

Namgung, R., Zhang, Y., Fang, Q. L., Singha, K., Lee, H. J., Kwon, I. K., Jeong, Y. Y., Park, I. K., Son, S. J. & Kim, W. J. (2011). Multifunctional silica nanotubes for dual-modality gene delivery and MR imaging. *Biomaterials*, 32, 11, pp. 3042-3052

Narayan, R. J., Kumta, P. N., Sfeir, C., Lee, D. H., Olton, D. & Choi, D. W. (2004). Nanostructured ceramics in medical devices: Applications and prospects. *Jom*, 56, 10, pp. 38-43

Neumann, S., Kovtun, A., Dietzel, I. D., Epple, M. & Heumann, R. (2009). The use of size-defined DNA-functionalized calcium phosphate nanoparticles to minimise intracellular calcium disturbance during transfection. *Biomaterials*, 30, 35, pp. 6794-6802

Niidome, T., Pissuwan, D. & Cortie, M. B. (2011). The forthcoming applications of gold nanoparticles in drug and gene delivery systems. *Journal of Controlled Release*, 149, 1, pp. 65-71

Nishikawa, M. & Huang, L. (2001). Nonviral vectors in the new millennium: Delivery barriers in gene transfer. *Human Gene Therapy*, 12, 8, pp. 861-870

Omahoney, J. V. & Adams, T. E. (1994). Optimization of Experimental-Variables Influencing Reporter Gene-Expression in Hepatoma-Cells Following Calcium-Phosphate Transfection. *DNA and Cell Biology*, 13, 12, pp. 1227-1232

Orrantia, E. & Chang, P. L. (1990). Intracellular-Distribution of DNA Internalized through Calcium-Phosphate Precipitation. *Experimental Cell Research*, 190, 2, pp. 170-174

Pantarotto, D., Singh, R., McCarthy, D., Erhardt, M., Briand, J. P., Prato, M., Kostarelos, K. & Bianco, A. (2004). Functionalized carbon nanotubes for plasmid DNA gene delivery. *Angewandte Chemie-International Edition*, 43, 39, pp. 5242-5246

Park, I. Y., Kim, I. Y., Yoo, M. K., Choi, Y. J., Cho, M. H. & Cho, C. S. (2008). Mannosylated polyethylenimine coupled mesoporous silica nanoparticles for receptor-mediated gene delivery. *International Journal of Pharmaceutics*, 359, 1-2, pp. 280-287

Roy, I., Ohulchanskyy, T. Y., Bharali, D. J., Pudavar, H. E., Mistretta, R. A., Kaur, N. & Prasad, P. N. (2005). Optical tracking of organically modified silica nanoparticles as DNA carriers: A nonviral, nanomedicine approach for gene delivery. *Proceedings of the National Academy of Sciences of the United States of America*, 102, 2, pp. 279-284

Sameti, M., Bohr, G., Kumar, M. N. V. R., Kneuer, C., Bakowsky, U., Nacken, M., Schmidt, H. & Lehr, C. M. (2003). Stabilisation by freeze-drying of cationically modified silica nanoparticles for gene delivery. *International Journal of Pharmaceutics*, 266, 1-2, pp. 51-60

Slowing, I. I., Vivero-Escoto, J. L., Wu, C. W. & Lin, V. S. Y. (2008). Mesoporous silica nanoparticles as controlled release drug delivery and gene transfection carriers. *Advanced Drug Delivery Reviews*, 60, 11, pp. 1278-1288

Sokolova, V. & Epple, M. (2008). Inorganic nanoparticles as carriers of nucleic acids into cells. *Angewandte Chemie-International Edition*, 47, 8, pp. 1382-1395

Sokolova, V. V., Radtke, I., Heumann, R. & Epple, M. (2006). Effective transfection of cells with multi-shell calcium phosphate-DNA nanoparticles. *Biomaterials*, 27, 16, pp. 3147-3153

Stow, N. D. & Wilkie, N. M. (1976). Improved Technique for Obtaining Enhanced Infectivity with Herpes-Simplex Virus Type-1 DNA. *Journal of General Virology*, 33, Dec, pp. 447-458

Tan, K., Cheang, P., Ho, I. A. W., Lam, P. Y. P. & Hui, K. M. (2007). Nanosized bioceramic particles could function as efficient gene delivery vehicles with target specificity for the spleen. *Gene Therapy*, 14, 10, pp. 828-835

Tang, M. X., Redemann, C. T. & Szoka, F. C. (1996). In vitro gene delivery by degraded polyamidoamine dendrimers. *Bioconjugate Chemistry*, 7, 6, pp. 703-714

Templeton, N. S. & Lasic, D. D. (1999). New directions in liposome gene delivery. *Molecular Biotechnology*, 11, 2, pp. 175-180

Templeton, N. S., Lasic, D. D., Frederik, P. M., Strey, H. H., Roberts, D. D. & Pavlakis, G. N. (1997). Improved DNA: Liposome complexes for increased systemic delivery and gene expression. *Nature Biotechnology*, 15, 7, pp. 647-652

Thamaraiselvi, T. V. & Rajeswari, S. (2004). Biological Evaluation of Bioceramic Materials - A Review. *Trends Biomater. Artif. Organs*, 18, 1, pp. 9-17

Toyoda, K., Andresen, J. J., Zabner, J., Faraci, F. M. & Heistad, D. D. (2000). Calcium phosphate precipitates augment adenovirus-mediated gene transfer to blood vessels in vitro and in vivo. *Gene Ther*, 7, 15, pp. 1284-1291

Trubetskoy, V. S., Torchilin, V. P., Kennel, S. J. & Huang, L. (1992). Use of N-Terminal Modified Poly(L-Lysine) Antibody Conjugate as a Carrier for Targeted Gene Delivery in Mouse Lung Endothelial-Cells. *Bioconjugate Chemistry*, 3, 4, pp. 323-327

Vallet-Regi, M. & Gonzalez-Calbet, J. M. (2004). Calcium phosphates as substitution of bone tissues. *Progress in Solid State Chemistry*, 32, 1-2, pp. 1-31

Van Der EB, A. J., Mulder, C., Graham, F. L. & Houweling, A. (1977). Transformation with Specific Fragments of Adenovirus Dnas .1. Isolation of Specific Fragments with Transforming Activity of Adenovirus-2 and 5 DNA. *Gene*, 2, 3-4, pp. 115-132

Wightman, L., Kircheis, R., Rossler, V., Carotta, S., Ruzicka, R., Kursa, M. & Wagner, E. (2001). Different behavior of branched and linear polyethylenimine for gene delivery in vitro and in vivo. *Journal of Gene Medicine*, 3, 4, pp. 362-372

Yang, Y. W. & Yang, J. C. (1996a). Characterization of Calcium Phosphate as a Gene Carrier (I): Electrochemical Properties. *Drug Delivery*, 3, pp. 173-179

Yang, Y. W. & Yang, J. C. (1996b). Characterization of Calcium Phosphate as a Gene Carrier (II): Zeta Potential and DNA Transfection. *Drug Delivery*, 3, pp. 181-186

Zhou, C., Yu, B., Yang, X., Huo, T., Lee, L. J., Barth, R. F. & Lee, R. J. (2010). Lipid-coated nano-calcium-phosphate (LNCP) for gene delivery. *Int J Pharm*, 392, 1-2, pp. 201-208

Zinselmeyer, B. H., Mackay, S. P., Schatzlein, A. G. & Uchegbu, I. F. (2002). The lower-generation polypropylenimine dendrimers are effective gene-transfer agents. *Pharmaceutical Research*, 19, 7, pp. 960-967

25

Modular Multifunctional Protein Vectors for Gene Therapy

Hugo Peluffo
Department of Histology and Embryology, Faculty of Medicine, University of the Republic (UDELAR) and Neurodegeneration Laboratory, Institut Pasteur de Montevideo Uruguay

1. Introduction

The introduction of genes into the organism or the regulation of the expression of endogenous genes has emerged in the last decade as a very potent strategy for correcting monogenic inherited diseases, treating acute disorders, and slowing down the progression of diseases without known cure. In addition it constitutes an important tool for research, which has been widely used and has contributed to show the mechanisms behind several physiological processes and pathologies.

Adequate carriers able to transfer DNA or RNA into target cells have been largely explored. However, this is an area under continuous expansion as there is no ideal vector suitable for all applications. In fact, no individual vector will meet all the characteristics for a perfect or ideal vector, as many of the needs are different and even contradictory. For example, immunogenicity is in most cases an undesirable side effect, while it is a valuable property when treating tumours as it contributes to their clearance. Another example of contradictory needs of one single vector would be the capacity of a vector to determine the overexpression of the transgenic protein for life. This would be an essential property for the treatment of inherited diseases produced by the lack of a particular protein, however for the treatment of acute injuries the lifelong expression of a therapeutic protein will probably be deleterious. Moreover, some vectors do not transduce post-mitotic cells like neurons or muscle fibres, which is a drawback for targeting these cell types but may be an advantage for the targeting of cancer cells. Thus, there is a need for diverse type of vectors for diverse therapeutic or experimental paradigms, and in particular versatile tuneable vectors would be very interesting. Moreover, several basic problems with the known vectors persist, like toxicity, oncogenicity, immunogenicity, low transfection efficiency, or poor bioavailability, which need further consideration and efforts.

Due to their natural efficiency, viruses have been modified to act as vectors, and they have shown a good degree of success. Non-viral vectors have also been developed by combining several properties necessary for transfection: nucleic acid attachment and condensation, cell attachment, cell entry, endosomal escape, intracellular trafficking, nuclear entry, and nucleic acid release. Some of these vectors are quite simple, as the ones formed by the combination of nucleic acids and lipid components or other carriers like polyethylene glycol (PEG). Others include the previous components but have in addition attached targeting molecules like antibodies, enabling these vectors to preferentially transfect a given tissue. In fact even

magnetic fields have been used to concentrate suitable engineered vectors to a given area (Corchero and Villaverde 2009).
An interesting type of non-viral vectors is the one based on multifunctional proteins (Aris and Villaverde 2004; Mastrobattista *et al.* 2006). The combination of functional domains in a single polypeptide is a simple yet powerful approach for the development of vectors suitable for gene therapy. In fact, this approach has generated the first prototypes of modular protein gene therapy vectors. Three general methods have been used for the engineering of these molecules: i) production of a recombinant protein by the direct fusion of the functional domains; ii) production of a recombinant protein by combining a known scaffold protein and several functional domains inserted into exposed regions of the scaffold protein; and iii) chemical conjugation of functional domains and proteins. Many of these vectors can be produced recombinantly, generating reproducible and stable stocks appropriate for the formulation of clinically usable drugs. Moreover, the modular nature of these versatile vectors enables the combination of different domains to fulfil the changing requirements of pathological end experimental situations.

2. Functional domains available

2.1 Nucleic acid attachment and condensation

Trans-membrane transport of DNA is an inefficient process, and thus the successful introduction of a transgene into a target cell must include two important steps regarding the plasmid or oligonucleotid DNA that is included in the vector. First, the extended DNA needs to be condensed into an ordered compact nano-particle, and second, once inside the nucleus, the DNA must be de-condensed and thus accessible to transcription. Basic peptides or polycations have been exploited for the interaction with the DNA backbone due to their electrostatic interactions (Bloomfield 1996; Saccardo *et al.* 2009)(see Table 1). When DNA is mixed with these condensing agents, smaller molecules of different shapes are formed mainly depending on DNA size (Vijayanathan *et al.* 2002). For instance, in the absence of DNA, the HNRK modular vector that uses poly-lysine for DNA condensation, self-organize as amorphous, polydisperse particulate entities ranging from a few nanometres up to around one micron. However, in the presence of DNA, protein-DNA complexes appear as tight and rather monodisperse spherical-like nanoparticles of around 80 nm in diameter (Domingo-Espín *et al.* 2011). The most widely used condensing agent is a poly-lysine chain (Saccardo *et al.* 2009). Poly-lysine polymers containing at least 6 lysines will efficiently condense DNA, however, additional 4 to 9 lysines are needed to fully condensate the DNA into smaller particles of 50-100nm, increasing in this way many folds the transfection capacity (Wadhwa *et al.* 1997). Other basic peptides used are the poly-arginine peptides, which not only induce DNA condensation, but also show membrane translocation potential (Futaki *et al.* 2001) and nuclear translocation capacity, determining in this way transgene expression (Kim *et al.* 2003; Vazquez *et al.*).
The condensed DNA by these peptides is partially protected from cellular acid nucleases of the lysosomal compartment (Krishnamoorthy *et al.* 2003; Ross *et al.* 1998; Wolfert and Seymour 1998) and serum nucleases, inducing an extended half-life in serum (Kumar *et al.* 2007) and in the circulation, making tissue targeting possible (Kawabata *et al.* 1995; Nishikawa *et al.* 2000a). For example, the addition of the acid nuclease inhibitor DMI-2 induced a 10-fold increase in receptor-mediated transfection in cultured cells exposed to a

Surfactant Protein A-poly-lysine modular vector or a transferrin-poly-lysine modular vector (Ross *et al.* 1998). Naturally DNA condensing proteins have also been used for the construction of modular vectors. For instance, Histones condense plasmid DNA and protects it from endonucleases, being the lysine-rich H1 Histone the most effective one (Pyhtila *et al.* 1976). Moreover, some nuclear localization signals like the NLS peptide from SV40 virus large T-antigen are lysine-rich peptides that when used as a tetramer can efficiently condense DNA without loosing its nuclear localization properties (Ritter *et al.* 2003).

2.2 Cell attachment and cell targeting

When a viral or non-viral gene therapy vector is injected intravenously, most of the vectors will localize mainly in the liver but also in the kidneys, lungs and spleen. While this is normally a problem to circumvent for most gene therapy applications, it constitutes an advantage for the expression of molecules in the liver. There are many fetal metabolic diseases resulting from a defect or a deficiency of hepatocyte-derived proteins. Moreover, the liver can be considered as a platform to produce various proteins secreted into the blood. Therefore, many pioneer studies focused on the development of more efficient gene delivery systems for the introduction of therapeutic genes selectively into hepatocytes (Wu and Wu 1988). Intravenously injected plasmids are cleared from the circulation by the liver non-parenchymal cells by a scavenging receptor mediated mechanism (Kawabata *et al.* 1995). When Nishikawa and colleagues administered naked ^{32}PDNA into the tail vein of mice, about 40% and 10% of the radioactivity rapidly accumulated in the liver and kidneys, respectively (Nishikawa *et al.* 2000b). Again, the main cell-types targeted were the liver non-parenchymal cells: Kupffer cells and endothelial cells. When they injected a vector composed of ^{32}PDNA/polyornithine, little effect on the distribution of the DNA was observed. However, the injection of the ^{32}PDNA/Gal-pOrn galactose-mediated hepatocyte-targeting vector induced a 60% hepatic accumulation of radioactivity, but more interestingly, most of the targeted cells were now hepatocytes instead of Kupffer or endothelial cells. The same effect was observed at the level of luciferase transgene expression, indicating that the DNA/Gal-pOrn vector was not only able to adhere and enter preferentially into hepatocytes, but it could also transfect them.

Many different domains of known proteins and sugars have been used for cell targeting of modular vectors, like galactose (Wu and Wu 1987), transferrin (Wagner *et al.* 1990), foot-and-mouth disease virus integrin interacting peptide (Aris *et al.* 2000; Aris and Villaverde 2003; Domingo-Espín *et al.* 2011), nerve growth factor (Ma *et al.* 2004; Zeng *et al.* 2004), surfactant protein A (Ross *et al.* 1995), rabies virus glycoprotein (Kumar *et al.* 2007), tetanus toxin fragment Hc (Box *et al.* 2003; Knight *et al.* 1999), cholera toxin b chain (Barrett *et al.* 2004), and neurotensin (Navarro-Quiroga *et al.* 2002). In an interesting study, Arango-Rodríguez and colleagues showed that they could target only substantia nigra neurotensin high affinity receptor positive neurons by means of a modular vector that displayed neurotensin, while no other neurons were transfected (Arango-Rodriguez *et al.* 2006). *In vivo*, many of these targeting systems have shown success (see Table 1). An additional interesting targeting strategy is the use of antibodies (Berhanu and Rush 2008; Buschle *et al.* 1995; Thurnher *et al.* 1994). For instance, the use of the 1E3 antibody against the Tn antigen expressed on many carcinomas coupled to polylysine induced an important increase in the transfection of a cancer cell line (Thurnher *et al.* 1994). Another vector, named fkAbp75-ipr, possess several

Name	Functional Domains	Production Method	Particle Size with nucleic acid (nm)	Gene	Target cells	Administration route	Time of transgene expression	Functional effect	Toxicity	Authors
ASOR-PL	Asialoorosomucoid glycoprotein, Poly-Lys	Chemical conjugation	ND	Human serum albumin	Asialoglyco-protein receptor+ Hepatocytes	i.v.	At least 4 weeks	Partial correction of analbuminemia and hypercholesterolemia	ND	(Wilson et al. 1992; Wu et al. 1991; Wu and Wu 1987)
F105-P	αHIV-gp160 Fab fragment, protamine	Expressed in COS cells	ND	c-myc, MDM2, VEGF siRNA	HIV-gp160 overexpressing cancer cells	i.v.	ND	Partial inhibition of tumour growth	No interferon response detected	(Song et al. 2005)
Gal-PL	Galactose, Poly-Lys	Chemical conjugation	10-12	Human Factor IX	Asialoglyco-protein receptor+ Hepatocytes	i.v.	At least 140 days	No, but increased blood human Facto IX	ND	(Perales et al. 1994)
Man-PL	Mannose, Poly-Lys	Chemical conjugation	220	Chloramphenicol acetyltransferase	Mannose receptor+ hepatic Kuppfer cells	i.v.	At least 2 days	ND	ND	(Nishikawa et al. 2000a)
PEI600/DNA/NL4-10K	PEI600, NGF loop4, Poly-Lys	Chemical synthesis and charge interaction assembly	180.4± 5.5	Luciferase	DRG neurons	i.t.	At least 2 days	ND	No	(Zeng et al. 2007)
MC192-P-L-l	MAB MC192 αp75NTR, Poly-Lys	Chemical conjugation	ND	GDNF	p75NTR+ cells	Gel foam at nerve transection site	Al least 8 weeks	Neuroprotection of motor neurons after peripheral nerve transection	ND	(Barati *et al.* 2006)
fkAbp75-ipr	MAB MC192 αp75NTR, HA2, Poly-Lys, SV40-NLS	Chemical conjugation	ND	TrkA siRNA	p75NTR+ cells	i.c.v. Osmotic pump	20 days	Impaired spatial memory after TrkA downregulation	ND	(Berhanu and Rush 2008)
249AL	β-Galactosidase scaffold, integrin binding FMDV RGD, Poly-Lys	Bacterial recombinant	20-40x100-200 filaments	GFP	αvβ3 and other αv integrin+ cells	i.c.	3 days	ND	No	(Aris et al. 2000; Peluffo et al. 2003)
NLSCt	β-Galactosidase scaffold, integrin binding FMDV RGD, Poly-Lys, SV40-NLS	Bacterial recombinant	ND but probably similar to 249AL	Cu/Zn SOD	αvβ3 and other αv integrin+ cells	i.c.	3 days	Neuroprotection from excitotoxic brain lesion after Cu/Zn SOD overexpression	No, in fact neuroprotective per se	(Aris and Villaverde 2003; Peluffo et al. 2006)

Name	Functional Domains	Production Method	Particle Size with nucleic acid (nm)	Gene	Target cells	Administration route	Time of transgene expression	Functional effect	Toxicity	Authors
LDL-DNA	Several domains of the Apo B100 protein of LDL	Isolated from human and rat plasma	ND	GFP and luciferase	Apoprotein B100 receptor+ cells	i.v.	2 days	ND	ND	(Guevara et al.)
RVG+9R	Rabies virus glycoprotein (29aa), Poly-Arg	Chemical synthesis	ND	GFP siRNA, Cu/ZnSOD siRNA, and FvEJ siRNA	Acetylcholine receptor+ cells	i.v.	2-3 days	Downregulation of genes, protection from mortal viral encephalitis	No inflammation nor specific antibodies produced	(Kumar et al. 2007)
Gal-pOrn-mHA2	Galactose, Poly-Orn, mHA2	Chemical synthesis	130.9 ± 22.6	Luciferase	Asialoglyco-protein receptor+ Hepatocytes	i.v.	2 days	ND	ND	(Nishikawa et al. 2000b)
Fusogenic-karyophilic-NT-polyplex	Neurotensin, HA2, Poly-Lys, SV40-NLS	Charge interaction assembly and chemical conjugation	<200	GFP, GDNF	High affinity Neurotensin receptor+ cells	i.c.	2 months	Neuroprotection and functional recovery in a model of Parkinson's Disease	ND	(Arango-Rodriguez *et al.* 2006; Gonzalez-Barrios *et al.* 2006; Navarro-Quiroga *et al.* 2002)
SPKR4NL1-2/PEI600	SPKR, NGF loops 1 and 2, poly-His	Recombinant and charge interaction assembly	100-200	Luciferase	TrkA and p75NTR+ cells	i.t.	3 days	ND	ND	(Ma et al. 2004)
DNA/TfPEI/PEG	Transferrin, PEI, PEG	Charge interaction assembly and chemical conjugation	200-400	Luciferase	Transferrin receptor+ cells	i.v.	2 days	Preferential tumour targeting	ND	(Ogris et al. 1999)
Tat-PTD-DRBD	Tat-PTD, DRBD, poly-His	Recombinant	ND	Luciferase siRNA	Non-selective	i.n.	3-4 days	No, but downregulation of luciferase	ND	(Eguchi *et al.* 2009)
Tf-HSV-TK	Biotinylated-DNA, streptavidin, biotinylated-transferrin	Chemical conjugation	ND	herpes simplex virus thymidine kinase	Transferrin receptor+ cells	i.v.	At least 7 days	Decreased metastasis and increased survival	ND	(Sato *et al.* 2000)

Abbreviations: RGD: Arg-Gly-Asp; NGF: Nerve growth factor; i.v.: intravenous; i.c.: intracerebral; i.t.: intrathecal; i.c.v.: intracerebroventricular; i.n.: intranasal; LDL: low-density lipoprotein; HA2: peptide from influenza virus hemagglutinin subunit HA-2; i.t. intrathecal; SPKR: DNA binding motif derived from Histone H1; FMDV: foot-and-mouth disease virus; PEG: poly (ethylene glycol); PEI: polyethyleneimine; Tat-PTD: Tat peptide transduction domain; DRBD: (ds)RNA-binding domain; GDNF: Glial derived neurotrophic factor; TK: thymidine kinase.

Table 1. Modular protein vectors effective in vivo

functional domains (see Table 1), being one of them the monoclonal antibody MC192 against $p75^{NTR}$, the low affinity neurotrophin receptor (Berhanu and Rush 2008). By injecting it intracerebroventricularly coupled to siRNA against TrkA, one of the high affinity neurotrophin receptors, Berhanu and Rush were able to down-regulate TrkA expression in $p75^{NTR}$ expressing cells and correlate this with functional alterations like impaired spatial memory.

2.3 Endosomal escape

A limiting step for receptor-mediated gene delivery is the escape from endosomes, as the vector needs to gain access to the cytosol to enter the nuclei. Fusogenic peptides are reported to strongly enhance *in vitro* gene transfer after being incorporated into carrier systems by chemical linkage (Box *et al.* 2003; Fisher and Wilson 1997; Navarro-Quiroga *et al.* 2002; Nishikawa *et al.* 2000b; Ogris *et al.* 2001; Wagner *et al.* 1992) or by ionic interaction (Gottschalk *et al.* 1996; Plank *et al.* 1994), but co-treatment of the cells with the vector and the fusogenic peptide may also be effective (Read *et al.* 2005). The most widely used method for endosome escape is based on the amino-terminal motif of influenza virus hemagglutinin subunit HA2 (Plank *et al.* 1994; Wagner *et al.* 1992). For example, Nishikawa and colleagues showed that when an acid-sensitive fusogenic peptide derived from HA2 was incubated with mouse erythrocytes at pH 5.0, it induced hemolysis while it did not show any significant hemolytic activity at pH 7.4 (Nishikawa *et al.* 2000b). Interestingly, the same study showed that the *in vivo* liver transgene expression obtained after intravenous injection of the vector DNA/Gal-pOrn-mHA2 was 300 fold higher than that obtained with the same vector lacking the HA2 domain (Nishikawa *et al.* 2000b).

Other domains used for DNA condensation or vector purification as polylysine or polyhistidine have shown endosome disrupting activities (Read *et al.* 2005; Zauner *et al.* 1997). The most effective ones were histidine rich polyplexes formed by the condensation of approximately 50 monomers of Cys-His_6-Lys_3-His_6-Cys and DNA (Read *et al.* 2005). In this study, the endosomolytic agent chloroquine, which normally enhance the transfection capacity of most non-viral vectors, did not enhance the transfection with the histidine rich polyplexes while it enhanced transfection with other non-viral vectors, suggesting that the poly-his domains are in fact endosomolytic. Though polycations like polylysine may be toxic to cells, especially if they have membrane-disrupting activity, this polyhistidine vector showed no toxicity. Histidine becomes positively charged when the pH decrease to less than 7 and thus becomes useful for the permeabilization of the endosomal membrane induced by acidification of endosomes, increasing cell transfection (Midoux *et al.* 1998). *In vivo*, many of these endosomal escape systems have shown success (see Table 1). For an extensive review on different strategies and domains used for endosomal escape please refer to Ferrer-Miralles et al. (Ferrer-Miralles *et al.* 2008).

For the introduction of siRNA and DNA into cells, several cationic peptide transduction domains or also called cell-penetrating domains have been used. TAT, 8xArg, Hph-1or Antp domains can deliver a wide variety of cargo into primary cells, to most tissues, and are in addition being evaluated in clinical trials (Gump and Dowdy 2007). For instance, when the Tat-domain was combined with a poly-His domain and the (ds)RNA-binding domain DRBD, the vector coupled to siRNA could successfully down-regulate Luciferase expression in the nasal and tracheal passages for 4 days after intranasal administration (Eguchi *et al.* 2009). An important characteristic of these systems using cell-penetrating peptides is that they are not cell-specific, and thus should be used for general non-selective transfection. A careful evaluation of the toxicity of this cell penetrating domains in *in vivo* settings has to be performed as toxicity of Tat protein has been reported (Cardozo *et al.* 2007), specially for the CNS (Bonavia *et al.* 2001; Nath *et al.* 1996). In addition, toxicity of the Antp domain has also been reported for many cell types (Cardozo *et al.* 2007).

2.4 Nuclear translocation

The transgene expression levels obtained after plasmid DNA injection into the cytoplasm or the nucleus showed that de nuclear double membrane and its pores are important barriers for naked DNA (Liu *et al.* 2003; Pollard *et al.* 1998). The selection of macromolecules that will be actively imported into the nucleus occurs at the nuclear pore complex, which is composed of more than 50 different proteins. The pore complex will recognise importin proteins bound to short (normally 4-8 amino acids) nuclear localization signals which can be located almost anywhere in the amino acid sequence of the protein, and which are rich in the positively charged amino acids lysine and arginine and usually contains proline (Pouton 1998). This mechanism has been exploited for the design of modular protein vectors, introducing nuclear localization sequences like the SV40 NLS peptide from the T antigen (Aris and Villaverde 2003; Fritz *et al.* 1996). For instance, Aris and co-workers introduced this nuclear localization sequence into the 249AL modular vector (see Table 1) and they observed an enhanced transgene expression with the resulting vector termed NLSCt (Aris and Villaverde 2003). However, studies performed in cells in culture show that even in the presence of nuclear localizations sequences, complexes of more than 60nm seem to be excluded (Chan *et al.* 2000). This data are in contrast to the high transfection efficiency obtained, even *in vivo*, with different modular protein vectors that exceeds this size, reaching 200nm (see Table 1). One can speculate that in fact some molecules of up to 200nm can be imported into the nucleus by being flexible, or that during the interaction of the vector with the nuclear import machinery the vector is disassembled and only the DNA is imported.
Another important step for efficient transgene expression may be the release of the nucleic acid from the vector once in the nucleus. Several studies have addressed the possible enhancement of the release of the DNA by the cellular reducing conditions. For example, histidine rich polyplexes were able to release the complexed DNA when exposed to the reducing agent Dithiothreitol (DTT), suggesting that in cells a similar mechanism would occur (Read *et al.* 2005). In fact, the increase in the cellular antioxidant and reducing agent glutathione, induced an important 200 fold increase in the transfection observed with the histidine rich polyplexes, but only a 3fold increase was observed with the PEI/DNA vector, another non-viral vector with no reduction-dependent release of DNA. Though this is an interesting phenomenon, it is difficult to understand why the cytosol reducing conditions do not disassemble the vector too early, determining that the DNA is released into the cytosol instead of inside the nucleus, not favouring the transfection process.

2.5 Trophic vectors/functional vectors

An attractive possibility is the combination of the effects mediated by the overexpression of a transgene and the direct effects of the vector per se. In fact, as modular vectors normally take advantage of a cell attaching motif for receptor mediated endocytosis, they tend to display intrinsic activities. More importantly, the use of trophic factors or toxin domains for cell attachment and internalization is ideal, as their natural mechanism of action includes the attachment to high affinity cell surface receptors, the endocytosis to early endosomes,

and even being transported to the cell soma in the case of neurons (Lalli and Schiavo 2002). An interesting modular vector was produced combining a polylysine tail with the loop 4 of the nerve growth factor (NGF) (Zeng *et al.* 2004; Zeng and Wang 2005). This "trophic vector" maintained the trophic effects of NGF, was able to condensate DNA, and when combined with polyethylenimine (PEI600), transfected cells in culture that expressed NGF receptors but not cells without these receptors. Interestingly, the DNA-PEI600 showed a size of 445nm and an zeta potential of 6,2mV, but the addition of the NGF loop4 poly-lysine peptide to the complex induced the formation of smaller 180nm particles with a zeta potential of 23,2mV (Zeng *et al.* 2007). This shows that the addition of targeting peptides to non-specific DNA/condensing products complexes may in fact contribute to enhance not only the targeted delivery but also to decrease the particle size and charge of the resulting vector. A somehow more complex trophic vector including NGF loops was also produced. It combined the loops 1 and 2 of NGF and the SPKR4 domain derived from histone H1 DNA binding motif, linked together by a α-helical linker (Ma *et al.* 2004). Both NGF-loop derived vectors could even transfer a transgene *in vivo* preferentially to dorsal root ganglia neurons (which express NGF receptors) after intrathecal spinal cord injection (Ma *et al.* 2004; Zeng *et al.* 2007). Several toxins have been used as cell attachment motifs (Andreu *et al.* 2008; Box *et al.* 2003; Knight *et al.* 1999), and some motifs of these toxins can in fact display trophic effects (Chaib-Oukadour *et al.* 2004), and have thus been used to design trophic vectors.
An important consideration regarding many acute injuries is that the therapeutic time window is short. In those cases, a direct trophic or functional effect of the vector per se could extend the therapeutic window, giving time for the transgene to be expressed and mediate its own effects. For example, the neuroprotection observed after an acute brain injury using the vector termed NLSCt was partially mediated by the transgene overexpressed, but also partially mediated by the RGD integrin-interacting motif of the vector itself (Peluffo *et al.* 2006; Peluffo *et al.* 2007). In this experimental setting the direct injection of the vector into the lesioned brain area was performed 4 hours after the lesion. The CNS is a tissue that tolerates injures very badly due to its high dependence on blood flow and oxygen consumption, and its poor regeneration capacity. This determines that the therapeutic window for the treatment of acute injuries is very short. Interestingly, even in this experimental paradigm, the modular recombinant NLSCt vector overexpressing the anti-oxidant enzyme Cu/Zn superoxide dismutase (SOD) could mediate neuroprotection (Peluffo *et al.* 2006). These studies shows the wide possibilities of combining the vectors themselves with active protein domains like trophic factors, which will exert rapid direct effects, which in turn may increase the therapeutic window or the potency of the effect of the transgene used.

3. Immunogenicity and inflammation

The introduction of modular protein vectors into the organism may be accompanied by a humoral or cell-mediated immune response against the inserted motifs, which in many cases are derived from viral molecules. However, when injected intravenously, the Rabies virus glycoprotein (29aa)-Poly-Arg vector (RVG-9R) (see Table 1) did not induce an antibody response or an increase in several pro-inflammatory cytokines evaluated (Kumar *et al.* 2007). In another example, when the recombinant 249AL vector (see Table 1) was injected into the normal postnatal brain, no changes were observed in glial activation, demyelination, recruitment of cytotoxic CD8 lymphocytes, or expression of IL1β. Interestingly, when a very similar vector termed NLSCt (see Table 1) was injected into the postnatal brain after an excitotoxic injury, an increase in macrophage/microglia number and in the levels of IL1β and Cox2 enzyme were observed in the lesion (Gonzalez *et al.* 2011). Most interesting, the same set of studies discovered that this vector, with or without accomplished control DNA, besides inducing an inflammatory response, also induced a decrease in the brain lesion volume and in the number of degenerating neurons (Peluffo *et al.* 2006; Peluffo *et al.* 2007), an effect that was mediated by the prototypic RGD-integrin interacting motif of the vector (Peluffo *et al.* 2007). These data may suggest that the modulation of the inflammation by the vector may be beneficial under some circumstances. Another vector termed Tat-PTD-DRBD (see Table 1) did not induce interferon (IFN)-α or tumour necrosis factor (TNF)-α responses when incubated with primary human peripheral blood mononuclear cells (Eguchi *et al.* 2009). Thus, the overall data suggests that these types of vectors are less immunogenic and pro-inflammatory than most viral and other non-viral vectors.

4. Administration routes and transgene expression

If these types of vectors are useful for gene therapy applications is still an open question, and adequate testing of these vectors in preclinical and actual clinical studies need to be performed. In fact, it has been well established that there is no ideal vector for all gene therapy applications, being the characteristics of each vector critical for each pathological paradigm. The use of modular protein vectors is limited to pathologies accepting an acute treatment, but would be ineffective for chronic ones as the transgene expression that they determine is normally short lived. The time of transgene expression varies from a few days to more than two months, depending on the doses and the method of administration. For instance, multifunctional recombinant vectors can induce the *in vivo* brain expression of a reporter gene after direct injection into the bran in a model of acute brain injury, lasting the transgenic protein in the brain for 3 days (Peluffo *et al.* 2003), but another vector was able to determine expression in normal brain for two months after intracerebral injection (Navarro-Quiroga *et al.* 2002). In the case of other administration routes and pathologies, as for example the intravenous administration of these vectors, the time for transgenic protein expression in the liver may range from a few days to more that 4 months (Perales *et al.* 1994). In another study, the liver-selective and transient overexpression of the therapeutic protein human coagulation factor IX could be achieved using a synthetic modular glycoprotein vector, and secreted factor IX into the serum could be detected for 30 days (Ferkol *et al.* 1993). This same paradigm could be used for vaccination, overexpressing transiently the desired immunogenic protein (Chen and Huang 2005). Even the use of modular vectors coupled to plasmids producing shRNA show potent downregulation of an endogenous gene during 20 days when infused with osmotic pumps into the nervous system (Berhanu and Rush 2008). In all this approaches, the transient expression of a protein by means of multifunctional vectors would be desirable when compared to viral vector inoculation, which present higher risks of oncogenic and inflammatory complications, may produce very high levels of transgenic protein, and will produce the transgenic protein for life or for extended periods.

5. Pharmacokinetics and biodistribution

Various approaches have been undertaken to overcome the interaction of vectors with blood components to avoid aggregation as well as embolisms. Moreover for most strategies, the phagocytic clearing system of the organism must be eluded. Pharmacokinetic analysis has shown that physicochemical properties of the vectors such as molecular weight, electrical charge and immunogenicity (or pre-existing antibodies in the organism) are important determinants for the *in vivo* success of the treatment. In addition, the volume and shape of the final vector is also important as it determines if the complex will be internalized into the cell and the cell nucleus. ^{P32}plasmid DNA is rapidly eliminated from the circulation after intra-venous injection in mice (Kawabata *et al.* 1995), mainly by a scavenger receptor mechanism-mediated uptake by hepatic phagocytes (Kawabata *et al.* 1995; Takakura *et al.* 1999). Thus, the *in vivo* plasmid delivery needs to modify its physicochemical properties by condensing carriers. One interesting example is the Mannose-Poly-Lysine vector (Man-PL), which was designed to accommodate plasmid DNA for the mannose receptor-mediated transfection of liver endothelial cells and Kuppfer phagocytes. After intravenous injection, the Man-PL-P32DNA vector disappeared from the plasma with a half-life of 1 minute, being 80% of the radioactivity recovered from the liver at 10 minutes (mainly in the mannose receptor+ target cells) and less than 1% at lungs or kidneys at 1 hour after (Nishikawa *et al.* 2000a). This vector had a size of 220nm and a zeta potential of 12,1mV, while the DNA alone had a size of 200nm and a zeta potential of -36,4. This type of study clearly shows the importance of the condensation of plasmid DNA into small less charged particles. In accordance, it has been described that positively charged DNA complexes can activate the alternative complement pathway (Plank *et al.* 1996). The conjugation of vectors with hydrophilic polymers has been shown to decrease their interaction with plasmatic proteins and blood cells, increasing their half-life in circulation. One of the most used polymers is poly (ethylene glycol) (PEG). In an interesting study, Ogris and colleagues compared the blood stability of DNA/transferrin/PEI vectors with or without covalently linked PEG. The non-PEGylated vectors aggregated in plasma, bound several plasmatic proteins like IgM, fibrinogen, fibronectin, and complement C3, and also induced erythrocyte aggregation (Ogris *et al.* 1999). Interestingly, the PEGylated vector showed stable complex size, reduced surface charge, reduced binding of plasmatic proteins and erythrocyte aggregation, and most important, increased *in vivo* circulation half-life combined with enhanced transfection selectivity towards tumours.

An interesting vector for improving pharmacokinetics could be the use of natural circulating molecules, like the low-density lipoprotein (LDL). In fact it has been shown that LDL can act as a vector when mixed with plasmid DNA and injected intravenously, reaching several organs including the brain, heart, kidneys and spleen (Guevara *et al.*). The LDL molecule is composed of a highly hydrophobic core, surrounded by a shell of phospholipids and unesterified cholesterol, as well as a single copy of Apo B100 protein (Segrest *et al.* 2001). The B100 protein contains several motifs that explain the vector profile of the LDL: i) a motif that enable nucleic acid binding, ii) a motif that mediate cellular uptake, and iii) a motif that is apparently involved in transferring DNA into the cell nucleus (Guevara *et al.*). Interestingly, low-density particles composed of lipid, Apo B100, RNA, and core protein of hepatitis C virus were reported in the plasmas of individuals infected with this virus (Andre *et al.* 2002). This and other studies suggested that virus might utilize the potential of the LDL particle to act as a vector as a mechanism for persistent chronic infection.

6. Preclinical studies

Many interesting preclinical studies have been performed with modular multifunctional protein vectors (see Table 1). The first studies showing *in vivo* functional effects using modular protein vectors were made by Wu and colleagues. By injecting intravenously the asialoorosomucoid glycoprotein-polylysine vector (ASOR-PL, see Table 1), they targeted hepatocytes and were able to partially and temporary correct analbuminemia and hypercholesterolemia by overexpressing human serum albumin or functional LDL receptor respectively (Wilson *et al.* 1992; Wu *et al.* 1991; Wu and Wu 1987). In another study, neuroprotection from an acute brain injury was achieved after direct intracerebral injection of the NLSCt vector overexpressing the antioxidant enzyme Cu/ZnSOD (see Table 1). In this experimental setting the overexpression of the therapeutic protein could not only induce reduced infarct volume but also functional improvement of the animals (Peluffo *et al.* 2006). Here, the vector was injected directly into the lesioned brain by a tightly controlled microinjector, using a similar protocol reported for the injection of cells into the human Parkinsonian brain (Brundin *et al.*), or for the intracerebral injection of adeno-associated viral vectors for the treatment of infantile lysosomal storage disease (Worgall *et al.* 2008). Thus, this direct intracerebral injection approach could show some benefits in clinical cases of focal traumatic or ischemic injuries, were a delimited area is lesioned and were in some cases even a decompressing craniectomy is needed leaving a direct entrance to the brain parenchyma. Modular protein vectors have also been used for neuroprotection after acute peripheral nerve transection. For example, Barati and colleagues (Barati *et al.* 2006) delivered a polylysine-based polyplex targeting $p75^{NTR}$ positive cells accomplishing the plasmid encoding for GDNF after a peripheral nerve transection (see Table 1). They showed an almost complete reversal in neuronal death caused by GDNF transgene expression. Though this is a very interesting study, the authors performed a subtle pre-lesion to the nerve one week before the nerve transection injury to upregulate $p75^{NTR}$ receptor, and thus the same experiment should be repeated but under more clinically relevant conditions. In another preclinical setting, the intravenous injection (once a day during 3 consecutive days) of the RVG-9R vector accomplished to the antiviral siRNA siFvEJ (see Table 1) was able to induce 80% survival of animals 30 days after their inoculation with a fatal flavivirus (Kumar *et al.* 2007). Thought many modular vectors have been shown to mediate over-expression or down-regulation of reporter genes, they need to be tested *in vivo* in clinically relevant models for the establishment of their real potential.

7. Conclusion

More complex modular protein vectors including all the important domains for efficient nucleic acid delivery need to be engineered. They should include domains for DNA attachment and condensation, cell attachment and endocytosis, endosomal escape, cytosol trafficking towards the nucleus, nuclear import, and DNA release. HNRK (Domingo-Espín *et al.* 2011), fkAbp75-ipr (Berhanu and Rush 2008), and the fusogenic-karyophilic-NT-polyplex (Navarro-Quiroga *et al.* 2002) (see Table 1) are three prototypes of this increasingly complex vectors, but additional domains have to be inserted. In addition, an interesting strategy could be the exploitation of several domains that have dual functions, like poly-his with DNA attachment and endosomal escape properties, like melittin with endosomal escape properties and nuclear import potential, or histones with DNA attachment and nuclear import potential. Considering the fact that for example several cellular nuclear proteins have several nuclear localization domains, the introduction of several domains with the same function in the same vector may further increase their efficiency. In fact, dual targeting of cancer cell lines using both transferrin and RGD domains showed synergistic effects (Nie *et al.*). Furthermore, the combination of engineered modular protein vectors with engineered plasmids for long term-regulated expression *in vivo* will be essential. For instance, the pEPI DNA vector was the first prototype of episomal vector whose function relies exclusively on chromosomal elements, replicating autonomously in low copy numbers in all cells tested (Piechaczek *et al.* 1999). This vector was further engineered to show regulated expression and to be removed from transduced cells when transgene expression is no longer needed (Rupprecht *et al.*). Finally, vectors have to be tested *in vivo,* but evaluating biological effects and not only reporter gene expression, and the comparison of different vectors in a same *in vivo* experimental setting will also contribute to the selection of the best prototypes.

8. Acknowledgments

This work was supported by the Comisión Sectorial de Investigación Cienctífica (CSIC) of the Universidad de la República (UDELAR) and by the Agencia Nacional de Investigación e Innovación (ANII) of the Ministerio de Cultura, Uruguay.

9. References

Andre, P., F. Komurian-Pradel, S. Deforges, M. Perret, J.L. Berland, M. Sodoyer, S. Pol, C. Brechot, G. Paranhos-Baccala and V. Lotteau. 2002. Characterization of low- and very-low-density hepatitis c virus rna-containing particles. J Virol 76, no. 14: 6919-28.

Andreu, A., N. Fairweather and A.D. Miller. 2008. Clostridium neurotoxin fragments as potential targeting moieties for liposomal gene delivery to the cns. Chembiochem 9, no. 2: 219-31.

Arango-Rodriguez, M.L., I. Navarro-Quiroga, J.A. Gonzalez-Barrios, D.B. Martinez-Arguelles, M.J. Bannon, J. Kouri, P. Forgez, W. Rostene, R. Garcia-Villegas, I. Jimenez and D. Martinez-Fong. 2006. Biophysical characteristics of neurotensin polyplex for *in vitro* and in vivo gene transfection. Biochim Biophys Acta 1760, no. 7: 1009-20.

Aris, A., J.X. Feliu, A. Knight, C. Coutelle and A. Villaverde. 2000. Exploiting viral cell-targeting abilities in a single polypeptide, non-infectious, recombinant vehicle for integrin-mediated DNA delivery and gene expression. Biotechnol Bioeng 68, no. 6: 689-96.

Aris, A. and A. Villaverde. 2003. Engineering nuclear localization signals in modular protein vehicles for gene therapy. Biochem Biophys Res Commun 304, no. 4: 625-31.

Aris, A. and A. Villaverde. 2004. Modular protein engineering for non-viral gene therapy. Trends Biotechnol 22, no. 7: 371-7.

Barati, S., P.R. Hurtado, S.H. Zhang, R. Tinsley, I.A. Ferguson and R.A. Rush. 2006. Gdnf gene delivery via the p75(ntr) receptor rescues injured motor neurons. Exp Neurol 202, no. 1: 179-88.

Barrett, L.B., M. Berry, W.B. Ying, M.N. Hodgkin, L.W. Seymour, A.M. Gonzalez, M.L. Read, A. Baird and A. Logan. 2004. Ctb targeted non-viral cdna delivery enhances transgene expression in neurons. J Gene Med 6, no. 4: 429-38.

Berhanu, D.A. and R.A. Rush. 2008. Targeted silencing of trka expression in rat forebrain neurons via the p75 receptor. Neuroscience 153, no. 4: 1115-25.

Bloomfield, V.A. 1996. DNA condensation. Curr Opin Struct Biol 6, no. 3: 334-41.

Bonavia, R., A. Bajetto, S. Barbero, A. Albini, D.M. Noonan and G. Schettini. 2001. Hiv-1 tat causes apoptotic death and calcium homeostasis alterations in rat neurons. Biochem Biophys Res Commun 288, no. 2: 301-8.

Box, M., D.A. Parks, A. Knight, C. Hale, P.S. Fishman and N.F. Fairweather. 2003. A multi-domain protein system based on the hc fragment of tetanus toxin for targeting DNA to neuronal cells. J Drug Target 11, no. 6: 333-43.

Brundin, P., R.A. Barker and M. Parmar. Neural grafting in parkinson's disease problems and possibilities. Prog Brain Res 184: 265-94.

Buschle, M., M. Cotten, H. Kirlappos, K. Mechtler, G. Schaffner, W. Zauner, M.L. Birnstiel and E. Wagner. 1995. Receptor-mediated gene transfer into human t lymphocytes via binding of DNA/cd3 antibody particles to the cd3 t cell receptor complex. Hum Gene Ther 6, no. 6: 753-61.

Cardozo, A.K., V. Buchillier, M. Mathieu, J. Chen, F. Ortis, L. Ladriere, N. Allaman-Pillet, O. Poirot, S. Kellenberger, J.S. Beckmann, D.L. Eizirik, C. Bonny and F. Maurer. 2007. Cell-permeable peptides induce dose- and length-dependent cytotoxic effects. Biochim Biophys Acta 1768, no. 9: 2222-34.

Chaib-Oukadour, I., C. Gil and J. Aguilera. 2004. The c-terminal domain of the heavy chain of tetanus toxin rescues cerebellar granule neurones from apoptotic death: Involvement of phosphatidylinositol 3-kinase and mitogen-activated protein kinase pathways. J Neurochem 90, no. 5: 1227-36.

Chan, C.K., T. Senden and D.A. Jans. 2000. Supramolecular structure and nuclear targeting efficiency determine the enhancement of transfection by modified polylysines. Gene Ther 7, no. 19: 1690-7.

Chen, W.C. and L. Huang. 2005. Non-viral vector as vaccine carrier. Adv Genet 54: 315-37.

Corchero, J.L. and A. Villaverde. 2009. Biomedical applications of distally controlled magnetic nanoparticles. Trends Biotechnol 27, no. 8: 468-76.

Domingo-Espín, J., E. Vazquez, J. Ganz, O. Conchillo, E. García-Fruitós, J. Cedano, U. Unzueta, V. Petegnief, N. Gonzalez-Montalbán, A.M. Planas, X. Daura, H. Peluffo, N. Ferrer-Miralles and A. Villaverde. 2011. The nanoparticulate architecture of protein-based artificial viruses is supported by protein-DNA interactions. Nanomedicine In Press.

Eguchi, A., B.R. Meade, Y.C. Chang, C.T. Fredrickson, K. Willert, N. Puri and S.F. Dowdy. 2009. Efficient sirna delivery into primary cells by a peptide transduction domain-dsrna binding domain fusion protein. Nat Biotechnol 27, no. 6: 567-71.

Ferkol, T., G.L. Lindberg, J. Chen, J.C. Perales, D.R. Crawford, O.D. Ratnoff and R.W. Hanson. 1993. Regulation of the phosphoenolpyruvate carboxykinase/human factor ix gene introduced into the livers of adult rats by receptor-mediated gene transfer. Faseb J 7, no. 11: 1081-91.

Ferrer-Miralles, N., E. Vazquez and A. Villaverde. 2008. Membrane-active peptides for non-viral gene therapy: Making the safest easier. Trends Biotechnol 26, no. 5: 267-75.

Fisher, K.J. and J.M. Wilson. 1997. The transmembrane domain of diphtheria toxin improves molecular conjugate gene transfer. Biochem J 321 (Pt 1): 49-58.

Fritz, J.D., H. Herweijer, G. Zhang and J.A. Wolff. 1996. Gene transfer into mammalian cells using histone-condensed plasmid DNA. Hum Gene Ther 7, no. 12: 1395-404.

Futaki, S., T. Suzuki, W. Ohashi, T. Yagami, S. Tanaka, K. Ueda and Y. Sugiura. 2001. Arginine-rich peptides. An abundant source of membrane-permeable peptides having potential as carriers for intracellular protein delivery. J Biol Chem 276, no. 8: 5836-40.

Gonzalez, P., H. Peluffo, L. Acarin, A. Villaverde, B. Gonzalez and B. Castellano. 2011. Il-10 overexpression does not synergize with the neuroprotective action of rgd-containing vectors after postnatal brain excitotoxicity, but modulates the main inflammatory cell responses. . Under second revision in the Journal of Neuroscience Research.

Gonzalez-Barrios, J.A., M. Lindahl, M.J. Bannon, V. Anaya-Martinez, G. Flores, I. Navarro-Quiroga, L.E. Trudeau, J. Aceves, D.B. Martinez-Arguelles, R. Garcia-Villegas, I. Jimenez, J. Segovia and D. Martinez-Fong. 2006. Neurotensin polyplex as an efficient carrier for delivering the human gdnf gene into nigral dopamine neurons of hemiparkinsonian rats. Mol Ther 14, no. 6: 857-65.

Gottschalk, S., J.T. Sparrow, J. Hauer, M.P. Mims, F.E. Leland, S.L. Woo and L.C. Smith. 1996. A novel DNA-peptide complex for efficient gene transfer and expression in mammalian cells. Gene Ther 3, no. 5: 448-57.

Guevara, J., Jr., N. Prashad, B. Ermolinsky, J.W. Gaubatz, D. Kang, A.E. Schwarzbach, D.S. Loose and N.V. Guevara. 2010. Apo b100 similarities to viral proteins suggest basis for ldl-DNA binding and transfection capacity. J Lipid Res 51, no. 7: 1704-18.

Gump, J.M. and S.F. Dowdy. 2007. Tat transduction: The molecular mechanism and therapeutic prospects. Trends Mol Med 13, no. 10: 443-8.

Kawabata, K., Y. Takakura and M. Hashida. 1995. The fate of plasmid DNA after intravenous injection in mice: Involvement of scavenger receptors in its hepatic uptake. Pharm Res 12, no. 6: 825-30.

Kim, H.H., W.S. Lee, J.M. Yang and S. Shin. 2003. Basic peptide system for efficient delivery of foreign genes. Biochim Biophys Acta 1640, no. 2-3: 129-36.

Knight, A., J. Carvajal, H. Schneider, C. Coutelle, S. Chamberlain and N. Fairweather. 1999. Non-viral neuronal gene delivery mediated by the hc fragment of tetanus toxin. Eur J Biochem 259, no. 3: 762-9.

Krishnamoorthy, G., B. Roques, J.L. Darlix and Y. Mely. 2003. DNA condensation by the nucleocapsid protein of hiv-1: A mechanism ensuring DNA protection. Nucleic Acids Res 31, no. 18: 5425-32.

Kumar, P., H. Wu, J.L. Mcbride, K.E. Jung, M.H. Kim, B.L. Davidson, S.K. Lee, P. Shankar and N. Manjunath. 2007. Transvascular delivery of small interfering rna to the central nervous system. Nature 448, no. 7149: 39-43.

Lalli, G. and G. Schiavo. 2002. Analysis of retrograde transport in motor neurons reveals common endocytic carriers for tetanus toxin and neurotrophin receptor p75ntr. J Cell Biol 156, no. 2: 233-9.

Liu, G., D. Li, M.K. Pasumarthy, T.H. Kowalczyk, C.R. Gedeon, S.L. Hyatt, J.M. Payne, T.J. Miller, P. Brunovskis, T.L. Fink, O. Muhammad, R.C. Moen, R.W. Hanson and M.J. Cooper. 2003. Nanoparticles of compacted DNA transfect postmitotic cells. J Biol Chem 278, no. 35: 32578-86.

Ma, N., S.S. Wu, Y.X. Ma, X. Wang, J. Zeng, G. Tong, Y. Huang and S. Wang. 2004. Nerve growth factor receptor-mediated gene transfer. Mol Ther 9, no. 2: 270-81.

Mastrobattista, E., M.A. Van Der Aa, W.E. Hennink and D.J. Crommelin. 2006. Artificial viruses: A nanotechnological approach to gene delivery. Nat Rev Drug Discov 5, no. 2: 115-21.

Midoux, P., A. Kichler, V. Boutin, J.C. Maurizot and M. Monsigny. 1998. Membrane permeabilization and efficient gene transfer by a peptide containing several histidines. Bioconjug Chem 9, no. 2: 260-7.

Nath, A., K. Psooy, C. Martin, B. Knudsen, D.S. Magnuson, N. Haughey and J.D. Geiger. 1996. Identification of a human immunodeficiency virus type 1 tat epitope that is neuroexcitatory and neurotoxic. J Virol 70, no. 3: 1475-80.

Navarro-Quiroga, I., J. Antonio Gonzalez-Barrios, F. Barron-Moreno, V. Gonzalez-Bernal, D.B. Martinez-Arguelles and D. Martinez-Fong. 2002. Improved neurotensin-vector-mediated gene transfer by the coupling of hemagglutinin ha2 fusogenic peptide and vp1 sv40 nuclear localization signal. Brain Res Mol Brain Res 105, no. 1-2: 86-97.

Nie, Y., D. Schaffert, W. Rodl, M. Ogris, E. Wagner and M. Gunther. Dual-targeted polyplexes: One step towards a synthetic virus for cancer gene therapy. J Control Release.

Nishikawa, M., S. Takemura, F. Yamashita, Y. Takakura, D.K. Meijer, M. Hashida and P.J. Swart. 2000a. Pharmacokinetics and in vivo gene transfer of plasmid DNA complexed with mannosylated poly(l-lysine) in mice. J Drug Target 8, no. 1: 29-38.

Nishikawa, M., M. Yamauchi, K. Morimoto, E. Ishida, Y. Takakura and M. Hashida. 2000b. Hepatocyte-targeted in vivo gene expression by intravenous injection of plasmid DNA complexed with synthetic multi-functional gene delivery system. Gene Ther 7, no. 7: 548-55.

Ogris, M., S. Brunner, S. Schuller, R. Kircheis and E. Wagner. 1999. Pegylated DNA/transferrin-pei complexes: Reduced interaction with blood components, extended circulation in blood and potential for systemic gene delivery. Gene Ther 6, no. 4: 595-605.

Ogris, M., R.C. Carlisle, T. Bettinger and L.W. Seymour. 2001. Melittin enables efficient vesicular escape and enhanced nuclear access of nonviral gene delivery vectors. J Biol Chem 276, no. 50: 47550-5.

Peluffo, H., L. Acarin, A. Aris, P. Gonzalez, A. Villaverde, B. Castellano and B. Gonzalez. 2006. Neuroprotection from nmda excitotoxic lesion by cu/zn superoxide dismutase gene delivery to the postnatal rat brain by a modular protein vector. BMC Neurosci 7: 35.

Peluffo, H., A. Aris, L. Acarin, B. Gonzalez, A. Villaverde and B. Castellano. 2003. Nonviral gene delivery to the central nervous system based on a novel integrin-targeting multifunctional protein. Hum Gene Ther 14, no. 13: 1215-23.

Peluffo, H., P. González, A. Arís, L. Acarin, A. Villaverde, B. Castellano and B. González. 2007. Rgd domains neuroprotect the immature brain by a glial dependent mechanism. Ann Neurol 62: 251-56.

Perales, J.C., T. Ferkol, H. Beegen, O.D. Ratnoff and R.W. Hanson. 1994. Gene transfer *in vivo*: Sustained expression and regulation of genes introduced into the liver by receptor-targeted uptake. Proc Natl Acad Sci U S A 91, no. 9: 4086-90.

Piechaczek, C., C. Fetzer, A. Baiker, J. Bode and H.J. Lipps. 1999. A vector based on the sv40 origin of replication and chromosomal s/mars replicates episomally in cho cells. Nucleic Acids Res 27, no. 2: 426-8.

Plank, C., K. Mechtler, F.C. Szoka, Jr. and E. Wagner. 1996. Activation of the complement system by synthetic DNA complexes: A potential barrier for intravenous gene delivery. Hum Gene Ther 7, no. 12: 1437-46.

Plank, C., B. Oberhauser, K. Mechtler, C. Koch and E. Wagner. 1994. The influence of endosome-disruptive peptides on gene transfer using synthetic virus-like gene transfer systems. J Biol Chem 269, no. 17: 12918-24.

Pollard, H., J.S. Remy, G. Loussouarn, S. Demolombe, J.P. Behr and D. Escande. 1998. Polyethylenimine but not cationic lipids promotes transgene delivery to the nucleus in mammalian cells. J Biol Chem 273, no. 13: 7507-11.

Pouton, C.W. 1998. Nuclear import of polypeptides, polynucleotides and supramolecular complexes. Adv Drug Deliv Rev 34, no. 1: 51-64.

Pyhtila, M.J., I. Miettola, T. Kurkela and A. Hoyhtya. 1976. Protection of deoxyribonucleic acid from nuclease action by histones. Acta Chem Scand B 30, no. 8: 797-8.

Read, M.L., S. Singh, Z. Ahmed, M. Stevenson, S.S. Briggs, D. Oupicky, L.B. Barrett, R. Spice, M. Kendall, M. Berry, J.A. Preece, A. Logan and L.W. Seymour. 2005. A versatile reducible polycation-based system for efficient delivery of a broad range of nucleic acids. Nucleic Acids Res 33, no. 9: e86.

Ritter, W., C. Plank, J. Lausier, C. Rudolph, D. Zink, D. Reinhardt and J. Rosenecker. 2003. A novel transfecting peptide comprising a tetrameric nuclear localization sequence. J Mol Med 81, no. 11: 708-17.

Ross, G.F., M.D. Bruno, M. Uyeda, K. Suzuki, K. Nagao, J.A. Whitsett and T.R. Korfhagen. 1998. Enhanced reporter gene expression in cells transfected in the presence of dmi-2, an acid nuclease inhibitor. Gene Ther 5, no. 9: 1244-50.

Ross, G.F., R.E. Morris, G. Ciraolo, K. Huelsman, M. Bruno, J.A. Whitsett, J.E. Baatz and T.R. Korfhagen. 1995. Surfactant protein a-polylysine conjugates for delivery of DNA to airway cells in culture. Hum Gene Ther 6, no. 1: 31-40.

Rupprecht, S., C. Hagedorn, D. Seruggia, T. Magnusson, E. Wagner, M. Ogris and H.J. Lipps. Controlled removal of a nonviral episomal vector from transfected cells. Gene 466, no. 1-2: 36-42.

Saccardo, P., A. Villaverde and N. Gonzalez-Montalban. 2009. Peptide-mediated DNA condensation for non-viral gene therapy. Biotechnol Adv 27, no. 4: 432-8.

Sato, Y., N. Yamauchi, M. Takahashi, K. Sasaki, J. Fukaura, H. Neda, S. Fujii, M. Hirayama, Y. Itoh, Y. Koshita, K. Kogawa, J. Kato, S. Sakamaki and Y. Niitsu. 2000. *In vivo* gene delivery to tumor cells by transferrin-streptavidin-DNA conjugate. Faseb J 14, no. 13: 2108-18.

Segrest, J.P., M.K. Jones, H. De Loof and N. Dashti. 2001. Structure of apolipoprotein b-100 in low density lipoproteins. J Lipid Res 42, no. 9: 1346-67.

Song, E., P. Zhu, S.K. Lee, D. Chowdhury, S. Kussman, D.M. Dykxhoorn, Y. Feng, D. Palliser, D.B. Weiner, P. Shankar, W.A. Marasco and J. Lieberman. 2005. Antibody mediated *in vivo* delivery of small interfering rnas via cell-surface receptors. Nat Biotechnol 23, no. 6: 709-17.

Takakura, Y., T. Takagi, M. Hashiguchi, M. Nishikawa, F. Yamashita, T. Doi, T. Imanishi, H. Suzuki, T. Kodama and M. Hashida. 1999. Characterization of plasmid DNA binding and uptake by peritoneal macrophages from class a scavenger receptor knockout mice. Pharm Res 16, no. 4: 503-8.

Thurnher, M., E. Wagner, H. Clausen, K. Mechtler, S. Rusconi, A. Dinter, M.L. Birnstiel, E.G. Berger and M. Cotten. 1994. Carbohydrate receptor-mediated gene transfer to human t leukaemic cells. Glycobiology 4, no. 4: 429-35.

Vazquez, E., M. Roldan, C. Diez-Gil, U. Unzueta, J. Domingo-Espin, J. Cedano, O. Conchillo, I. Ratera, J. Veciana, X. Daura, N. Ferrer-Miralles and A. Villaverde. Protein nanodisk assembling and intracellular trafficking powered by an arginine-rich (r9) peptide. Nanomedicine (Lond) 5, no. 2: 259-68.

Vijayanathan, V., T. Thomas and T.J. Thomas. 2002. DNA nanoparticles and development of DNA delivery vehicles for gene therapy. Biochemistry 41, no. 48: 14085-94.

Wadhwa, M.S., W.T. Collard, R.C. Adami, D.L. Mckenzie and K.G. Rice. 1997. Peptide-mediated gene delivery: Influence of peptide structure on gene expression. Bioconjug Chem 8, no. 1: 81-8.

Wagner, E., C. Plank, K. Zatloukal, M. Cotten and M.L. Birnstiel. 1992. Influenza virus hemagglutinin ha-2 n-terminal fusogenic peptides augment gene transfer by transferrin-polylysine-DNA complexes: Toward a synthetic virus-like gene-transfer vehicle. Proc Natl Acad Sci U S A 89, no. 17: 7934-8.

Wagner, E., M. Zenke, M. Cotten, H. Beug and M.L. Birnstiel. 1990. Transferrin-polycation conjugates as carriers for DNA uptake into cells. Proc Natl Acad Sci U S A 87, no. 9: 3410-4.

Wilson, J.M., M. Grossman, C.H. Wu, N.R. Chowdhury, G.Y. Wu and J.R. Chowdhury. 1992. Hepatocyte-directed gene transfer *in vivo* leads to transient improvement of hypercholesterolemia in low density lipoprotein receptor-deficient rabbits. J Biol Chem 267, no. 2: 963-7.

Wolfert, M.A. and L.W. Seymour. 1998. Chloroquine and amphipathic peptide helices show synergistic transfection *in vitro*. Gene Ther 5, no. 3: 409-14.

Worgall, S., D. Sondhi, N.R. Hackett, B. Kosofsky, M.V. Kekatpure, N. Neyzi, J.P. Dyke, D. Ballon, L. Heier, B.M. Greenwald, P. Christos, M. Mazumdar, M.M. Souweidane, M.G. Kaplitt and R.G. Crystal. 2008. Treatment of late infantile neuronal ceroid lipofuscinosis by cns administration of a serotype 2 adeno-associated virus expressing cln2 cdna. Hum Gene Ther 19, no. 5: 463-74.

Wu, G.Y., J.M. Wilson, F. Shalaby, M. Grossman, D.A. Shafritz and C.H. Wu. 1991. Receptor-mediated gene delivery *in vivo*. Partial correction of genetic analbuminemia in nagase rats. J Biol Chem 266, no. 22: 14338-42.

Wu, G.Y. and C.H. Wu. 1987. Receptor-mediated *in vitro* gene transformation by a soluble DNA carrier system. J Biol Chem 262, no. 10: 4429-32.

Wu, G.Y. and C.H. Wu. 1988. Receptor-mediated gene delivery and expression *in vivo*. J Biol Chem 263, no. 29: 14621-4.

Zauner, W., A. Kichler, W. Schmidt, K. Mechtler and E. Wagner. 1997. Glycerol and polylysine synergize in their ability to rupture vesicular membranes: A mechanism for increased transferrin-polylysine-mediated gene transfer. Exp Cell Res 232, no. 1: 137-45.

Zeng, J., H.P. Too, Y. Ma, E.S. Luo and S. Wang. 2004. A synthetic peptide containing loop 4 of nerve growth factor for targeted gene delivery. J Gene Med 6, no. 11: 1247-56.

Zeng, J. and S. Wang. 2005. Enhanced gene delivery to pc12 cells by a cationic polypeptide. Biomaterials 26, no. 6: 679-86.

Zeng, J., X. Wang and S. Wang. 2007. Self-assembled ternary complexes of plasmid DNA, low molecular weight polyethylenimine and targeting peptide for nonviral gene delivery into neurons. Biomaterials 28, no. 7: 1443-51.

26

Peptides as Promising Non-Viral Vectors for Gene Therapy

Wei Yang Seow and Andrew JT George
Imperial College London, England
United Kingdom

1. Introduction

In its most simplistic sense, gene therapy involves the delivery and expression of DNA by target cells so as to produce a therapeutic protein. In the case of RNA interference (RNAi), it is to shut off or silence the expression of a particular target protein. In order to exert its effects, the nucleic acid must first reach its intended site of action. DNA molecules (frequently as plasmids, which are circularised DNA) have to gain nuclear entry to access the transcription machinery. Conversely, RNAi molecules such as small interfering RNA (siRNA), short hairpin RNA (shRNA) and micro RNA (miRNA) will need to accumulate within the cytoplasm, although shRNA-encoding plasmids will require prior nuclear access before transcription into shRNA. However, if administered alone, a great majority of the nucleic acids will be degraded en route, leading to a lost of therapeutic potential. This then necessitates the development of vectors that protect and deliver nucleic acids to their target site. Arguably, it is the lack of safe and efficient delivery systems, rather than suitable therapeutic molecules that is limiting the success of gene therapy.

In this chapter, we start by examining how issues at the cellular level have shaped the design of modern, multifunctional vectors. We then briefly review the various types of gene delivery system, focusing on peptides as a promising class of non-viral vector. We will concentrate on the delivery of plasmids since the phenomenon of RNAi is relatively recent (Fire et al., 1998). As such, many strategies for RNAi delivery are adapted from DNA delivery technology.

2. Intracellular barriers in gene therapy: Problems and potential solutions

Ensuring the arrival of a plasmid at its site of action in a transcriptional state is the entire aim of gene delivery systems. However, plasmids face a constant threat of being degraded. The challenge begins as soon as they are introduced into the extracellular milieu (Figure 1). In most experimental setups, cells/tissues are maintained at 37°C in serum-supplemented medium where serum nucleases can extensively damage a naked plasmid. The plasmid therefore needs protection. Next, the plasmid needs to be internalised. However, both DNA (phosphate groups within the backbone) and plasma membrane (glycoproteins with their sialic acid groups, glycerophosphates with their phosphate groups and proteoglycans which contain sulphate groups) are negatively charged. Electrostatic repulsion then ensures that there is little chance of the plasmid being naturally taken up by a cell.

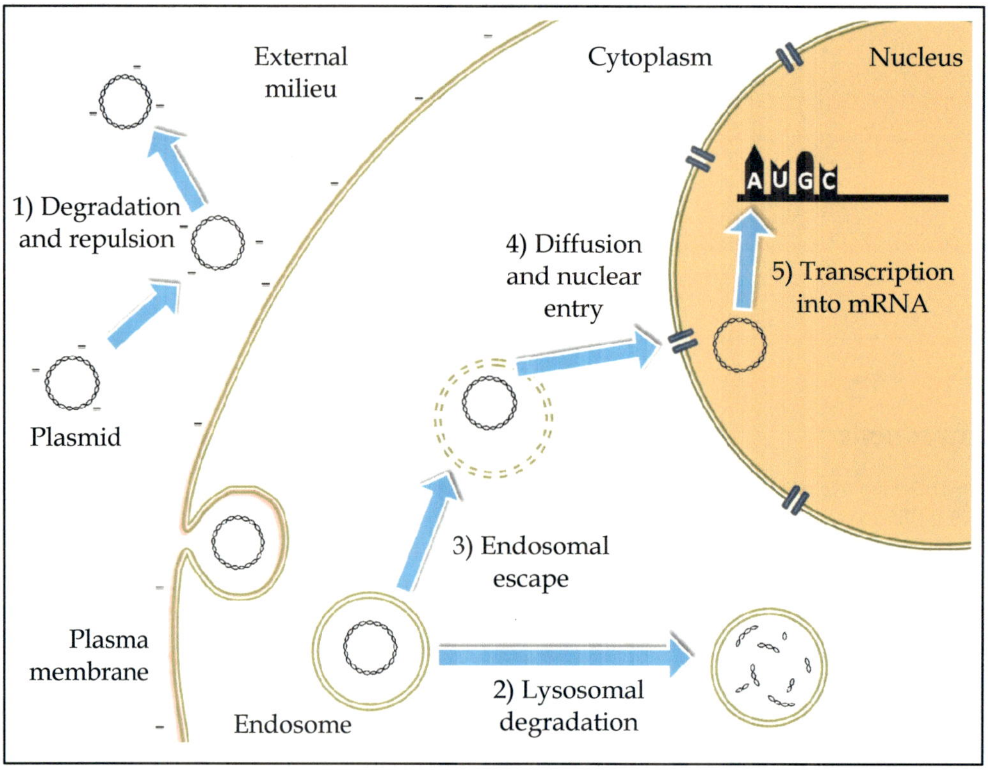

Fig. 1. Chronological sequence of events and challenges that a plasmid faces during its treacherous journey towards the nucleus. 1) A naked plasmid is susceptible to degradation by nucleases and is likely to be repelled from the plasma membrane. 2) Assuming successful endocytosis, the plasmid has to avoid trafficking into lysosomes where it will be degraded. 3) The plasmid has to escape into the cytoplasm. 4) It now has to diffuse through the viscous cytoplasm towards the nucleus while avoiding degradation and penetrate the nuclear membrane. 5) Transcription into mRNA can then occur if the plasmid is still intact.

For these reasons, gene delivery systems are frequently designed to be cationic in character and this fulfils several functions. First, the carrier can use its positive charges to mask the negative charges on the plasmid and package itself as a carrier/DNA complex with an overall positive charge. As expected, positively charged particles are internalised much more readily, as confirmed by an elegant study using PRINT (Particle Replication In Non-wetting Templates) technology to fabricate particles with exquisite control over their size, shape and surface charge (Gratton et al., 2008b). By keeping size and shape constant, positively charged particles were found in 84% of cells after an hour of incubation compared to the <5% uptake of negatively charged particles, proving that surface charge alone can influence uptake dramatically. Second, due to a charge screening effect, the macromolecular plasmid is collapsed (or condensed) into a compact structure more amendable for cellular uptake. This condensing process was clearly demonstrated using transmission electron microscopy which showed an elongated plasmid (long-axis diameter of ~470 nm) being compacted into tight, 80-100 nm toroid-shaped complexes by polylysine carriers (Wagner et al., 1991). Third, the carrier protects its cargo against degradation by nucleases, presumably by steric obstruction. This was shown by first exposing the complexes to DNase and then using gel electrophoresis to validate the physical integrity of the plasmid upon its release from the carrier. Control plasmids that were unprotected gave no bands in the subsequent gel electrophoresis experiment.

A problem with cationic carriers is that negatively charged serum protein can be non-specifically bound. As a result, targeting signals on the carrier can become blocked or complexes can start to aggregate. Reducing or removing serum from the media during *in vitro* transfection can mitigate such effects and improve transfection (Moore et al., 2009; Moulton et al., 2004). However, this strategy fails during *in vivo* experiments where serum proteins are unavoidably present. Another approach is to mix DNA and carrier in precise stoichiometric ratio so as to result in electro-neutral complexes (Funhoff et al., 2005). Along similar lines, zwitterionic (McManus et al., 2004) or anionic (Liang et al., 2005) lipids have been proposed in which binding between carrier and plasmid is dependant on hydrophobic forces and the presence of divalent cations such as Ca^{2+}, Zn^{2+} and Mg^{2+} to screen the disruptive repulsion between like charges. Neutral water-soluble polymers such as polyvinyl alcohol (PVA) and polyvinyl pyrolidone (PVP) similarly exploit non-electrostatic forces such as hydrogen bonding and van der Waal's attraction to condense plasmids (Park et al., 2006). These particles are however less popular because the lack of positive charge is expected to adversely impact cellular uptake. The PEGylation of carriers is another option. PEGylation refers to the surface decoration of carriers with flexible chains of polyethylene glycol (PEG), which is a highly hydrophilic polymer capable of making a surface less susceptible to protein adsorption (Duncan, 2006). Having said that, a major concern is that PEGylation obstructs the positive charges, resulting in carriers which are less efficient in DNA binding and transfection (Lin et al., 2008; Meyer et al., 2008). Moreover, while PEGylated drug formulations are already in clinical use, PEG is non-biodegradable and its chronic use may be a concern (Urakami & Guan, 2008).

The positive charges on cationic carriers have also been implicated in the formation of pores on the membrane, leading to cytotoxicity (Rimann et al., 2008). The observation that carrier/DNA complexes are less toxic to the cells compared to the carrier alone can be interpreted as partial evidence that charge compensation on the carrier may be a reason, albeit a non-exclusive one, for the reduced toxicity (Niidome et al., 1997). However, the exact mechanism is not totally clear. It may be due to the high rate of uptake of cationic carriers - and not the positive charges *per se* - that is to blame for pore formation. Herein lies a dilemma of the gene therapist: a high rate of internalisation can increase transfection efficiency but is also frequently paralleled by toxicity (Gabrielson & Pack, 2006; Pouton & Seymour, 2001). Fortunately, cells do have membrane repair mechanisms. One example is the membrane repair response (MRR) where the influx of Ca^{2+} ions directs lysosomes to donate their vesicular membrane in a concerted effort to plug the hole (Palm-Apergi et al., 2009). As always, the challenge is to strike a fine balance between two counter-acting events.

Assume the plasmid has been successfully taken up by a cell via endocytosis and now resides within an endosome. Another degradative fate awaits as endosomes eventually acidify into lysosomes and activate a broth of acid hydrolases capable of degrading nucleic acids. For this reason, a high rate of uptake may not necessarily translate into high transfection efficiency if, for example, most of the plasmids are degraded in lysosomes (Lundin et al., 2008). To avoid degradation, the plasmid/carrier complex will need to escape from the confines of the endosome into the cytosol. A popularly cited mechanism by which cationic carriers can achieve this is the proton-sponge hypothesis, so called because it relies on the buffering capability of the carrier to absorb H^+ ions and thus function as a proton sink. This model assumes that as the H^+-ATPase endosomal membrane pump injects protons into the vesicle during acidification, a build-up of positive charges will result due to the ability of the carrier to protonate and absorb the protons. This then triggers a concomitant influx of compensatory negative ions (e.g., Cl^-) and water, leading to the osmotic swelling of the vesicle and its eventual rupture. Consistent with this line of argument, carriers must thus contain chemical groups that are capable of undergoing protonation within the pH range of the endo/lysosomal transition, i.e., a pK_a of 7 to 4. This has motivated investigators to design carriers with a large buffering capacity. The polymer polyethylenimine (PEI), for instance, has a combination of protonated amines to bind plasmids at pH 7 and a stockpile of unprotonated amines that can still undergo protonation during the endo/lysosomal transition (Boussif et al., 1995). As such, PEI has a large buffering capacity and this feature is frequently cited as a main reason for PEI's status as one of the most efficient non-viral vector commercially available for *in vitro* transfection (Putnam, 2006).

Another common strategy to promote endosomal escape is to coincubate cells with a lysosomotropic agent such as chloroquine. Traditionally used as an anti-malaria drug, chloroquine is also a weak base capable of buffering the acidification of endosomes. In reality, however, chloroquine is pleiotropic in nature – besides its lysosomotropic property, chloroquine has been reported to be able to aid in the release of plasmid from its carrier and also to inhibit DNase activity (Yang et al., 2009) – and its actual mechanism of action remains controversial. Nevertheless, chloroquine does generally improve the transfecting capability of many carriers (Pouton & Seymour, 2001). A caveat, though, is that chloroquine at the dose normally used (100 μM) is toxic to cells (Wadia et al., 2004; Zauner et al., 1998). Glycerol is another agent reported to augment transfection due to its ability to weaken and make vesicular membrane more susceptible to disruption (Zauner et al., 1997). Interestingly, the more obvious effect of adding glycerol – its osmotic property – was ruled out as the main cause of vesicle escape. Finally, carriers can be functionalised with membrane-disruptive peptides, a strategy which will be reviewed in later sections.

The proton-sponge hypothesis is the most commonly cited explanation to account for the positive correlation between increased buffering capacity and transfection ability. It is hence easy to overlook that no study has provided any convincing evidence in direct support of its mechanism (Won et al., 2009). In fact, discrediting observations exist. For instance, it was reported that ammonium sulphate, also a weak base and should theoretically be able to provide buffering effects, does not boost transfection (Pouton & Seymour, 2001). Recent calculations have also revealed that the amount of strain that lipid vesicles can withstand before rupture is significantly larger than that which can be induced by endosomal buffering (Won et al., 2009). This suggests that the proton-sponge hypothesis can at best contribute, but cannot be the only cause of endosomal escape. Moreover, increased buffering and endosomal escaping properties do not always produce an accompanying increase in transfection (Akita et al., 2010; Moore et al., 2009). This implies that, while important, cytosolic access is not the only bottleneck of the transfection process. Further, it has to be pointed out that of the multiple pathways which a cell can use for internalisation, only the clathrin-mediated one is widely-accepted to involve vesicle acidification (Won et al., 2009; Zauner et al., 1997). Vesicle acidification is, of course, an inherent requirement of the proton-sponge hypothesis but whether vesicles from other pathways acidify is equivocal. Some researchers believe that macropinocytosis (Akita et al., 2010; Pelkmans & Helenius, 2002) and caveolae-mediated endocytosis (Lundin et al., 2008; Sahay et al., 2010) produce vesicles that do not undergo acidification, while others claim that macropinosomes do acidify (Räägel et al., 2009; Wadia et al., 2004). Furthermore, is it safe to assume that vesicles which do not acidify remain distinct from endo/lysosomes? On this, opinion is also polarised, with some claiming that caveosomes (Pelkmans & Helenius, 2002; Sahay et al., 2010) and macropinosomes (Wadia et al., 2004) remain distinct from endo/lysosomes; and others arguing that vesicles from different pathways can eventually interact (Sahay et al., 2010). Thus, the proton-sponge hypothesis even if true, may not always be relevant and on top of that, definitive trafficking studies of the various modes of uptake are required.

In the cytosol, the plasmid continues its migration towards the nucleus. Current dogma suggests that this proceeds via passive diffusion and that nuclear localisation is a hit-or-miss event. The viscous cytosolic environment makes diffusion extremely inefficient. The diffusion coefficient of bovine serum albumin (BSA) in human fibroblasts, for example, is about 70× lower than in buffer (Wojcieszyn et al., 1981). Protecting the plasmid during migration is also important as cytosolic nucleases restrict the half life of naked DNA to about 90 minutes (Belting et al., 2005).

During migration, another feature of the carrier becomes important - the release of its plasmid cargo. To undergo transcription, the plasmid must first be unpackaged from its carrier and the trick here, is one of timing. A plasmid that gets released too early will risk degradation while one that binds too strongly is not accessible for transcription. For this reason, lower molecular weight chitosan transfects better because their higher molecular weight counterpart interacts too strongly with their plasmid cargo (Koping-Hoggard et al., 2004). Another example involves PEI, where acetylation of its polymeric chains (which removes the amines) reduced both its buffering capacity and binding strength, but improved its transfection (Gabrielson & Pack, 2006). This suggests that vector unpackaging can indeed be a rate-limiting step and a carrier that binds in moderation is ideal. Fluorescence resonance energy transfer (FRET) is a powerful technique to study the process of vector unpackaging. It depends on the excitation of an acceptor dye by a donor dye in close physical proximity, which is the case when the plasmid is being tightly condensed. Using FRET, plasmid-release in the perinuclear region has been observed; alternatively, the plasmid/carrier can enter the nucleus as an associated complex (Seow et al., 2009).

Nuclear entry is believed to be achieved in two ways: either via the ~10 nm wide nuclear pores or during mitosis when the nuclear envelope momentarily disintegrates (Luo & Saltzman, 2000a). The latter appears to be a more efficient method for the large-scale accumulation of complexes. It further provides a possible explanation for why amitotic cells or primary cells which proliferate slower are more difficult to transfect than cancer-derived cell lines. A dilution effect after mitotic cell division also accounts for the transient nature of gene expression mediated by non-integrating vectors. Having said that, mitosis is not a pre-requisite (Won et al., 2009) as amitotic cells have been successfully transfected - it merely provides a convenient window of opportunity for nuclear entry. A proposed method to improve nuclear penetration is to attach a nuclear localisation signal (NLS) to the carrier. The quintessential example of a NLS is the short peptide sequence corresponding to the Simian virus 40 (SV40) T antigen. However, responses regarding the benefits of including a NLS have been mixed, with some investigators (Trentin et al., 2005) more convinced than others (Zauner et al., 1998). A key issue pointed out was that studies involving the use of NLS failed to examine the effect of including a NLS on nuclear import *per se* (Lam & Dean, 2010). Instead, reporter gene expression was frequently used as a proxy and an improved expression was simply accepted to be due to the inclusion of NLS. Given that most NLS are cationic, it is debatable if the observed increase in transfection is strctly the result of improved nuclear import *per se*, or due to other non-specific effects such as enhanced plasmid association and uptake. Moreover, the fact that a NLS can be sterically hindered by plasmids upon binding also contradicts the requirement of NLS to be freely accessible for interaction with importins, the nuclear entry regulating proteins.

In light of the many obstacles that nucleic acids and their carriers have to surmount, it is perhaps understandable that less than 10% of the pool of plasmids that made it into a cell will go on to accumulate in the nucleus (Lam & Dean, 2010). The challenge is to design a multifunctional vector that can address the issues highlighted above and yet, remain safe to use in a human body.

3. Overview and classification of gene delivery systems

3.1 Physical systems

Gene delivery systems can be classified based on their means of achieving transfection (Figure 2). There are systems that utilise physical forces, mostly with the aim of disrupting the plasma membrane, to facilitate nucleic acids delivery. For instance, electroporation and sonoporation (Frenkel, 2008) uses electrical and sonication forces respectively to transiently compromise the plasma membrane. The ballistic gene gun method, on the other hand,

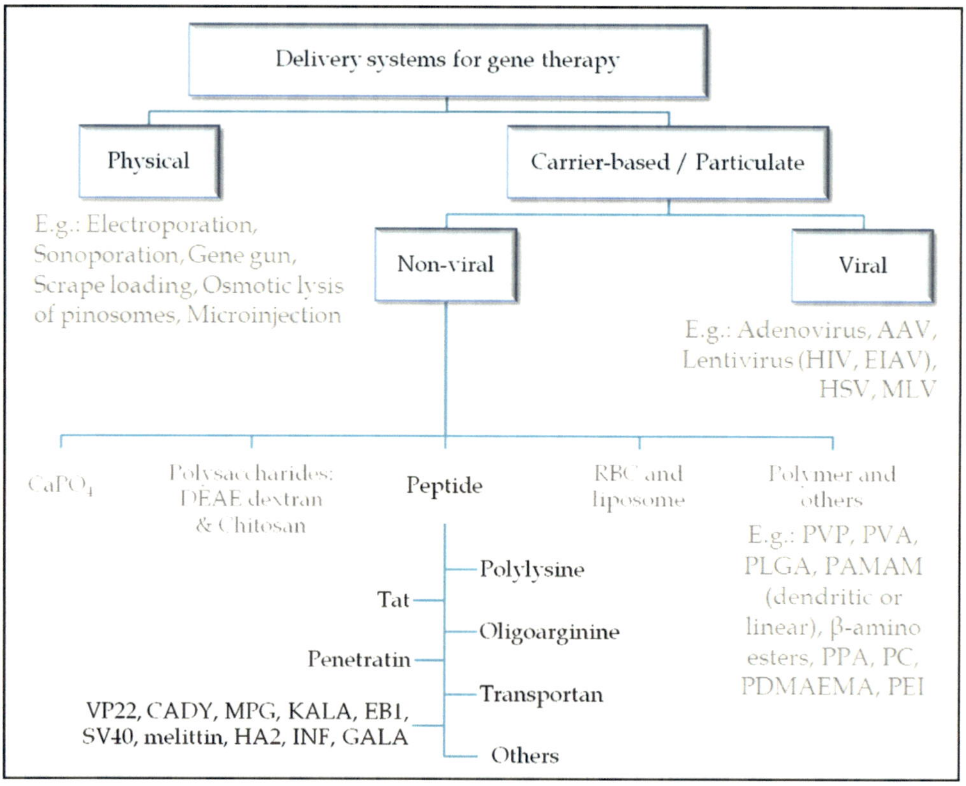

Fig. 2. The different classes and examples of gene delivery systems. This chapter will concentrate on peptide-derived vectors.

directly shoots DNA-coated metal particles (frequently gold) into cells (Merediz et al., 2000). Expectedly, such aggressive methods can irreversibly damage the cell membrane and cause widespread cell death. Scrape loading, first described in 1984, requires the forceful scraping of cells attached to their culture dishes, thereby creating pores on their membranes for plasmid entry (McNeil et al., 1984). This technique, however, is only applicable to adherent cells. The osmotic lysis of pinosomes was proposed in 1982 and requires that cells capable of pinocytosis be initially exposed to a hypertonic medium of sucrose, PEG and the plasmid of interest (Okada & Rechsteiner, 1982). Subsequent exchange to a hypotonic medium then released the pinosomal content. Although cells are constitutively capable of pinocytosis, such wild fluctuations in osmotic conditions can cause cell death. Finally, microinjection refers to the piecemeal injection of plasmids directly into the cell. This technique, while relatively gentle, is extremely laborious. As such, it is prone to failure and the number of cells that can be processed is limited.

3.2 Viral vectors

There are systems that function as particulate carriers by ferrying nucleic acids into or near to their site of action. Such systems can be viral or non-viral in nature. Viral vectors such as adenovirus, adeno-asociated virus (AAV), human immunodeficiency virus (HIV), equine infectious anaemia virus (EIAV), herpes simplex virus (HSV) and murine leukaemia virus (MLV) have been used and comprehensively reviewed elsewhere (Kay et al., 2001). The prime advantage of viral vectors is their transfection efficiency which has benefitted from centuries of selective evolutionary pressure. As a result, viruses are several orders of magnitude more efficient than non-viral vectors (Kircheis et al., 1997) and account for about 70% of all clinical trials involving gene therapy so far (Won et al., 2009). A recent success for viral gene therapy involved the use of lentiviruses to deliver a correct copy of a therapeutic gene to an adult patient suffering from β-thalassaemia (Cavazzana-Calvo et al., 2010). Such patients suffer from defective haemoglobin production and require chronic blood transfusion for survival. Upon reinfusing the patient with his own bone-marrow haematopoietic stem cells that had earlier been transduced *ex vivo*, the patient became transfusion free 1 year after treatment and has been doing well, according to the most recent report at 33 months after treatment. The longer-term outcome, of course, remains to be seen. Having said that, investigators have not abandoned all forms of non-viral research as there are limitations in the use of viral vectors. For example, the technical difficulty of scaling up virus production compliant to good manufacturing practices (GMP) may prevent such therapy from being cheaply accessible (Sheridan, 2011). The size of the construct that can be delivered is also limited. Above all, toxicity and immunogenicity (reviewed by Nayak & Herzog, 2010) provoked by the viral vectors can and have brought clinical trials to premature ends. Repeated administration is also not possible if the body has mounted a systemic immune response. The danger of viral gene therapy was first illustrated about a decade ago by the death of Jesse Gelsinger (Hollon, 2000). Researchers were using experimental adenoviruses to correct his partial ornithine transcarbamylase deficiency affecting the ability of his body to metabolise nitrogen. Unfortunately, the systemic inflammatory response syndrome was triggered and he succumbed, rather rapidly, to multiple organ failure. In another high-profile example, stem cells transduced *ex vivo* with MLV were used to treat children suffering from X-linked severe combined immunodeficiency (Hacein-Bey-Abina et al., 2003). However, MLV is an integrating retrovirus and can cause insertional mutagenesis, which is a phenomenon where random viral integration can trigger the activation of an oncogene or disrupt genes with tumor-suppressive properties. Consequently, several patients became leukemic and at least one has died so far (Sheridan, 2011). More recently, retroviruses were also used to treat two patients diagnosed with X-linked chronic granulomatous disease which affected the ability of their phagocytes to clear bacterial infections (Ott et al., 2006). Insertional mutagenesis was again responsible for a clone of cells whose genes responsible for growth were activated, prompting fears that such cells may turn cancerous. Having said that, viral gene therapy is not expected to be perfect and its success should be assessed relative to existing treatments. Nonetheless, researchers have not completely mastered the use of viruses and there is still a need for alternative non-viral vectors with safer profiles.

3.3 Non-viral vectors

Diethylaminoethyl (DEAE)-dextran and calcium phosphate ($CaPO_4$) were two of the earliest systems popular in the 1970s and 80s. DEAE-dextran has a cationic polysaccharide backbone and one of the earliest reports in 1965 used this polymer in a 1:1 mixture with nucleic acids to transfect rhesus monkey kidney cells (Vaheri & Pagano, 1965). Authors of this study also insightfully commented that DEAE-dextran, like histones, could bind and protect nucleic acids from degradation. Although these are now fundamental concepts in modern carrier design, it may not have been as obvious in the past. The co-precipitation of $CaPO_4$ with DNA was first described in 1973, when it was observed that Ca^{2+} (not Mg^{2+} or Na^+) and PO_4^{2-} ions, at high enough concentrations, could enhance DNA uptake by cells (Graham & Eb, 1973). This technique was further shown to be sensitive to pH, amount of DNA used and even the level of CO_2 in the incubator (Chen & Okayama, 1987). Using an optimised protocol, $CaPO_4$-mediated transfection achieved up to 50% efficiency with a murine L cell line (Chen & Okayama, 1987).

Chitosan is a polysaccharide obtained by the deacetylation of chitin, an exoskeletal component of crustaceans. Each deacetylation site contains a primary amine (pK_a~6.5) which allows chitosan to bind nucleic acids. The degree of deacetylation also determines its biodegradability and transfection efficiency. Chitosan was first described as a plasmid carrier by Mumper and colleagues in 1995 and is known to be biocompatible, mucoadhesive and virtually non-toxic (MacLaughlin et al., 1998). As such, chitosan has been evaluated in rabbits, although reporter gene expression in that study was low (MacLaughlin et al., 1998). Strong interactions between high molecular chitosan and DNA were blamed for the overly-stable complexes that could not release their plasmid cargos. Using lower molecular weight chitosan, *in vitro* transfection efficiency was improved by up to 24 fold (Koping-Hoggard et al., 2004). Adding histidine (pK_a~6) residues to chitosan further improved buffering capacity and overall transfection efficiency (Chang et al., 2010). Recently, it was also shown that the introduction of thiol groups in *N,N,N*-trimethylated chitosan improved its efficiency as a siRNA carrier (Varkouhi et al., 2010).

Red blood cells (RBC) were used for the delivery of macromolecules before liposomes became popular. To function as carriers, RBC were first loaded up with the macromolecule under hypotonic conditions to induce mild lysis. A fusogen was then used to cause fusion with target cells. Using this technique, thymidine kinase and BSA were introduced into 3T3-4E mouse cells using Sendai virus as a fusogen (Schlegel & Rechsteiner, 1975). In another study, horseradish peroxidase (HRP) and immunoglobulins (IgG) were delivered into cells expressing hemagglutinin derived from influenza virus by exploiting the fusogenic activity of hemagglutinin under mildly acidic conditions (Doxsey et al., 1985). Fluorescent IgG and

BSA were also delivered into human fibroblast cells using PEG as a fusogen (Wojcieszyn et al., 1981). Dehydration may play a role in PEG-mediated fusion and intriguingly, purification by recrystallisation removed the fusogenic ability of PEG, suggesting that other ingredients in commercial PEG was essential (Wojcieszyn et al., 1983).

Plasmids were initially delivered by synthetic liposomes using concepts adapted from RBC technology. In an early study, plasmids were encapsulated within anionic liposomes and fused with tobacco mesophyll protoplasts using PEG (Deshayes et al., 1985). Since 1987, however, surface binding became popular when liposomes made of *N*-[1-(2,3,-dioleyloxy)propyl]-*N,N,N*-trimethylammonium chloride (DOTMA) were synthesised for the first time (Felgner et al., 1987). DOTMA contains cationic quaternary ammonium groups which can be used for DNA binding. Lipofectin®, the prototypical lipid formulation and a workhorse for transfection experiments today, is a 1:1 mixture of DOTMA and the neutral lipid, dioleoyl phosphatidylethanolamine (DOPE). In this formulation, DOPE functions as a fusogen to aid cellular uptake. Several other formulations of liposomes have been reported. Gao and Huang prepared liposomes made out of DOPE and a novel cationic cholesterol derivative, 3*β*-[*N*-(*N′*,*N′*-dimethylamino)ethane-carbamoyl] cholesterol (DC-chol), and used it to transfect several cell lines with high efficiency (Gao & Huang, 1996). A mixture of *N′*,*N′*-dioctadecyl-*N*-4,8-diaza-10-aminodecanoylglycine amide (DODAG) and DOPE was also proposed to be a novel liposomal formulation that is good for both DNA and siRNA delivery (Mével et al., 2010). In another study, the cationic lipid 1,2-dilinoleyloxy-3-dimethylaminopropane (DLinDMA) was used as a starting template and systematically modified to yield an optimised construct (Semple et al., 2010). Although toxicity remains one of the chief complaints, liposomes are definitely one of the most successful non-viral vectors around. Already, several sustained-release liposomal drug formulations have been approved for human use and thermosensitive liposomes are being evaluated in clinical trials (Hossann et al., 2010). Lipids also dominate in gene therapy trials aimed at using non-viral vectors to treat cystic fibrosis (Griesenbach & Alton, 2009).

An advantage of polymeric carriers is that they offer so much structural diversity that their potential should, theoretically, be limited only by the imagination of chemists. Two of the more archaic examples including PVP and PVA have been mentioned. Poly(D,L-lactic-co-glycolic acid) (PLGA), a polymer originally developed for controlled drug release, has also been used to encapsulate plasmids for delivery (Wang et al., 1999). Most polymeric carriers, however, are cationic in nature. Dendritic poly(amido amine) (PAMAM) which contained primary amines for DNA binding was further decorated with PEG and sugars (Wood et al., 2005) or peptide (Wood et al., 2008) for targeting purposes. Linear PAMAM was functionalised with disulfide bonds to make the polymer biodegradable and various chemical side-groups were attached to test for its impact on transfection efficiency (Lin et al., 2007). A large library of poly(β-amino ester)s has been synthesised and systematically screened for transfection efficiency (Green et al., 2006). The effects of molecular weight and charge density of polyphosphoramidates (PPA) on DNA binding and buffering capacity have been reported (Ren et al., 2010). A series of novel enzyme-degradable polycarbonates (PC) with various aliphatic side-chains attached were prepared and shown to effectively transfect cells with virtually no toxicity (Seow & Yang, 2009a). Poly(2-(dimethyl-amino)ethylmethacrylate) (PDMAEMA) was also shown to transfect cells with high efficiency (Lin et al., 2008). Indeed, there are so many other classes of polymers being developed that it is impossible to do all justice with this paragraph. Nonetheless, amongst all, the most notable polymer must be PEI. PEI was first developed in 1995 (Boussif et al.,

1995) and is frequently used in its branched, high molecular weight (usually 25 kDa) form. Together with liposomes, they are widely acknowledged to be the best non-viral vectors currently available (Putnam, 2006) and frequently serve as standards to which other novel carriers are referenced. A key feature of PEI is that nitrogen (in a mixture of primary, secondary and tertiary amines) accounts for a third of its molecular weight. Since different classes of amines possess characteristic pK_a, this ensures that not all the nitrogen will be protonated at a given pH. Furthermore, the proximity of the nitrogen atoms also means that a protonated amine can suppress the protonation of its neighbours due to the energetic penalty that gets incurred by situating like charges adjacent to one another (Suh et al., 1994). This blend of protonated and yet-to-be protonated amines is then suggested to endow PEI with its strong DNA binding and buffering abilities. The intracellular trafficking properties of PEI/DNA complexes has been studied (Godbey et al., 1999) and targeting moieties such as mannose (Diebold et al., 1999) and transferrin (Kircheis et al., 1997) were also coupled onto PEI. However, two of the main problems of PEI are its toxicity and non-biodegradability. In response to the latter, PEI was functionalised with reducible disulfide bonds (Lee et al., 2007) or hydrolysable ester bonds (Liu et al., 2008) to facilitate biodegradation and at the same time, to aid its intracellular plasmid release.

4. Peptide-derived vectors for gene therapy

Peptide chains can be fabricated from any of the 20 naturally occurring L-amino acids, which are referred to by their single- or three-lettered code (e.g., R or arg for arginine). Peptides are thus biocompatible and often degradable. Peptide synthesis also does not involve harmful catalysts, which is a concern in the synthesis of some polymeric carriers. Furthermore, synthesis can now be automated, courtesy of advances in solid phase peptide synthesis, which makes the manufacturing process amendable to up-scaling.

Before peptides were seen as proper DNA carriers, studies conducted in the 1960s with histones had already suggested that cationic amino acids such as lysine and arginine can be useful (Akinrimisi et al., 1965). Today, peptide vectors are given fanciful names such as "cell penetrating peptides" (CPP) or "protein transduction domains" (PTD) to celebrate their ability to efficiently penetrate the plasma membrane and mediate the entry of nucleic acids or other macromolecules. Such CPP can be derived from proteins existing in nature (e.g., viral proteins or venom proteins of bees and wasps) or designed *de novo*. There is little in common among CPP and the only unifying theme seems to be the significant presence of cationic residues (mainly lysine and arginine). Amphipathicity has been suggested to be another common feature. However, this is only true for most CPP – oligoarginine being an exception. There are two methods by which peptide vectors carry their cargoes. Nucleic acids are usually non-covalently (electrostatically) attached, while proteins and other macromolecules are typically covalently coupled (chemical cross-linking or by plasmid fusion). The advantages of electrostatic attachment include convenience and the largely unaltered chemical properties of the cargo. However, charge interactions are non-specific and excess peptides are usually needed to completely bind the plasmid. On the other hand, covalent attachment requires chemical modification of the cargo and usually results in stable complexes which, as discussed earlier, may not be desirable. In the following sections, we will review the key classes of peptide vectors and provide non-exhaustive examples of strategies that have been used to improve their efficiency as vectors.

Peptide	Sequence (single letter code)	Short description
Poly-L-lysine	K_n	Frequently, n = 50-400
Tat	YGRK KRRQ RRRP PQ	HIV-derived, sequence 47-60
Oligoarginine	R_n	Frequently, n = 7-9
Penetratin	RQIK IWFQ NRRM KWKK	3rd helix of Antennapedia homeodomain
Tp	GWTL NSAG YLLG KINL KALA ALAK KIL	Galanin + mastoparan (wasp venom)
Tp10	AGYL LGKI NLKA LAAL AKKI L	First 6 residues deleted from Tp
VP22	300-residue long sequence given in (Elliott & O'Hare, 1997)	HSV-1 structural protein
MPG	GALF LGFL GAAG STMG AWSQ PKSK RKV	HIV gp41 + SV40 T-antigen
CADY	GLWR ALWR LLRS LWRL LWRA	Peptide carrier PPTG1-derived
KALA	WEAK LAKA LAKA LAKH LAKA LAKA LKAC EA	Membrane disruptive peptide, also a carrier
GALA	WEAA LAEA LAEA LAEH LAEA LAEA LEAL AA	Membrane disruptive peptide
EB1	LIRL WSHL IHIW FQNR RLKW KKK	Penetratin analogue
HA2	GLFG AIAG FIEN GWEG MIDG	Influenza virus hemagglutinin protein
INF5	$(GLFE AIEG FIEN GWEG nIDG)_2K$	HA2-derived, lysine-connected dimer. n = norleucine
INF7	GLFE AIEG FIEN GWEG MIDG WYG	HA2-derived, monomer
SV40	PKKK RKV	Simian virus 40 T antigen NLS
Melittin	GIGA VLKV LTTG LPAL ISWI KRKR QQ	Bee venom

Table 1. The amino acid sequences of all the peptides discussed in this chapter.

4.1 Poly-L-lysine (PLL)

The amino acid sequence of PLL and all other peptides subsequently discussed can be found in Table 1. PLL is the first peptide-based vector to be studied intensively. The molecular weight of PLL spans a wide range and depends on the number of repeating units within a chain, or its degree of polymerisation (DP). For the sake of discussion, the molecular weight of PLL is arbitrarily classified as follows: oligolysine (DP<20), low (20≤DP<50), medium (50≤DP≤400) or high (DP>400). Most studies use PLL of medium molecular weight.

PLL has been successfully employed to deliver a host of different cargos. By covalently coupling human serum albumin or HRP to PLL via amide bonds in a 1-ethyl-3-(3-dimethylaminopropyl) carbodiimide (EDC) catalysed reaction, proteins were delivered into L929 mouse fibroblasts for the first time using such a PLL-mediated strategy (Shen & Ryser, 1978). More recently, streptavidin-conjugated quantum dots (QD) were also attached to biotin-tagged PLL and delivered into HeLa cells (Mok et al., 2008). However, PLL is most frequently used to deliver nucleic acids where the electrostatic attachment is preferred. Although polylysine made out of D-amino acids has been suggested to work better - presumably because they are more resistant to enzymatic degradation (Mitchell et al., 2000) - PLL continues to be favoured in transfection studies. Wu and partner provided one of the earliest examples of PLL being used to condense plasmids for receptor-mediated delivery (Wu & Wu, 1987). In that study, asialoorosomucoid (ASOR) was first covalently attached to PLL with *N*-succinimidyl 3-(2-pyridyldithio) propionate (SPDP) as a linker and then used to bind a reporter plasmid. Complexes then accumulated within HepG2 cells (ASOR receptor positive) but not in SK-Hep1 cells (ASOR receptor negative).

Plasmids dissociated more slowly if bound to a higher molecular weight PLL and this can negatively affect transfection (Schaffer et al., 2000). To facilitate plasmid release, cysteine residues were added to oligolysine, which was then cross-linked using disulfide bonds (McKenzie et al., 2000). The intention was to make use of the intracellular environment - which is much more reductive due to its elevated levels of glutathione (Lee et al., 2007) - to break down the disulfide bonds for polymer disintegration and plasmid release. The number of lysine, cysteine and histidine (for buffering capacity) residues used and the spacing and ordering between the residues were found to influence the final performance of the vector. Upon optimisation, some constructs transfected at levels that were comparable or even higher than LipofectAce, a commercial reagent used as a positive control (McKenzie et al., 2000). Disulfide-linked oligolysine was then further functionalised with triantennary N-glycan signals to target hepatocytes and evaluated *in vivo* (Kwok et al., 2003). However, contrary to results *in vitro*, the particles were not stable enough in the reductive intracellular liver environment and premature plasmid release ultimately limited gene expression.

PLL by itself is generally not considered to be an efficient vector (Meyer et al., 2008) and is frequently coupled with other agents. The imidazole headgroup of histidine (pK_a~6) can provide endosomal buffering and has been added to PLL to boost transfection (Midoux & Monsigny, 1999). Histidine was also added onto a K15-based oligopeptide which was then self assembled for drug and gene co-delivery (Wiradharma et al., 2009). The HA2 subunit of the hemagglutinin glycoprotein present on the surface of influenza virus plays an important role in the endosomal escape of viruses. To do this, HA2 exhibits a pH-dependent membrane fusion activity. HA2 is not normally lytic at neutral pH. However, protonation of its acidic residues during endo/lysosomal transition triggers HA2 to adopt a more α-helical secondary conformation. At the same time, it exposes a highly-conserved hydrophobic sequence which then interacts and destabilises the endosomal membrane (Wagner et al., 1992a). To exploit this membrane-disrupting mechanism, 20 amino acids corresponding to the N-terminus of HA2 were attached to PLL via cysteine-mediated disulfide bonds. The HA2-functionalised PLL was then shown to induce pH-dependent liposomal leakage (Wagner et al., 1992a) and to augment transfection to a greater extent than the use of chloroquine (Midoux et al., 1993). Melittin, a major component of bee venom, is another peptide with fusogenic activity but unlike HA2, melittin is unresponsive to pH. As such, it remains fusogenic at pH 7 and can indiscriminately disrupt plasma membranes (Chen et al., 2006). To confine fusogenic activity within the endosomes, dimethylmaleic anhydride protecting groups were attached to mask the activity of melittin at neutral pH. Upon cleavage of the protecting groups under acidic conditions, the activity of melittin was restored (Meyer et al., 2008). This protected form of melittin was then coupled to PLL via a cysteine-mediated disulfide bond and the entire construct mediated siRNA knockdown more efficiently than PEI. Adenovirus, known to display pH-dependent membrane disruption as part of its infectious cycle (Curiel et al., 1991), has also been coupled to PLL to improve transfection efficiency. Human adenovirus type 5 (dl312) was either biotinylated and coupled to a streptavidinylated PLL (Wagner et al., 1992b), or simply added as free viral particles into the culture medium to be taken up together with the PLL complexes (Curiel et al., 1991). In another study, chicken embryo lethal orphan virus, an adenovirus from chicken, was attached to PLL and augmented transfection as well as human adenovirus (Cotten et al., 1993).

Various signals have also been added onto PLL to improve its uptake or target specificity. For instance, galactose containing an isothiocyanate group was reacted with the amine groups on PLL to form a thiourea bond and used to mediate gene expression in the livers of rats for up to 140 days (Perales et al., 1994). Mannose and lactose were also used to target cell lines that have receptors for the specific sugar (Midoux et al., 1993). ASOR was coupled onto PLL in an EDC catalysed reaction and intravenously injected into rats (Wu et al., 1989). However, reporter gene expression by liver cells disappeared by day four. Transferrin was coupled to PLL via disulfide bonds in a SPDP-mediated reaction to increase its accumulation within cells (Wagner et al., 1991). Insulin was also coupled to PLL in an SPDP-mediated reaction and used with adenovirus (biotin-streptavidin conjugated) to deliver plasmids into pre-implantation mammalian embryos (Ivanova et al., 1999). PEG was grafted onto PLL via amide bonds in an *N*-hydroxysuccinimide (NHS) catalysed reaction and helped in preventing particle aggregation (Rimann et al., 2008). Stearyl-PLL mixed with a low density lipoprotein was also used to condense plasmids (~600 nm) into ~100 nm complexes, as measured by atomic force microscopy (Kim et al., 1998). Further, the lipoprotein was found to be essential for efficient uptake. Finally, peptides themselves can serve as targeting signals. For example, a short peptide sequence (GACRRETAWACG) suggested to target $\alpha5\beta1$ integrins was linked to K_{16} and mixed with Lipofectin® to transfect neuroblastoma cells (Lee et al., 2003). Several groups have also used the RGD motif to target integrins. A recent example involved RGD being linked to K_{16} peptides, which were then used with an intracellularly cleavable PEG-lipid formulation to deliver plasmids into mice bearing subcutaneous tumors (Tagalakis et al., 2011). The integrin-targeting signal was shown to be important. Upon augmentation by the enhanced permeation and retention effect, the complexes were mainly distributed to the tumor.

4.2 Tat

Full length tat has 86 amino acids (sequence 1-86) and it is a regulatory protein encoded by HIV-1 that transactivates viral gene expression. The ability of tat to cross cell membrane was initially observed by two groups independently in 1988 (Frankel & Pabo, 1988; Green & Loewenstein, 1988). In one study, tat was simply added to a culture of HL3T1 cells modified to contain an integrated copy of chloramphenicol acetyltransferase (CAT, a reporter gene) under the control of the HIV-1 LTR (long terminal repeat) promoter and CAT expression was unexpectedly detected (Frankel & Pabo, 1988). Crucially, the amount of CAT expression was dependent on the dosage of tat. Unlike earlier experiments, tat did not require any help from the scrape loading technique to enter cells. Tat 1-86 was further dissected into five regions and region II and III, together spanning roughly residues 38-62, were identified to be essential and sufficient for transactivation activity (Green & Loewenstein, 1988). Region III (roughly residues 49-62), in particular, was interesting and was rich in arginine and lysine. Furthermore, replacing the three arginines at position 55-57 with alanines drastically reduced transactivation activity. Tat was also observed to localise in the nucleus and thought to be a NLS (Green & Loewenstein, 1988).

The region surrounding the arginine- and lysine-rich domain of tat was keenly evaluated as a gene carrier. Today, full length tat is seldom used and among the many truncated versions being studied (Table 2), tat 47-57 and 48-60 are the two most popular sequences. The *in vivo* half life of free tat 47-57 was calculated to be ~3.5 minutes (Grunwald et al., 2009) and tat 48-60 exists as an unstructured random coil in buffer solutions or when bound to lipid vesicles (Caesar et al., 2006). The secondary structure of a carrier has been suggested to affect its membrane translocation ability. However, it remains unclear if it is better for a structure to be rich in α-helices or unordered. On the one hand, structures rich in α-helices have been suggested to be more efficient in inserting themselves and crossing lipid bilayers (Almeida & Pokorny, 2009). This is consistent with the view that α-helical structures are responsible for the membrane disrupting property of fusogenic peptides such as HA2 (Wagner et al., 1992a), melittin (Chen et al., 2006) and GALA (Subbarao et al., 1987). On the other, α-helices has also been negatively correlated with uptake (Ye et al., 2010). Instead, an unordered structure was preferred as it afforded the flexibility needed to adopt the most energetically favourable conformation during membrane translocation (Caesar et al., 2006).

Entry	Sequence	Reference
1	1-86	(Green & Loewenstein, 1988)
2	1-72	(Frankel & Pabo, 1988)
3	37-72	(Fawell et al., 1994)
4	37-57	(Leonetti et al., 2010)
5	43-60	(Eguchi et al., 2001)
6	47-57	(Wang et al., 2010)
7	48-57	(Wadia et al., 2004)
8	48-58	(Fittipaldi et al., 2003)
9	48-59	(Richard et al., 2005)
10	48-60	(Eiriksdottir et al., 2010)
11	49-57	(Saleh et al., 2010)
12	49-60	(Astriab-Fisher et al., 2000)

Table 2. Heterogeneity in tat sequences being reported in the literature. All sequences are with respect to the original sequence 1-86 in the first entry. Only one reference is provided for each entry, although there may be more discussed in text.

Proteins have been delivered by tat and are usually covalently attached. Fawell and colleagues were the first to chemically conjugate several different proteins onto tat 37-72 (Fawell et al., 1994). One of the model proteins used was β-galactosidase (β-gal), which was grafted onto tat using succinimidyl 4-(N-maleimidomethyl)-cyclohexane-1-carboxylate (SMCC) as a heterobifunctional cross-linker. The β-gal/tat conjugate was then intravenously injected into mice and found to accumulate mainly in the heart, liver and spleen. In a separate study, β-gal/tat 47-57 conjugates were generated by plasmid fusion and injected intraperitoneally into mice (Schwarze et al., 1999). The conjugates were then found to be distributed to all tissues, even across the tight blood-brain-barrier. GFP/tat 47-57 fusion protein was also delivered into cells and uptake was discovered to increase if the cells had been pretreated with 10% dimethylsulfoxide (DMSO) for one hour prior to transfection (Wang et al., 2010). Other macromolecules delivered by tat include peptide nucleic acid (PNA), which are artificial nucleic acid-mimicking polymers. PNA was either conjugated to tat 48-59 using 2-aminoethoxy-2-ethoxyacetic acid as a cross-linker (Richard et al., 2003) or linked via a disulfide bond to a cysteine-modified tat 48-60 (Lundin et al., 2008).

Nucleic acids, on the other hand, are mostly electrostatically carried by tat. For instance, tat 48-60 was used to deliver reporter plasmids into HeLa cells and it was shown that its efficiency can be further improved by adding the SV40 NLS and a dendrimer of seven lysine residues (Yang et al., 2009). A short membrane active peptide, LK15 (KLLKLLLKLLLKLLK) was also conjugated onto tat 49-57 and used for plasmid transfection (Saleh et al., 2010). Antisense oligonucleotides were linked via disulfide bonds to cysteine-modified tat 49-60 and delivered into cells to inhibit the expression of P-glycoprotein, a transmembrane pump that is responsible for the multidrug resistance phenotype of tumor cells (Astriab-Fisher et al., 2000). siRNA has also been delivered by tat 47-57 and interestingly, photostimulation promoted the escape of tat complexes into the cytosol (Endoh et al., 2008). Reactive oxygen species produced during laser illumination was postulated to damage the endosomal vesicles for the enhanced cytosolic access. Finally, tat has also played the role of a helper. As an internalisation enhancer, tat 43-60 was displayed on the surfaces of phage particles to augment the delivery of plasmids encapsulated within the phages (Eguchi et al., 2001). In another study, tat 47-57 was used more as a NLS during the transfection of CHO cells (Moore et al., 2009). Unlike many other systems, the presence of serum augmented tat-mediated transfection (Astriab-Fisher et al., 2000; Eguchi et al., 2001).

Although tat can bring nucleic acids and other macromolecules into a cell, the pathway(s) which tat exploits to do so is ambiguous. There is little consensus in the literature, except for the observation that heparan sulphate, an anionic cell membrane glycosaminoglycan, is crucial for uptake (Sandgren et al., 2002; Tyagi et al., 2001). Besides being rapidly internalised via endocytosis (Tyagi et al., 2001), heparan sulphate is probably also involved in the initial binding step before internalisation (Ferrari et al., 2003). It can also act as a co-receptor for endocytosis (Leonetti et al., 2010). Interestingly, other glycosaminoglycans such as chondroitin sulphate and dermatan sulphate have been ruled out in the binding/internalisation of full length tat 1-86 (Tyagi et al., 2001) and tat 37-57 (Leonetti et al., 2010), but not for the shorter tat 48-60 (Sandgren et al., 2002).

Classical endocytosis is an energy- and ATP-dependent mechanism. For the sake of discussion, endocytosis can be further classified into clathrin-mediated endocytosis, caveolae-mediated endocytosis, macropinocytosis and other forms of clathrin- and caveolae-independent endocytosis. Prompted by the observation that tat 48-60 was internalised at 4°C, a temperature normally considered inhibitory for endocytosis, an energy-independent pathway was initially suggested to be responsible (Futaki et al., 2001b). Another group similarly detected low-temperature internalisation of tat 43-60 and reported that uptake was independent of endocytosis but required the presence of caveolae (Eguchi et al., 2001). The ability of free tat 47-57 to enter cells in the presence of sodium azide, which blocks intracellular ATP synthesis, also led the authors to preclude endocytosis as the uptake mechanism (Ignatovich et al., 2003).

Several models of energy-independent uptake have been proposed. A common theme seems to involve the peptide sticking to the cell membrane and creating a local mass imbalance. At the same time, it transforms itself into a more non-polar compound either due to charge neutralisation (Su et al., 2009) or hydrogen bonding (Rothbard et al., 2004) with the anionic membrane proteins. The peptide then partitions into the hydrophobic lipid bilayer (Rothbard et al., 2002) and translocates through the membrane in a process that is driven by the voltage potential across membrane (Rothbard et al., 2004) and/or the need to relieve membrane curvature stress caused by the mass imbalance in the initial step (Su et al., 2009).

In stark contrast, Richard and colleagues reported that the uptake of tat 48-59, in both its free and PNA-conjugated forms were sensitive to low temperature and sodium azide, indicative of classical endocytosis (Richard et al., 2003). Endocytosis is also believed to be responsible for the uptake of protein-conjugated tat 37-72 in another study (Fawell et al., 1994). Having agreed that the uptake of tat requires energy, opinions are once again divided regarding which of the specific endocytosis pathways involved. For instance, a study singled out clathrin-mediated endocytosis as the pathway responsible for the uptake of unconjugated tat 48-59 (Richard et al., 2005). In others, caveolae-mediated endocytosis was suggested to be the dominant form of uptake for GFP/tat 48-60 fusion protein (Ferrari et al., 2003), and also for GFP/tat 48-58 and GFP/tat 1-86 fusion proteins (Fittipaldi et al., 2003). To confound matters, macropinocytosis was reported to be mainly responsible for the uptake of PNA-conjugated tat 48-60 (Lundin et al., 2008) and tat 48-57 fusion protein (Wadia et al., 2004). In yet another twist, multiple pathways involving both clathrin-mediated endocytosis and macropinocytosis were proposed for the internalisation of unconjugated tat 48-60 (Räägel et al., 2009).

With this amount of confusion in the literature, is there hope of reconciliation? It seems that the first step is to recognise that there may not be a single mechanism responsible for the uptake of tat or indeed, other CPP that will be discussed. CPP thus cannot be taken in the same light as transferrin (Rejman et al., 2004) or cholera toxin (Torgersen et al., 2001), which are accepted to be internalised exclusively via the clathrin- and caveolae-mediated pathway respectively in a wide variety of cells. The outcome being observed therefore depends on the combination of cell/peptide/detection method chosen for that experiment and heterogeneity in conclusion can be expected due to the following reasons.

Cell: Different cell lines can use different pathways to internalise tat (Ignatovich et al., 2003). The nature of cells (primary versus immortalised or adherent versus suspension) (Eiriksdottir et al., 2010) and culture conditions such as the type of growth medium (Moulton et al., 2004), passage number of cells or even the Young's modulus (Kong et al., 2005) of the substrate were suggested to influence plasmid transfection and uptake.

Peptide: As can be seen from Table 2, there are at least 12 distinct sequences under the same umbrella name of tat - more if one takes into account chain-end modifications. Considering that simply modifying a few residues can drastically affect the property of tat, as discussed earlier, it is understandable why the literature cannot seem to agree. The concentration of peptide used was also shown to be important. For instance, it was reported that below 10 mM, unconjugated tat 47-57 exploited both macropinocytosis and caveolae-mediated endocytosis to gain entry but once above 10 mM, a non-endocytosis mechanism seemed to operate (Duchardt et al., 2007). Perhaps there is a concentration threshold above which there is sufficient amount of surface-bound peptide to cause the mass imbalance and trigger direct transport through the membrane. Finally, the absence or presence and the nature of the cargo can also influence the mechanism of uptake. For example, unconjugated tat 47-57 was reported to enter cells using an energy-independent mechanism but endocytosis was responsible after a plasmid was bound (Ignatovich et al., 2003).

Detection method: The majority of experiments aimed at studying the endocytosis pathways of peptides uses one or both of the following techniques: 1) assaying the effects of drugs that are known to inhibit specific endocytosis pathways at the uptake (by flow cytometry or confocal microscopy) and/or the gene expression level, or 2) using a confocal microscope to trace for any co-localisation with known markers for endocytosis pathways, e.g., transferrin (clathrin), cholera toxin (caveolae) or dextran (macropinocytosis). While both are sensible experiments, one must also be aware of their limitations. Inhibitory drugs are usually pleiotropic and affect more than one pathway concurrently. For instance, dynasore has been used to shut down the clathrin-mediated pathway (Gratton et al., 2008a). However, dynasore is a drug that interferes with the activity of dynamin, an enzyme that is needed in both clathrin- and caveolae-mediated pathway to pinch off vesicles from the cell membrane

(Macia et al., 2006). The same is true for methyl-β-cyclodextrin, which depletes cholesterol from the membrane (Richard et al., 2005) and cytochalasin, which disrupts actin formation (Belting et al., 2005). Both drugs can affect all three forms of endocytosis. Moreover, any drug that interferes with uptake is usually toxic and a safe effective dosage must be established in order not to affect the conclusion. There is also possible redundancy in the uptake mechanisms whereby shutting off one pathway may activate another (Rodal et al., 1999), further complicating interpretation.

Both flow cytometry and confocal microscopy are fluorescent-based techniques and rely on either the carrier or/and its cargo to be labelled with a dye. However, the process of tagging the peptide with a dye can already affect its property. For example, results from isothermal titration calorimetry showed that unlabelled tat 47-57 binds to heparan sulphate much more strongly that tat 47-57 labelled with fluorescein isothiocyanate (FITC), a florescent dye whose hydrophobicity has been implicated in the weakening of binding affinity (Ziegler et al., 2005). In another study, FITC labelling was also observed to alter the trafficking property of an octaarginine conjugate (Puckett & Barton, 2009). Significantly, fixing of cells has been shown to be undesirable and even mild fixing can cause artifactual intracellular accumulation (Richard et al., 2003). As a result of this revelation, the validity of earlier publications has been challenged, especially in studies where cells were fixed and intracellular accumulation could still be observed despite low temperature incubation. Surface-bound peptides are another source of confusion which must be separated from those which have been truly internalised (Richard et al., 2003). A brief trypsin wash is typically enough to digest and remove most of the surface-bound peptides.

Above all, it is fair to say that our understanding of endocytosis is still not perfect. As mentioned earlier, it is still not clear which other pathways, besides the clathrin-mediated one, can produce vesicles that undergo acidification. Whether vesicles from different origin eventually merge is another unresolved issue. Furthermore, both the size (Choi et al., 2006) and shape (Sharma et al., 2010) can affect the uptake of a particle and its *in vivo* distribution (Decuzzi et al., 2010). However, these physical parameters of tat or other CPP complexes are seldom reported. Great care must also be taken when reporting particle sizes based on light scattering as a recent survey has estimated that up to 90% of the published figures can be erroneous due to inappropriate assumptions being made during measurements (Keck & Muller, 2008). With such a plethora of factors that can affect outcome, it seems more realistic to accept that the uptake of tat or its conjugates cannot be ascribed any particular route.

4.3 Oligoarginine (Arg_n, usually n = 7 to 9)

The potential of using arginine for gene delivery was firmly established when it was shown that replacing most of the arginine residues in tat 1-86 with alanine drastically reduced internalisation (Tyagi et al., 2001). Replacing the arginine residues within tat 48-60 with lysine had a similar effect and abolished internalisation (Thoren et al., 2004). Clearly, arginine residues are crucial. However, another important (but less obvious) message from these experiments is that arginine is more than just a cationic residue as replacing it with lysine, another cationic residue, is not good enough.

Oligoarginine of various lengths have been evaluated. In one study, oligoarginine with 4, 6, 8, 10, 12 or 16 residues were compared and it was found that both arg_4 and arg_{16} were poorly taken up by cells (Futaki et al., 2001b). Instead, arg_8 exhibited the highest rate of internalisation both in its free form or when linked via a disulfide bond to a model carbonic anhydrase protein. This demonstrated that cationic charge was not sufficient to afford efficient uptake. Consistent with this, another study showed that arg_7 was internalised much more efficiently into Jurkat cells than lys_7 and his_7 (Mitchell et al., 2000). There was therefore something unique about the chemical structure of arginine that cannot be explained simply by it carrying a cationic charge. Indeed, the guanidine (pK_a~12) sidegroup of arginine was determined to be key as replacing it with a urea (pK_a~0.1) sidegroup removed internalisation. Urea differs from guanidine by only a single nitrogen atom, which in the former is replaced by an oxygen atom. However, this simple modification removed not only the ability of urea to protonate at neutral pH, but also its ability to form hydrogen bonds. This ability to form stable hydrogen bonds with the anionic phosphates and sulphates on cell membrane was then suggested to be the feature that distinguished arginine from lysine and histidine in terms of translocation efficiency (Mitchell et al., 2000).

The spacing between arginine residues can also influence internalisation (Rothbard et al., 2002). To study this, a library of oligoarginines was synthesised, all with seven residues but separated by 1-6 spacers at all the possible permutations. It was argued that the addition of spacers imparted flexibility to the arginine backbone which was important for better membrane translocation.

A length of 7-9 arginines is usually preferred and the chains exist as random coils in buffer solutions and when bound to lipid vesicles (Caesar et al., 2006). Both D- and L-arginines have been explored with some authors preferring D-arginines (Hyun et al., 2010; Puckett & Barton, 2009) and others finding no difference between the stereoisomers (Mitchell et al., 2000; Nakase et al., 2004). Cargoes of different nature have been delivered. Negatively charged QCs were electrostatically bound to arg_8 and delivered into adipose tissue-derived stem cells for imaging purposes (Yukawa et al., 2010). The anti-cancer drug, taxol was covalently bound to arg_8 via disulfide bonds using a novel linker to increase its water solubility and uptake. The drug was also designed to be released intracellularly so as to combat multidrug resistant cell lines which otherwise have limited accumulation of chemotherapeutic drugs (Dubikovskaya et al., 2008). The immunosuppressive drug, cyclosporine A, was coupled with arg_7 using a novel pH-sensitive linker and used for topical delivery in a skin inflammation model (Rothbard et al., 2000). Phosphorodiamidate morpholino oligomers (PMO) are antisense molecules that interfere with mRNA translation but structurally differ from nucleic acids in several aspects. In one study, PMO was electrostatically carried by an arg_9-based carrier, but the efficiency was not as good as covalently linked ones (Moulton et al., 2004). In another study, a short peptide sequence corresponding to the C-terminus of the cystic fibrosis transmembrane regulator was joined to arg_7 during synthesis and laser illumination was used to trigger the release of the conjugate into the cytosol of U2OS cells (Maiolo-III et al., 2004). siRNA was electrostatically carried by an arg_8-based vector and used to transfect mouse bone marrow-derived dendritic cells (Akita et al., 2010). Finally, D-arg_9 with cysteines added on both terminals (i.e., cys-arg_9-cys) was crosslinked via disulfide bonds to form a mesh of reducible poly(oligoarginine) (Hyun et al., 2010). The carrier was then used to deliver plasmids encoding for heme oxygenase-1 (useful for the treatment of ischemia/reperfusion-induced brain stroke) by direct injection into the brain of mice.

Several modifications have been made to oligoarginine to improve its transfection efficiency. For example, arg_8 has been combined with GALA, a pH sensitive fusogenic peptide to enhance its endosomal escaping property (Akita et al., 2010). The addition of a hydrophobic stearyl chain to arg_8 was also shown to greatly increase its transfection ability (Futaki et al., 2001a). This was suggested to be due to a better association between the hydrophobic moieties on the vector and the lipid bilayer (Putnam, 2006). Indeed, a certain degree of hydrophobicity is a common feature of many efficient vectors and this was clearly shown in a recent study where a novel triblock peptide, phobic$_5$-his$_4$-arg$_8$, was developed (Seow & Yang, 2009b; Seow et al., 2009). This design featured a block of five hydrophobic residues (tryptophan, phenylalanine or isoleucine, in order of increasing hydrophobicity) for enhanced uptake, a middle block of four histidines for buffering capacity and a third block of arg$_8$ for DNA binding and membrane penetration. Removing the hydrophobic block drastically reduced the efficiency of the carrier at both the uptake and gene expression level. Transfection efficiency can also be modulated just by changing the hydrophobicity of the hydrophobic block. The buffering capacity of the carriers was also assessed in a series of acid-base titration experiments and shown to vary with the length of the histidine block used. Each block was then systematically studied and an optimised sequence was used to mediate reporter plasmid expression by direct local injection into mice bearing 4T1 tumors. In another study, cholesterol was added as the hydrophobic end of a his5/10-arg10 vector for gene delivery (Guo et al., 2008).

The internalisation of oligoarginine is sharply inhibited by the presence of heparin, which competes with heparan sulphate for binding (Seow et al., 2009). This shows that heparan sulphate is crucial for uptake. Low-temperature internalisation was observed and energy-independence was originally proposed to characterise the uptake of oligoarginine (Futaki et al., 2001b). However, those observation was made with fixed cells. In response to studies that had exposed the flaws of using fixed cells (Richard et al., 2003), authors of the original study re-evaluated the uptake mechanism using live cells. Consequently, they reported macropinocytosis to be a major, but not exclusive pathway for the uptake of oligoarginine (Nakase et al., 2004). Macropinocytosis was also proposed to be the main form of uptake for protein-conjugated (Takayama et al., 2009) and siRNA-bound arg$_8$ (Akita et al., 2010). Nonetheless, an energy-independent form of uptake was still suggested if the concentration of unconjugated arg$_9$ exceeded 10 mM - otherwise, macropinocytosis and caveolae-mediated, but not clathrin-mediated endocytosis seemed to be important (Duchardt et al., 2007). Another study reported that both clathrin-mediated endocytosis and macropinocytosis play a role for the uptake of unconjugated arg$_9$ (Räägel et al., 2009). On the other hand, all three forms of endocytosis (clathrin-mediated, caveolae-mediated and macropinocytosis) were found to be responsible for the uptake of plasmid-bound oligoarginine complexes (Seow et al., 2009). Finally, an energy-dependent but non-endocytosis mechanism was also proposed to be responsible for uptake (Mitchell et al., 2000). Like tat, there is little consensus over the internalisation pathway(s) of oligoarginine, although endocytosis is generally accepted to play a key role in most cases (Richard et al., 2003; Rothbard et al., 2000).

4.4 Penetratin

Homeoproteins are regulatory proteins essential for proper physical development. The DNA binding domain of these proteins is made up of a highly conserved sequence known as the homeobox. The homeobox of the *Drosophila* antennapedia gene (pAntp) is 60-amino acid long (sequence 1-60) and contains three α-helices (Derossi et al., 1994). pAntp was first discovered to effectively translocate into nerve cells and accumulate within their nuclei (Joliot et al., 1991). To demonstrate the usefulness of pAntp as a carrier, a 33-residue peptide cargo corresponding to the C-terminus of rab3, a GTP-binding protein in human, was linked to pAntp via plasmid fusion and shown to translocate into the nuclei of myoblasts and neurons (Perez et al., 1992). A study later revealed that the third helix was actually the domain driving internalisation (Roux et al., 1993). Based on this, penetratin, a 16-residue peptide within the third helix (sequence 43-58 of the original pAntp) was described (Derossi et al., 1994). Penetratin demonstrated membrane penetrating ability but was prone to aggregation. Aggregated particles can enjoy better internalisation due to a sedimentation effect which promotes a more intimate particle-cell contact (Luo & Saltzman, 2000b). While this may have helped the internalisation of penetratin, aggregation alone was excluded as the dominant reason for its efficient internalisation (Derossi et al., 1994).

The secondary structure of penetratin in buffer is unstructured but becomes α-helical when bound to lipid vesicles (Caesar et al., 2006). Raman microscopy on live cells further showed that penetratin within the cytosol was either unstructured or in the β-sheet conformation (Ye et al., 2010). The arginine residues within penetratin are important as replacing them with lysine greatly reduced its translocation ability (Caesar et al., 2006). Various cargoes have been carried by penetratin. Antisense oligonucleotides (Astriab-Fisher et al., 2000), PNA (Lundin et al., 2008) and luciferin protein (Eiriksdottir et al., 2010) have all been coupled onto a cysteine-modified penetratin via disulfide bonds and delivered into cells. siRNA was electrostatically bound to penetratin and although the complexes accumulated favourably within cells, there was limited silencing activity (Lundberg et al., 2007). HA2 was then added to enhance endosomal escape but produced only a modest improvement. Penetratin has been evaluated *in vivo*. In one study, penetratin was directly injected into a rat's brain and the peptide was observed to spread away from the site of injection (Bolton et al., 2000). However, dosage-dependent cell death and inflammatory responses were also provoked.

Penetratin was initially suggested to enter cells using energy-independent mechanisms (Derossi et al., 1994; Perez et al., 1992; Roux et al., 1993), but a caveat is that fixed cells were used in those studies. Nonetheless, an energy-independent mechanism was still suggested to be possible past a concentration threshold of 40 mM, below which all three forms of endocytosis should dominate (Duchardt et al., 2007). Endocytosis was also reported to be responsible for the uptake of siRNA-bound penetratin (Lundberg et al., 2007) while macropinocytosis was suggested to be the main form of uptake for PNA-conjugated penetratin (Lundin et al., 2008).

4.5 Transportan (Tp) and Tp10

Tp uses a lysine residue to join the first 12 N-terminus residues of the neuropeptide, galanin, to the 14 C-terminus residues of the wasp venom, mastoparan. Tp is thus 27 residues long (sequence 1-27) and was first shown to penetrate Bowes' melanoma cells rapidly and efficiently (Pooga et al., 1998). However, Tp at a high concentration was found to inhibit the GTPase activity of cells. To overcome this side effect, a series of Tp analogues was prepared (Soomets et al., 2000). This led to the identification of Tp10 which, upon deleting the first 6 residues of Tp (i.e., sequence 7-27 remaining), was internalised as efficiently as Tp but did not have any effect on the GTPases.

PNA (Lundin et al., 2008) and luciferin (Eiriksdottir et al., 2010) were conjugated to both cysteine-modified Tp and Tp10 via disulfide bonds. siRNA was also electrostatically bound to Tp10 but had little silencing effects when transfected into cells (Lundberg et al., 2007). This was surprising insofar as Tp10 was shown earlier to mediate good levels of plasmid expression. This however resonates with comments made by other researchers (Mahon et al., 2010; unpublished observation) who had observed that a carrier's efficiency in plasmid delivery may not automatically apply to the delivery of the shorter and stiffer siRNA molecules. Earlier studies with fixed cells reported low temperature internalisation of Tp

(Pooga et al., 1998) but more recent observations have linked endocytosis to the uptake of both Tp and Tp10 (Lundin et al., 2008).

4.6 Other notable peptide sequences

VP22 is a 300-residue long peptide derived from the structural protein of HSV-1 and has been used successfully to deliver GFP as a fusion protein (Elliott & O'Hare, 1997). When COS-1 cells were microinjected with plasmids encoding for VP22, an interesting pattern was observed in which a central cell would first express VP22 and exhibit cytosolic staining when probed with anti-VP22 antibodies. The VP22 peptide was then excreted and could infect neighbouring cells before eventually localising to their nuclei. CADY is a 20-residue long peptide evaluated for siRNA delivery (Crombez et al., 2009). It changes from unordered to being α-helical in the presence of lipid vesicles which then drives its internalisation independently of the endosomal pathway (Konate et al., 2010). MPG is a 27-residue peptide designed to have a hydrophobic domain (sequence 1-17) derived from HIV gp41 and a NLS domain (sequence 21-27) derived from SV40 separated by a "trp-ser-gln" unit (Morris et al., 1997). The uptake of MPG/oligonucleotide complexes was shown to be rapid and independent of the endosomal pathway. Other carriers explored for delivery include KALA (Wyman et al., 1997) and EB1 (Lundberg et al., 2007).

Throughout the discussion, various peptides with fusogenic and nuclear localising properties were introduced. SV40 is the classical NLS and different sequences exist. The most commonly used sequence for SV40 is provided in Table 1. Other sequences include "glu-asp-pro-tyr" (Trentin et al., 2005) and "glu-pro-tyr-cys" (Moore et al., 2009) being added onto the C-terminus and an even longer form of SV40 has been described (Eguchi et al., 2001). INF 5 and INF 7 are examples of two commonly used fusogenic peptide and both are derived from the parent HA2 peptide (Plank et al., 1994). GALA is a 30-amino acid long pH-sensitive fusogenic peptide (Subbarao et al., 1987). Upon protonation of its glu residues, its secondary structure changes from unordered at neutral pH to being α-helical in acidic environments. Both the amphipathicity and degree of α-helicity have been correlated with the ability of GALA to interact and destabilise membranes (Parente et al., 1990).

5. Conclusion

This chapter started by discussing the challenges and intracellular barriers associated with the delivery of nucleic acids. Strategies used to overcome these hurdles were next examined, mainly in the context of peptide-derived vectors. It is clear that peptide carriers are not characterised by any typical sequences, although the majority of current designs rely on cationic residues to bind nucleic acids. This strategy, nonetheless, may be problematic during *in vivo* applications. An area that deserves more attention is the development of vectors that can bind nucleic acids using non-electrostatic forces, e.g., by including more hydrophobic residues. The stability and *in vivo* behaviour of such vectors then need to be thoroughly evaluated. Another challenge is to further improve strategies that are already in place to shield the cationic charges, e.g., by attaching PEG chains that are intracellularly cleavable so as to increase the circulation time of the complexes without compromising excessively on transfection efficiency. Advances in either will enable peptides to further realise their potential as a class of non-viral vector.

6. References

Akinrimisi, E. O., Bonner, J. & Ts'o, P. O. P. (1965). Binding of basic proteins to DNA. *Journal of Molecular Biology*, Vol. 11, pp. 128-136.

Akita, H., et al. (2010). Nanoparticles for *ex vivo* siRNA delivery to dendritic cells for cancer vaccines: programmed endosomal escape and dissociation. *Journal of Controlled Release*, Vol. 143, pp. 311-317.

Almeida, P. F. & Pokorny, A. (2009). Mechanisms of antimicrobial, cytolytic, and cell-penetrating peptides: from kinetics to thermodynamics. *Biochemistry*, Vol. 48, pp. 8083-8093.

Astriab-Fisher, A., et al. (2000). Antisense inhibition of P-glycoprotein expression using peptide-oligonucleotide conjugates. *Biochemical Pharmacology*, Vol. 60, pp. 83-90.

Belting, M., Sandgren, S. & Wittrup, A. (2005). Nuclear delivery of macromolecules: barriers and carriers. *Advanced Drug Delivery Reviews*, Vol. 57, pp. 505-527.

Bolton, S. J., et al. (2000). Cellular uptake and spread of the cell-permeable peptide penetratin in adult rat brain. *European Journal of Neuroscience*, Vol. 12, pp. 2847-2855.

Boussif, O., et al. (1995). A versatile vector for gene and oligonucleotide transfer into cells in culture and in vivo: polyethylenimine. *Proceedings of the National Academy of Sciences*, Vol. 92, pp. 7297-7301.

Caesar, C. E. B., et al. (2006). Membrane interactions of cell-penetrating peptides probed by tryptophan fluorescence and dichroism techniques: correlations of structure to cellular uptake. *Biochemistry*, Vol. 45, pp. 7682-7692.

Cavazzana-Calvo, M., et al. (2010). Transfusion independence and HMGA2 activation after gene therapy of human β-thalassaemia. *Nature*, Vol. 467, pp. 318-323.

Chang, K.-L., et al. (2010). Efficient gene transfection by histidine-modified chitosan through enhancement of endosomal escape. *Bioconjugate Chemistry*, Vol. 21, pp. 1087-1095.

Chen, C.-P., et al. (2006). Gene transfer with poly-melittin peptides. *Bioconjugate Chemistry*, Vol. 17, pp. 1057-1062.

Chen, C. & Okayama, H. (1987). High-efficiency transformation of mammalian cells by plasmid DNA. *Molecular and Cellular Biology*, Vol. 7, pp. 2745-2752.

Choi, H. S., et al. (2006). An insight into the gene delivery mechanism of the arginine peptide system: role of the peptide/DNA complex size. *Biochimica et Biophysica Acta*, Vol. 1760, pp. 1604-1612.

Cotten, M., et al. (1993). Chicken adenovirus (CELO virus) particles augment receptor-mediated DNA delivery to mammalian cells and yield exceptional levels of stable transformants. *Journal of Virology*, Vol. 67, pp. 3777-3785.

Crombez, L., et al. (2009). A new potent secondary amphipathic cell–penetrating peptide for siRNA delivery into mammalian cells. *Molecular Therapy*, Vol. 17, pp. 95-103.

Curiel, D. T., et al. (1991). Adenovirus enhancement of transferrin-polylysine-mediated gene delivery. *Proceedings of the National Academy of Sciences*, Vol. 88, pp. 8850-8854.

Decuzzi, P., et al. (2010). Size and shape effects in the biodistribution of intravascularly injected particles. *Journal of Controlled Release*, Vol. 141, pp. 320-327.

Derossi, D., et al. (1994). The third helix of the antennapedia homeodornain translocates through biological membranes. *Journal of Biological Chemistry*, Vol. 269, pp. 10444-10450.

Deshayes, A., Herrera-Estrella, L. & Caboche, M. (1985). Liposome-mediated transformation of tobacco mesophyll protoplasts by an Escherichia coli plasmid. *EMBO Journal*, Vol. 4, pp. 2731-2737.

Diebold, S. S., et al. (1999). Mannose polyethylenimine conjugates for targeted DNA delivery into dendritic cells. *Journal of Biological Chemistry*, Vol. 274, pp. 19087-19094.

Doxsey, S. J., et al. (1985). An efficient method for introducing macromolecules into living cells. *Journal of Cell Biology*, Vol. 101, pp. 19-27.

Dubikovskaya, E. A., et al. (2008). Overcoming multidrug resistance of small-molecule therapeutics through conjugation with releasable octaarginine transporters. *Proceedings of the National Academy of Sciences*, Vol. 105, pp. 12128-12133.

Duchardt, F., et al. (2007). A comprehensive model for the cellular uptake of cationic cell-penetrating peptides. *Traffic*, Vol. 8, pp. 848-866.

Duncan, R. (2006). Polymer conjugates as anticancer nanomedicines. *Nature Reviews Cancer*, Vol. 6, pp. 688-701.

Eguchi, A., et al. (2001). Protein transduction domain of HIV-1 tat protein promotes efficient delivery of DNA into mammalian cells. *Journal of Biological Chemistry*, Vol. 276, pp. 26204-26210.

Eiriksdottir, E., et al. (2010). Cellular internalization kinetics of (luciferin-)cell-penetrating peptide conjugates. *Bioconjugate Chemistry*, Vol. 21, pp. 1662-1672.

Elliott, G. & O'Hare, P. (1997). Intercellular trafficking and protein delivery by a herpesvirus structural protein. *Cell*, Vol. 88, pp. 223-233.

Endoh, T., Sisido, M. & Ohtsuki, T. (2008). Cellular siRNA delivery mediated by a cell-permeant RNA-binding protein and photoinduced RNA interference. *Bioconjugate Chemistry*, Vol. 19, pp. 1017-1024.

Fawell, S., et al. (1994). Tat-mediated delivery of heterologous proteins into cells. *Proceedings of the National Academy of Sciences*, Vol. 91, pp. 664-668.

Felgner, P. L., et al. (1987). Lipofection: a highly efficient, lipid-mediated DNA-transfection procedure. *Proceedings of the National Academy of Sciences*, Vol. 84, pp. 7413-7417.

Ferrari, A., et al. (2003). Caveolae-mediated internalization of extracellular HIV-1 tat fusion proteins visualized in real time. *Molecular Therapy*, Vol. 8, pp. 284-294.

Fire, A., et al. (1998). Potent and specific genetic interference by double-stranded RNA in Caenorhabditis elegans. *Nature*, Vol. 391, pp. 806-811.

Fittipaldi, A., et al. (2003). Cell membrane lipid rafts mediate caveolar endocytosis of HIV-1 tat fusion proteins. *Journal of Biological Chemistry*, Vol. 278, pp. 34141-34149.

Frankel, A. D. & Pabo, C. O. (1988). Cellular uptake of the tat protein from human immunodeficiency virus. *Cell*, Vol. 55, pp. 1189-1193.

Frenkel, V. (2008). Ultrasound mediated delivery of drugs and genes to solid tumors. *Advanced Drug Delivery Reviews*, Vol. 60, pp. 1193-1208.

Funhoff, A. M., et al. (2005). PEG shielded polymeric double-layered micelles for gene delivery. *Journal of Controlled Release*, Vol. 102, pp. 711-724.

Futaki, S., et al. (2001a). Stearylated arginine-rich peptides: a new class of transfection systems. *Bioconjugate Chemistry*, Vol. 12, pp. 1005-1011.

Futaki, S., et al. (2001b). Arginine-rich Peptides: an abundant source of membrane-permeable peptides having potential as carriers for intracellular protein delivery. *Journal of Biological Chemistry*, Vol. 276, pp. 5836-5840.

Gabrielson, N. P. & Pack, D. W. (2006). Acetylation of polyethylenimine enhances gene delivery via weakened polymer/DNA interactions. *Biomacromolecules*, Vol. 7, pp. 2427-2435.

Gao, X. & Huang, L. (1996). Potentiation of cationic liposome-mediated gene delivery by polycations. *Biochemistry*, Vol. 35, pp. 1027-1036.

Godbey, W. T., Wu, K. K. & Mikos, A. G. (1999). Tracking the intracellular path of poly(ethylenimine)/DNA complexes for gene delivery. *Proceedings of the National Academy of Sciences*, Vol. 96, pp. 5177-5181.

Guo, X. D., et al. (2008). Cationic micelles self-assembled from cholesterol-conjugated oligopeptides as an efficient gene delivery vector. *Biomaterials*, Vol. 29, pp. 4838-4846.

Graham, F. L. & Eb, A. J. V. D. (1973). A new technique for the assay of infectivity of human adenovirus 5 DNA. *Virology*, Vol. 52, pp. 456-467.

Gratton, S. E. A., et al. (2008a). Microfabricated particles for engineered drug therapies: elucidation into the mechanisms of cellular internalization of PRINT particles. *Pharmaceutical Research*, Vol. 25, pp. 2845-2852.

Gratton, S. E. A., et al. (2008b). The effect of particle design on cellular internalization pathways. *Proceedings of the National Academy of Sciences*, Vol. 105, pp. 11613-11618.

Green, J. J., et al. (2006). Biodegradable polymeric vectors for gene delivery to human endothelial cells. *Bioconjugate Chemistry*, Vol. 17, pp. 1162-1169.

Green, M. & Loewenstein, P. M. (1988). Autonomous functional domains of chemically synthesized human immunodeficiency virus tat trans-activator protein. *Cell*, Vol. 55, pp. 1179-1188,.

Griesenbach, U. & Alton, E. W. F. W. (2009). On behalf of the UK Cystic Fibrosis Gene Therapy Consortium. Gene transfer to the lung: lessons learned from more than 2 decades of CF gene therapy. *Advanced Drug Delivery Reviews*, Vol. 61, pp. 128-139.

Grunwald, J., et al. (2009). Tat peptide and its conjugates: proteolytic stability. *Bioconjugate Chemistry*, Vol. 20, pp. 1531-1537.

Hacein-Bey-Abina, S., et al. (2003). LMO2-associated clonal T cell proliferation in two patients after gene therapy for SCID-X1. *Science*, Vol. 302, pp. 415-419.

Hollon, T. (2000). Researchers and regulators reflect on first gene therapy death. *Nature Medicine*, Vol. 6, p. 6.

Hossann, M., et al. (2010). Size of thermosensitive liposomes influences content release. *Journal of Controlled Release*, Vol. 147, pp. 436-443.

Hyun, H., et al. (2010). Therapeutic effects of a reducible poly (oligo-D-arginine) carrier with the heme oxygenase-1 gene in the treatment of hypoxic-ischemic brain injury. *Biomaterials*, Vol. 31, pp. 9128-9134.

Ignatovich, I. A., et al. (2003). Complexes of plasmid DNA with basic domain 47–57 of the HIV-1 tat protein are transferred to mammalian cells by endocytosis-mediated pathways. *Journal of Biological Chemistry*, Vol. 278, pp. 42625-42636.

Ivanova, M. M., et al. (1999). Receptor-mediated transport of foreign DNA into preimplantation mammalian embryos. *Molecular Reproduction and Development*, Vol. 54, pp. 112-120.

Joliot, A., et al. (1991). Antennapedia homeobox peptide regulates neural morphogenesis. *Proceedings of the National Academy of Sciences*, Vol. 88, pp. 1864-1868.

Kay, M. A., Glorioso, J. C. & Naldini, L. (2001). Viral vectors for gene therapy: the art of turning infectious agents into vehicles of therapeutics. *Nature Medicine*, Vol. 7, pp. 33-40.

Keck, C. M. & Muller, R. H. (2008). Size analysis of submicron particles by laser diffractometry—90% of the published measurements are false. *International Journal of Pharmaceutics*, Vol. 355, pp. 150-163.

Kim, J.-S., et al. (1998). A new non-viral DNA delivery vector: the terplex system. *Journal of Controlled Release*, Vol. 53, pp. 175-182.

Kircheis, R., et al. (1997). Coupling of cell-binding ligands to polyethylenimine for targeted gene delivery. *Gene Therapy*, Vol. 4, pp. 409-418.

Konate, K., et al. (2010). Insight into the cellular uptake mechanism of a secondary amphipathic cell-penetrating peptide for siRNA delivery. *Biochemistry*, Vol. 49, pp. 3393-3402.

Kong, H. J., et al. (2005). Non-viral gene delivery regulated by stiffness of cell adhesion substrates. *Nature Materials*, Vol. 4, pp. 460-464.

Koping-Hoggard, M., et al. (2004). Improved chitosan-mediated gene delivery based on easily dissociated chitosan polyplexes of highly defined chitosan oligomers. *Gene Therapy*, Vol. 11, pp. 1441-1452.

Kwok, K. Y., et al. (2003). In vivo gene transfer using sulfhydryl cross-linked PEG-peptide/glycopeptide DNA co-condensates. *Journal of Pharmaceutical Sciences*, Vol. 92, pp. 1174-1185.

Lam, A. P. & Dean, D. A. (2010). Progress and prospects: nuclear import of nonviral vectors. *Gene Therapy*, Vol. 17, pp. 439-447.

Lee, L. K., et al. (2003). Biophysical characterization of an integrin-targeted non-viral vector. *Medical Science Monitor*, Vol. 9, pp. BR54-61.

Lee, Y., et al. (2007). Visualization of the degradation of a disulfide polymer, linear poly(ethylenimine sulfide), for gene delivery. *Bioconjugate Chemistry*, Vol. 18, pp. 13-18.

Leonetti, M., Gadzinski, A. & Moine, G. (2010). Cell surface heparan sulfate proteoglycans influence MHC class II-restricted antigen presentation. *Journal of Immunology*, Vol. 185, pp. 3847-3856.

Liang, H., Harries, D. & Wong, G. C. L. (2005). Polymorphism of DNA–anionic liposome complexes reveals hierarchy of ion-mediated interactions. *Proceedings of the National Academy of Sciences*, Vol. 102, pp. 11173-11178.

Lin, C., et al. (2007). Novel bioreducible poly(amido amine)s for highly efficient gene delivery. *Bioconjugate Chemistry*, Vol. 18, pp. 138-145.

Lin, S., et al. (2008). An acid-labile block copolymer of PDMAEMA and PEG as potential carrier for intelligent gene delivery systems. *Biomacromolecules*, Vol. 9, pp. 109-115.

Liu, X., Yang, J. W. & Lynn, D. M. (2008). Addition of "charge-shifting" side chains to linear poly(ethyleneimine) enhances cell transfection efficiency. *Biomacromolecules*, Vol. 9, pp. 2063–2071.

Lundberg, P., et al. (2007). Delivery of short interfering RNA using endosomolytic cell-penetrating peptides. *The FASEB Journal*, Vol. 21, pp. 2664-2671.

Lundin, P., et al. (2008). Distinct uptake routes of cell-penetrating peptide conjugates. *Bioconjugate Chemistry*, Vol. 19, pp. 2535-2542.

Luo, D. & Saltzman, W. M. (2000a). Synthetic DNA delivery systems. *Nature Biotechnology*, Vol. 18, pp. 33-37.

Luo, D. & Saltzman, W. M. (2000b). Enhancement of transfection by physical concentration of DNA at the cell surface. *Nature Biotechnology*, Vol. 18, pp. 893-895.

Macia, E., et al. (2006). Dynasore, a cell-permeable inhibitor of dynamin. *Developmental Cell*, Vol. 10, pp. 839-850.

MacLaughlin, F. C., et al. (1998). Chitosan and depolymerized chitosan oligomers as condensing carriers for in vivo plasmid delivery. *Journal of Controlled Release*, Vol. 56, pp. 259-272.

Mahon, K. P., et al. (2010). Combinatorial approach to determine functional group effects on lipidoid-mediated siRNA delivery. *Bioconjugate Chemistry*, Vol. 21, pp. 1448-1454.

Maiolo-III, J. R., Ottinger, E. A. & Ferrer, M. (2004). Specific redistribution of cell-penetrating peptides from endosomes to the cytoplasm and nucleus upon laser illumination. *Journal of the American Chemical Society*, Vol. 126, pp. 15376-15377.

McKenzie, D. L., et al. (2000). Low molecular weight disulfide cross-linking peptides as nonviral gene delivery carriers. *Bioconjugate Chemistry*, Vol. 11, pp. 901-909.

McManus, J. J., Radler, J. O. & Dawson, K. A. (2004). Observation of a rectangular columnar phase in a DNA-calcium-zwitterionic lipid complex. *Journal of the American Chemical Society*, Vol. 126, pp. 15966-15967.

McNeil, P. L., et al. (1984). A method for incorporating macromolecules into adherent cells. *Journal of Cell Biology*, Vol. 98, pp. 1556-1564.

Merediz, S. A. K., et al. (2000). Ballistic transfer of minimalistic immunologically defined expression constructs for IL4 and CTLA4 into the corneal epithelium in mice after orthotopic corneal allograft transplantation. *Graefe's Archive for Clinical and Experimental Ophthalmology*, Vol. 238, pp. 701-707.

Mével, M., et al. (2010). DODAG; a versatile new cationic lipid that mediates efficient delivery of pDNA and siRNA. *Journal of Controlled Release*, Vol. 143, pp. 222-232.

Meyer, M., et al. (2008). Breathing life into polycations: functionalization with pH-responsive endosomolytic peptides and polyethylene glycol enables siRNA delivery. *Journal of the American Chemical Society*, Vol. 130, pp. 3272-3273.

Midoux, P., et al. (1993). Specific gene transfer mediated by lactosylated poly-L-lysine into hepatoma cells. *Nucleic Acids Research*, Vol. 21, pp. 871-878.

Midoux, P. & Monsigny, M. (1999). Efficient gene transfer by histidylated polylysine/pDNA complexes. *Bioconjugate Chemistry*, Vol. 10, pp. 406-411.

Mitchell, D. J., et al. (2000). Polyarginine enters cells more efficiently than other polycationic homopolymers. *Journal of Peptide Research*, Vol. 56, pp. 318-325.

Mok, H., Park, J. W. & Park, T. G. (2008). Enhanced intracellular delivery of quantum dot and adenovirus nanoparticles triggered by acidic pH via surface charge reversal. *Bioconjugate Chemistry*, Vol. 19, pp. 797-801.

Moore, N. M., Sheppard, C. L. & Sakiyama-Elbert, S. E. (2009). Characterization of a multifunctional PEG-based gene delivery system containing nuclear localization signals and endosomal escape peptides. *Acta Biomaterialia*, Vol. 5, pp. 854-864.

Morris, M. C., et al. (1997). A new peptide vector for efficient delivery of oligonucleotides into mammalian cells. *Nucleic Acids Research*, Vol. 25, pp. 2730-2736.

Moulton, H. M., et al. (2004). Cellular uptake of antisense morpholino oligomers conjugated to arginine-rich peptides. *Bioconjugate Chemistry*, Vol. 15, pp. 290-299.

Nakase, I., et al. (2004). Cellular uptake of arginine-rich peptides: roles for macropinocytosis and actin rearrangement. *Molecular Therapy*, Vol. 10, pp. 1011-1022.

Nayak, S. & Herzog, R. W. (2010). Progress and prospects: immune responses to viral vectors. *Gene Therapy*, Vol. 17, pp. 295-304.

Niidome, T., et al. (1997). Binding of cationic α-helical peptides to plasmid DNA and their gene transfer abilities into cells. *Journal of Biological Chemistry*, Vol. 272, pp. 15307-15312.

Okada, C. Y. & Rechsteiner, M. (1982). Introduction of macromolecules into cultured mammalian cells by osmotic lysis of pinocytic vesicles. *Cell*, Vol. 29, pp. 33-41.

Ott, M. G., et al. (2006). Correction of X-linked chronic granulomatous disease by gene therapy, augmented by insertional activation of *MDS1-EVI1*, *PRDM16* or *SETBP1*. *Nature Medicine*, Vol. 12, pp. 401-409.

Palm-Apergi, C., et al. (2009). The membrane repair response masks membrane disturbances caused by cell-penetrating peptide uptake. *The FASEB Journal*, Vol. 23, pp. 214-223.

Parente, R. A., et al. (1990). Association of a pH-sensitive peptide with membrane vesicles: role of amino acid sequence. *Biochemistry*, Vol. 29, pp. 8713-8719.

Park, T. G., Jeong, J. H. & Kim, S. W. (2006). Current status of polymeric gene delivery systems. *Advanced Drug Delivery Reviews*, Vol. 58, pp. 467-486.

Pelkmans, L. & Helenius, A. (2002). Endocytosis via caveolae. *Traffic*, Vol. 3, pp. 311-320.

Perales, J. C., et al. (1994). Gene transfer in vivo: sustained expression and regulation of genes introduced into the liver by receptor-targeted uptake. *Proceedings of the National Academy of Sciences*, Vol. 91, pp. 4086-4090.

Perez, F., et al. (1992). Antennapedia homeobox as a signal for the cellular internalization and nuclear addressing of a small exogenous peptide. *Journal of Cell Science*, Vol. 102, pp. 717-722.

Plank, C., et al. (1994). The influence of endosome-disruptive peptides on gene transfer using synthetic virus-like gene transfer systems. *Journal of Biological Chemistry*, Vol. 269, pp. 12918-12924.

Pooga, M., et al. (1998). Cell penetration by transportan. *The FASEB Journal*, Vol. 12, pp. 67-77.

Pouton, C. W. & Seymour, L. W. (2001). Key issues in non-viral gene delivery. *Advanced Drug Delivery Reviews*, Vol. 46, pp. 187-203.

Puckett, C. A. & Barton, J. K. (2009). Fluorescein redirects a ruthenium-octaarginine conjugate to the nucleus. *Journal of the American Chemical Society*, Vol. 131, pp. 8738-8739.

Putnam, D. (2006). Polymers for gene delivery across length scales. *Nature Medicine*, Vol. 5, pp. 439-451.

Räägel, H., et al. (2009). CPP–protein constructs induce a population of non-acidic vesicles during trafficking through endo-lysosomal pathway. *Journal of Controlled Release*, Vol. 139, pp. 108-117.

Rejman, J., et al. (2004). Size-dependent internalization of particles via the pathways of clathrin and caveolae-mediated endocytosis. *Biochemical Journal*, Vol. 377, pp. 159-169.

Ren, Y., et al. (2010). Charge density and molecular weight of polyphosphoramidate gene carrier are key parameters influencing its DNA compaction ability and transfection efficiency. *Biomacromolecules*, Vol. 11, pp. 3432-3439.

Richard, J. P., et al. (2005). Cellular uptake of unconjugated tat peptide involves clathrin dependent endocytosis and heparan sulfate receptors. *Journal of Biological Chemistry*, Vol. 280, pp. 15300-15306.

Richard, J. P., et al. (2003). Cell-penetrating peptides: a reevaluation of the mechanism of cellular uptake. *Journal of Biological Chemistry*, Vol. 278, pp. 585-590.

Rimann, M., et al. (2008). Characterization of PLL-g-PEG-DNA nanoparticles for the delivery of therapeutic DNA. *Bioconjugate Chemistry*, Vol. 19, pp. 548-557.

Rodal, S. K., et al. (1999). Extraction of cholesterol with methyl-β-cyclodextrin perturbs formation of clathrin-coated endocytic vesicles. *Molecular Biology of the Cell*, Vol. 10, pp. 961-974.

Rothbard, J. B., et al. (2000). Conjugation of arginine oligomers to cyclosporin A facilitates topical delivery and inhibition of inflammation. *Nature Medicine*, Vol. 6, pp. 1253-1257.

Rothbard, J. B., et al. (2004). Role of membrane potential and hydrogen bonding in the mechanism of translocation of guanidinium-rich peptides into cells. *Journal of the American Chemical Society*, Vol. 126, pp. 9506-9507.

Rothbard, J. B., et al. (2002). Arginine-rich molecular transporters for drug delivery: role of backbone spacing in cellular uptake. *Journal of Medicinal Chemistry*, Vol. 45, pp. 3612-3618.

Roux, I. L., et al. (1993). Neurotrophic activity of the Antennapedia homeodomain depends on its specific DNA-binding properties. *Proceedings of the National Academy of Sciences*, Vol. 90, pp. 9120-9124.

Sahay, G., Alakhova, D. Y. & Kabanov, A. V. (2010). Endocytosis of nanomedicines. *Journal of Controlled Release*, Vol. 145, pp. 182-195.

Saleh, A. F., et al. (2010). Improved Tat-mediated plasmid DNA transfer by fusion to LK15 peptide. *Journal of Controlled Release*, Vol. 143, pp. 233-242.

Sandgren, S., Cheng, F. & Belting, M. (2002). Nuclear targeting of macromolecular polyanions by an HIV-Tat derived peptide role for cell-surface proteoglycans. *Journal of Biological Chemistry*, Vol. 277, pp. 38877-38883.

Schaffer, D. V., et al. (2000). Vector unpacking as a potential barrier for receptor-mediated polyplex gene delivery. *Biotechnology and Bioengineering*, Vol. 67, pp. 598-606.

Schlegel, R. A. & Rechsteiner, M. C. (1975). Microinjection of thymidine kinase and bovine serum albumin into mammalian cells by fusion with red blood cells. *Cell*, Vol. 5, pp. 371-379.

Schwarze, S. R., et al. (1999). In vivo protein transduction: delivery of a biologically active protein into the mouse. *Science*, Vol. 285, pp. 1569-1572.

Semple, S. C., et al. (2010). Rational design of cationic lipids for siRNA delivery. *Nature Biotechnology*, Vol. 28, pp. 172-178.

Seow, W. Y. & Yang, Y.-Y. (2009a). Functional polycarbonates and their self-assemblies as promising non-viral vectors. *Journal of Controlled Release*, Vol. 139, pp. 40-47.

Seow, W. Y. & Yang, Y.-Y. (2009b). A class of cationic triblock amphiphilic oligopeptides as efficient gene delivery vectors. *Advanced Materials*, Vol. 21, pp. 86-90.

Seow, W. Y., Yang, Y.-Y. & George, A. J. T. (2009). Oligopeptide-mediated gene transfer into mouse corneal endothelial cells: expression, design optimization, uptake mechanism and nuclear localization. *Nucleic Acids Research*, Vol. 37, pp. 6276-6289.

Sharma, G., et al. (2010). Polymer particle shape independently influences binding and internalization by macrophages. *Journal of Controlled Release*, Vol. 147, pp. 408-412.

Shen, W.-C. & Ryser, H. J.-P. (1978). Conjugation of poly-L-lysine to albumin and horseradish peroxidase: a novel method of enhancing the cellular uptake of proteins. *Proceedings of the National Academy of Sciences*, Vol. 75, pp. 1872-1876.

Sheridan, C. (2011). Gene therapy finds its niche. *Nature Biotechnology*, Vol. 29, pp. 121-128.

Soomets, U., et al. (2000). Deletion analogues of transportan. *Biochimica et Biophysica Acta*, Vol. 1467, pp. 165-176.

Su, Y., et al. (2009). Roles of arginine and lysine residues in the translocation of a cell-penetrating peptide from ^{13}C, ^{31}P, and ^{19}F solid-state NMR. *Biochemistry*, Vol. 48, pp. 4587-4595.

Subbarao, N. K., et al. (1987). pH-dependent bilayer destabilization by an amphipathic peptide. *Biochemistry*, Vol. 26, pp. 2964-2912.

Suh, J., Paik, H.-J. & Hwang, B. K. (1994). Ionization of poly(ethylenimine) and poly(allylamine) at various pH's. *Bioconjugate Chemistry*, Vol. 22, pp. 318-327.

Tagalakis, A. D., et al. (2011). Integrin-targeted nanocomplexes for tumour specific delivery and therapy by systemic administration. *Biomaterials*, Vol. 32, pp. 1370-1376.

Takayama, K., et al. (2009). Enhanced intracellular delivery using arginine-rich peptides by the addition of penetration accelerating sequences (Pas). *Journal of Controlled Release*, Vol. 138, pp. 128-133.

Thoren, P. E. G., et al. (2004). Membrane binding and translocation of cell-penetrating peptides. *Biochemistry*, Vol. 43, pp. 3471-3489.

Torgersen, M. L., et al. (2001). Internalization of cholera toxin by different endocytic mechanisms. *Journal of Cell Science*, Vol. 114, pp. 3737-3747.

Trentin, D., Hubbell, J. & Hall, H. (2005). Non-viral gene delivery for local and controlled DNA release. *Journal of Controlled Release*, Vol. 102, pp. 263-275.

Tyagi, M., et al. (2001). Internalization of HIV-1 tat requires cell surface heparan sulfate proteoglycans. *Journal of Biological Chemistry*, Vol. 276, pp. 3254-3261.

Urakami, H. & Guan, Z. (2008). Living ring-opening polymerization of a carbohydrate-derived lactone for the synthesis of protein-resistant biomaterials. *Biomacromolecules*, Vol. 9, pp. 592-597.

Vaheri, A. & Pagano, J. S. (1965). Infectious poliovirus RNA: a sensitive method of assay. *Virology*, Vol. 27, pp. 434-436.

Varkouhi, A. K., et al. (2010). Gene silencing activity of siRNA polyplexes based on thiolated *N,N,N*-trimethylated chitosan. *Bioconjugate Chemistry*, Vol. 21, pp. 2339-2346.

Wadia, J. S., Stan, R. V. & Dowdy, S. F. (2004). Transducible TAT-HA fusogenic peptide enhances escape of TAT-fusion proteins after lipid raft macropinocytosis. *Nature Medicine*, Vol. 10, pp. 310-315.

Wagner, E., et al. (1991). Transferrin-polycation-DNA complexes: the effect of polycations on the structure of the complex and DNA delivery to cells. *Proceedings of the National Academy of Sciences*, Vol. 88, pp. 4255-4259.

Wagner, E., et al. (1992a). Influenza virus hemagglutinin HA-2 N-terminal fusogenic peptides augment gene transfer by transferrin-polylysine-DNA complexes: toward a synthetic virus-like gene-transfer vehicle. *Proceedings of the National Academy of Sciences*, Vol. 89, pp. 7934-7938.

Wagner, E., et al. (1992b). Coupling of adenovirus to transferrin-polylysine/DNA complexes greatly enhances receptor-mediated gene delivery and expression of transfected genes. *Proceedings of the National Academy of Sciences*, Vol. 89, pp. 6099-6103.

Wang, D., et al. (1999). Encapsulation of plasmid DNA in biodegradable poly(D,L-lactic-co-glycolic acid) microspheres as a novel approach for immunogene delivery. *Journal of Controlled Release*, Vol. 57, pp. 9-18.

Wang, H., et al. (2010). Enhancement of TAT cell membrane penetration efficiency by dimethyl sulphoxide. *Journal of Controlled Release*, Vol. 143, pp. 64-70.

Wiradharma, N., Tong, Y. W. & Yang, Y.-Y. (2009). Self-assembled oligopeptide nanostructures for co-delivery of drug and gene with synergistic therapeutic effect. *Biomaterials*, Vol. 30, pp. 3100-3109.

Wojcieszyn, J. W., et al. (1983). Studies on the mechanism of polyethylene glycol-mediated cell fusion using fluorescent membrane and cytoplasmic probes. *Journal of Cell Biology*, Vol. 96, pp. 151-159.

Wojcieszyn, J. W., et al. (1981). Diffusion of injected macromolecules within the cytoplasm of living cells. *Proceedings of the National Academy of Sciences*, Vol. 78, pp. 4407-4410.

Won, Y.-Y., Sharma, R. & Konieczny, S. F. (2009). Missing pieces in understanding the intracellular trafficking of polycation/DNA complexes. *Journal of Controlled Release*, Vol. 139, pp. 88-93.

Wood, K. C., et al. (2008). Tumor-targeted gene delivery using molecularly engineered hybrid polymers functionalized with a tumor-homing peptide. *Bioconjugate Chemistry*, Vol. 19, pp. 403-405.

Wood, K. C., et al. (2005). A family of hierarchically self-assembling linear-dendritic hybrid polymers for highly efficient targeted gene delivery. *Angewandte Chemie International Edition*, Vol. 44, pp. 6704-6708.

Wu, C. H., Wilson, J. M. & Wu, G. Y. (1989). Targeting genes: delivery and persistent expression of a foreign gene driven by mammalian regulatory elements in vivo. *Journal of Biological Chemistry*, Vol. 264, pp. 16985-16987.

Wu, G. Y. & Wu, C. H. (1987). Receptor-mediated in vitro gene transformation by a soluble DNA carrier system. *Journal of Biological Chemistry*, Vol. 262, pp. 4429-4432.

Wyman, T. B., et al. (1997). Design, synthesis, and characterization of a cationic peptide that binds to nucleic acids and permeabilizes bilayers. *Biochemistry*, Vol. 36, pp. 3008-3017.

Yang, S., et al. (2009). Cellular uptake of self-assembled cationic peptide–DNA complexes: multifunctional role of the enhancer chloroquine. *Journal of Controlled Release*, Vol. 135, pp. 159-165.

Ye, J., et al. (2010). Determination of penetratin secondary structure in live cells with raman microscopy. *Journal of the American Chemical Society*, Vol. 132, pp. 980-988.

Yukawa, H., et al. (2010). Quantum dots labeling using octa-arginine peptides for imaging of adipose tissue-derived stem cells. *Biomaterials*, Vol. 31, pp. 4094-4103.

Zauner, W., et al. (1997). Glycerol and polylysine synergize in their ability to rupture vesicular membranes: a mechanism for increased transferrin-polylysine-mediated gene transfer. *Experimental Cell Reasearch*, Vol. 232, pp. 137-145.

Zauner, W., Ogris, M. & Wagner, E. (1998). Polylysine-based transfection systems utilizing receptor-mediated delivery. *Advanced Drug Delivery Reviews*, Vol. 30, pp. 97-113.

Ziegler, A., et al. (2005). The cationic cell-penetrating peptide CPP^{TAT} Derived from the HIV-1 protein tat is rapidly transported into living fibroblasts: optical, biophysical, and metabolic evidence. *Biochemistry*, Vol. 44, pp. 138-148.

27

Binding of Protein-Functionalized Entities onto Synthetic Vesicles

Federica De Persiis[1], Ramon Pons[2], Carlotta Pucci[1], Franco Tardani[1] and Camillo La Mesa[1,3]
[1]*Dept. of Chemistry, La Sapienza University, Rome, Italy*
[2]*Institut de Química Avançada de Catalunya, IQAC-CSIC*
[3]*SOFT-INFM-CNR Research Centre, La Sapienza University, Rome*
[1,3]*Italy*
[2]*Spain*

1. Introduction

Mono-disperse silica nano-particles with pending functional acid groups lying on their surface were reacted with coupling agents and, then, with lysozyme, to get protein-functionalized entities. The synthetic procedure reported therein gives tiny amounts of protein functionalized sites; surface coverage by the protein is, thus, moderate. The amount of covalently bound lysozyme was estimated from *UV*-vis methods and resulted to be about <5> molecules per nano-particle. Electro-phoretic mobility experiments indicate the occurrence of significant variations in surface charge density of functionalized nano-particles compared to the original ones and ensure a significant binding efficiency onto reconstructed, or synthetic, vesicles.

Protein-functionalized nano-particles form clusters and are readily re-dispersed by application of shear methods. Thereafter, they remain in disperse form for long times. According to *DLS*, protein-functionalized nano-particles interact with either cationic or cat-anionic synthetic vesicles. Care was made to ensure that nano-particles and vesicles have comparable sizes. The above procedure ensures to determine the fate of the reactive pathways by *DLS*. At room temperature and moderate ionic strength, the binding of protein-functionalized entities onto the aforementioned vesicles is completed in about one hour. The nano-particle vesicle complexes precipitate as fine powders, or form large floating objects, depending on vesicle size, relative concentrations of protein-functionalized particles and their net charge (which is related to the *pH* of the dispersing medium).

The binding efficiency for the above processes is controlled by the overlapping of repulsive and attractive interactions between particles and vesicles. The kinetic pathways relative to the interactions between vesicles and nano-particles were investigated, and significant differences were met in the two cases. Some technological implications of the above systems are preliminarily discussed. For instance, it is stated that interactions between nano-particles and vesicles mimic those occurring between cells and solid particles, or viral vectors, located in the medium surrounding vesicles.

Graphical Abstract

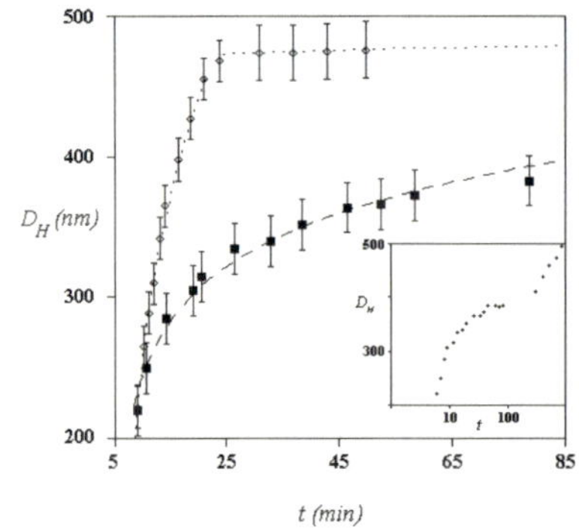

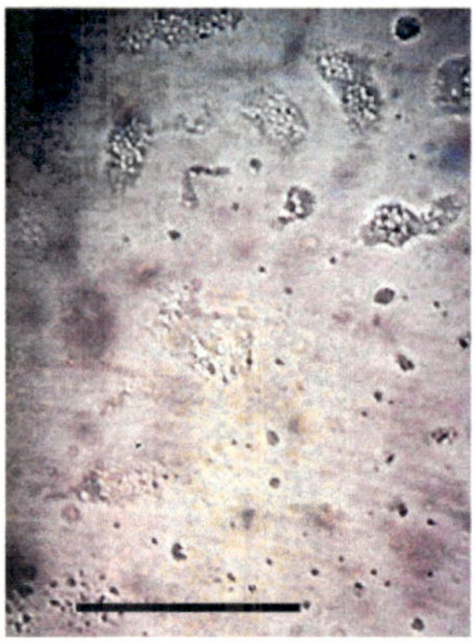

Left, Dependence of the size of nano-particle/vesicle clusters on reaction time, inferred by DLS methods.
Right, Clusters of vesicles and protein-functionalized nano-particles obtained by mixing DDAB vesicles and nano-particles in number ratio 300/1. Images were visualized through a Zeiss optical microscope using normal light. The bar size in the left bottom of the figure is 100 mm large.

Nanotechnologies deal with the synthesis, the characterization, the production and the application of objects and devices operating at the nano-scale level (1). As a consequence of substantial interest in this field, many scientific journals and books are progressively addressing attention to nano-technologically oriented items. The same holds for the number of patents relative to these subjects. This is because the demand on the possible applications of the above materials is drastically increasing in the last few years. Practical applications are manifold and find use in electronics, in the preparation of magnetic devices, in chemistry (mostly in the field of heterogeneous catalysis), but also in biotechnology and biomedicine.
Materials at the nano-scale are widely different each from the other in chemical composition, size and surface functionalities. Particles properties depend on the preparation procedures and can be tailored accordingly. Nano-particles can be made of metals, oxides, polymers and/or a combination thereof. Properly functionalized particles, such as quantum dots, spheres, disks, filaments, tubes and composite objects (all in the nano-meter size range) find substantial application in the aforementioned fields.
In this contribution, we report on silica nano-particles, onto which a protein, lysozyme, was covalently bound (2,3). The synthetic part of the work is reported below. The same holds for the characterization of the resulting hybrid composites. A substantial amount of work was needed to ensure the required performances to nano-particles, which were tailored in terms of state of the dispersion, size, stability and net charge. Obviously, the above effects are strongly interrelated each other. The reasons for using protein-functionalized entities arise by the need to have objects at the nano-scale level, characterized by a significant number of bound proteins. Apart from intrinsic interest towards the structural properties of hybrid nano-composites, the advantages of protein-functionalized particles are manifold compared to other bio-medical formulations, since:

i. the surface area of the resulting nano-composites can be properly controlled,
ii. the number of covalently bound proteins can be modulated accordingly, and,
iii. the conformation of proteins adsorbed therein can be somehow predicted (4).

Silica was used as an anchoring site because of its good bio-compatibility, which is substantially higher compared to polymer-based nano-particles. It is particularly useful since blood and other bio-fluids contain markers adsorbing on the surface of hydrophobic carriers, and indicating to *RES* (the *Reticulum Endothelial System*) the urgency to remove them from the target tissue (5). Conversely, silica nano-particles (*NPs*) are of friendly use with biological tissues. As most inorganic oxides, SiO_2 is strongly hydrophilic in character. Such property increases its compatibility and ensures a safe circulation in bio-fluids. In addition, it is possible to anchor efficiently proteins or other biologically active substances onto mono-dispersed silica.

Lysozyme was chosen to test the covalent binding efficiency onto nano-particles because of its ubiquitary nature. In the following, we report on anchoring efficiency and do not explicitly account for the effect that *pH*, salts or other substances have on the fate of protein-functionalized *NPs* in biological matrices. The present communication only focuses on the synthesis and characterization of such materials.

In the second part of this contribution the interactions between protein-functionalized silica *NPs* and synthetic vesicles were experienced. The synthetic vesicles dealt with in this contribution are also relatively mono-dispersed, thermodynamically, or kinetically, stable and are characterized, in some cases, by a bi-layer structure (6). Hence, they can be considered the synthetic analogues of cell membranes. Were the interactions between vesicles and *NPs* effective, the possibility of surface adhesion, or encapsulation, can be realized. Perspectives of these complex systems as composite drug-delivery carriers are, thus, at hand.

We choose different vesicle-forming materials based on a synthetic double-chain surfactant and mixtures of different surface active species. The performances of the former class, based on quaternary ammonium salts, were extensively characterized by Barenholz and coworkers (7,8). Such species, however, are of questionable utility for biomedical applications, since most quaternary ammonium salts have strong anti-bacterial character. In addition, the vesicles they form are intrinsically meta-stable and progressively coagulate into large entities.

Recently, alternatives to the above lipido-mimetic systems were proposed; they rely on systems obtained by mixing oppositely charged surfactants, or lipids, in due amounts. Such mixtures are currently defined by the acronym cat-anionic. These systems came in use since when Kaler and Khan independently characterized some of them (9,10). In cat-anionic systems the vesicle size and net charge are tuned by modulating the ratio between the two components, provided one of them is in excess. (N.B. If not, the 1/1 mixtures precipitate out.) It is possible, thus, to get negatively or positively charged vesicles. This can be relevant in case vesicles should selectively interact through electrostatic interactions with proteins (11) or *DNA* (12) and form complexes, or lipo-plexes, with the above substances.

In the following we report on the synthetic procedures we have followed, on the optimization required getting stable dispersions of hybrid protein-silica colloids, and on their interactions with vesicles. For reasons to be discussed later, the characterization of the above protein-silica composite material is based on the combination of optical (*UV-vis* or *CD*), dynamic light scattering, *DLS*, and electro-phoretic mobility methods. Some relevant results are briefly reported in the forthcoming sections. Biomedical applications, which are surely relevant, require dedicated formulation work and need substantial studies on the cyto-toxicity of vesicles, lysozyme-bound *NP*s and of the related adducts. The former systems were previously characterized on this regard by some of us (13), but almost nothing is known on the latter ones.

2. Experimental section

Materials. 3-aminopropyl-(3-oxobutanoic acid)-functionalized silica *NP*s, termed *APOB*, contain significant amounts of carboxylic acids on their surface. They are given from the purveyor (Sigma Aldrich) as 2.5% (w/v) dispersions in dimethylformamide, *DMF*. Their nominal density is 0.927 g ml^{-1} at 25°C (14). *NP*s were dialyzed against aqueous Borax (50 millimol, pH 8.5) under stirring, sonicated and recovered. The resulting dispersions are relatively stable, since *APOB* nano-particles bear negative charges on their surface.

Hen yolk lysozyme, *LYS*, (Sigma Aldrich) was dialyzed, crystallized, lyophilized and dried over P_2O_5. Its purity was confirmed by ionic conductance, density and viscosity of the corresponding aqueous solutions, at 25.00 °*C* (15,16).

Sodium dodecylsulfate, *SDS*, cetyltrimethylammonium bromide, *CTAB*, and didodecyl-dimethylammonium bromide, *DDAB*, (Sigma Aldrich) were individually dissolved in ethanol and precipitated by addition of cold acetone. The products were vacuum dried at 70°C. Their purity was confirmed by conductometric determination of the critical micellar concentration, *CMC*, at 25.00 °C. *Pluronic F-127* (Sigma Aldrich), a surface active block co-polymer, forming micelles at high temperatures (17), was used as dispersant, when required.

A water soluble carbodiimide, termed *EDAC*, hydroxysuccynimide, *NHS*, triethylamine, $N(Et)_3$, and glycine, (Sigma Aldrich), were used as such.

3. Materials preparation

LYS-ABOP nano-particles. 20 mg of *APOB* in 50 millimolar kg^{-1} (*mmol*) aqueous Borax were added with 13.0 mg *EDAC,* 10.0 mg *NHS* and7.27 mg $N(Et)_3$, at 25°C (7), and homogenized upon stirring. 44.13 mg solid *LYS* was added and the reaction proceeded for 5 hours, at 40°C. The reaction between *ABOP* and *LYS* is concomitant to an increase in opalescence of the dispersions, due to both a decreased surface charge density (because of the reaction of *COOH* groups with *EDAC),* and to protein covalent binding. The final dispersion was centrifuged at 12000 rpm for 10 minutes, at 4°C. Thereafter, 10 mmol glycine was added, to quench un-reacted groups that were eventually bound onto *NP*s. The latter procedure significantly reduces the dispersion turbidity. A summary of the whole synthetic procedure, in four stages, is sketched in *Scheme 1,* where are indicated the different preparation steps.

Prolonged sonication, dialysis, with pH and/or ionic strength adjustment significantly tailors the average size of *NP*s and reduces their size. Substantial characterization is required to ensure the attainment of equilibrium conditions, since the size of particles increases with aging, *Figure 1.* The dispersions were extensively dialyzed against the buffer, until no more lysozime, *EDAC* and/or *NHS* was determined in the supernatant. To avoid the occurrence of clusters, the dispersions must be sheared (18) or forced to flow in tilted long syringe steel needles (19), as indicated in *Figure 2A.*

Synthesis of Lys-ABOP nano-particles: a reactive scheme

Step 1

P-NH-R-COOH ***(in DMF)*** —*dialysis* / *Borax 50 mmol pH 8.5*→ ***P-NH-R-COOH*** ***(in Borax buffer)***

Step 2

P-NH-R-COOH ***(in Borax buffer)*** —*+ EDAC + N-suc + N(Et)$_3$* / *Borax 50 mmol, 25° C*→ ***Active***

Step 3

Active + Lyso —*10 mmol Glycine* / *Borax 50 mmol*→ ***Lys-ABOP nano-particles***

Step 4

Dialisys + pH conditioning + ionic strength control + centrifugation

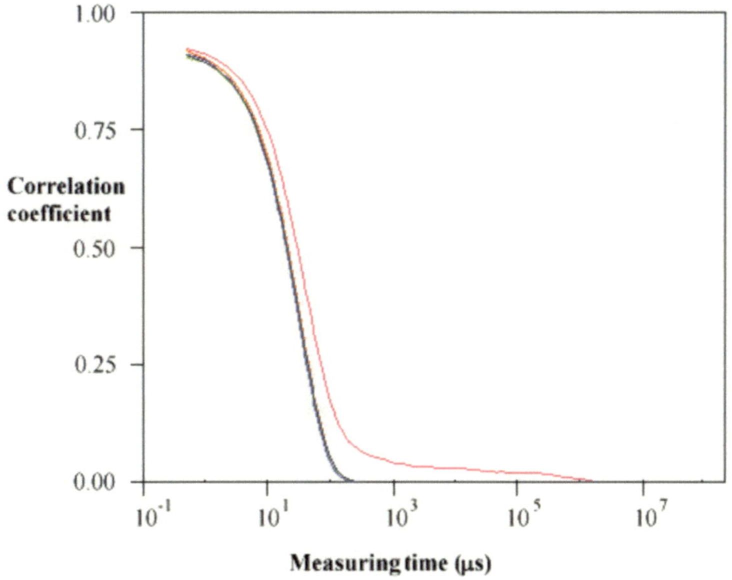

Fig. 1. Plots of the correlation coefficient (in arbitrary units) versus the measuring time, in μs, for a 0.20 wt/vol % dispersion of Lysozyme-ABOP nano-particles (in 50 mmol Borax buffer, pH 8.5, at 25°C) one day after preparation, in blue, one week, in orange, and one month, in cyan.

When particles are subjected to shear forces during flow, large aggregates break down. This procedure decreases the size of *LYS/ABOP NPs*, *Figure 2B*.
Cat-anionic vesicles were prepared by mixing 6.00 *mmol* aqueous *SDS* with 6.00 *mmol CTAB*, in due proportions. Optimal sizes and surface charge density occur when the mole ratio between *SDS* and *CTAB* is in the range 1.5-2.5. The dispersions are milky, because multi-lamellar, and size-poly-disperse, vesicles occur. It was formerly observed, however, that heating them to temperatures close to 50°C reduces the average size of multi-lamellar vesicles, with formation of truly bi-layered entities [20]. Thereafter, vesicles remain in such state for over two months, even when they are kept at room temperature.

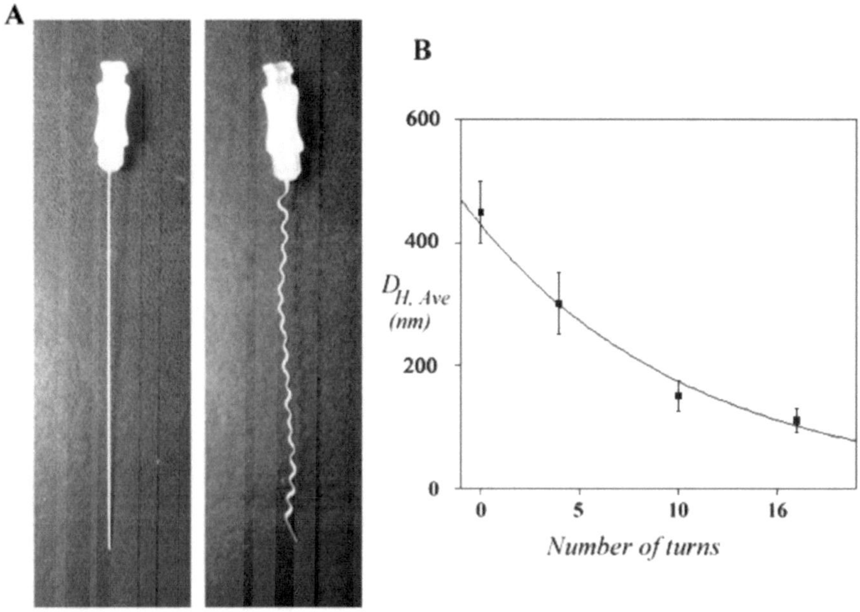

Fig. 2. A; View of iron steel needles, tilted to increase the number of turns. B; Reduction in size of 0.12 w/v % LYS-ABOP nano-particles obtained by coupling (and dispersed in 50 mmol Borax, pH 8.5, at 25°C) when forced to flow in tilted needles. Data are reported as average particles size (nm) versus number of turns in the needle. Each sample was forced to flow in the needles for 50 times.

DDAB vesicles are multi-layered entities and their properties were tailored by extrusion and/or thermal cycling. Both vesicular dispersions were thermally equilibrated at 25.0°C soon after the preparation procedures and controlled over a long-time scale. Temperatures lower than 20°C were avoided, since they imply partial surfactant precipitation in the *SDS-CTAB* system.

4. Methods

Dynamic Light Scattering. A Zeta Nanosizer unit, Malvern, performed measurements at 632.8 nm, in back scattering mode (*BSM*), at 173°. This configuration minimizes multiple scattering and allows measuring poly-disperse systems. The unit performances were checked by standard procedures [21]. Thermal equilibrium was controlled by a Peltier unit, at

25.0°C. The dispersions were passed through 0.80 μm Millipore filters and equilibrated at 25.0° or 37.0°C for some minutes. Correlation fits of the light scattering intensity were elaborated by *CONTIN* algorithms (22). The auto-correlation decay function, $g_1(\tau)$, determined the self-diffusion coefficient, and the hydrodynamic radii were evaluated by the Stokes-Einstein equation ($D_{app} = K_BT/6\pi\eta R_H$). The uncertainty on vesicles sizes is to 10-20 nm, depending on their size.

ζ-potential measurements. ζ-potential methods determined the surface charge density, σ, of particles moving under the effect of an applied electric field, $\bar{E}$ (23). A laser-Doppler utility performed measurements, at 25.0°C, in cells equipped with gold electrodes. The scattered light passing in the medium, subjected to the action of $\bar{E}$, shifts in frequency compared to unperturbed conditions. Data manipulation of the signal gives the ζ-potential ($\zeta = 4\pi\sigma\tau/\varepsilon°$, where τ the double layer thickness and $\varepsilon°$ the static dielectric constant of the medium). The uncertainty on ζ-potentials is 0.5-1.0 mV. Data are reported in *Figure 3*.

Ionic Conductivity. The electrical conductance, κ ($S\ cm^{-1}$), was determined by a Wayne-Kerr impedance bridge, at 1 *KHz*, using a Daggett-Krauss cell thermostated to 25.00±0.01°C.

CD. Measurements were run on a Jasco J-715 unit, working with 1 nm resolution. 0.100 cm quartz cells were used. Spectra are the average of three independent runs in the 190-300 nm range. Signals due to native *LYS*, at 208 and 222 nm, respectively, were determined.

UV-Vis Light Absorbance. Light absorption spectra, *A*, were recorded in the range 190-300 nm by a Jasco V-570 unit, at 25.0±0.1 °C; the cell path length was 0.100 cm.

Microscopy. Optical microscopy, in normal or polarized light, was performed through a Zeiss optical microscope.

Density. The particles density was determined by a DMA-60 Anton Paar vibrating densimeter, and thermally controlled by a water circulation bath working at 25.00 ± 0.01 °C.

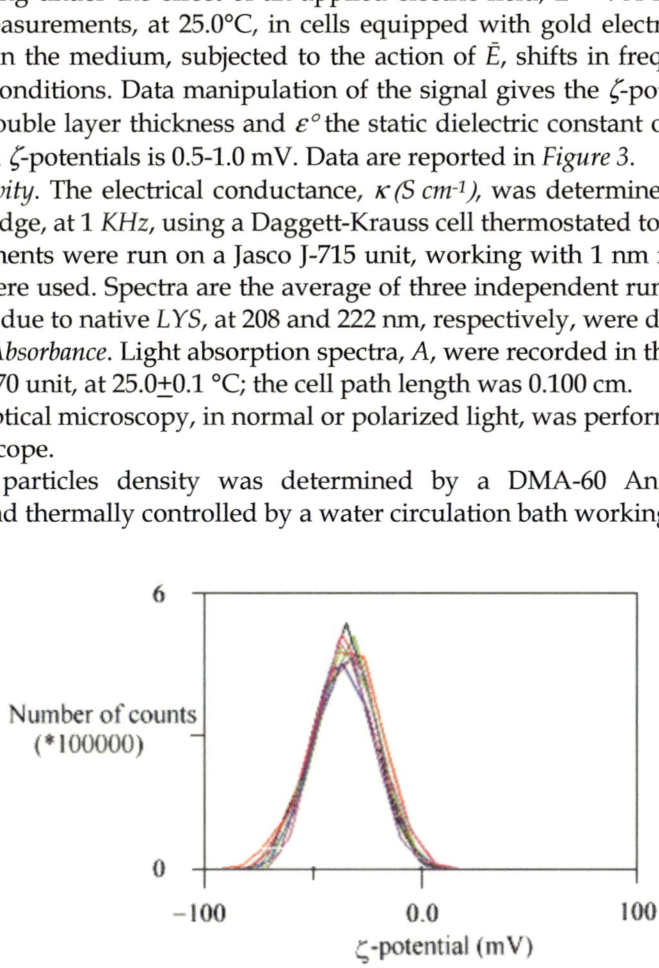

Fig. 3. Plot of ζ-potential values for different dispersions of nominal concentration in LYS-ABOP nano-particles equal to 0.12 w/v %. Measurements were run in 50 mmol Borax, at 25.0°C. Data are reported as number of counts (*10^5) vs. measured ζ-potential value.

5. Results and discussion

Nano-particles characterization. Nano-particles made of *LYS* and *APOB* (termed as *LYS-ABOP*) were characterized by *DLS, CD, UV-vis* and ζ-potential methods. A substantial amount of work was required to stabilize the resulting dispersions, because of their tendency to agglomerate and/or phase separate. The optimal conditions for an effective stabilization (i.e. stirring, temperature, *pH* and/or ionic strength) were determined. The surface charge density, σ, plays a pivotal role in the stability of these dispersions and depends on the medium ionic strength. In buffers with 50 mmol Borax and 10 mmol *NaCl* the dispersions remain stable for about two weeks; usually, they were used one day after preparation. Care was taken to get macroscopic homogeneity and to avoid the presence of clusters or sediments.

In the characterization by *DLS*, a proper selection of the elaborating functions, taking into account the particles sizes and poly-dispersity, was necessary. The cumulant method was applied and the scattering equation, $g_1(t)$, was expressed as a power-law series, according to the well-known relation

$$\ln g_1(t) = \sum_{n=1}^{\infty} \Gamma_n \frac{(-t)^n}{n!} = -\Gamma_1 t + \frac{1}{2!}\Gamma_2 t^2 - \frac{1}{3!}\Gamma_3 t^3 + \ldots\ldots\ldots \quad (1)$$

Eq. (1) gives information on the average value of the distribution function, (that is $\Gamma_1 = \langle \Gamma \rangle = q^2 \langle D_{app} \rangle$), and on poly-dispersity index, *PdI* (Γ_2/Γ_1^2). Minor terms are also present.

Even when the particles number is moderate, a prolonged aging of the dispersions must be avoided, since a significant shift of the correlation functions is observed, *Figure 1*. That is, both Γ_1 (related to the particles self-diffusion, D_{app}) and Γ_2 (related to *PdI*) depend on aging. This implies the presence of reactive terms. Data were analyzed accounting for the diffusive contributions pertinent to nano-particles and for the respective reactive terms, respectively. The results are expressed in terms of the relation

$$I_2(t) = \left[|I_1(0)|^2 + |I_1(t)|^2 \right] \quad (2)$$

where $I_2(t)$, $I_1(0)$ and $I_1(t)$ are the scattering intensity at time *t*, the original value at time zero and the reactive part, respectively.

DLS data were interpreted according to Berne and Pecora (24). Attractive terms, due to particles coagulation, and electrostatic ones, due to the presence of repulsive or attractive forces between colloid entities, are introduced in the time-dependent scattering functions. The relation contains a reactive term, related to the formation of large particles, and is balanced by a flux, in which mobility and diffusive terms are accounted for (24). Accordingly,

$$\left(\frac{\partial c_a}{\partial t} \right) + \nabla \bullet J_a = k_b c_b - k_a c_a \quad (3)$$

where (dc_a/dt) indicates the production, or disappearance, of particles with time. The second term in the right hand side of the equation is expressed as

$$J_a = \mu_a \bar{E} c_a - D_{app,a} \nabla c_a \quad (4)$$

where μ_a is the electro-phoretic mobility of a class of particles, at concentration c_a, under the effect of and applied electric field, $\bar{E}$, and D_{app} is the self diffusion times the concentration gradient, ∇c_a. K_a and K_b are the kinetic constants of reactants, *a*, and products, *b*, respectively.

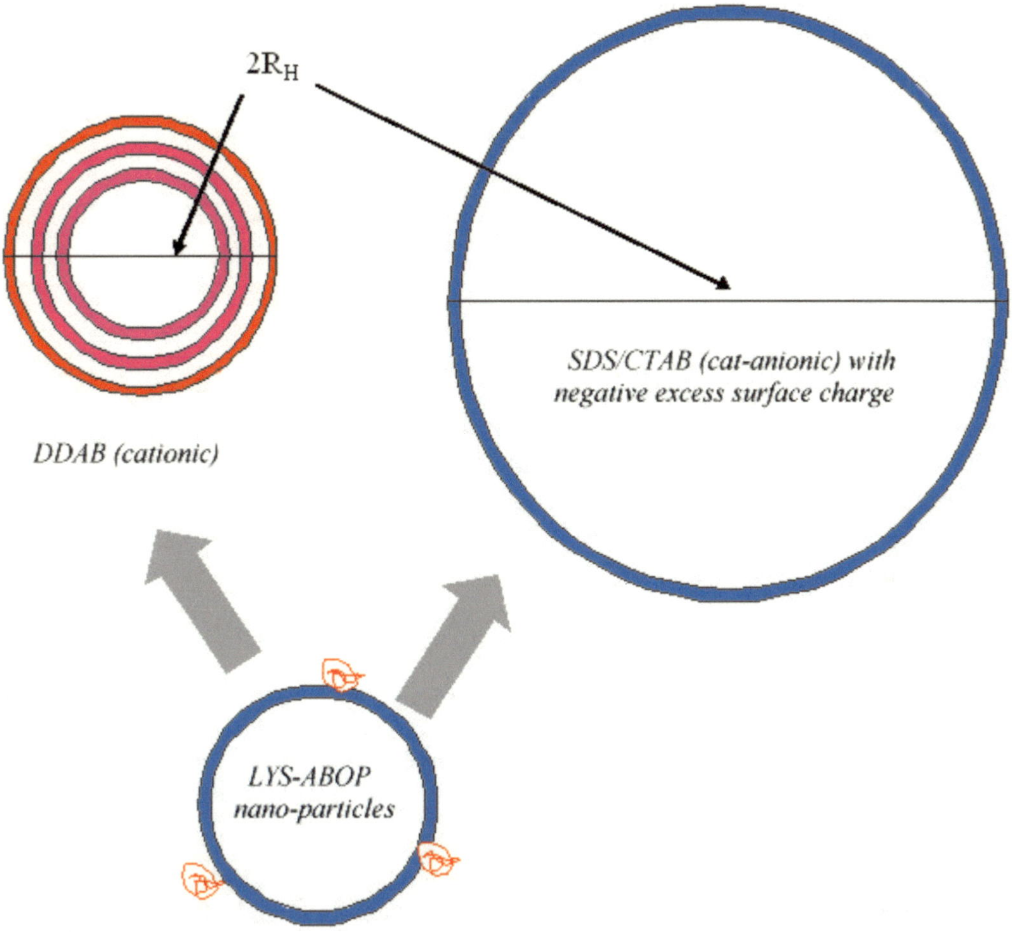

Fig. 4. In the top is reported a schematic representation of vesicle structure. On the upper left is reported a picture relative to multi-lamellar DDAB vesicles (in red/cyan colors, to distinguish the different layers), on the upper right the one related to bi-layered SDS/CTAB vesicles (in blue color). Sizes scale with the average hydrodynamic vesicle radius, inferred from DLS. In the bottom is indicated a cartoon of ABOP nano-particles with surface-bound LYS molecules. As before, regions in red indicate the dominance of positive charges (around the protein), when the blue color of the corona indicates an excess of negative charges.

The above approach helps determining the kinetic features of interactions between different *LYS-ABOP* particles. It will also be used to account for the interactions taking place between vesicles and *LYS-ABOP*. It is expected that attractions are experienced in the interaction between *LYS-ABOP* and cat-anionic vesicles (bearing a negative charge), and repulsions in the other case, *Figure 4*.

DLS alone does not allow to asses any firm statement on lysozyme binding, since the sizes of functionalized *NP*s is only slightly higher than before the reaction. That's why combination of optical absorbance with *DLS*, *CD* and electro-phoretic mobility is helpful.

The former method quantifies the amount of *ABOP*-bound protein (in native or denatured state) and whether binding is effective. The second gives information on the conformational state of *LYS*. Electro-phoretic mobility, finally, indicates an effective surface modification of silica upon protein binding. Binding will reduce in modulus the ζ-potential values, as observed.

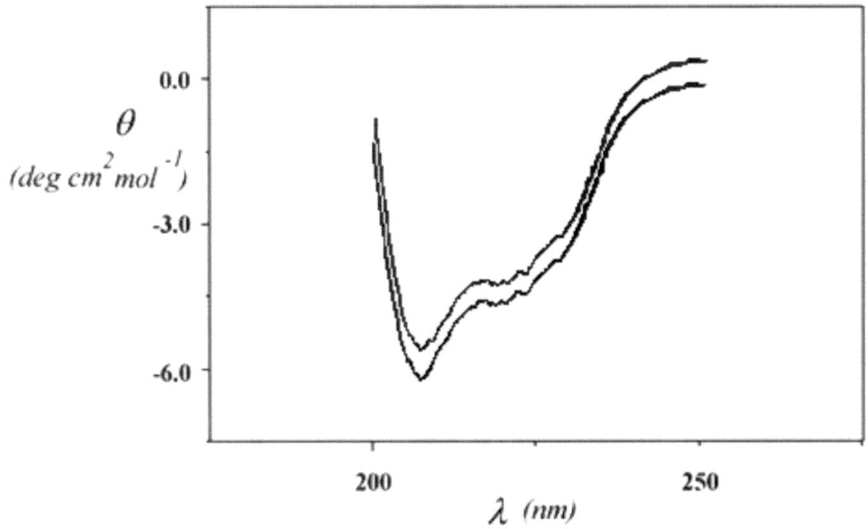

Fig. 5. CD spectrum, in molal ellipticity (θ, in deg cm^2 mol^{-1}) vs. the measuring wavelength (λ, in nm) of LYS-ABOP nano-particles, in grey color, compared to the corresponding value for bulk LYS, in black. The signal intensities were rescaled to allow for a comparison. In both cases data refer to pH 8.5, with 50.0 mmol Borax buffer, and 25.0° C. The former was upward shifted, to avoid overlapping.

Optical absorbance, performed in the 220-230 nm range, determined the presence and number of *LYS* molecules bound onto *ABOP* particles. The average value is <5±1> molecules. The uncertainty is high since the number of *NP*s in the medium is low, and scattering effects reduce the datum quality. *CD* data, *Figure 5*, indicate that the conformation of covalently bound protein is very close to its native form. Thus, the presence of bound protein was inferred by optical absorbance (and elemental analysis, as well), whereas a conformation close to the native one was inferred by *CD*.

Finally, the ζ-potential of *LYS-ABOP* particles decreases from -36 mV of the bare ones to -20, in case of protein-bound entities. Data indicate a significant *LYS* binding and surface modification, but a significant reduction of surface charge density compared to the native particles. This is because some *COOH* units are linked with *LYS* and the charge density of the particle as a whole is substantially reduced. The reduction in ζ-potential also explains why *LYS-ABOP* adducts are less kinetically stable compared to bare *ABOP*.

The optimal conditions leading to stabilization are fulfilled for *pH* values between 7.0 and 8.5. Below *pH* 7.0 the particles sizes increase significantly and such conditions were avoided. Substantial amounts of salt must be used to stabilize the dispersions in such *pH* conditions.

A scheme representing all particles considered here is in *Figure 4*. There is indicated the structure of vesicles and *LYS-ABOP* complexes, with charge distribution in evidence. It is expected that the charge distribution is responsible for interactions with both negatively or positively charged vesicles. It is expected that the kinetic features inherent to vesicle-*LYS-ABOP* particles interactions should behave accordingly.

The analysis of kinetic data, performed by *DLS* methods, is essentially based on the supposed dominance of electrostatic interactions between particles. Were this hypothesis absolutely unrealistic, different kinetic approaches should be considered. For instance the elecctro-phoretic term in the flux equation should be critically reconsidered. Very presumably, however, binding is due to the combined effect of dominant electrostatic contributions plus hydrophobic and ancillary (osmotic?) ones into an as yet undefined mechanism.

Kinetic features. Processes related to vesicles-*NPs* interactions are dealt with in this part. Dispersions of *DDAB* and (*SDS-CTAB*), at the same nominal concentration in lipid, were mixed with tiny amounts of *LYS-ABOP* particles. The number ratio between the latter and vesicles is moderate. This allows measuring the kinetic features inherent to the interactions between *LYS-ABOP NP*s and vesicles. An eye-view to the results, *Figure 6* and *Figure 7*, indicates that the interactive processes can be rationalized on volume fraction statistics. The kinetic pathways scale with the *VES-NP* number ratio. Vesicles sizes are different each from the other, but are reasonably close to *NP*s. That means that changes in size of the scattering entities are mostly due to vesicles-*NPs* adducts. The respective kinetic pathways and the size of particles obtained at the end of the respective reactive processes are different in the two cases. In the [*DDAB*+(*LYS-ABOP*)] system sizes at equilibrium are lower compared to the [(*SDS-CTAB*)+(*LYS-ABOP*)] one. These effects are a sound indication of clustering between

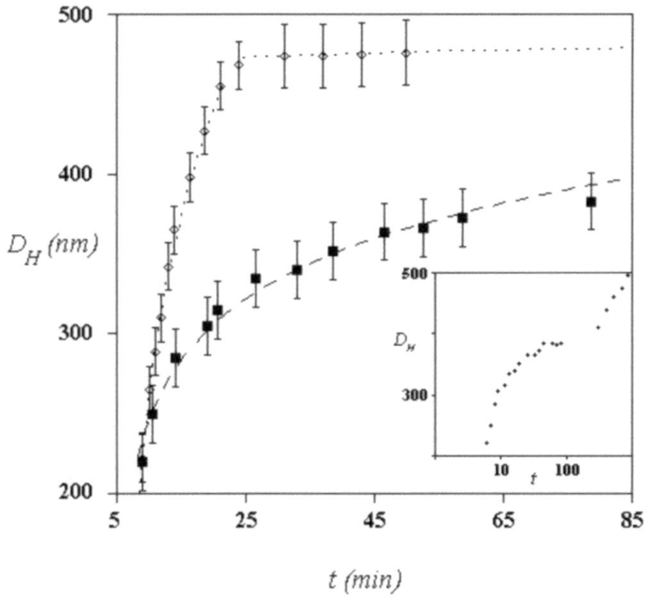

Fig. 6. Kinetics of vesicle-NP interaction inferred from DLS plots of average particles size, D_H, as a function of measuring time, t (min), for two different vesicles to LYS-ABOP nano-particles number ratios. Data refer to systems buffered with 50 mmol Borax, at 25°C. Black symbols refer to a number ratio between NP's and cat-anionic SDS-CTAB vesicles (having mole ratio between the two of 1.7/1.0) equal to 1/60 and 1/150 in the other case. In the inset is reported the long term behavior observed in the former system.

objects similar in size, driven by electrostatic interactions between the two entities. Differences in the size of super-colloids formed in these mixtures are the consequences of the interaction mechanisms and result in significant changes in size and shape (presumably) of the resulting entities. Similar features were observed in the [*DDAB*+(*LYS-ABOP*)] system, *Figure 7*. There a marked tendency to sedimentation is observed after the interactions took place. Presumably, part of the observed decrease in size may be due to sedimentation processes, occurring at the early stages of the process.

The interactions between *DDAB* and *LYS-ABOP NP*'s show a different kinetic behavior compared to the former system, with a significant increase in size at low times, followed by a substantial decrease at long ones. This behavior is controlled by the net charge of the reacting objects and indicates that electrostatic terms are significant. According to *Figure 7*, there is a pronounced redistribution of particles sizes after about 40 minutes. Such features are, very presumably, related to a structural rearrangement and eventual rupture of vesicle-*NP* adducts with time.

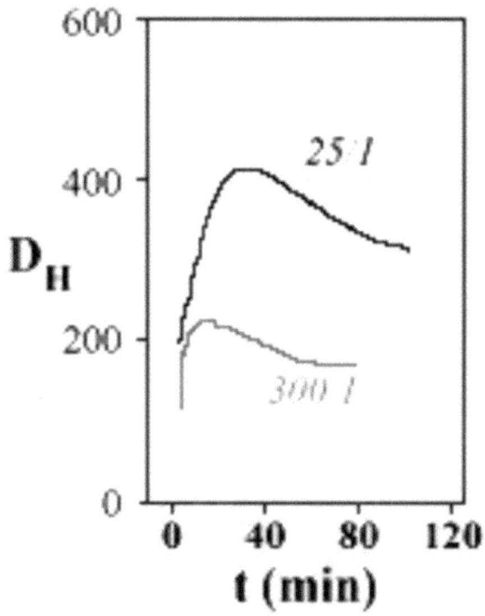

Fig. 7. Plot of the average vesicle/Lys-ABOP adducts size (in nm) with time, in minutes, upon interaction between DDAB vesicles and LYS-ABOP nano-particles. The nominal number ratio between the colloidal objects is indicated in the figure. Experimental conditions refer to the same pH and temperature values reported above.

It is also possible that adducts sedimentation takes place after some time. In words, the formation of composites colloids implies a progressive saturation mechanism in case of *SDS-CTAB* vesicles. Conversely, a significantly different behavior occurs in the *DDAB* containing system. This is put in evidence by the macroscopic appearance of the super-colloid entities formed in this way. In some instances sediments are found at the bottom of vials, in others large floating particles are observed in the medium. That means that the super-colloids formed upon interaction between vesicles and nano-particles differ each from the other in packing density and surface charge, to mind but a few effects.

According to *Figure 8*, for instance, it is evident that entities made of *DDAB* and *LYS-ABOP* particles do form small aggregates, held together by significant forces, presumably electrostatic in nature. According to optical microscopy, it results that these composite objects are made of different sub-domains, differing each from the other in optical appearance and color. Apparently, there is no significant relation between the average stoichiometry of adducts made by vesicles and nano-particles and that pertinent to mother solution. In words, there is no direct proportionality between number of particles in the medium and composition of the precipitates.

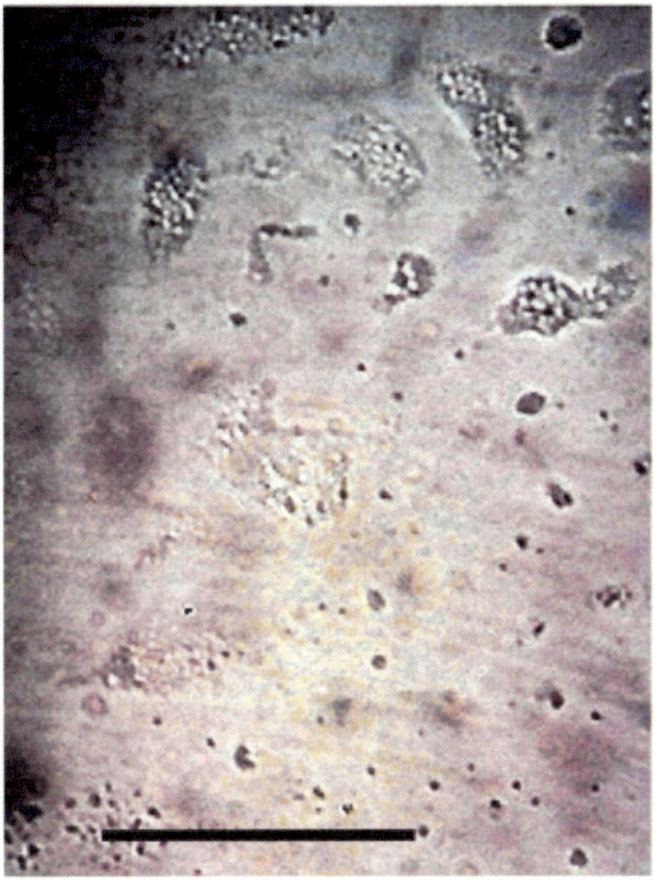

Fig. 8. Vesicle- PFNP clusters, obtained by mixing DDAB and PFNP in number ratios 300/1 and recovering the precipitates. They are visualized through a Zeiss Optical Microscope using normal light. The bar size in the bottom is 100 μm large.

6. Conclusions

The results reported here indicate the possibility to get *"hybrid"* colloid composites from the interactions between *LYS-NPs* complexes and vesicles. The reported results refer to the phenomenological aspects of the interaction process, as it was inferred from *DLS*. Very

presumably, the observed features are related to structural rearrangements and to eventual rupture of vesicle-*NP* adducts with time. In one case, apparently, the sedimentation of adducts takes place after some time. In others, large floating objects are present in the dispersing medium.
Depending on the forces active between vesicles and *LYS-NPs*, it is possible that the kinetics of adducts formation follows different pathways. In the case of *SDS-CTAB* cat-anionic vesicles (bearing a substantial negative charge), the interaction mechanism obeys a pseudo first-order mechanism, controlled by the number ratio between the components. In the interaction between *DDAB* vesicles and *LYS-NPs*, conversely, the situation is more cumbersome to be rationalized. In this latter case, it is presumed that the interaction mechanism implies the formation of a transient state (characterized by a maximum in *DLS* plots); after some time the mixed colloid particles rearrange and change in size and shape. It is also possible that the large increase in size observed in this system is due to the incipient nucleation of particles, which precipitate after some time.
Some questions are still under debate on the biological implications of the above systems. However, when *LYS-ABOP* particles interact with cells, it is expected that the reactive behavior (mostly the one relative to surface adsorption) will be close to that reported in case of cat-anionic surfactant mixtures. In fact, cells are negatively charged and are generally composed by mixtures of oppositely charged lipids. On this regard, thus, cat-anionic systems are much more effective as bio-mimetic models compared to other currently used lipid dispersions. It must be also considered that the mechanisms controlling the pynocytosis of particles adsorbed onto cells require the deformation of the latter. In fact, vesicles made by different lipids are more prone to be deformed and envaginate (25), as a consequence of local changes in composition associated to adsorption of charged and bulky entities onto them. This implies the migration of the lipid components in the bi-layer and induces a local deformation of vesicles, making possible particles uptake into cells. More dedicated investigation is required to clarify such aspects.
Another relevant question deals with use of the above systems in modeling bio-mimetic processes. In nature there are cases of interactions between "*hard*" and "*soft*" particles, as, for instance, in the interactions between viruses and other viral vectors and cells (26,27). From such a point of view, the ones presented here are excellent mimetic models of the above interactions, because viruses are generally covered with enzymes attaching onto the surface of cells and tissues. Preparing nano-particles sharing some properties in common to viruses (having, for instance, a similar surface coverage) would help understanding the physical grounds underlying the interactions between viruses and cells.

7. Acknowledgments

This work was made possible through a financial support from La Sapienza University. F.D.P. wishes to acknowledge the Ministry of Education for financing her stay in Barcelona, where she completed the characterization of the above mixtures.
Financial support from MICIN CTQ2010-14897, Generalitat de Catalunya, through the 2009SGR1331 grant and COST Action Project on Chemistry at Interfaces, D36, are gratefully acknowledged.
Thanks to A. Scipioni, Dept. of Chemistry at La Sapienza, for help in performing *CD* spectra, and for fruitful discussions on some aspects of the manuscript. Thanks also to G. Risuleo,

Dept. of Molecular Biology at La Sapienza, for suggestions on the biological implications of these systems.

8. References

[1] F. Feng, F. Le, L. An, S. Wang, Y. Li, D. Zhu, *Adv. Mater.*, 2008, *20*, 2959.

[2] H.K. Valo; P.H. Laaksonen; L.J. Peltonen; M.B. Linder; J.T. Hirvonen; T.J. Laaksonen, *ACS Nano*, 2010, *4*, 1750.

[3] C. Mateo; J.M. Palomo; G. Fernàndez-Lorente; J.M. Guisàn; R. Fernàndez-Lafuente, *Enzyme Microbial Technol.*, 2007, *40*, 1451.

[4] J.L. Brash; T.A. Horbett, *ACS Symp. Ser.* (*Proteins at Interfaces*), 1995, Vol. *602*, p. 1.

[5] E. Soussan; S. Cassel; M. Blanzat; I. Rico-Lattes, *Angew. Chem. Int. Ed.*, 2009, *48*, 274.

[6] C. Letizia, P. Andreozzi, A. Scipioni, C. La Mesa, A. Bonincontro, E. Spigone, *J. Phys. Chem. B*, 2007, *111*, 898.

[7] J. Szebeni; L. Baranyi; S. Savay; J. Milosevits; R. Bunger; P. Laverman; J.M. Metselaar; G. Storm; A. Chanan-Khan; L. Liebes; F.M. Muggia; R. Cohen; Y. Barenholz; C.R. Alving, *J. Liposome Res.*, 2002, *12*, 165.

[8] D. Simberg; S. Weisman; Y. Talmon; Y. Barenholz, *Crit. Rev. Ther. Drug Carrier Syst.*, 2004, *21*, 257.

[9] H.T. Jung; B. Coldren; J.A. Zasadzinski,; D.J. Iampietro; E.W. Kaler, *Proc. Nat. Acad. Sci. U.S.A.*, 2001, *98*, 1353.

[10] E.F. Marques; O. Regev; A. Khan; B. Lindman, *Adv. Colloid Interface Sci.*, 2003, *100-102*, 83.

[11] A. Bonincontro; E. Spigone; M. Ruiz Peña; C. Letizia; C. La Mesa, *J. Colloid Interface Sci.*, 2006, *304*, 342.

[12] A. Bonincontro; C. La Mesa; C. Proietti; G. Risuleo, *Biomacromolecules*, 2007, 8, 1824.

[13] C. Aiello; P. Andreozzi; C. La Mesa; G. Risuleo, *Colloids Surf. B: Biointerfaces*, 2010, *78*, 149.

[14] T.H. Galow; K. Boal; V.M. Rotello, *Adv. Mater.*, 2000, *12*, 576.

[15] A. Zielenciewicz, *J. Therm. Anal. Calor.* 2001, *65*, 467.

[16] K. Monkos, *Biochim. Biophys. Acta: Prot. Struct. Mol. Enzymol.*, 1997, *1339*, 304.

[17] G. Gente; A. Iovino; C. La Mesa, *J. Colloid Interface Sci.*, 2004, *274*, 458.

[18] A. Budhian; S.J. Siegel; K.I. Winey, *Intern. J. Pharmaceutics*, 2007, *336*, 367.

[19] F. De Persiis; P. Andreozzi; C. La Mesa; R. Pons, *submitted.*

[20] P. Andreozzi; S.S. Funari; C. La Mesa; P. Mariani; M.G. Ortore; R. Sinibaldi; F. Spinozzi, *J. Phys. Chem. B*, 2010, *114*, 8056.

[21] P. Andreozzi; A. Bonincontro; C. La Mesa, *J. Phys. Chem. B*, 2008, *112*, 3339.

[22] S. W. Provencher, *Comput. Phys. Comm.* 1982, *27*, 213.

[23] A.W. Adamson, *Physical Chemistry of Surfaces*, 5th ed.; Wiley & Sons: New York, 1990; Chapt. *V*, p. 203.

[24] J.B. Berne; R. Pecora, *Dynamic Light Scattering*; Wiley & Sons: New York, 1976; Chapt. *VI*, p. 96.

[25] D. Fennel Evans; H. Wennerstroem, *The Colloidal Domain: where Physics, Chemistry, Biology and Technology meet*, VCH Publishers, Inc.; New York, 1994, *Chapt. VI*, p. 239.

[26] M.F. Hagan, *J. Chem. Phys.*, 2009, *130*, 114902/1.

[27] X. Huang; L.M. Bronstein; J. Retrum; C. Dufort; I. Tsvetkova; S. Aniagyei; B. Stein; G. Stucky; M. McKenna; N. Remmes; D. Baxter; C.C. Kao; B. Dragnea, *Nano Lett.*, 2007, 7, 2407.

28

Targeting TRAIL Receptors with Genetically-Engineered CD34+ Hematopoietic Stem Cells

Carmelo Carlo-Stella, Arianna Giacomini, Silvia L. Locatelli,
Cristiana Lavazza and Alessandro M. Gianni
Medical Oncology, Fondazione IRCCS Istituto Nazionale Tumori and University of Milano
Italy

1. Introduction

Dysregulated apoptosis plays a key role in the pathogenesis and progression of neoplastic disorders, allowing tumor cells to survive beyond their normal life-span, and to eventually acquire chemo-radioresistance (Laconi et al., 2000; Pommier et al., 2004). Thus, targeting either the intrinsic or the extrinsic pathways of apoptosis represent attractive therapeutic strategies for restoring apoptosis sensitivity of malignant cells, or activating agonists of apoptosis (Waxman & Schwartz, 2003). Due to the ability of death receptor ligands to induce cell death, there has been considerable interest in the physiological roles and therapeutic potential of these cytokines as anti-cancer agents. Death receptor ligands of the tumor necrosis factor α (TNFα) superfamily are type II transmembrane proteins that signal to target cells upon cell-cell contact, or after protease-mediated release to the extracellular space (Ashkenazi, 2002). Members of this family, including Fas ligand (FasL), TNFα, and tumor necrosis factor-related apoptosis-inducing ligand (TRAIL), stand out because of their ability to induce cell death (Wajant, 2003; Wiley et al., 1995).

2. Soluble TRAIL

Unlike other apoptosis-inducing TNF family members, soluble TRAIL appears to be inactive against normal healthy tissue (Ashkenazi et al., 1999; Lawrence et al., 2001). A variety of preclinical data clearly show that soluble TRAIL is a cancer cell-specific molecule exerting a remarkable antitumor activity both in vitro (Ashkenazi et al., 1999; Gazitt, 1999; Jin et al., 2004; Mitsiades et al., 2001; Pollack et al., 2001; Rieger et al., 1998) as well as in vivo in athymic nude mice or in non-obese diabetic/severe combined immunodeficient (NOD-SCID) mice (Ashkenazi et al., 1999; Daniel et al., 2007; Kelley et al., 2001).
The physiological functions of TRAIL are not yet fully understood, but mouse gene knockout studies indicate that this agent has an important role in antitumor surveillance by immune cells, mediates thymocyte apoptosis, and is important in the induction of autoimmune diseases (Cretney et al., 2002; Lamhamedi-Cherradi et al., 2003; Smyth et al., 2003).
TRAIL signals by interacting with its receptors. So far, five receptors have been identified, including the two agonistic receptors TRAIL-R1 (Pan et al., 1997b) and TRAIL-R2 (Walczak et al., 1997), and the three antagonistic receptors (Sheridan et al., 1997) TRAIL-R3 (Pan et al.,

1997a), TRAIL-R4 (Degli-Esposti et al., 1997), and osteoprotegerin (OPG) (Emery et al., 1998). Both TRAIL-R1 and TRAIL-R2 are type I transmembrane proteins containing a cytoplasmic death domain (DD) motif that engage apoptotic machinery upon ligand binding (Almasan & Ashkenazi, 2003), whereas the other three receptors either act as decoys or transduce antiapoptotic signals (Wang & El-Deiry, 2003). TRAIL-R3 and TRAIL-R4 have close homology to the extracellular domains of agonistic receptors. TRAIL-R4 has a truncated, nonfunctional cytoplasmic DD, while TRAIL-R3 exists on the plasma membrane as a glycophospholipid-anchored protein lacking the cytosolic tail. The physiological relevance of OPG as a soluble receptor for TRAIL is unclear, but a recent study suggests that cancer-derived OPG may be an important survival factor in hormone-resistant prostate cancer cells (Holen et al., 2002).

3. TRAIL-induced apoptosis signaling

Soluble TRAIL forms homotrimers that bind three receptor molecules, each at the interface between two of its subunits. A Zn atom bound to cysteine residues in the trimeric ligand is essential for trimer stability and optimal biologic activity. Binding of TRAIL to the extracellular domain of agonistic receptors results in trimerization of the receptors and clustering of the intracellular DDs, which leads to the recruitment of the adaptor molecule Fas-associated protein with death domain (FADD). Subsequently, FADD recruits initiator caspase-8 and -10, leading to the formation of the death-inducing signaling complex (DISC), where initiator caspases are autoactivated by proteolysis. Once they become enzymatically active, caspase-8 and/or -10 are released from the DISC and signal through two different proteolytic pathways that converge on caspase-3 and lead to cellular disassembly (Kaufmann & Steensma, 2005). In type I cells, activation of initiator caspases upon death receptors ligation is sufficient to directly activate downstream effector caspases, such as caspase-3 and/or -7 (Scaffidi et al., 1998). This extrinsic pathway is independent of the mitochondria and is not blocked by overexpression of Bcl-2. In type II cells, the commitment from death receptor ligation to apoptosis is less direct (Scaffidi et al., 1998). The amount of initially cleaved caspase-8 and/or -10 is not enough to directly trigger effector caspases activation. Consequently, apoptotic signaling requires an amplification loop by mithocondrial pathway engagement through caspase 8-mediated cleavage of Bid (BH3 interacting death domain agonist), which, in turn, induces the cytosolic Bcl-2 family member Bax (Bcl-2-associated X protein) and/or the loosely bound mitochondrial homolog Bak (Bcl-2 antagonist/killer) to insert into the mitochondrial membrane, where they contribute to the mitochondrial release of cytochrome c (Lucken-Ardjomande & Martinou, 2005). In the cytosol, cytochrome c binds the adaptor protein Apaf-1 (apoptotic protease activating factor 1) to form an apoptosome with recruitment and activation of the apoptosis-initiating caspase-9, which proteolytically activates additional caspase-3. These events are further amplified by apoptogenic factors released from the mitochondrial space, including Smac/DIABLO (second mitochondrial activator of caspases/direct IAP-binding protein with low pI) (Verhagen & Vaux, 2002).

4. Enhancing the antitumor efficacy of soluble TRAIL

Despite very promising preclinical in vitro and in vivo antitumor evidences, phase I/II clinical trials have demonstrated limited antitumor activity of soluble TRAIL likely due to its short half-life and the consequent short exposure of tumor cells to the molecule (Ashkenazi et al., 2008). Because of soluble TRAIL's short half-life (Ashkenazi et al., 1999; Kelley et al., 2001; Walczak et al., 1999), it seems unlikely that the recommended soluble TRAIL dose of 8 mg/kg body weight will allow adequate exposure of tumor cells at high drug concentrations (Ashkenazi et al., 2008). Strategies to enhance the therapeutic activity of soluble TRAIL include combining it with conventional chemotherapy (Ballestrero et al., 2004) or with new agents such as histone deacetylase inhibitors that upregulate TRAIL-R1 and/or TRAIL-R2 (Inoue et al., 2004).

Gene therapy approaches have also been proposed to enhance TRAIL-mediated tumor cell targeting. Recently, a TRAIL-expressing adenoviral vector (Ad-TRAIL) has been shown to cause direct tumor cell killing, as well as a potent bystander effect through presentation of TRAIL by transduced normal cells (Lee et al., 2002). Thus, using Ad-TRAIL might be an alternative to systemic delivery of soluble TRAIL possibly resulting in better tumor cell targeting and increased tumoricidal activity (Armeanu et al., 2003; Griffith et al., 2000; Griffith & Broghammer, 2001; Kagawa et al., 2001; Lee et al., 2002). However, systemic Ad-TRAIL-based gene therapy requires efficient infection of target tumor cells as well as avoidance of immune clearance, and is limited by several safety and toxicity issues related to intravenous adenovector administration (Harrington et al., 2002). Intratumoral injection of TRAIL-encoding adenovectors has been successfully explored in a number of experimental models; however, this approach results in local antitumor activity and has little, if any, value in the treatment of disseminated tumors.

Alternatively, cell-based vehiculation of the full-length, membrane-bound (m)TRAIL (Griffith et al., 2009) has been proposed to achieve an optimal systemic delivery. Indeed, genetically modified stem/progenitor cells represent an innovative approach for delivery of anticancer molecules (Harrington et al., 2002; Introna et al., 2004). Due to their homing properties, systemically injected stem/progenitor cells could infiltrate both primary and metastatic tumor sites, thus allowing tumor-specific targeting (Burger & Kipps, 2006; Jin et al., 2006; Kaplan et al., 2007; Kucia et al., 2005; Loebinger et al., 2009; Najbauer et al., 2007; Rafii et al., 2002), and potentially overcoming limitations inherent to the pharmacokinetic profile of soluble drugs (Aboody et al., 2008; Griffith et al., 2009; Sasportas et al., 2009). Neural or mesenchymal stem cell-mediated mTRAIL delivery has been investigated in solid tumors (Grisendi et al., 2010; Kim et al., 2008; Loebinger et al., 2009; Menon et al., 2009; Mohr et al., 2008; Uzzaman et al., 2009).

In order to optimize the use of TRAIL-encoding adenovectors for the treatment of systemic tumors, we have recently investigated a cell-based approach using mobilized CD34+ hematopoietic cells transduced with a replication-deficient Ad-TRAIL (CD34-TRAIL+) encoding a full-length mTRAIL under the control of the CMV promoter (Carlo-Stella et al., 2006; Griffith et al., 2000). Several lines of evidence support the use of gene-modified CD34+ cells as optimal vehicles of antitumor molecules. In fact, CD34+ cells are already widely used in the clinical setting. Additionally, they can migrate from the bloodstream into tumor tissues due to the expression of adhesion receptors that specifically interact with counter-receptors on endothelial cells in the tumor microenvironment (Burger & Kipps, 2006; Kaplan et al., 2005; Verfaillie, 1998). Moreover, up-regulation of inflammatory chemo-attractants in the tumor microenvironment provides with a permissive milieu that potentially allows for homing of systemically delivered CD34-TRAIL+ cells and efficient tumor targeting (Jin et al., 2006). Using a multiplicity of infection (MOI) of 500, the transduction protocol optimized for the transduction of CD34+ cells consistently results in a transduction efficiency higher than 80% (range 70% - 96%), a high level expression of mTRAIL, and a cell viability ≥85%. Flow cytometry analysis of CD34-TRAIL+ cells shows significant levels of transgene expression for at least 96 hours after transduction, and Western blot analysis reveals the presence of 32- and 55-kDa proteins, which are the expected products for full-length monomer and dimer TRAIL, respectively (Carlo-Stella et al., 2006).

5. Antitumor activity of mTRAIL-expressing cells

The antitumor activity of CD34-TRAIL+ cells has been investigated in a variety of localized and disseminated tumor models in NOD/SCID mice. Using a localized, subcutaneous multiple myeloma model (KMS-11 cell line), intravenously-injected mTRAIL-expressing cells significantly reduced tumor growth over controls as well as soluble TRAIL.[1] In fact, compared with untreated controls, both CD34-TRAIL+ cells and soluble TRAIL significantly inhibited tumor growth by day 28 after tumor injection, when tumor volumes were reduced by 38% ($P < .05$) and 31% ($P < .05$), respectively. However, on day 35, CD34-TRAIL+ cells induced a 40% reduction in tumor growth over controls (4.2 ± 1.2 vs 7.0 ± 2.0 g, $P < .001$), whereas a 29% reduction of tumor growth was detected in mice receiving soluble TRAIL (5.0 ± 1.7 g vs 7.0 ± 2.0 g, $P < .001$) (Lavazza et al., 2010). Even more importantly, an efficient antitumor activity of intravenously injected mTRAIL-expressing CD34+ cells was also detected in NOD/SCID mice bearing disseminated, systemic multiple myeloma and non-Hodgkin lymphoma xenografts (Carlo-Stella et al., 2006; Carlo-Stella et al., 2007; Carlo-Stella et al., 2008). Using KMS-11 as model system, treatment of advanced-stage disease with CD34-TRAIL+ cells resulted in a significant increase of median survival over controls (83 vs 55 days, $P \leq 0.0001$), with 28% of NOD/SCID mice alive and disease-free at the end of the 150-day observation period (Carlo-Stella et al., 2006).[2]

6. In vivo homing of CD34-TRAIL+ cells

Homing properties of transduced cells in healthy tissues as well as tumor nodules were extensively investigated in tumor-bearing NOD/SCID mice who received a single

[1] Six- to eight-week-old female NOD/SCID mice with body weight of 20 to 25 g were purchased from Charles River (Milano, Italy, EU). Mice were housed under standard laboratory conditions according to our institutional guidelines. Animal experiments were performed according to the Italian laws (D.L. 116/92 and following additions), and were approved by the institutional Ethical Committee for Animal Experimentation. KMS-11 cells (5×10^6 cells/mouse) were inoculated subcutaneosuly in the left flank of each mouse. When tumor reached approximately 7 - 10 mm in diameter (usually 10–12 days after tumor inoculation), mice were randomly assigned to planned treatments consisting of daily injections of either CD34-TRAIL+ cells or mock-transduced CD34+ cells (1×10^6 cells/mouse/injection/day, intravenous, days 12–15), or a 4-day course of recombinant soluble TRAIL (30 mg/kg/day, intraperitoneal, days 12–15). Mice were checked twice weekly for tumor appearance, tumor dimensions, body weight, and toxicity. Tumor volumes were measured with calipers and their weights calculated using the formula: $(a \times b^2)/2$, where a and b represented the longest and shortest diameters, respectively. Mice were followed up for 3 weeks after the end of the treatments. The endpoint of the subcutaneous model was tumor weight. Each experiment was performed on at least two separate occasions, using five mice per treatment group.

[2] KMS-11 (0.5×10^6 cells/mouse) cell line was inoculated intravenously. CD34-mock or CD34-TRAIL+ cells (1×10^6 cells/mouse/injection) were inoculated intravenously weekly for 4 weeks starting either on day 7 (early-stage tumor model), or 14 (advanced-stage tumor model) after tumor cell injection.

intravenous injection of CD34-TRAIL+ cells (3 × 10^6 cells/mouse) (Lavazza et al., 2010). Tumor and healthy tissue sections were immunostained with an anti-human CD45 antibody and digitally recorded to count transduced cells on entire tissue sections.[3] Early following injection, transduced cells were detected at high frequencies in the lung, liver and spleen (**Figure 1**). CD34-TRAIL+ cells progressively decreased and were no longer detectable in these tissues 24 hours after injection. Bone marrow CD34-TRAIL+ cells peaked 5 hours after injection and were detectable up to 24 hours. Low frequencies of transduced cells were detected within tumors as early as 30 minutes following injection. They progressively increased and peaked 48 hours post-injection when on average 188 ± 25 CD45+ cells per 10^5 tumor cells (i.e., 0.2 ± 0.03%) were recorded (**Figure 1**). Overall, kinetics data suggest that transduced cells transiently circulate through healthy tissues, whereas they are preferentially recruited within tumor nodules, allowing to hypothesize that homing signals by tumor endothelial cells actively promote intratumor homing of transduced cells.

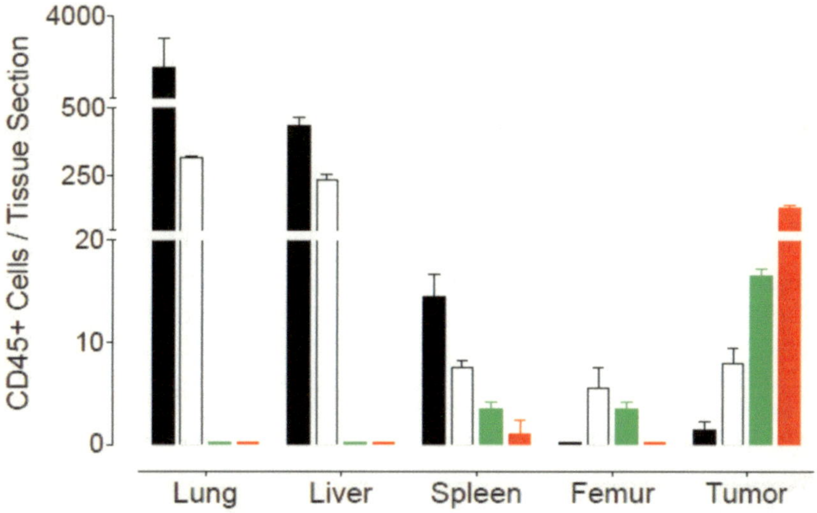

Fig. 1. Tissue kinetics of CD34-TRAIL+ cells. Lung, liver, spleen, femur, and tumor nodules were harvested from tumor-bearing NOD/SCID mice 0.5 (■), 5 (□), 24 (■), and 48 (■) hours after a single intravenous injection of CD34-TRAIL+ cells (3 × 10^6 cells/mouse). Shown is the quantification of CD34-TRAIL+ cells on digitally acquired tissue sections stained with anti-CD45. Frequency of CD34-TRAIL+ cells is expressed as the mean (± SD) number of CD45+ cells per tissue section.

---

[3] Images of tissue sections were acquired at 20× magnification with an automatic high-resolution scanner (dotSlide System, Olympus, Tokyo, Japan) and subdivided into a collection of non-overlapping red, green, and blue (RGB) images in TIFF format (final resolution 3.125 pixels/μm). Image analysis was carried out using the open-source ImageJ software (http://rsb.info.nih.gov/ij/). Routines for image analysis were coded in ImageJ macro language and executed on RGB images without further treatment. Per each experimental condition, at least three sections from different tumor nodules or healthy tissues were analyzed. Intratumor frequency of CD34-TRAIL+ cells was expressed as the number of CD45+ cells per total cells per tisue section. Total cells were counted by the ImageJ internal function for particle analysis, whereas CD45+ cells were manually counted in all images from whole scanning of histochemically stained tissue sections.

7. Vascular signals involved in tumor homing

This issue was investigated by evaluating the expression of homing receptors on tumor vasculature. Confocal microscopy[4] revealed that 30% of tumor vessels expressed high levels of VCAM-1 on the luminal surface (**Figure 2$_{b\text{-}c}$**) (Jin et al., 2006), whereas SFD-1 was ubiquitously expressed on tumor vessels and tumor cells (**Figure 2$_{e\text{-}f}$**). Thus, α4β1 integrins and the CXCR4 chemokine (De Raeve et al., 2004; Peled et al., 1999) seem to play a critical role in regulating intratumor homing of mTRAIL-expressing cells. To further investigate the functional relevance of SDF-1/CXCR4 and VCAM-1/VLA-4 pathways in mediating tumor homing of transduced cells, inhibitory experiments with an anti–VCAM-1 antibody and the CXCR4 antagonist AMD3100 were performed.[5] As compared to controls, tumor homing of CD34-TRAIL+ cells was significantly reduced in mice administered with anti–VCAM-1 antibody [0.2 ± 0.03% vs 0.09 ± 0.01% (P = .001)] or the CXCR4 antagonist AMD3100 (Fricker et al., 2006) [0.2 ± 0.03% vs 0.05 ± 0.006% (P = .0003)]. Tumor vasculature was also analyzed for the expression of TRAIL-R2 receptor. Indeed, confocal microscopy revealed that approximately 8 - 12% of tumor endothelial cells expressed TRAIL-R2 receptor on their luminal surface (**Figure 2$_{h\text{-}i}$**), suggesting that mechanisms other than SDF-1/CXCR4 and VCAM-1/VLA-4, such as the mTRAIL/TRAIL-R2 interactions, might be involved in regulating intratumor homing as well as functional activity of CD34-TRAIL+ cells (Lavazza et al., 2010).

8. CD34-TRAIL+ cells induce tumor cell apoptosis and hemorrhagic necrosis

Tumor-homing of CD34-TRAIL+ cells is associated with significant levels of tumor cell apoptosis (Carlo-Stella et al., 2006). To obtain an objective quantification of apoptosis, a computer-aided image analysis using ImageJ software was performed.[6] As compared to controls, TUNEL+ cells were increased by 8- (2.4 ± 1.4% vs 0.3 ± 0.3%, P < .0001) and 4-fold (1.2 ± 0.7% vs 0.3 ± 0.3%, P < .0001) following treatment with CD34-TRAIL+ cells and soluble TRAIL, respectively (**Figure 3A**). Interestingly, apoptotic effects of CD34-TRAIL+ cells resulted significantly more potent than those exerted by soluble TRAIL (P < .0001). Additionally, TUNEL staining of tumor sections from untreated, mock- and soluble TRAIL-

---

[4] Cryosections were fixed with cold acetone, rinsed with PBS, and then blocked with 2% BSA. Sections were first incubated with the appropriate primary antibody, including mouse anti-human stromal cell-derived factor-1 (SDF-1) (R&D Systems), rat anti-mouse VCAM-1 (Southern Biotech), or hamster anti-mouse TRAIL-R2 (BD Pharmingen). After washing, sections were incubated with the appropriate Alexa Fluor 568-conjugated secondary antibody (Invitrogen). Biotinylated tumor vessels were revealed with Alexa Fluor 488-conjugated streptavidin (Invitrogen). Sections were examined under an epifluorescent microscope equipped with a laser confocal system (MRC-1024, Bio-Rad Laboratories). Image processing was carried out using LaserSharp computer software (Bio-Rad Laboratories).

[5] To inhibit intratumor homing of CD34-TRAIL+ cells, mice received either one single intraperitoneal dose of anti–VCAM-1 (vascular cell adhesion molecule-1) antibody (clone M/K-2; Southern Biotech, Birmingham, AL, USA) at 0.5 mg/mouse, 3 hours before cell administration, or two doses of AMD3100 (5 mg/kg, subcutaneous, 1 hour prior to and 3 hours after cell administration).

[6] The number of total and TUNEL+ cells per section was counted as follows. Briefly, the dynamic range of images was expanded to full by contrast enhancement, and cells were identified by appropriate filtering in the red, green, and blue (RGB) channels. Resulting black and white images were combined to represent only pixels selected in every color channel. For each image, both total and TUNEL+ cells were counted by the ImageJ internal function for particle analysis.

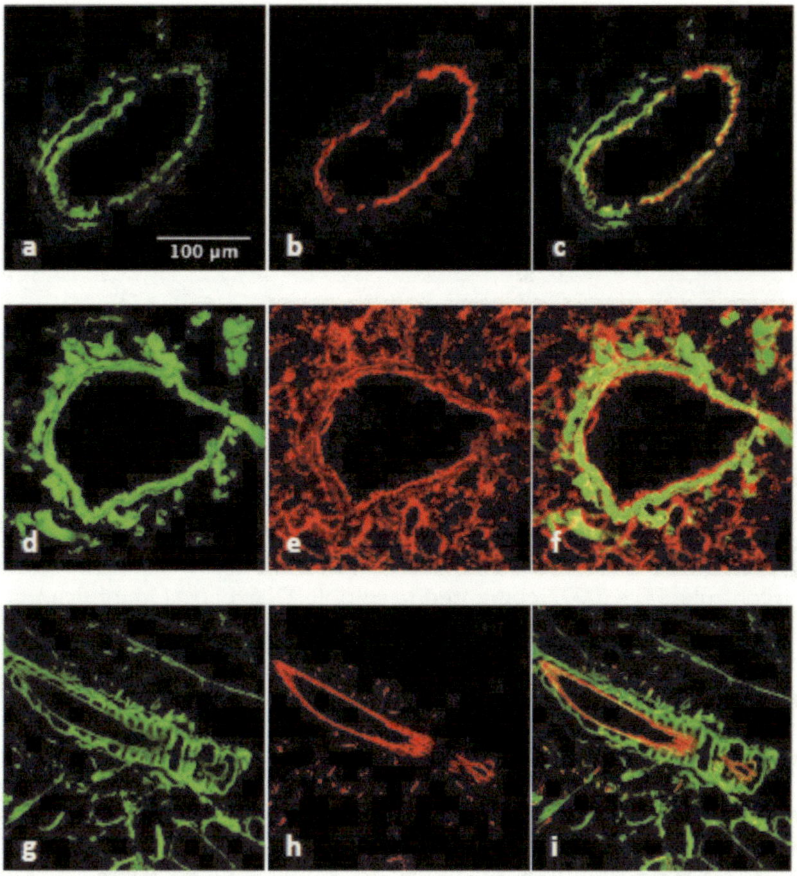

Fig. 2. Vascular molecules involved in intratumor homing of CD34-TRAIL+ cells. Confocal microscopy analysis of intratumor recruiting signals was carried out on 4-μm cryosections from in vivo biotinylated tumors. Cryosections were stained with Alexa Fluor 488-conjugated streptavidin (*green*) to detect tumor vasculature (*a, d, g*). Cryosections were also stained with anti–VCAM-1 (*b*), anti–SDF-1 (*e*), or anti–TRAIL-R2 (*h*) followed by the appropriate Alexa Fluor 568-conjugated secondary antibody for indirect detection of the corresponding antigen (*red*). Merged images demonstrate VCAM-1 (*c*), SDF-1 (*f*), or TRAIL-R2 (*i*) expression by endothelial cells. Objective lens, 40×.

treated mice revealed a homogeneous mass of viable cells with necrotic areas accounting only for 1.4 ± 1.0%, 1.8 ± 1%, and 2.9 ± 1% of total tissue, respectively (**Figure 3B**). In contrast, tumors from CD34-TRAIL-treated mice displayed a significant increase of necrotic areas as compared to controls, with percentages of necrotic areas per tissue section ranging from 6% to 18%, and a mean 8-fold increase over controls (11 ± 3.8% vs 1.4 ± 1.0%, $P < .0001$), and 4-fold increase over soluble TRAIL-treated mice (11 ± 3.8% vs 2.9 ± 1%, $P = .0001$) (**Figure 3B**). Pharmacological inhibition of intratumor recruitment of CD34-TRAIL+ cells using AMD3100, or anti-VCAM-1 antibody significantly reduced necrotic areas by 37% ($P = .02$) and 56% ($P = .002$), respectively (**Figure 3C**), suggesting that intratumor recruitment of CD34-TRAIL+ cells specifically triggered tumor necrosis.

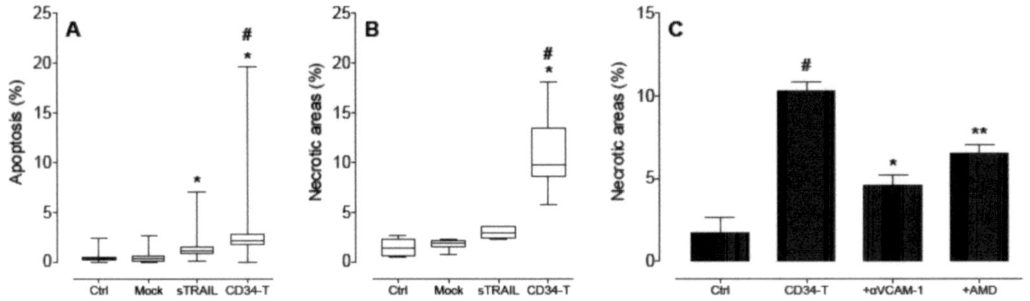

Fig. 3. Pro-apoptotic and necrotic effects of CD34-TRAIL+ cells. NOD/SCID mice bearing subcutaneous tumor nodules 10 mm in diameter were randomly assigned to receive CD34-TRAIL+ cells, mock-transduced CD34+ cells (3×10^6 cells/mouse, intravenous), recombinant soluble TRAIL (500 μg/mouse, IP), or control vehicle. (A) Percentages of apoptotic cells in tumors from untreated or treated animals were computationally calculated on digitally acquired images (objective lens, 20×) using ImageJ. At least three sections from different animals were analyzed. The boxes extend from the 25th to the 75th percentiles, the lines indicate the median values, and the whiskers indicate the range of values. * $P < .0001$, compared to controls. # $P < .0001$, compared to soluble TRAIL. (B) Quantification of necrotic areas by ImageJ analysis on tissue sections stained with TUNEL. At least six sections from different animals were analyzed per treatment group. * $P < .0001$, compared to controls. # $P = .0001$, compared to soluble TRAIL. (C) Anti-VCAM-1 and AMD3100 reduced tumor necrosis in mice treated with CD34-TRAIL+ cells. # $P < .0001$, compared to control. * $P = .002$, compared with CD34-TRAIL+ cells. ** $P = .02$, compared with CD34-TRAIL+ cells.

A distinctive and prominent feature of tumors treated with CD34-TRAIL+ cells was represented by hemorrhagic phenomena within necrotic areas close to damaged vessels which were detected by immunohistochemical staining with glycophorin A (**Figure 4A**). Hemorrhagic phenomena exactly matched TUNEL+ necrotic areas and closely associated with apoptotic endothelial cells (**Figure 4B$_L$**). In striking contrast, apoptotic vessels and hemorrhagic phenomena could not be detected neither in tumors from mice treated with soluble TRAIL (**Figure 4B$_K$** and **4A**), nor in healthy tissues (**Figure 5**), suggesting a tumor-restricted antivascular activity by CD34-TRAIL+ cells.

9. Antivascular effects of CD34-TRAIL+ cells

To better understand the relationship between the antitumor effects of CD34-TRAIL+ cells and apoptosis of endothelial cells, an extensive vascular analysis[7] was performed on

[7] Tumor vasculature was analyzed on cryosections using the open-source ImageJ software (http://rsb.info.nih.gov/ij/) from in vivo biotinylated mice stained with HRP-conjugated streptavidin. To calculate endothelial area, i.e., the percentage of tissue section occupied by endothelium, endothelial cells were identified by contrast enhancement and appropriate filtering. Background signal was removed considering only structures larger than an arbitrary minimal value. To analyze vessel wall thickness, we manually selected rectangular regions of RGB input images containing at least a hollow vessel. An automatic routine computed vessel thickness according to the formula: Thickness = 2 × (vessel area)/[(vessel perimeter) + (lumen perimeter)]. At first, endothelial tissue was identified applying a threshold on the blue channel and obtaining a binary image representative of its

histological sections from tumors treated with transduced cells and subsequently in vivo biotinylated to detect tumor vasculature (Lavazza et al., 2010; Rybak et al., 2005). In untreated mice, tumor vasculature was abundant, tortuous, and evenly distributed throughout the tumor (**Figure 6A**). In striking contrast, in NOD/SCID mice treated with CD34-TRAIL+ cells, viable tumor cells surrounding necrotic areas appeared deficient in capillaries and small-caliber blood vessels, which were less tortuous and had fewer branches and sprouts (**Figure 6A**). Globally, mean percentages of endothelial areas from control and mock-treated tumors were 8.8 ± 5.6% and 8.2 ± 3.3%, respectively (**Figure 6B**). Administration of soluble TRAIL did not affect endothelial area compared to controls (8.1 ± 2.9% vs 8.8 ± 5.6%, P = ns). In contrast, a single intravenous injection of 3×10^6 CD34-TRAIL+ cells caused a 37% decrease of endothelial area compared to control (5.6 ± 3.2% vs 8.8 ± 5.6%, $P < .0001$) (**Figure 6B**). Additionally, blood vessels from tumors treated with CD34-TRAIL+ cells were thicker than those observed in untreated or soluble TRAIL-treated animals (**Figure 6A**). Based on these findings, we isolated images of transversally oriented vessels in streptavidin-HPR stained sections and calculated vessel wall thickness by processing images with ImageJ and specifically written macros. As shown in **Figure 6C**, wall thickness was 1.7-fold increased compared to control (5.5 ± 1.4 vs 3.2 ± 0.8 µm, $P < .0001$), whereas no increases emerged after soluble TRAIL administration (3.3 ± 0.7 vs 3.2 ± 0.8 µm).

10. Conclusions

Experimental data obtained in a variety of preclinical models of both localized and disseminated disease strongly suggest that TRAIL-expressing CD34+ cells can efficiently vehiculate mTRAIL within the tumors where they exert potent antivascular and antitumor activities resulting in a significant reduction of tumor growth. Analysis of tumor nodules obtained 48 hours after a single administration of transduced cells showed that TRAIL-expressing cells were 2-fold more effective than soluble TRAIL in inducing apoptosis of tumor cells. Broad necrotic events, involving up to 18% of tumor tissue, were detected only after administration of CD34-TRAIL+ cells and were associated with a hemorrhagic component which was not detectable after soluble TRAIL administration. Hemorrhagic

---

distribution. Then, the lumen of each vessel in the image was identified as a non-endothelial area, ringed by endothelial tissue and greater than an arbitrary threshold. This procedure rejected smaller artifacts and allowed for recognition of hollow vessels even when erythrocytes or other cells occupied the lumen. Subsequently, we identified the endothelium surrounding a given lumen by an iterative procedure. At first, we subdivided the binary representation of stained tissue into areas by means of a watershed algorithm. Then we selected only those regions adjacent to the lumen, obtaining a minimal image of the vessel wall. This minimal image was used to compute a working thickness according to the previously stated formula. Then, to avoid arbitrary removal of bona fide portions of the walls, we calculated a theoretical vessel contour expanding the lumen outline by a number of pixels equivalent to the working thickness. We next turned back to the watershedded image of endothelium distribution, selecting only those areas connected with the new, theoretical contour. Inclusion of the new regions in the minimal image produced the final vessel image. Both images were saved to allow for manual appreciation of proper vessel identification. At last, the final vessel thickness was calculated after assessment of the final vessel area and external perimeter. Per each parameter, the accuracy and appropriate cut-off levels were determined by comparing processed images to the RGB originals. In all instances, automatic routines were validated by comparing results with those obtained by visual counting of up to 10% of the total images by two independent pathologists.

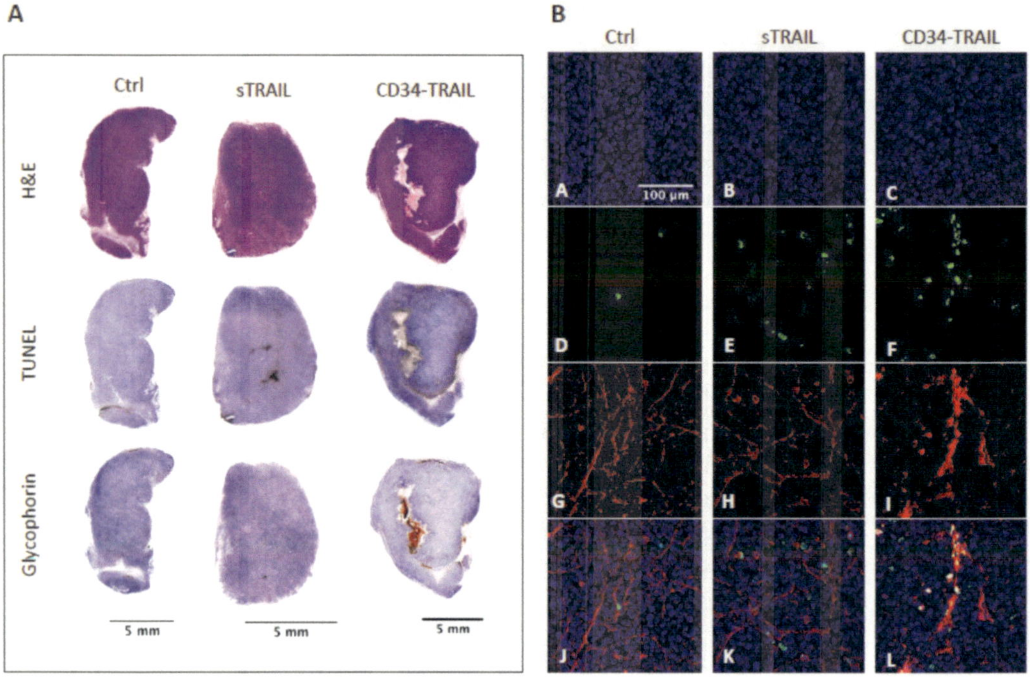

Fig. 4. Tumor hemorrhagic necrosis and endothelial cell apoptosis induced by CD34-TRAIL+ cells. NOD/SCID mice bearing subcutaneous tumor nodules 10 mm in diameter were randomly assigned to receive CD34-TRAIL+ cells, recombinant TRAIL (500 µg/mouse, IP), or control vehicle. Tumors were harvested forty-eight hours after treatment. (**A**) Hematoxylin and eosin (H&E), TUNEL and glycophorin A staining were performed. Objective lens, 2×. (**B**) Just before sacrifice NOD/SCID mice were intravenously injected with sulfo-NHS-LC-biotin to biotinylate tumor vasculature. Representative confocal images of tumors from untreated and treated animals processed by triple immunofluorescence staining. (*A–C*) Cell nuclei were detected in blue by TO-PRO-3; (*D–F*) apoptotic cells were detected in green by TUNEL staining; (*G–I*) tumor endothelial cells were detected in red by Alexa 568-conjugated streptavidin. (*J–L*) After merging of single-color images, apoptotic nuclei (*green*) were detectable throughout tumor parenchyma after treatment with either soluble TRAIL or CD34-TRAIL+ cells, whereas endothelial cells with apoptotic nuclei (*yellow*) could be detected only in CD34-TRAIL+ cell-treated animals. Objective lens, 40×.

necrosis was localized near TUNEL+ blood vessels, suggesting that apoptosis of tumor endothelial cells represents an early event triggered by CD34-TRAIL+ cells. Overall, these findings support the hypothesis that CD34-TRAIL+ cells exert their cytotoxic activity not only by targeting parenchymal tumor cells but also by targeting tumor vasculature (Carlo-Stella et al., 2006; Lavazza et al., 2010). Indeed, the vascular-disrupting activity of mTRAIL might represent a major concern in view of clinical applications. Notwithstanding the intratumor vascular-disrupting activity of mTRAIL, extensive analysis of healthy tissues failed to detect any evidence of hemorrhagic necrosis, suggesting that vascular damage was tumor-restricted.

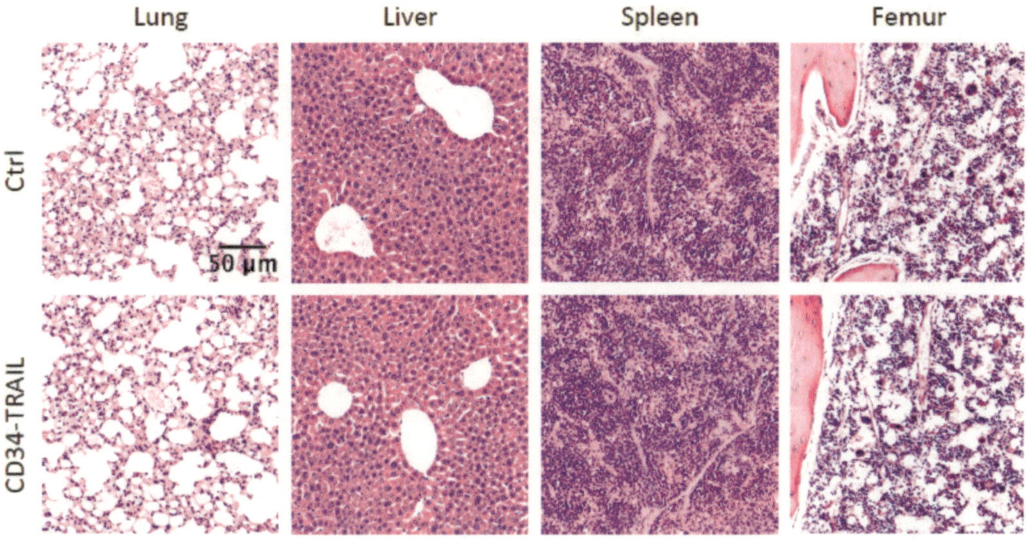

Fig. 5. Tissue and vascular toxicity in healthy tissue after CD34-TRAIL+ cells administration. NOD/SCID mice bearing subcutaneous tumor nodules received a single intravenous injection of CD34-TRAIL+ cells (3×10^6 cells/mouse), or control vehicle. Forty-eight hours after treatment, lung, liver, spleen, and femur were harvested and analyzed. Hematoxylin and eosin staining demonstrated the absence of tissue or vascular damage. Representative histological images are shown. Objective lens, 10x.

Increasing evidences suggest that recruitment of CD34+ cells in the tumor microenvironment is due to homing signals similar to those found in the bone marrow hematopoietic niches (Jin et al., 2006; Kaplan et al., 2007; Rafii et al., 2002; Wels et al., 2008). Both SDF-1/CXCR4 and VCAM-1/VLA-4 pathways play a key role in regulating bone marrow homing of transplanted hematopoietic stem cells (Aiuti et al., 1997; Peled et al., 1999) as well as intratumor recruitment of CXCR4-expressing cells and neovascularization during acute ischemia and tumor growth (Burger & Kipps, 2006; Jin et al., 2006; Petit et al., 2007). Kinetics data obtained in our models clearly show that intravenously injected transduced cells circulate in normal tissues up to 24 hours, but they progressively and preferentially home at tumor sites where they can be detected up to 48 hours after injection. Lack of intratumor detection of CD34-TRAIL+ cells beyond 48 hours after injection (data not shown) may be due to destruction of mTRAIL-expressing cells in the context of antitumor activities (i.e., disruption of tumor vasculature, hemorrhagic necrosis, tumor necrosis, etc.). Pharmacological manipulation of adhesion receptor expression using either AMD3100 or anti-VCAM-1 antibodies significantly reduced both the frequency and the antitumor efficacy of CD34-TRAIL+ cells strongly suggesting that SDF-1 and VCAM-1 expressed by tumor vasculature efficiently recruit transduced CD34+ cells within tumors by challenging their trafficking and homing properties. The role of additional binding systems, such as mTRAIL/TRAIL-R2, in mediating tumor tropism of CD34-TRAIL+ cells may be hypothesized on the basis of our data. Binding of CD34-TRAIL+ cells to TRAIL-R2 expressed by tumor vasculature could significantly contribute to initiation of a cascade of events that induce early endothelial damage, leading to extensive tumor cell death (Arafat et al., 2000).

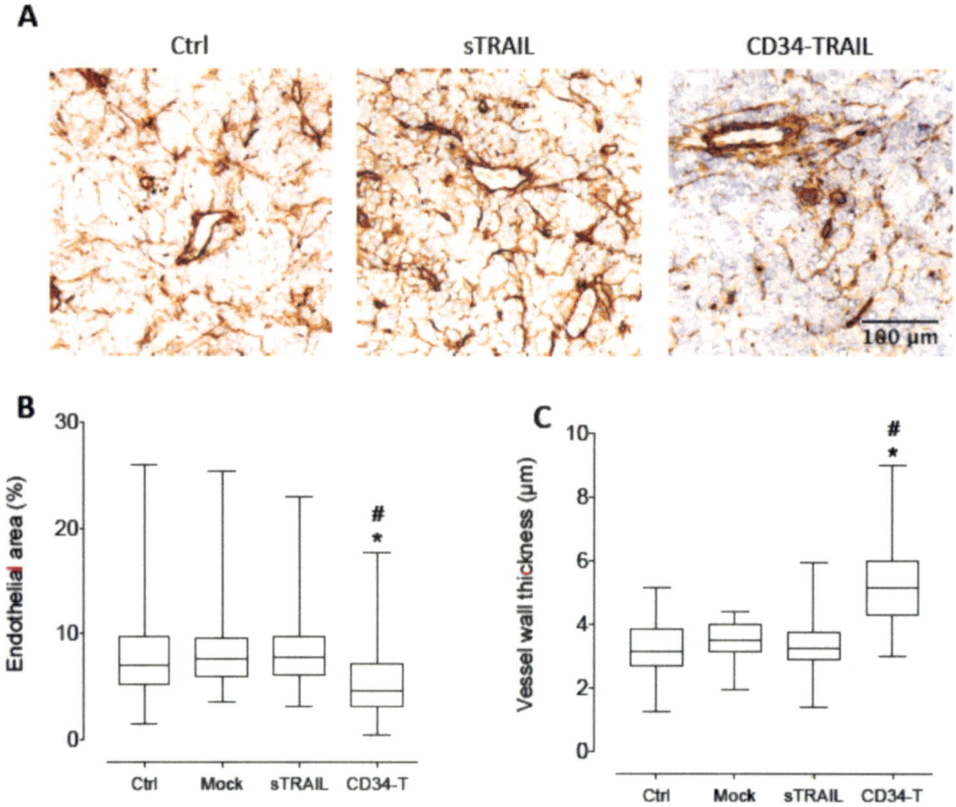

Fig. 6. Antivascular effects of CD34-TRAIL+ cells. NOD/SCID mice bearing subcutaneous tumor nodules 10 mm in diameter were randomly assigned to receive CD34-TRAIL+ cells, mock-transduced CD34+ cells (3×10^6 cells/mouse, intravenous), recombinant soluble TRAIL (500 µg/mouse, IP), and control vehicle. (**A**) Forty-eight hours after treatment, NOD/SCID mice were intravenously injected with 0.2 mL of sulfo-NHS-LC-biotin (5 mg/mL) to biotinylate tumor vasculature. Tumors were then excised, and biotinylated endothelium was revealed by HRP-streptavidin and 3,3′-diaminobenzidine for light microscopy analysis. Representative histological images of in vivo biotinylated mice receiving the different treatments are shown. (**B**) Sections were analyzed using ImageJ for quantification of vascular parameters. Endothelial area was calculated on whole tissue sections as (streptavidin-HRP stained area)/(total tissue area) × 100. * $P < .0001$, compared to controls. # $P < .0001$, compared to soluble TRAIL . (**C**) Vessel wall thickness was calculated on transversally oriented vessels. * $P < .0001$, compared to controls. # $P < .0001$, compared to soluble TRAIL .

In conclusion, under our experimental conditions the use of transduced CD34+ cells as a vehicle of mTRAIL resulted in an antitumor effect greater than that exerted by soluble TRAIL, likely because of an antivascular action. Our findings appear to be of outstanding interest in the context of the increasing need for therapeutic strategies targeting not only tumor cells but also the tumor microenvironment (De Raeve et al., 2004; Joyce, 2005; Rafii et al., 2002). Finally, the clinical feasibility of such a systemic CD34+ cell-based gene therapy approach could be exploited to develop effective autologous or allogeneic anticancer treatments.

11. Acknowledgements

This work was supported in part by grants from Special Program Molecular Clinical Oncology of Associazione Italiana per la Ricerca sul Cancro (Milano, Italy), Ministero dell'Istruzione, dell'Università e della Ricerca (MIUR, Rome, Italy), Ministero della Salute (Rome, Italy), Alleanza Contro il Cancro (Rome, Italy), and the Michelangelo Foundation for Advances in Cancer Research and Treatment (Milano, Italy).

12. References

Aboody, K.S., Najbauer, J., and Danks, M.K. (2008). Stem and progenitor cell-mediated tumor selective gene therapy. *Gene Ther,* Vol.15, No.10, (May 2008), pp. 739-752

Aiuti, A., Webb, I.J., Bleul, C., Springer, T., and Gutierrez-Ramos, J.C. (1997). The chemokine SDF-1 is a chemoattractant for human CD34+ hematopoietic progenitor cells and provides a new mechanism to explain the mobilization of CD34+ progenitors to peripheral blood. *J Exp Med,* Vol.185, No.1, (Jan 6 1997), pp. 111-120

Almasan, A., and Ashkenazi, A. (2003). Apo2L/TRAIL: apoptosis signaling, biology, and potential for cancer therapy. *Cytokine Growth Factor Rev,* Vol.14, No.3-4, (Jun-Aug 2003), pp. 337-348

Arafat, W.O., Casado, E., Wang, M., Alvarez, R.D., Siegal, G.P., Glorioso, J.C., Curiel, D.T., and Gomez-Navarro, J. (2000). Genetically modified CD34+ cells exert a cytotoxic bystander effect on human endothelial and cancer cells. *Clin Cancer Res,* Vol.6, No.11, (Nov 2000), pp. 4442-4448

Armeanu, S., Lauer, U.M., Smirnow, I., Schenk, M., Weiss, T.S., Gregor, M., and Bitzer, M. (2003). Adenoviral gene transfer of tumor necrosis factor-related apoptosis-inducing ligand overcomes an impaired response of hepatoma cells but causes severe apoptosis in primary human hepatocytes. *Cancer Res,* Vol.63, No.10, (May 15 2003), pp. 2369-2372

Ashkenazi, A., Pai, R.C., Fong, S., Leung, S., Lawrence, D.A., Marsters, S.A., Blackie, C., Chang, L., McMurtrey, A.E., Hebert, A., DeForge, L., Koumenis, I.L., Lewis, D., Harris, L., Bussiere, J., Koeppen, H., Shahrokh, Z., and Schwall, R.H. (1999). Safety and antitumor activity of recombinant soluble Apo2 ligand. *J. Clin. Invest.,* Vol.104, No.2, (July 15 1999), pp. 155-162

Ashkenazi, A. (2002). Targeting death and decoy receptors of the tumour-necrosis factor superfamily. *Nat Rev Cancer,* Vol.2, No.6, (Jun 2002), pp. 420-430

Ashkenazi, A., Holland, P., and Eckhardt, S.G. (2008). Ligand-based targeting of apoptosis in cancer: the potential of recombinant human apoptosis ligand 2/Tumor necrosis factor-related apoptosis-inducing ligand (rhApo2L/TRAIL). *J Clin Oncol,* Vol.26, No.21, (Jul 20 2008), pp. 3621-3630

Ballestrero, A., Nencioni, A., Boy, D., Rocco, I., Garuti, A., Mela, G.S., Van Parijs, L., Brossart, P., Wesselborg, S., and Patrone, F. (2004). Tumor necrosis factor-related apoptosis-inducing ligand cooperates with anticancer drugs to overcome chemoresistance in antiapoptotic Bcl-2 family members expressing jurkat cells. *Clin Cancer Res,* Vol.10, No.4, (Feb 15 2004), pp. 1463-1470

Burger, J.A., and Kipps, T.J. (2006). CXCR4: a key receptor in the crosstalk between tumor cells and their microenvironment. *Blood,* Vol.107, No.5, (Mar 1 2006), pp. 1761-1767

Carlo-Stella, C., Lavazza, C., Di Nicola, M., Cleris, L., Longoni, P., Milanesi, M., Magni, M., Morelli, D., Gloghini, A., Carbone, A., and Gianni, A.M. (2006). Antitumor activity of human CD34+ cells expressing membrane-bound tumor necrosis factor-related apoptosis-inducing ligand. *Human gene therapy,* Vol.17, No.12, (Dec 2006), pp. 1225-1240

Carlo-Stella, C., Lavazza, C., Locatelli, A., Vigano, L., Gianni, A.M., and Gianni, L. (2007). Targeting TRAIL Agonistic Receptors for Cancer Therapy. *Clin Cancer Res,* Vol.13, No.8, (Apr 15 2007), pp. 2313-2317

Carlo-Stella, C., Lavazza, C., Carbone, A., and Gianni, A.M. (2008). Anticancer cell therapy with TRAIL-armed CD34+ progenitor cells. *Adv Exp Med Biol,* Vol.610, (2008), pp. 100-111

Cretney, E., Takeda, K., Yagita, H., Glaccum, M., Peschon, J.J., and Smyth, M.J. (2002). Increased susceptibility to tumor initiation and metastasis in TNF-related apoptosis-inducing ligand-deficient mice. *J Immunol,* Vol.168, No.3, (Feb 1 2002), pp. 1356-1361

Daniel, D., Yang, B., Lawrence, D.A., Totpal, K., Balter, I., Lee, W.P., Gogineni, A., Cole, M.J., Yee, S.F., Ross, S., and Ashkenazi, A. (2007). Cooperation of the proapoptotic receptor agonist rhApo2L/TRAIL with the CD20 antibody rituximab against non-Hodgkin lymphoma xenografts. *Blood,* Vol.110, No.12, (Dec 1 2007), pp. 4037-4046

De Raeve, H., Van Marck, E., Van Camp, B., and Vanderkerken, K. (2004). Angiogenesis and the role of bone marrow endothelial cells in haematological malignancies. *Histol Histopathol,* Vol.19, No.3, (Jul 2004), pp. 935-950

Degli-Esposti, M.A., Dougall, W.C., Smolak, P.J., Waugh, J.Y., Smith, C.A., and Goodwin, R.G. (1997). The novel receptor TRAIL-R4 induces NF-kappaB and protects against TRAIL-mediated apoptosis, yet retains an incomplete death domain. *Immunity,* Vol.7, No.6, (Dec 1997), pp. 813-820

Emery, J.G., McDonnell, P., Burke, M.B., Deen, K.C., Lyn, S., Silverman, C., Dul, E., Appelbaum, E.R., Eichman, C., DiPrinzio, R., Dodds, R.A., James, I.E., Rosenberg, M., Lee, J.C., and Young, P.R. (1998). Osteoprotegerin is a receptor for the cytotoxic ligand TRAIL. *J Biol Chem,* Vol.273, No.23, (Jun 5 1998), pp. 14363-14367

Fricker, S.P., Anastassov, V., Cox, J., Darkes, M.C., Grujic, O., Idzan, S.R., Labrecque, J., Lau, G., Mosi, R.M., Nelson, K.L., Qin, L., Santucci, Z., and Wong, R.S. (2006). Characterization of the molecular pharmacology of AMD3100: a specific antagonist of the G-protein coupled chemokine receptor, CXCR4. *Biochem Pharmacol,* Vol.72, No.5, (Aug 28 2006), pp. 588-596

Gazitt, Y. (1999). TRAIL is a potent inducer of apoptosis in myeloma cells derived from multiple myeloma patients and is not cytotoxic to hematopoietic stem cells. *Leukemia,* Vol.13, No.11, (Nov 1999), pp. 1817-1824

Griffith, T.S., Anderson, R.D., Davidson, B.L., Williams, R.D., and Ratliff, T.L. (2000). Adenoviral-mediated transfer of the TNF-related apoptosis-inducing ligand/Apo-2 ligand gene induces tumor cell apoptosis. *J Immunol,* Vol.165, No.5, (Sep 1 2000), pp. 2886-2894

Griffith, T.S., and Broghammer, E.L. (2001). Suppression of tumor growth following intralesional therapy with TRAIL recombinant adenovirus. *Mol Ther,* Vol.4, No.3, (Sep 2001), pp. 257-266

Griffith, T.S., Stokes, B., Kucaba, T.A., Earel, J.K., Jr., VanOosten, R.L., Brincks, E.L., and Norian, L.A. (2009). TRAIL gene therapy: from preclinical development to clinical application. *Curr Gene Ther,* Vol.9, No.1, (Feb 2009), pp. 9-19

Grisendi, G., Bussolari, R., Cafarelli, L., Petak, I., Rasini, V., Veronesi, E., De Santis, G., Spano, C., Tagliazzucchi, M., Barti-Juhasz, H., Scarabelli, L., Bambi, F., Frassoldati, A., Rossi, G., Casali, C., Morandi, U., Horwitz, E.M., Paolucci, P., Conte, P., and Dominici, M. (2010). Adipose-derived mesenchymal stem cells as stable source of tumor necrosis factor-related apoptosis-inducing ligand delivery for cancer therapy. *Cancer Research,* Vol.70, No.9, (May 1 2010), pp. 3718-3729

Harrington, K., Alvarez-Vallina, L., Crittenden, M., Gough, M., Chong, H., Diaz, R.M., Vassaux, G., Lemoine, N., and Vile, R. (2002). Cells as vehicles for cancer gene therapy: the missing link between targeted vectors and systemic delivery? *Hum Gene Ther,* Vol.13, No.11, (Jul 20 2002), pp. 1263-1280

Holen, I., Croucher, P.I., Hamdy, F.C., and Eaton, C.L. (2002). Osteoprotegerin (OPG) is a survival factor for human prostate cancer cells. *Cancer Res,* Vol.62, No.6, (Mar 15 2002), pp. 1619-1623

Inoue, S., Macfarlane, M., Harper, N., Wheat, L.M., Dyer, M.J., and Cohen, G.M. (2004). Histone deacetylase inhibitors potentiate TNF-related apoptosis-inducing ligand (TRAIL)-induced apoptosis in lymphoid malignancies. *Cell Death Differ,* Vol.11 Suppl 2, (December 2004), pp. S193-206

Introna, M., Barbui, A.M., Golay, J., and Rambaldi, A. (2004). Innovative cell-based therapies in onco-hematology: what are the clinical facts ? *Haematologica,* Vol.89, No.10, (Oct 2004), pp. 1253-1260

Jin, H., Aiyer, A., Su, J., Borgstrom, P., Stupack, D., Friedlander, M., and Varner, J. (2006). A homing mechanism for bone marrow-derived progenitor cell recruitment to the neovasculature. *J Clin Invest,* Vol.116, No.3, (Mar 1 2006), pp. 652-662

Joyce, J.A. (2005). Therapeutic targeting of the tumor microenvironment. *Cancer Cell,* Vol.7, No.6, (Jun 2005), pp. 513-520

Kagawa, S., He, C., Gu, J., Koch, P., Rha, S.-J., Roth, J.A., Curley, S.A., Stephens, L.C., and Fang, B. (2001). Antitumor activity and bystander effects of the tumor necrosis factor-related apoptosis-inducing ligand (TRAIL) gene. *Cancer Res,* Vol.61, No.8, (April 1, 2001 2001), pp. 3330-3338

Kaplan, R.N., Riba, R.D., Zacharoulis, S., Bramley, A.H., Vincent, L., Costa, C., MacDonald, D.D., Jin, D.K., Shido, K., Kerns, S.A., Zhu, Z., Hicklin, D., Wu, Y., Port, J.L., Altorki, N., Port, E.R., Ruggero, D., Shmelkov, S.V., Jensen, K.K., Rafii, S., and Lyden, D. (2005). VEGFR1-positive haematopoietic bone marrow progenitors initiate the pre-metastatic niche. *Nature,* Vol.438, No.7069, (Dec 8 2005), pp. 820-827

Kaplan, R.N., Psaila, B., and Lyden, D. (2007). Niche-to-niche migration of bone-marrow-derived cells. *Trends Mol Med,* Vol.13, No.2, (Feb 2007), pp. 72-81

Kaufmann, S.H., and Steensma, D.P. (2005). On the TRAIL of a new therapy for leukemia. *Leukemia,* Vol.19, No.12, (Dec 2005), pp. 2195-2202

Kelley, S.K., Harris, L.A., Xie, D., Deforge, L., Totpal, K., Bussiere, J., and Fox, J.A. (2001). Preclinical studies to predict the disposition of Apo2L/tumor necrosis factor-related apoptosis-inducing ligand in humans: characterization of in vivo efficacy, pharmacokinetics, and safety. *J Pharmacol Exp Ther,* Vol.299, No.1, (Oct 2001), pp. 31-38

Kim, S.M., Lim, J.Y., Park, S.I., Jeong, C.H., Oh, J.H., Jeong, M., Oh, W., Park, S.H., Sung, Y.C., and Jeun, S.S. (2008). Gene therapy using TRAIL-secreting human umbilical cord blood-derived mesenchymal stem cells against intracranial glioma. *Cancer Res,* Vol.68, No.23, (Dec 1 2008), pp. 9614-9623

Kucia, M., Reca, R., Miekus, K., Wanzeck, J., Wojakowski, W., Janowska-Wieczorek, A., Ratajczak, J., and Ratajczak, M.Z. (2005). Trafficking of normal stem cells and metastasis of cancer stem cells involve similar mechanisms: pivotal role of the SDF-1-CXCR4 axis. *Stem Cells,* Vol.23, No.7, (Aug 2005), pp. 879-894

Laconi, E., Pani, P., and Farber, E. (2000). The resistance phenotype in the development and treatment of cancer. *Lancet Oncol,* Vol.1, (Dec 2000), pp. 235-241

Lamhamedi-Cherradi, S.E., Zheng, S.J., Maguschak, K.A., Peschon, J., and Chen, Y.H. (2003). Defective thymocyte apoptosis and accelerated autoimmune diseases in TRAIL-/-mice. *Nat Immunol,* Vol.4, No.3, (Mar 2003), pp. 255-260

Lavazza, C., Carlo-Stella, C., Giacomini, A., Cleris, L., Righi, M., Sia, D., Di Nicola, M., Magni, M., Longoni, P., Milanesi, M., Francolini, M., Gloghini, A., Carbone, A., Formelli, F., and Gianni, A.M. (2010). Human CD34+ cells engineered to express membrane-bound tumor necrosis factor-related apoptosis-inducing ligand target both tumor cells and tumor vasculature. *Blood,* Vol.115, No.11, (Mar 18 2010), pp. 2231-2240

Lawrence, D., Shahrokh, Z., Marsters, S., Achilles, K., Shih, D., Mounho, B., Hillan, K., Totpal, K., DeForge, L., Schow, P., Hooley, J., Sherwood, S., Pai, R., Leung, S., Khan, L., Gliniak, B., Bussiere, J., Smith, C.A., Strom, S.S., Kelley, S., Fox, J.A., Thomas, D., and Ashkenazi, A. (2001). Differential hepatocyte toxicity of recombinant Apo2L/TRAIL versions. *Nat Med,* Vol.7, No.4, (Apr 2001), pp. 383-385

Lee, J., Hampl, M., Albert, P., and Fine, H.A. (2002). Antitumor activity and prolonged expression from a TRAIL-expressing adenoviral vector. *Neoplasia (New York, N.Y.),* Vol.4, No.4, (2002), pp. 312-323

Loebinger, M.R., Eddaoudi, A., Davies, D., and Janes, S.M. (2009). Mesenchymal stem cell delivery of TRAIL can eliminate metastatic cancer. *Cancer Res,* Vol.69, No.10, (May 15 2009), pp. 4134-4142

Lucken-Ardjomande, S., and Martinou, J.C. (2005). Newcomers in the process of mitochondrial permeabilization. *J Cell Sci,* Vol.118, No.Pt 3, (Feb 1 2005), pp. 473-483

Menon, L.G., Kelly, K., Wei Yang, H., Kim, S.K., Black, P.M., and Carroll, R.S. (2009). Human Bone Marrow Derived Mesenchymal Stromal Cells Expressing S-TRAIL as a Cellular Delivery Vehicle for Human Glioma Therapy. *Stem Cells,* (May 28 2009), pp.

Mitsiades, C.S., Treon, S.P., Mitsiades, N., Shima, Y., Richardson, P., Schlossman, R., Hideshima, T., and Anderson, K.C. (2001). TRAIL/Apo2L ligand selectively induces apoptosis and overcomes drug resistance in multiple myeloma: therapeutic applications. *Blood,* Vol.98, No.3, (2001/8/1 2001), pp. 795-804

Mohr, A., Lyons, M., Deedigan, L., Harte, T., Shaw, G., Howard, L., Barry, F., O'Brien, T., and Zwacka, R. (2008). Mesenchymal Stem Cells expressing TRAIL lead to tumour growth inhibition in an experimental lung cancer model. *J Cell Mol Med,* (Mar 28 2008), pp.

Najbauer, J., Danks, M., Schmidt, N., Kim, S., and Aboody, K. (2007). Neural stem cell-mediated therapy of primary and metastatic solid tumors. *Progress in Gene Therapy, Autologous and Cancer Stem Cell Gene Therapy. World Scientific: Singapore,* (2007), pp.

Pan, G., Ni, J., Wei, Y.F., Yu, G., Gentz, R., and Dixit, V.M. (1997a). An antagonist decoy receptor and a death domain-containing receptor for TRAIL. *Science,* Vol.277, No.5327, (Aug 8 1997a), pp. 815-818

Pan, G., O'Rourke, K., Chinnaiyan, A.M., Gentz, R., Ebner, R., Ni, J., and Dixit, V.M. (1997b). The receptor for the cytotoxic ligand TRAIL. *Science,* Vol.276, No.5309, (Apr 4 1997b), pp. 111-113

Peled, A., Petit, I., Kollet, O., Magid, M., Ponomaryov, T., Byk, T., Nagler, A., Ben-Hur, H., Many, A., Shultz, L., Lider, O., Alon, R., Zipori, D., and Lapidot, T. (1999). Dependence of human stem cell engraftment and repopulation of NOD/SCID mice on CXCR4. *Science,* Vol.283, No.5403, (Feb 5 1999), pp. 845-848

Petit, I., Jin, D., and Rafii, S. (2007). The SDF-1-CXCR4 signaling pathway: a molecular hub modulating neo-angiogenesis. *Trends Immunol,* Vol.28, No.7, (Jul 2007), pp. 299-307

Pollack, I.F., Erff, M., and Ashkenazi, A. (2001). Direct stimulation of apoptotic signaling by soluble Apo2L/tumor necrosis factor-related apoptosis-inducing ligand leads to selective killing of glioma cells. *Clinical Cancer Research,* Vol.7, No.5, (2001), pp. 1362-1369

Pommier, Y., Sordet, O., Antony, S., Hayward, R.L., and Kohn, K.W. (2004). Apoptosis defects and chemotherapy resistance: molecular interaction maps and networks. *Oncogene,* Vol.23, No.16, (Apr 12 2004), pp. 2934-2949

Rafii, S., Lyden, D., Benezra, R., Hattori, K., and Heissig, B. (2002). Vascular and haematopoietic stem cells: novel targets for anti-angiogenesis therapy? *Nat Rev Cancer,* Vol.2, No.11, (Nov 2002), pp. 826-835

Rieger, J., Naumann, U., Glaser, T., Ashkenazi, A., and Weller, M. (1998). APO2 ligand: a novel lethal weapon against malignant glioma? *FEBS Lett,* Vol.427, No.1, (May 1 1998), pp. 124-128

Rybak, J.N., Ettorre, A., Kaissling, B., Giavazzi, R., Neri, D., and Elia, G. (2005). In vivo protein biotinylation for identification of organ-specific antigens accessible from the vasculature. *Nat Methods,* Vol.2, No.4, (Apr 2005), pp. 291-298

Sasportas, L.S., Kasmieh, R., Wakimoto, H., Hingtgen, S., van de Water, J.A., Mohapatra, G., Figueiredo, J.L., Martuza, R.L., Weissleder, R., and Shah, K. (2009). Assessment of therapeutic efficacy and fate of engineered human mesenchymal stem cells for cancer therapy. *Proc Natl Acad Sci U S A,* Vol.106, No.12, (Mar 24 2009), pp. 4822-4827

Scaffidi, C., Fulda, S., Srinivasan, A., Friesen, C., Li, F., Tomaselli, K.J., Debatin, K.M., Krammer, P.H., and Peter, M.E. (1998). Two CD95 (APO-1/Fas) signaling pathways. *Embo J,* Vol.17, No.6, (Mar 16 1998), pp. 1675-1687

Sheridan, J.P., Marsters, S.A., Pitti, R.M., Gurney, A., Skubatch, M., Baldwin, D., Ramakrishnan, L., Gray, C.L., Baker, K., Wood, W.I., Goddard, A.D., Godowski, P., and Ashkenazi, A. (1997). Control of TRAIL-induced apoptosis by a family of signaling and decoy receptors. *Science,* Vol.277, No.5327, (Aug 8 1997), pp. 818-821

Smyth, M.J., Takeda, K., Hayakawa, Y., Peschon, J.J., van den Brink, M.R., and Yagita, H. (2003). Nature's TRAIL--on a path to cancer immunotherapy. *Immunity,* Vol.18, No.1, (Jan 2003), pp. 1-6

Uzzaman, M., Keller, G., and Germano, I.M. (2009). In vivo gene delivery by embryonic-stem-cell-derived astrocytes for malignant gliomas. *Neuro Oncol,* Vol.11, No.2, (Apr 2009), pp. 102-108

Verfaillie, C.M. (1998). Adhesion Receptors as Regulators of the Hematopoietic Process. *Blood,* Vol.92, No.8, (October 15, 1998 1998), pp. 2609-2612

Verhagen, A.M., and Vaux, D.L. (2002). Cell death regulation by the mammalian IAP antagonist Diablo/Smac. *Apoptosis,* Vol.7, No.2, (Apr 2002), pp. 163-166

Wajant, H. (2003). Death receptors. *Essays Biochem,* Vol.39, (2003), pp. 53-71

Walczak, H., Degli-Esposti, M.A., Johnson, R.S., Smolak, P.J., Waugh, J.Y., Boiani, N., Timour, M.S., Gerhart, M.J., Schooley, K.A., Smith, C.A., Goodwin, R.G., and Rauch, C.T. (1997). TRAIL-R2: a novel apoptosis-mediating receptor for TRAIL. *Embo J,* Vol.16, No.17, (Sep 1 1997), pp. 5386-5397

Walczak, H., Miller, R.E., Ariail, K., Gliniak, B., Griffith, T.S., Kubin, M., Chin, W., Jones, J., Woodward, A., Le, T., Smith, C., Smolak, P., Goodwin, R.G., Rauch, C.T., Schuh, J.C., and Lynch, D.H. (1999). Tumoricidal activity of tumor necrosis factor-related apoptosis-inducing ligand in vivo. *Nat Med,* Vol.5, No.2, (Feb 1999), pp. 157-163

Wang, S., and El-Deiry, W.S. (2003). TRAIL and apoptosis induction by TNF-family death receptors. *Oncogene,* Vol.22, No.53, (Nov 24 2003), pp. 8628-8633

Waxman, D.J., and Schwartz, P.S. (2003). Harnessing apoptosis for improved anticancer gene therapy. *Cancer Res,* Vol.63, No.24, (Dec 15 2003), pp. 8563-8572

Wels, J., Kaplan, R.N., Rafii, S., and Lyden, D. (2008). Migratory neighbors and distant invaders: tumor-associated niche cells. *Genes Dev,* Vol.22, No.5, (Mar 1 2008), pp. 559-574

Wiley, S.R., Schooley, K., Smolak, P.J., Din, W.S., Huang, C.P., Nicholl, J.K., Sutherland, G.R., Smith, T.D., Rauch, C., and Smith, C.A. (1995). Identification and characterization of a new member of the TNF family that induces apoptosis. *Immunity,* Vol.3, No.6, (Dec 1995), pp. 673-682

29

Pyrrole-Imidazole Polyamides for Gene Therapy: Bioanalytical Methods and Pharmacokinetics

Tomonori Kamei[1], Takahiko Aoyama[1], Takahiro Ueno[2],
Noboru Fukuda[2,3], Hiroki Nagase[3,4] and Yoshiaki Matsumoto[1]
[1]*Department of Clinical Pharmacokinetics, School of Pharmacy, Nihon University*
[2]*Department of Medicine, Division of Nephrology and Endocrinology*
Nihon University School of Medicine
[3]*Advanced Research Institute for the Science and Humanities, Nihon University*
[4]*Division of Cancer Genetics, Department of Advanced Medical Science*
Nihon University School of Medicine
Japan

1. Introduction

Pyrrole(Py)-imidazole(Im)(PI) polyamides are small synthetic molecules composed of aromatic rings of *N*-methylpyrrole and *N*-methylimidazole amino acids (Trauger et al., 1996). Synthetic polyamides recognize and bind to specific nucleotide sequences in the minor groove of double-helical DNA with high affinity (Pilch et al., 1996). Various sequence-specific DNA-binding PI polyamides have been developed to regulate gene expression by targeting the promoter regions of enhancer and transcription factor-binding elements in vitro (Murty et al., 2004). PI polyamides were first identified from duocarmycin A and distamycin A, which bind in the minor groove of DNA (Tao et al., 1999; Trauger et al., 1996). Sequence-specific DNA recognition by PI polyamide depends on the sequence of side-by-side amino acid pairs. A pair of Py opposite Im targets the CG base pair, whereas Im opposite Py recognizes the GC base pair, and the Py/Py combination binds to both AT and TA base pairs (White et al., 1997). PI polyamides designed to bind to the transcription factors Ets-1, lymphoid-enhancer binding factor 1, and the TATAbox-binding protein DNA binding site have been shown to inhibit virus replication in isolated human peripheral blood lymphocytes (Dickinson et al., 1998).

PI polyamides can easily enter into the nucleus and bind to chromosomal DNA. Many promising observation for gene therapy using PI polyamides have been reported. PI polyamide targeting rat transforming growth factor (TGF)-β_1 has been reported to inhibit the expressions of TGF-β_1 mRNA and protein in the renal cortex of Dahl-S rats. The targeted PI polyamide also reduced glomerulosclerosis and interstitial fibrosis without side effects. These observations indicate that PI polyamides will be effective for TGF-β_1-related diseases, including progressive renal injury (Matsuda et al., 2011; Matsuda et al., 2006). PI polyamides targeting human aurora kinase-A (AURKA) and -B (AURKB) promoters significantly inhibited the promoter activities, and mRNA and protein expression levels of AURKA and

AURKB. They also demonstrated a marked antiproliferative synergy in human tumor cell lines as a result of induction of apoptosis-mediated severe catastrophe of cell-cycle progression (Takahashi et al., 2008). PI polyamides specifically inhibited lectin-like oxidized low-density lipoprotein receptor-1 mRNA expression and apoptosis induced by oxidized low-density lipoprotein and angiotensin II in human umbilical vein endothelial cells (Ueno et al., 2009). From these observations, PI polyamides have been identified as novel candidates for gene therapy.

Pharmacokinetics is the science that studies the behavior of a circulating drug administered to a body, mainly focusing on absorption, distribution, metabolism, and excretion (ADME) of a drug (Jang et al., 2001). The concentration of a drug in a body can be obtained by a bioanalytical method which includes sample extraction and detection of a drug, and the obtained data are analyzed to evaluate the pharmacokinetics of the drug. Needless to say, a robust bioanalytical procedure is crucial for evaluating the appropriate pharmacokinetic profile of a drug.

In this chapter, we show the bioanalytical procedure, pharmacokinetics, and modeling of PI polyamides A and B. PI polyamides A and B are illustrated in Fig. 1. PI polyamide A was composed of Ac-ImPyPy-ImPyPy-β-Dp (β, β-alanine; Dp, *N*, *N*-dimethylaminopropylamide). PI polyamide B was composed of Ac-PyPy-β-PyImPy-PyPyPy-β-ImPy-β-Dp. The molecular weights of PI polyamides A and B were calculated from the sum of the standard atomic weights of all the atoms (Wieser, 2006). The molecular weights of PI polyamides A and B are 1035.12 and 1665.78, respectively. PI polyamide B was designed to bind to the activator protein-1 (AP-1)-binding site of the TGF-β_1 promoter, whereas PI polyamide A also, with a hairpin structure, was designed for comparing with other types of PI polyamide with a hairpin structure and a higher molecular weight.

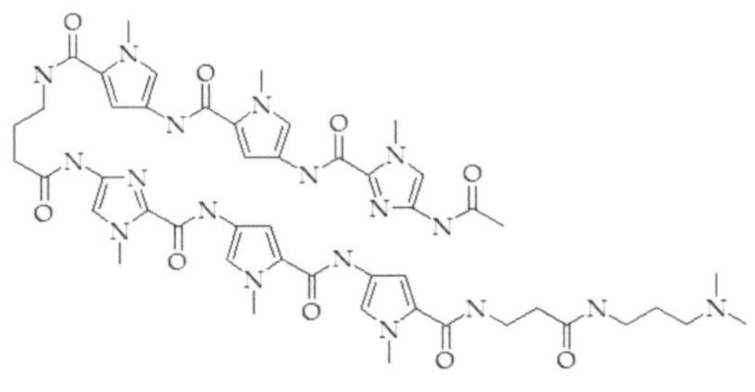

PI polyamide A

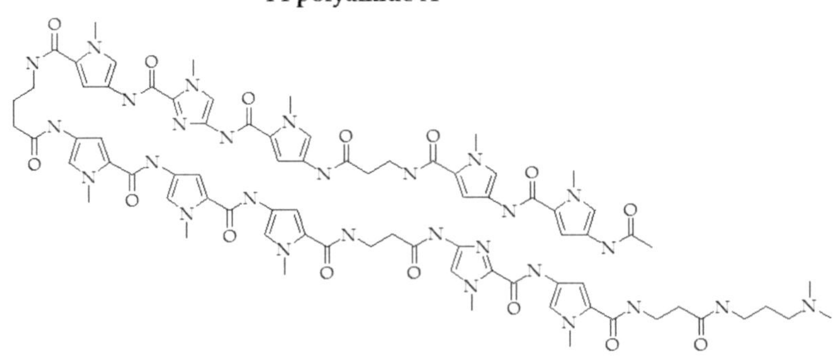

PI polyamide B

Fig. 1. Chemical structures of PI polyamides A and B.

2. Bioanalytics

High-performance liquid chromatography (HPLC) has been used for many years as a useful and conventional tool for the analysis of a drug. Bioanalytical methods by HPLC with UV detection were developed for the determination of PI polyamides A and B in the rat matrix. Sample extraction is one of the important steps and key to success in constructing a robust method. A simple protein precipitation method was developed for the extraction of PI polyamides A and B from rat plasma, whereas solid phase extraction was carried out to extract PI polyamides A and B from rat urine and bile, because a large number of urinary and biliary matrices can interfere with the compounds. It is important to determine the rates of urinary and biliary excretions because these excretions play pivotal roles in the elimination pathway of a drug. The developed methods were successively validated for selectivity, sensitivity, linearity, accuracy, and precision, following the guideline for Bioanalytical Method Validation published by Food and Drug Administration in 2001.

Chromatographic separation was conducted using a reversed-phase TSK-GEL ODS-80T_M (4.6 mm x 150 mm) column maintained at 40 °C. The mobile phase of solvent A was 0.1% acetic acid and that of solvent B was acetonitrile (a linear increase from 0 to 80% B over 10 min (plasma and urine) or 35 min (bile) and an isocratic flow at 60% B for 5 min). The flow rate was set at 1.0 mL/min (plasma and urine) or 0.75 mL/min (bile). The detection wavelength was set at 310 nm. PI polyamides A and B were well separated from the coextracted material under the described chromatographic conditions at approximate retention times of 9.7 (25.0 in bile) and 10.5 min, respectively. The peak shapes were satisfactory and completely resolved from one another. No interference from rat matrices was observed (Fukasawa et al., 2007).

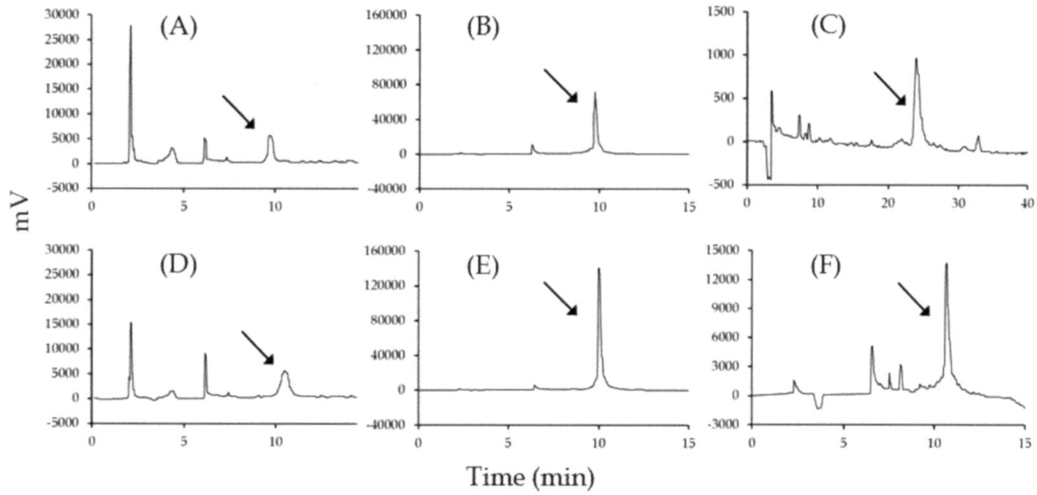

Fig. 2. Representative chromatograms of blank rat plasma (A), blank rat urine (B) and blank rat bile (C) spiked with PI polyamide A, and blank rat plasma (D), blank rat urine (E) and blank rat bile (F) spiked with PI polyamide B. The concentrations of PI polyamides were 5 (A), 20 (B), 1 (C), 5 (D), 20 (E) and 5 (F) μg/mL.

Table 1 shows the intra- and inter-assay precision and accuracy of PI polyamides A and B. The intra- and inter-assay accuracies (RE) were within ± 20% for the lower limit of quantitation (LLOQ) and ± 15% for the other QC samples. The intra- and inter-assay precisions (CV) were also within the acceptable ranges of 20% for the LLOQ and 15% for the other QC samples. The LLOQ was determined as 1 μg/mL for both PI polyamides A and B. All of the methods were successfully applied to evaluate the pharmacokinetics of the PI polyamides (Fukasawa et al., 2009; Fukasawa et al., 2007; Nagashima et al., 2009b).

Matrix		Nominal concentration (μg/mL)	Intra-assay		Inter-assay	
			RE (%)	CV (%)	RE (%)	CV (%)
Plasma	PI polyamide A	1	2.2	5.3	6.7	14.4
		20	1.4	1.4	-8.7	9.7
		100	7.7	3.7	3.6	3.5
	PI polyamide B	1	2.8	10.0	2.2	15.0
		20	-2.5	0.6	-9.2	7.9
		100	3.7	2.6	3.2	3.2
Urine	PI polyamide A	1	13.4	1.2	4.6	7.9
		20	-0.9	0.7	-4.7	3.6
		200	0.4	0.3	-2.6	4.5
	PI polyamide B	1	7.3	1.9	11.9	4.4
		10	1.9	1.2	0.1	2.3
		20	0.4	0.5	0.1	0.8

Table 1. Intra- and inter-assay accuracy and precision for the determination of PI polyamides A and B in rat plasma and urine.

Although HPLC with UV detection is a useful tool for the determination of a drug, the sensitivity is a limitation factor for evaluating pharmacokinetic characteristic for many hours. Recently, liquid chromatography-tandem mass spectrometry (LC-MS/MS) has been used for the determination of a drug, especially when a sensitivity higher than that of HPLC is required. A bioanalytical method for the determination of PI polyamide A in rat plasma was successfully developed and validated by ultra-performance liquid chromatography (UPLC)-MS/MS with electrospray ionization (Nagashima et al., 2009a).

An MS scan was conducted in the positive ion mode to obtain the precursor ion of PI polyamide A. The mass spectra of PI polyamide A showed significant ions at the *m/z* of 1036, 519, and 346, which corresponds to $[M+H]^+$, $[M+2H]^{2+}$, and $[M+3H]^{3+}$, respectively (Fig. 3). The doubly charged polyamide showed the highest sensitivity during ionization. The product ion spectra of the doubly charged PI polyamide A are shown in Fig. 4. The multiple reaction monitoring (MRM) transition was selected at the *m/z* of 519 and 288.

Chromatographic separation was performed using an ACQUITY UPLC HSS T3 (1.8 μm, 2.1×50 mm) column with an in-line filter and maintained at 40 °C. The liquid flow rate was set at 0.3 mL/min. The mobile phase of solvent A was acetonitrile/water/acetic acid (5/95/0.1, v/v/v) and that of solvent B was acetonitrile/water/acetic acid (95/5/0.1, v/v/v). The gradient started at the mobile phase A-B (95:5%), changed linearly to A-B (45:55%) until 2 min, washed with A-B (0:100%) until 3.5 min, and equilibrated under the initial condition until 5.5 min. PI polyamide A was well separated from the coextracted material under the described conditions at an approximate retention time of 1.5 min. No interference from rat matrices was observed (Fig. 5).

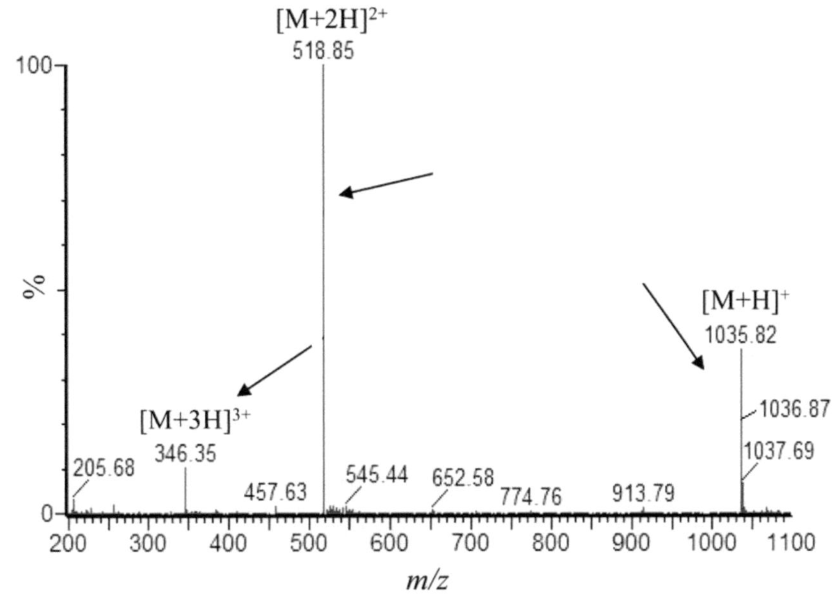

Fig. 3. Representative mass spectra of precursor ions (m/z, 1036 $[M+H]^+$, 519 $[M+2H]^{2+}$, and 346 $[M+3H]^{3+}$) of PI polyamide A.

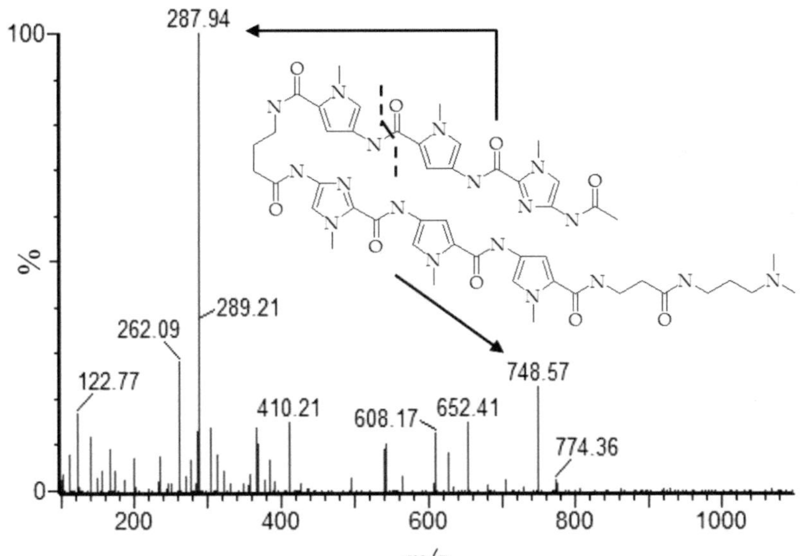

Fig. 4. Representative product ion mass spectra (*m/z*, 519) of PI polyamide A.

Table 2 shows the intra- and inter-assay precision and accuracy of PI polyamide A. The intra- and inter-assay accuracies (RE) were within ± 20% for the LLOQ and ± 15% for the other QC samples. The intra- and inter-assay precisions (CV) were also within the acceptable ranges of 20% for the LLOQ and 15% for the other QC samples. The LLOQ was

10 ng/mL, which means it has a sufficient sensitivity to evaluate the pharmacokinetics of PI polyamides.

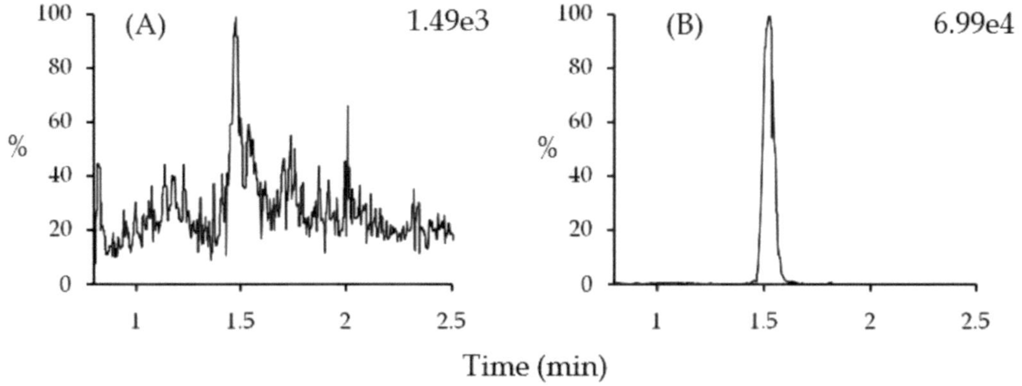

Fig. 5. Representative MRM chromatograms (*m/z*, 519>288) of (A) blank rat plasma, (B) blank rat plasma spiked with PI polyamide A (10 ng/mL).

Nominal concentration (ng/mL)	Intra-assay		Inter-assay	
	RE (%)	CV (%)	RE (%)	CV (%)
10	-10.6	3.3	3.7	11.2
1000	-11.7	1.5	-2.1	9.2
10000	-0.6	4.6	-5.0	8.9

Table 2. Intra- and inter-assay accuracy and precision for the determination of PI polyamide A in rat plasma.

3. Pharmacokinetics of PI polyamides A and B

3.1 Plasma and lung concentrations of PI polyamides A and B

PI polyamide B significantly inhibited the expressions of TGF-β_1 mRNA and protein in the renal cortex of the Dahl-S rats and reduced the rates of increases in the amounts of urinary protein and albumin in the Dahl-S rats independent of blood pressure at a dose of 1.0 mg (Matsuda et al., 2006). From these observations, the doses of PI polyamides were selected on the basis of 1.0 mg dose of PI polyamide B per rat (about 3.0 mg/kg). PI polyamide B had a lower water solubility than PI polyamide A. The doses of PI polyamides A and B were determined to be in the ranges of 1.3-15.0 mg/kg and 1.0-5.0 mg/kg, respectively.

The mean plasma concentration-time profiles after the intravenous administration of PI polyamide A at 1.3, 2.0, 7.5, and 15.0 mg/kg and after that of PI polyamide B at 1.0, 2.0, 3.0, and 5.0 mg/kg are shown in Fig. 6. The plasma concentrations of PI polyamides A and B declined in a polyexponential manner for the four doses studied. The plasma concentration-time profiles of PI polyamides were analyzed by a non-compartmental method. The area under the plasma concentration-time curve ($AUC_{(0\text{-}Tlast)}$) and the area under the first moment curve ($AUMC_{(0\text{-}Tlast)}$) were obtained using the linear trapezoidal rule. $AUC_{(Tlast\text{-}\infty)}$ and $AUMC_{(Tlast\text{-}\infty)}$ were respectively calculated using C_n/λ_z and $t_nC_n/\lambda_z + C_n/\lambda_z{}^2$, where C_n is the last quantifiable concentration. Terminal-phase rate constant (λ_z) was calculated by the regression of the terminal log-linear portion of the plasma concentration curve. Terminal elimination half-life ($t_{1/2}$) was calculated to be $0.693/\lambda_z$. Systemic clearance (CL_t), mean residence time (MRT), and the volume of distribution in the steady state (V_{ss}) were calculated as dose/AUC, AUMC/AUC, and $CL_t \bullet MRT$, respectively. The plasma concentrations of PI polyamides A and B were extrapolated to time zero (C_0). The maximum plasma concentration (C_{max}) of PI polyamide B was directly obtained from the observed data.

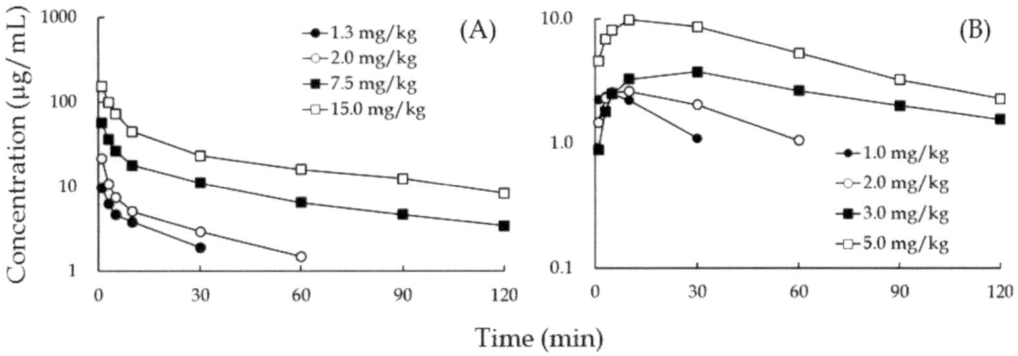

Fig. 6. Mean plasma concentration–time profiles of PI polyamides in rats after intravenous administration. (A) and (B) show PI polyamides A and B.

The pharmacokinetic parameters of PI polyamides A and B obtained in rats using non-compartmental analysis are summarized in Table 3. After the intravenous administration of PI polyamide A at 1.3, 2.0, 7.5, and 15.0 mg/kg, the average $t_{1/2}$, CL_t, and V_{ss} values were in the ranges of 42.3-74.8 min, 4.6-6.4 mL/min/kg, and 244-412 mL/kg, respectively. After the intravenous administration of PI polyamide B at 1.0, 2.0, 3.0, and 5.0 mg/kg, the average $t_{1/2}$, CL_t, and V_{ss} values were in the ranges of 27.5-58.7 min, 7.3-11.9 mL/min/kg, and 407-667 mL/kg, respectively. The CL_t and V_{ss} of PI polyamides A and B showed no significant differences as functions of administration dose. The pharmacokinetics of PI polyamides A and B are linear in the intravenous dose ranges of 1.3-15.0 mg/kg and 1.0-5.0 mg/kg, respectively as revealed by the fact that AUC increased linearly as a function of dose, and CL_t and V_{ss} remained unaltered.

The plasma concentration-time profiles after the intravenous administration of PI polyamide B resembled those after the oral administration. After the intravenous administration of PI polyamide B at 1.0, 2.0, 3.0, and 5.0 mg/kg, C_{max} gradually increased. The concentrations of PI polyamide B in the lungs, liver, heart, kidney and spleen were measured. The mean concentrations of PI polyamide B in the lungs were the highest among those in other tissues, and the mean concentrations 10, 30, and 60 min after injection were 134.7, 97.0, and 73.9 μg/g, respectively. Among various tissues, the concentration of PI polyamide B was observed to be highest in the lungs. The mean lung concentration of PI polyamide B decreased with time.

PI polyamide A

Parameter	Dose			
	1.3 mg/kg	2.0 mg/kg	7.5 mg/kg	15.0 mg/kg
Body weight (kg)	0.267	0.291	0.243	0.26
$t_{1/2}$ (min)	54.8	42.3	74.8	45.3
C_0 (μg/mL)	14.1	22.9	77.1	227.5
AUC (μg min/kg)	259.6	316.8	1528.6	3331.9
Cl (mL/min/kg)	5.6	6.4	5.1	4.6
Vss (mL/kg)	305.8	274.6	411.8	243.7
MRT (min)	68.1	42.6	80.5	54

PI polyamide B

Parameter	Dose			
	1.0 mg/kg	2.0 mg/kg	3.0 mg/kg	5.0 mg/kg
Body weight (kg)	0.313	0.317	0.317	0.317
$t_{1/2}$ (min)	139.1	165.8	207.3	359.3
C_0 (μg/mL)	1.5	4	3.8	4
AUC (μg min/kg)	108.1	205.2	326.8	508.3
Cl (mL/min/kg)	9.9	8.9	9.2	10.3
Vss (mL/kg)	2170.5	1990.1	2602.2	4567
MRT (min)	194.7	222.5	289.7	492.1

Table 3. Mean non-compartmental pharmacokinetic parameters of PI polyamides after intravenous administration at various doses into rats (n = 3).

3.2 Urinary and biliary excretions

Determination of the urinary and biliary excretion rates is crucial for the evaluation of the pharmacokinetics of a drug, because drugs are usually eliminated from the body into urine and/or bile (Ullrich, 1997; van Montfoort et al., 2003). The urinary and biliary excretion rate-time profiles are shown in Figs. 7 and 8, respectively. The urinary excretion rates of PI polyamides A and B showed a linear elimination. The biliary excretion rate of PI polyamide A showed saturation at the early period, while PI polyamide B was not detected in the bile. The cumulative urinary excretion rates of PI polyamides A and B at 48 h were 72.4 ± 11.6 and 4.8 ± 0.5% (mean ± SD, n = 3) of the administered dose, respectively. The cumulative biliary excretion rate of PI polyamide A at 24 h was 4.3 ± 0.4% (n = 4) of the administered dose. These observations indicated that unchanged PI polyamides A and B were slowly eliminated from the body. As observed from the plasma concentration-time profile, it is considered that most of the PI polyamide B remained in the lungs. No peaks of metabolites were detected for all the samples.

The differences in the molecular weights of compounds affect their eliminations (Hirom et al., 1976). The molecular weight thresholds for the excretion of organic cations into rat bile were found to be in the ranges of 200 ± 50 for monovalent organic cations and 500-600 for bivalent organic cations. (Hughes et al., 1973a; b) PI polyamide with a molecular weight of

1422.51 was excreted at 2% into rat urine 24 h after administration and was not detected in rat bile (data not shown). These findings suggested that PI polyamides with high molecular weights tend to be poorly excreted in both rat urine and bile, whereas those with molecular weights less than that of PI polyamide A can be readily eliminated. As described above, the differences in the elimination pathway between PI polyamides A and B may be attributed to the differences in their molecular weights.

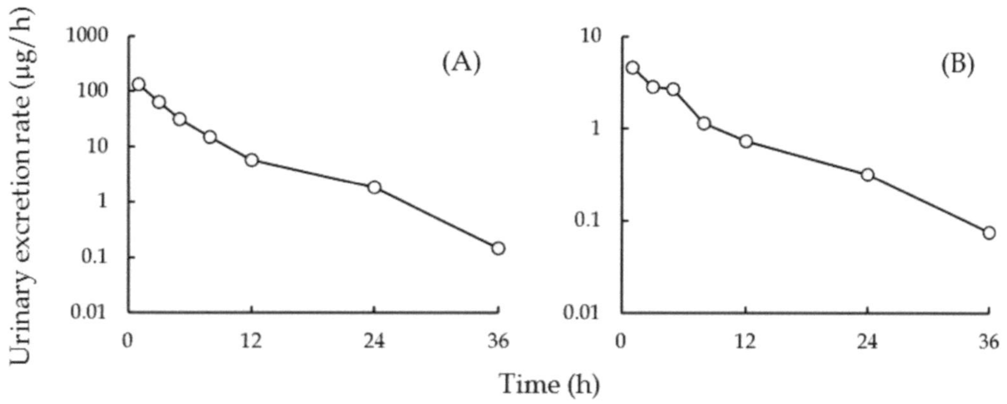

Fig. 7. Urinary excretion rate versus time profile of PI polyamides A (A) and B (B) in rats.

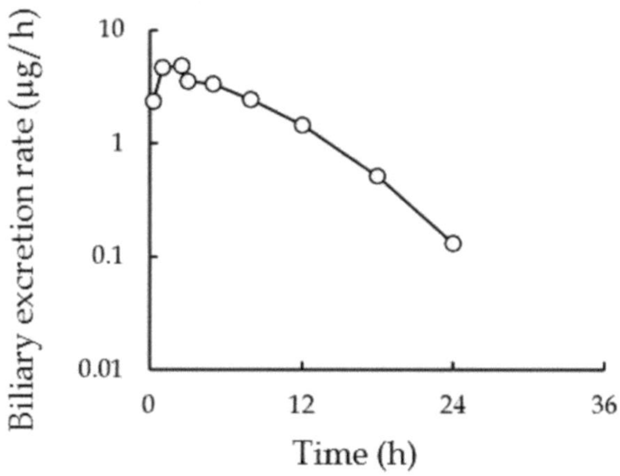

Fig. 8. Biliary excretion rate versus time profile of PI polyamide A in rats.

4. Pharmacokinetic modeling and simulations

4.1 Pharmacokinetic modeling

The plasma concentration-time profiles after the intravenous administration of PI polyamide A was fitted well by a two-compartment model. The estimated pharmacokinetic parameters using the model are summarized in Table 4. After the intravenous administration of PI polyamide A at 1.3, 2.0, 7.5, and 15.0 mg/kg, the average CL_t and V_{ss} values were in the ranges of 4.9-7.0 mL/min/kg and 245-335 mL/kg, respectively. The CL_t and V_{ss} values estimated using a two-compartment model and a non-compartment model are thought to be identical.

Parameter	Dose			
	1.3 mg/kg	2.0 mg/kg	7.5 mg/kg	15.0 mg/kg
CL_t (mL/min/kg)	5.8	7	5.8	4.9
V_{ss} (mL/kg)	335	250	323	245
V_c (mL/kg)	90.5	89.6	96.6	69.7

Table 4. Estimated pharmacokinetic parameters of PI polyamide A obtained using two-compartment model.

The plasma concentration-time profiles after the intravenous administration of PI polyamide B increased in the early phase and resembled those after the oral administration. The slope of the decline in the lung concentration-time profiles of PI polyamide B was nearly equal to that in the plasma concentration-time profiles of PI polyamide B. To describe the increasing phase of PI polyamide B after the intravenous administration, the lung and plasma concentration-time profiles of PI polyamide B were fitted using a catenary two-compartment model (Fig. 9) (Brown et al., 1981).

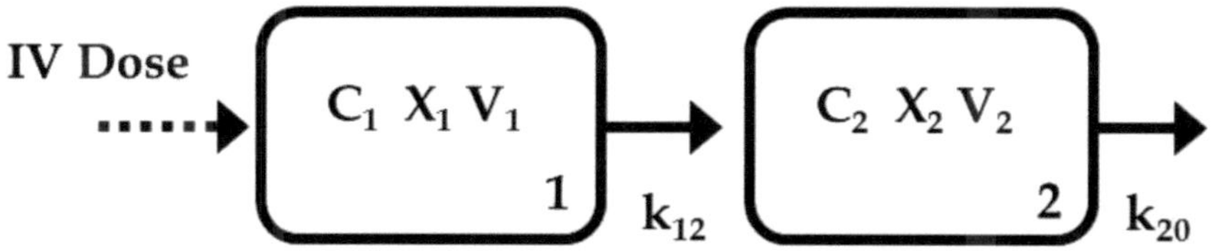

Fig. 9. Pharmacokinetic model of PI polyamide B.

C_1, X_1, and V_1 represent the concentration of PI polyamide B in the lungs, the amount of PI polyamide B in the lungs, and the distribution volume of the lung compartment, respectively. C_2, X_2, and V_2 represent the concentration of PI polyamide B in plasma, the amount of PI polyamide B in plasma, and the distribution volume of the plasma compartment, respectively. The pharmacokinetic parameters were calculated using the NONMEM program.

Figure 10 shows the simulation curves for PI polyamide B based on the catenary two-compartment model. The plasma and lung concentrations were fitted well by the model. The estimated pharmacokinetic parameters after the intravenous administration of PI polyamide B are summarized in Table 5. The estimated coefficients of variation (CV%) were small, the catenary two-compartment model better fitted the concentration-time profile after the intravenous administration of PI polyamide B. The model-estimated clearance (6.8 mL/min/kg) calculated as k_{20} multiplied by V_2 was nearly equal to CL_t (7.3 mL/min/kg). In this study, lung concentrations of first-point were measured at 10 min. It is thought that the concentration in the lungs immediately after the intravenous administration of PI polyamide B is higher than the calculated value. The early-plasma concentration-time profiles after the intravenous administration of a hairpin polyamide-chlorambucil conjugate, duocarmycin, and nitroglycerin are similar to that of PI polyamide B (Alberts et al., 1998; Chou et al., 2008; Wester et al., 1983) Recently, the biodistribution of a hairpin polyamide-chlorambucil conjugate administered into mice has been reported (Chou et al., 2008). The predominant occupancy of the polyamide-chlorambucil conjugate was observed in the lungs, spleen, small intestine, and pancreas 2 and 24 h after the injection. The concentration of polyamide-chlorambucil conjugate in the lungs at 2 h was higher than that of the polyamide-chlorambucil conjugate at 24 h. These findings are consistent with our results. PI polyamide B is distributed in the aorta and localizes in the nuclei of aortic midlayer smooth muscle (Matsuda et al., 2006). The lungs consist of pulmonary alveoli, which are surrounded by capillary vessels. It has been reported that weak basic drugs accumulate in the lungs and that such accumulation is attributable to lysosomal trapping (MacIntyre et al., 1988; Rodgers et al., 2005). A high concentration of PI polyamide B in the lungs was thought to be caused by PI polyamide B being distributed in capillary vessels of the lungs and by PI polyamide B being a weak base compared with PI polyamide with a molecular weight of 1422.51. It is also conceivable that PI polyamide B accumulated in the lungs owing to its high molecular weight, as suggested in a previous study (Wiseman et al., 2000). From these considerations, the proposed catenary two-compartment model may be applicable to describing PI polyamide B in detail.

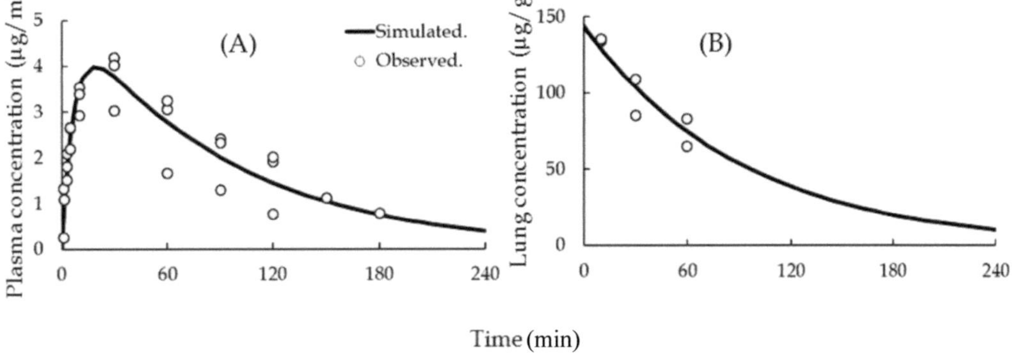

Fig. 10. Model fitted PI polyamide B concentration-time profiles in plasma and lungs. A is plasma concentration–time profiles and B is lung concentration-time profiles. The middle bold line indicates the 50th percentiles for 1000 simulations. Symbols depict the observed data after the intravenous administration of PI polyamide B at 3.0 mg/kg.

4.2 Pharmacokinetic modeling with excretion data in addition to plasma concentration

To predict the plasma concentration-time profile in the elimination phase of PI polyamide A after intravenous administration, two pharmacokinetic models (i.e., one- and two-compartment models with the linear output compartment interpreted as the urine compartment and the non-linear output compartments interpreted as the bile compartment) using the plasma concentration-time profile and cumulative urinary and biliary excretion

Parameter	Estimates
k_{12} (L/min)	0.0109
k_{20} (L/min)	0.1476
V_1 (mL/kg)	20.88
V_2 (mL/kg)	45.86

Table 5. Pharmacokinetic parameters of PI polyamide B from model fitting.

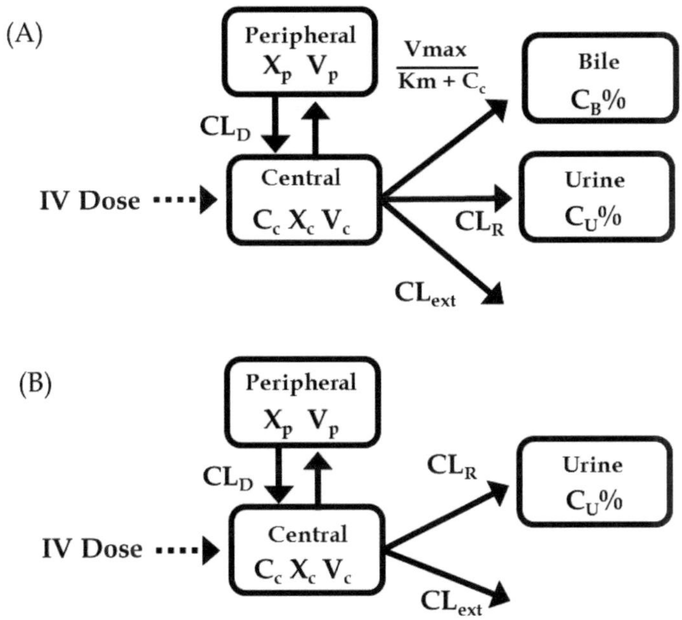

Fig. 11. Scheme of pharmacokinetic model describing the disposition and elimination of PI polyamides A (A) and B (B)

rates of PI polyamide A were tested. A scheme of the two-compartment model, with the linear output compartment interpreted as the urine compartment and the non-linear output compartment interpreted as the bile compartment, is shown in Fig. 11A.

X and V are the amount and volume of distribution in the corresponding compartments designated by the subscripts C, P, U, and B representing central, peripheral, urine, and bile compartments, respectively. CL_D is the distribution clearance, CL_R is the renal clearance, CL_{ext} is the clearance excluding renal and biliary clearances, V_{MAX} is the maximum velocity for excretion into bile, and Km is the Michaelis constant for excretion into bile. Cc represents the plasma concentration of PI polyamide A. C_U% and C_B% represent the cumulative urinary and biliary excretion rates (percentage of administered dose), respectively.

The residual error model of the plasma concentration was assumed to be the proportional error model because the plasma concentration was measured by HPLC. The model of the cumulative urinary and biliary excretions was assumed to be the additive error model because the percentage of the administered dose was calculated from the urine and bile concentrations, urine and bile volumes, and administered dose. The choice of model was based on model fitting criteria such as visual inspection of the fitted curves, objective function value of NONMEM (OFV), and CV% of the parameter estimates (Hazra et al., 2007; Matsumoto et al., 2005).

The plasma concentration and cumulative urinary and biliary excretion-time profiles after intravenous administration of PI polyamide A were fitted well by the two-compartment model with the linear output compartment interpreted as the urine compartment and the non-linear output compartment interpreted as the bile compartment (Fig. 12). The 50th percentiles of the model-based prediction for plasma concentrations and cumulative urinary and biliary excretions are presented together with the observed value. To obtain 50th percentiles of the model estimations, 10000 simulations were performed using the estimated model parameters, variability in the estimated parameters, and residual variability of the data. Compared with a one-compartment model using only plasma data, more accurate data can be obtained from the two-compartment model including urine and bile data because PI polyamide A was excreted into urine and bile until at least 36 and 18 h, respectively, after administration. The plasma concentration-time profile in the elimination phase could also be described better using both the linear and non-linear compartments than using plasma data only.

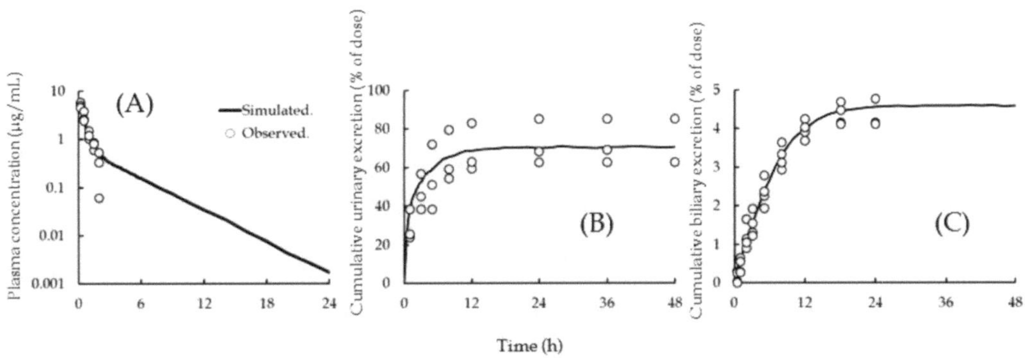

Fig. 12. Plasma concentration–time profile (A), cumulative urinary excretion rate (B), and cumulative biliary excretion rate (C) of PI polyamide A after intravenous administration at 2.0 mg/kg to rats. Each data point represents observed data from three (for plasma and urine) and four rats (for bile). The solid line indicates 50th percentiles from model estimations of 10000 simulations.

To predict the plasma concentration-time profile in the elimination phase of PI polyamide B after intravenous administration, two pharmacokinetic models (i.e., one- and two-compartment models with the linear output compartment interpreted as the urine compartment) using the plasma concentration-time profile and cumulative urinary excretions of PI polyamide B were tested. A scheme of the two-compartment model with the linear output compartment interpreted as the urine compartment is shown in Fig. 11B. The residual error models of the plasma concentration of PI polyamide B were the same as described in the part of PI polyamide A.

The plasma concentration and cumulative urinary excretion-time profiles after intravenous administration of PI polyamide B were fitted well by the two-compartment model with the linear output compartment interpreted as the urine compartment (Fig. 13). The 50th percentiles of the model-based prediction for plasma concentrations and cumulative urinary excretions are presented together with the observed value. To obtain 50th percentiles of the model estimations, 10000 simulations were performed using the estimated model parameters, variability in the estimated parameters, and residual variability of the data.

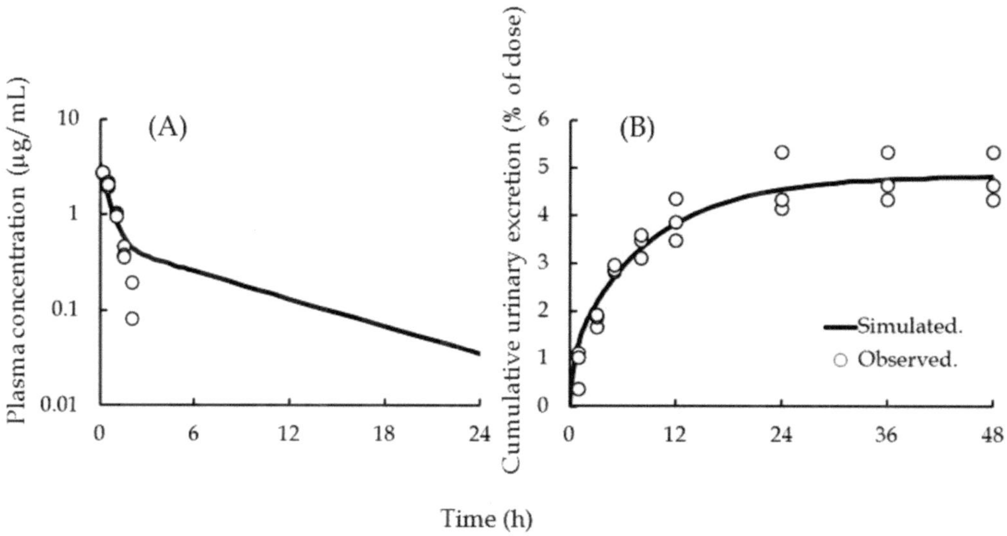

Fig. 13. Plasma concentration–time profile (A) and cumulative urinary excretion (B) of PI polyamide B after intravenous administration at 2.0 mg/kg to rats. Each data point represents observed data from three rats (for plasma and urine). The solid line indicates 50th percentiles from model estimations of 10000 simulations.

To predict the effective dose of PI polyamide B in Dahl-S rats administered at 1 mg every 2 or 3 days for 4 weeks, pharmacokinetic simulations of PI polyamide B were performed using a slightly modified pharmacokinetic model (Nagashima et al., 2009b) by NONMEM program. The average plasma concentrations of PI polyamide B after the administration at 1 mg every 3 and 2 days were 0.18 and 0.28 μg/mL, respectively, which were calculated by the area under the concentration-time curves between 0 and 27 days, divided by 27 days. PI polyamide B did not accumulate following multiple-dose administration.

5. Conclusion

PI polyamides show a remarkable potential for use in non viral gene therapy as many attractive results were obtained. The novel compounds could provide a promising impact on gene therapy for diseases not treatable by current remedies. To obtain the maximum therapeutic effect of the PI polyamide, it is crucial to evaluate the pharmacokinetics of the compounds for designing appropriate dosage regimens. Bioanalytical procedures for PI polyamides A and B were successfully developed and validated by HPLC or LC-MS/MS, and applied to sample assay. The pharmacokinetic profiles of PI polyamides show interesting results, which are thought to be related to their molecular weights (Brown et al.,

1981). It was suggested that the features of various compositions of Py and Im were related to their unique pharmacokinetic profiles. Further examination will be conducted using other PI polyamides that have unique Py and Im combinations for gene therapy.

6. Acknowledgements

This work was supported in part by a Grand-in-Aid from the High-Tech Research Center Project for 2007-2011 and the Academic Frontier Project for 2006-2010 for Private Universities: matching fund subsidy from the Ministry of Education, Culture, Sports, Science and Technology. We thank Takashi Nagashima, Ph.D. and Akiko Fukawasa, Ph.D. for their help.

7. References

Alberts, S. R.; Erlichman, C.; Reid, J. M.; Sloan, J. A.; Ames, M. M.; Richardson, R. L. & Goldberg, R. M. (1998). Phase I study of the duocarmycin semisyntheticderivative KW-2189 given daily for five days every six weeks. *Clin Cancer Res*, Vol. 4, No. 9, pp. 2111-2117, ISSN 1078-0432 (Print) 1078-0432 (Linking).

Brown, P. H.; Krishnamurthy, G. T.; Bobba, V. V. & Kingston, E. (1981). Radiation dose calculation for Tc-99m HIDA in health and disease. *J Nucl Med*, Vol. 22, No. 2, pp. 177-183, ISSN 0161-5505 (Print) 0161-5505 (Linking).

Chou, C. J.; Farkas, M. E.; Tsai, S. M.; Alvarez, D.; Dervan, P. B. & Gottesfeld, J. M. (2008). Small molecules targeting histone H4 as potential therapeutics for chronic myelogenous leukemia. *Mol Cancer Ther*, Vol. 7, No. 4, pp. 769-778, ISSN 1535-7163 (Print) 1535-7163 (Linking).

Dickinson, L. A.; Gulizia, R. J.; Trauger, J. W.; Baird, E. E.; Mosier, D. E.; Gottesfeld, J. M. & Dervan, P. B. (1998). Inhibition of RNA polymerase II transcription in human cells by synthetic DNA-binding ligands. *Proc Natl Acad Sci U S A*, Vol. 95, No. 22, pp. 12890-12895, ISSN 0027-8424 (Print) 0027-8424 (Linking).

Fukasawa, A.; Aoyama, T.; Nagashima, T.; Fukuda, N.; Ueno, T.; Sugiyama, H.; Nagase, H. & Matsumoto, Y. (2009). Pharmacokinetics of pyrrole-imidazole polyamides after intravenous administration in rat. *Biopharm Drug Dispos*, Vol. 30, No. 2, pp. 81-89, ISSN 1099-081X (Electronic) 0142-2782 (Linking).

Fukasawa, A.; Nagashima, T.; Aoyama, T.; Fukuda, N.; Matsuda, H.; Ueno, T.; Sugiyama, H.; Nagase, H. & Matsumoto, Y. (2007). Optimization and validation of a high-performance liquid chromatographic method with UV detection for the determination of pyrrole-imidazole polyamides in rat plasma. *J Chromatogr B Analyt Technol Biomed Life Sci*, Vol. 859, No. 2, pp. 272-275, ISSN 1570-0232 (Print) 1570-0232 (Linking).

Hazra, A.; Pyszczynski, N.; DuBois, D. C.; Almon, R. R. & Jusko, W. J. (2007). Pharmacokinetics of methylprednisolone after intravenous and intramuscular administration in rats. *Biopharm Drug Dispos*, Vol. 28, No. 6, pp. 263-273, ISSN 0142-2782 (Print) 0142-2782 (Linking).

Hirom, P. C.; Millburn, P. & Smith, R. L. (1976). Bile and urine as complementary pathways for the excretion of foreign organic compounds. *Xenobiotica*, Vol. 6, No. 1, pp. 55-64, ISSN 0049-8254 (Print) 0049-8254 (Linking).

Hughes, R. D.; Millburn, P. & Williams, R. T. (1973a). Biliary excretion of some diquaternary ammonium cations in the rat, guinea pig and rabbit. *Biochem J*, Vol. 136, No. 4, pp. 979-984, ISSN 0264-6021 (Print) 0264-6021 (Linking).

Hughes, R. D.; Millburn, P. & Williams, R. T. (1973b). Molecular weight as a factor in the excretion of monoquaternary ammonium cations in the bile of the rat, rabbit and guinea pig. *Biochem J*, Vol. 136, No. 4, pp. 967-978, ISSN 0264-6021 (Print) 0264-6021 (Linking).

Jang, G. R.; Harris, R. Z. & Lau, D. T. (2001). Pharmacokinetics and its role in small molecule drug discovery research. *Med Res Rev*, Vol. 21, No. 5, pp. 382-396, ISSN 0198-6325 (Print) 0198-6325 (Linking).

MacIntyre, A. C. & Cutler, D. J. (1988). The potential role of lysosomes in tissue distribution of weak bases. *Biopharm Drug Dispos*, Vol. 9, No. 6, pp. 513-526, ISSN 0142-2782 (Print) 0142-2782 (Linking).

Matsuda, H.; Fukuda, N.; Ueno, T.; Katakawa, M.; Wang, X.; Watanabe, T.; Matsui, S.; Aoyama, T.; Saito, K.; Bando, T.; Matsumoto, Y.; Nagase, H.; Matsumoto, K. & Sugiyama, H. (2011). Transcriptional inhibition of progressive renal disease by gene silencing pyrrole-imidazole polyamide targeting of the transforming growth factor-beta1 promoter. *Kidney Int*, Vol. 79, No. 1, pp. 46-56, ISSN 1523-1755 (Electronic) 0085-2538 (Linking).

Matsuda, H.; Fukuda, N.; Ueno, T.; Tahira, Y.; Ayame, H.; Zhang, W.; Bando, T.; Sugiyama, H.; Saito, S.; Matsumoto, K.; Mugishima, H. & Serie, K. (2006). Development of gene silencing pyrrole-imidazole polyamide targeting the TGF-beta1 promoter for treatment of progressive renal diseases. *J Am Soc Nephrol*, Vol. 17, No. 2, pp. 422-432, ISSN 1046-6673 (Print) 1046-6673 (Linking).

Matsumoto, Y.; Fujita, T.; Ishida, Y.; Shimizu, M.; Kakuo, H.; Yamashita, K.; Majima, M. & Kumagai, Y. (2005). Population pharmacokinetic-pharmacodynamic modeling of TF-505 using extension of indirect response model by incorporating a circadian rhythm in healthy volunteers. *Biol Pharm Bull*, Vol. 28, No. 8, pp. 1455-1461, ISSN 0918-6158 (Print) 0918-6158 (Linking).

Murty, M. S. & Sugiyama, H. (2004). Biology of N-methylpyrrole-N-methylimidazole hairpin polyamide. *Biol Pharm Bull*, Vol. 27, No. 4, pp. 468-474, ISSN 0918-6158 (Print) 0918-6158 (Linking).

Nagashima, T.; Aoyama, T.; Fukasawa, A.; Watabe, S.; Fukuda, N.; Ueno, T.; Sugiyama, H.; Nagase, H. & Matsumoto, Y. (2009a). Determination of pyrrole-imidazole polyamide in rat plasma by liquid chromatography-tandem mass spectrometry. *J Chromatogr B Analyt Technol Biomed Life Sci*, Vol. 877, No. 11-12, pp. 1070-1076, ISSN 1873-376X (Electronic) 1570-0232 (Linking).

Nagashima, T.; Aoyama, T.; Yokoe, T.; Fukasawa, A.; Fukuda, N.; Ueno, T.; Sugiyama, H.; Nagase, H. & Matsumoto, Y. (2009b). Pharmacokinetic modeling and prediction of plasma pyrrole-imidazole polyamide concentration in rats using simultaneous urinary and biliary excretion data. *Biol Pharm Bull*, Vol. 32, No. 5, pp. 921-927, ISSN 0918-6158 (Print) 0918-6158 (Linking).

Pilch, D. S.; Poklar, N.; Gelfand, C. A.; Law, S. M.; Breslauer, K. J.; Baird, E. E. & Dervan, P. B. (1996). Binding of a hairpin polyamide in the minor groove of DNA: sequence-specific enthalpic discrimination. *Proc Natl Acad Sci U S A*, Vol. 93, No. 16, pp. 8306-8311, ISSN 0027-8424 (Print) 0027-8424 (Linking).

Rodgers, T.; Leahy, D. & Rowland, M. (2005). Tissue distribution of basic drugs: accounting for enantiomeric, compound and regional differences amongst beta-blocking drugs in rat. *J Pharm Sci*, Vol. 94, No. 6, pp. 1237-1248, ISSN 0022-3549 (Print) 0022-3549 (Linking).

Takahashi, T.; Asami, Y.; Kitamura, E.; Suzuki, T.; Wang, X.; Igarashi, J.; Morohashi, A.; Shinojima, Y.; Kanou, H.; Saito, K.; Takasu, T.; Nagase, H.; Harada, Y.; Kuroda, K.; Watanabe, T.; Kumamoto, S.; Aoyama, T.; Matsumoto, Y.; Bando, T.; Sugiyama, H.; Yoshida-Noro, C.; Fukuda, N. & Hayashi, N. (2008). Development of pyrrole-imidazole polyamide for specific regulation of human aurora kinase-A and -B gene expression. *Chem Biol*, Vol. 15, No. 8, pp. 829-841, ISSN 1074-5521 (Print) 1074-5521 (Linking).

Tao, Z. F.; Fujiwara, T.; Saito, I. & Sugiyama, H. (1999). Sequence-specific alkylation of DNA by duocarmycin A and its novel derivatives bearing PY/IM polyamides. *Nucleosides Nucleotides*, Vol. 18, No. 6-7, pp. 1615-1616, ISSN 0732-8311 (Print) 0732-8311 (Linking).

Trauger, J. W.; Baird, E. E. & Dervan, P. B. (1996). Recognition of DNA by designed ligands at subnanomolar concentrations. *Nature*, Vol. 382, No. 6591, pp. 559-561, ISSN 0028-0836 (Print) 0028-0836 (Linking).

Ueno, T.; Fukuda, N.; Tsunemi, A.; Yao, E. H.; Matsuda, H.; Tahira, K.; Matsumoto, T.; Matsumoto, K.; Matsumoto, Y.; Nagase, H.; Sugiyama, H. & Sawamura, T. (2009). A novel gene silencer, pyrrole-imidazole polyamide targeting human lectin-like oxidized low-density lipoprotein receptor-1 gene improves endothelial cell function. *J Hypertens*, Vol. 27, No. 3, pp. 508-516, ISSN 1473-5598 (Electronic) 0263-6352 (Linking).

Ullrich, K. J. (1997). Renal transporters for organic anions and organic cations. Structural requirements for substrates. *J Membr Biol*, Vol. 158, No. 2, pp. 95-107, ISSN 0022-2631 (Print) 0022-2631 (Linking).

van Montfoort, J. E.; Hagenbuch, B.; Groothuis, G. M.; Koepsell, H.; Meier, P. J. & Meijer, D. K. (2003). Drug uptake systems in liver and kidney. *Curr Drug Metab*, Vol. 4, No. 3, pp. 185-211, ISSN 1389-2002 (Print) 1389-2002 (Linking).

Wester, R. C.; Noonan, P. K.; Smeach, S. & Kosobud, L. (1983). Pharmacokinetics and bioavailability of intravenous and topical nitroglycerin in the rhesus monkey: estimate of percutaneous first-pass metabolism. *J Pharm Sci*, Vol. 72, No. 7, pp. 745-748, ISSN 0022-3549 (Print) 0022-3549 (Linking).

White, S.; Baird, E. E. & Dervan, P. B. (1997). On the pairing rules for recognition in the minor groove of DNA by pyrrole-imidazole polyamides. *Chem Biol*, Vol. 4, No. 8, pp. 569-578, ISSN 1074-5521 (Print) 1074-5521 (Linking).

Wieser, M. (2006). Atomic weights of the elements 2005. *Pure Appl. Chem.*, Vol. 78, No. 11, pp. 2051-2066,

Wiseman, G. A.; White, C. A.; Stabin, M.; Dunn, W. L.; Erwin, W.; Dahlbom, M.; Raubitschek, A.; Karvelis, K.; Schultheiss, T.; Witzig, T. E.; Belanger, R.; Spies, S.; Silverman, D. H.; Berlfein, J. R.; Ding, E. & Grillo-Lopez, A. J. (2000). Phase I/II 90Y-Zevalin (yttrium-90 ibritumomab tiuxetan, IDEC-Y2B8) radioimmunotherapy dosimetry results in relapsed or refractory non-Hodgkin's lymphoma. *Eur J Nucl Med*, Vol. 27, No. 7, pp. 766-777, ISSN 0340-6997 (Print) 0340-6997 (Linking).